Clinical Obstetrics

The Fetus & Mother

Fourth Edition

Clinical Obstetrics
The Fetus & Mother

Fourth Edition

EDITORS

E. Albert Reece, MD, PhD, MBA
Executive Vice President for Medical Affairs,
 UM Baltimore
John Z. and Akiko K. Bowers Distinguished
 Professor and Dean
Professor, Departments of Obstetrics, Gynecology &
 Reproductive Sciences, Biochemistry &
 Molecular Biology, and Medicine
University of Maryland School of Medicine
Baltimore, Maryland

Gustavo F. Leguizamón, MD
Postgraduate Professor
Director, Maternal Fetal Medicine Division
Department of Obstetrics and Gynecology
Principal Investigator, Rene Baron Institute

CEMIC University
Buenos Aires, Argentina

George A. Macones, MD, MSCE
Professor and Chairman
Department of Women's Health
Dell Medical School
University of Texas at Austin
Austin, Texas

Arnon Wiznitzer, MD
Professor and Chairman
Women's Hospital
Deputy Director, Rabin Medical Center
Vice Dean, Sackler Faculty of Medicine, Tel Aviv
 University
Tel Aviv, Israel

ASSISTANT PUBLICATION EDITOR

Julie A. Rosen, PhD
Assistant Professor, Department of Obstetrics,
 Gynecology & Reproductive Sciences
Executive Director, Medical Research & Scientific
 Publications
University of Maryland School of Medicine
Baltimore, Maryland

FOREWORD BY

Charles Lockwood, MD, MHCM
Dean, Morsani College of Medicine
Senior Vice President, USF Health
Professor of Obstetrics & Gynecology, and Public
 Health
University of South Florida
Tampa, Florida

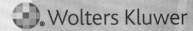
. Wolters Kluwer

Philadelphia • Baltimore • New York • London
Buenos Aires • Hong Kong • Sydney • Tokyo

Acquisitions Editor: Chris Teja
Development Editors: Carole Wonsiewicz, Thomas Celona
Senior Editorial Coordinator: Lindsay Ries
Editorial Assistant: Maribeth Wood
Marketing Manager: Kirsten Watrud
Production Project Manager: Kirstin Johnson
Design Coordinator: Stephen Druding
Art Director, Illustration: Jennifer Clements
Manufacturing Coordinator: Beth Welsh

Prepress Vendor: TNQ

9 8 7 6 5 4 3 2 1

Printed in China.

Library of Congress Cataloging-in-Publication Data

ISBN-13: 978-1-975141-46-2

Cataloging in Publication data available on request from publisher.

shop.lww.com

DEDICATIONS

To Sharon, Kelie, Brynne, Sharon-Andrea, Perceval, and Samantha Rose with greatest love and gratitude.
—E. Albert Reece, MD, PhD, MBA

To the memory of my father for teaching me the meaning of joy, grit, and striving for excellence.
To my mother for sowing the seeds of trust leading me to believe and to find happiness.
To my loving and unique wife Tamy, best friend, unconditional partner, and wonderful mother.
To my son Tomy, for his love that changed my life forever.
—Gustavo F. Leguizamón, MD

To Alison, my best friend and partner.
—George A. Macones, MD, MSCE

To my wife Miri and my children Lior, Nimrod, and Michal with love and appreciation for your support in the long journey.
—Arnon Wiznitzer, MD

Contents

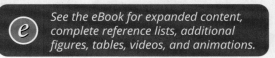

See the eBook for expanded content, complete reference lists, additional figures, tables, videos, and animations.

Part I
Early Pregnancy Complications

Part II
Fetal Infections and Teratogenesis

Part III
Prenatal Diagnosis

Part IV
Methods of Evaluation of Fetal Development and Well-being

Contributors

Horacio Aiello, MD
Professor, Division of Obstetrics
Department of Obstetrics and Gynecology
Instituto Universitario Hospital Italiano de Buenos Aires
Buenos Aires, Argentina

Ali Alhousseini, MD
Assistant Professor
Department of Obstetrics and Gynecology
Oakland University William Beaumont School of Medicine
Royal Oak, Michigan

Cande V. Ananth, PhD, MPH
Professor and Vice Chair of Academic Affairs
Chief, Division of Epidemiology and Biostatistics
Department of Obstetrics, Gynecology, and Reproductive
    Sciences
Rutgers Robert Wood Johnson Medical School
New Brunswick, New Jersey

Maria Andrikopoulo, MD, PhD
Maternal Fetal Medicine Fellow
Division of Maternal Fetal Medicine
Department of Obstetrics and Gynecology
Columbia University Irving Medical Center
New York, New York

Erol Arslan, MD
Visiting Researcher
Department of Obstetrics and Gynecology
University of Utah Health
Salt Lake City, Utah

Perceval Bahado-Singh, PhD, MSc
Director, System Integration & Chief of Staff (Former)
Corporate Office
University of Maryland Medical System
Baltimore, Maryland

Ray Oliver Bahado-Singh, MD, MBA
Professor
Department of Obstetrics and Gynecology
Oakland University William Beaumont School of Medicine
Royal Oak, Michigan

Limor Besser, MD, PhD
Division of Obstetrics and Gynecology
Soroka University Medical Center, School of Medicine
Faculty of Health Sciences
Ben Gurion University of the Negev
Beer Sheva, Israel

David Ware Branch, MD
Professor
Department of Obstetrics and Gynecology
Division of Maternal Fetal Medicine
University of Utah
Salt Lake City, Utah

Alexis Bridges, DO
Resident Physician
Department of Obstetrics and Gynecology
University of Utah Health
Salt Lake City, Utah

Dana R. Canfield, MD
Resident Physician
Department of Obstetrics and Gynecology
University of Utah
Salt Lake City, Utah

Steven James Cassady, MD
Assistant Professor
Division of Pulmonary & Critical Care Medicine
Department of Medicine
University of Maryland School of Medicine
Baltimore, Maryland

Victoria Lindstrom Chase, MD
Assistant Professor
Maternal Fetal Medicine
Intermountain Healthcare
Provo, Utah

Frank A. Chervenak, MD
Chair, Obstetrics & Gynecology
Lenox Hill Hospital
Professor and Chair, Obstetrics & Gynecology
Associate Dean for International Medicine
Zucker School for Medicine at Hofstra/Northwell
New York, New York

Ramen H. Chmait, MD
Associate Professor
Department of Obstetrics and Gynecology
University of Southern California
Los Angeles, California

Andrew H. Chon, MD
Fellow
Department of Obstetrics and Gynecology
University of Southern California
Los Angeles, California

Janaki Deepak, MBBS, FACP
Assistant Professor
Department of Medicine
University of Maryland School of Medicine
Baltimore, Maryland

Meagan Elise Deming, MD, PhD
Infectious Disease Fellow
Department of Medicine
Institute of Human Virology
University of Maryland School of Medicine
Baltimore, Maryland

Neal Dodia, MD
Chief Fellow
Division of Pulmonary and Critical Care
Department of Medicine
University of Maryland School of Medicine
Baltimore, Maryland

Marcia S. Driscoll, MD, PharmD
Associate Professor
Department of Dermatology
University of Maryland School of Medicine
Baltimore, Maryland

Jose R. Duncan, MD
Assistant Professor
Department of Obstetrics and Gynecology
University of South Florida, Morsani College of Medicine
Tampa Florida

Tara Dutta, MD
Assistant Professor
Department of Neurology
University of Maryland School of Medicine
Baltimore, Maryland

Offer Erez, MD
Professor
Division of Obstetrics and Gynecology
Soroka University Medical Center, School of Medicine
Faculty of Health Sciences
Ben Gurion University of the Negev
Beer Sheva Israel

Adjunct Professor
Department of Obstetrics and Gynecology
Hutzek Women's Hospital
School of Medicine
Wayne State University
Detroit, Michigan

Anna G. Euser, MD, PhD
Assistant Professor
Department of Obstetrics and Gynecology
Division of Maternal-Fetal Medicine
University of Colorado School of Medicine
Aurora, Colorado

Mark I. Evans, MD
Professor
Department of Obstetrics and Gynecology
Icahn School of Medicine at Mount Sinai
President, Fetal Medicine Foundation of America
New York, New York

Yinon Gilboa, MD
Associate Professor
Sackler Faculty of Medicine, Tel Aviv University
Tel Aviv, Israel

James D. Goldberg, MD
Chief Medical Officer
Myriad Women's Health
South San Francisco, California

Cornelia R. Graves, MD
Professor
University of Tennessee
Clinical Professor
Vanderbilt University
Adjunct Professor
Meharry Medical College
Department of Obstetrics and Gynecology
Division of Maternal Fetal Medicine
Nashville, Tennessee

Amos Grünebaum, MD
Associate Director of Obstetric Safety
Northwell Health
Professor of Obstetrics & Gynecology
Zucker School of Medicine at Hofstra/Northwell
New York, New York

Eran Hadar, MD
Associate Professor
Sackler Faculty of Medicine, Tel Aviv University
Department of Obstetrics and Gynecology, Rabin Medical
  Center
Tel Aviv, Israel

Jeffrey D. Hasday, MD
Dr. Herbert Berger Professor in Medicine
University of Maryland School of Medicine
Baltimore, Maryland

Barbara B. Head, MD
Associate Professor
Department of Obstetrics and Gynecology
Medical University of South Carolina
Charleston, South Carolina

Alison D. Hermann, MD
Assistant Professor in Clinical Psychiatry
Department of Psychiatry
Weill Cornell Medicine
New York, New York

Washington C. Hill, MD
Faculty Affiliate
Department of Obstetrics and Gynecology
Division of Maternal Fetal Medicine
University of South Florida College of Medicine
Tampa, Florida

Sarasota Memorial HealthCare System
CenterPlace Health
Obstetrics, Gynecology and Maternal-Fetal Medicine
Sarasota, Florida

John C. Hobbins, MD
Distinguished Professor
Department of Obstetrics and Gynecology
University of Colorado School of Medicine
Aurora, Colorado

Conisha M. Holloman, MD
Fellow
Maternal-Fetal Medicine
McGovern Medical School
University of Texas Health Science Center
Houston, Texas

Carol J. Homko, RN, PhD
Associate Research Professor (Retired),
Department of Medicine
Temple University, Lewis Katz School of Medicine
Philadelphia, Pennsylvania

Charles C. Hong, MD, PhD
Melvin Sharoky, MD Professor in Medicine
Director of Cardiology Research, Co-Chief of
    Cardiovascular Medicine
Department of Medicine, Division of Cardiovascular
    Medicine
University of Maryland School of Medicine
Baltimore, Maryland

Susie N. Hong, MD, MSc
Assistant Professor
Medical Director, Echocardiography
Department of Medicine, Division of Cardiovascular
    Medicine
Department of Diagnostic Radiology and Nuclear Medicine
University of Maryland, School of Medicine
Baltimore, Maryland

Brenna L. Hughes, MD
Associate Professor
Department of Obstetrics and Gynecology
Duke University
Durham, North Carolina

Mohamed Ibrahim, MD
Obstetric Anesthesiology Fellowship Program Director
Assistant Professor
Department of Anesthesiology
University of Texas Medical Branch
Galveston, Texas

Laura Igarzábal, MD
Associate Professor of Medical Genetics
Genetics Section, Department of Obstetrics and Gynecology
Medical Genetics Residency Program
CEMIC University Hospital
Buenos Aires, Argentina

William Brian Karkowsky, MD
Fellow
Department of Medicine
Division of Pulmonary and Critical Care
University of Maryland Medical Center
Baltimore, Maryland

Jeannie C. Kelly, MD, MS
Assistant Professor
Division of Maternal-Fetal Medicine
Department of Obstetrics and Gynecology
Washington University in St. Louis
St. Louis, Missouri

Sun Kwon Kim, MD, PhD
Attending Physician
Department of Maternal-Fetal Medicine
Henry Ford Health System
Detroit, Michigan

Bhavani Shankar Kodali, MD
Professor
Department of Anesthesiology
Division Chief of Obstetric Anesthesiology
University of Maryland School of Medicine
Baltimore, Maryland

Effichia Kontopoulos, MD, PhD, FACOG
The Fetal Institute
Miami, Florida

Shyam Kottilil, MBBS, PhD
Professor
Department of Medicine
Institute of Human Virology
University of Maryland School of Medicine
Baltimore, Maryland

Eyal Krispin, MD
Helen Schneider Hospital for Women
Rabin Medical Center
Tel Aviv, Israel

Texas Children's Hospital
Baylor College of Medicine
Houston, Texas

Jeffrey A. Kuller, MD
Professor
Division of Maternal-Fetal Medicine
Department of Obstetrics and Gynecology
Duke University School of Medicine
Durham, North Carolina

Allison Lankford, MD
Assistant Professor
Department of Obstetrics, Gynecology and Reproductive
    Sciences
Division of Maternal Fetal Medicine
University of Maryland School of Medicine
Anesthesia Critical Care Medicine in R Adams Cowley
    Shock Trauma Program
Baltimore, Maryland

Talia Lanxberg, MD
Division of Obstetrics and Gynecology
Soroka University Medical Center, School of Medicine
Faculty of Health Sciences
Ben Gurion University of the Negev
Beer Sheva, Israel

Denise Araujo Lapa, MD, PhD
Maternal-Fetal Medicine Specialist
Hospital Israelita Albert Einstein
Sao Paulo, Brazil

Elad Laron, MD
Lecturer
Division of Obstetrics and Gynecology
Soroka University Medical Center, School of Medicine
Faculty of Health Sciences
Ben Gurion University of the Negev
Beer Sheva, Israel

Gustavo F. Leguizamón, MD
Postgraduate Professor
Director, Maternal Fetal Medicine Division
Department of Obstetrics and Gynecology
Principal Investigator, Rene Baron Institute
CEMIC University
Buenos Aires, Argentina

Nicole Leistikow, MD
Assistant Professor
Department of Psychiatry
University of Maryland School of Medicine
Baltimore, Maryland

Charles J. Lockwood, MD, MHCM
Dean, Morsani College of Medicine
Senior Vice President, USF Health
Professor of Obstetrics & Gynecology and Public Health
University of South Florida
Tampa, Florida

Thanh Ha Luu, MD
Fellow of Reproductive Endocrinology and Infertility
Department of Obstetrics and Gynecology
University of Colorado School of Medicine
Denver, Colorado

George A. Macones, MD, MSCE
Professor and Chairman
Department of Women's Health
Dell Medical School
University of Texas at Austin
Austin, Texas

Mercedes Negri Malbrán, MD
Fellow
Maternal Fetal Medicine
Department of Obstetrics and Gynecology
CEMIC University Institute
Buenos Aires, Argentina

Rana Malek, MD
Associate Professor
Department of Medicine
Division of Endocrinology, Diabetes, and Nutrition
University of Maryland School of Medicine
Baltimore, Maryland

Andrew M. Malinow, MD
Professor
Department of Anesthesiology, and Department of
    Obstetrics, Gynecology, and Reproductive Sciences
University of Maryland School of Medicine
Baltimore, Maryland

Divya Mallampati, MD, MPH
Clinical Instructor and Fellow
Division of Maternal Fetal Medicine
Department of Obstetrics and Gynecology
University of North Carolina at Chapel Hill
Chapel Hill, North Carolina

Katrina Schafer Mark, MD, FACOG
Associate Professor
Department of Obstetrics, Gynecology, and Reproductive
    Sciences
University of Maryland School of Medicine
Baltimore, Maryland

Laurence B. McCullough, PhD
Ethics Scholar, Obstetrics and Gynecology
Lenox Hill Hospital
Professor of Obstetrics and Gynecology
Zucker School of Medicine at Hofstra/Northwell
New York, New York

César Meller, MD, MSc
Assistant Professor
Department of Obstetrics and Gynecology
Instituto Universitario Hospital Italiano de Buenos Aires
Buenos Aires, Argentina

Audrey A. Merriam, MD, MS
Assistant Professor
Department of Obstetrics, Gynecology, and Reproductive
    Sciences
Yale University
New Haven, Connecticut

Torri D. Metz, MD, MS
Associate Professor
Department of Obstetrics and Gynecology
University of Utah Health
Salt Lake City, Utah

Alex S. Miller, MD
Instructor
Department of Obstetrics, Gynecology, and Reproductive
    Sciences
Yale School of Medicine
New Haven, Connecticut

Courtney J. Mitchell, MD, PhD
Maternal-Fetal Medicine Fellow
Department of Obstetrics and Gynecology
Duke University
Durham, North Carolina

Jason K. Molitoris, MD, PhD
Assistant Professor
Department of Radiation Oncology
University of Maryland School of Medicine
Baltimore, Maryland

Kashif M. Munir, MD
Associate Professor
Department of Medicine
Division of Endocrinology, Diabetes and Nutrition
University of Maryland School of Medicine
Medical Director, University of Maryland Center for
    Diabetes and Endocrinology
Baltimore, Maryland

Liesl Nel-Themaat, PhD, HCLD
IVF Lab Director
Assistant Professor
Department of Obstetrics and Gynecology
University of Colorado
CU Advanced Reproductive Medicine
Denver, Colorado

Chloe M. Nielsen, MD
Fellow
Department of Obstetrics and Gynecology
University of Colorado School of Medicine
Aurora, Colorado

Anthony O. Odibo, MD, MSCE
Professor of Obstetrics and Gynecology
Director, Fetal Care Center of Tampa Bay
Division of Maternal Fetal Medicine
Department of Obstetrics and Gynecology
University of South Florida, Morsani College of Medicine
Tampa, Florida

Dotun Ogunyemi, MD
Associate Dean of Faculty Affairs
Multicultural Diversity & Inclusion
Professor of Medical Education
Department of Obstetrics and Gynecology
California University of Science & Medicine
Colton, California

Lucas Otaño, MD, PhD
Professor, Head of Maternal-Fetal Medicine Section,
    Division of Obstetrics
Department of Obstetrics and Gynecology
Instituto Universitario Hospital Italiano de Buenos Aires
Universidad de Buenos Aires
Buenos Aires, Argentina

Michelle Y. Owens, MD
Professor and Chief, Fellowship Director
Division of Maternal Fetal Medicine
Department of Obstetrics and Gynecology
University of Mississippi Medical Center
Jackson, Mississippi

Yinka Oyelese, MD
Chief
Maternal Fetal Medicine
Atlantic Health System
Morristown, New Jersey

Luis D. Pacheco, MD
Professor
Department of Obstetrics and Gynecology and
    Anesthesiology
Maternal Fetal Medicine/ Critical Care
University of Texas Medical Branch
Galveston, Texas

Michael J. Paidas, MD
Professor and Chair
Department of Obstetrics, Gynecology and Reproductive
    Sciences
Miller School of Medicine
University of Miami
Miami, Florida

Ji Eun Park, MD, MA
Fellow
Division of Cardiovascular Medicine
Department of Internal Medicine
University of Maryland School of Medicine
Baltimore, Maryland

W. Tony Parks, MD
Professor
Laboratory Medicine and Pathobiology
University of Toronto
Toronto, Canada

Juan A. Peña, MD, MPH
Fellow, Maternal-Fetal Medicine
Department of Obstetrics and Gynecology
Icahn School of Medicine at Mount Sinai
New York, New York

Juan Ignacio Pereira, MD
Assistant Professor
Division of Maternal Fetal Medicine
Department of Obstetrics and Gynecology
CEMIC University Institute
Buenos Aires, Argentina

Florencia Petracchi, MD
Chief of Clinical Genetics
Department of Obstetrics and Gynecology
CEMIC (Centro de educación médica e investigaciones
    clínicas, Instituto Universitario)
Buenos Aires, Argentina

Christian M. Pettker, MD
Professor and Chief of Obstetrics
Department of Obstetrics, Gynecology, and Reproductive
    Sciences
Yale School of Medicine
New Haven, Connecticut

Ashish Premkumar, MD
Fellow
Department of Obstetrics and Gynecology
Northwestern University
Chicago, Illinois

Tabitha Morgan Quebedeaux, MD, PhD
Assistant Professor
Department of Obstetrics and Gynecology
Division of Maternal Fetal Medicine
LSUHSC School of Medicine
New Orleans, Louisiana

Ruben Quintero, MD
The Fetal Institute
Miami, Florida

Patrick S. Ramsey, MD, MSPH
H. Frank Connally, Jr Professor in Obstetrics & Gynecology
Chief, Division of Maternal-Fetal Medicine
Director, Maternal-Fetal Medicine Fellowship
University of Texas Health Science Center at San Antonio
Center for Pregnancy and Newborn Research
San Antonio, Texas

Gautam Gorantla Rao, MD
Assistant Professor
Department of Obstetrics, Gynecology, and Reproductive
    Sciences
University of Maryland School of Medicine
Baltimore, Maryland

Uma M. Reddy, MD, MPH
Professor
Department of Obstetrics, Gynecology, and Reproductive
    Sciences
Division Chief, Maternal Fetal Medicine
Yale University
New Haven, Connecticut

E. Albert Reece, MD, PhD, MBA
Executive Vice President for Medical Affairs, UM Baltimore
John Z. and Akiko K. Bowers Distinguished Professor and
    Dean
Professor, Departments of Obstetrics, Gynecology &
    Reproductive Sciences, Biochemistry & Molecular
    Biology, and Medicine
University of Maryland School of Medicine
Baltimore, Maryland

Kathryn S. Robinett, MD
Assistant Professor
Department of Medicine
University of Maryland School of Medicine
Baltimore, Maryland

Tania Roman, MD
Fellow
Maternal Fetal Medicine
Department of Obstetrics and Gynecology
University of Texas Health Science Center
San Antonio, Texas

Julie A. Rosen, PhD
Assistant Professor, Department of Obstetrics, Gynecology &
    Reproductive Sciences
Executive Director, Medical Research & Scientific
    Publications
University of Maryland School of Medicine
Baltimore, Maryland

Michael G. Ross, MD, MPH
Distinguished Professor of Obstetrics and Gynecology and
    Public Health
Department of Obstetrics and Gynecology, and Department
    of Community Health Sciences
Geffen School of Medicine at UCLA
Fielding School of Public Health at UCLA
Los Angeles, California

Antonio F. Saad, MD
Associate Professor
MFM and Critical Care Specialist
Associate MFM Fellowship Program Director
The University of Texas Medical Branch
Department of OB-GYN & Anesthesia
Galveston, Texas

Yoel Sadovsky, MD
Executive Director, Magee-Womens Research Institute
Elsie Hilliard Hillman Chair of Women's Health Research
Distinguished Professor of OBGYN, Microbiology and
 Molecular Genetics
Vice Chair (research), Department of OBGYN and
 Reproductive Sciences
Associate Dean, Women's Health Research and
 Reproductive Sciences
University of Pittsburgh
Pittsburgh, Pennsylvania

Nanette Santoro, MD
Professor and E. Stewart Taylor Chair
Department of Obstetrics and Gynecology
University of Colorado School of Medicine
Aurora, Colorado

Eyal Sheiner, MD, PhD
Chairman, Department of Obstetrics and Gynecology
Soroka University Medical Center
Vice Dean, Faculty of Health Sciences
Ben-Gurion University of the Negev
Beer Sheva, Israel

Anat Shmueli, MD
Sackler Faculty of Medicine, Tel Aviv University
Tel Aviv, Israel

Baha M. Sibai, MD
Professor
Fellowship Director
Maternal-Fetal Medicine
Department of Obstetrics, Gynecology, and Reproductive
 Sciences
McGovern Medical School
University of Texas Health Science Center
Houston, Texas

Robert M. Silver, MD
Professor
Maternal Fetal Medicine
Department of Obstetrics and Gynecology
University of Utah
Salt Lake City, Utah

Melissa A. Simon, MD, MPH
Vice Chair of Research
Department of Obstetrics and Gynecology
Northwestern University
Feinberg School of Medicine and Robert H. Lurie
 Comprehensive Cancer Center
Chicago, Illinois

Silvina Sisterna, MD
Staff Member of Clinical Genetics
Department of Obstetrics and Gynecology
Hospital Privado de Comunidad
Mar del Plata, Argentina

Maria Jacqueline Small, MD, MPH
Associate Professor
Department of Obstetrics and Gynecology
Division of Maternal-Fetal Medicine
Duke University School of Medicine
Durham, North Carolina

James W. Snider, MD
Assistant Professor
Department of Radiation Oncology
University of Maryland School of Medicine
Baltimore, Maryland

Rebecca Sokal, MD
Staff Psychiatrist
Center for Eating Disorders
Sheppard Pratt Hospital
Towson, Maryland

Joanne Stone, MD, MS
Professor
Department of Obstetrics and Gynecology
Icahn School of Medicine at Mount Sinai
New York, New York

Scott A. Sullivan, MSCR
Professor
Department of Obstetrics and Gynecology
Medical University of South Carolina
Charleston, South Carolina

Marta Szymanska, MD
Research Assistant
Department of Obstetrics and Gynecology
Beaumont Research Institute
Royal Oak, Michigan

Katherine Johansen Taber, PhD
Senior Director, Clinical Development
Department of Medical Affairs
Myriad Women's Health
South San Francisco, California

Nandor Gabor Than, MD, PhD
First Department of Pathology and Experimental Cancer
 Research
Semmelweis University, Budapest, Hungary
Systems Biology of Reproduction Lendulet Research Group
Institute of Enzymology
Research Centre for Natural Sciences
Hungarian Academy of Sciences
Budapest, Hungary
Maternity Private Department
Kutvolgyi Clinical Block
Semmelweis University
Budapest, Hungary

Denise Trigubo, MD
Assistant Professor
Division of Maternal Fetal Medicine
Department of Obstetrics and Gynecology
CEMIC University Institute
Buenos Aires, Argentina

Ozhan M. Turan, MD, PhD
Professor
Department of Obstetrics, Gynecology, and Reproductive
 Sciences
University of Maryland School of Medicine
Baltimore, Maryland

Shifa Turan, MD, RDMS
Associate Professor
Department of Obstetrics, Gynecology, and Reproductive
 Sciences
University of Maryland School of Medicine
Baltimore, Maryland

Anthony M. Vintzileos, MD
Professor and Chair
Department of Obstetrics and Gynecology
NYU Langone Hospital—Long Island
NYU Long Island School of Medicine
Mineola, New York

Carl P. Weiner, MD, MBA, FACOG
Professor, Obstetrics and Gynecology
Professor, Molecular and Integrative Physiology
University of Kansas School of Medicine
Kansas City, Kansas

Patricia F. Widra, MD
Assistant Professor
Department of Psychiatry
University of Maryland School of Medicine
Baltimore, Maryland

Mae-Lan Winchester, MD
Division of Maternal Fetal Medicine
Department of Obstetrics and Gynecology
University of Kansas Medical Center
Kansas City, Kansas

Arnon Wiznitzer, MD
Professor and Chairman
Women's Hospital
Deputy Director Rabin Medical Center
Vice Dean, Sackler Faculty of Medicine Tel-Aviv University
Tel Aviv, Israel

Kellie Woodfield, MD
Resident
Department of Obstetrics and Gynecology
University of Utah
Salt Lake City, Utah

Tal Rafaeli Yehudai, MD
Department of Obstetrics and Gynecology
Shamir Medical Center, School of Medicine
Tel Aviv University
Tel Aviv, Israel

Omri Zamstein, MD
Medical Doctor
Department of Obstetrics and Gynecology B
Soroka University Medical Center
Be'er Sheva, Israel

Foreword to *Clinical Obstetrics: The Fetus & Mother, Fourth Edition*

Keeping up with the exponential expansion of medical knowledge is perhaps the greatest challenge faced by contemporary physicians. Obstetricians and maternal-fetal medicine subspecialists are clearly not immune from this "age of data acceleration." Moreover, what was once a specialty focused almost exclusively on the mother and then gradually transitioned to a principal focus on the fetus has now reached an equipoise wherein the obstetrician must be dedicated to the care of both patients. Fortunately, such care is greatly enhanced by the remarkable genomic, imaging, pharmacological, and surgical advances we have witnessed over the last two decades. However, therein lies the challenge of keeping up with these advances.

Although the acceleration of medical knowledge demands lifelong learning, there remains an essential need to build such learning on a solid foundation of core knowledge. That is precisely why this fourth edition of *Clinical Obstetrics: The Fetus & Mother* is so important. In one textbook, the authors elucidate for both trainees and practitioners core information with nuanced details and a vast array of recent clinical developments. Chapter by chapter, the authors blend evidenced-validated traditional data with emerging discoveries. The text covers both the predicted progress of uncomplicated pregnancy and the unexpected, sometimes life-threatening, conditions that can complicate pregnancy and birth.

As a maternal-fetal medicine researcher and obstetric practitioner committed to finding solutions for preterm birth, recurrent pregnancy loss, venous thromboembolism, and maternal mortality, among other conditions faced by mother and fetus, I commend the editors and authors for rendering coherent such vast amounts of pertinent information. Major themes covered include early pregnancy complications, fetal infections and teratogenesis, prenatal diagnosis, fetal assessment and therapy, maternal and obstetrical conditions complicating pregnancy, and the puerperium.

This updated volume also addresses new topics that have witnessed rapid scientific advances such as expanded carrier screening and preimplantation genetic diagnosis in assisted reproductive technology and reflects the growing importance of the social determinants of health such as obesity and health disparities, or the preventative health window presented by the so-called fourth trimester. This edition also adds new chapters with fresh insights on older topics such as maternal thrombophilias, fetal demise, radiation in pregnancy, invasive diagnostic procedures, neonatal alloimmune thrombocytopenia, fetal malpresentation, placental abruption, and cervical insufficiency.

What could be more relevant to today's practice than the impact of obesity on pregnancy? Clearly this public health crisis touches every demographic group and region of our country and is sadly pervasive within our obstetrics practices. Many of the comorbidities seen in older adults with obesity are the same for women of reproductive age including heart disease, diabetes, cancer, and hypertension, to name a few. However, obesity also offers discrete obstetrical challenges including an increased risk of birth defects, macrosomia, preterm birth, stillbirth, preeclampsia, and gestational diabetes. Moreover, lifelong adverse sequelae accrue in both the mother and fetus when obesity complicates pregnancy.

The new chapter addressing the fourth trimester brings to light a topic found in today's consumer news and, thus, into the vernacular of our patients. As a critical transition for every new mother, the fourth trimester is a period when we must address both the postpartum issues faced by the mother, including lactation and postpartum depression, and common problems of the newborn as well as prevention of long-term adverse health outcomes presaged by complications of pregnancy. Not nearly enough research has been done for this crucial time in caring for both the mother and the newborn. This new chapter offers the kind of in-depth detail we need about the postpartum period, a time when many obstetricians might think their work is done, but, in fact, marks the start of a lifetime of care for which we are responsible.

Both foundational and groundbreaking work fills this updated volume of *Clinical Obstetrics: The Fetus & Mother*. Trainees and experienced practitioners alike should take in every word as it presents both a solid foundation and an essential update of knowledge on the current state of obstetric health care.

The demand on obstetricians to know more will continue as the pace of scientific discovery continues to accelerate. Our challenge is not to fall behind. This fourth edition of *Clinical Obstetrics: The Fetus & Mother* is a welcome companion on this race.

Charles J. Lockwood, MD, MHCM
Dean, Morsani College of Medicine
Senior Vice President, USF Health
Professor, Obstetrics & Gynecology, and Public Health
University of South Florida, Tampa, Florida

Preface

The first edition of this book was introduced as the fulfillment of a concept: to combine into one source for maternal medicine—an established field focusing primarily on medical complications of pregnancy—and the rapidly evolving field of fetal medicine. At the time, a single-source book was overwhelmingly embraced not only by obstetricians but also by maternal-fetal medicine specialists, resident physicians in training, medical students, and others who used the book for its comprehensive obstetrical coverage. A second edition followed as a straight revision of the first.

The third edition was entirely reengineered to contain a strong clinical emphasis, while maintaining a scholarly orientation. However, the third edition was published in 2007, nearly 14 years ago. In the intervening years, substantive changes have occurred in the fields of obstetrics and maternal-fetal medicine. Practice guidelines have been updated, and discoveries made through biomedical research have provided new insights into gestation, perinatal development, treatments, and care. In addition, conditions which were prevalent in the general population but not yet at epidemic levels, such as obesity and diabetes, have required practitioners to broaden their knowledge base as they manage patients with a confluence of chronic health disorders. Therefore, the emphasis of this updated book is on diagnosis and management, which are changing rapidly with technological advances in the medical profession, as well as on rigorously conducted biomedical research.

Recognizing that the continuous updates to medical practice far outpace the speed of traditional print publications, the primary text of this fourth edition is an online electronic book (ebook), with a companion print book. The complete ebook curates the most up-to-date research studies, clinical practice guidelines, and opinions from authoritative sources as these pertain to the chapter topics, with commensurate illustrations, images, and videos. The companion print book will provide trainees and practitioners with easy access to the most relevant diagnostic and management information from the complete online text—a veritable "pocket guide" which can be referenced between patient consults when a quick review is necessary.

Although comprehensive, this book is designed to provide readily accessible information based on the most up-to-date clinical guidelines, algorithms, and evidence for clinical practice. The overall balance, scope, content, and design fully serve the needs of academic subspecialists, obstetricians, and house staff physicians, as well as other keen students of medicine.

E. Albert Reece, MD, PhD, MBA
Gustavo F. Leguizamón, MD
George A. Macones, MD
Arnon Wiznitzer, MD
2021

Tribute to John C. Hobbins, MD

I write this tribute to John Hobbins, former coeditor of this text, my mentor, colleague, and dear friend. Following my residency at Columbia University Medical Center, I was privileged to be accepted by Dr. Hobbins into the Yale maternal-fetal medicine (MFM) fellowship. Working with John Hobbins during my fellowship and as a faculty for nearly 10 years was the desire of most candidates as John was, and is, a super star and a very innovative and active physician-scientist. His contributions to the field of obstetric sonography and the advancement of the art and science of prenatal diagnosis are legendary. Over the course of his distinguished career, he led teams which discovered and invented various aspects of the discipline—from fetoscopy, to intraperitoneal transfusion, to fetal biometry, to *in utero* fetal weight estimation, to prenatal diagnosis of congenital anomalies, and more. His first book with Fred Winsberg in 1978, "*Ultrasonography in Obstetrics and Gynecology*," was one of the very earliest textbooks on sonography in this specialty. Under his leadership, Yale launched one of the first advanced and comprehensive prenatal diagnosis programs in the United States.

In 2018, the *American Journal of Obstetrics and Gynecology* profiled John in its "Giants in Obstetrics and Gynecology" feature column[a]. An anecdote from that column, which bears mention here as it is incredibly relevant to the primary purpose of this text as a teaching and educational tool, is that in the early days of ultrasonography at Yale, John would often wheel the ultrasound equipment—the only one available at that time and, therefore, extremely precious—to labor and delivery to encourage its broad use. His willingness to share his unique knowledge and insight, as well as take responsibility of anything that was broken, with the trainees was indicative of both his magnanimous nature as a physician-scientist, as well as his staunch dedication to teaching.

Indeed, John was a juggernaut who never seemed to slow down. I do not ever recall a moment when he was not off seeing patients, teaching, meeting with his trainees, or out of the office giving an invited lecture at some national or international conference. In fact, back then, we used to joke that he was a "visiting professor at Yale," because he was in such high demand elsewhere. However, regardless of his schedule, John could return to the office and not miss a beat. He always knew what was going on at Yale. He took time to interact with each of us, his academic "offspring." He put himself on regular clinical rotations. He frequently checked in with us to see how our work in the clinic or in the research laboratory was going.

However, it was not all work, work, work. John is a great jazz pianist. He also recognized the importance of morale building. On several occasions, I clearly remember him popping his head into my office to announce that, "We're having a meeting tomorrow at the beach. You create the agenda, and I'll bring the food!"

John had high expectations of himself and for his fellows and faculty. Hence, he recruited people with equally high aspirations. Many of the research fellows and faculty he mentored have become celebrated names in the field of fetal medicine and prenatal diagnosis. Part of his success was that he valued clinical training as well as time spent in the laboratory. Years ahead of today's push to provide research-based patient management, John recognized that bench science lays the groundwork for the best possible care. He was a staunch advocate for protecting time spent in the laboratories so that his mentees could fully engage in both clinical training and scientific investigations.

In addition, he trusted us to succeed. When we did deliver, John would always acknowledge our contributions. The confidence that he placed in us pushed us to thrive.

I was pleased and privileged to be part of his extraordinary team for a decade in New Haven and delighted when he joined me to work on prior editions of this textbook. John has left an indelible imprint on an entire generation of students, residents, fellows, and faculty members. He is a luminary, a scholar, and a leader well ahead of his time.

Our goal with this revised book is to provide a guide for the next generation of clinicians and academicians who approach obstetric practice with the same rigor as my great mentor, John Hobbins.

E. Albert Reece, MD, PhD, MBA
2021

Acknowledgments

The editors are deeply indebted to all of the contributors, who have invested an enormous amount of time and energy in this project. We count ourselves extremely fortunate to have colleagues and friends who are willing to make this type of investment. The collective efforts have resulted in an entirely revised and most up-to-date book series.

We truly appreciate the invaluable effort of our colleagues from the University of Maryland School of Medicine, especially our Assistant Publication Editor, Dr. Julie A. Rosen, who assisted in editing and managing this entire project, and Ms. Lisa Joseph for helping to coordinate chapters of this book.

Finally, we are greatly appreciative of the editorial team at Wolters Kluwer, especially Mses. Lindsay Ries and Carole Wonsiewicz, for their time, insight, and excellent project management, and Mr. Chris Teja, whose vision helped shepherd this project along.

The collective efforts of all who contributed to this revised edition are a true testimony of scholarship, commitment, and selflessness. Our lives have been touched by the willingness of everyone to be so generous in sharing their time and talents. Thank you very kindly.

E. Albert Reece, MD, PhD, MBA
Gustavo F. Leguizamón, MD
George A. Macones, MD
Arnon Wiznitzer, MD
2021

Historical Development on Fetal Medicine and the Fetus as a Patient

Amos Grünebaum, Laurence B. McCullough, and Frank A. Chervenak

Introduction

It was not until the mid-20th century that the fetus was considered a patient.[1] Until Cesarean deliveries became somewhat safer for the mother, Cesarean deliveries and forceps were done mostly to save a woman's life, for example, if the pelvis was contracted, labor was too long, or there was sepsis present.[2] Even early fetal diagnoses, such as auscultation of the fetal heart rate or x-rays of the fetus, limited the diagnosis of fetal conditions until the early 1950s.

Auscultation of the Fetal Heart Rate and Diagnosis of Fetal Distress

Auscultation of the fetal heart rate was the first method for evaluating the fetus. In 1818,[3] a Swiss surgeon reported the presence of fetal heart tones; 3 years later, Lejuma[4] suggested auscultation would be helpful in the diagnosis of twins and the fetal lie and its position. In 1833, Kennedy[5] suggested that the fetal heart rate was indicative of "fetal distress." Such distress, if diagnosed late in pregnancy, could be treated using forceps for delivery. However, it was not until relatively recent times that Cesarean delivery was used to manage fetal distress in labor.

In 1870, Schwartz[6] described fetal bradycardia following compression of the fetal head, and in 1885, Schatz[7] had provided detailed descriptions of umbilical cord compression.

In 1903, Van Winkel[8] was the first to postulate that a fetal heart rate over 160 or below 100 beats per minute was presumptive evidence of "fetal distress." However, Lund[9] believed that tachycardia is not as important as bradycardia. In a series of 250 cases, he found a transient tachycardia during labor in 17.6% and persistent tachycardia in 5.6% without any correlation with fetal distress. In addition to fetal bradycardia, passage of meconium *in utero* was also considered a sign of "fetal distress" for a long time. In 1927, Freed[10] reported on clinical signs of fetal distress during labor.

Perhaps the first time that "fetal indication" for performing a Cesarean delivery was used in the literature was in 1953.[11] Thus, the fetus did not become a "patient" worthwhile of intervention and treatment prior to delivery until the mid-20th century when Cesarean deliveries and anesthesia were deemed safe enough and potential benefits of Cesarean deliveries for the fetus and baby outweighed potential maternal risks. Douglas and Stromme,[12] in their 1957 text *Operative Obstetrics*, state that "fetal distress was virtually nonexistent as a cause for Cesarean section on our service [New York Hospital] until 10 years ago."

In 1953 McCall[13] reviewed 8,785 deliveries with 173 cases of "fetal distress." He said that, "…one or more signs commonly accepted as evidence of fetal distress…[were] fetal heart changes, or meconium, or both." Fitzgerald and McFarland[14] emphasized the significance of bradycardia, arrhythmia, and the expulsion of frank meconium as signs of "fetal distress." Goodlin[15] in 1979 provided an extensive review of the history of fetal monitoring

Amniocentesis

In 1923, Boursier and Gautret[16] reported on a patient with polyhydramnios who was treated with "abdominal puncture" removing two liters of amniotic fluid for relief of the polyhydramnios.

In 1964, Goodlin[17] reviewed diagnostic abdominal amniocentesis and removal of amniotic fluid. He said that visual inspection of the fluid would be informative: yellow fluid could indicate erythroblastosis, green fluid could indicate "fetal distress," and dark or reddish black fluid could indicate fetal death. In addition, he said that amniotic fluid analysis could be helpful in estimating fetal age and fetal oxidation. In 1982, Romero[18] diagnosed umbilical cord lesions by ultrasound, and in 1985, he confirmed that sonographically monitored amniocentesis was safe to decrease intraoperative complications.[19] The same year Hobbins reported on percutaneous blood sampling.[20]

Rh Disease

A major diagnostic step of diagnosing fetal and subsequent neonatal disease was made by Bevis in 1952.[21] He documented a correlation between amniotic fluid nonheme iron (obtained by amniocentesis) and the severity of fetal anemia. This pioneering work was amplified by Liley,[22] who in 1961 demonstrated that the spectral peak at 450 mU reflected the severity of hemolysis. This gave the obstetrician a method with which to follow the patient with Rh sensitization and, in some cases, deliver the fetus prematurely for fetal salvage. The next major step in the treatment of these Rh-sensitized fetuses was also made by Liley, who in 1963 demonstrated that one could successfully treat these anemic fetuses *in utero* by transfusing blood into the fetal abdomen.[23,24]

Amnioscopy and Meconium-Stained Amniotic Fluid

Saling[25] was the first in 1962 to publish on the use of amnioscopy to diagnose "hazardous conditions to the fetus" by identifying meconium-stained amniotic fluid through intact fetal membranes. In 1968, Kornacki[26] said: "...appearance of meconium in the amniotic fluid without other warning clinical signs forecast fetal asphyxia in 5 of 13 cases." In 1973, Vujić[27] reported on his experience with diagnosis meconium in the amniotic fluid prior to rupture of fetal membranes as a sign of "fetal distress."

Intrauterine Fetal Blood Sampling

In 1962, Saling[28,29] published a report of sampling fetal blood by amnioscopy from the scalp or other presenting part during the course of labor, thus overcoming centuries of ethical and emotional barriers to access the fetus inside the uterus. This was the first documented direct approach to the human fetus before delivery. In his report, "New procedures for examining the fetus during labor: introduction, technique, and basics," Saling described his pioneering approach to obtaining a fetal scalp blood sample and championed the concept of combining pH with abnormal fetal heart rate pattern to assess the fetal condition shortly after cardiotocography had been introduced for clinical routine use in 1968.

Electronic Fetal Heart Rate Monitoring

In 1951, Caldeyro-Barcia and Alvarez[30], from Montevideo, Uruguay, first reported on measuring uterine contractions in labor, and in 1958, they developed a method to measure the effect of uterine contractions on fetal heart rate, which would later become the basis of fetal monitoring. They defined normal and abnormal responses of the fetus through the continuous monitoring of fetal heart rate. During approximately this same period,

Hon[31,32] was developing methods for continuous recording of the fetal heart rate and, more important, the factors acting in the fetus that altered the fetal heart rate in response to uterine contractions. He identified three basic patterns, early, late, and variable decelerations, which were due to head compression, uteroplacental insufficiency, and umbilical cord compression, respectively. This permitted the attending obstetrician to assign a cause for the fetal heart rate decelerations that had already been described in the 1800s. It also permitted a more individualized therapy for the deceleration: change of position for the variable decelerations and maternal oxygen for the late decelerations. Baseline heart rate change and heart rate variability were also related to specific fetal or maternal conditions.

The association of late decelerations and fetal oxygen deficiency was carried into the antepartum period by Hammacher[33] in 1966. He observed that those infants who had late decelerations of their fetal heart rate in association with spontaneous uterine contractions had lower Apgar scores at birth and a higher stillbirth rate. In 1967, Pose and Escarcena[34] induced the contractions with oxytocin and found a similar correlation.

Biochemical Monitoring

Fetal heart rate changes are best characterized as biophysical changes. During this same period, fetal biochemical changes related to fetal well-being were being observed. The initial biochemical change associated with fetal health was its ability to make estriol.

Although Spielman[35] in 1933 and Smith[36] in 1941 demonstrated the association between maternal urinary estriol excretion and fetal health, the test was not used extensively until the 1950s, owing to the lack of a reliable and easily performed chemical assay. Brown[37] developed such an assay, and the test was used for many years, finally succumbing to less expensive, more accurate biophysical tests. Another biochemical marker of fetal distress was the acid-base balance of the fetal scalp blood introduced by Saling[38,39] in 1963.

Genetic Testing

The development of a method of culturing and examining the chromosomes of the fetal cells residing in the amniotic fluid of the first- and early second-trimester fetus permitted the diagnosis of chromosomal abnormalities when pregnancy could be safely terminated. In 1949, Barr[40] identified the sex chromatin that allowed several investigators to use amniotic fluid to determine whether a sex-linked genetic aberration was a possibility in a given pregnancy. Culture of amniotic fluid cells was reported by Jacobson[41] in 1967. They used available techniques to search for chromosomal abnormalities in 56 pregnancies before 20 weeks of gestation, with a greater than 90% success rate in obtaining adequate chromosomal patterns. Knowledge of chromosomal abnormalities has increased as new techniques such as banding allowed the geneticist a more detailed look at the chromosomal structure; more recently, the development of genetic probes has significantly widened the field of genetic diagnosis. Chromosomal abnormalities were not the only fetal problems that could be determined using amniotic fluid. Biochemical determinations allowed the diagnosis of such inheritable diseases as Tay-Sachs disease and many others.

Although amniotic sac puncture to obtain fluid had relatively few risks, there were some. This, coupled with the significant work and cost associated with analyzing amniotic fluid for chromosomal abnormalities, has led to restricting the test to those most at risk: older pregnant patients (aged 35 years and older) and patients who have a genetic problem in the family or had an abnormal prior pregnancy. The development of maternal blood markers for fetal abnormalities was extremely important because, using the criteria described above, one would miss a significant proportion of fetal problems. For example, although the risk of trisomy 21 is much greater in infants of patients older than 35 years, screening only these patients failed to detect 75% of the trisomy 21 fetuses, because patients were younger than 35 years.

In 1944, Pederson[42] described a protein, "fetuin," found only in the fetus. This was the first specific fetal protein identified. Bergstrand and Czar[43] found another fetal-specific protein, which migrated between the albumin and α-globulin fraction. This was named α-fetoprotein by Gitlin and Boesman[44] in 1966. In 1972, Brock and Sutcliffe[45] reported elevated levels of α-fetoprotein in the amniotic fluid surrounding fetuses with neural tube defects, and in 1984, Merkatz[46] noted that pregnant patients with a trisomy 21 fetus had lower than expected maternal levels of α-fetoprotein. This marker allows all pregnant patients to be offered screening for neural tube defects and some trisomies based on analysis of placental and fetal cells, which enter the maternal circulation, albeit in small numbers. Investigators are currently working on methods of harvesting and culturing these cells, which would obviate the need for amniocentesis.

Sonography

Until the mid-20th century, x-ray was the only methodology to diagnose intrauterine fetal abnormalities such as anencephaly.[47,48]

In 1958, Ian Donald[49] introduced a technical innovation to obstetrics and gynecology that brought the fetus to the obstetrician's fingertips. Ultrasound changed the way obstetrics was practiced because, for the first time, the fetus, placenta, and umbilical cord were visualized with increasing clarity.[50] One could assess fetal position, fetal growth, fetal weight, and fetal structure for anomalies, as well as placental and umbilical cord location and vessel number. As ultrasound improved technologically, it became possible to perform fetal echocardiograms and evaluate fetal blood flow through umbilical, uterine, and numerous fetal vessels. This clarity of observation allowed the obstetrician fetal access in terms of placing needles in the umbilical vessels to perform fetal diagnostic studies or therapy such as transfusion. In 1974, Campbell[51] was among the first to diagnose anencephaly by ultrasound *in utero*, and Chervenak[52] in 1985 reviewed the diagnosis and treatment of holoprosencephaly using ultrasound.

Although the fetus could be very accurately visualized and sometimes treated, using ultrasound, there were some conditions, such as diaphragmatic hernia, that required a surgical approach during the second trimester if pulmonary hypoplasia was to be avoided. Removal of the fetus from the uterus had been tried since 1980, but it was not successful owing to premature labor or fetal death *in utero*. In 1990, Harrison and his colleagues[53] reported the successful repair of a diaphragmatic hernia on a midtrimester fetus that was placed back into the uterus. The pregnancy continued into the third trimester, with delivery of a live fetus.

Development of Maternal-Fetal Medicine

In the decades after introduction of ultrasound and fetal monitoring, the fetus was ultimately considered a patient on its own right.[1]

Especially with the arrival of updated ultrasound equipment, by the 1980s, the fetus had become a patient whom the obstetrician could diagnose and treat. This is recognized in a variety of ways. The American Board of Obstetrics and Gynecology developed certification for the specialist in maternal-fetal medicine in 1974. Centers of excellence in care of the fetus have developed throughout the country, receiving referrals for difficult maternal and fetal management problems from the generalist obstetrician-gynecologist. Texts such as this stress fetal diagnostic and therapeutic approaches.

The Fetus as a Patient

McCullough, Coverdale, and Chervenak recently provided a brief account of the development of the discourse of the "fetal patient" and of the "fetus as a patient" in the medical literature[1], which started as early as the early 1970s when Liley[54] referred to the fetus as a "personality." At this time, the editors of the 14th edition of *Williams Obstetrics*[55] wrote:

"Since World War II and especially in the last decade, knowledge of the fetus and his environment has increased remarkably. As an important consequence, the fetus has acquired the status as a patient to be cared for by the physician as he has long been accustomed to caring for the mother."

The discourse of the fetus as a patient was motivated by advances in fetal diagnosis, e.g., ultrasound imaging and karyotyping, and by initial efforts of medical and surgical maternal-fetal intervention. From these investigations, there emerged the prediction that "prenatal diagnosis of a fetal malformation may now lead to treatment rather than abortion."[56]

Harrison and Adzick[57] embraced this new discourse in their review titled, "The Fetus as a Patient," and finally a textbook on "the unborn patient."[58]

In conjunction with the paper by Harrison and colleagues, John Fletcher, a pioneer in bioethics, addressed the ethical challenges of maternal-fetal intervention.[59] These centered on how to balance the health and life of the fetus with the health and life of the pregnant woman, how to implement respect for her autonomy in this balancing, and the potential incompatibility between offering treatment for a fetus with an abnormality and abortion. Fletcher set out an ethical framework for guiding clinical investigators and policy makers.

This decades-long discourse of the fetus as a patient culminates in the most current edition of *Williams Obstetrics*, which makes the notable claim that obstetrics practice concerns both the pregnant patient and "our second patient—the fetus."[60]

In 1985, Chervenak and McCullough presented for the first time an ethical framework based on the obligations of the obstetrician to both the pregnant and fetal patient.[61] This framework, they argued, should guide clinical judgment and decision-making and counseling of the pregnant patient when the fetus is a patient. Three ethical obligations must in all cases be considered: beneficence-based and autonomy-based ethical obligations to the pregnant patient and beneficence-based (*not* rights-based) ethical obligations to the fetal patient. In subsequent work, they explored the implications of the ethical concept of the fetus as a patient for a range of ethical challenges, including the intrapartum management of fetal hydrocephalus and the management of fetal anomalies detected during the third trimester.[62-65]

The discourse of the fetus as a patient has become international, indicating acceptance of the ethical concept of the fetus as a patient in diverse cultural contexts. The International Academy of Perinatal Medicine (IAPM) and the World Association of Perinatal Medicine (WAPM) have an important affiliated society, the International Society of the Fetus as a Patient, which sponsors a scientific congress annually.[66]

References

1. McCullough LB, Coverdale JH, Chervenak FA. *Professional Ethics in Obstetrics and Gynecology.* Cambridge University Press; 2020.
2. Waters EG. Disputed indications and technics for cesarean section. *N Engl J Med.* 1946;234:849-853.
3. Mayor H. *Biblioth Univ. de Geneve. November 9, 1818,* quoted by *Thomas, H.* In: *Classical Contributions to Obstetrics and Gynecology.* Charles C Thomas, Publisher; 1935.
4. de Kergaradec DLA. *Memoire sur l'Auscultation, applique a l'Etude de la Grossesse, Paris.* Méquignon-Marvis; 1822.
5. Kennedy E. *Observations on Obstetric Auscultation.* Hodges and Smith; 1833.
6. Schwartz H. *Arch Gynaekol.* 1870;1:361.
7. Schatz F. *Arch Gyiaekol.* 1885;25:159.
8. Von Winkel F. *Handbuch der Geburtshulfe.* J. F. Bergmann; 1903.
9. Lund CJ. Fetal tachycardia during labor: A fallible sign of fetal distress *Am J Obstet Gynecol.* 1943;45(4):636-645.

10. Freed FC. Clinical signs of fetal distress during labor. *Am J Obstet Gynecol.* 1927;14(5):659-666.

11. Noack H. Fetal indications of cesarean section; lessons from 50,000 obstetric cases during 15 years. *Geburtshilfe Frauenheilkd.* 1953;13(9):778-786.

12. Douglas RG, Stromme WB. *Operative Obstetrics.* Appleton-Century-Crofts; 1957:413.

13. McCall JO, Fulsher RW. A study of fetal distress, its interpretation and significance. *Am J Obstet Gynecol.* 1953;65(5):1006-1019.

14. Fitzgerald TB, McFarlane CN. Foetal distress and intrapartum foetal death. *Br Med J.* 1955;2(4935):358-361.

15. Goodlin R. History of fetal monitoring. *Am J Obstet Gynecol.* 1979;33:325.

16. Societe de Gynecologie et d'Obstetrique de Paris. *Boursier and Gautret from Paris. Bulletin de la Societe d'Obstetrique et Gynecologie de Paris.* Vol 12. Masson et Cie; 1923:389.

17. Goodlin RC. Diagnostic abdominal amniocentesis. *Am J Obstet Gynecol.* 1964;88:1090-1091.

18. Romero R, Chervenak FA, Coustan D, Berkowitz RL, Hobbins JC. Antenatal sonographic diagnosis of umbilical cord laceration. *Am J Obstet Gynecol.* 1982;143(6):719-720.

19. Romero R, Jeanty P, Reece EA, Grannum P, Bracken M, Berkowitz R, Hobbins JC. Sonographically monitored amniocentesis to decrease intraoperative complications. *Obstet Gynecol.* 1985;65(3):426-430.

20. Hobbins JC, Grannum PA, Romero R, Reece EA, Mahoney MJ. Percutaneous umbilical blood sampling. *Am J Obstet Gynecol.* 1985;152(1):1-6.

21. Bevis DCA. The prenatal prediction of antenatal disease of the newborn. *Lancet.* 1952;1:395.

22. Liley AW. Liquor amnii analysis in the management of the pregnancy complicated by rhesus sensitization. *Am J Obstet Gynecol.* 1961;82:1359.

23. Liley AW. Intrauterine transfusion of fetus in hemolytic disease. *Br Med J.* 1963; 2:1107-1109.

24. Liley AW. Technique of fetal transfusion in treatment of severe hemolytic disease. *Am J Obstet Gynecol.* 1964;89:817.

25. Saling E. Amnioscopy, a new method for diagnosis of conditions hazardous to the fetus when membranes are intact. *Geburtshilfe Frauenheilkd.* 1962;22:830-845.

26. Kornacki Z, Biczysko R, Jakubowski A. Amnioscopy as a routine obstetric examination in the later stages of pregnancy and at the beginning of labor. *Am J Obstet Gynecol.* 1968;101(4):539-541.

27. Vujić J. Time determination of the occurrence of meconium staining of amniotic fluid during the last weeks of normal pregnancy. *J Perinat Med.* 1973;1(4):263-267.

28. Saling E. Neue Untersuchungsmoglichkeiten des Kindes unter der Geburt. *Zentralbl Gynakol.* 1961;83:1906-1907.

29. Saling E. A new method for examination of the fetus during labor: introduction, technic and basics. Article in German. *Arch Gynak.* 1962;197:108-122.

30. Alavarez H, Caldeyro Barcia R, Amador Fernandez R. Uterine contractions in labor. *Ginecol Obstet Mex.* 1951;6(2):113-134.

31. Hon EH. The electronic evaluation of the fetal heart rate (preliminary report). *Am J Obstet Gynecol.* 1958;75:1215.

32. Hon EH, Hess OW. The clinical value of fetal electrocardiography. *Am J Obstet Gynecol.* 1960;79(5):1012-1023.

33. Hammacher K. Fruherkennung intrauteriner gefahrenzustande durch electrophonocardiographie und focographie. In: Elert R, Hates KA, eds. *Prophylaxe frunddkindicher hirnschaden.* Georg Thieme Verlag; 1966:120.

34. Pose SV, Escarcena L. The influence of uterine contractions on the partial pressure of oxygen in the human fetus. In: Calderyo-Barcia R, ed. *Effects of Labor on the Fetus and Newborn.* Pergamon Press; 1967:48.

35. Spielman F, Goldberger MA, Frank RT. Hormonal diagnosis of viability of pregnancy. *J Am Med Assoc.* 1933;101:266.

36. Smith GV, Smith OW. Estrogen and progestin metabolism in pregnancy: endocrine imbalance of preeclampsia and eclampsia. Summary of findings to February 1941. *Endocrinology.* 1941;1:470.

37. Brown JB. Chemical method for determination of oestriol, oestrone, and oestradiol in human urine. *Biochem J.* 1955;60:185.

38. Saling E, Schneider D. Biochemical supervision of the fetus during labor. *Br J Obstet Gynecol.* 1967;74:799.

39. Saling E. Fetal blood analysis during labor. *Am J Obstet Gynecol.* 2006;194(3):896-899.

40. Barr ML, Bertram LF. A morphologic distinction between neurons of the male and the female and the behavior of the nuclear satellite during accelerated nucleoprotein synthesis. *Nature.* 1949;163:676.

41. Jacobson CB, Barter RH. Intrauterine diagnosis and management of genetic defects. *Am J Obstet Gynecol.* 1967;99:796.

42. Pedersen K. Fetuin, a new globulin isolated from serum. *Nature.* 1944;154:575.

43. Bergstrand CG, Czar B. Demonstration of a new protein fraction in the serum from the human fetus. *Scand J Clin Lab Invest.* 1956;8:174.

44. Gitlin D, Boesman M. Serum alpha-fetoprotein albumen and gamma G-globulin in the human conceptus. *J Clin Invest.* 1966;45:1826.

45. Brock DJH, Sutcliffe RG. Alpha-fetoprotein in the diagnosis of anencephaly and spine bifida. *Lancet.* 1972;2:197.

46. Merkatz IR, Nitowsky IJM, Macri JN, Johnson WE. An association between low serum alpha-fetoprotein and fetal chromosomal abnormalities. *Am J Obstet Gynecol.* 1984;148:886.

47. Hensel E. Beitrag zur Röntgendiagnostik anenzephaler Missbildungen ante partum. *Klin Med Osterr Z Wiss Prakt Med.* 1948;3(5):181-184.

48. Ferrario E. Radiological diagnosis of fetal malformation and action of roentgen rays on the fetus. *Minerva Ginecol.* 1950;2(6):251-254.

49. Donald I, MacVicar J, Brown TG. Investigation of abdominal masses by pulsed ultrasound. *Lancet.* 1958;1:1188.

50. Donald I. On launching a new diagnostic science. *Am J Obstet Gynecol.* 1969;103:609.

51. Campbell S, Johnstone FD, Holt EM, May P. Anencephaly: early ultrasonic diagnosis and active management. *Lancet.* 1972;2(7789):1226-1227.

52. Chervenak FA, Isaacson G, Hobbins JC, Chitkara U, Tortora M, Berkowitz RL. Diagnosis and management of fetal holoprosencephaly. *Obstet Gynecol.* 1985;66(3):322-326.

53. Harrison MR, Odzick NS, Longaker MT, et al. Successful repair in-utero of a fetal diaphragmatic hernia after removal of herniated viscera from the left thorax. *N Engl J Med.* 1990;322:1582.

54. Liley AW. The fetus as personality. *Austr N Z J Psych.* 1972;6:99-105.

55. Williams JW, Hellman LM, Pritchard JA. *Williams Obstetrics.* 14th ed. Appleton-Century-Crofts; 1971.

56. Harrison MR, Golbus MS, Filly RA. Management of the fetus with a correctable congenital defect. *J Am Med Assoc.* 1981;246:774-777.

57. Harrison MR, Adzick NS. The fetus as a patient: surgical considerations. *Ann Surg.* 1991;213:279-291.

58. Harrison MR, Golbus MS, Filly RA, eds. *The Unborn Patient: Prenatal Diagnosis and Treatment.* Saunders; 1984.

59. Fletcher JC. The fetus as a patient: ethical issues. *J Am Med Assoc.* 1981;246:773

60. Cunningham GF, Leveno KJ, Bloom SL, et al. *Williams Obstetrics.* 25th ed. McGraw-Hill Education; 2018.

61. Chervenak FA, McCullough LB. Perinatal ethics: a practical method of analysis of obligations to mother and fetus. *Obstet Gynecol.* 1985;66(3):442-446.

62. Chervenak FA, McCullough LB. The fetus as a patient: an essential ethical concept for maternal-fetal medicine. *J Matern Fetal Med.* 1996;5(3):115-119.

63. Chervenak FA, McCullough LB. Nonaggressive obstetric management. An option for some fetal anomalies during the third trimester. *J Am Med Assoc.* 1989;261(23):3439-3440.

64. Chervenak FA, McCullough LB. Ethical analysis of the intrapartum management of pregnancy complicated by fetal hydrocephalus with macrocephaly. *Obstet Gynecol.* 1986;68(5):720-725.

65. Chervenak FA, McCullough LB. The fetus as patient: implications for directive versus nondirective counseling for fetal benefit. *Fetal Diagn Ther.* 1991;6(1-2):93-100.

66. International Academy of Perinatal Medicine. Accessed June 2, 2019. https://iaperinatalmedicine.org/

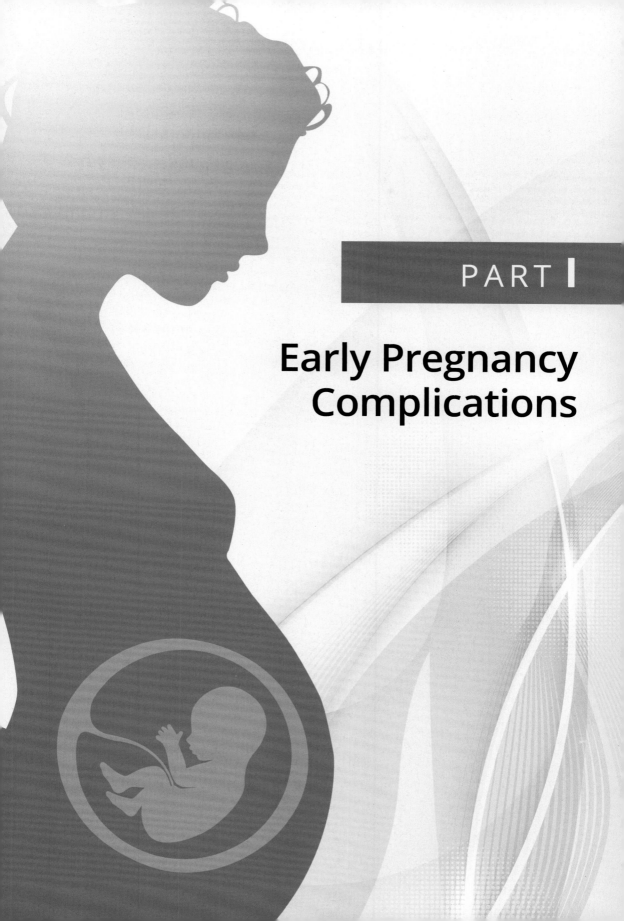

PART I

Early Pregnancy Complications

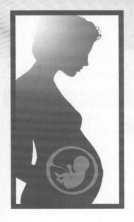

CHAPTER 1

Early Pregnancy Loss and Fetal Death

Erol Arslan, Kellie Woodfield, and David Ware Branch

Introduction and Definitions

Although various definitions of pregnancy losses are in use, a current and practical categorization that also recognizes distinct, albeit overlapping, periods in embryo-fetal development is shown in **Table 1.1**.[3]

In this chapter, the term *early pregnancy loss (EPL)* will be used to refer to clinically recognized pregnancies that fail prior to 10 weeks' gestation—in clinical practice, these are predominantly pre-embryonic and embryonic pregnancy losses but may include peri-implantation losses. We will group *early fetal death* (between 10 and 15 6/7 weeks) and *late fetal death* (between 16 and 19 6/7 weeks) together.

Sporadic Early Pregnancy Loss

Sporadic early pregnancy loss (SEPL), or sporadic miscarriage, is the occasional, nonconsecutive pregnancy loss that occurs in a woman who has (or will have) her desired number of children. Reasonable estimates suggest that up to 30% of pregnancies in otherwise healthy women are lost after implantation.[4]

The clinical presentation of SEPL is classified into several well-known (though sometimes ill-defined) categories: threatened abortion, inevitable abortion, incomplete abortion, missed abortion known as early pregnancy failure, complete abortion, and septic abortion (**Table 1.2**).

The etiology of SEPL can be divided into fetal, maternal, and paternal factors. Fetal factors, primarily genetic, play a prominent role in the etiology of SEPL, with aneuploid abortions occurring in an estimated 50% to 70% of cases.[10] The incidence of aneuploid abortions decreases with advancing gestational age, accounting for less than one-third of second-trimester losses and 5% or less of third-trimester losses.[11]

Chromosomal abnormalities responsible for SEPL are most often the result of errors in maternal gametogenesis; errors in paternal gametogenesis occur in only 5% of cases.[11] The most common chromosomal abnormality in sporadic miscarriages is single autosomal trisomy, which account for well over half of the abnormal karyotypes in SEPL.[12] This is usually the result of isolated nondisjunction or the failure of homologous chromosomes to separate. Among these, trisomy 16, 22, and 15 account for over one-third of the single autosomal trisomies.[13] Other abnormal karyotypes include X monosomy, autosomal monosomy, triploidy, tetraploidy, and chromosomal structural abnormalities such as balanced and unbalanced translocations.[12] Autosomal monosomy, or the presence of an unpaired, nonsex chromosome, is incompatible with life. Triploidy pregnancies frequently abort early and are associated with molar gestations. Tetraploidy, or the presence of two extra sets of chromosomes, also abort early.[14,15]

A wide array of maternal factors also contributes to a tendency for SEPL.[11] Age plays particularly prominent role; the incidence of abortions, both aneuploid and euploid, significantly increases after age 35 years. Endocrine abnormalities, most notably insulin-dependent diabetes, are associated with an increased risk of SEPL. Other less common contributing factors are frank intrauterine infections (infrequent), environmental factors such a radiation exposure in doses used to treat malignancy, and the presence of an intrauterine device (IUD) (associated with septic abortions). Paternal factors are generally less studied and, when present, likely arise from chromosomal abnormalities found in sperm.

See the eBook for expanded content and a complete reference list.

Table 1.1 Suggested Classification of Pregnancy Loss by Periods in Embryo-Fetal Development

Term	Definition
Peri-implantational loss	Failed pregnancy as shown by abnormal human chorionic gonadotropin progression <5 wk gestation and before the formation of an intrauterine gestational sac discernible by modern ultrasound methods
Pre-embryonic loss	Pregnancy loss in which ultrasonographic evaluation shows a gestational sac with no distinct embryo apparent, although a yolk sac may be present
Embryonic loss	Embryonic death defined as an ultrasonographically detectable, nonviable embryonic form measuring less than 10 wk in size on ultrasonography; or detectable embryonic cardiac activity with subsequent loss before the beginning of the fetal period (<10 wk); or loss of a formed embryo detected by visual inspection of the products of conception
Fetal loss	Death of the conceptus after the beginning of the 10th week of gestation or after the fetus has reached a crown rump length of more than 30 mm or after the detection of fetal heart motion beyond 10 wk

Recurrent Early Pregnancy Loss

Recurrent early pregnancy loss (REPL), most commonly defined as the loss of two or more clinically recognized pregnancies, is one of the most common reproductive health problems. It is estimated to occur in up to several percent of couples desiring to have a family, and approximately 0.5% to 1% of such couples suffer three or more consecutive REPLs.[16] The incidence of REPL varies according to a number of factors, including maternal age, number of prior EPLs, and self-selection factors.[17-19] The rate of miscarriage per recognized conception rises in women above age 35 years, owing in part to increasing rates of aneuploidy associated with older oocytes.[17]

In most couples with REPL, an identifiable, dominant etiologic factor amenable to evidence-based treatment will not be found. Fortunately, most couples with REPL will have one or more successful pregnancies. Best clinical practice calls for a fundamental understanding of the current status of REPL and an evidence-based approach to evaluation and management.

Known or Suspected Etiologic Factors for REPL

Lifestyle and Environmental Factors

Whether maternal smoking or alcohol consumption is associated with REPL is uncertain, although

Table 1.2 Types of Spontaneous Abortion by Clinical Presentation

Threatened abortion	Vaginal bleeding without diagnostic criteria for abortion as yet met. Although bleeding increases the risk of pregnancy loss, it is not an uncommon occurrence in early pregnancy, with an estimated incidence of 20%-25%.[5,6] Approximately 20% of women with threatened abortion in early pregnancy will miscarry.[5]
Inevitable abortion	Vaginal bleeding and uterine cramping with a dilated cervix and evidence of products of conception discernible by visual or digital inspection of the cervical os or rupture of membranes.
Incomplete abortion	Vaginal bleeding and uterine cramping with a dilated cervix and products of conception in the cervical canal.
Missed abortion	Diagnosis of failed pregnancy, typically by ultrasound, without symptoms of abortion and with a closed cervix.
Complete abortion	Products of conception have been passed through the cervix, continued bleeding is minimal, uterine cramping has largely resolved, and the uterus is contracted down on examination.
Septic abortion	Uterine infection associated with a miscarriage or elective termination. Endomyometritis is most common, but parametritis, peritonitis, and even endocarditis and septic emboli may develop.[7,8] Septic abortion may lead to severe sepsis, acute respiratory distress syndrome, or disseminated intravascular coagulation. Responsible pathogens are often native vaginal flora, including *Clostridium perfringens* and *Clostridium sordellii*.[9]

each has been associated with SEPL in retrospective studies.[22] General physical activity levels have not been associated with REPL and are not linked to sporadic miscarriage.

Obesity (body mass index [BMI] > 30 kg/m^2) is associated with REPL, with a recent systematic review noting an odds ratio (OR) of 1.75 (95% confidence interval [CI] of 1.24-2.47).[24] In a prospective study, women with obesity were found to have a higher frequency of euploid miscarriages,[25] and another study showed that women with obesity having REPL were more likely to have a subsequent miscarriage.[26] Although being underweight has been linked to sporadic miscarriage, its relationship to REPL is unknown.

Genetic Abnormalities

Emerging evidence suggests that EPLs are, at least in some cases, associated with gain or loss of subchromosomal amounts of genetic material, discernible using such techniques as microarray.[30] Given that most of these so-called microdeletions or microduplications are of uncertain pathological significance, they are referred to as copy number changes (CNCs). To be sure, some CNCs are more likely to represent a causative factor in pregnancy loss, including those of large CNC size, deletions (rather than duplications), CNCs including genes described in the Online Mendelian Inheritance in Man database, and changes not described in databases of healthy individuals.

In 3% to 5% of couples with REPL, one of the partners is found to have a balanced chromosomal rearrangement, a figure that is at least severalfold higher than in the general population.[31] Most mutations are reciprocal balanced translocations; Robertsonian translocations, sex chromosome mosaicisms, and chromosomal inversions are less commonly found.[32] In REPL couples, balanced translocations are more commonly found in the female partner, and it appears that the risk of subsequent EPL is increased if the translocation originates from maternal side.

Moreover, a woman with a first-degree relative with REPL has a two- to sixfold increased risk of REPL herself.[33,34] Although there is some evidence that otherwise unexplained REPL is associated with an increased rate of aneuploid sperm and apoptosis, the role of such paternal gamete meiotic errors in REPL is uncertain; this is an area that deserves

further, more sophisticated study. A case-controlled study investigated the additional risk factors in REPL couples that increased the risk of parental karyotype abnormalities.[36] Younger maternal age at second miscarriage, history of ≥3 miscarriages, or having a sibling or parent with >2 miscarriages were found to be associated with higher prevalence of parental karyotype abnormalities.

In addition to numerical and structural chromosomal abnormalities, some single gene disorders are known to be associated with REPL. The most common ones are metabolic disorders and hemoglobinopathies, although they contribute to a very small proportion of REPL cases.[32] Skewed X inactivation, a phenomenon of preferential inactivation of one X chromosome instead of random inactivation of either, has been considered as a cause of REPL. One study found that the rate of skewed X inactivation was threefold higher in women with REPL compared to those in the general population,[37] while another did not find any association between skewed X inactivation and REPL.[38]

Uterine Factors

Interpretations of the studies that examine an association between REPL and uterine malformations are limited by variation in the definition of recurrent loss and the use of different malformation classifications systems.[39] That said, most experts would accept that uterine malformations are found in 10% to 25% of women with REPL[40] with a mean of 12.6% based on results from various studies.[22] By comparison, a malformed uterus (including arcuate uterus) is found in approximately 4% to 8% of women seeking gynecologic care for a variety of reasons other than pregnancy loss.[39,41] It also has been shown that in women undergoing three dimensional (3D) ultrasound screening for reasons other than pregnancy loss, a history of pregnancy loss was more common in women with uterine malformations than in women with a structurally normal uterus[42]; a history of first-trimester loss was found in 42% of women with a subseptate uterus and 16% of women with arcuate uterus. The most common malformations found in women with REPL are septate, subseptate, or arcuate anomalies, followed by bicornuate uterus (**Figure 1.1**). Unicornuate uterus is uncommon.

The cause of REPL in women with uterine malformations may be implantation on a poorly vascularized septum, although this mechanism is

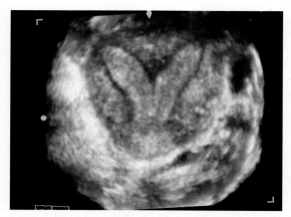

Figure 1.1 Antiphospholipid syndrome.

supported only by indirect evidence. Whether the degree of uterine cavity distortion, for example, the length of the uterine septum or the reduction in the length of the remaining cavity, is associated with a higher likelihood of pregnancy loss is debatable.

Whether acquired uterine abnormalities, such as leiomyomata, intrauterine adhesions, or endometrial polyps, are associated with REPL is not well established.

Antiphospholipid syndrome (APS) is a widely accepted cause of REPL. International consensus criteria[49] recognize three clinically relevant aPLs: lupus anticoagulant (LAC), anticardiolipin (aCL), and anti–β_2-glycoprotein 1 (aβ_2GP1) antibodies. Some experts also test for immunoglobulin (Ig) G and IgM antibodies to phosphatidylserine.

Pathogenic aPL antibodies recognize β_2GP1, a glycoprotein constitutively expressed on the cell surface of trophoblast cells, as well as on many other cells, including maternal decidual endothelial cells. In extravillous trophoblasts, aPL antibodies promote pro-inflammatory, antimigratory, and antiangiogenic effects. aPL antibodies also displace annexin V, an inhibitor of coagulation, from the surface of trophoblastic cells.[51] aPL antibody–induced immune activation, including complement activation, at the maternal-fetal interface results in pregnancy loss in animal models.

Hypocomplementemia and increased complement activation products have been reported in women with APS and in association with adverse pregnancy outcomes, including miscarriage.[54,55]

The association of aPL antibodies with REPL is not without controversy.[56] Overall, the published studies are highly heterogeneous, with many flawed by the inclusion of subjects with either poorly characterized pregnancy losses, especially regarding gestational age of loss, or the admixture of subjects with pre-embryonic, embryonic, and fetal deaths. Many studies also used nonstandard aPL antibody tests and/or "positive" results that do not meet international criteria definitions of positive. Some studies did not perform repeat testing to confirm positive aPL antibodies in accord with expert guidelines. Over the course of nearly a decade, two experienced groups of investigators have found fewer than 25 women with REPL as an isolated chief complaint (ie, without thrombosis, systemic lupus erythematosus, or fetal death), and with repeatedly positive aPL antibody titers, meeting international criteria.[57,58]

Endocrine Abnormalities

Thyroid Disorders

Retrospective studies suggest that recurrent pregnancy loss may be associated with overt hypothyroidism.[59] A link between REPL and subclinical or mild thyroid disease is debated because of conflicting findings among available studies.[60-62]

Thyroid autoantibodies may be associated with REPL, and both anti–thyroid peroxidase antibodies (TPOAbs) and antithyroglobulin antibodies (TGAbs) have been implicated, although the evidence is stronger for TPOAbs. A meta-analysis found an increased risk of miscarriage in women with REPL and TPOAbs, even if the mother was euthyroid.[63] However, a 2019 randomized trial of women with TPOAbs antibodies used very early urine pregnancy test screening and found that, of the women who became pregnant, the pregnancy loss rate prior to 24 weeks was 30%, a figure that may not be remarkably different than the rate of pregnancy loss in the general obstetric population if pregnancy is identified at 3 to 4 weeks' gestation.[64]

Diabetes

Poorly controlled overt diabetes is associated with miscarriage at both high and low extremes of glycemic control.[65] However, the relationship between overt glucose intolerance and REPL is poorly defined; the same is true for mild glucose intolerance or prediabetes. One case-controlled study found that serum fructosamine levels, an indication of average blood glucose over 1 to 3 weeks, were higher in women with REPL even after adjusting for BMI.[66] Likewise, some studies showed an association between REPL and insulin resistance.

Polycystic Ovary Syndrome

Polycystic ovary syndrome (PCOS) has been showed to have an association with REPL.

However, the association of PCOS with REPL is complicated by the tendency of PCOS to be associated with other conditions (ie, increased BMI, insulin resistance, hyperandrogenism, and poor endometrial receptivity) that might contribute to increased risk of miscarriage.[70]

Luteal Phase Deficiency

Historically, luteal phase deficiency (LPD) has been defined as a condition in which endogenous progesterone production is insufficient to support the secretory endometrium and foster normal implantation. However, whether LPD exists as an independent entity affecting consecutive menstrual cycles has been questioned,[71] and there is no consensus on the best method to make a diagnosis. Basal body temperature assessment, urinary luteinizing hormone detection kits, luteal progesterone levels, and endometrial biopsy interpretation are poorly reproducible, physiologically irrelevant, or clinical impractical.

Prolactin Abnormalities

Both low and elevated levels of prolactin have been associated with REPL by some,[72,73] but not all,[74] investigators.

Other Possible Etiologies

Inherited Thrombophilias

Thrombophilias are discussed in Chapter 2, but a brief overview is warranted here. Factor V Leiden (FVL) is the best-studied inherited thrombophilia with regard to REPL, but findings are inconsistent.[75]

The prothrombin mutation (G20210A) is somewhat less well studied, although the available evidence suggests no more than a weak association between G20210A and REPL.[76,77] Protein C deficiency, protein S deficiency, and antithrombin deficiency are each infrequently seen that there are not enough data to show possible associations with REPL.

The relatively common methylenetetrahydrofolate reductase mutations (C677T and A1298C) are now widely considered to not be associated with thromboembolism.[75] Contrary findings notwithstanding,[85] many, if not most, experts also do not consider these mutations to be associated with REPL.[76,86,87]

Immunologic Abnormalities

A causative role for immunological abnormalities in REPL remains a subject of ongoing study and considerable debate. Polymorphism of human leukocyte antigen (HLA) G and three or more REPL with an OR of 1.5 (95% CI 1.16-1.99).[91]

Circulating tumor necrosis factor alpha (TNF-alpha) levels have been found in women with REPL,[93] and elevated levels of TNF-alpha increase the likelihood of miscarriage in women with REPL.[95] Experts currently conclude that methodological concerns limit the interpretation of a possible role for cytokines as a causative factor in REPL.[96]

Some,[98] but not all, studies[99] have found that women with REPL have a higher percentage of peripheral NK cells compared to controls. Similarly, increased peripheral NK cell cytotoxicity has been demonstrated in women with REPL by some,[100] but not all,[101] investigators. Finally, increased NK cell cytotoxicity has been associated with subsequent pregnancy loss in women with REPL by some,[102] but not others.[101] The story is much the same for endometrial and decidual NK cells.[96]

Evaluation of Patients With REPL

Our recommended evaluation of couples with REPL is summarized in **Table 1.3**. Importantly, evaluation should initially involve screening for conditions that (1) identify a credible etiology for REPL, (2) aid in determining the prognosis for future pregnancy, and (3) are amenable to a management or treatment that will improve next pregnancy outcome for the couple. We favor evaluating couples using a standardized approach based on the existing professional organization guidelines. Unfortunately, few diagnoses serve all three goals and, in particular, solid evidence of effective treatment for REPL in a majority of cases is lacking.

Prognosis and Treatment of REPL

It is imperative that clinicians counseling couples with REPL recognize that, in most cases, a single, credible cause of pregnancy loss *amenable to a management or treatment that will improve the outcome of the next pregnancy* is unlikely to be found. It is reassuring in most of these cases, though, that the prognosis for successful pregnancy is relatively good (**Table 1.4**).[105,106]

Table 1.3 Recommended Evaluations in Couples With Recurrent Early Pregnancy Loss

Known or Suspected Cause	Specific Tests or Assessments	Comments	
		ASRM Guidelines	ESHRE Guidelines
History and select physical examination	Maternal age; details of and number of prior losses; BMI; social habits	—	—
Uterine anomalies or defects	Options: • 3D ultrasound of uterus • Sonohysterography • Hysterosalpingography • MRI	Recommended	• Transvaginal 3D ultrasound preferred due to high sensitivity and specificity and can distinguish between septate uterus and bicorporeal uterus with normal cervix (former AFS bicornuate uterus).
Cytogenetic	• Parental karyotypes	Recommended	• Parental karyotyping is not routinely recommended in couples due to low yield in couples with without a history of a genetically abnormal fetus/newborn or a child with congenital anomalies. Individual risk assessment recommended.
	• Products of conception array-CGH	Cytogenetic analysis of subsequent losses can be employed to evaluate whether the event was random and may be of psychological value to the couple.	• Genetic analysis of pregnancy tissue is not routinely recommended, but it may be performed for explanatory purposes.
Autoimmune	Antiphospholipid antibodies: • Lupus anticoagulant (LA) • Anticardiolipin (aCL) IgG and IgM • Anti–β_2-glycoprotein 1 (aβ_2GP1) IgG and IgM	Recommended. Other autoantibody tests, eg, ANA are not generally recommended.	• Screening for LA and aCL IgG and IgM recommended. Screening for aβ_2GP1 may be considered. Other autoantibody tests such as ANA and celiac disease markers not recommended.
Endocrinologic disorders	• TSH	TSH recommended. Testing for antithyroid antibodies not recommended.	• TSH and TPO antibodies recommended. Abnormal TSH and TPO antibody levels should be followed up by T4 testing.
	• Diabetes screen	Hemoglobin A1c recommended.	• Assessment of fasting glucose (or insulin) not recommended.
	• Prolactin	Recommended	• Prolactin testing is not recommended in women with RPL in the absence of clinical symptoms of hyperprolactinemia (oligo/amenorrhea).

AFS, American Fertility Society; ANA, antinuclear antibody; ASRM, American Society of Reproductive Medicine; BMI, body mass index; CGH, comparative genomic hybridization; ESHRE, European Society of Human Reproduction and Embryology; Ig, immunoglobulin; MRI, magnetic resonance imaging; TPO, thyroid peroxidase; TSH, thyroid-stimulating hormone.

Table 1.4 Predicted Pregnancy Success Rates According to Age and Previous Miscarriage

| | History in Patient With Idiopathic Recurrent Pregnancy Loss | | | |
| | No. of Prior Miscarriages | | | |
Age (y)	2	3	4	5
20	92% (86-98)	90% (83-97)	88% (79-96)	85% (74-96)
25	89% (82-95)	86% (79-93)	82% (75-91)	79% (68-90)
30	84% (77-90)	80% (74-86)	76% (69-83)	71% (61-81)
35	77% (69-85)	73% (66-80)	68% (60-75)	62% (51-74)
40	69% (57-82)	64% (52-76)	58% (45-71)	52% (37-67)
45	60% (41-79)	54% (35-72)	48% (29-67)	42% (22-62)

95% confidence interval shown in parentheses.
Modified from Brigham SA, Conlon C, Farquharson RG. A longitudinal study of pregnancy outcome following idiopathic recurrent miscarriage. *Hum Reprod.* 1999;14(11):2868-2871.

Lifestyle and Environmental Factors

Whether altering behaviors, such as smoking or alcohol or caffeine intake, will reduce the likelihood of subsequent EPL in couples with REPL is unknown. It is our practice to use the opportunity afforded by consultation to make reasonable recommendations regarding healthy behaviors. It is also currently unknown whether weight management to achieve a relatively normal BMI will reduce the likelihood of EPL, although we routinely make recommendations that women seeking our advice should strive to achieve a BMI less than 30 kg/m². It is worth emphasizing that smoking, alcohol intake, and obesity are each associated with well-recognized complications of pregnancy beyond the first trimester.

The prognosis for couples in which one member carries a balance chromosomal abnormality depends upon the nature of the abnormality, as well as other factors such as maternal age. Given the risk for a chromosomally imbalanced conceptus, preconceptional genetic counseling is advisable, and antenatal cytogenetic studies should be recommended once the patient is pregnant.

Uterine Factors

Treatment of uterine malformations to improve pregnancy outcome in women with RPL is not based on properly designed trials. Although it is tempting to speculate that hysteroscopic metroplasty in women with REPL and a septate uterus may be beneficial, claims of improved pregnancy outcomes after hysteroscopic resection of a uterine septum are based on analyses of retrospective data or case series.

Guidelines of the American Society of Reproductive Medicine (ASRM) conclude that there is limited (Grade C) evidence to support hysteroscopic septum resection to reduce the rate of miscarriages in women with REPL.[113] At the time of this publication a randomized trial of uterine septum take down is apparently underway.[114] Despite the controversial results in uterine septum surgery, it is more likely that the arcuate uterus is not plausibly amenable to a surgical correction.

Hysteroscopic surgery to address submucosal leiomyomata, uterine polyps, or uterine synechiae is also of unproven benefit in terms of reducing the miscarriage rate in subsequent pregnancy. The paucity of quality evidence should remind practitioners to approach corrective procedures with the knowledge that surgery may not always improve a patient's chances for successful pregnancy. Surgical injury to the uterus poses potential risks for further intrauterine scarring in the case of inadvertent transmural injury and uterine rupture in subsequent pregnancy.

Antiphospholipid Syndrome

Currently recommended therapy for women with REPL who are diagnosed with APS and no history of prior thrombosis is prophylactic or intermediate-dose unfractionated heparin or a prophylactic dose of low-molecular-weight heparin in combination with low-dose aspirin (LDA).[22] The LDA may be started preconceptionally, and the heparin agent is started once a potentially viable pregnancy is identified (usually around 6 or 7 weeks' gestation). Women with APS and a history of thrombosis, most of whom are maintained on long-term anticoagulation, require transitioning from their long-term anticoagulation agent to therapeutic levels of a heparin agent prior to or very early in pregnancy. These recommendations notwithstanding, the use of a heparinoid to treat RPL in women diagnosed with APS has been questioned.[56,117]

The most recent American College of Obstetricians and Gynecologists (ACOG) Practice Bulletin acknowledges that for women with APS without a preceding thrombotic event, "expert consensus suggests that clinical surveillance or prophylactic heparin" may be used in the antepartum period, although that "prophylactic doses of heparin and low-dose aspirin during pregnancy...should be considered."[126]

Endocrine Disorders

Clinically apparent endocrine disorders, such as overt hypothyroidism or diabetes, require treatment to avoid the detrimental impact on pregnancy. Whether the treatment of subclinical hypothyroidism found in women with REPL reduces the likelihood of EPL is uncertain. A recent meta-analysis concluded that levothyroxine supplementation of women with subclinical hypothyroidism was associated with a significant decrease in the rate of pregnancy loss,[63] although the included studies did not target women with REPL. One small, observational study in which women with two or more early losses were treated with levothyroxine if their thyroid-stimulating hormone (TSH) was >2.5 found no difference in subsequent pregnancy outcomes.[60]

The American Thyroid Association recommends that euthyroid women with TPOAb or TGAb should be tested in early pregnancy for evidence of subclinical hypothyroidism and advises thyroid supplementation for those with a TSH >2.5 mU/L but within the normal range.[127] It is unknown, however, if this reduces miscarriage risks. Both ASRM and European Society of Human Reproduction and Embryology (ESHRE) recognize the absence of evidence for treatment of euthyroid women to reduce the likelihood of EPL.

Just as it is medically prudent to treat overt thyroid disease, it is also medically prudent to do so for diabetes and impaired glucose tolerance, with or without PCOS. However, whether the treatment of mild glucose intolerance in women with REPL improves pregnancy outcomes is uncertain.

Thus, both ASRM and ESHRE guidelines conclude that there is insufficient evidence to recommend metformin supplementation in pregnancy to prevent pregnancy loss in women with REPL and glucose metabolism defects.

Progesterone treatment of women with REPL has been popular and is widely considered to be without significant risk of harm. A major randomized trial in the United Kingdom, however, has shown that this approach is without benefit with regard to live birth rates or other outcomes.[131]

One small randomized trial of 64 women with hyperprolactinemia and REPL showed that bromocriptine treatment was associated with a higher live birth rate compared to no treatment.[73] Therefore, it seems medically appropriate to treat hyperprolactinemia, a view supported by both ASRM and ESHRE.

Other Possible Etiologies

Inherited Thrombophilias

Systematic reviews have found no benefit of anticoagulant treatment for the prevention of pregnancy loss[132] or the promotion of live birth[133] in women with inherited thrombophilia and REPL. Neither the ASRM nor ESHRE recommends antithrombotic treatment of women with inherited thrombophilia and REPL to prevent subsequent pregnancy loss outside of a research protocol.

Immunologic Abnormalities

Various immunomodulatory treatments have been studied in women with REPL, and proponents of such treatments tend to be adamant that these treatments are beneficial.

Neither the ASRM nor the ESHRE recommends such treatments, in part because uncertainties related to testing for immunologic abnormalities would serve to identify a population that might benefit. In addition, immunization with allogeneic cells and intravenous immune globulin treatment each carry risks of adverse events.

Prednisone treatment of women with REPL and autoantibodies, such as antinuclear and anti-DNA antibodies, is without significant benefit with regard to EPL and is associated with later pregnancy complications.[137] In addition, a small randomized trial of women with REPL and elevated endometrial NK cell counts found no benefit to treatment with prednisolone in early pregnancy.[138] The ASRM and ESHRE do not recommend glucocorticoids for women with REPL.

Idiopathic Causes

Despite the improvement in diagnosis and treatment options, the cause of RPL remains unknown in over 50% of patients.[139] The idiopathic etiology of RPL increases patient anxiety, and some may look to unproven treatments that have no clear benefits on improving pregnancy outcomes but may have side effects as well as higher costs. Therefore, psychological support for couples with RPL may be important for achieving a pregnancy resulting in a live birth.[140] Indeed, Lund et al found that referral to a tertiary center for RPL resulted in two-thirds of couples having a live birth within 5 years.[106]

Fetal Death

Early and late fetal death (10-19 6/7 weeks' gestation), herein referred to as fetal death, is estimated to occur in 0.5% to 1% of pregnancies and is the topic of Chapter 4. The exact incidence is uncertain, in part because early and late fetal deaths are very often classified as miscarriages, along with EPLs. Focused studies of carefully dated fetal deaths are very few; studies of early fetal death >10 weeks and before 15 to 16 weeks are scant. Late fetal death (between 16 and 19 6/7 weeks) has been better evaluated, particularly in the context of patients being considered for genetic amniocentesis.

Known or Suspected Etiologic Factors for Fetal Death

The known and suspected causes of fetal death were shown in **Table 1.5**. But they likely overlap somewhat with those of EPL and very likely overlap with those of stillbirth at or beyond 20 weeks' gestation. Fetal death may be due to conditions for which the presentation leads to an established and

Table 1.5 Known or Suspected Etiologies of Fetal Death

Etiology	Comments
Lifestyle, environmental factors, and endocrine disorders	Very little is known regarding a relationship between fetal death and maternal smoking, maternal weight, or endocrine disorders of mild to moderate severity in otherwise asymptomatic patients. Both smoking and obesity are associated with an increased likelihood of fetal death after 20 weeks' gestation.[141]
Genetic abnormalities	Approximately 5%-10% of stillbirths are chromosomally abnormal.[142] The rate in fetal death between 10 and 20 wk is less well studied, but in practice, those with genetic abnormalities are often associated with obvious fetal anomalies discovered by ultrasound or autopsy. The role of parental karyotype abnormalities in fetal death is less well studied than in recurrent early pregnancy loss.
Uterine factors	In one retrospective study, 4% of women attending a consultation practice who had experienced one or more fetal deaths had a uterine malformation.[143]
Antiphospholipid syndrome (APS)	APS is associated with otherwise unexplained fetal death. In our experience, fetal death secondary to APS typically occurs after 16-18 wk and is classically associated with signs or features of severe placental insufficiency.
Placental abnormalities	Abnormalities of the umbilical cord, membranes, or placenta have been found in more than 50% of fetal deaths <20 wk.[144] These include maternal vascular malperfusion features as seen in preeclampsia, fetal vascular occlusion, chronic histiocytic intervillositis (CHI), massive perivillous fibrin deposition, villitis of unknown etiology, and features of infection. In many cases, the implications of these abnormalities are primarily explanatory, but CHI is known to recur.[145]
Fetal abnormalities	Fetal death may be associated with subtle or non-diagnostic fetal abnormalities may be detected via prenatal ultrasound or fetal autopsy. One prospective study in which targeted midtrimester fetal ultrasound was performed between 13 and 17 weeks' gestation found abnormalities in 72% of 61 fetal death cases, with fetal nuchal edema, cystic hygroma, or gross edema being the most common abnormal findings.[146]
Infection	A variety of bacteria, viruses, and protozoa have been documented to cause fetal death, and with diligent evaluation, many are associated with placental or fetal ultrasonographic or autopsy findings, positive maternal serologies, or positive cultures.
Inherited thrombophilias	The relationship between inherited thrombophilias and fetal death is a subject of ongoing debate. The most recent American College of Obstetricians and Gynecologists Practice Bulletin[75] suggests there is no association, and large prospective studies of women with heterozygous for Factor V Leiden[81] or for the prothrombin mutation[147] were negative.

credible diagnosis. Examples include gross hydrops fetalis in a case of Kell alloimmunization or characteristic structural anomalies in a case of trisomy 18. However, in perhaps 50% or more of cases of fetal death between 10 and 19 6/7 weeks' gestation, a definitive diagnosis is not found.

Evaluation of Patients With Fetal Death

Our recommended evaluation of couples with one or more fetal deaths not obviously due to chromosomal and/or structural abnormalities is summarized in **Table 1.6**.

Prognosis and Treatment of Subsequent Pregnancies in Cases of Prior Fetal Death

The prognosis for subsequent fetal death ultimately depends upon the nature of the etiology, and if an etiology is suspected or found. APS associated with fetal death is treated with a heparin agent and LDA, as discussed above under REPL. Favorable outcomes may be expected in most cases, but women with repeatedly positive tests for lupus anticoagulant or those that are positive for LAC, aCL, and $a\beta_2GP1$ are at risk of

Table 1.6 Recommended Evaluations in Couples With One or More Fetal Deaths (10 to 19 6/7 Weeks) Not Obviously Due to Chromosomal and/or Structural Abnormalities

Known or Suspected Cause	Specific Tests or Assessments	Comments
History and selected physical examination	Maternal age; details of and number of prior losses; BMI; social habits	—
Uterine anomalies or defects	Options: • 3D ultrasound of uterus • Sonohysterography • Hysterosalpingography • MRI	—
Cytogenetic	Parental karyotypes	**Individual risk assessment recommended.** Likely of low yield in couples without a history of a genetically abnormal fetus/newborn or a fetus/child with congenital anomalies.
	Products of conception array-CGH	Likely of low yield in morphologically normal fetus.
Autoimmune	Antiphospholipid antibodies • Lupus anticoagulant (LA) • Anticardiolipin (aCL) IgG and IgM • Anti–β_2-glycoprotein 1 ($a\beta_2GP1$) IgG and IgM	Screening for LA and aCL IgG and IgM recommended. Screening for $a\beta_2GP1$ may be considered.
Placental abnormalities	Placental pathology examination	High yield with regard to explanatory value; potential for prognostic value in some cases.
Fetal abnormalities	Fetal autopsy	High yield with regard to explanatory value; potential for prognostic value in some cases.
Infections	Bacterial and viral cultures/serology	Placental pathology and fetal autopsy findings may point to an infectious etiology.
Endocrinologic disorders	Diabetes screen	Mechanistic relationship in absence of frank diabetes uncertain. Testing very inexpensive.

BMI, body mass index; CGH, comparative genomic hybridization; MRI, magnetic resonance imaging.

recurrent fetal death or early delivery for severe preeclampsia or placental insufficiency in spite of a heparin agent and LDA.[148]

The recurrence risk for the most common placental abnormalities, maternal vascular malperfusion/fetal thrombotic vasculopathy and perivillous fibrin deposition are not well understood, but clinicians should search for predispositions to early-onset gestational hypertensive disease in such patients, for example, maternal chronic hypertensive disease, underlying chronic renal disease, or APS. Similarly, the recurrence rate for (VUE) is uncertain. Chronic histiocytic intervillositis has a high recurrence risk, probably in excess of 60% to 70%,[145] and there is no known treatment. The recurrence rate for VUE is uncertain.

Fetal death due to a maternal-fetal viral infection, for example, primary cytomegalovirus or parvovirus infection, does not recur. The rate of recurrence for fetal death due to bacterial infections as well as fetal death due to bacterial infections such as group B streptococcus is unknown. In women with prior fetal death, it would seem clinically prudent to be certain that routine immunizations are up-to-date and to immunize against influenza. Screening for and treating sexually transmitted infections is the best clinical practice. In practice, many fetal deaths between 10 and 19 6/7 weeks will not have an obvious etiology.

KEY POINTS

- Approximately 20% of all pregnancies are lost as peri-implantational events. Another 10% to 12% are lost after clinically recognized, early pregnancy events before the 10th week. Finally, 0.5% to 1% are lost as fetal deaths at or beyond 10 weeks but before the 20th week.
- Approximately 50% to 70% of SEPLs are due conceptus aneuploidy. The most common chromosomal abnormality is single autosomal trisomy, which accounts for 50% of cases.
- Maternal risk factors for SEPL are increased age, endocrine abnormalities (thyroid diseases, diabetes, PCOS), environmental factors such as radiation exposure, presence of an IUD (associated with septic abortions), and intrauterine infections.
- Approximately 0.5% to 1% of couples suffer three or more consecutive REPLs. In the majority of couples, the etiology of REPL is very likely multifactorial, and despite recommended assessments, the etiology remains unknown in over half of the patients.
- Given the frustration and anxiety, most couples seek for unproven, often costly, evaluations and remedies. We recommend an evidence-based approach based on professional guidelines.
- Evaluations of couples with REPL should aim to (1) identify a credible etiology for REPL, (2) aid in determining the prognosis for future pregnancy, and (3) determine if there is an evidence-based management or treatment that will improve next pregnancy outcome.
- The known or suspected causes of fetal death between 10 and 20 weeks overlap with those of REPL, but the prognosis in otherwise unexplained cases is less favorable. Those are environmental and endocrine factors, genetic abnormalities, uterine factors, APS, placental and fetal abnormalities, infection and inherited thrombophilias.

REFERENCES

(only references cited in synoptic print chapter; for a complete reference list, see ebook)

3. Silver RM, Branch DW, Goldenberg R, Iams JD, Klebanoff MA. Nomenclature for pregnancy outcomes: time for a change. *Obstet Gynecol.* 2011;118(6):1402-1408.
4. Larsen EC, Christiansen OB, Kolte AM, Macklon N. New insights into mechanisms behind miscarriage. *BMC Med.* 2013;11:154.
5. Coomarasamy A, Devall AJ, Cheed V, et al. A randomized trial of progesterone in women with bleeding in early pregnancy. *N Engl J Med.* 2019;380(19):1815-1824.
6. Pillai RN, Konje JC, Tincello DG, Potdar N. Role of serum biomarkers in the prediction of outcome in women with threatened miscarriage: a systematic review and diagnostic accuracy meta-analysis. *Hum Reprod Update.* 2016;22(2):228-239.
7. Rouse CE, Eckert LO, Munoz FM, et al. Postpartum endometritis and infection following incomplete or complete abortion: case definition & guidelines for data collection, analysis, and presentation of maternal immunization safety data. *Vaccine.* 2019;37(52):7585-7595.
8. Piedimonte S, Almohammadi M, Lee TC. Group B Streptococcus tricuspid valve endocarditis with subsequent septic embolization to the pulmonary artery: a case report following elective abortion. *Obstet Med.* 2018;11(1):39-44.

9. Udoh A, Effa EE, Oduwole O, Okusanya BO, Okafo O. Antibiotics for treating septic abortion. *Cochrane Database Syst Rev.* 2016;7:Cd011528.

10. Romero ST, Geiersbach KB, Paxton CN, et al. Differentiation of genetic abnormalities in early pregnancy loss. *Ultrasound Obstet Gynecol.* 2015;45(1):89-94.

11. Cunningham FG, Leveno KJ, Bloom SL, et al. *Williams Obstetrics.* 25th ed. McGraw-Hill Education; 2018.

12. Blue NR, Page JM, Silver RM. Genetic abnormalities and pregnancy loss. *Semin Perinatol.* 2019;43(2):66-73.

13. Hardy K, Hardy PJ. 1(st) trimester miscarriage: four decades of study. *Transl Pediatr.* 2015;4(2):189-200.

14. Stefanova I, Jenderny J, Kaminsky E, et al. Mosaic and complete tetraploidy in live-born infants: two new patients and review of the literature. *Clin Dysmorphol.* 2010;19(3):123-127.

15. Toufaily MH, Roberts DJ, Westgate MN, Holmes LB. Triploidy: variation of phenotype. *Am J Clin Pathol.* 2016;145(1):86-95.

16. Branch DW, Gibson M, Silver RM. Clinical practice. Recurrent miscarriage. *N Engl J Med.* 2010;363(18):1740-1747.

17. Marquard K, Westphal LM, Milki AA, Lathi RB. Etiology of recurrent pregnancy loss in women over the age of 35 years. *Fertil Steril.* 2010;94(4):1473-1477.

18. Egerup P, Kolte AM, Larsen EC, Krog M, Nielsen HS, Christiansen OB. Recurrent pregnancy loss: what is the impact of consecutive versus nonconsecutive losses? *Hum Reprod.* 2016;31(11):2428-2434.

19. Rasmark Roepke E, Matthiesen L, Rylance R, Christiansen OB. Is the incidence of recurrent pregnancy loss increasing? A retrospective register-based study in Sweden. *Acta Obstet Gynecol Scand.* 2017;96(11):1365-1372.

22. Practice Committee of the American Society for Reproductive Medicine. Evaluation and treatment of recurrent pregnancy loss: a committee opinion. *Fertil Steril.* 2012;98(5):1103-1111.

24. Cavalcante MB, Sarno M, Peixoto AB, Araujo Junior E, Barini R. Obesity and recurrent miscarriage: a systematic review and meta-analysis. *J Obstet Gynaecol Res.* 2019;45(1):30-38.

25. Boots CE, Bernardi LA, Stephenson MD. Frequency of euploid miscarriage is increased in obese women with recurrent early pregnancy loss. *Fertil Steril.* 2014;102(2):455-459.

26. Metwally M, Saravelos SH, Ledger WL, Li TC. Body mass index and risk of miscarriage in women with recurrent miscarriage. *Fertil Steril.* 2010;94(1):290-295.

30. Rajcan-Separovic E, Diego-Alvarez D, Robinson WP, et al. Identification of copy number variants in miscarriages from couples with idiopathic recurrent pregnancy loss. *Hum Reprod.* 2010;25(11):2913-2922.

31. Royal College of Obstetricians & Gynaecologists. *Green-Top Guideline No. 17: Recurrent Miscarriage, Investigation and Treatment.* RCOG; 2011.

32. Page JM, Silver RM. Genetic causes of recurrent pregnancy loss. *Clin Obstet Gynecol.* 2016;59(3):498-508.

33. Christiansen OB, Mathiesen O, Lauritsen JG, Grunnet N. Idiopathic recurrent spontaneous abortion. Evidence of a familial predisposition. *Acta Obstet Gynecol Scand.* 1990;69(7-8):597-601.

34. Zhang BY, Wei YS, Niu JM, Li Y, Miao ZL, Wang ZN. Risk factors for unexplained recurrent spontaneous abortion in a population from southern China. *Int J Gynaecol Obstet.* 2010;108(2):135-138.

36. Franssen MT, Korevaar JC, Leschot NJ, et al. Selective chromosome analysis in couples with two or more miscarriages: case-control study. *Br Med J.* 2005;331(7509):137-141.

37. Robinson WP, Beever C, Brown CJ, Stephenson MD. Skewed X inactivation and recurrent spontaneous abortion. *Semin Reprod Med.* 2001;19(2):175-181.

38. Sullivan AE, Lewis T, Stephenson M, et al. Pregnancy outcome in recurrent miscarriage patients with skewed X chromosome inactivation. *Obstet Gynecol.* 2003;101(6):1236-1242.

39. Grimbizis GF, Campo R. Congenital malformations of the female genital tract: the need for a new classification system. *Fertil Steril.* 2010;94(2):401-407.

40. van Dijk MM, Kolte AM, Limpens J, et al. Recurrent pregnancy loss: diagnostic workup after two or three pregnancy losses? A systematic review of the literature and meta-analysis. *Hum Reprod Update.* 2020;26(3):356-367.

41. Chan YY, Jayaprakasan K, Zamora J, Thornton JG, Raine-Fenning N, Coomarasamy A. The prevalence of congenital uterine anomalies in unselected and high-risk populations: a systematic review. *Hum Reprod Update.* 2011;17(6):761-771.

42. Woelfer B, Salim R, Banerjee S, Elson J, Regan L, Jurkovic D. Reproductive outcomes in women with congenital uterine anomalies detected by three-dimensional ultrasound screening. *Obstet Gynecol.* 2001;98(6):1099-1103.

49. Miyakis S, Lockshin MD, Atsumi T, et al. International consensus statement on an update of the classification criteria for definite antiphospholipid syndrome (APS). *J Thromb Haemost.* 2006;4(2):295-306.

51. Rand JH, Wu XX, Quinn AS, Taatjes DJ. The annexin A5-mediated pathogenic mechanism in the antiphospholipid syndrome: role in pregnancy losses and thrombosis. *Lupus.* 2010;19(4):460-469.

54. Breen KA, Seed P, Parmar K, Moore GW, Stuart-Smith SE, Hunt BJ. Complement activation in patients with isolated antiphospholipid antibodies or primary antiphospholipid syndrome. *Thromb Haemost.* 2012;107(3):423-429.

55. Mankee A, Petri M, Magder LS. Lupus anticoagulant, disease activity and low complement in the first trimester are predictive of pregnancy loss. *Lupus Sci Med.* 2015;2(1):e000095.

56. de Jesus GR, Benson AE, Chighizola CB, Sciascia S, Branch DW. Sixteenth international congress on antiphospholipid antibodies task force. Report on obstetric antiphospholipid syndrome. *Lupus.* 2020;29(12):1601-1615. doi:10.1177/0961203320954520

57. Bowman ZS, Wunsche V, Porter TF, Silver RM, Branch DW. Prevalence of antiphospholipid antibodies and risk of subsequent adverse obstetric outcomes in women with prior pregnancy loss. *J Reprod Immunol.* 2015;107:59-63.

58. Clark CA, Davidovits J, Spitzer KA, Laskin CA. The lupus anticoagulant: results from 2257 patients attending a high-risk pregnancy clinic. *Blood.* 2013;122(3):341-347; quiz 466.

59. Rao VR, Lakshmi A, Sadhnani MD. Prevalence of hypothyroidism in recurrent pregnancy loss in first trimester. *Indian J Med Sci.* 2008;62(9):357-361.

60. Bernardi LA, Cohen RN, Stephenson MD. Impact of subclinical hypothyroidism in women with recurrent early pregnancy loss. *Fertil Steril.* 2013;100(5):1326-1331.

61. Uchida S, Maruyama T, Kagami M, et al. Impact of borderline-subclinical hypothyroidism on subsequent pregnancy outcome in women with unexplained recurrent pregnancy loss. *J Obstet Gynaecol Res.* 2017;43(6):1014-1020.

62. van Dijk MM, Vissenberg R, Bisschop PH, et al. Is subclinical hypothyroidism associated with lower live birth rates in women who have experienced unexplained recurrent miscarriage? *Reprod Biomed Online.* 2016;33(6):745-751.

63. Rao M, Zeng Z, Zhou F, et al. Effect of levothyroxine supplementation on pregnancy loss and preterm birth in women with subclinical hypothyroidism and thyroid autoimmunity: a systematic review and meta-analysis. *Hum Reprod Update.* 2019;25(3):344-361.

64. Dhillon-Smith RK, Middleton LJ, Sunner KK, et al. Levothyroxine in women with thyroid peroxidase antibodies before conception. *N Engl J Med.* 2019;380(14):1316-1325.

65. Jovanovic L, Knopp RH, Kim H, et al. Elevated pregnancy losses at high and low extremes of maternal glucose in early normal and diabetic pregnancy: evidence for a protective adaptation in diabetes. *Diabetes Care.* 2005;28(5):1113-1117.

66. Romero ST, Sharshiner R, Stoddard GJ, Ware Branch D, Silver RM. Correlation of serum fructosamine and recurrent pregnancy loss: case-control study. *J Obstet Gynaecol Res.* 2016;42(7):763-768.

70. Krog MC, Nielsen HS, Christiansen OB, Kolte AM. Reproductive endocrinology in recurrent pregnancy loss. *Clin Obstet Gynecol.* 2016;59(3):474-486.

71. Practice Committee of the American Society for Reproductive Medicine. Current clinical irrelevance of luteal phase deficiency: a committee opinion. *Fertil Steril.* 2015;103(4):e27-32.

72. Li W, Ma N, Laird SM, Ledger WL, Li TC. The relationship between serum prolactin concentration and pregnancy outcome in women with unexplained recurrent miscarriage. *J Obstet Gynaecol.* 2013;33(3):285-288.

73. Hirahara F, Andoh N, Sawai K, Hirabuki T, Uemura T, Minaguchi H. Hyperprolactinemic recurrent miscarriage and results of randomized bromocriptine treatment trials. *Fertil Steril.* 1998;70(2):246-252.

74. Triggianese P, Perricone C, Perricone R, De Carolis C. Prolactin and natural killer cells: evaluating the neuroendocrine-immune axis in women with primary infertility and recurrent spontaneous abortion. *Am J Reprod Immunol.* 2015;73(1):56-65.

75. American College of Obstetricians and Gynecologists' Committee on Practice Bulletins–Obstetrics. ACOG Practice Bulletin No. 197: inherited thrombophilias in pregnancy. *Obstet Gynecol.* 2018;132(1):e18-e34.

76. Rey E, Kahn SR, David M, Shrier I. Thrombophilic disorders and fetal loss: a meta-analysis. *Lancet.* 2003;361(9361):901-908.

77. Bradley LA, Palomaki GE, Bienstock J, Varga E, Scott JA. Can Factor V Leiden and prothrombin G20210A testing in women with recurrent pregnancy loss result in improved pregnancy outcomes?: results from a targeted evidence-based review. *Genet Med.* 2012;14(1):39-50.

81. Dizon-Townson D, Miller C, Sibai B, et al. The relationship of the factor V Leiden mutation and pregnancy outcomes for mother and fetus. *Obstet Gynecol.* 2005;106(3):517-524.

85. Zhang Y, He X, Xiong X, et al. The association between maternal methylenetetrahydrofolate reductase C677T and A1298C polymorphism and birth defects and adverse pregnancy outcomes. *Prenat Diagn.* 2019;39(1):3-9.

86. Pritchard AM, Hendrix PW, Paidas MJ. Hereditary thrombophilia and recurrent pregnancy loss. *Clin Obstet Gynecol.* 2016;59(3):487-497.

87. Dell'Edera D, L'Episcopia A, Simone F, Lupo MG, Epifania AA, Allegretti A. Methylenetetrahydrofolate reductase gene C677T and A1298C polymorphisms and susceptibility to recurrent pregnancy loss. *Biomed Rep.* 2018;8(2):172-175.

91. Fan W, Li S, Huang Z, Chen Q. Relationship between HLA-G polymorphism and susceptibility to recurrent miscarriage: a meta-analysis of non-family-based studies. *J Assist Reprod Genet.* 2014;31(2):173-184.

93. Mueller-Eckhardt G, Mallmann P, Neppert J, et al. Immunogenetic and serological investigations in nonpregnant and in pregnant women with a history of recurrent spontaneous abortions. German RSA/IVIG Study Group. *J Reprod Immunol.* 1994;27(2):95-109.

95. Choi YK, Kwak-Kim J. Cytokine gene polymorphisms in recurrent spontaneous abortions: a comprehensive review. *Am J Reprod Immunol.* 2008;60(2):91-110.

96. Wang NF, Kolte AM, Larsen EC, Nielsen HS, Christiansen OB. Immunologic abnormalities, treatments, and recurrent pregnancy loss: what is real and what is not? *Clin Obstet Gynecol.* 2016;59(3):509-523.

98. King K, Smith S, Chapman M, Sacks G. Detailed analysis of peripheral blood natural killer (NK) cells in women with recurrent miscarriage. *Hum Reprod.* 2010;25(1):52-58.

99. Azargoon A, Mirrasouli Y, Shokrollahi Barough M, Barati M, Kokhaei P. The state of peripheral blood natural killer cells and cytotoxicity in women with recurrent pregnancy loss and unexplained infertility. *Int J Fertil Steril.* 2019;13(1):12-17.

100. Karami N, Boroujerdnia MG, Nikbakht R, Khodadadi A. Enhancement of peripheral blood CD56(dim) cell and NK cell cytotoxicity in women with recurrent spontaneous abortion or *in vitro* fertilization failure. *J Reprod Immunol.* 2012;95(1-2):87-92.

101. Katano K, Suzuki S, Ozaki Y, Suzumori N, Kitaori T, Sugiura-Ogasawara M. Peripheral natural killer cell activity as a predictor of recurrent pregnancy loss: a large cohort study. *Fertil Steril.* 2013;100(6):1629-1634.

102. Ebina Y, Nishino Y, Deguchi M, Maesawa Y, Nakashima Y, Yamada H. Natural killer cell activity in women with recurrent miscarriage: etiology and pregnancy outcome. *J Reprod Immunol.* 2017;120:42-47.

105. Brigham SA, Conlon C, Farquharson RG. A longitudinal study of pregnancy outcome following idiopathic recurrent miscarriage. *Hum Reprod.* 1999;14(11):2868-2871.

106. Lund M, Kamper-Jorgensen M, Nielsen HS, Lidegaard O, Andersen AM, Christiansen OB. Prognosis for live birth in women with recurrent miscarriage: what is the best measure of success? *Obstet Gynecol.* 2012;119(1):37-43.

113. Practice Committee of the American Society for Reproductive Medicine. Electronic address: ASRM@asrm.org; Practice Committee of the American Society for Reproductive Medicine. Uterine septum: a guideline. *Fertil Steril.* 2016;106(3):530-540.

114. Rikken JFW, Kowalik CR, Emanuel MH, et al. The randomised uterine septum transsection trial (TRUST): design and protocol. *BMC Womens Health.* 2018;18(1):163.

117. Clark CA, Laskin CA, Spitzer KA. Anticardiolipin antibodies and recurrent early pregnancy loss: a century of equivocal evidence. *Hum Reprod Update.* 2012;18(5):474-484.

126. Committee on Practice Bulletins—Obstetrics, American College of Obstetricians and Gynecologists. Practice Bulletin No. 132: antiphospholipid syndrome. *Obstet Gynecol.* 2012;120(6):1514-1521.

127. Alexander EK, Pearce EN, Brent GA, et al. 2017 guidelines of the American Thyroid Association for the diagnosis and management of thyroid disease during pregnancy and the postpartum. *Thyroid.* 2017;27(3):315-389.

131. Coomarasamy A, Williams H, Truchanowicz E, et al. A randomized trial of progesterone in women with recurrent miscarriages. *N Engl J Med.* 2015;373(22):2141-2148.

132. Skeith L, Carrier M, Kaaja R, et al. A meta-analysis of low-molecular-weight heparin to prevent pregnancy loss in women with inherited thrombophilia. *Blood.* 2016;127(13):1650-1655.

133. de Jong PG, Kaandorp S, Di Nisio M, Goddijn M, Middeldorp S. Aspirin and/or heparin for women with unexplained recurrent miscarriage with or without inherited thrombophilia. *Cochrane Database Syst Rev.* 2014;(7):CD004734.

137. Laskin CA, Bombardier C, Hannah ME, et al. Prednisone and aspirin in women with autoantibodies and unexplained recurrent fetal loss. *N Engl J Med.* 1997;337(3):148-153.

138. Tang AW, Alfirevic Z, Turner MA, Drury JA, Small R, Quenby S. A feasibility trial of screening women with idiopathic recurrent miscarriage for high uterine natural killer cell density and randomizing to prednisolone or placebo when pregnant. *Hum Reprod.* 2013;28(7):1743-1752.

139. Jaslow CR, Carney JL, Kutteh WH. Diagnostic factors identified in 1020 women with two versus three or more recurrent pregnancy losses. *Fertil Steril.* 2010;93(4):1234-1243.

140. Green DM, O'Donoghue K. A review of reproductive outcomes of women with two consecutive miscarriages and no living child. *J Obstet Gynaecol.* 2019;39(6):816-821.

141. Silver RM. Fetal death. *Obstet Gynecol.* 2007;109(1):153-167.

142. Wapner RJ. Genetics of stillbirth. *Clin Obstet Gynecol.* 2010;53(3):628-634.

143. Drakeley AJ, Quenby S, Farquharson RG. Mid-trimester loss – Appraisal of a screening protocol. *Hum Reprod.* 1998;13(7):1975-1980.

144. Man J, Hutchinson JC, Heazell AE, Ashworth M, Jeffrey I, Sebire NJ. Stillbirth and intrauterine fetal death: role of routine histopathological placental findings to determine cause of death. *Ultrasound Obstet Gynecol.* 2016;48(5):579-584.

145. Contro E, deSouza R, Bhide A. Chronic intervillositis of the placenta: a systematic review. *Placenta.* 2010;31(12):1106-1110.

146. Blumenfeld Z, Khatib N, Zimmer EZ, Bronshtein M. Fetal demise in the early second trimester: sonographic findings. *J Clin Ultrasound.* 2015;43(2):109-112.

147. Silver RM, Zhao Y, Spong CY, et al. Prothrombin gene G20210A mutation and obstetric complications. *Obstet Gynecol.* 2010;115(1):14-20.

148. Lockshin MD, Kim M, Laskin CA, et al. Prediction of adverse pregnancy outcome by the presence of lupus anticoagulant, but not anticardiolipin antibody, in patients with antiphospholipid antibodies. *Arthritis Rheum.* 2012;64(7):2311-2318.

CHAPTER 2

Thrombophilias

Alexis Bridges and Torri D. Metz

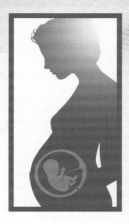

Introduction

Avoidance of thrombosis and disseminated intravascular coagulation requires a synergistic balance between the coagulation cascade and local anticoagulation molecules, including antithrombin, protein C, and protein S.

Normal physiologic changes of pregnancy result in a prothrombotic state by affecting all aspects of Virchow triad (hypercoagulability, venous stasis, and tissue damage). Hormonal alterations create a hypercoagulable environment by increasing levels of VWF and clotting factors, decreasing anticoagulant properties of protein C, protein S, and antithrombin, all while increasing plasminogen activator inhibitors 1 and 2, resulting in a decrease in fibrinolysis and platelet activation. Venous stasis occurs throughout pregnancy from progesterone-mediated vasodilation and peaks in the late third trimester.[15] In addition, the gravid uterus applies pressure to the inferior vena cava and pelvic veins causing decreased flow in the lower extremities. Vessel injury from venous distention, surgery, trauma, and venipuncture can occur anytime but are especially prevalent around the time of delivery. Physiologic changes alter the coagulation pathway in favor of clotting with the purpose of limiting delivery-related blood loss, but it comes at the cost of predisposing women to venous thromboembolism (VTE). Pregnancy-associated risk factors such as obesity, immobilization, and the postsurgical state, can further increase risk of thromboembolic events peripartum.[16]

ⓔ *See the eBook for expanded content and a complete reference list.*

Screening and Diagnosis of Inherited Thrombophilias

An evaluation for thrombophilia in pregnancy can be considered in the following clinical situations:

1. First-degree relative (parent or sibling) with history of high-risk thrombophilia[18]; or
2. Personal history of VTE with no prior thrombophilia testing.

An inherited thrombophilia evaluation includes testing for factor V Leiden (FVL) mutation, prothrombin G20210A mutation, antithrombin deficiency, protein C deficiency, and protein S deficiency (**Table 2.1**). It is best to postpone testing until 6 weeks after a VTE event and when the woman is not pregnant or on any anticoagulation or hormonal therapy.

During pregnancy, testing is reliable for FVL mutation, prothrombin G20210A mutation, protein C deficiency, and antithrombin deficiency. Screening for FVL can be completed using a "second-generation" functional assay for activated protein C resistance or via DNA analysis. Prothrombin G20210A testing is completed by DNA analysis. Testing for protein C and antithrombin deficiency is completed via activity level assays, with levels <65% and <60% being diagnostic, respectively.[20]

Women should not be evaluated for protein S deficiency during pregnancy as plasma levels drop significantly. Outside of pregnancy, an activity level less than 55% is consistent with a diagnosis of protein S deficiency.[20]

Antithrombin, protein C, and protein S levels are all reduced during an acute thrombotic event or when on anticoagulation therapy. Antithrombin

Table 2.1 Appropriate Screening Tests for Inherited Thrombophilias

Thrombophilia	Testing Method
Factor V Leiden mutation	Functional assay: Second-generation activated protein C resistance assay If abnormal, then DNA analysis
Prothrombin G20210A mutation	DNA analysis
Protein C deficiency	Protein C activity <65%
Protein S deficiency	Protein S activity <55% If tested in pregnancy, <30% and <24% in second and third trimesters, respectively
Antithrombin deficiency	Antithrombin activity <60%

DNA, deoxyribonucleic acid.

concentration is affected by heparin[21], and as protein C and S are vitamin K dependent, their concentrations are altered by warfarin.[22]

Thrombophilia and VTE Risk Classification

Experts typically classify thrombophilias as low or high risk based predominantly on the likelihood of the patient developing a VTE.

Recommendations are limited by the quality of evidence, which is highly reliant on case-controlled studies. Decisions for anticoagulation use should always be individualized and influenced by multiple risk factors, such as a personal history of VTE, a family history of VTE, severity of thrombophilia, as well as factors such as obesity and cesarean delivery.

In 2016, experts formed the Anticoagulation Forum, where guidelines from the American College of Obstetricians and Gynecologists (ACOG), Society of Obstetricians and Gynaecologists of Canada (SOGC), Royal College of Obstetricians and Gynaecologists (RCOG), and American College of Chest Physicians (ACCP) were reviewed in an effort to clarify the current clinical recommendations. A consensus was reached that pharmacologic prophylaxis should be recommended for a patient with a VTE risk of 3% or greater antepartum and postpartum.[23]

Medication Regimens for VTE Prevention

Unfractionated heparin (UFH) and low-molecular-weight heparin (LMWH) are the preferred therapeutic agents in pregnancy as neither crosses the placenta. In general, LMWH is considered superior because of its ease of use, dosing predictability, safety, and side effect profile.[24] For simplicity, enoxaparin is the only LMWH discussed here.

Prophylactic dosing regimens include enoxaparin 40 mg injected subcutaneously once daily and 5000 to 7000 units UFH subcutaneously every 12 hours in the first trimester, 7500 to 10,000 units every 12 hours in the second trimester, and 10,000 units every 12 hours in the third trimester. An intermediate dosing regimen is 40 mg enoxaparin injected subcutaneously every 12 hours. Therapeutic, or adjusted-dose, dosing regimens include 1 mg/kg of enoxaparin injected subcutaneously every 12 hours or 10,000 units or more of UFH injected subcutaneously every 12 hours in doses adjusted to achieve a target activated partial thromboplastin time range 6 hours after injection, which is 1.5 to 2.5× the laboratory control.[24]

LOW-RISK THROMBOPHILIAS

FVL Heterozygosity

FVL is the most common inherited thrombophilia, accounting for approximately 50% of all individuals with a thrombophilia.[25] In pregnancy, this low-risk thrombophilia accounts for approximately 40% of VTE episodes; however, in women with no history of VTE (identified by family history), the annual VTE risk in pregnancy is only 0.2% to 2.1%.[28,29]

FVL Heterozygosity and Adverse Pregnancy Outcomes

Historically, case-controlled studies have alluded to a predominantly positive, albeit variable, association between first-trimester pregnancy loss and FVL.

Neither anticoagulation therapy nor screening for the sole indication of prevention of adverse pregnancy outcomes in women with FVL mutations is recommended.

FVL Heterozygosity and VTE Prevention

The risk of VTE in pregnancy among women who are heterozygous for FVL is stratified based on personal history prior VTE.

For women heterozygous for FVL without personal or family history of VTE, we do not recommend prophylaxis antepartum. Instead, we recommend close clinical surveillance. In the postpartum period, we recommend close surveillance or prophylactic anticoagulation if the patient has additional risk factors. Notable additional risk factors include first-degree relative with a history of VTE, obesity, prolonged immobility, and cesarean delivery.

We recommend close surveillance or prophylactic anticoagulation therapy antepartum for women heterozygous for FVL with a family history of a first-degree relative with VTE. Postpartum management for these women should include prophylactic- or intermediate-dose anticoagulation therapy.

Women heterozygous for FVL with a single prior VTE should receive prophylactic- or intermediate-dose anticoagulation both during antepartum and postpartum periods.

Prothrombin Gene Mutation Heterozygosity

Similar to FVL, findings are inconsistent for an association between prothrombin gene mutation (PGM) and adverse pregnancy outcomes with positive associations only found in small, retrospective studies that have not been confirmed in larger prospective studies.

The relationship between a PGM and preeclampsia has been studied by many investigators, and historically results are mixed.

Anticoagulation therapy for the sole indication of prevention of adverse pregnancy outcomes for women with PGM is not recommended.

PGM Heterozygosity and VTE Prevention

Without personal or family history of VTE, we do not recommend prophylaxis antepartum. It is reasonable for postpartum management to include either close surveillance or prophylactic anticoagulation therapy if the patient has additional risk factors. For women with a family history of VTE (first degree), we recommend close surveillance or prophylactic anticoagulation therapy antepartum and prophylactic- or intermediate-dose anticoagulation postpartum. For those with a personal history of VTE, prophylactic- or intermediate-dose anticoagulation therapy should be administered antepartum and postpartum.

Protein C Deficiency

There are two types of the heterozygous form of protein C deficiency that both result in decreased protein C activity levels. Individuals with the homozygous form, however, generate little to no protein C activity resulting in neonatal purpura fulminans, which is often fatal.[45]

There is consistent evidence demonstrating no association between protein C deficiency and adverse pregnancy outcomes (ie, early, late or recurrent pregnancy loss, preeclampsia, or placental abruption).

Anticoagulation therapy for the sole indication of prevention of adverse pregnancy outcomes is not recommended.

Protein C Deficiency and VTE Prevention

Without personal or family history of VTE, we do not recommend prophylaxis antepartum. Postpartum management can include close surveillance or prophylactic anticoagulation therapy if the patient has additional risk factors such as first-degree family history of VTE, obesity, prolonged immobility, or cesarean delivery. If women have a family history of VTE, we recommend close surveillance or prophylactic anticoagulation therapy antepartum and prophylactic- or intermediate-dose anticoagulation therapy postpartum. For those with a personal history of VTE, prophylactic- or intermediate-dose anticoagulation therapy should be administered antepartum and postpartum.

Protein S Deficiency

Protein S deficiency affects the overall number of free or total protein S.

The low prevalence of protein S deficiency limits the available evidence related to adverse pregnancy outcomes. Anticoagulation therapy and screening for the sole indication of prevention of adverse pregnancy outcomes is not recommended.

Without personal or family history of VTE, we do not recommend prophylaxis antepartum. Postpartum management can include close surveillance or prophylactic anticoagulation therapy if the patient has additional risk factors such as first-degree family history of VTE, obesity, prolonged immobility, or cesarean delivery. If women have a family history of VTE (first-degree relative), we recommend either close surveillance or prophylactic anticoagulation therapy antepartum and prophylactic- or intermediate-dose anticoagulation

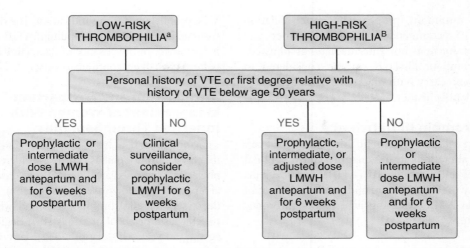

VTE, venous thromboembolism; LMWH, low molecular weight heparin
a Low-risk thrombophilias include heterozygosity for factor V Leiden or prothrombin gene mutation, protein C and
    protein S deficiency.
b High-risk thrombophilias include homozygosity for factor V Leiden or prothrombin gene mutation, heterozygosity
    for both factor V Leiden or prothrombin gene mutation, and antithrombin III deficiency.

Algorithm 2.1 Algorithm for use of low molecular weight heparin in women with inherited thrombophilias.

postpartum. For those with a personal history of VTE, prophylactic- or intermediate-dose anticoagulation therapy should be administered antepartum and postpartum (**Algorithm 2.1**).

INHERITED HIGH-RISK THROMBOPHILIAS

High-risk thrombophilias are rare in the general population.

FVL Homozygosity

The relationship between homozygosity for FVL and adverse pregnancy outcomes has not been sufficiently studied. Therefore, the majority of management approaches in pregnancy stem from a desire to prevent VTE in at-risk women rather than to prevent pregnancy complications.

FVL Homozygosity and VTE Prevention

The risk of thrombosis in women who are homozygous for FVL is on the order of 1% to 2%; this risk increases to approximately 17% in women with homozygosity and a personal or family history of VTE. Women who are homozygous for FVL mutation who have no history of clot typically receive prophylactic doses of LMWH during pregnancy and for 6 weeks postpartum.[24,40] Among women who are homozygous for FVL who also have a history of VTE, intermediate- or adjusted-dose LMWH can be considered.[24]

PGM Homozygosity

There are no observed associations between homozygosity for PGM and adverse pregnancy outcomes.

PGM Homozygosity and VTE Prevention

Management of pregnancy among women who are homozygous for PGM is aimed predominantly at prevention of thrombosis.

Women who are homozygous for PGM who have no history of clot typically receive prophylactic doses of LMWH during the pregnancy and for 6 weeks postpartum. Among women who are homozygous for PGM and have a history of VTE, intermediate- or adjusted-dose LMWH can be considered (**Algorithm 2.1**).[24]

Heterozygous for FVL and PGMs

Women who are heterozygous for both FVL and PGM mutations are at higher risk of VTE than either of these mutations alone.[23]

At a minimum, prophylactic anticoagulation therapy is recommended during pregnancy and for 6 weeks postpartum. Intermediate- or adjusted-dose thromboprophylaxis can be considered in women who carry both mutations and have a personal or family history of VTE.[24]

Antithrombin III Deficiency

There are numerous genetic mutations that can result in alterations in the quantity and functional quality of antithrombin III (ATIII). Homozygous deficiency for ATIII is rare and results in a lack of functional ATIII, resulting in a highly thrombogenic state.

ATIII Deficiency and Adverse Pregnancy Outcomes

Data regarding ATIII deficiency and adverse pregnancy outcomes are essentially nonexistent. Management of women with ATIII deficiency during pregnancy is, therefore, based on the risk of VTE.

ATIII Deficiency and VTE Prevention

ATIII deficiency (inclusive of both heterozygous and homozygous forms) is a hereditary thrombophilia that varies in classification as low or high risk depending on which expert opinion is considered. ATIII deficiency is classified as a high-risk thrombophilia in the ACOG and National Partnership for Maternal Safety (NPMS) guidelines but does not meet high-risk criteria according to other expert consensus documents.[23]

Women with ATIII deficiency typically receive prophylaxis with LMWH antepartum and for 6 weeks postpartum. In women with a history of VTE and known ATIII deficiency, intermediate- or adjusted-dose heparin can be considered.[24] In women with ATIII who are refractory to anticoagulants, the use of antithrombin concentrates can be considered.[52,53] A decision to use antithrombin concentrate would likely be made in consultation with hematology and maternal-fetal medicine.

Women can develop a relative acquired ATIII deficiency in the setting of massive proteinuria (>8 g/24 h). This situation occurs most frequently in women with preeclampsia. There is no good consensus as to whether women with large volume proteinuria require anticoagulation therapy to prevention of VTE. Different practice patterns exist with some practitioners initiating pharmacologic VTE prophylaxis for women with more than 5 g of protein, others at 8 or 10 g, and still others who do not initiate

VTE prophylaxis for this indication. The risk of VTE from an acquired (protein-spilling) ATIII deficiency is unknown. In the absence of data, clinical practice patterns will likely continue to vary.

Antepartum and Postpartum Management of Women With Inherited Thrombophilias

Women with a history of VTE and high-risk inherited thrombophilias can be considered for prophylactic-, intermediate-, or adjusted-dose LMWH antepartum and for 6 weeks postpartum. Dosing is dependent on the thrombophilia and whether the patient has a personal or family (first-degree relative aged < 50 years) history of VTE. Many women in this category will also be on lifelong anticoagulation therapy. For women requiring lifelong anticoagulation therapy with warfarin or an alternative newer oral anticoagulant, adjusted-dose (therapeutic) LMWH is preferred during pregnancy. Transition back to warfarin should be encouraged in the early postpartum period. Warfarin is safe with breastfeeding, as is LMWH and UFH. Direct thrombin inhibitors and factor Xa inhibitors should not be used during pregnancy or while breastfeeding as the safety of these agents remains unknown in pregnant and lactating women.

As inherited thrombophilias have not been associated with any specific adverse pregnancy outcomes, increased surveillance with growth scans and nonstress tests for the presence of an inherited thrombophilia alone is not warranted. Similarly, anticoagulants can be given for VTE prevention if the anticipated risk is unacceptably high for the patient and clinician following a discussion of the risks and benefits. When counseling women with an inherited thrombophilia about LMWH prophylaxis, it is important to also consider other risk factors for VTE, such as obesity or cesarean delivery, which will modify the patient's overall risk of thrombosis. There may be instances in which women do not receive anticoagulation during pregnancy but do receive anticoagulants in the postpartum period (see **Algorithm 2.1**).

Anticoagulation therapy and screening have not been demonstrated to reduce the risk of adverse pregnancy outcomes among women with inherited thrombophilias and is currently not recommended for the sole indication of preventing such outcomes.

Essentially all women with a high-risk thrombophilia, and some women with a low-risk thrombophilia, will receive anticoagulation therapy in the peripartum period.

ACQUIRED THROMBOPHILIAS

Antiphospholipid Syndrome

Antiphospholipid syndrome (APS) is an acquired thrombophilia that occurs predominantly in women.[58] APS is diagnosed in women who meet both laboratory and clinical criteria (**Table 2.2**).

Although women likely have a genetic predisposition for APS, this is not an inherited coagulation disorder. APS is acquired and is frequently observed in women with other autoimmune disorders such as systemic lupus erythematosus (SLE). The risk of thromboembolism is high among women with a diagnosis of APS. There is consistent evidence of an association between APS and venous and arterial thrombotic events.

APS and Adverse Pregnancy Outcomes

APS is associated with recurrent pregnancy loss. Similarly, APS is associated with stillbirth. Although early-onset (<32 weeks) severe fetal growth restriction and preeclampsia are clinical criteria for the diagnosis of APS, and women with APS have a high incidence of these adverse pregnancy outcomes, testing for APS in these cases remains controversial.[58,63]

Given the increased risk of adverse pregnancy outcomes, women with APS require more intensive pregnancy monitoring. Based on expert opinion, serial growth ultrasounds are typically performed beginning at 24 weeks' gestation and continued at 3- to 6-week intervals throughout gestation. In addition, women with APS generally start antenatal surveillance with nonstress tests or biophysical profiles beginning at 32 weeks' gestation. Delivery is recommended at 37 to 39 weeks if no other complications of pregnancy prompting delivery are detected before that time.

Table 2.2 Diagnostic Criteria for Antiphospholipid Syndrome

Clinical Criteria for Antiphospholipid Syndrome

- Deep venous thrombosis or arterial thrombosis
- Three or more unexplained consecutive pregnancy losses (<10 wk)
- Unexplained fetal death (>10 wk)
- Severe, earlyonset (<34 wk) preeclampsia or features of placental insufficiency such as fetal growth restriction

Laboratory Criteria for Antiphospholipid Syndrome[a]

- Lupus anticoagulant positive
- Anticardiolipin antibody, IgG or IgM (>40 GPL or MPL or > 99% tile)
- Beta-2-glycoprotein-1 IgG or IgM (titer > 99% tile for normal population)

GPL, result is from IgG isotype; Ig, immunoglobulin; MPL, result is from IgM isotype.
[a]Laboratory testing must be repeated in 12 weeks for confirmation of abnormal results to make the diagnosis of antiphospholipid syndrome.

APS and VTE Prevention

Pharmaceutical prophylaxis with LMWH is recommended in women with APS to prevent VTE as well as to reduce the risk of adverse pregnancy outcomes.[58] Based on this and other studies, most experts recommend prophylactic-dose LMWH and 81 mg aspirin daily for women with APS and no history of VTE. Prophylactic- or intermediate-dose anticoagulation and 81 mg aspirin daily is recommended in women with APS and a history of VTE for prevention of recurrent thromboembolism.[58]

KEY POINTS

- Women with both inherited and acquired thrombophilias are at increased risk of VTE in pregnancy.
- Management is dictated by the degree of risk associated with the patient's thrombophilia and the presence or absence of other risk factors for VTE.
- While there is no consistent evidence to associate inherited thrombophilias with adverse pregnancy outcomes, the acquired thrombophilia, APS, has been associated with adverse outcomes and treatment with heparin likely improves pregnancy outcomes.
- For inherited thrombophilias, treatment and screening should be based on the risk of VTE rather than prevention of adverse outcomes.

REFERENCES

(only references cited in synoptic print chapter; for a complete reference list, see ebook)

15. Macklon NS, Greer IA, Bowman AW. An ultrasound study of gestational and postural changes in the deep venous system of the leg in pregnancy. *Br J Obstet Gynaecol.* 1997;104:191-197.

16. Kupferminc MJ. Thrombophilia and pregnancy. *Reprod Biol Endocrinol.* 2003;1:111.

18. Vossen CY, Conard J, Fontcuberta J. et al. Risk of a first venous thrombotic event in carriers of a familial thrombophilic defect. The European Prospective Cohort on Thrombophilia (EPCOT). *J Thromb Haemost.* 2005;3(3):459-464.

20. Paidas MJ, Ku DH, Lee MJ, et al. Protein Z, protein S levels are lower in patients with thrombophilia and subsequent pregnancy complications. *J Thromb Haemost.* 2005;3:497-501.

21. Marciniak E, Gockerman JP. Heparin-induced decrease in circulating antithrombin-III. *Lancet.* 1977;2:581-584.

22. Stirling Y. Warfarin-induced changes in procoagulant and anticoagulant proteins. *Blood Coagul Fibrinolysis.* 1995;6(5):361-373.

23. Bates SM, Middeldorp S, Rodger M, James AH, Greer I. Guidance for the treatment and prevention of obstetric-associated venous thromboembolism. *J Thromb Thrombolysis.* 2016;41(1):92-128.

24. American College of Obstetricians and Gynecologists' Committee on Practice Bulletins—Obstetrics. ACOG Practice Bulletin No. 197: inherited thrombophilias in pregnancy. *Obstet Gynecol.* 2018;132: e18-e34.

25. Rosendaal FR, Koster T, Vandenbroucke JP, Reitsma PH. High risk of thrombosis in patients homozygous for factor V Leiden (activated protein C resistance). *Blood.* 1995;85:1504-1508.

28. Gerhardt A, Scharf RE, Beckmann MW, et al. Prothrombin and factor V mutations in women with a history of thrombosis during pregnancy and the puerperium. *N Engl J Med.* 2000;342:374-380.

29. Middeldorp S, Henkens CM, Koopman MM. et al. The incidence of venous thromboembolism in family members of patients with factor V Leiden mutation and venous thrombosis. *Ann Intern Med.* .1998;128(1):15-20.

40. Bates SM, Greer IA, Middeldorp S, Veenstra DL, Prabulos AM, Vandvik PO. VTE, thrombophilia, antithrombotic therapy, and pregnancy: antithrombotic therapy and prevention of thrombosis, 9th ed. American College of Chest Physicians evidence-based clinical practice guidelines. *Chest.* 2012;141:e691S-e736S.

45. Marlar RA, Neumann A. Neonatal purpura fulminans due to homozygous protein C or protein S deficiencies. *Semin Thromb Hemost.* 1990;16:299-309.

52. James AH, Konkle BA, Bauer KA. Prevention and treatment of venous thromboembolism in pregnancy in patients with hereditary antithrombin deficiency. *Int J Womens Health.* 2013;5:233-241.

53. Refaei M, Xing L, Lim W, Crowther M, Boonyawat K. Management of venous thromboembolism in patients with hereditary antithrombin deficiency and pregnancy: case report and review of the literature. *Case Rep Hematol.* 2017;2017:9261351.

58. American College of Obstetricians and Gynecologists. ACOG Practice Bulletin No. 132: antiphospholipid syndrome. *Obstet Gynecol.* 2012;120:1514-1521.

63. Branch DW, Silver RM, Blackwell JL, Reading JC, Scott JR. Outcome of treated pregnancies in women with antiphospholipid syndrome: an update of the Utah experience. *Obstet Gynecol.* 1992;80:614-620.

69. Empson M, Lassere M, Craig JC, Scott JR. Recurrent pregnancy loss with antiphospholipid antibody: a systematic review of therapeutic trials. *Obstet Gynecol.* 2002;99:135-144.

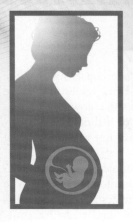

CHAPTER 3

Ectopic and Heterotopic Pregnancies

Omri Zamstein, Eyal Sheiner, and Arnon Wiznitzer

Ectopic Pregnancy

Incidence

Ectopic pregnancy, ie, implantation of a fertilized ovum outside the uterus (**Figure 3.1**), is a major health problem for women of reproductive age and is a leading cause of pregnancy-related death during the early stages of gestation.[1] Ectopic pregnancy is currently believed to account for 2% of all pregnancies, with an annual rate of up to 0.6% among women of reproductive age.[2] Importantly, ruptured ectopic pregnancy accounts for around 3% of all pregnancy-related mortality, and thus, accurate diagnosis and management of ectopic pregnancy decrease this risk and additionally optimize subsequent fertility outcomes.[1]

Etiology and Risk Factors

The leading site of ectopic pregnancy is the fallopian tube, although implantation may take place in the abdominal cavity or the adjacent pelvic viscera (ie, ovary, cervix, broad ligament, and cesarean scar) with less frequency.[5] The most commonly cited risk factors for ectopic pregnancy share a common etiology of tubal obstruction and injury. Previous episodes of pelvic inflammatory disease, especially when caused by *Chlamydia trachomatis*, are also major risk factors for ectopic pregnancy.[6] Other factors associated with an increased risk of ectopic pregnancy include prior ectopic pregnancy (which increases the risk for subsequent ectopic pregnancy 10-fold), a history of infertility (and specifically *in vitro* fertilization), cigarette smoking (causing alterations in tubal motility and ciliary activity), prior tubal surgery, diethylstilbestrol exposure (which alters fallopian tube morphology), and advanced maternal age (>35 years old).

Intrauterine contraceptive devices (IUDs), progesterone-only contraceptives, estrogen/progestin contraceptives, and sterilization hinder conception at any location and thus protect women against developing an ectopic pregnancy.[9-11] However, if a woman using these contraception methods becomes pregnant, her risk for an ectopic pregnancy is increased, as these methods of contraception provide greater protection against intrauterine pregnancy than against ectopic pregnancy.

Although the risk of ectopic pregnancy for women who undergo assisted reproductive technology treatments has generally declined throughout the years,[12] these women are still at increased risk for ectopic pregnancy as fallopian tube pathology underlies both the need for *in vitro* fertilization and the tendency for abnormal implantation.[13] Other contributing factors include transfer of multiple embryos, fresh versus frozen cycles, and implanting cleavage state compared to blastocyst transfer.[12,14]

Hormonal alterations during ovulation induction have been suggested to affect tubal function

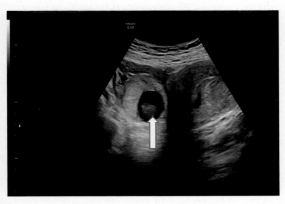

Figure 3.1 Transvaginal scan shows a left tubal pregnancy at 6 weeks of gestation demonstrating a fetus with heartbeat (arrow).

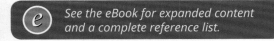

See the eBook for expanded content and a complete reference list.

and peristalsis and increase uterine contractility, thus promoting a retrograde movement of the embryo toward the fallopian tube.[12] Other less common causes of ectopic pregnancy include salpingitis isthmica nodosa (anatomic thickening of the fallopian tube with epithelium leading to multiple lumen diverticula), and possibly vaginal douching and multiple sexual partners, which both lead to a higher risk of pelvic infections.[15,16]

Signs and Symptoms

Clinical manifestations of ectopic pregnancy vary and depend on whether rupture has occurred. Historically, the triad of amenorrhea, irregular vaginal bleeding, and lower abdominal pain would raise suspicion for ectopic pregnancy.[17] However, these symptoms are present in only one-half of all patients, while a significant portion of women with unruptured ectopic pregnancy have no symptoms at all. When present, symptoms are often nonspecific, overlapping with other common abdominal and pelvic conditions such as appendicitis, urological disorders, miscarriage, and adnexal torsion.[18] Typical symptoms of pregnancy, such as nausea and breast tenderness, may occur as well. Initial physical examination should include measurements of vital signs to assess hemodynamic stability, as tubal rupture can lead to life-threatening hemorrhage.[19] Abdominal and pelvic tenderness, especially cervical motion tenderness, is common when rupture has occurred and present in approximately 75% of patients. A palpable pelvic mass on bimanual examination is noticeable in less than one-half of all cases.[17] Thus, additional tests are required in order to differentiate ectopic pregnancy from early intrauterine pregnancy (**Algorithm 3.1**).

Laboratory Assessment

β-Human Chorionic Gonadotropin

The first stage in the evaluation of women with a suspected ectopic pregnancy is to determine if the patient is pregnant. The β-human chorionic gonadotropin (β-hCG) enzyme immunoassay, with a sensitivity of 25 mIU/mL, is an accurate screening test and is positive in virtually all cases of normal as well as ectopic pregnancies.[20]

The level of β-hCG in normal pregnancies usually doubles every 2 days, and thus clinicians rely on a normal "doubling time" to characterize a viable gestation. Although there is a consensus that the predictable rise in serial β-hCG values in a viable pregnancy is different from the slow rise or plateau of an ectopic pregnancy, it should be remembered that a slower rise does not rule out normal pregnancy.

The discriminatory threshold is a level of β-hCG above which intrauterine gestation is expected to be visualized. If no intrauterine gestation is seen, it is often assumed to be ectopic and treated accordingly. However, given the overlap of the discriminatory threshold of β-hCG in viable intrauterine pregnancies and ectopic pregnancies, the chance of unintended termination of a normal pregnancy, and the treatment consequences of nonviable pregnancy, β-hCG alone cannot accurately determine the viability and location of pregnancy.[22] Further complicating laboratory evaluation based on β-hCG alone is the presence of a multifetal gestation, which is associated with elevated rates of β-hCG.[23] Therefore, choosing a higher discriminatory threshold of β-hCG >3500 mIU/mL[24] and carrying out additional testing, if hemodynamic status permits, can help consolidate the diagnosis.[25]

Serum Progesterone

Serum progesterone levels are of limited clinical value in the diagnosis of ectopic pregnancy, but can be useful in evaluating the chances of early pregnancy failure. A baseline serum progesterone level of >60 nmol/L usually indicates a normal pregnancy, whereas levels <20 nmol/L can be used to identify abnormal pregnancy (either intra- or extrauterine) with a positive predictive value (PPV) of ≥95%.[26,27] However, although not routinely obtained in adjunct, low progesterone levels combined with low β-hCG levels can suggest spontaneous resolution of ectopic pregnancy.[29] In summary, serum progesterone levels cannot distinguish ectopic pregnancy from spontaneous abortion. Thus, progesterone levels at defined times can be used to predict the immediate viability of a pregnancy, but cannot be used reliably to predict its location.[30]

Ultrasonography

Transvaginal ultrasound is the most sensitive tool for determining the location of pregnancy[1] and is especially useful for the diagnosis of ectopic pregnancy.[31] Unfortunately, although ultrasonographic visualization of extrauterine pregnancy with a yolk

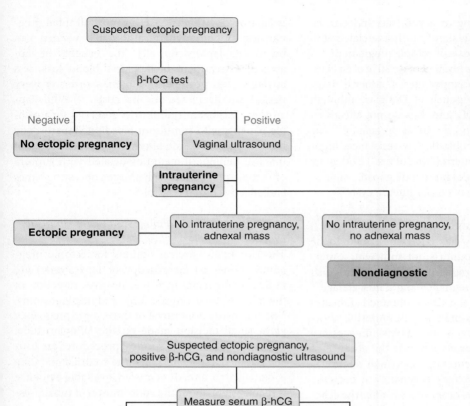

Algorithm 3.1
Diagnostic management of ectopic pregnancy. β-hCG, β-human chorionic gonadotropin; EP, ectopic pregnancy.

sac or embryo has a specificity and PPV approaching 100% in detecting ectopic pregnancy,[32] it is not seen at all events, and up to 31% of suspected cases do not exhibit radiological signs of either uterine or extrauterine pregnancy.[25] Factors that may impede visualization of ectopic pregnancy include lower gestational age, smaller ectopic mass, large body habitus, and uterine or ovary anatomical pathology that obscure the adnexa.[31] It is generally agreed that a normal intrauterine pregnancy should be seen by transvaginal ultrasound beginning 5 weeks of gestation or when β-hCG levels reach between 1000 and 2000 mIU/mL, although higher β-hCG levels have been suggested as the discriminatory threshold for ultrasound, thus avoiding injury to a not yet visualized but viable pregnancy.[24,33] When the β-hCG level exceeds the transvaginal discriminatory zone, the absence of an intrauterine gestational sac is suggestive of ectopic pregnancy, but the differential diagnosis includes failed intrauterine pregnancy.

If an intrauterine pregnancy is detected, this is taken to exclude a diagnosis of ectopic pregnancy because coexistent intra- and extrauterine pregnancies (heterotopic) following spontaneous cycles are rare.

The double decidual sign is useful to the physician for early diagnosis of intrauterine pregnancy and for the exclusion of ectopic pregnancy. However, the appearance of an intrauterine sac can be seen in up to 15% cases of ectopic pregnancy owing to intrauterine fluid or blood collection, ie, a pseudosac. A pseudosac is a uterine sac without a double decidual ring or a yolk sac. Indeed, the report of a pseudosac is significantly associated with a false-positive diagnosis of ectopic pregnancy.[35]

Other sonographic findings suggestive of an ectopic pregnancy are an empty uterus, adnexal mass, and free fluid in the pouch of Douglas, although all have poor sensitivity and thus do not effectively rule out the possibility of a tubal pregnancy.[36] The presence of peritrophoblastic low-resistance, high-velocity blood flow pattern ("ring of fire") evident by Doppler ultrasound is of limited diagnostic value as it also a typical feature of corpus luteum cysts.[37]

Dilation and Curettage

When the pregnancy has been confirmed to be nonviable and ultrasound is not sufficient, a uterine dilation and curettage can help distinguish between an ectopic pregnancy and a miscarriage.[38] Detection of villi in the tissue obtained indicates the occurrence of spontaneous intrauterine abortion with high accuracy and avoids unnecessary exposure to methotrexate, whereas the absence of chorionic villi in the curettage specimen reinforces the possibility of an ectopic pregnancy. A decrease in β-hCG levels of 15% or more a day after the evacuation indicates a complete abortion.[39] A plateau or a rise in the β-hCG levels is diagnostic for ectopic pregnancy. Once the possibility of an abortion is excluded, medical or surgical treatment for ectopic pregnancy should be pursued.

Culdocentesis

Culdocentesis was used as a diagnostic technique for ectopic pregnancy before the widespread availability of the vaginal ultrasound and β-hCG assay. Culdocentesis is positive in around 80% of women with ectopic pregnancy who have hemoperitoneum. In the remaining 20% of cases, the results are nondiagnostic. A nondiagnostic finding cannot be used to exclude ectopic pregnancy, and the test alters management only when it is positive. Thus, it is rarely indicated and is performed only in places where facilities for pregnancy testing and ultrasound are limited.[40]

Management of Ectopic Pregnancy

Surgical Treatment

Laparoscopy Versus Laparotomy

The standard operative procedure for the treatment of ectopic pregnancy in the developed world is laparoscopy (**Figure 3.2**). Almost all tubal pregnancies in hemodynamically stable women can be treated laparoscopically. The benefits of laparoscopic treatment include less blood loss, less analgesia, less postoperative pain, shorter recovery period, and decreased hospital costs.[44,45] While laparotomy has been traditionally reserved for unstable patients with significant bleeding,[1] laparoscopy has emerged as a safe alternative even in cases of massive hemoperitoneum associated with rupture of ectopic pregnancy, with shorter operating times and effective blood control.[47]

Salpingectomy and Salpingostomy and Fimbrial Evacuation

The two main surgical options for ectopic pregnancy (either by laparoscopy or laparotomy) are radical salpingectomy, which involves resection of the affected tube (**Figure 3.3**), and salpingostomy, which consists of removal of the ectopic pregnancy *via* a small incision made on the fallopian tube. Although conservative surgical procedures are usually pursued, especially when the contralateral tube is damaged or already removed, available evidence is inconsistent about the contribution of tubal preservation for future fertility.

Factors such as extensive tubal injury, uncontrolled bleeding, large ectopic pregnancy, undesired fertility, or recurrent ectopic pregnancy in the same location may favor complete removal of the tube. In addition, given the compelling evidence regarding the role of the fallopian tube in the carcinogenesis of many high-grade ovarian carcinomas,[51,52] salpingectomy offers a potential benefit of reducing the risk of malignancy.[53,54] However, salpingectomy for unruptured ectopic pregnancy is rarely performed, and linear salpingostomy remains the procedure of choice. During this procedure, the ectopic pregnancy is removed through a linear incision of 10 to 15 mm made into the tube on its antimesenteric border. The products will extrude from the incision and can be flushed out and evacuated. Meticulous irrigation and occasionally a short course of methotrexate are needed to effectively remove any remaining trophoblastic tissue.[55-58]

The practice of fimbrial evacuation has largely been abandoned.

Medical Treatment With Methotrexate

Methotrexate interferes with DNA synthesis, repair, and cellular replication; therefore, actively

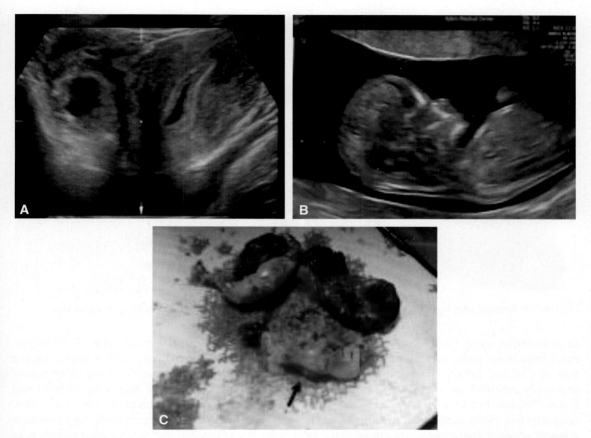

Figure 3.2 Ultrasonography (**A and B**) and gross anatomy (**C**) of tubal ectopic pregnancy. A rare care of tubal pregnancy at 11.5 weeks mistaken for abdominal pregnancy in an asymptomatic patient, diagnosed by transabdominal and transvaginal sonography adjacent to an empty uterus. A crown-rump length measuring 50 mm of a normal-appearing fetus was noted (**A and B**). **C,** Laparoscopy salpingectomy of a right fallopian tube harboring the fetus (black arrow).

proliferating cells, such as the trophoblasts of an ectopic pregnancy, are generally more sensitive to treatment.[60,61] Although methotrexate is associated with wide array of adverse reactions, severe toxicity during short-duration treatment for ectopic pregnancy is rarely encountered, and carefully selected patients can benefit from this noninvasive option with similar efficacy and fertility outcomes as compared to the various surgical approaches.[58,62]

Candidates for Medical Therapy

Hemodynamically stable patients without active bleeding or signs of hemoperitoneum are candidates for medical therapy. Contraindications for methotrexate treatment are summarized in **Table 3.1**.

During treatment, patients should be counseled to promptly report any signs and symptoms associated with tubal rupture such as abdominal pain, dizziness, weakness, and syncope. Sexual intercourse, alcohol consumption, and use of nonsteroidal anti-inflammatory drugs, folic acid supplements, or prenatal vitamins are prohibited until serum β-hCG levels are undetectable. Avoidance from sunlight during treatment is advised as well to minimize the risk of dermatitis.[1,66]

The main factor in predicting successful medical treatment of ectopic pregnancy is rigorous patient selection. Several parameters aimed at the suitable choice of patients have already been established, such as the presence of fetal cardiac activity, size of the ectopic pregnancy, and initial levels of β-hCG. Other ultrasonographic findings, such

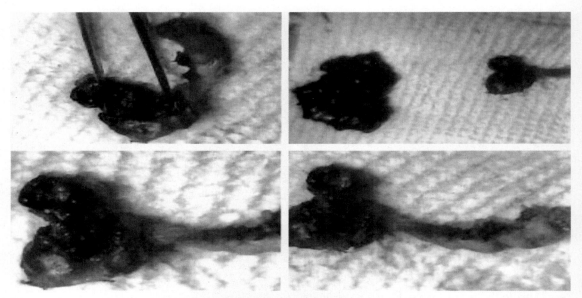

Figure 3.3 Radical salpingectomy (removal of the affected tube) for ruptured ectopic pregnancy.

as endometrial stripe thickness and vascularity of the ectopic mass, play a certain role in the prediction of effective therapy.[67] Interestingly, although previously regarded as a predictor of treatment failure,[68,69] prior history of ectopic pregnancy may not adversely affect medical treatment; however, repeated doses of methotrexate may be required in these patients.[70]

Treatment Protocols
Methotrexate is most commonly administered using a single-dose method, based on 50 mg/m^2

Table 3.1 Relative and Absolute Contraindications for Methotrexate Treatment

Absolute Contraindications	Relative Contraindications
Shock, hemodynamic instability	Embryonic cardiac activity
Known sensitivity to methotrexate	Gestational sac of 3.5 cm or more
Breastfeeding	
Immunodeficiency	
Alcoholism	
Hepatic, pulmonary, renal, or hematological dysfunction	
Blood dyscrasias	
Peptic ulcer disease	

of body surface area, without the need for leucovorin rescue.[71] Alternatively, methotrexate is given using a multidose regimen of 1 mg/kg intramuscularly once every 2 days, alternating with 0.1 mg/kg of leucovorin intramuscularly, for up to a total of four doses of each drug. Overall, both protocols have been demonstrated to have good success rates in the treatment of ectopic pregnancy, although the single-dose protocol is usually preferred as it is easier to administer and monitor and appears to result in fewer side effects.[1] Although currently there are no predefined indications to guide selection of one protocol over the other, pretreatment levels of β-hCG may be predictive of treatment success.[75]

Monitoring Efficacy of Therapy
The overall success rate of methotrexate treatment is almost 90%.[72,76]

Patient monitoring continues until β-hCG levels are nondetectable. It usually takes a month or longer until β-hCG levels disappear from the plasma.[72] With the single-dose treatment, levels of β-hCG may increase during the first week of treatment, peaking 4 days following administration, due to residual production by the resistant syncytiotrophoblast.[78] Levels are expected to decline 1 week after injection. If a response is observed and the fall in β-hCG levels is greater than 15%, weekly serum β-hCG levels should be measured until it is documented as undetectable. Failure of the β-hCG levels to decline requires a second dose of methotrexate and may imply a need for surgical intervention.[79] An additional dose of methotrexate may also be given if β-hCG levels plateau or increase 1 week after treatment.

When applying the multidose regimen, β-hCG measurements are drawn every other day before drug administration (eg, days 1, 3, 5, and 7 prior to methotrexate treatment). Similar to the single-dose regimen, a drop of more than 15% in β-hCG levels indicate adequate response to treatment and allows weekly laboratory evaluation until complete resolution is established.

Side Effects
High doses can cause bone marrow suppression, hepatotoxicity, stomatitis, pulmonary fibrosis, alopecia, and photosensitivity.[61] Toxic effects are usually related to the amount and duration of therapy. Most side effects during regular treatment for ectopic pregnancy are minor and are generally limited to a transient increase in hepatic transaminases, conjunctivitis, mild stomatitis, and gastrointestinal disturbances.[80]

One of the more familiar phenomena of methotrexate treatment for ectopic pregnancy is the development of acute abdominal pain that is believed to result from the process of tubal abortion or hematoma formation that stretches the fallopian tube. It can be effectively controlled using nonsteroidal anti-inflammatory drugs or acetaminophen. Nonetheless, the clinical presentation can be difficult to distinguish from that of intra-abdominal hemorrhage secondary to tubal rupture, which requires emergent surgical intervention. Thus, a high index of suspicion is essential to spot the development of severe complications, and patients are counseled regarding the potential side effects and the continuing risk of tubal rupture during treatment. However, it is important to note that the development of side effects is generally associated with higher rates of resolution of the ectopic pregnancy without the need for surgical intervention.[72]

Reproductive Outcomes After Methotrexate Treatment
Methotrexate treatment does not seem to impair ovarian function and future fertility outcomes.

However, it is not well established in the literature what is the optimal interval from completion of medical treatment to subsequent conception attempts. Nonetheless, given the teratogenic potential of methotrexate and its delayed clearance from liver cells, women are usually advised to avoid pregnancy for a safety period of 3 months after the last methotrexate treatment.[1,66,86]

Expectant Management
Candidates for successful expectant management must be asymptomatic with no evidence of tubal rupture or hemodynamic compromise and exhibit satisfactory decrease in β-hCG during repeated measurements. Fetal cardiac activity, adnexal mass of greater than 4 cm, and β-hCG levels greater than 2000 mIU/mL are all contraindications for expectant management.

Lower β-hCG levels may correlate with successful spontaneous resolution and are, therefore, the preferred selection criteria by some clinicians.[89] Initial serum β-hCG level was the best predictor for the successful outcome of expectant management.

Specific Forms of Ectopic Pregnancy

Interstitial Pregnancy
Interstitial implantation of the blastocyst is the rarest form of tubal ectopic pregnancy.[92] The term cornual pregnancy is occasionally used as a synonym, but the latter refers to a different ectopic location—the horn of a bicornuate uterus. Because of their proximity to the highly vascularized area supplied by uterine and the ovarian arteries, late diagnosis and treatment of interstitial pregnancies can result in deleterious outcomes, including uterine rupture, hemorrhagic shock, and maternal death, with reported mortality rate that is twofold higher compared to other types of ectopic pregnancies.[93-95]

Several distinctive sonographic features can aid in the diagnosis of an interstitial ectopic pregnancy: an empty uterine cavity with an eccentrically located or a lateral gestational sac, thin myometrial line surrounding the gestational sac (myometrial mantle sign), echogenic line bordering the interstitial gestational sac (interstitial line sign), and abnormal contour of the adjacent myometrium.[97]

The traditional treatments of interstitial pregnancy are hysterectomy or cornual resection by laparotomy (**Figure 3.4**), but these surgical approaches are usually reserved for symptomatic and hemodynamically unstable patients.[99] The progress in diagnostic and surgical techniques has

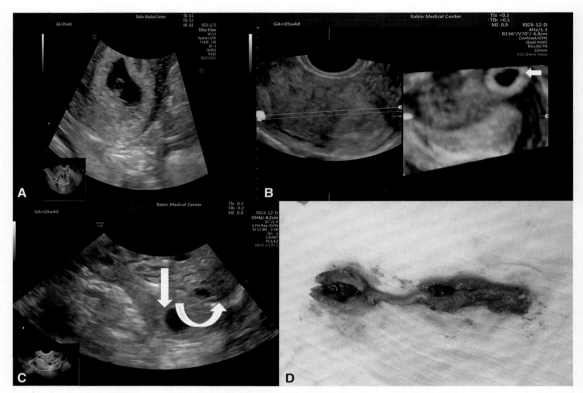

Figure 3.4 Cornual pregnancy at 15 weeks' gestation, after cornual resection. A combined cornual and a tubal ectopic pregnancy after *in vitro* fertilization treatment. Transvaginal probe of a viable pregnancy 5.4 weeks of gestation was suspected to be a cornual pregnancy (**A**). Using volume contrast imaging a cornual pregnancy in the interstitial part of the fallopian tube was diagnosed (short arrow) (**B**). Note no communication between the endometrial cavity and the cornual pregnancy (long arrow). In addition, a tubal ring (curved arrow) was noted in close proximity to the left ovary and suspected to be a tubal pregnancy (**C**). The patient was operated on with resection of the left cornual and the tubal pregnancies (**D**).

allowed for utilization of more conservative surgical approaches, including laparoscopic cornual resection, cornuostomy, salpingostomy or salpingectomy, and even transcervical evacuation of the pregnancy.[96,100,101] The role of medical treatment for interstitial pregnancy remains unresolved, with wide variation in the reported success rates.[102,103] Systemic administration or ultrasound-guided injection of methotrexate can serve as an alternative for surgery in early intact pregnancies but requires intensive clinical and laboratory surveillance.

Nontubal Ectopic Pregnancy (Figure 3.5)
Ovarian Pregnancy
Ovarian pregnancy is an infrequent variant of ectopic pregnancy with an incidence of 0.5% to 3% of all ectopic pregnancies.[105] It is likely, however, that the frequency is underestimated as some of

the suspected tubal pregnancies that are treated conservatively with methotrexate are in fact early ovarian pregnancies. In addition, several cases of ovarian pregnancy have been retrospectively confirmed by a pathologist as these cases had been mistakenly considered as ruptured corpus luteum. Improvements in ultrasonography and operative laparoscopy have led to earlier and a more accurate diagnosis of ovarian pregnancies, although preoperative identification and timely treatment before rupture occurs remain major clinical challenges.[106]

Specific predisposing factors for ovarian pregnancies are not fully understood, although the use of an IUD and ovarian hyperstimulation during artificial reproductive technology may correlate with the increasing incidence.[107]

The major presenting symptom is abdominal pain.[108] Other findings include vaginal bleeding and

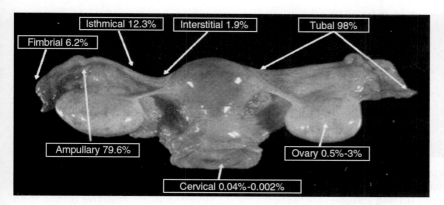

Figure 3.5 Sites of ectopic pregnancy and approximate incidence rates.

amenorrhea. It is not uncommon for ovarian pregnancy to first manifest with significant hemoperitoneum and hemodynamic instability secondary to rupture of the gestational sac.[109,110]

Historically, oophorectomy was considered the treatment of choice for ovarian pregnancies. However, improvements in operative laparoscopic skills and instrumentation have led to a more conservative approach, and laparoscopic wedge resection (**Figure 3.6**) and ovarian cystectomy have become the preferred treatment modalities.[111] Successful treatment with methotrexate has also been reported.[112,113] In patients with circulatory collapse, however, immediate laparotomy is mandatory.

Cervical Pregnancy
Cervical pregnancy is a rare complication with incidence rates of less than 1% of all ectopic pregnancies.[114]

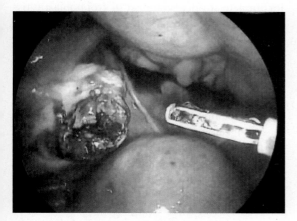

Figure 3.6 Laparoscopic wedge resection for ovarian ectopic pregnancy.

Presenting symptoms include significant vaginal bleeding accompanied by abdominal pain,[118] which can easily be confused with incomplete abortion.[119] On physical examination, the cervix is usually enlarged, global (barrel shaped), and distended. Occasionally, the external cervical os is dilated.

Accurate diagnosis can be performed by vaginal ultrasound and magnetic resonance imaging, demonstrating an intracervical ectopic sac below a closed internal cervical os (**Figure 3.7**). Transvaginal demonstration of an intact part of the cervical canal between the endometrium and gestational sac is also suggestive of cervical pregnancy.

Conservative medical management with systemic or local methotrexate injection has been reported to be successful, obviating the need for surgical treatment, which entails a risk of hysterectomy.[120] Dilation and evacuation followed by cervical tamponade can be successfully applied using Foley catheter tamponade.[121] Other treatment options include arterial embolization and Shirodkar cerclage placement in order to reduce bleeding.[122] However, in cases of massive and uncontrolled vaginal bleeding, abdominal hysterectomy is necessary (**Figure 3.8**).[123]

Abdominal Ectopic Pregnancy
Abdominal pregnancies can be classified as primary, as a result of intra-abdominal fertilization and peritoneal implantation, or secondary, as a result of reimplantation following tubal abortion or rupture.

The incidence of abdominal pregnancy is increased in women with *in vitro* fertilization, history of pelvic infections, previous ectopic

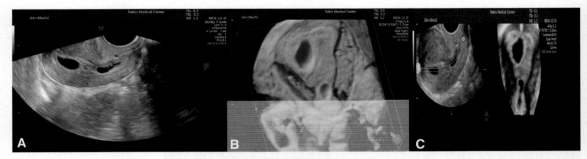

Figure 3.7 Sonographic image of a heterotopic pregnancy involving the cervix. Transvaginal sonography demonstrating a viable 6-week-old intrauterine and cervical pregnancy using two-dimensional **(A)** and three-dimensional ultrasound **(B)** and volume contrast imaging **(C)**. An attempt for selective termination of the cervical pregnancy by needle aspiration was done. Spontaneous abortion of the intrauterine pregnancy occurred at 8 weeks of gestation.

pregnancy, and endometriosis.[129] As with the other sites of unusual ectopic implantation, diagnosis is relatively difficult and demands a high level of clinical suspicion. Diagnosis is established ultrasonographically, when an ectopic pregnancy is suspected and a gestational sac with surrounding echogenic margins and peritrophoblastic flow is visualized inside the peritoneal cavity.[97] Although abdominal pregnancy has the potential to progress beyond the second trimester and reach viability,[132,133] conservative management in an attempt to extend gestation is generally not recommended because of the continuously growing risk for serious maternal complications and the poor outcomes expected to the newborn in case of survival.[134]

The main goal of treatment is safe removal the pregnancy from the adjacent friable anatomic structures, with or without removal of the placenta.[135] Laparotomy is the preferred surgical approach owing to fast hemostatic control, although laparoscopy can be performed at earlier gestational stages.[136] The placenta can be detached if its vascular supply is recognized and ligated. If the vascular supply cannot be adequately identified, the cord is ligated, and the placenta is left *in situ*. In cases where the placenta is left in place, complications related to the remaining senescent placental tissue, such as sepsis, abscess formation, hemorrhage, and intestinal obstruction, may develop. On the other hand, incautious removal of the placenta can provoke significant hemorrhage as the main mechanism to prevent blood loss, myometrial contraction, is absent. Administration of methotrexate to hasten involution of the retained placenta carries its own risks for infectious complications and thus remains controversial.

Persistent Ectopic Pregnancy

Incomplete surgical removal of trophoblastic tissue can lead to persistent ectopic pregnancy, a condition that is estimated to occur following salpingostomy in 5% to 20% of cases.[137] Several studies have reported higher incidence of persistent ectopic pregnancy after laparoscopic surgery than after laparotomy,[44] and it is also more likely to occur following salpingostomy as compared to salpingectomy owing to the residual section of the fallopian tube.[48] Other associated risk factors for persistency include surgical inexperience and elevated pretreatment β-hCG levels. Methotrexate is an effective treatment for the majority of cases, although additional surgery is occasionally required to ensure definite removal of the implicated tube.[138]

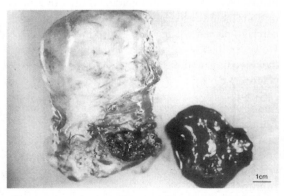

Figure 3.8 Cervical ectopic pregnancy ruptured in the cervical area (left) with hemorrhagic placental tissue (right).

Heterotopic Pregnancy

Incidence

Coexistent intrauterine and extrauterine pregnancies are referred to as a heterotopic pregnancy. The occurrence of a heterotopic pregnancy following spontaneous cycles is rare. However, incidence has risen by a factor of 10 in the era of assisted reproductive technology,[140] particularly following ovulation induction with gonadotropins and multiple embryo transfer techniques.[141]

Clinical Features and Diagnosis

Heterotopic pregnancy poses a diagnostic dilemma. Serial β-hCG levels are not helpful because of the intrauterine pregnancy, and ultrasound can be misleading in cases of simultaneous viable intrauterine pregnancy, as the ectopic pregnancy may be mistakenly regarded as a benign corpus luteum cyst.[142] In cases of nonviable intrauterine pregnancy, the presence of chorionic villi in the curettage specimen serves consistently to delay the correct diagnosis. For these reasons, many patients suffer from late diagnosis and arrive at the hospital after tubal rupture has occurred.[143,144] There are no specific features to guide the physician to make an accurate, early diagnosis of heterotopic pregnancy other than a general awareness of such a possibility. This is particularly important in cases of abdominal pain and tenderness accompanying normal intrauterine pregnancy or following uterine curettage for a nonviable intrauterine pregnancy among patients who conceived by methods of assisted reproductive technology. In addition, in cases of persistent or rising β-hCG levels following uterine curettage for a nonviable intrauterine pregnancy, the possibility of heterotopic pregnancy should be considered.

Treatment of Heterotopic Pregnancy

Treatment consists of removal of the ectopic pregnancy by surgery, and avoidance of intrauterine instrumentation and systemic methotrexate treatment in cases when the pregnancy is desirable (especially following assisted reproductive technology). In hemodynamically unstable patients, an explorative laparotomy is necessary. Expectant management is problematic as β-hCG levels cannot be monitored effectively owing to the intrauterine pregnancy. The prognosis for the intrauterine pregnancy is generally good, and many are carried to term.[146,147]

Other complex treatment modalities are usually reserved for cases where the ectopic pregnancy is implanted in sites other than the fallopian tube.

KEY POINTS

- Ectopic pregnancy is a major cause of maternal mortality during early stages of pregnancy.
- The most common risk factor for ectopic pregnancy is prior tubal obstruction and injury.
- The β-hCG levels in normal pregnancy double every 2 days (48 hours); thus, clinicians rely on a normal "doubling time" to characterize a viable gestation.
- The accuracy of the initial clinical evaluation before rupture is less than optimal, and additional tests are required in order to differentiate ectopic pregnancy from early intrauterine pregnancy.
- The risk of ectopic pregnancy is increased among women undergoing assisted reproductive technology and specifically *in vitro* fertilization.
- The most common complaint in ectopic pregnancy is severe abdominal pain that may be accompanied by vaginal bleeding.
- Pelvic examination before rupture is usually nonspecific, and a palpable pelvic mass on bimanual examination is noticeable in less than half of all cases.
- A baseline serum progesterone level of <20 nmol/L can be used to identify abnormal pregnancy (either intra- or extrauterine) with a PPV of ≥95%. However, serum progesterone levels cannot distinguish ectopic pregnancy from spontaneous abortion.
- Accurate diagnosis of ectopic pregnancy is based on visualization of an extrauterine pregnancy.
- At β-hCG levels between 1000 and 2000 mIU/mL, or at 5 weeks' gestation, a viable intrauterine pregnancy should be seen by transvaginal ultrasound.

- Coexistent intra- and extrauterine pregnancies (heterotopic) following spontaneous cycles are rare, with estimated incidence of 1 in 30,000 normal pregnancies.
- Methotrexate is a cost-effective, nonsurgical fallopian tube-sparing treatment for ectopic pregnancy.
- Absolute contraindications to methotrexate include breastfeeding; immunodeficiency; alcohol consumption; hepatic, pulmonary, renal, or hematologic dysfunction; known sensitivity to methotrexate; blood dyscrasias; or peptic ulcer disease.
- The overall success rate of methotrexate treatments is almost 90%.
- Candidates for successful expectant management must be asymptomatic with an objective evidence of resolution (generally manifested by declining levels of β-hCG).

REFERENCES

(only references cited in synoptic print chapter; for a complete reference list, see ebook)

1. Committee on Practice Bulletins—Gynecology. ACOG practice bulletin no. 191: tubal ectopic pregnancy. *Obstet Gynecol.* 2018;131(2):e65-e77.
2. Marion LL, Meeks GR. Ectopic pregnancy: history, incidence, epidemiology, and risk factors. *Clin Obstet Gynecol.* 2012;55(2):376-386.
5. Dolinko AV, Vrees RA, Frishman GN. Non-tubal ectopic pregnancies: overview and treatment via local injection. *J Minim Invasive Gynecol.* 2018;25(2):287-296.
6. Davies B, Turner KME, Frolund M, et al. Risk of reproductive complications following chlamydia testing: a population-based retrospective cohort study in Denmark. *Lancet Infect Dis.* 2016;16(9):1057-1064.
9. Backman T, Rauramo I, Huhtala S, Koskenvuo M. Pregnancy during the use of levonorgestrel intrauterine system. *Am J Obstet Gynecol.* 2004;190(1):50-54.
10. Li C, Zhao WH, Meng CX, et al. Contraceptive use and the risk of ectopic pregnancy: a multi-center case-control study. *PLoS One.* 2014;9(12):e115031.
11. Malacova E, Kemp A, Hart R, Jama-Alol K, Preen DB. Long-term risk of ectopic pregnancy varies by method of tubal sterilization: a whole-population study. *Fertil Steril.* 2014;101(3):728-734.
12. Perkins KM, Boulet SL, Kissin DM, Jamieson DJ. Risk of ectopic pregnancy associated with assisted reproductive technology in the United States, 2001-2011. *Obstet Gynecol.* 2015;125(1):70-78.
13. Malak M, Tawfeeq T, Holzer H, Tulandi T. Risk factors for ectopic pregnancy after in vitro fertilization treatment. *J Obstet Gynaecol Can.* 2011;33(6):617-619.
14. Bu Z, Xiong Y, Wang K, Sun Y. Risk factors for ectopic pregnancy in assisted reproductive technology: a 6-year, single-center study. *Fertil Steril.* 2016;106(1):90-94.
15. Cottrell BH. An updated review of of evidence to discourage douching. *MCN Am J Matern Child Nurs.* 2010;35(2):102-107; quiz 8-9.
16. Kurtoglu E, Kokcu A, Celik H, Kefeli M. Salpingitis isthmica nodosa and recurrent ectopic pregnancy. *J Obstet Gynaecol.* 2015;35(2):217-218.
17. Weckstein LN, Boucher AR, Tucker H, Gibson D, Rettenmaier MA. Accurate diagnosis of early ectopic pregnancy. *Obstet Gynecol.* 1985;65(3):393-397.
18. Kirk E, Bottomley C, Bourne T. Diagnosing ectopic pregnancy and current concepts in the management of pregnancy of unknown location. *Hum Reprod Update.* 2014;20(2):250-261.
19. Murray H, Baakdah H, Bardell T, Tulandi T. Diagnosis and treatment of ectopic pregnancy. *Can Med Assoc J.* 2005;173(8):905-912.
20. Davies S, Byrn F, Cole LA. Human chorionic gonadotropin testing for early pregnancy viability and complications. *Clin Lab Med.* 2003;23(2):257-264.
22. Shaunik A, Kulp J, Appleby DH, Sammel MD, Barnhart KT. Utility of dilation and curettage in the diagnosis of pregnancy of unknown location. *Am J Obstet Gynecol.* 2011;204(2):130.e1-6.
23. Doubilet PM, Benson CB, Bourne T, Blaivas M. Diagnostic criteria for nonviable pregnancy early in the first trimester. *N Engl J Med.* 2013;369(15):1443-1451.
24. Connolly A, Ryan DH, Stuebe AM, Wolfe HM. Reevaluation of discriminatory and threshold levels for serum beta-hCG in early pregnancy. *Obstet Gynecol.* 2013;121(1):65-70.
25. Barnhart KT. Clinical practice. Ectopic pregnancy. *N Engl J Med.* 2009;361(4):379-387.
26. Memtsa M, Jurkovic D, Jauniaux E. Diagnostic biomarkers for predicting adverse early pregnancy outcomes: Scientific Impact Paper No. 58. *Br J Obstet Gynaecol.* 2019;126(3):e107-e113.
27. Banerjee S, Aslam N, Woelfer B, Lawrence A, Elson J, Jurkovic D. Expectant management of early pregnancies of unknown location: a prospective evaluation of methods to predict spontaneous resolution of pregnancy. *Br J Obstet Gynaecol.* 2001;108(2):158-163.
29. Rana P, Kazmi I, Singh R, et al. Ectopic pregnancy: a review. *Arch Gynecol Obstet.* 2013;288(4):747-757.
30. Rausch ME, Barnhart KT. Serum biomarkers for detecting ectopic pregnancy. *Clin Obstet Gynecol.* 2012;55(2):418-423.
31. Kirk E, Bourne T. Diagnosis of ectopic pregnancy with ultrasound. *Best Pract Res Clin Obstet Gynaecol.* 2009;23(4):501-508.
32. Barnhart KT, Fay CA, Suescum M, et al. Clinical factors affecting the accuracy of ultrasonography in symptomatic first-trimester pregnancy. *Obstet Gynecol.* 2011;117(2 pt 1):299-306.
33. Goldstein SR, Snyder JR, Watson C, Danon M. Very early pregnancy detection with endovaginal ultrasound. *Obstet Gynecol.* 1988;72(2):200-204.
35. Richardson A, Hopkisson J, Campbell B, Raine-Fenning N. Use of double decidual sac sign to confirm intrauterine pregnancy location prior to sonographic visualization of embryonic contents. *Ultrasound Obstet Gynecol.* 2017;49(5):643-648.
36. Richardson A, Gallos I, Dobson S, Campbell BK, Coomarasamy A, Raine-Fenning N. Accuracy of first-trimester ultrasound in diagnosis of tubal ectopic pregnancy in the absence of an obvious extrauterine embryo: systematic review and meta-analysis. *Ultrasound Obstet Gynecol.* 2016;47(1):28-37.
37. Aydogmus S, Aydogmus H, Gencdal S, Kelekci S. Density of tubal ring vascularization: a new marker for prediction of success of medical treatment in tubal ectopic pregnancy. *Eur J Obstet Gynecol Reprod Biol.* 2017;217:113-118.
38. Chung K, Chandavarkar U, Opper N, Barnhart K. Reevaluating the role of dilation and curettage in the diagnosis of pregnancy of unknown location. *Fertil Steril.* 2011;96(3):659-662.
39. Seeber BE, Barnhart KT. Suspected ectopic pregnancy. *Obstet Gynecol.* 2006;107(2 pt 1):399-413.
40. Givens VM, Lipscomb GH. Diagnosis of ectopic pregnancy. *Clin Obstet Gynecol.* 2012;55(2):387-394.
44. Hajenius PJ, Mol F, Mol BW, Bossuyt PM, Ankum WM, van der Veen F. Interventions for tubal ectopic pregnancy. *Cochrane Database Syst Rev.* 2007;(1):Cd000324.
45. Snyman L, Makulana T, Makin JD. A randomised trial comparing laparoscopy with laparotomy in the management of women with ruptured ectopic pregnancy. *S Afr Med J.* 2017;107(3):258-263.
47. Cohen A, Almog B, Satel A, Lessing JB, Tsafrir Z, Levin I. Laparoscopy versus laparotomy in the management of ectopic pregnancy with massive hemoperitoneum. *Int J Gynaecol Obstet.* 2013;123(2):139-141.
48. Mol F, van Mello NM, Strandell A, et al. Salpingotomy versus salpingectomy in women with tubal pregnancy (ESEP study): an open-label, multicentre, randomised controlled trial. *Lancet.* 2014;383(9927):1483-1489.

51. Erickson BK, Conner MG, Landen Jr CN. The role of the fallopian tube in the origin of ovarian cancer. *Am J Obstet Gynecol.* 2013;209(5):409-414.

52. Kurman RJ, Shih IM. The origin and pathogenesis of epithelial ovarian cancer: a proposed unifying theory. *Am J Surg Pathol.* 2010;34(3):433-443.

53. ACOG Committee Opinion No. 774: opportunistic salpingectomy as a strategy for epithelial ovarian cancer prevention. *Obstet Gynecol.* 2019;133(4):e279-e284.

54. Long Roche KC, Abu-Rustum NR, Nourmoussavi M, Zivanovic O. Risk-reducing salpingectomy: let us be opportunistic. *Cancer.* 2017;123(10):1714-1720.

55. Al-Sunaidi M, Tulandi T. Surgical treatment of ectopic pregnancy. *Semin Reprod Med.* 2007;25(2):117-122.

56. Zhang Y, Chen J, Lu W, Li B, Du G, Wan X. Clinical characteristics of persistent ectopic pregnancy after salpingostomy and influence on ongoing pregnancy. *J Obstet Gynaecol Res.* 2017;43(3):564-570.

57. Gracia CR, Brown HA, Barnhart KT. Prophylactic methotrexate after linear salpingostomy: a decision analysis. *Fertil Steril.* 2001;76(6):1191-1195.

58. Mol F, Mol BW, Ankum WM, van der Veen F, Hajenius PJ. Current evidence on surgery, systemic methotrexate and expectant management in the treatment of tubal ectopic pregnancy: a systematic review and meta-analysis. *Hum Reprod Update.* 2008;14(4):309-319.

60. Berlin NI, Rall D, Mead JA, et al. Folic acid antagonist. Effects on the cell and the patient. Combined clinical staff conference at the National Institutes of Health. *Ann Intern Med.* 1963;59:931-956.

61. Stika CS. Methotrexate: the pharmacology behind medical treatment for ectopic pregnancy. *Clin Obstet Gynecol.* 2012;55(2):433-439.

62. Juneau C, Bates GW. Reproductive outcomes after medical and surgical management of ectopic pregnancy. *Clin Obstet Gynecol.* 2012;55(2):455-460.

66. Practice Committee of American Society for Reproductive Medicine. Medical treatment of ectopic pregnancy: a committee opinion. *Fertil Steril.* 2013;100(3):638-644.

67. Czuczwar P. The role of ultrasonography in methotrexate therapy for ectopic pregnancy. *J Ultrason.* 2018;18(73):158-161.

68. Laibl V, Takacs P, Kang J. Previous ectopic pregnancy as a predictor of methotrexate failure. *Int J Gynaecol Obstet.* 2004;85(2):177-178.

69. Lipscomb GH, Givens VA, Meyer NL, Bran D. Previous ectopic pregnancy as a predictor of failure of systemic methotrexate therapy. *Fertil Steril.* 2004;81(5):1221-1224.

70. Cirik DA, Kinay T, Keskin U, Ozden E, Altay M, Gelisen O. Success rates of single-dose methotrexate and additional dose requirements among women with first and previous ectopic pregnancies. *Int J Gynaecol Obstet.* 2016;133(1):49-52.

71. Tabatabaii Bafghi A, Zaretezerjani F, Sekhavat L, Dehghani Firouzabadi R, Ramazankhani Z. Fertility outcome after treatment of unruptured ectopic pregnancy with two different methotrexate protocols. *Int J Fertil Steril.* 2012;6(3):189-194.

72. Barnhart KT, Gosman G, Ashby R, Sammel M. The medical management of ectopic pregnancy: a meta-analysis comparing "single dose" and "multidose" regimens. *Obstet Gynecol.* 2003;101(4):778-784.

75. Kim J, Jung YM, Lee DY, Jee BC. Pretreatment serum human chorionic gonadotropin cutoff value for medical treatment success with single-dose and multi-dose regimen of methotrexate in tubal ectopic pregnancy. *Obstet Gynecol Sci.* 2017;60(1):79-86.

76. Panelli DM, Phillips CH, Brady PC. Incidence, diagnosis and management of tubal and nontubal ectopic pregnancies: a review. *Fertil Res Pract.* 2015;1:15.

78. Visconti K, Zite N. hCG in ectopic pregnancy. *Clin Obstet Gynecol.* 2012;55(2):410-417.

79. Cohen A, Bibi G, Almog B, Tsafrir Z, Levin I. Second-dose methotrexate in ectopic pregnancies: the role of beta human chorionic gonadotropin. *Fertil Steril.* 2014;102(6):1646-1649.

80. Lipscomb GH. Medical management of ectopic pregnancy. *Clin Obstet Gynecol.* 2012;55(2):424-432.

86. Nurmohamed L, Moretti ME, Schechter T, et al. Outcome following high-dose methotrexate in pregnancies misdiagnosed as ectopic. *Am J Obstet Gynecol.* 2011;205(6):533.e1-533.e3.

89. Craig LB, Khan S. Expectant management of ectopic pregnancy. *Clin Obstet Gynecol.* 2012;55(2):461-470.

92. Garavaglia E, Quaranta L, Redaelli A, Colombo G, Pasi F, Candiani M. Interstitial pregnancy after in vitro fertilization and embryo transfer following bilateral salpingectomy: report of two cases and literature review. *Int J Fertil Steril.* 2012;6(2):131-134.

93. Di Tizio L, Spina MR, Gustapane S, D'Antonio F, Liberati M. Interstitial pregnancy: from medical to surgical approach-report of three cases. *Case Rep Obstet Gynecol.* 2018;2018:2815871.

94. Garretto D, Lee LN, Budorick NE, Figueroa R. Interstitial twin pregnancy: a unique case presentation. *J Clin Ultrasound.* 2015;43(7):447-450.

95. Grindler NM, Ng J, Tocce K, Alvero R. Considerations for management of interstitial ectopic pregnancies: two case reports. *J Med Case Rep.* 2016;10(1):106.

96. Moawad NS, Mahajan ST, Moniz MH, Taylor SE, Hurd WW. Current diagnosis and treatment of interstitial pregnancy. *Am J Obstet Gynecol.* 2010;202(1):15-29.

97. Chukus A, Tirada N, Restrepo R, Reddy NI. Uncommon implantation sites of ectopic pregnancy: thinking beyond the complex adnexal mass. *Radiographics.* 2015;35(3):946-959.

98. Valsky DV, Yagel S. Ectopic pregnancies of unusual location: management dilemmas. *Ultrasound Obstet Gynecol.* 2008;31(3):245-251.

100. Zuo X, Shen A, Chen M. Successful management of unruptured interstitial pregnancy in 17 consecutive cases by using laparoscopic surgery. *Aust N Z J Obstet Gynaecol.* 2012;52(4):387-390.

101. Thakur Y, Coker A, Morris J, Oliver R. Laparoscopic and ultrasound-guided transcervical evacuation of cornual ectopic pregnancy: an alternative approach. *J Obstet Gynaecol.* 2004;24(7):809-810.

102. Hiersch L, Krissi H, Ashwal E, From A, Wiznitzer A, Peled Y. Effectiveness of medical treatment with methotrexate for interstitial pregnancy. *Aust N Z J Obstet Gynaecol.* 2014;54(6):576-580.

103. Kim MJ, Cha JH, Bae HS, et al. Therapeutic outcomes of methotrexate injection in unruptured interstitial pregnancy. *Obstet Gynecol Sci.* 2017;60(6):571-578.

105. Choi HJ, Im KS, Jung HJ, Lim KT, Mok JE, Kwon YS. Clinical analysis of ovarian pregnancy: a report of 49 cases. *Eur J Obstet Gynecol Reprod Biol.* 2011;158(1):87-89.

106. Melcer Y, Maymon R, Vaknin Z, et al. Primary ovarian ectopic pregnancy: still a medical challenge. *J Reprod Med.* 2016;61(1-2):58-62.

107. Seo MR, Choi JS, Bae J, et al. Preoperative diagnostic clues to ovarian pregnancy: retrospective chart review of women with ovarian and tubal pregnancy. *Obstet Gynecol Sci.* 2017;60(5):462-468.

108. Alalade A, Mayers K, Abdulrahman G, Oliver R, Odejinmi F. A twelve year analysis of non-tubal ectopic pregnancies: do the clinical manifestations and risk factor for these rare pregnancies differ from those of tubal pregnancies? *Gynecol Surg.* 2016;13(2):103-109.

109. Begum J, Pallavee P, Samal S. Diagnostic dilemma in ovarian pregnancy: a case series. *J Clin Diagn Res.* 2015;9(4):QR01-QR03.

110. Resta S, Fuggetta E, D'Itri F, Evangelista S, Ticino A, Porpora MG. Rupture of ovarian pregnancy in a woman with low beta-hCG levels. *Case Rep Obstet Gynecol.* 2012;2012:213160.

111. Papillon-Smith J, Krishnamurthy S, Mansour FW. Ovarian pregnancy. *J Obstet Gynaecol Can.* 2016;38(1):1-2.

112. Birge O, Erkan MM, Ozbey EG, Arslan D. Medical management of an ovarian ectopic pregnancy: a case report. *J Med Case Rep.* 2015;9:290.

113. Di Luigi G, Patacchiola F, La Posta V, Bonitatibus A, Ruggeri G, Carta G. Early ovarian pregnancy diagnosed by ultrasound and successfully treated with multidose methotrexate. *Clin Exp Obstet Gynecol.* 2012;39(3):390-393.

114. Shan N, Dong D, Deng W, Fu Y. Unusual ectopic pregnancies: a retrospective analysis of 65 cases. *J Obstet Gynaecol Res.* 2014;40(1):147-154.

118. Vela G, Tulandi T. Cervical pregnancy: the importance of early diagnosis and treatment. *J Minim Invasive Gynecol.* 2007;14(4):481-484.

119. Kumar N, Agrawal S, Das V, Agrawal A. Cervical pregnancy masquerading as an incomplete abortion- A learning lesson. *J Clin Diagn Res.* 2017;11(3):QD04-QD05.

120. Uludag SZ, Kutuk MS, Aygen EM, Sahin Y. Conservative management of cervical ectopic pregnancy: single-center experience. *J Obstet Gynaecol Res.* 2017;43(8):1299-1304.

121. Fylstra DL. Cervical pregnancy: 13 cases treated with suction curettage and balloon tamponade. *Am J Obstet Gynecol.* 2014;210(6):581.e1-581.e5.

122. Ding W, Zhang X, Qu P. An efficient conservative treatment option for cervical pregnancy: transcatheter intra-arterial methotrexate infusion combined with uterine artery embolization followed by curettage. *Med Sci Monit.* 2019;25:1558-1565.

123. Saeng-anan U, Sreshthaputra O, Sukpan K, Tongsong T. Cervical pregnancy with massive bleeding after treatment with methotrexate. *BMJ Case Rep.* 2013;2013:bcr2013200440.

129. Parker VL, Srinivas M. Non-tubal ectopic pregnancy. *Arch Gynecol Obstet.* 2016;294(1):19-27.

132. Marcellin L, Menard S, Lamau MC, et al. Conservative management of an advanced abdominal pregnancy at 22 weeks. *AJP Rep.* 2014;4(1):55-60.

133. Nassali MN, Benti TM, Bandani-Ntsabele M, Musinguzi E. A case report of an asymptomatic late term abdominal pregnancy with a live birth at 41 weeks of gestation. *BMC Res Notes.* 2016;9:31.

134. Lee C. Abdominal pregnancy in a low-resource setting. *Obstet Gynecol.* 2015;125(5):1039-1041.

135. Rohilla M, Joshi B, Jain V, Neetimala, Gainder S. Advanced abdominal pregnancy: a search for consensus. Review of literature along with case report. *Arch Gynecol Obstet.* 2018;298(1):1-8.

136. Cosentino F, Rossitto C, Turco LC, et al. Laparoscopic management of abdominal pregnancy. *J Minim Invasive Gynecol.* 2017;24(5):724-725.

137. Kayatas S, Demirci O, Kumru P, Mahmutoglu D, Saribrahim B, Arinkan SA. Predictive factors for failure of salpingostomy in ectopic pregnancy. *J Obstet Gynaecol Res.* 2014;40(2):453-458.

138. Farquhar CM. Ectopic pregnancy. *Lancet.* 2005;366(9485):583-591.

140. Chadee A, Rezai S, Kirby C, et al. Spontaneous heterotopic pregnancy: dual case report and review of literature. *Case Rep Obstet Gynecol.* 2016;2016:2145937.

141. Clayton HB, Schieve LA, Peterson HB, Jamieson DJ, Reynolds MA, Wright VC. A comparison of heterotopic and intrauterine-only pregnancy outcomes after assisted reproductive technologies in the United States from 1999 to 2002. *Fertil Steril.* 2007;87(2):303-309.

142. Singhal M, Ahuja CK, Saxena AK, Dhaliwal L, Khandelwal N. Sonographic appearance of heterotopic pregnancy with ruptured ectopic tubal pregnancy. *J Clin Ultrasound.* 2010;38(9):509-511.

143. Kumar R, Dey M. Spontaneous heterotopic pregnancy with tubal rupture and pregnancy progressing to term. *Med J Armed Forces India.* 2015;71(suppl 1):S73-S75.

144. Shetty SK, Shetty AK. A case of heterotopic pregnancy with tubal rupture. *J Clin Diagn Res.* 2013;7(12):3000-3001.

146. Guan Y, Ma C. Clinical outcomes of patients with heterotopic pregnancy after surgical treatment. *J Minim Invasive Gynecol.* 2017;24(7):1111-1115.

147. Maciel N, Lima AF, Cruz R, Ponte C. Advanced abdominal pregnancy in a spontaneous heterotopic pregnancy. *BMJ Case Rep.* 2017;2017:bcr2017222098.

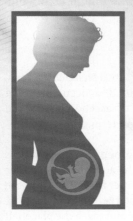

CHAPTER 4

Evaluation of Stillbirth

Alex S. Miller and Uma M. Reddy

Introduction

Epidemiology

Stillbirth, defined as fetal death at 20 weeks or more of gestation, remains a common adverse pregnancy outcome worldwide, affecting 2.6 million third-trimester pregnancies in 2015.[1] Significant disparities exist with 98% of stillbirths occurring in low-income and middle-income countries: 77% in South Asia and sub-Saharan Africa.[2] As of 2015, the global rate of stillbirth was approximately 18 per 1000 births, exceeding the target set by the World Health Organization's (WHO's) Every Newborn Action Plan of 12 or fewer stillbirths per 1000 births in every country by 2030.[2,3]

In the United States, approximately 24,000 stillbirths occur annually, a rate of 5.96 per 1000 births in 2013, evenly dispersed between "early" stillbirth (20-27 weeks' gestation) and "late" stillbirth (≥28 weeks' gestation).[4] This rate has changed minimally since 2006, while infant mortality has declined by 11%.[4]

Risk Factors for Stillbirth

In the United States, there is significant racial/ethnic variation among stillbirth rates. In 2013, the highest stillbirth rate occurred among non-Hispanic black women of 10.53 per 1000 births compared with 4.88 per 1000 births for non-Hispanic white women.[4] In order to understand the reasons for this racial/ethnic disparity, the Stillbirth Collaborative Research Network (SCRN) conducted a population-based, case-controlled study involving 59 tertiary care and community hospitals across five geographic catchment areas. Compared with non-Hispanic white women, non-Hispanic black women were significantly more likely to have stillbirth occur prior to 24 weeks, intrapartum, and secondary to an infection or obstetric complication.[5] Because

of the shared pathophysiology with spontaneous preterm birth (see Chapter 49), a condition with well-documented racial disparity, interventions that reduce rates of early spontaneous preterm birth may also address this subset of stillbirths.

Stillbirth rates vary by maternal age in a parabolic distribution, with the lowest occurring in women aged 25 to 29 years (5.34 per 1000 births) and highest occurring in women younger than 15 years (15.88 per 1000 births).[4] Advanced maternal age (AMA) also increases the risk of stillbirth—increases 2-fold from ages 40 to 44 years and 2.5-fold with maternal age 45 years and older (13.76 per 1000 births).[4] This association persists after adjusting for maternal medical disease, race/ethnicity, and parity.[6,7] A meta-analysis evaluating the effect of AMA on pregnancy outcomes noted that the increased risk of stillbirth parallels an increased risk of placental abruption, preeclampsia, and fetal growth restriction, highlighting placental dysfunction as a possible contributor to the age-related increase in stillbirth.[8]

Obesity also increases the risk of stillbirth in a dose-dependent fashion with a meta-analysis of 38 cohort studies revealing a relative risk of 1.21 for every increase of 5 units of maternal body mass index (BMI).[9] Women with a BMI over 30 kg/m^2 are twice as likely to experience stillbirth. Causes of obesity-related stillbirth include placental diseases, hypertension, fetal anomalies, and cord abnormalities (see Chapter 32).[10]

Other obstetric risk factors, such as increased parity, are associated with an increased risk of stillbirth, with rates more than doubled in women with four or more prior pregnancies.[11] Stillbirth also occurs more frequently in multifetal gestations, with approximately a 2.5-fold increased risk in twins and 5.5-fold increased risk in triplet or higher order gestations (see Chapter 5).[4] Smoking, alcohol use, illicit drug use (see Chapter 8), low education, and inadequate prenatal care (see Chapter 54) are also associated with elevated risks of stillbirth.[12]

In the SCRN review of 512 stillbirths, 17% occurred intrapartum. These are generally secondary to preterm labor, premature prelabor rupture of membranes, cervical insufficiency, intra-amniotic infection, or placental abruption at a previable or periviable gestational age.[5]

Classification of Stillbirth

Accurate, consistent reporting of causes of stillbirth is needed to guide further efforts aiming to reduce the risk of stillbirth. Over 80 classification systems have been proposed with no current uniformly used system for stillbirth reporting.[13] The SCRN developed a classification system based on the evidence in the existing literature entitled "Initial Causes of Fetal Death" or INCODE.[14] This system assigned levels of certainty to causes of stillbirth, ranging from "probable," to "possible," and "present." Using INCODE to analyze 512 stillbirths that had a complete evaluation, including autopsy and placental pathology, the SCRN assigned a probable cause of death in 60.9% of cases and a possible or probable cause in 76.2% of cases, with multiple probable or possible causes in 31.4% of cases.[5] The most frequent cause of stillbirth (29.3% of cases) was obstetric complications, a category that included abruption, complications of multiple gestations, preterm labor, preterm rupture of membranes, and cervical insufficiency predominantly at a pre- or periviable gestation. The second most frequent category (23.6% of cases) was placental complications, which included uteroplacental insufficiency and maternal vascular disorders.[5] Other etiologies of stillbirth included fetal genetic or structural anomalies (13.7% of cases), infection (12.9% of cases), umbilical abnormalities (10.4% of cases), hypertensive disorders (9.2% of cases), and maternal medical complications (7.8% of cases).[5]

Causes of Stillbirth

Infection

Maternal infections increase the risk of stillbirth by causing severe maternal illness, direct fetal infection, placental dysfunction, or preterm labor at a previable gestation. Worldwide, maternal infections, including syphilis and malaria, are associated with a substantial number of stillbirths, up to 50%

depending on the area.[1,15,16] In developed nations, this rate decreases to 10% to 20%, occurring most commonly in the setting of ascending bacterial infections in the setting of preterm premature rupture of membranes.[5,17]

Pathogens, including group B *Streptococcus* and *Escherichia coli*, enter the amniotic fluid either after membrane rupture or after ascension from the vagina.[16] Alternatively, bacteria, such as *Listeria*, may spread hematogenously and reach the placental villi causing microabscesses and villous necrosis.[16] Viral pathogens, such as enteroviruses, cytomegalovirus, Zika virus, and parvovirus, have also been implicated in stillbirth through both placental and fetal mechanisms.[16,18] A more detailed discussion of infectious diseases affecting pregnancy is presented in Chapter 39.

Maternal Medical Conditions

Hypertension

Hypertension is a significant cause of stillbirth, contributing to 9.2% of stillbirths identified by the SCRN.[5] In the United States in 2017, 8.6% of pregnancies were complicated by hypertensive disorders of pregnancy: 1.9% by chronic hypertension and 6.45% by preeclampsia or gestational hypertension.[19] Stillbirth risk is highest in the setting of preeclampsia that is superimposed on chronic hypertension and lowest in uncomplicated chronic and gestational hypertension.[20,21] A detailed discussion of hypertensive diseases in pregnancy is presented in Chapter 27.

Diabetes

In the United States in 2017, 7.3% of pregnancies were complicated by gestational or preexisting diabetes mellitus: 0.9% prepregnancy and 6.4% gestational diabetes.[19] Preexisting diabetes increases the risk of stillbirth by a factor of 2.9.[12] In a study of 5000 pregnant women with type 1 diabetes, the rate of stillbirth was five times higher than the nondiabetic population.[22] Stillbirth occurs most frequently in the setting of poor glycemic control secondary to congenital abnormalities, placental insufficiency, growth restriction, macrosomia, or obstructed labor. Unlike preexisting diabetes, gestational diabetes does not have an increased stillbirth rate in most large studies.[23] Perinatal outcomes are improved in the setting of improved glycemic control.[24] A detailed discussion of diabetes in pregnancy is presented in Chapter 30.

Thyroid Disease

Maternal hyperthyroidism is rare in pregnancy, complicating 0.1% to 0.4% of births.[25] Hyperthyroidism secondary to Graves disease is associated with fetal thyrotoxicosis in approximately 1% of cases secondary to thyroid-stimulating immunoglobulins.[26] Untreated, this may cause growth restriction, hydrops, and fetal death.

Hypothyroidism is more prevalent, occurring in approximately 2% of women.[27] Overt hypothyroidism places women at an increased risk for stillbirth; the risk for fetal or neonatal death increasing 1.6-fold for each doubling of the thyroid-stimulating hormone concentration.[28] However, treatment of hypothyroidism is associated with a return to the baseline risk of stillbirth.[29] Treatment of subclinical hypothyroidism with levothyroxine has not been associated with a reduction in stillbirth rate.[30]

Systemic Lupus Erythematosus

Systemic lupus erythematosus (SLE) is associated with stillbirth in the setting of active disease, renal involvement, and antiphospholipid syndrome. In a review of 554 women with SLE, the presence of antiphospholipid antibodies increased the risk of fetal death from 16% to 38%.[31] Rarely, stillbirth may be secondary to congenital atrioventricular block, occurring secondary to transplacental passage of SS-A/Ro and SS-B/La antibodies, which cause scarring of the endocardium and permanent destruction of the atrioventricular conduction system.[32] This may cause hydrops in up to 40% of cases with one-third of these cases resulting in stillbirth.[32] SLE and its effects on pregnancy are discussed in Chapter 40.

Renal Disease

Approximately 4% of women of childbearing age are affected by chronic kidney disease.[33] Perinatal mortality is 7% in stages 1 and 2 chronic kidney disease (glomerular filtration rate ≥ 60 mL/min) and 14% in stages 3 to 5 (glomerular filtration rate < 60 mL/min).[34] Hypertension is often associated with maternal kidney disease and is associated with an additional two- to tenfold increase in adverse fetal outcomes including stillbirth.[33] Altering dialysis schedules to optimize maternal and fetal outcomes has increased live birth rates to 50% to 87%.[35] Kidney transplantation performed prior to pregnancy with normalization of renal function results

in the most significant improvement of pregnancy outcomes. Pregnancy complicated by renal disorders is discussed in Chapter 35.

Intrahepatic Cholestasis of Pregnancy

Intrahepatic cholestasis of pregnancy (ICP), characterized by pruritus and elevated serum bile acid concentration, is associated with an increased rate of stillbirth. A prospective study in Sweden involving 45,000 pregnant women screened for ICP noted that women with bile acids greater than 40 μmol/L experienced significantly higher rates of fetal complications including asphyxia, spontaneous preterm labor, and presence of meconium.[36] Increased stillbirth rates are theorized to be secondary to bile acid associated damage to the fetal cardiomyocytes causing fatal arrhythmias and vasoconstriction of the chorionic veins.[37] Antenatal testing does not appear to reduce the risk of stillbirth.[38] Liver diseases in pregnancy are discussed in Chapter 34.

Inherited/Acquired Thrombophilias

Antiphospholipid antibody syndrome, the most common acquired thrombophilia, is associated with an increased risk of stillbirth. The SCRN noted that elevated levels of anticardiolipin and anti-β2 glycoprotein antibodies were associated with a threefold increased risk of stillbirth.[39] In contrast, the SCRN did not find an association between most heritable coagulopathies or thrombophilias with stillbirth rates with the exception of maternal homozygous factor V Leiden.[40] However, prospective studies do not demonstrate a link between inherited thrombophilias and stillbirth, including factor V Leiden.[41] Thrombophilias are discussed in Chapter 2.

Fetal Conditions

Genetic Abnormalities

Fetal cytogenetic abnormalities account for approximately 10% of stillbirths, and this percentage is elevated in the setting of fetal structural abnormalities.[42,43] A Dutch study of 1025 stillbirths with a 68% rate of cytogenetic testing detected an overall rate of 11.9% of chromosomal abnormalities. The distribution of chromosomal abnormalities was as follows: trisomy 21 accounted for 37% of cases, trisomy 18 accounted for 23% of cases, monosomy (45,X) accounted for 16% of cases, and trisomy 13 accounted for 5% of cases.[42] In addition to aneuploidy, other chromosomal abnormalities, such as copy number variants (ie, microdeletions or duplications), likely contribute to stillbirth.[44]

Confined placental mosaicism (CPM), a condition where the fetus is euploid but the placenta carries an abnormal cell line, also increases the risk of stillbirth and other adverse pregnancy outcomes. CPM is identified in approximately 1% of first-trimester chorionic villus samples.[45] Type 3 CPM, where the chromosomal abnormality is found in the cytotrophoblast and the mesenchymal core, is the genetic abnormality most associated with adverse pregnancy outcomes, including preterm birth (56%), fetal growth restriction (74%), and a composite of adverse pregnancy outcomes including fetal death (35%).[45] These pregnancies may be associated with a low first-trimester pregnancy-associated plasma protein A (PAPP-A) and a variety of chromosomal abnormalities (most commonly trisomy 16).[45,46]

Stillbirth may also result from fetal single-gene disorders. Numerous autosomal recessive disorders are associated with stillbirth, including hemoglobinopathies, metabolic disorders, peroxisomal disorders, glycogen storage disorders, and amino acid disorders.[47] X-linked disorders, such as incontinentia pigmenti, and autosomal dominant disorders, including skeletal dysplasias and familial long QT syndrome, also have an elevated risk of stillbirth.[47] A discussion of fetal genetic disorders appears in Chapter 11.

Fetal Structural Abnormalities

Approximately 10% of stillbirths can be directly attributed to a fetal structural abnormality.[48,49] These may occur in isolation or as a part of a chromosomal abnormality or syndrome. More than 90 conditions have been associated with stillbirth with no condition accounting for more than 1.5% of cases.[50]

Fetomaternal Hemorrhage

Fetomaternal hemorrhage, the transplacental passage of fetal blood cells to the maternal circulation, likely contributes to approximately 4% of stillbirths.[5] Fifty percent of women will have detectable fetal cells following delivery. However, massive fetomaternal hemorrhage is rare and occurs in less than 1% of women.[51] Risk factors for significant hemorrhage include abruption, trauma, and multiple gestation.[52]

The volume of fetomaternal hemorrhage sufficient to cause stillbirth is unknown. However, volumes greater than 20 mg/kg (>25% fetal blood volume) are associated with an elevated risk of stillbirth (26%)[53] (see Chapter 22).

Fetal Growth Restriction

Fetal growth restriction occurs when the fetus is unable to meet its growth potential and is generally a symptom of an underlying condition. These conditions may include uteroplacental insufficiency, fetal genetic abnormalities, multifetal pregnancies, cord abnormalities, and maternal conditions including infection, hypertension, malnutrition, and tobacco use (see Chapter 18). Customized growth curves that adjust for physiologic maternal variations, including height, weight, parity, and ethnic origin, may assist in differentiating normal and pathologic growth patterns.

Using these customized growth curves, a Swedish study demonstrated a sixfold increase in stillbirth if the fetus was less than the 10th percentile, an association that did not persist with population-based curves.[54] The SCRN study of 527 stillbirths also demonstrated strong associations of stillbirth not only with small for gestational age stillborn infants (<fifth percentile) but also with large for gestational age stillborn infants(>95th percentile); ultrasound and individualized norms performed better than population norms.[55]

Placental Abnormalities

In addition to uteroplacental insufficiency, placental abnormalities, such as placenta previa, vasa previa, neoplasms, and placental abruption, may also increase the risk of stillbirth. Vasa previa, the coursing of fetal vessels across the endocervical os, may result in rupture of the fetal vessels during labor or rupture of membranes, triggering exsanguination of the fetus.[56] Placental abruption, based on clinical signs or histopathologic examination of the placenta, increases the risk of stillbirth approximately ninefold, with the adjusted relative risk increasing to 31 if at least 75% of the placenta was involved.[57] Other histologic placental findings associated with stillbirth as determined by the SCRN include single umbilical artery, velamentous cord insertion, diffuse terminal villous immaturity, inflammation, vascular degenerative changes in the chorionic plate, retroplacental hematoma, intraparenchymal thrombi, parenchymal infarction, fibrin deposition, fetal vascular thrombi, avascular villi, and hydrops.[58]

Umbilical cord pathologies are associated with up to 15% of stillbirths.[59] Umbilical cord events that may lead to stillbirth include umbilical cord prolapse, cord hemorrhage, intrinsic cord abnormalities, and entanglement of the cords in the case of monochorionic twin gestation.[59] Umbilical cord torsion, resulting in interruption of blood flow to the fetus, has also been reported as a cause of stillbirth. This generally occurs at the fetal end of the cord and is marked by a congested and edematous cord with evidence of cord vessel thrombosis.[60]

Nuchal cords and true knots occur frequently in pregnancies that result in live birth. The presence of single or multiple nuchal cords has not been associated with an increased risk of stillbirth.[61] True knots are also commonly noted during live births; however, pathologic demonstration of edema, congestion, and thrombosis in the cord may signal the knot as likely causal.[62]

A detailed discussion of the placenta is found in Chapters 6 and 47.

Multifetal Gestations

Multiple gestations have an eight- to tenfold increased risk of stillbirth, predominately due to placental abnormalities in monochorionic placentation. Twin-to-twin transfusion occurs in 10% of monochorionic diamniotic pregnancies as a result of shared arteriovenous anastomoses with a risk of fetal loss that remains elevated even in the setting of treatment.[63] Additional potentially lethal complications of monochorionic gestation include selective fetal growth restriction and twin anemia polycythemia sequence.[64] Multifetal gestations are also at an increased risk of preterm labor, premature prelabor rupture of membranes, preeclampsia, and fetal growth restriction, conditions that independently increase the risk of stillbirth.

Monochorionic monoamniotic gestations additionally have an elevated risk of death due to cord entanglement, although cord entanglement can occur frequently without resulting in stillbirth.[65] The increased risk in monochorionic monoamniotic gestations may alternatively be increased in the case of twin reverse arterial perfusion sequence, conjoined twins, and discordant anomalies.[65] Multifetal gestations are discussed in Chapter 5.

Evaluation of Stillbirth

Rates of evaluation of stillbirth vary widely. Fetal autopsy rates vary across the United States, generally falling under 50% with lower rates at community hospitals versus tertiary care centers.[66] Objection to autopsy may be secondary to lack of adequate information among family and healthcare professionals, lack of resources, and beliefs that no new information will be found.[67]

Offering and encouraging an evaluation for stillbirth is imperative. The identification of possible or probable cause in approximately 75% of stillbirths can provide a sense of closure.[68] In addition, modifiable findings may help guide care in subsequent pregnancies.[69] Prior to autopsy, families should be provided sufficient time to spend with the baby and to allow for the performance of desired religious or cultural traditions.

The first step in evaluation of stillbirth is obtaining a thorough medical and obstetric history. Maternal medical conditions, symptoms, events during the pregnancy, and the obstetric history will help guide a focused and cost-effective workup.

Placental evaluation is recommended for all stillbirths and includes an evaluation of the placenta, umbilical cord, and fetal membranes by a trained pathologist.[42] Placental weight should be noted in relation to the gestational age. A placenta less than the 5% of the expected weight for gestational age may be associated with reduced uteroplacental blood flow and impaired villous growth. Placental growth may also be impaired in the setting of aneuploidy or infection. Placental weights of 95% or greater of expected weight for gestational age are more common in hydrops fetalis, maternal diabetes, and some infections such as syphilis.[70] Signs of abruption, umbilical cord thrombosis, velamentous cord insertion, and vasa previa should be documented if present. Placental infarcts and decidual vasculopathy may be noted in the setting of maternal hypertensive disorders. The placenta should be evaluated for signs of infection, genetic abnormalities, and anemia. In the setting of a multifetal gestation, chronicity and any vascular anastomoses should be documented.

The umbilical cord should be examined for knots and tangling. However, findings should be interpreted with caution considering 25% of normal pregnancies have evidence of cord entanglement and true knots are frequently found at the time of live birth.[59,65] To consider a diagnosis of cord accident, histologic findings should include vascular ectasia and thrombosis in the umbilical cord, chorionic plate, and stem villi. For probable diagnosis, avascular villi or villi showing stromal karyorrhexis is required.[71]

Fetal autopsy is also an integral step in the evaluation of stillbirth. This should be performed in accordance with published guidelines from the College of American Pathologists.[72] Examination may identify gross anomalies or more subtle findings of infection, anemia, hypoxia, or metabolic abnormalities.[73] In the case of reluctance by the family to pursue autopsy, a combination of gross examination and imaging with either ultrasound or magnetic resonance imaging may aid in diagnosis.[74]

Genetic evaluation should be offered in most cases of stillbirth. A detailed pedigree and evaluation for consanguinity should be performed to assess for single-gene or autosomal recessive disorders. Arrhythmias and sudden cardiac death may reveal presence of familial prolonged QT syndromes.[75] Regarding genetic testing, an abnormal fetal karyotype is found in 6% to 13% of stillbirths, a percentage that increases the setting of structural anomalies or growth restriction.[47] Microarray improves diagnosis of genetic causes of stillbirth beyond karyotype by detecting smaller deletions and duplications (as small as 50 kilobases) and does not require viable tissue. In the SCRN study of 532 stillbirths, microarray analysis yielded results more often when compared to karyotype (87.4% vs 70.5%) and provided better detection of genetic abnormalities (eg, aneuploidy or pathogenic copy number variants) (8.3% vs 5.8%; $P = .007$).[44] Acceptable specimens for cytogenetic testing include amniotic fluid, a placental block from below the cord insertion that includes the chorionic plate, an umbilical cord segment, or an internal fetal tissue specimen such as patellar tissue or fascia lata. Cultured amniocytes provide the highest yield (85% vs 28% for postpartum tissue analysis), so amniocentesis may be considered prior to the delivery.[76]

Antiphospholipid testing is frequently warranted in the setting of stillbirth, especially in the setting of growth restriction, preeclampsia with severe features, and signs of placental insufficiency.[77] Laboratory evaluation should include lupus anticoagulant as well as anticardiolipin and anti-β2 glycoprotein immunoglobulin (Ig) M and IgG. Titers >99th percentile or >40 M phospholipid

(MPL) units or G phospholipid (GPL) units are considered positive but should be confirmed with repeat testing after 12 weeks. Routine testing for heritable thrombophilias is not recommended.[78]

Evaluation for fetomaternal hemorrhage should occur prior to the onset of induction of labor. Although flow cytometry may provide a more accurate quantitative assessment of fetomaternal hemorrhage than Kleihauer-Betke, given that stillbirth likely only results from significant hemorrhage (>25% of fetal blood volume), either test may be used.[53]

Evaluation for illicit substances with a maternal urine toxicology screen may be warranted based on history or population risk. This testing may also be performed on fetal tissues including meconium, hair, and umbilical cord.

Testing for bacterial, viral, protozoal, and fungal pathogens should be based on clinical history and findings on evaluation of the placenta, autopsy, or relevant imaging findings. If clinical or histologic suspicion is lacking, testing for infection beyond evaluation of the placenta and autopsy is of low yield. Serologic testing for syphilis is recommended if not performed as part of routine prenatal care. Routine parvovirus testing was found to be of low yield in stillbirth.[79] TORCH (toxoplasmosis, rubella, cytomegalovirus, herpes simplex) titers have historically been recommended for evaluation; however, their usefulness in routine testing is unproven.

Maternal testing for possible associated medical conditions should be guided by history, physical examination, and circumstances surrounding the stillbirth. This includes testing for thyroid abnormalities, diabetes, and ICP. Routine screening for subclinical maternal disease is not recommended.

Using the INCODE classification system, the SCRN evaluated the components of the stillbirth evaluation in achieving a probable or possible cause of stillbirth. Placental pathology aided in diagnosis in 64.6% of cases, fetal autopsy in 42.4%, genetic testing in 11.9%, antiphospholipid antibodies in 11.1%, fetomaternal hemorrhage assessment in 6.4%, glucose screen in 1.6%, parvovirus testing in 0.4%, and syphilis in 0.2%.[79] Further stratified by clinical scenario (**Algorithm 4.1**), stillbirths in the setting of both growth restriction and hypertensive disorders achieved probable or possible causes most often with the assistance of placental pathology, fetal autopsy, and antiphospholipid testing. In

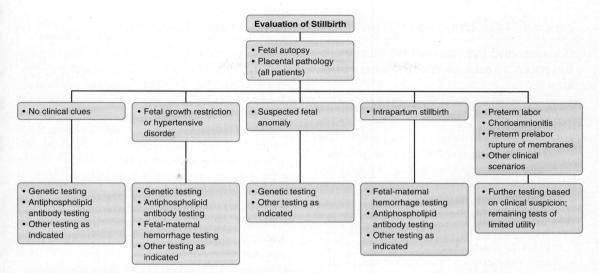

Algorithm 4.1 Evaluation of stillbirth based on test utility in a variety of clinical scenarios.

(From Page JM, Christiansen-Lindquist L, Thorsten V, et al. Diagnostic tests for evaluation of stillbirth: results from the Stillbirth Collaborative Research Network. *Obstet Gynecol.* 2017;129(4):699-706.)

the case of suspected fetal anomalies, fetal autopsy and genetic testing were most helpful with additional benefit from placental evaluation.

Delivery/Bereavement

Following diagnosis of stillbirth, timing and mode of delivery may vary by gestational age, clinical circumstances, and patient preference. See **Box 4.1** for protocols for various stillbirth delivery clinical scenarios. Consumptive coagulopathy rarely complicates expectant management. Approximately 80% to 90% of women will experience spontaneous labor within 2 weeks of stillbirth.[80] Chronic consumptive coagulopathy occurs secondary to release of tissue factor from the decidua or placenta into the maternal circulation in approximately 3% to 4% of patients over 4 to 8 weeks.[81] This risk increases in the setting of placental abruption or uterine perforation.[81]

In the second trimester, dilation and evacuation (D&E) is associated with a lower rate of maternal complications, including failure of the initial method for delivery or retained products of conception when compared to induction of labor (4% vs 29%).[82] However, D&E may limit the quality of perinatal autopsy given the reduced likelihood of an intact fetus. In addition, this option does not permit the family to hold their baby to facilitate bereavement, although a prospective cohort study did not

show a difference in grief response after induction of labor or D&E in women undergoing termination for fetal anomalies.[83] Either option should be offered as long as there is a skilled operator available to perform second-trimester D&E.

Based on studies of midtrimester termination, prior to 28 weeks, misoprostol is the most efficient method of induction.[78,84] After 28 weeks, standard obstetric protocols should be used for induction of labor. In the setting of prior cesarean delivery, women with a prior low transverse uterine incision and less than 28 weeks' gestation may undergo induction with misoprostol.[78] Beyond 28 weeks, mechanical cervical ripening with a Foley balloon and oxytocin may be used.[78] Cesarean delivery should be avoided unless strongly desired by the patient after counseling regarding the risks and benefits. In the SCRN study of 611 cases of stillbirth, 15% of women opted for cesarean delivery. Of women without a prior cesarean delivery undergoing induction, 98.5% had a vaginal delivery and 91.1% of women with a prior cesarean delivery had a vaginal delivery with two cases of uterine rupture.[85]

Families should be provided the opportunity to see and hold their baby as well as receive keepsake items such as handprints or footprints, blankets or clothing, and photos.[86] Bereavement services, counseling, and stillbirth advocacy and support

BOX 4.1 PROTOCOL FOR VARIOUS STILLBIRTH DELIVERY SCENARIOS

Dilation and Evacuation for Uterus Between 13 and 22 Weeks' Gestation Size

- On admission, obtain hematocrit and type and screen.
- Administer doxycycline (100 mg orally) 1 hour before procedure and 200 mg after procedure, or postoperative metronidazole (500 mg orally twice a day for 5 days).
- To facilitate cervical dilation.
  - Administer misoprostol (200 µg) in the posterior fornix 4 hours before procedure OR.
  - Place laminaria in cervix.
- Perform dilation and evacuation under ultrasound guidance.
- Discharge to home after anesthesia has worn off and vaginal bleeding is minimal.
- Administer RhD immune globulin if patient is Rh negative.
- Schedule a follow-up visit in 2 weeks.
- Prescribe nonsteroidal anti-inflammatory drugs or mild narcotics.

Induction of Labor

- Upon admission to labor and delivery department, obtain complete blood count and type and screen. Consider fibrinogen level if fetus has been dead for more than 4 weeks.
- Administer induction medications:
  - For uterus less than 28 weeks' size: misoprostol (200-400 µg) vaginally or orally every 4 hours until delivery of the fetus.

- For uterus greater than 28 weeks' size: misoprostol (25-50 µg) vaginally or orally every 4 hours OR oxytocin infusion per usual protocol.
- To minimize retained placenta, allow spontaneous placental delivery, avoid pulling on umbilical cord, and consider further doses of misoprostol at appropriate intervals.
- Options for anesthesia include epidural, intravenous narcotics via patient-controlled analgesia (PCA) pump, or intermittent doses.
- Parents should be encouraged to spend time with the infant and offered keepsake items (eg, pictures, hand/footprints).
- Administer RhD immune globulin to Rh-negative mothers.
- Consider postpartum care on a nonmaternity ward.
- Offer bereavement services.
- Schedule a follow-up visit in 2 to 6 weeks.

History of Previous Cesarean Delivery

- Previous low transverse incision and uterus less than 28 weeks' size—use misoprostol, dosing for induction at less than 28 weeks.
- Previous low transverse incision and a uterus greater than 28 weeks' size—use oxytocin protocols and cervical ripening with Foley bulb.
  - Repeat cesarean delivery is an option after discussing risks and benefits.
- Previous classic uterine incision—repeat cesarean delivery is appropriate.

groups should be discussed. The parents should be monitored closely for development of depression. A subsequent visit to discuss the findings of the stillbirth evaluation and preconception planning is recommended.

Management of Subsequent Pregnancy

In women with a history of stillbirth, the risk of recurrence is increased almost fivefold (odds ratio [OR] 4.83, 95% confidence interval [CI] 3.77-6.18).[87,88] Unfortunately, there is very limited evidence in guidance for care in the subsequent pregnancy. A 2018 Cochrane review examining possible interventions in subsequent pregnancy including use of antiplatelet agents, leukocyte immunization, intravenous immunoglobulin, and progestogens in subsequent pregnancies was unable to provide recommendations regarding these interventions given the limited data.[89] Growth ultrasounds can be considered starting at 28 weeks given the association of stillbirth with growth restriction. Antepartum fetal testing starting at 32 weeks is recommended but should be balanced against the risk of prematurity in the setting of interventions for false-positive results.[90]

Prevention of Stillbirth

The risk of stillbirth is decreased with optimization of maternal comorbidities, including improved glycemic control in cases of maternal diabetes, and heparin and low-dose aspirin for antiphospholipid antibody syndrome.[91] A meta-analysis of 40 trials evaluating 33,098 women at risk of developing preeclampsia also noted a 14% reduction in fetal or neonatal deaths with use of low-dose aspirin; however, its use has not been proven outside of this indication.[92]

Antepartum fetal testing should first be based on medical indications such as diabetes and chronic hypertension. Testing for women at increased risk for stillbirth due to such conditions as AMA, women ≥ 35 years old, has been debated. A retrospective cohort study evaluated the risk of stillbirth in women who were AMA undergoing weekly antepartum testing from 36 to 41 weeks gestation, noting equivalent stillbirth rates to non-AMA women not receiving testing. The authors concluded that routine antepartum testing should be considered in the setting of AMA.[93] Currently, neither the America College of Obstetricians and Gynecologists nor the Society for Maternal-Fetal Medicine recommend antepartum fetal surveillance for AMA without additional risk factors.

Induction of labor has been considered as a strategy to reduce risk of stillbirth. A randomized controlled trial of 619 women with AMA evaluated induction of labor at 39 weeks compared with expectant management, noting no differences in the cesarean delivery rate or adverse maternal and neonatal outcomes rates between both arms. However, it was not powered to allow for assessment of stillbirth risk reduction.[94] The Maternal-Fetal Medicine Units Network ARRIVE trial compared induction of labor at 39 weeks with expectant management in low-risk nulliparous women and found the rates of cesarean delivery, hypertensive disorders, and neonatal respiratory morbidity were all reduced in the induction arm.[95]

KEY POINTS

- Stillbirth, defined as fetal death at 20 weeks or more of gestation, remains a common adverse pregnancy outcome worldwide.
- Stillbirth rates vary by race/ethnicity, maternal age, and parity. Other obstetric risk factors include multifetal gestation; smoking, alcohol use, or illicit drug use; education level; and adequacy of prenatal care.
- Maternal infections increase the risk of stillbirth by causing severe maternal illness, direct fetal infection, placental dysfunction, or preterm labor at a previable gestation.
- Stillbirth risk is highest in the setting of preeclampsia that is superimposed on chronic hypertension and lowest in uncomplicated chronic and gestational hypertension.
- Maternal comorbidities that increase the risk for fetal demise include preexisting diabetes, thyroid disorders, SLE, renal or liver disease, and thrombophilias.
- Fetal conditions that increase the risk of stillbirth include genetic, structural, and placental abnormalities; fetomaternal hemorrhage; growth restriction; and presence of multifetal gestation.

- The first step in evaluation of stillbirth is obtaining a thorough medical and obstetric history.
- Evaluation of the placenta and umbilical cord and a fetal autopsy are also useful.
- Following diagnosis of stillbirth, timing and mode of delivery may vary by gestational age, clinical circumstances, and patient preference.
- If spontaneous delivery does not occur, either labor induction or D&E performed by a skilled operator should be offered.
- Families should be provided the opportunity to see and hold their baby as well as receive keepsake items to facilitate bereavement and should be monitored closely for signs of depression.
- There is very limited evidence in guidance for care in the subsequent pregnancy, although the risk of loss recurrence is almost fivefold in women with a history of stillbirth.
- The risk of stillbirth is decreased with optimization of maternal comorbidities.
- Antepartum fetal testing for women with AMA and no additional risk factors is not recommended.
- Induction of labor has been considered as a strategy to reduce risk of stillbirth.

REFERENCES

1. Lawn JE, Blencowe H, Waiswa P, et al. Stillbirths: rates, risk factors, and acceleration toward 2030. *Lancet*. 2016;387:587-603.
2. Blencowe H, Cousens S, Jassir FB, et al. National, regional, and worldwide estimates of stillbirth rates in 2015, with trends from 2000: a systematic analysis. *Lancet Glob Health*. 2016;4:e98-e108.
3. World Health Organization. *Every Newborn: An Action Plan to End Preventable Newborn Deaths*. WHO Press; 2014.
4. MacDorman MF, Gregory EC. Fetal and perinatal mortality: United Sates, 2013. *Natl Vital Stat Rep*. 2015;64:1-24.
5. Stillbirth Collaborative Research Network Writing Group. Causes of death among stillbirths. *J Am Med Assoc*. 2011;306:2459-2468.
6. Balayla J, Azoulay L, Assayag J, Benjamin A, Abenhaim HA. Effect of maternal age on the risk of stillbirth: a population-based cohort study on 37 million births in the United States. *Am J Perinatol*. 2011;28:643-650.
7. Waldenstrom U, Cnattingius S, Normal M, et al. Advanced maternal age and stillbirth risk in nulliparous and parous women. *Obstet Gynecol*. 2015;126:355-362.
8. Lean SC, Derricott H, Jones RL, Heazell AEP. Advanced maternal age and adverse pregnancy outcomes: a systematic review and meta-analysis. *PLoS One*. 2017;12:e0186287.
9. Stothard KJ, Tennant PW, Bell R, Rankin J. Maternal overweight and obesity and the risk of congenital anomalies: a systematic review and meta-analysis. *J Am Med Assoc*. 2009;301:636-650.
10. Bodnar LM, Parks WT, Perkins K, et al. Maternal prepregancy obesity and cause-specific stillbirth. *Am J Clin Nutr*. 2015;102:858-864.
11. MacDorman MF, Kirmeyer S. *The Challenge of Fetal Mortality. NCHS Data Brief, No 16*. National Center for Health Statistics; 2009.
12. Flenady V, Koopmans L, Middleton P, et al. Major risk factors for stillbirth in high-income countries: a systematic review and metaanalysis. *Lancet*. 2011;377:1331-1340.
13. Flenady V, Wojcieszek AM, Ellwood D, et al. Classification of causes and associated conditions for stillbirths and neonatal deaths. *Semin Fetal Neonatal Med*. 2017;22:176-185.
14. Dudley DJ, Goldenberg R, Conway D, et al. A new system for determining the causes of stillbirth. *Obstet Gynecol*. 2010;116:254-260.
15. DiMario S, Say L, Lincetto O. Risk factors for stillbirth in developing countries: a systematic review of the literature. *Sex Transm Dis*. 2007;34:S11-S21.
16. Goldenberg RL, McClure EM, Saleem S, Reddy UM. Infection-related stillbirths. *Lancet*. 2010;375:1482-1490.
17. Flenady V, Middleton P, Smith GC, et al. Stillbirths: the way forward in high-income countries. *Lancet*. 2011;377:1703-1717.
18. Chibueze EC, Tirado V, Lopes KD, et al. Zika virus infection in pregnancy: a systematic review of disease course and complications. *Reprod Health*. 2017;14:28.
19. Martin JA, Hamilton BE, Osterman MJK, Driscoll AK, Drake P. Births: final data for 2017. *Natl Vital Stat Rep*. 2018;67:1-50.
20. Ray JG, Burrows RF, Burrows EA, Vermeulen MJ. MOSHIP: McMaster outcome study of hypertension in pregnancy. *Early Hum Dev*. 2001;64:129-143.
21. Xiong T, Mu Y, Liang J, et al. Hypertensive disorders in pregnancy and stillbirth rates: a facility-based study in China. *Bull World Health Organ*. 2018;96:531-539.
22. Persson M, Norman M, Hanson U. Obstetric and perinatal outcomes in type 1 diabetic pregnancies: a large, population-based study. *Diabetes Care*. 2009;32:2005-2009.
23. Lapolla A, Dalfra MG, Bonomo M, et al. Gestational diabetes mellitus in Italy: a multicenter study. *Eur J Obstet Gynecol Reprod Biol*. 2009;145:149-153.
24. Owens LA, Egan AM, Carmody L, Dunne F. Ten years of optimizing outcomes for women with type 1 and type 2 diabetes in pregnancy- the Atlantic DIP experience. *J Clin Endocrinol Metab*. 2016;101:1598-1605.
25. Uenaka M, Tanimura K, Tairaku S, et al. Risk factors for neonatal thyroid dysfunction in pregnancies complicated by Graves' disease. *Eur J Obstet Gynecol Reprod Biol*. 2014;177:89-93.
26. Labadzhyan A, Brent GA, Hershman JM, Leung AM. Thyrotoxicosis of pregnancy. *J Clin Transl Endocrinol*. 2014;1:140-144.
27. Allan WC, Haddow JE, Palomaki GE, et al. Maternal thyroid deficiency and pregnancy complications: implications for population screening. *J Med Screen*. 2000;7:127-130.
28. Benhadi N, Wiersinga WM, Reitsma JB, Vrijkotte TG, Bonsel GJ. Higher maternal TSH levels in pregnancy are associated with increased risk for miscarriage, fetal or neonatal death. *Eur J Endocrinol*. 2009;160:985-991.
29. Wolfberg AJ, Lee-Parritz A, Peller AJ, Lieberman ES. Obstetric and neonatal outcomes associated with maternal hypothyroid disease. *J Matern Fetal Neonatal Med*. 2005;17:35-38.
30. Casey BM, Thom EA, Peaceman AM, et al. Treatment of subclinical hypothyroidism or hypothyroxinemia in pregnancy. *N Engl J Med*. 2017;376:815-825.
31. McNeil HP, Chesterman CN, Krilis SA. Immunology and clinical importance of antiphospholipid antibodies. *Adv Immunol*. 1991;49:193-280.
32. Breur JM, Kapusta I, Stoutenbeck P, Visser GH, van den Berg P, Meijboom EJ. Isolated congenital atrioventricular block diagnosed in utero: natural history and outcome. *J Matern Fetal Neonatal Med*. 2008;21:469-476.
33. Fischer MJ. Chronic kidney disease and pregnancy: maternal and fetal outcomes. *Adv Chronic Kidney Dis*. 2007;14:132-145.
34. Davidson NL, Wolski P, Callaway LW, et al. Chronic kidney disease in pregnancy: maternal and fetal outcomes and progression of kidney disease. *Obstet Gynecol*. 2015;8:92-98.
35. Nadeau-Fredette AC, Hladunewich M, Hui D, et al. End-stage renal disease and pregnancy. *Adv Chronic Kidney Dis*. 2013;20:246-252.
36. Glantz A, Marschall HU, Mattson LA. Intrahepatic cholestasis of pregnancy: relationships between bile acid levels and fetal complication rates. *Hepatology*. 2004;40:467-474.
37. Brouwers L, Koster MPH, Page-Christiaens GC, et al. Intrahepatic cholestasis of pregnancy: maternal and fetal outcomes associated with elevated bile acid levels. *Am J Obstet Gynecol*. 2015;212:100.e1-100.e7.
38. Herrera CA, Manuck TA, Stoddard GJ, et al. Perinatal Outcomes associated with intrahepatic cholestasis of pregnancy. *J Matern Fetal Neonatal Med*. 2018;31:1913-1920.
39. Silver RM, Parker C, Reddy U, et al. Antiphospholipid antibodies in stillbirth. *Obstet Gynecol*. 2013;122:641-657.
40. Silver RM, Saade GR, Thorsten V, et al. Factor V Leiden, prothrombin G20210A, and methylene tetrahydrofolate reductase mutations and stillbirth: the Stillbirth Collaborative Research Network. *Am J Obstet Gynecol*. 2016;215:468.e1-468.e17.
41. Werner EF, Lockwood CJ. Thrombophilias and stillbirth. *Clin Obstet Gynecol*. 2010;53(3):617-627.
42. Korteweg FJ, Erwich JJ, Timmer A, et al. Evaluation of 1025 fetal deaths: proposed diagnostic workup. *Am J Obstet Gynecol*. 2012;206:53.e1-53.e12.
43. Sahlin E, Gustavsson P, Lieden A, et al. Molecular and cytogenetic analysis in stillbirth: results from 481 consecutive cases. *Fetal Diagn Ther*. 2014;36:326-332.
44. Reddy UM, Page GP, Saade GR, et al. Karyotype versus microarray testing for genetic abnormalities after stillbirth. *N Engl J Med*. 2012;367:2185-2193.
45. Toutain J, Goutte-Gattat D, Horvitz J, et al. Confined placental mosaicism revisited: impact on pregnancy characteristics and outcome. *PLoS One*. 2018;13:e0195905.
46. Toutain J, Labeau-Gauzere C, Barnetche T, et al. Confined placental mosaicism and pregnancy outcome: a distinction needs to be made between types 2 and 3. *Prenat Diagn*. 2010;30:1155-1164.
47. Wapner RJ. Genetics of stillbirth. *Clin Obstet Gynecol*. 2010;53:628-634.
48. Miller ES, Minturn L, Linn R, Weese-Mayer DE, Ernst LM. Stillbirth evaluation: a stepwise assessment of placental pathology and autopsy. *Am J Obstet Gynecol*. 2016;214:115.e1-115.e6.
49. Smith GC, Fretts RC. Stillbirth. *Lancet*. 2007;370:1715-1725.
50. Pauli RM. Stillbirth: fetal disorders. *Clin Obstet Gynecol*. 2010;53:646-655.
51. Cohen E, Zuelzer WW, Gustafson DC, Evans MM. Mechanisms of isoimmunization. I. The transplacental passage of fetal erythrocytes in homospecific pregnancies. *Blood*. 1964;23:621-646.
52. Sebring ES, Polesky HF. Fetomaternal hemorrhage: incidence, risk factors, time of occurrence, and clinical effects. *Transfusion*. 1990;30:344-357.
53. Rubod C, Deruelle P, Le Goueff F, et al. Long-term prognosis for infants after massive fetomaternal hemorrhage. *Obstet Gynecol*. 2007;110:256-260.
54. Gardosi J, Mul T, Mongelli M, Fagan D. Analysis of birthweight and gestational age in antepartum stillbirths. *Br J Obstet Gynaecol*. 1998;105:524-530.
55. Bukowski R, Hansen NI, Willinger M, et al. Fetal growth and risk of stillbirth: a population-based case-control study. *Plos Med*. 2014;11:e1001633.
56. Nohuz E, Boulay E, Gallot D, et al. Can we perform a prenatal diagnosis of vasa previa to improve its obstetrical and neonatal outcomes? *J Gynececol Obstet Hum Reprod*. 2017;46:373-377.

57. Anath CV, Berkowitz GS, Savitz DA, Lapinski RH. Placental abruption and adverse perinatal outcomes. *J Am Med Assoc.* 1999;282:1646-1651.

58. Pinar H, Goldenberg RL, Koch MA, et al. Placental findings in singleton stillbirths. *Obstet Gynecol.* 2014;123:325-336.

59. Collins JH. Umbilical cord accidents: human studies. *Semin Perinatol.* 2002;26:79-82.

60. Bakotic BW, Boyd T, Poppiti R, Pflueger S. Recurrent umbilical cord torsion leading to fetal death in 3 subsequent pregnancies: a case report and review of the literature. *Arch Pathol Lab Med.* 2000;124:1352-1355.

61. Carey JC, Rayburn WF. Nuchal cord encirclements and the risk of stillbirth. *Int J Gynaecol Obstet.* 2000;69:173-174.

62. Ryan WD, Trivedi N, Benirschke K, Lacoursiere DY, Parast MM. Placental histologic criteria for diagnosis of cord accident: sensitivity and specificity. *Pediatr Dev Pathol.* 2012;15:275-280.

63. Lewi L, Jani J, Blickstein I, et al. The outcome of monochorionic diamniotic twin gestations in the era of invasive fetal therapy: a prospective cohort study. *Am J Obstet Gynecol.* 2008;199:514.e1-514.e8.

64. Moldenhauer JS, Johnson MP. Diagnosis and management of complicated monochorionic twins. *Clin Obstet Gynecol.* 2015;58:632-642.

65. Dias T, Mahsud-Dornan S, Bhide A, Papageorghiou AT, Thilaganathan B. Cord entanglement and perinatal outcome in monoamniotic pregnancies. *Ultrasound Obstet Gynecol.* 2010;35:201-204.

66. Forsberg K, Christiansen-Lindquist L, Silver RM. Factors associated with stillbirth autopsy in Georgia and Utah, 2010-2014: the importance of delivery location. *Am J Perinatol.* 2018;35:1271-1280.

67. Horey D, Flenady V, Heazell AEP, et al. Interventions for supporting parent's decisions about autopsy after stillbirth. *Cochrane Database Syst Rev.* 2013;(2):CD009932.

68. Samuelsson M, Radestad I, Segesten RN. A waste of life: fathers' experience of losing a child before birth. *Birth.* 2001;28:124-130.

69. Reddy UR. Prediction and prevention of recurrent stillbirth. *Obstet Gynecol.* 2007;110:1151-1164.

70. Sheffield JS, Sanchez PJ, Wendel GD, et al. Placental histopathology of congenital syphilis. *Obstet Gynecol.* 2002;100:126-133.

71. Parast MM, Crum CP, Boyd TK. Placental histologic criteria for umbilical blood flow restriction in unexplained stillbirth. *Hum Pathol.* 2008;39:948-953.

72. Bove KE. Practice guidelines for autopsy pathology: the perinatal and pediatric autopsy. Autopsy committee of the College of American Pathologists. *Arch Pathol Lab Med.* 1997;121:368-376.

73. Faye-Petersen OM, Guinn DA, Wenstrom KD. Value of perinatal autopsy. *Obstet Gynecol.* 1999;94:915-920.

74. Thayyil S, Cleary JO, Sebire NJ, et al. Post-mortem examination of human fetuses: a comparison of whole-body high-field MRI at 9.4 T with conventional MRI and invasive autopsy. *Lancet.* 2009;374:467-475.

75. Crotti L, Tester DJ, White WM, et al. Long QT syndrome-associated mutations in intrauterine fetal death. *J Am Med Assoc.* 2013;309:1473-1482.

76. Korteweg FJ, Bouman K, Erwich JJ, et al. Cytogenetic analysis after evaluation of 750 fetal deaths: proposal for diagnostic workup. *Obstet Gynecol.* 2008;111:865-874.

77. American College of Obstetricians and Gynecologists Committee on Practice Bulletins-Obstetrics. ACOG Practice Bulletin No. 118: antiphospholipid syndrome. *Obstet Gynecol.* 2011;117:192-199.

78. American College of Obstetricians and Gynecologists. ACOG practice bulletin No. 102: management of stillbirth. *Obstet Gynecol.* 2009;113:748-761.

79. Page JM, Christiansen-Lindquist L, Thorsten V, et al. Diagnostic tests for evaluation of stillbirth: results from the Stillbirth Collaborative Research Network. *Obstet Gynecol.* 2017;129:699-706.

80. Goldstein DP, Reid DE. Circulating fibrinolytic activity- a precursor of hypofibrinogenemia following fetal death in utero. *Obstet Gynecol.* 1963;22:174-180.

81. Maslow AD, Breen TW, Sarna MC, Soni AK, Watkins J, Oriol NE. Prevalence of coagulation abnormalities associated with intrauterine fetal death. *Can J Anaesth.* 1996;43:1237-1243.

82. Autry AM, Hayes EC, Jacobson GF, Kirby RS. A comparison of medical induction and dilation and evacuation for second-trimester abortion. *Am J Obstet Gynecol.* 2002;187:393-397.

83. Burgoine GA, Van Kirk SD, Romm J, Edelman AB, Jacobson SL, Jensen JT. Comparison of perinatal grief after dilation and evacuation or labor induction in second trimester terminations for fetal anomalies. *Am J Obstet Gynecol.* 2005;192:1928-1932.

84. Wildschut H, Both MI, Medema S, Thomee E, Wildhagen MF, Kapp N. Medical methods for mid-trimester termination of pregnancy. *Cochrane Database Syst Rev.* 2011;(1):CD005216.

85. Boyle A, Preslar JP, Hogue CJ, et al. Route of delivery in women with stillbirth: results from the Stillbirth Collaborative Research Network. *Obstet Gynecol.* 2017;129:693-698.

86. Gold KJ, Dalton VK, Schwenk TL. Hospital care for patents after perinatal death. *Obstet Gynecol* 2007;109:1156-1166.

87. Lamont K, Scott NW, Jones GT, et al. Risk of recurrent stillbirth: systematic review and metaanalysis. *Br Med J.* 2015;350:h3080.

88. Varner MW, Silver RM, Rowland Hogue CJ, et al. Association between stillbirth and illicit drug use and smoking during pregnancy. *Obstet Gynecol.* 2014;123:113-125.

89. Wojcieszek AM, Shepherd E, Middleton P, et al. Care prior to and during subsequent pregnancies following stillbirth for improving outcomes. *Cochrane Database Syst Rev.* 2018;(12):CD012203.

90. American College of Obstetricians and Gynecologists. Practice Bulletin No. 145: antepartum fetal surveillance. *Obstet Gynecol.* 2014;124:182-192.

91. Chaturvedi S, McCrae KR. Diagnosis and management of antiphospholipid syndrome. *Blood Rev.* 2017;31:406-417.

92. Duley L, Henderson-Smart DJ, Meher S, King JF. Antiplatelet agents for preventing pre-eclampsia and its complications. *Cochrane Database Syst Rev.* 2007;(18):CD004659.

93. Fox NS, Rebarber A, Silerstein M, Roman AS, Klauser CK, Saltzman DH. The effectiveness of antepartum surveillance in reducing the risk of stillbirth in patients with advanced maternal age. *Eur J Obstet Gynecol Reprod Biol.* 2013;170:387-390.

94. Walker KF, Bugg GJ, Macpherson M, et al. Randomized trial of labor induction in women 35 Years of age or older. *N Engl J Med.* 2016;374:813-822.

95. Grobman WA, Rice MM, Reddy UM, et al. Labor induction versus expectant management in low-risk nulliparous women. *N Engl J Med.* 2018;379:513-523.

CHAPTER 5

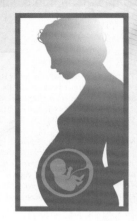

Multifetal Pregnancies: Epidemiology, Clinical Characteristics, and Management

Lucas Otaño, César Meller, and Horacio Aiello

Epidemiology

The twin birth rate has significantly increased in most regions of the world during the last decades. In the United States, it rose around 75% in 35 years, from 19/1000 births in 1980 to 334/1000 births in 2016.[3] The main reasons for this are delayed childbirth, advanced maternal age at conception, and the widespread use of assisted reproduction techniques (ART).

Classification

Multifetal pregnancies can be classified according to the number of fetuses, zygosity, or chorionicity. According to the *number of fetuses*, multiple pregnancies can be twins, triplets, quadruplets, etc. In clinical practice, most are twins. According to *zygosity*, multiple pregnancies can be classified as dizygotic or monozygotic. Dizygotic twins result from the fertilization of two oocytes by two sperms that produce two genetically different embryos. Monozygotic twins result from the fertilization of one oocyte and one sperm and the early splitting of the resulting embryo in two genetically identical twins.[6]

According to *chorionicity* and *amnionicity*, twin pregnancies can be dichorionic (DC) or monochorionic (MC). In DC twins, each fetus has its own placenta and its own amniotic sac (diamniotic [DA]), whereas in MC both fetuses shared the same placenta and can be DA (~99%) or monoamniotic (MA; ~1%) (**Algorithm 5.1**).[7]

See the eBook for expanded content, a complete reference list, and additional figures and tables.

Ultrasound Diagnosis and Surveillance

The ultrasound assessment of multiple pregnancies includes

- Determining gestational age (dating of the pregnancy)
- Determining chorionicity and amnionicity
- Twin labeling
- Ultrasound surveillance
- Detection and management of complications

Determining Gestational Age

As in singletons, gestational age of multifetal pregnancies conceived spontaneously should be dated ideally during the first trimester, based on the fetus with the larger crown-rump length (CRL) at the 11 to 14-week scan. In cases of twins conceived by ART, dating should be based on the embryonic age from fertilization.[8] For spontaneous twin pregnancies with first consultation after 14 weeks, gestational age is estimated based on the fetus with the larger head circumference.[8]

Determining Chorionicity and Amnionicity

Algorithm 5.2A and **B** and **Figure 5.1** summarize the most important features for chorionicity and amnionicity assessment.

Twin Labeling

Labeling the fetuses is a major process in the prenatal care of multifetal pregnancies. Labeling includes a description of each twin's location (left-right, superior-inferior, anterior-posterior) and any other information that could help discriminate both

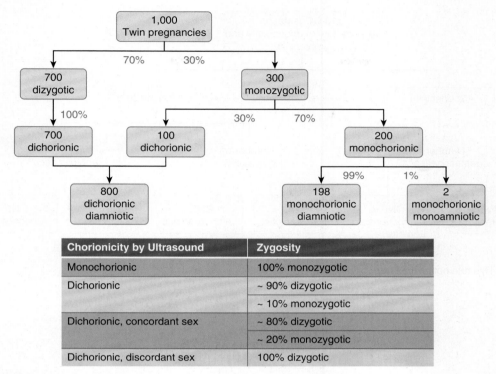

Chorionicity by Ultrasound	Zygosity
Monochorionic	100% monozygotic
Dichorionic	~ 90% dizygotic
	~ 10% monozygotic
Dichorionic, concordant sex	~ 80% dizygotic
	~ 20% monozygotic
Dichorionic, discordant sex	100% dizygotic

Algorithm 5.1 Relationship between zygosity, chorionicity, and amnionicity.

twins: discordant sex, cord insertion sites, any discordant ultrasound marker, or anomaly. Usually, the lower twin is labeled as "A" or "1," and the other as "B" or "2."

However, if during the pregnancy one twin changes position, it is useful to keep the original nomenclature.[8]

Ultrasound Surveillance of Twin Pregnancies

Ideally, every pregnant woman should undergo an ultrasound examination between 11 and 13 6/7 weeks. This is the optimal time for dating the pregnancy, establishing chorionicity and amnionicity, estimating aneuploidy risk, and screening for major structural anomalies (**Figure 5.1A** and **B**).

Current recommendations for first-trimester combined screening are as follows: in DC twins, an individual risk for each fetus is estimated according to nuchal translucency (NT) measurement and eventually according to other secondary markers such as nasal bone, ductus venosus, or mitral valve regurgitation. In MC twins (always monozygotic),

a unique risk is estimated for both fetuses based on the average NT of each fetus.[8]

The ultrasound surveillance in second and third trimesters will depend on chorionicity.

The minimal contents in the ultrasound surveillance in MC twins vary among the different guidelines, but there is consensus that (**Figure 5.1**)

- Every MC has to be assessed every 2 weeks, beginning at 16 weeks until delivery.
- Every scan must include the maximum vertical pocket (MVP) of amniotic fluid of each sac for early diagnosis of twin-to-twin transfusion syndrome (TTTS), and the estimated fetal weight (EFW) of each fetus for detection of selective intrauterine growth restriction (sIUGR) or discordant growth.
- Every MC twin pregnancy should have a detailed scan at 20 to 22 weeks, including a cardiac screening assessment.
- Women with uncomplicated MC twins should be delivered around 36 to 37 weeks—34-376/7 weeks—according to the 2014 American College of Obstetricians and Gynecologists (**ACOG**) Practice Bulletin.

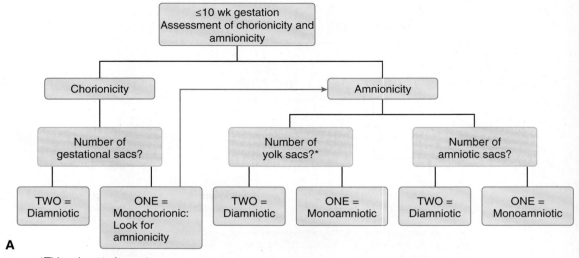

*This rule not always true

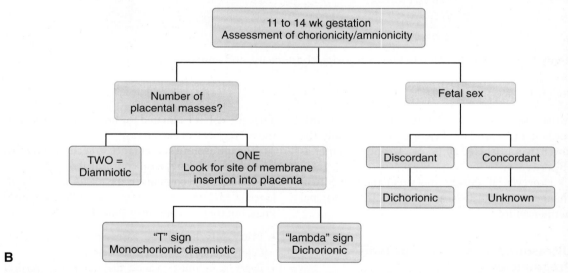

Algorithm 5.2 **A,** Assessment of chorionicity and amnionicity before 11 weeks of gestation. **B,** Assessment of chorionicity and amnionicity between 11 and 14 weeks of gestation.

There are some other aspects that differ among guidelines, like the use of Doppler and CL measurement. Regarding the use of Doppler in uncomplicated twins, there is no consensus on when, how often and which vessels should be assessed. The measurement of CL is also suggested in the second trimester in the International Society of Ultrasound in Obstetrics and Gynecology (ISUOG) guidelines,[8] but it is not recommended in the ACOG Practice Bulletin[1] or in the Royal College of Obstetricians and Gynaecologists (RCOG) guidelines.[16]

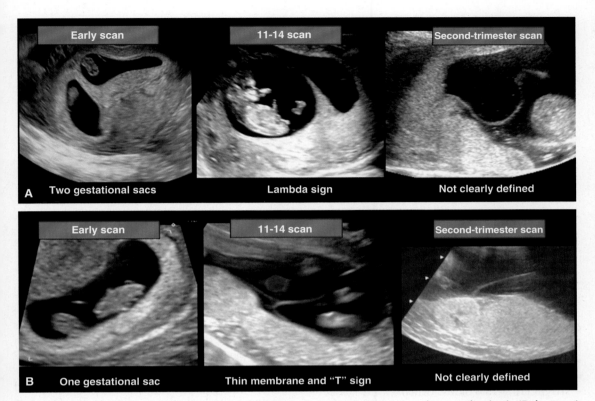

Figure 5.1 Ultrasound assessment of chorionicity in dichorionic (**A**, top) and monochorionic (**B**, bottom) pregnancies.

Complications in Multifetal Pregnancies

Complications in multiple pregnancies, either maternal or fetal, are more frequent than in singletons. In addition, the higher the number of fetuses, the higher the complication rate.

Maternal Complications

Maternal complications are more common in patients with twins than in singletons[1] and include a higher incidence of gestational hypertension and preeclampsia, gestational diabetes mellitus, acute fatty liver of pregnancy, intrahepatic cholestasis of pregnancy, hyperemesis, anemia, urinary tract infections, postpartum hemorrhage, cesarean delivery, and postpartum depression.[1,18]

Fetal Complications

There is increased incidence of

- Vanishing twin
- Prematurity
- Intrauterine growth restriction (IUGR)
- Fetal malformations
- Fetal death
- Placental anomalies

MC Twin Pregnancy

Around 30% of MC twin pregnancies will have major complications with high risk of perinatal mortality and short- and long-term morbidity.[23,45]

Complications Present From the Beginning of the Gestation

- Gene disorders and chromosome aberrations occur in 1% to 2% of MC twins and, when present, usually affect both fetuses.[39]
- MC twins have higher risks of major congenital malformations (1%-3%) such as neural tube defects and congenital heart diseases. When present, these multifactorial anomalies usually affect only one fetus.[23]

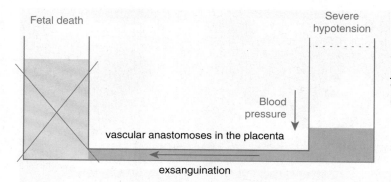

Figure 5.11 Intrauterine death of one twin in monochorionic pregnancies: exsanguination of the survivor into the dead fetus just before or at the time of death when its blood pressure drops dramatically.

- Conditions exclusive to MC twin pregnancies include:
  - MA twins (1 in 25,000 pregnancies);
  - Acardiac twin or twin-reversed arterial perfusion (TRAP) (1 in 35,000 pregnancies); and
  - Conjoined twins (1 in 25,000-80,000 pregnancies).

Complications That Occur During Pregnancy

- Death of one twin (see below)
- TTTS (10%-15% of MC twins)
- sIUGR (10%-15% of MC twins)
- Twin anemia-polycythemia sequence (TAPS) (3%-5% of MC twins)

Single Fetal Demise in MC Twins

The risk of intrauterine fetal death in MC twin pregnancies is around 12%.[27] This event is usually associated to a complication of the MC placentation, like TTTS or sIUGR, but it may occur in an otherwise uncomplicated pregnancy. In the case of one twin's death, the co-twin is at an increased risk of fetal demise or severe morbidity owing to acute fetal exsanguination into the low-pressure circulation of the demised fetus through the placental vascular anastomoses[7,10,46,47] (**Figure 5.11**).

Twin-to-Twin Transfusion Syndrome

TTTS is a severe complication of MC twin pregnancies and occurs in 10% to 15% of MC twin pregnancies.[10,16,51-54] It is diagnosed by ultrasound, and requires the presence of polyhydramnios, MVP ≥8 cm, in the recipient twin's sac and oligohydramnios, MVP of ≤2 cm, in the donor's sac.

Management of TTTS is based on staging, and staging is performed according to the Quintero classification[1,10,16,27,50,51,59]:

- **Stage I**: The optimal management of stage-I TTTS is not clear; however, these patients are often managed expectantly, as around 75% of cases remain stable or regress spontaneously.[10,51,60]
- **Stages II, III, and IV**: The natural history of severe TTTS results in a perinatal mortality of 80% to 100%, and neurological morbidity in 15% to 50% of survivors.[53] The management strategies for stages II, III, and IV include

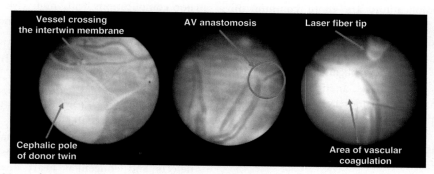

Figure 5.16 Monochorionic twin pregnancy complicated with twin-to-twin transfusion syndrome stage III. Note the cephalic pole of the donor twin and one vessel crossing the dividing membrane (left), and the laser coagulation of an arteriovenous (AV) anastomosis (center and right).

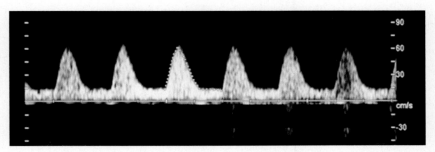

Figure 5.18 Type-I selective intrauterine growth restriction: positive end-diastolic flow in the umbilical artery of the smaller twin.

amnioreduction of the excess fluid in the recipient's sac, intentional septostomy of the intervening membrane to equalize the fluid in both sacs, FLC of placental anastomoses (**Figure 5.16**), selective reduction of one twin by cord coagulation (in countries where it is legal), and elective premature delivery.[53]

- **Stage V:** Stage-V TTTS occurs when there is a single fetal death. Patients should be counseled regarding co-twin's risk of death (10%-12% of cases) and risk of neurological complications (around 25%).

Selective Intrauterine Growth Restriction

Currently the most accepted definition of sIUGR is *EFW of one twin <10th percentile and EFW discordance of 25% or more in the absence of TTTS.*[8,27] EFW discordance is calculated as[66]:

$$\left(\left[\frac{\text{EFW of the larger twin} -}{\text{EFW of the smaller twin}}\right] \Big/ \frac{\text{EFW of the}}{\text{larger twin}}\right) \times 100$$

The classification of sIUGR is based on the pattern of end-diastolic velocity in the umbilical artery in the smallest fetus[70] (**Table 5.1**).

In **type I**, the umbilical artery Doppler waveform has positive end-diastolic flow. In **type II**, there is absent or reversed end-diastolic flow (AREDF). In **type III**, there is a cyclical/intermittent pattern of AREDF[8,70] (**Figures 5.18-5.20**).

There is consensus that optimum treatment of type-I sIUGR is expectant management. However, in contrast to TTTS where fetal therapy is standardized, the better strategy to treat from randomized controlled trials, prenatal management of sIUGR should be individualized.[65]

Twin Anemia-Polycythemia Sequence

First described by Lopriore et al,[74] TAPS is a rare form of fetofetal transfusion[75] that can occur spontaneously or after fetoscopic laser coagulation for TTTS cases. TAPS occurs in MC twins and is characterized by the presence of large intertwin hemoglobin difference between donor and recipient (**Figure 5.21**),

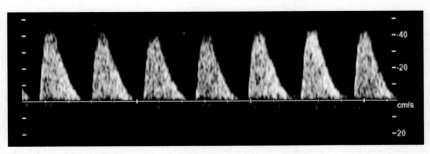

Figure 5.19 Type-II selective intrauterine growth restriction. Pulsed Doppler showing persistently absent end-diastolic flow in the umbilical artery of the smaller fetus. The sign is more prominent near the placental cord insertion. If required, maternal breathing must be held during Doppler recording, to rule out any influence of maternal movements.

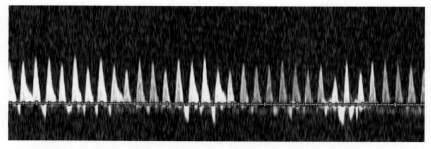

Figure 5.20 Type-III selective intrauterine growth restriction. Pulsed Doppler showing intermittent absent or reversed end-diastolic flow in the umbilical artery of the smaller twin. A low sweep speed of the spectral Doppler is recommended to identify the diastolic changes and the characteristic oscillation of the systolic peak velocities, reflecting the collision of the opposite systolic waveforms of either fetus.

without the degree of amniotic fluid discordance that is required for the diagnosis of TTTS.[10,75-77]

Prenatal diagnosis of TAPS is based on Doppler measurement of fetal middle cerebral artery peak systolic velocity (MCA-PSV), a noninvasive prenatal test described by Mari et al[78] that can identify anemic fetuses.

Postnatal diagnosis is based on hemoglobin differences between twins.

Other Complications

Infrequent complications of MC multifetal pregnancies include twin-reversed arterial TRAP sequence, MA twins, and conjoined twins.

TRAP is a condition in which one twin (pump twin) is usually morphologically normal and the other is a true parasite that receives blood from the pump twin and has an absent, rudimentary, or nonfunctioning heart (acardiac twin) (**Figure 5.22**).

TRAP includes four types: acardius *anceps* (poorly developed head), acardius *acephalus* (absent head, upper extremities usually absent, but the trunk and lower extremities are present), acardius *acormus* (head only), and acardius *amorphous* (no recognizable anatomy)[85] (**Figure 5.23**).

Conjoined twins has an incidence rate between 1 in 25,000 and 1 in 500,000 births[84,92] (**Figure 5.24**).

- *Thoracopagus twins* are connected in or near the sternal region. Twins lie face-to-face. Around 70% may have conjoined hearts.
- *Omphalopagus or xiphopagus twins* are connected in the umbilical region. They also lie face-to-face

Table 5.1 Main Characteristics of the Different Types of sIUGR According to the Classification Described by Gratacos et al

	Noncomplicated MC Twins	Type I	Type II	Type III
End-diastolic velocity in the umbilical artery	Present	Present	AREDF	Intermittent
Mean GA at delivery (weeks)	35,5	~34	~30	~32
Mean birth weight discordance	10%	29%	38%	36%
Mean Placental sharing, larger/smaller	1,3	1,8	2,6	4,4
Risk of deterioration of the IUGR twin	—	Low	High (90%)	Low
Risk of IUD of the IUGR twin	—	Low	Low	~15%
Risk of brain injury in the larger twin	—	Low	Low	~20%
AA anastomoses >2 mm	55%	70%	18%	98%
Perinatal outcomes	—	Better	Worst	±

AA, arterioarterial; AREDF, absent or reversed end-diastolic flow; GA, gestational age; IUD, intrauterine death; IUGR, intrauterine growth restriction; MC, monochorionic; sIUGR, selective intrauterine growth restriction.
Adapted from Gratacós E, Lewi L, Muñoz B, et al. A classification system for selective intrauterine growth restriction in monochorionic pregnancies according to umbilical artery Doppler flow in the smaller twin. *Ultrasound Obstet Gynecol.* 2007;30(1):28-34.

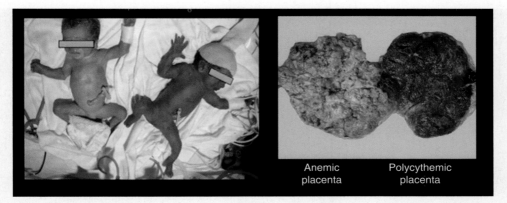

Figure 5.21 Monochorionic twin pregnancy complicated with twin anemia-polycythemia sequence (TAPS) with large intertwin hemoglobin differences (>11 g/dL) at birth (left). Maternal side of the placenta showing the difference in color between the white pale part for the anemic twin and a plethoric part for the polycythemic twin (right).

and usually have the least complicated union of all conjoined twins.

- *Pygopagus twins* represent about 20% of cases, are joined at the buttocks and perineum, and face away from each other.
- *Ischiopagus twins* account for 5% of cases. They are united at a single bony pelvis.
- *Craniopagus twins* account for 2% of cases and there is fusion of the skull.

Triplets and Higher Order Multiple Pregnancy

Triplets and higher order multiple pregnancies have higher risks of complications, as fetal morbidity and mortality increase with the number of fetuses.

A higher incidence of sIUGR, fetal anomalies, and above all, prematurity and its consequences represent the main causes of adverse outcomes in multifetal pregnancies and cause the greatest

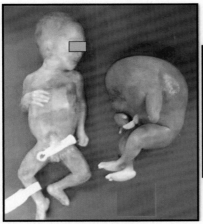
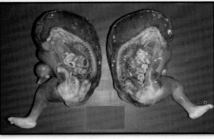

Figure 5.22 Twin reversal arterial perfusion (TRAP) sequence: The pump twin is usually morphologically normal (left). The acardiac twin (right) presents recognizable torso and lower extremities, but no identifiable cranial structures, and the presence and structure of upper extremities are extremely variable. Internal malformation includes absent lungs and heart, gastrointestinal atresia, omphalocele, gastroschisis, and absent liver, pancreas, spleen, and kidneys.

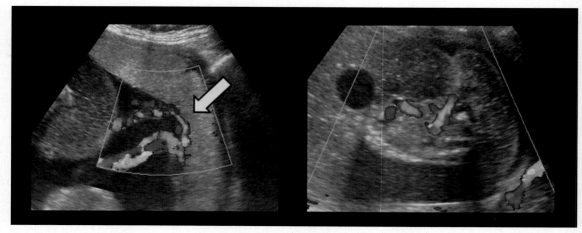

Figure 5.23 Twin reversed arterial perfusion (TRAP) sequence. Note the superficial artery-to-artery placental anastomosis (arrow) connecting the three-vessel cord of the pump twin with the two-vessel cord of the acardiac twin (left). Color Doppler detects the umbilical cord entering the second twin with intact blood flow, and pulsed Doppler study reveals reversal of the flow on the spectral pattern (right).

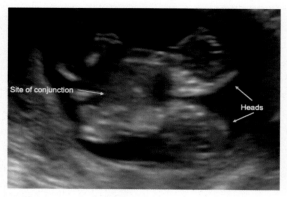

Figure 5.24 Conjoined twins.

impact on healthcare costs.[101] Moreover, similar to twins, fetal morbidity and mortality vary with chorionicity.

Timing and Mode of Delivery in Twins

The optimal mode of delivery for twin pregnancies depends on the type of twins, fetal presentations, gestational age, and experience of the clinician performing the delivery.[1] Uncomplicated DC twins can be delivered at 38 weeks' gestation,[4] and uncomplicated MC twins from 34 to 36 6/7 weeks.[1,16,52] In both cases, if the first twin is in cephalic presentation, it is appropriate to aim for a vaginal birth unless there is an indication for cesarean delivery.[16,110]

KEY POINTS

- A multifetal gestation is a high-risk pregnancy because it is associated with an increased rate of maternal, perinatal, and infant morbidity and mortality. One of the main problems is preterm birth and its short- and long-term consequences.
- Multifetal pregnancies can be classified according to the number of fetuses (twins, triplets, quadruplets, etc), zygosity (dizygotic or monozygotic), or chorionicity (DC or MC).
- DC twins have their own placentas and amniotic sacs (DA); MC twins share the same placenta but can be MA or DA.

- The ultrasound assessment of multiple pregnancies includes determining gestational age (dating of the pregnancy), determining chorionicity and amnionicity, twin labeling, ultrasound surveillance, and detection and management of complications.
- Complications in multiple pregnancies, either maternal or fetal, are more frequent than in singletons. In addition, the higher the number of fetuses, the higher the complication rate.

- Maternal complications include a higher incidence of gestational hypertension and preeclampsia, gestational diabetes mellitus, acute fatty liver of pregnancy, intrahepatic cholestasis of pregnancy, hyperemesis, anemia, urinary tract infections, postpartum hemorrhage, cesarean delivery, and postpartum depression.
- Fetal complications include vanishing twin, prematurity, IUGR, fetal malformations, fetal death, and placental anomalies.
- Fetal complications are more frequent in MC twins than in DC twins (ie, mortality, neurologic morbidity), and there are complications that are exclusive to MC twins (ie, TTTS, TAPS, TRAP sequence, MA twins, conjoined twins).

- Triplets and higher order multiple pregnancies have higher risks of complications. Prematurity and its consequences represent the main causes of adverse outcomes in higher order multifetal pregnancies.
- Fetal reduction in the first trimester can reduce risks of maternal and perinatal complications; selective fetal termination in the second and third trimesters is usually performed in cases of an abnormal co-twin.
- The optimal mode of delivery for twin pregnancies depends on the type of twins, fetal presentations, gestational age, and experience of the clinician performing the delivery.

REFERENCES

(only references cited in synoptic print chapter; for a complete reference list, see ebook)

1. Committee on Practice Bulletins—Obstetrics; Society for Maternal–Fetal Medicine. Practice bulletin No. 169: multifetal gestations. Twin, triplet, and higher-order multifetal pregnancies. *Obstet Gynecol.* 2016;128(4):e131-46.
3. Martin JA, Osterman MJK. Describing the increase in preterm births in the United States, 2014-2016. *NCHS Data Brief.* 2018;312:1-8.
4. American College of Obstetricians and Gynecologists. ACOG practice bulletin no.144: multifetal gestations. Twin, triplet, and higher-order multifetal pregnancies. *Obstet Gynecol.* 2014;123(5):1118-1132.
6. Bender W, Dugoff L. Screening for aneuploidy in multiple gestations: the challenges and options. *Obstet Gynecol Clin North Am.* 2018;45(1):41-53.
7. Bajoria R, Kingdom J. The case for routine determination of chorionicity and zygosity in multiple pregnancy. *Prenat Diagn.* 1997;17(13):1207-1225.
8. Khalil A, Rodgers M, Baschat A, et al. ISUOG Practice Guidelines: role of ultrasound in twin pregnancy. *Ultrasound Obstet Gynecol.* 2016;47:247-263.
10. Emery SP, Bahtiyar MO, Moise KJ; North American Fetal Therapy Network. The North American fetal therapy network consensus statement: management of complicated monochorionic gestations. *Obstet Gynecol.* 2015;126(3):575-584.
16. Kilby MD, Bricker L; on behalf of the Royal College of Obstetricians and Gynaecologists. Management of monochorionic twin pregnancy. *BJOG.* 2016;124(1):e1-e45. doi:10.1111/1471-0528.14188
18. Chasen S, Chervenak FA. *Twin Pregnancy: Prenatal Issues.* UpToDate. Accessed July 20, 2019. https://www.uptodate.com/contents/twin-pregnancy-prenatal-issues.
23. Gratacós E, Ortiz JU, Martinez JM. A systematic approach to the differential diagnosis and management of the complications of monochorionic twin pregnancies. *Fetal Diagn Ther.* 2012;32:145-155.
27. Townsend R, Khalil A. Ultrasound screening for complications in twin pregnancy. *Semin Fetal Neonatal Med.* 2018;23(2):133-141.
39. Weber MA, Sebire NJ. Genetics and developmental pathology of twinning. *Semen Fetal Neonatal Med.* 2010;15(6):313-318.
45. Lewi L, Gucciardo L, van Mieghem T, et al. Monochorionic diamniotic twin pregnancies: natural history and risk stratification. *Fetal Diagn Ther.* 2010;27(3):121-133.
46. van Klink JM, van Steenis A, Steggerda SJ, et al. Single fetal demise in monochorionic pregnancies: incidence and patterns of cerebral injury. *Ultrasound Obstet Gynecol.* 2015;45(3):294-300.

47. Lewi L, Deprest J, Hecher K. The vascular anastomoses in monochorionic twin pregnancies and their clinical consequences. *Am J Obstet Gynecol.* 2013;208(1):19-30.
50. Morin L, Lim K. No. 260-Ultrasound in twin pregnancies. *J Obstet Gynaecol Can.* 2017;39(10):e398-e411.
51. Simpson LL; Society for Maternal-Fetal Medicine. Twin-twin transfusion syndrome. *Am J Obstet Gynecol.* 2013;208(1):3-18.
52. Bahtiyar MO, Emery SP, Dashe JS, et al; North American Fetal Therapy Network. The North American Fetal Therapy Network consensus statement: prenatal surveillance of uncomplicated monochorionic gestations. *Obstet Gynecol.* 2015;125(1):118-123.
53. Djaafri F, Stirnemann J, Mediouni I, et al. Twin-twin transfusión syndrome - what we have learned from clinical trials. *Semin Fetal Neonatal Med.* 2017;22(6):367-375.
54. Hecher K, Gardiner HM, Diemert A, et al. Long-term outcomes for monochorionic twins after laser therapy in twin-to-twin transfusion syndrome. *Lancet Child Adolesc Health.* 2018;2(7):525-535.
59. Quintero RA, Morales WJ, Allen MH, et al. Staging of twin-twin transfusion syndrome. *J Perinatol.* 1999;19:550-555.
60. Washburn EE, Sparks TN, Gosnell KA, et al. Stage I twin-twin transfusion syndrome: outcomes of expectant management and prognostic features. *Am J Perinatol.* 2018;35(14):1352-1357.
65. Townsend R, D'Antonio F, Sileo FG, et al. Perinatal outcome of monochorionic twin pregnancy complicated by selective fetal growth restriction according to management: systematic review and meta-analysis. *Ultrasound Obstet Gynecol.* 2019;53(1):36-46.
66. Valsky DV, Eixarch E, Martinez JM, et al. Selective intrauterine growth restriction in monochorionic diamniotic twin pregnancies. *Prenat Diagn.* 2010;30(8):719-726.
70. Gratacós E, Lewi L, Muñoz B, et al. A classification system for selective intrauterine growth restriction in monochorionic pregnancies according to umbilical artery Doppler in the smaller twin. *Ultrasound Obstet Gynecol.* 2007;30:28-34.
74. Lopriore E, Middeldorp J, Oepkes D, et al. Twin anemia-polycythemia sequence in two monochorionic twin pairs without oligo-polyhydramnios sequence. *Placenta.* 2007;28:47-51.
75. Bahtiyar MO, Ekmekci E, Demirel E, et al. In utero partial exchange transfusion combined with in utero blood transfusion for prenatal management of twin anemia-polycythemia sequence. *Fetal Diagn Ther.* 2019;45(1):28-35.
76. Lopriore E, Slaghekke F, Oepkes D, et al. Hematological characteristics in neonates with twin anemia-polycythemia sequence (TAPS). *Prenat Diagn.* 2010;30(3):251-255.

77. Tollenaar LSA, Lopriore E, Middeldorp JM, et al. Improved antenatal prediction of twin anemia-polycythemia sequence by delta middle cerebral artery peak systolic velocity: a new antenatal classification system. *Ultrasound Obstet Gynecol.* 2019;53(6):788-793.

78. Mari G, Adrignolo A, Abuhamad AZ, et al. Diagnosis of fetal anemia with Doppler ultrasound in the pregnancy complicated by maternal blood group immunization. *Ultrasound Obstet Gynecol.* 1995;5:400-405.

84. Bianchi DW, Crombleholme TM, D'Alton ME, Malone FD. *Fetology: Diagnosis & Management of the Fetal Patient.* McGraw-Hill, Medical Pub. Division; 2010.

85. Steffensen TS, Gilbert-Barness E, Spellacy W, et al. Placental pathology in trap sequence: clinical and pathogenetic implications. *Fetal Pediatr Pathol.* 2008;27(1):13-29.

92. Arnold J, Luton A, Davies J. Introduction: unique challenges in the care of conjoined twins. *Semin Perinatol.* 2018;42(6):319-320.

101. Stone J, Kohari K. Higher-order multiples. *Clin Obstet Gynecol.* 2015;58:668-675.

110. Sentilhes L, Lorthe E, Marchand-Martin L, et al. Planned mode of delivery of preterm twins and neonatal and 2-year outcomes. *Obstet Gynecol.* 2019;133(1):71-80.

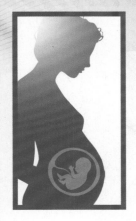

CHAPTER 6

The Normal and Abnormal Placenta

Yoel Sadovsky and W. Tony Parks

Introduction and a Historical Perspective

In eutherian mammals, the placenta forms the interface between the fetus and the mother, providing essential functions for fetal survival, development, and growth. These functions include regulation of gas exchange, supply of nutrients, removal of waste products, production of essential hormones, and establishment of immunological and mechanical defense.

The term placenta means "cake" in Latin and is derived from *plakous*, which means "flat cake" in Greek. Although the role of the placenta in supporting the developing fetus was probably recognized as early as the fifth century BCE, the term placenta was coined in the 16th century by Realdo Columbo at the University of Padua in Italy.[1]

A more detailed account of key milestones in the history of placental research was provided by Boyd and Hamilton.[1] Please refer to the e-book.

Anatomy and Morphology

The placenta comprises cells that originated from the conceptus; hence, it shares its genetic origin with the fetus. Maternal cells within the placenta are circulating red and white blood cells and their derivatives, which may become more abundant during a maternal inflammatory response. The placenta is usually round or slightly elliptical, and until 17 weeks, it is larger than the fetus. At term, the placenta weighs approximately 500 g, its mean diameter is 18 to 22 cm, and its thickness is 2.4 cm. These dimensions are fairly variable, and small deviations usually lack clinical significance. The mother-facing

See the eBook for expanded content, a complete reference list, and additional figures.

plate is called the *basal plate*, which directly interfaces with the maternal decidua (**Figure 6.1**).

The basal plate is characterized by grooves that divide the basal plate into 10 to 40 lobes and lobules, called cotyledons. Each groove contains interlobular septa that are directly attached to the decidua basalis. Importantly, each lobe or lobule is not a distinct developmental unit, but each is connected to one or more villous trees. At the center of the fetus-facing *chorionic plate* is the umbilical cord (UC), which delivers oxygen and nutrients from the placenta to the fetus through its vein, and delivers unoxygenated blood and waste products through the two arteries (**Figure 6.1**). The chorionic plate is covered by the amnion.

The human placenta is defined as chorioallantoic, which implies that the placental vessels originate in the allantois, the hindgut diverticulum that develops into the UC, and not in the extraembryonic mesoderm that covers the yolk sac, as is found in the marsupial's choriovitelline placenta. Villous interdigitations also define the human placenta, unlike the labyrinthine interface that defines the placenta of mice and many other rodents. Placental species are also defined by their maternal-fetal barrier interface, which plays a pivotal role in defining the placental transport function. In the noninvasive epitheliochorial interface (**Figure 6.2A**), the trophoblast is attached to the uterine epithelium, but does not invade into it, or the fetal trophoblast may fuse with the maternal epithelium, yet without invasion (endotheliochorial interface, **Figure 6.2B**). In contrast, trophoblast invasion leads to destruction of the uterine epithelium, thus reducing the barrier between the fetal and maternal vessels. The invasive hemochorial interface, characterized by direct contact between trophoblasts and the maternal vessels, is further defined by the number of cell layers separating the maternal and fetal blood: a hemotrichorial interface (**Figure 6.2C**) characterizes the mouse placenta, and a hemodichorial interface

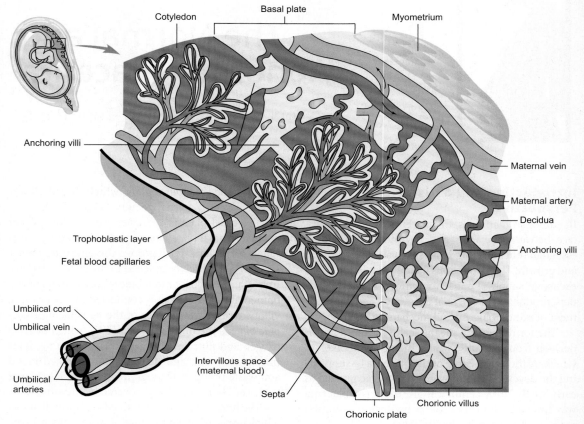

Figure 6.1 A general schematic diagram of the human placental structure and circulation.
(Modified from Pillitteri A. *Maternal and Child Nursing.* 4th ed. Wolters Kluwer; 2003.)

(**Figure 6.2D**) characterizes the human placenta in early pregnancy. In late human pregnancy, however, the cytotrophoblast cell layer is discontinuous, and the placenta is, therefore, considered a hemomonochorial interface[2,3] (**Figure 6.2E**).

The Placental Villus

The main functional unit within the placenta is the villus, with maternal blood cells perfusing the area around the villi, termed the intervillous space. The number of villi in the placenta is highly variable, ranging from several hundreds to the low thousands. They are organized as bifurcating branches that emanate from a stem villus to the terminal villi (**Figure 6.1**). The outermost layer of each villus, which is directly bathed in maternal blood, comprises the multinucleated syncytiotrophoblast (**Figures 6.1 and 6.3**). Like most epithelial cells, they exhibit polarity, with a microvillous ("brush border") membrane facing the maternal blood on the apical side

and a basal membrane on the opposite side. Thus, the maternal blood–facing microvillous membrane harbors receptors, channels, and proteins that transmit maternal molecules and signals to the placental villus. Immediately subjacent to this layer are mononucleated cytotrophoblasts (**Figure 6.3**), constituting 10% to 15% of the total trophoblastic volume.[4] The cytotrophoblasts serve as progenitor cells for the syncytiotrophoblast. Cytotrophoblasts may differentiate to replenish the syncytium, proliferate, or undergo programmed cell death. Each of these processes is highly regulated by intricate signals (eg, hypoxia, epidermal growth factor, cyclic adenosine monophosphate).[5-7] The process of cytotrophoblast fusion into syncytiotrophoblast involves membrane breakdown. Specific proteins, such as the fusogenic protein syncytin, play key roles in syncytiotrophoblast formation.[8] The cytotrophoblasts are separated from the villous core by a basement membrane, which is mainly composed of type IV collagen,

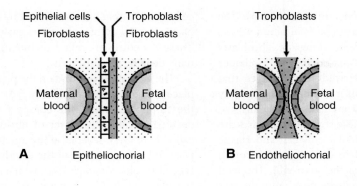

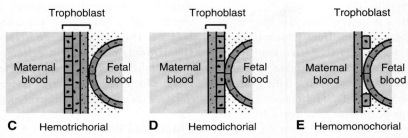

Figure 6.2 Examples of the placental maternal-fetal barrier interface. A, Epitheliochorial placenta, with six layers separating the maternal and fetal blood: (from left) maternal capillary endothelium, maternal endometrial connective tissue, maternal endometrial epithelium, fetal trophoblasts, chorionic connective tissue, and fetal capillary endothelium. **B,** Endotheliochorial placenta, where the trophoblast is in direct contact with maternal capillary endothelium. **C,** Hemotrichorial placenta, where the three-layered trophoblast is bathed in maternal blood. **D,** Hemodichorial placenta, which is the same as **(C)** but with only two layers of trophoblasts (early human pregnancy). **E,** Hemomonochorial placenta, which is the same as **(D)** but with only one layer of syncytiotrophoblast and interspersed cytotrophoblasts (late human pregnancy).

(Reprinted with permission from Sadovsky Y, Jansson T. Placenta and placental transport function. In: Plant TM, Zeleznik AJ, eds. *Knobil and Neill's Physiology of Reproduction*. 4th ed. Academic Press; 2015.)

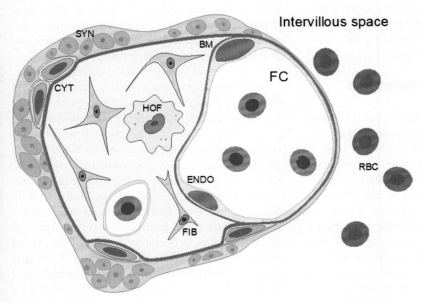

Figure 6.3 The basic structure of a terminal villus. BM, basement membrane; CYT, cytotrophoblast; ENDO, endothelial cell; FC, fetal capillary; FIB, fibroblast; HOF, Hofbauer cell; RBC, red blood cell; SYN, syncytiotrophoblast.

heparin sulfate, and fibronectin (**Figure 6.3**). The villus stroma contains sinusoidal fetal blood vessels lined with endothelial cells, alongside fibroblasts and speciated placental macrophages (Hofbauer cells), which are fetus-derived macrophages that likely originate from villous mesenchymal cells early in gestation and, later, from fetal bone marrow–derived macrophages.[9] These stromal structures are further supported by reticular collagen and elastic fibers that are connected to extravascular smooth muscle cells at the base of the stem villi. The fetal villous blood sinusoids coalesce into larger arteries and veins in stem villi.

Villi formation is defined as branching morphogenesis, where villous trees emanate from chorionic plate trabeculae that give rise to villous trunks.[10] These trunks bifurcate to either free-floating villi or to anchoring villi that are anchored to the basal plate. The majority of the villi gradually grow in size to form a bifurcating "villous tree"[10] (**Figure 6.1**), from the largest *stem villi* that mainly provide tensile support to the villous tree; to *mesenchymal and immature intermediate villi*, characterized by less compact stromal and vascular structures; to *mature intermediate villi*, which are more differentiated and comprise nearly half the villous volume; to the *terminal villi*, where most of the maternal-fetal exchange occurs and which is characterized by areas of very thin membranes as well as areas of cell bodies and stromal tissue[10] (**Figure 6.3**). The thin area, which is devoid of cell nuclei and measures only 0.5 to 2 μm between the intervillous space and fetal capillary, is termed the *vasculo-syncytial membrane*[11] and comprises the main functional maternal-fetal exchange unit.

The Chorionic and Basal Plates and Nonvillous Support

The entire maternal-fetal interface extends from the chorionic plate and the base of villous tree, across the basal plate, and into junctional zone at the decidua and the inner third of the maternal myometrium. The *extravillous trophoblasts* are trophoblasts that do not contribute to placental villi. They include the *interstitial trophoblasts* within the junctional zone and the *endovascular trophoblasts* within the decidual and myometrial vessels. They are also located within the chorion and chorionic plate, the placental septa in the basal plate, and the placental cell islands. The large stem villi are connected to the basal plate through the trophoblastic cell columns that are established by invasion of the basal plate by cytotrophoblasts early in pregnancy. These structures are called anchoring villi and gradually degenerate until term.

The basal plate is found on the placental side after placental separation at delivery.[12] At the junction of the trophoblasts and the compact portion of the decidua basalis is the layer of fibrin-type fibrinoid called *Rohr layer*. Deeper, at the junction of the compact and spongy layers of the decidua is the fibrin-type fibrinoid, *Nitabuch layer*, which normally forms the placenta-decidua separation layer. The deeper part of the junctional zone, closer to the maternal uterine wall, is termed the "placental bed" and harbors a mixture of necrotic decidual cells and extravillous trophoblasts. Lastly, extensions of the basal plate into the intervillous space are termed placental septa, which harbor maternal components, including decidual cells and even small maternal veins.[12]

Placental Blood Flow

At term, the placental bed is perfused by an average of 100 spiral arteries and drained by 50 to 200 veins. Remodeling of the feeding spiral arteries to maintain their full dilation is essential for optimal flow even in the face of vasoconstricting signals. Prior to extravillous trophoblast invasion toward the decidual maternal vessels, there is already marked vascular smooth muscle disorganization, endothelial vacuolization, and lumen dilation. These changes are bolstered by interstitial trophoblast invasion toward spiral vessels in the decidua and the inner third of the myometrium,[13] causing deposition of fibrinoid and further replacement of the vessel endothelial intima and muscularis with endovascular trophoblasts,[14] thus converting the narrow, high-resistance vessels to dilated, low-resistance vessels.

The intervillous space receives arterial blood through openings of the maternal spiral arteries within the basal plate (**Figure 6.1**), with flow initiated at the lobular center and progressing peripherally. When compared to intravascular flow, blood flow in the intervillous space is characteristically very slow, with multiple irregularly shaped lakes, clefts, and fusions among neighboring villi, and influenced by villous fetal capillary flow. Within each lobule, uterine veins drain blood from the intervillous space to the uterine veins. In the intravillous, fetal side, blood perfusion is initiated by differentiation of hemangiogenic cells within mesenchymal villi, which takes place in a hypoxic environment and is regulated by vascular endothelial growth factor (VEGF), placental growth factor (PlGF), and their receptors.[15,16] Villus arterioles and venules transform into coiled capillary loops within mature intermediate villi and terminal villi, and capillary sinusoids form at interspersed regions and reduce blood flow resistance.

Changes in oxygen levels may impact the development and maintenance of the villous tree.[17] Placental hypoxia is normal in early pregnancy (see below) and promotes the invasion and migration of extravillous trophoblasts toward the oxygen-enriched environment near decidual blood vessels.[13,17,18] Hypoxia after weeks 12 to 14 of pregnancy has been implicated in diverse villous injury pathways. Villous cell hypoxia may also stem from hypobaric (eg, high-altitude) hypoxia, maternal heart or lung diseases, maternal vascular disease, hypoxia-reperfusion injury, or reduced exchange surface area stemming from a damaged trophoblastic interface.[19] Although knowledge of the precise mechanisms underlying such injuries is lacking, it is clear that such injuries may result in altered villous architecture and cellular morphology, culminating in cellular dysfunction.[20] For example, first-trimester injury may lead to reduced villous terminal bifurcation, enhanced cytotrophoblast proliferation, and reduced trophoblast fusion, resulting in histological changes consistent with villous ischemia and infarct.[21] Injury later in gestation may lead to localized damage and scarring. Chronic hypoxia throughout gestation elicits an adaptive response that consists of increased vascularization of terminal villi, cytotrophoblast proliferation, villous membrane thinning, and reduced deposition of perivillous fibrin, all contributing to maintenance of maternal-fetal exchange.[22]

Placental Development

Our understanding of the pivotal steps that shape placental development is central to our grasp of placental function and dysfunction in clinically relevant diseases. Whereas descriptive and observational embryology studies have been performed in humans and other primates, mechanistic molecular and metabolic studies commonly depend on rodent and other animal models.

For information about placental development, please refer to the e-book.

Placental Hormones and Other Signals

The placenta is the most active site of steroid and protein hormone synthesis, which are vital for placental development and function.[37-39]

Progesterone

After 8 to 10 weeks' gestation, the placenta takes over the role of the corpus luteum as the main source of progesterone. At term, placenta-derived progesterone reaches a daily production of 250 mg/day. Placental progesterone is synthesized predominantly from maternal cholesterol and pregnenolone, similar to its production in the ovaries. Progesterone is particularly important for the maintenance of pregnancy and the relaxation of the myometrium and other smooth muscles.[37,38,40]

Estrogen

The production of estrogen in pregnancy shifts from the ovary to the placenta early in the first trimester, with placental estrogen production rapidly increasing during pregnancy until term. In the absence of 17α-hydroxylase, the placenta cannot produce estrogen precursors from progesterone and relies on the formation of estrogen from the C19 steroids dehydroepiandrosterone and dehydroepiandrosterone sulfate from the fetal adrenal and, to a lesser degree, the maternal adrenal. This is achieved by the serial action of placental steroid sulfatase, 3β-hydroxysteroid dehydrogenase, aromatase (CYP19) and 17β-hydroxysteroid dehydrogenase type 1.[40-42]

Human Chorionic Gonadotropin

Human chorionic gonadotropin (hCG) is produced nearly exclusively in the trophoblasts. It is composed of two noncovalently linked subunits, alpha and beta, with the alpha subunit shared with other glycoproteins: follicle-stimulating hormone, luteinizing hormone (LH), and adrenocorticotropic hormone, each with a distinct beta subunit. hCG is a highly glycosylated peptide, which serves to enhance its half-life. Intact hCG peaks in the middle of the first trimester, with variation among pregnant women. There is a gradual decline early in the second trimester, and hCG levels remain low until term. The most important function of hCG in the first trimester is the maintenance of the corpus luteum until the placenta starts producing progesterone. hCG acts like fetal LH and stimulates early fetal testosterone production. It also binds to maternal thyroid-stimulating hormone receptors to stimulate the production of T4.[43,44]

Human Placental Lactogen

Human placental lactogen (hPL) is similar to human growth hormone and is composed of one polypeptide chain. Although it is detectable as early as 1 week after implantation, its level gradually rises during pregnancy, with accelerated production and release in the second trimester. The major function of hPL is the promotion of maternal adaptation to gestational fetal needs, primarily maternal lipolysis and the release of free fatty acids, as well as insulin resistance. hPL also promotes fetal angiogenesis.[45]

Other Hormones and Signaling Molecules

The placenta produces other peptide hormones, including hypothalamic releasing hormones such as gonadotropin-releasing hormone, thyrotropin-releasing hormone, growth hormone–releasing hormone, and corticotropin-releasing hormone, growth hormone variant, parathyroid hormone–related protein, leptin, relaxin, serotonin, activin, and inhibin. Oxytocin is also produced by syncytiotrophoblasts, with levels far exceeding those produced by the mother. In addition, trophoblasts produce growth factors: insulin-like growth factor 2, PlGF, and VEGF. The role of many of these signaling molecules is assumed to be related to diverse homeostatic functions during pregnancy, but their precise activity and regulation have not been fully clarified.[37,46-51]

Maternal-Fetal Exchange

General Principles

As with other epithelial surfaces, the transport of ions, molecules, or protein complexes across the placental barriers can take place either between cells, *via* intercellular water-filled channels, or through cells,[52,53] where small or large molecules can traverse the placental surface by the hydrostatic and osmotic pressure gradients. Temporary cellular breaks of the thin vasculosyncytial membranes that result from the action of spiral artery blood jets entering the intervillous space may also add to the transplacental water pathway. Yet, together, these channels and breaks occupy a relatively small part of the placental surface area.

Most transplacental transport is achieved through diffusion, transport mechanisms, and endocytosis/exocytosis. Simple diffusion through the placenta follows Fick law, where diffusion is directly proportional to the exchange surface area, the concentration gradient, and the diffusion capacity of the molecule and inversely proportional to the membrane thickness. The transfer of small,

noncharged lipid-soluble molecules (ie, oxygen) across the placental barrier is commonly characterized by *flow-limited*, receptor-independent pathways, which are also influenced by blood flow, differences in concentrations or electrical gradients, and membrane thickness and composition.[54] Larger, water-soluble molecules (ie, proteins) are commonly transported by *diffusion-limited*, receptor-mediated pathways. When receptor-mediated transport does not require energy expenditure, the transport is termed "facilitated transport" or "facilitated diffusion." The term "active transport" implies that energy is consumed directly or indirectly. Transport proteins are commonly located in the syncytiotrophoblast's maternal blood–facing microvillous membrane, the cytoplasm, and the villous core–facing basal membrane. In general, for most substances, the movement across the microvillous membrane and/or basal membrane is the rate-limiting step in transplacental transfer. During gestation, the thickness of the microvillous membrane gradually declines, principally due to expansion of the fetal capillary bed, a process that is associated with increased diffusing capacity.[55] Large molecules, such as immunoglobulin G or cholesterol, are transported by endocytic pathways.[56] For information about transplacental maternal-fetal exchange, please refer to the e-book, and references therein.

Placental Dysfunction and Obstetrical Diseases—A Pathophysiological Approach

Diverse gestational diseases are associated with placental disorders or affect placental function, with important implications for maternal-fetal health. Even distinctly defined diseases (eg, preeclampsia, fetal growth restriction [FGR])[81,82] share many placental histopathological features, suggesting that these diseases may be a manifestation of an underlying placental maldevelopment or impairment of villous perfusion and trophoblast function.[83,84] It is also possible that shared placental lesions predispose or contribute to a clinical syndrome, yet additional factors, such as disruption of maternal homeostasis, shape the clinical presentation and its severity. Thus, our current grasp of placental pathology might not be sufficient to fully elucidate the pathogenesis of a specific disease phenotype.

A number of pathological processes, including villous maldevelopment, genetic or epigenetic aberrations, hypoperfusion and hypoxia, infections, immune responses, and environmental exposures, have been implicated in placental damage and clinical syndromes. Some of these conditions share common pathogenetic pathways. One example is oxidative stress, which likely plays a role in the pathophysiology of many obstetrical disorders associated with placental dysfunction.[83,85,86] As discussed earlier, the first-trimester placental villi develop in a hypoxic environment, and trophoblasts during that period are, therefore, well adapted to a low-oxygen environment. Premature oxygenation in the first trimester, sustained or intermittent hypoperfusion, and consequent fluctuating oxygen concentrations in the second or third trimesters may cause villous injury.[84,87] These conditions, which have been implicated in common obstetrical diseases such as preeclampsia, FGR and preterm birth,[83] are associated with syncytial injury, with the ultimate consequence of oxidative damage, depending on the balance between syncytial degeneration, cytotrophoblast proliferation, and repair of villus lesions.[87]

FGR is most directly linked to placental dysfunction.[52,88] Abnormal transport of nutrients has been commonly implicated in placental injury–related FGR. For example, the activity of system A amino acid transporters is decreased in microvillous membrane, and the activity of transporters of essential amino acids, including system beta and system L, is reduced in microvillous membrane and/or basal membrane isolated from placentas associated with FGR.[89] The activity of lipoprotein lipase (LPL) at the microvillous membrane, which mediates the first critical step in transplacental transfer of free fatty acids, is also reduced in FGR.[72,74,90] Other studies suggest that placentas from growth-restricted fetuses exhibit retained lipids within trophoblastic lipid droplets.[75] These findings are in line with studies showing lower fetal/maternal plasma ratios for lipids—specifically, long-chain polyunsaturated fatty acids—in FGR.[91] Some growth-restricted fetuses are hypoglycemic *in utero*, attributed to decreased glucose transport capacity.[92] Placental ion transporters are also subjected to regulation in FGR. For example, the activity of Na^+/K^+-ATPase, the Na^+/H^+ exchanger, and lactate transporters is decreased in the microvillous membrane isolated from placentas of growth-restricted fetuses. The reduced Na^+/K^+-ATPase activity may increase intracellular Na^+ concentrations, affecting all Na^+-dependent transport processes.

Although obesity increases the risk of macrosomic fetuses, the effect of maternal overweight and obesity on placental function remains largely unknown. System A amino acid transport activity is increased in microvillous membrane isolated from placentas of obese women giving birth to large babies, and this activity is associated with increased placental insulin/insulin-like growth factor 1 and the mammalian target of rapamycin signaling.[82,88] Placental LPL activity and CD36 expression are increased, while placental expression of fatty acid transport protein 4 (FATP4) and FABP1 and FABP3 are decreased in obese women.[93] The data with regard to the effect of diabetes on nutrient transporters are also unclear, with some amino acid transporters being upregulated in macrosomic newborns born to diabetic mothers and other transporters trending in the opposite direction. Glucose transport (GLUT) activity and GLUT1 expression in the basal membrane, and the expression of GLUT9 in the microvillous membrane and basal membrane, are increased in placentas of women with diabetes, supporting a link to fetal overgrowth. Diabetes is also associated with enhanced activity of placental membrane–bound LPL and endothelial lipase, in association with fetal overgrowth.[94] In addition, the expression of FABP1 and FABP4 is upregulated in the diabetic placenta,[95] supporting the hypothesis of a higher supply of bioenergetic fuels delivered to the fetus in pregnant women with diabetes.

Lastly, placental transport can be viewed as an integration of signals based on fetal demands[96,97] and maternal supply. At times of scarce resources, as has commonly been the case in human history, these may result in conflicting signals, leading to either a stable supply of resources to the fetoplacental unit at the cost of depleted maternal resources, or preservation of maternal resources with FGR and other sequelae for the fetus. Maternal and fetal responses may be differentially adaptive, dominated by fetal demand signals when the nutritional challenge is moderate or brief or by maternal supply if the nutritional challenge is severe or prolonged.[88]

Histopathology of the Placenta
Until recently, placental pathology has often been underappreciated and consequently left out of clinical consideration, leading to variable and often inconsistent diagnostic terminology, excessive reliance on small retrospective studies and

expert opinion, and suboptimal communication of research findings with obstetricians. Increased emphasis on larger, more definitive studies, ideally prospective, to clearly define the significance of various placental lesions—and the landmark 2014 Amsterdam Placental Workshop initiative to reach a consensus on standardized diagnostic criteria and the terminology of placental lesions—has changed the course of the placental pathology field.[98,99]

Placental Shape Abnormalities

Irregularly shaped placentas have been associated with reduced placental efficiency,[100] and a more elliptical placenta (shorter width measurement) has been associated with the development of pre-eclampsia.[101] The defining feature of a multilobated placenta is the presence of detached placental lobes connected to the main placental disc by fetal chorionic plate vessels. The extra lobe is termed an accessory or succenturiate lobe, identified in 5% to 6% of placentas.[102] More unusual shapes may also be seen, including bilobed placenta (two equal lobes with the UC inserting into the membranes between them), ring placenta (also called a zonary or annular placenta), and placenta membranacea, with nearly the entirety of the gestational sac covered by an extremely thin placenta.[102]

Under normal conditions, the extraplacental membranes insert at the periphery of the placental disc. In both circummarginate and circumvallate placentas, the membranes insert on the chorionic plate, away from the placental disc margin. This abnormality can be partial or span the entire placental circumference. In circumvallate placentas, the insertion point of the membranes has an abnormal ("plication") fold.[102] The membrane insertion point for circummarginate placentas lacks plication. Circummarginate membrane insertion occurs in up to 25% of placentas, whereas circumvallate membrane insertion is found in only 1% to 6.5%.[102]

Multifetal Gestation

The majority of multifetal gestations are twin gestations. Overall, the placental pathologies in twin placentas are similar to those of singleton placentas. Twin placentas are more likely to have marginal or velamentous cord insertions[103] and accelerated villous maturation (**Figure 6.5**). Monochorionic twin placentas more commonly have vascular thromboses than dichorionic twin or singleton placentas.[104] In twins with separate placental discs, or in

twins with a single amniotic sac, the determination of chorionicity is usually simple. Twins sharing a single placental disc require examination of the dividing membranes that separate the two amniotic sacs. By microscopy, the dividing membrane of dichorionic twin placentas is thicker, with readily identifiable chorionic tissue from each twin (**Figure 6.5**). Dividing membranes from monochorionic twin placentas consist only of two adjacent thin amniotic membranes. Monoamniotic twins often have closely spaced UC insertion sites with large arterial-arterial (A-A) anastomoses connecting the two circulations (**Figure 6.5**). These anastomoses allow ready redistribution of excess blood accumulation in one of the placentas, decreasing the likelihood of twin-twin transfusion syndrome (TTTS) or related clinical disorders. Monochorionic, diamniotic twin gestations usually have vascular connections between the two circulations,[105] which may include A-A, venous-to-venous (V-V), and arterial-to-venous (A-V) anastomoses. Blood may flow in either direction through A-A and V-V anastomoses. Flow through A-V anastomoses is unidirectional. In the absence of compensatory vascular anastomoses, A-V anastomoses may foster the development of TTTS. A detailed discussion of multifetal gestations is covered in Chapter 5.

UC Structural Abnormalities

As a long, thin tubular structure free floating within a confined environment, the UC is susceptible to mechanical trauma and obstruction throughout the pregnancy. Structural abnormalities of the UC may increase the risk of damage. Aberrant UC insertion is a frequent UC abnormality. In most placentas, the UC inserts roughly centrally into the placental disc. Although placentas with a UC displaced from the center show reduced transport efficiency and a lower infant birth weight, the effect is small.[106] More significant is a marginally inserted UC or a UC inserted into the extraplacental membranes (velamentous insertion). For both insertions, the UC vessels are susceptible to bending or twisting, with the potential for intermittent obstruction or thrombosis. A furcate UC insertion occurs when the UC vessels lose their covering of Wharton jelly prior to their insertion into the placenta, which renders the UC vessels more susceptible to obstruction or thrombosis.

True UC knots occur in up to 1.25% of placentas.[107] Although most true knots remain loose while

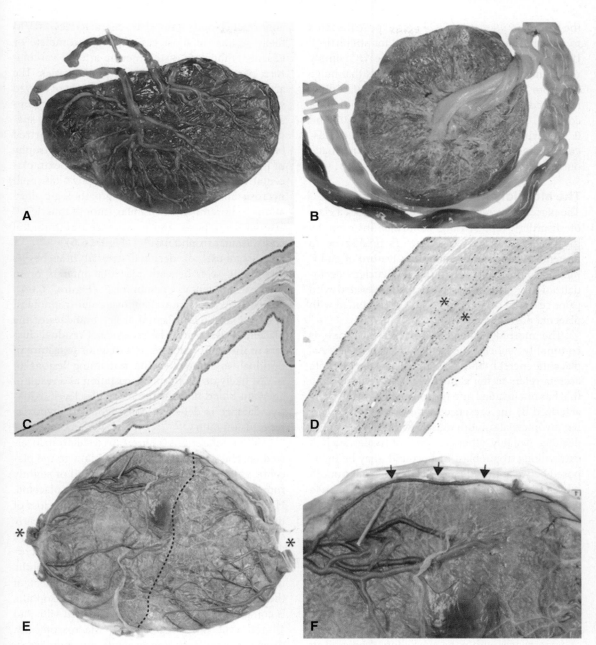

Figure 6.5 A-F, Twin placentas. A, Monochorionic, monoamniotic twin placenta. The vessels have been injected to help delineating the vascular distributions of each twin. **B,** Monochorionic, monoamniotic twin placenta with cord entanglement and knotting. The cords of these twins were extensively entangled. True knots are also present. **C,** Dichorionic, diamniotic dividing membranes. This dividing membrane is thin, with the amnion from one twin immediately adjacent to the amnion of the other twin, with no intervening chorion. **D,** Monochorionic, diamniotic dividing membranes. This dividing membrane is thick, containing not only the amnion from each twin but also the chorion from each. Typically, the layer of trophoblast that lies at the bottom of the chorion is also found in the dividing membranes (indicated here by the asterisks). **E,** Monochorionic, diamniotic twin placenta. The vessels from each twin have been injected with dye. The vascular equator is roughly traced by the dotted line. The cord insertion for each twin was marginal (indicated by the asterisks). **F,** Vascular anastomosis. This image is a higher power view of the placenta in panel E. The arrows point to a large arterial vessel connecting the two placental circulations.

the baby is *in utero*, true UC knots expose the fetus to a nearly four-fold increased risk for stillbirth.[107] Unlike true knots, false knots in the UC simply represent varicosities in the cord vessels that bulge out from the cord contour. The degree of coiling, measured by the coiling index (total number of coils/UC length in cm), ranges between 0.07 and 0.3. A hypercoiled UC is associated with fetal vascular malperfusion (FVM)[12] and adverse perinatal outcomes.

The Morbidly Adherent Placenta

The placenta accreta spectrum encompasses a class of disorders representing abnormal invasion by the placenta. Multiple risk factors predispose to placenta accreta, with a common feature of endometrial abnormality, resulting in deficient decidualization.[108] The risk is particularly elevated with prior cesarean delivery, especially if combined with placenta previa.

The morbidly adherent placenta spectrum is commonly subclassified into placenta accreta, placenta increta, and placenta percreta. Placenta accreta refers to the abnormally adherent placenta that has not invaded into the myometrium and characterized by the presence of chorionic villi overlying myometrial smooth muscle without intervening decidua. Notably, other cell types or tissues, such as extravillous trophoblast or fibrinoid, may be interposed between the villi and the myometrial smooth muscle. Unlike placenta accreta, placenta increta is more of a macroscopic diagnosis, with placental tissue bulging into and thinning the overlying myometrium. Placenta percreta is characterized by extension of the placental to the uterine serosa and typically requires a macroscopic examination to define the thinnest part of the myometrial wall and the absence of smooth muscle. Despite the marked changes, in cases of placenta percreta, the placenta generally remains unaffected, yet a higher incidence of hemorrhages within the intervillous space and an increased incidence of accelerated villous maturation have been documented.[109]

Maternal Vascular Malperfusion

Maternal vascular malperfusion (MVM) is the overarching term for a constellation of common placental abnormalities that foster or result from aberrant maternal blood flow to the placenta.[98,99] These lesions are commonly associated with preeclampsia, FGR, and preterm birth.[110-112] The abnormal blood flow that characterizes MVM likely results, in most cases, from incomplete or absent remodeling of the uterine arterial vasculature, particularly the maternal spiral arteries. The arterial lesions that develop in the context of altered vascular remodeling are termed decidual vasculopathy. Different types are characterized by the specific arterial lesion, persistence of a muscularized basal plate artery,[113] thickening and hypertrophy of the arterial smooth muscle wall in the extraplacental membranes (mural hypertrophy), fibrinoid necrosis and atherosis (reflecting pathologic alterations to unremodeled vascular smooth muscle),[114] arterial thrombosis, and persistence of intramural endovascular trophoblast[98,99] (**Figure 6.6**).

Thrombosis of decidual arterial branches is commonly seen beneath placental infarcts or in the extraplacental membranes (**Figure 6.6A**). Persistence of intramural endovascular trophoblast is only found within spiral artery branches of the placental basal plate. The presence of residual clusters in the third trimester is a diagnostic feature of decidual vasculopathy. The remaining lesions of MVM likely develop later in gestation as a result of aberrant blood flow. At the molecular level, oxidative damage is detected, consistent with hypoxia-reperfusion injury.[113]

Villous infarctions (**Figure 6.6**) result from localized obstruction of maternal blood flow to the placenta. Villous infarcts are wedge shaped or slightly rounded and abut the basal surface of the placenta. Histologically, recent infarcts show smudgy loss of nuclear basophilia in the trophoblast. At this early stage, erythrocytes remain within the fetal vessels, imparting a deep red color to the infarct macroscopically (**Figure 6.6**). A limited neutrophilic infiltrate may be present around the periphery of the infarct. With time, loss of nuclear basophilia is complete in all cells within the affected villi, and all red cells have degenerated. Macroscopically, these remote infarcts appear white-tan and densely firm. Whereas one to two small peripheral infarcts at term may be observed in normal pregnancies, infarcts are particularly significant in a preterm placenta or in the central placenta involving more than 5% of the placental volume.[98,99]

One of the most common features of MVM is accelerated villous maturation, which may develop in response to hypoxia and manifest as large numbers of villi that are more mature than expected for the gestational age, with smaller villous size, greater

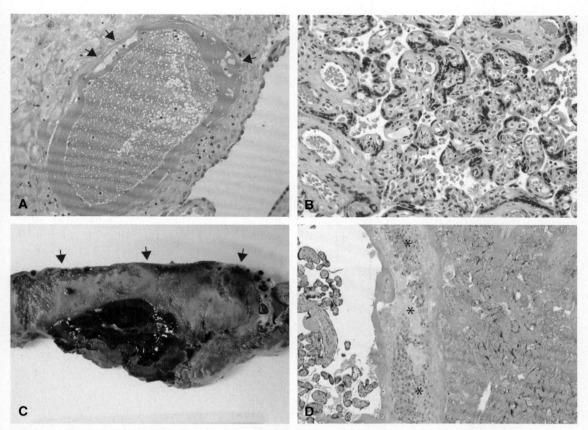

Figure 6.6 Maternal vascular malperfusion. A, Fibrinoid necrosis with atherosis. The wall of this spiral has been replaced by dense, brightly eosinophilic fibrinoid. Scattered foamy macrophages are also present (arrows). **B,** Increased syncytial knots. This section of term placenta shows large numbers of syncytial knots, present on the majority of the smaller villi. **C,** Retroplacental hemorrhage. Dark red-black gelatinous blood clot underlies a significant fraction of this placental slice, compressing the overlying parenchyma. Much of the overlying placental parenchyma is infarcted (light orange-red discoloration, indicated by arrows). Normal placental parenchyma is present to the left. **D,** Remote infarct. The right half of this image shows old infarction of the placental parenchyma. A vertical septum (marked with asterisks) separates the infarcted placenta from the adjacent uninvolved placenta.

vascular cross section, and increased syncytial knots (**Figure 6.6B**). Syncytial knots are aggregates of at least five syncytiotrophoblast nuclei that bulge above the surface of a villus. They are more common with advancing gestational age.[115] MVM lesions are also associated with distal villous hypoplasia,[98] which generally occurs late in the course of MVM, and may reflect a lengthy period of fetal hypoxia. Of all MVM lesions, distal villous hypoplasia is most directly associated with adverse clinical parameters, including abnormal umbilical artery Doppler flow[116] and FGR.[116] Distal villous hypoplasia is characterized by thin, elongated villi with limited branching, imparting an empty appearance to the placenta.

Retroplacental hemorrhage is the accumulation of blood beneath the placenta, usually due to premature separation of the placenta from the uterine wall, and is the pathologic diagnosis that supports placental abruption (**Figure 6.6C**; covered in Chapter 47). Clinically significant retroplacental hemorrhage is associated with secondary changes in the placental tissue, with compression and infarction of the overlying placental parenchyma and, at times, hemorrhage of fetal blood into the overlying villi (villous stromal hemorrhage).[113] Finally, MVM is characterized by a small placental size, which is usually defined as a weight below the 10th percentile for the gestational age.[98]

Fetal Vascular Malperfusion

FVM, previously termed fetal thrombotic vasculopathy, represents abnormal perfusion in the fetal circulation.[98,99] Although the etiology of FVM is not entirely clear, partial or intermittent obstruction of the UC and fetal hypercoagulability have been proposed.[117] FVM is characterized by thromboses and fibrin deposition in the fetal vascular system and secondary villous damage (**Figure 6.7**). Adherence of the fibrin aggregate to the vessel wall, with destruction of the underlying vascular endothelium, also defines FVM (**Figure 6.7A,B**). The segments of larger fetal vessels downstream of a thrombus show characteristic stem vessel obliteration, with degeneration of the endothelium and

vascular smooth muscle (**Figure 6.7C**), red blood cell migration into the degenerating vascular wall, and even fibroblast growth into the vessel lumen, sometimes dividing the vessel lumen into several small channels (luminal septation). Diffuse stem vessel obliteration is characteristic of the stillbirth placenta.

Once a fetal vessel is obstructed, the downstream villi begin to degenerate (**Figure 6.7D**). The villi first develop a histologic appearance, termed villous stromal-vascular karyorrhexis, with damage to endothelial cells and adjacent stromal cells, endothelial sloughing, and endothelial and stromal cell karyorrhexis, with subsequent villous stroma fibrosis (avascular villi). In contrast, the

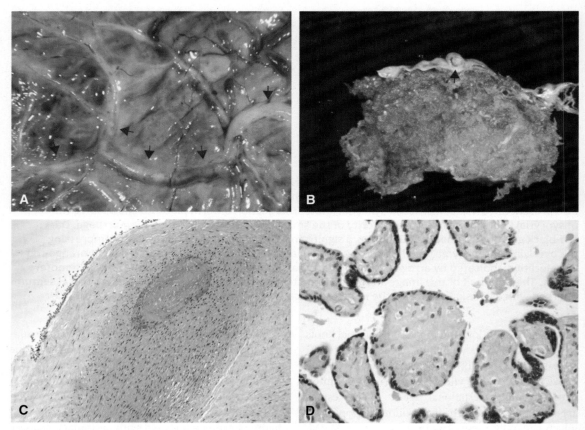

Figure 6.7 Fetal vascular malperfusion. A, Macroscopic photograph of a thrombosed chorionic plate vessel (arrows). The vessel is distended, and the surface is dull and white. **B,** Cross section of the vessel shown in A. The lumen is entirely occluded by old, white thrombus (arrow). **C,** Microscopic photograph of the thrombus shown in A and B. The lumen is nearly entirely occupied by dense remote thrombus. **D,** Avascular villi, showing complete loss of their vasculature. The stroma is densely collagenized, with some remaining stromal cells. The surrounding villous trophoblast remains viable. In the absence of blood-filled spaces in the villi, the contrast between the dark trophoblast and the pink villous stroma is stark.

villous trophoblasts, which obtain their nutrients from the maternal intervillous space blood, survive.

Perivillous Fibrinoid Deposition

Placental fibrinoid is composed of a mixture of extracellular matrix material, including fibronectin, collagen, and laminin; molecules of the coagulation cascade, including fibrin and fibrinogen; and major basic proteins.[99] Small foci of fibrinoid may be deposited within or adjacent to chorionic villi; this is known as intervillous fibrin deposition. Larger deposits, in a process called perivillous fibrinoid deposition, may surround and encase broad zones of villi. Although the significance of mildly increased amounts of fibrinoid of either pattern is unclear, excessive deposition of perivillous fibrinoid may obstruct maternal blood flow through the intervillous space and smother large numbers of chorionic villi. This most severe form of increased perivillous fibrinoid deposition is termed massive perivillous fibrinoid deposition (formerly called maternal floor infarction).[118] This rare lesion is highly recurrent, ranging from 12% to 78% in several small series,[118] and is associated with severe adverse pregnancy outcomes, including FGR, demise, preterm birth, and poor neurologic outcome.[99,118]

Placental Infection and Inflammation

Inflammation can affect any of the placental compartments, including the fetal membranes, chorionic villi, placental vasculature, and decidua. Inflammatory infiltrates are classified as acute or chronic, but, unlike elsewhere in the body, mixed inflammatory infiltrates are rare. Moreover, each type of inflammation corresponds to a limited subset of underlying etiologies. Although these etiologies are often infectious in origin, both maternal-fetal alloimmune responses and sterile inflammation are commonly encountered.

Acute Inflammation

Acute inflammation manifests most frequently as the cluster of pathologic findings termed histologic acute chorioamnionitis (HCA, **Figure 6.8**). The adjective "histologic" is included in the diagnostic terminology to distinguish this entity from the clinical syndrome of acute chorioamnionitis. The etiology for HCA is usually bacterial infection, ascending through the cervix to infect the amniotic fluid.

HCA consists of both a maternal and fetal response to the bacterial products found in infected amniotic fluid. The maternal response consists nearly entirely of neutrophils, which first accumulate within the fibrin along the underside of the chorionic plate or within the trophoblast layer beneath the chorion of the extraplacental membranes. As the inflammatory process continues, maternal neutrophils migrate through the subchorionic fibrin layer or through the trophoblast layer and into the chorion itself. As the process advances, it involves extensive neutrophil degeneration, necrosis of the amnion, and/or thickening of the amniotic basement membrane. Only the maternal inflammatory response leads to macroscopically identifiable changes in the placenta. As the maternal neutrophils accumulate within the fetal membranes, they decrease the translucence of the membranes that, instead, become opaque and white to yellow-tan (**Figure 6.8A** and **B**).

The fetal response is similar, with migration of fetal inflammatory cells out from the fetal vessels on the chorionic plate surface and in the UC. Vasculitis of the fetal vessels then develops as acute inflammatory cells migrate out of the fetal circulation in response to the infection. In addition to the predominating neutrophils, the fetal response may include other cell types such as eosinophils and occasionally chronic inflammatory cells. With longstanding infection, necrotizing funisitis develops, defined by the presence of a circumferential ring of neutrophils, debris, or calcification around the umbilical vessels (**Figure 6.8C** and **D**). For a small number of bacterial species, such as *Listeria monocytogenes*, Group B *Streptococcus*, *Klebsiella*, *Escherichia coli*, *Campylobacter*, and *Hemophilus*,[99] the infection may extend beyond the membranes into the underlying chorionic villi, resulting in acute villitis. It has long been known that the overlap among HCA, clinical chorioamnionitis, and proven intra-amniotic infection is limited, which led to the emergence of the concept of "sterile" placental inflammation,[119] where clear evidence for amniotic fluid inflammation is not associated with microbial involvement.[119-121]

Chronic Inflammation

Whereas acute inflammation in the placenta is largely confined to the fetal membranes, chronic inflammation is more widely dispersed, appearing in the chorionic villi, the fetal membranes, and the decidua. Of these, involvement of the chorionic

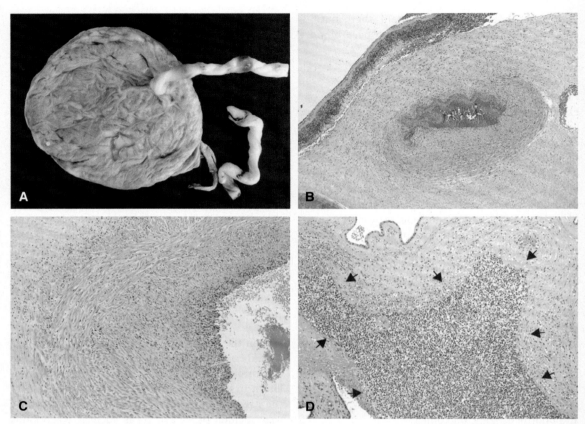

Figure 6.8 Acute chorioamnionitis. A, A placenta with acute chorioamnionitis. The surface membranes are opaque and have a yellow-tan discoloration. **B,** Acute chorioamnionitis, stage 3. In this severe acute chorioamnionitis, a thick band of densely packed neutrophils fills the amnion. The basement membrane of the overlying amniotic epithelium is thickened, forming a bright pink band above the dense blue of the neutrophils (upper right corner of image). The chorionic plate vessel shows early thrombus formation along the portion of the vessel nearest to the amnion. **C,** Acute funisitis involving the umbilical vein. Large numbers of neutrophils invade the vessel wall and spill into Wharton jelly. **D,** Microabscess, denoted by arrows. The microabscess nearly fills the entirety of this image.

villi (chronic villitis) is the most likely to affect the fetus.[122] The causes of chronic placental inflammation are different from those of acute inflammation. Infection has been associated with less than 10% of the cases and usually stems from infection with TORCH (*Toxoplasma gondii*, others, including *Treponema pallidum*, *Listeria*, varicella, and parvovirus B19, rubella virus, cytomegalovirus [CMV], and herpes simplex virus) pathogens, most commonly CMV.[99,118,123] In most chronic villitis cases, no infectious etiology is identified, and hence, these are defined as chronic villitis of unknown etiology (VUE) and assumed to reflect maternal alloimmune response against the fetus.

Histologically, chronic villitis is defined by the presence of an increased number of lymphocytes and histiocytes within the villous stroma, often with accompanying local tissue destruction. When histiocytes accumulate in maternal blood spaces adjacent to the affected villi, the process is termed intervillitis or intervillositis. VUE may involve stem villi, leading to stem vessel obliteration and the formation of clusters of avascular villi. Whereas VUE that affects a small proportion of the chorionic villi is likely to be clinically insignificant, extensive villous involvement may result in perinatal complications such as FGR, stillbirth, and poor neurologic outcomes.[118,122] For information on disorders of vascular proliferation, meconium, gestational trophoblastic disease and additional placental pathologies, please refer to the e-book.

The Placental Origins of Childhood and Adult Diseases

Work by David Barker and his associates, as well as by other scholars who have correlated the health of adult populations with their pregnancy and birth data, has linked abnormal fetal development and intrauterine diseases with chronic diseases during childhood or adulthood.[131] Studies that have focused specifically on the placenta have identified putative pathways that link intrauterine fetal disorders, possibly as a reflection of placental dysfunction, and chronic disorders later in life (reviewed in Refs 132 and 133). In general, the placental-to-fetal weight (P/E) ratio is a reactively crude, yet commonly used measure of placental efficiency, with a higher P/E ratio representing a less efficient placenta. Both high and low P/E ratios have been associated with adult coronary heart disease, and smaller or larger placentas have been associated with lung cancer.[134] Small placentas have been associated with adult chronic hypertension and adult heart failure. Similarly, deviations of placental shape from the typical circular perimeter (eg, more elliptical) have been associated with aberrant fetal growth and body composition and adult coronary heart disease,[135] hypertension,[136] and even colon cancer. Although the mechanisms underlying these associations remain unclear, it seems that placental response to adverse intrauterine influences may change placental function, leading to a reduced supply of oxygen, hormones, growth factors, and other homeostatic signals from the placenta and the fetus, which adversely impacts fetal/organ development and metabolic functions. Consequently, these changes in fetal development may predispose to diseases in childhood and adulthood.

KEY POINTS

- The placenta comprises cells that originated from the conceptus; hence, it shares its genetic origin with the fetus. Maternal cells within the placenta are circulating red and white blood cells and their inflammatory derivatives.

- The term placenta weighs approximately 500 g, its mean diameter is 18 to 22 cm, and its thickness is 2.4 cm. These dimensions are fairly variable, and small deviations usually lack clinical significance. The mother-facing plate is called the basal plate and is divided to cotyledons, which are not distinct developmental units. The fetus-facing chorionic plate is covered by the amnion. The UC connects to the chorionic plate and delivers oxygen and nutrients to the fetus, and unoxygenated blood and waste products to the mother.

- The main functional unit within the placenta is the villus, with maternal blood cells perfusing the area around the villi, termed the intervillous space. The outermost layer of each villus, which is directly bathed in maternal blood, comprises the multinucleated syncytiotrophoblast. Immediately subjacent to this layer are the less differentiated, mononucleated cytotrophoblasts. The cytotrophoblasts are separated from the villous core by a basement membrane.

- The villus stroma contains sinusoidal fetal blood vessels lined with endothelial cells, alongside fibroblasts and speciated Hofbauer placental macrophages. The vasculosyncytial membranes, where most of the maternal-fetal exchange occurs, define the functional maternal-fetal exchange unit.

- The extravillous trophoblasts, including the interstitial trophoblasts and the endovascular trophoblasts, are essential for remodeling the spiral arteries and supporting maximal dilation.

- Blood flow in the intervillous space is slow, with multiple irregularly shaped lakes, clefts, and fusions among neighboring villi, and influenced by villous fetal capillary flow.

- Placental hypoxia is normal in early pregnancy and promotes the invasion and migration of extravillous trophoblasts toward the oxygen-enriched decidual blood vessels. Hypoxia after weeks 12 to 14 of pregnancy has been implicated in diverse villous injuries.

- The placenta is an active site of steroid and protein hormone synthesis, which are vital for placental development and function. Key hormones are progesterone, estrogen, hCG, hPL, and many other releasing hormones, peptides, and growth factors.

- The transport of ions, molecules, or proteins across the placental barriers can take place either *via* intercellular water-filled channels or through cells, where molecules can traverse the placental surface by the hydrostatic and osmotic pressure gradients. Most transplacental transport is achieved through diffusion, transport mechanisms, and endocytosis/exocytosis.

- Diverse gestational diseases are associated with placental disorders or affect placenta function. Even distinctly defined diseases (eg, preeclampsia, FGR) share many placental histopathological features, suggesting that these diseases may be a manifestation of an underlying placental maldevelopment or impaired function. Additional factors, such as disruption of maternal homeostasis, shape the disease manifestation.

- A number of placental pathologies, including villous maldevelopment, genetic or epigenetic aberrations, hypoperfusion and hypoxia, infections, immune responses, and environmental exposures, have been implicated in placental damage and related clinical syndromes.

- Irregularly shaped placentas, unusually thick or thin placentas, or abnormal membrane insertion have been associated with reduced placental efficiency.

- Placental pathologies in multifetal placentas are generally similar to those of singleton placentas, with a higher incidence of marginal or velamentous cord insertions and accelerated villous maturation. Monochorionic twin placentas exhibit more anastomoses and vascular thromboses than dichorionic placentas.

- The placenta accreta spectrum represents abnormal placental invasion, commonly linked to endometrial abnormality, deficient decidualization, and is associated with placenta previa.

- MVM includes lesions related to altered decidual vascular remodeling. Villous infarctions result from localized obstruction of maternal blood flow to the placenta and commonly result in accelerated villous maturation or distal villous hypoplasia. FVM, in turn, is characterized by thromboses and fibrin deposition in the fetal vascular system and secondary villous damage.

- Acute histologic chorioamnionitis usually stems from bacterial infection, ascending through the cervix to infect the amniotic fluid, with the reciprocal fetal inflammatory response. Chronic inflammation is more commonly associated with TORCH infections, or with villitis, which may be of unknown cause. Extensive villous involvement may result in perinatal complications such as FGR, stillbirth, and poor neurologic outcomes.

- Abnormalities in placental size, shape, or function have been associated with chronic diseases during childhood or adulthood. This likely reflects placental response to adverse intrauterine influences that impact placental function, leading to reduced supply to the fetoplacental unit, adversely impacting fetal development and metabolic functions.

REFERENCES

(only references cited in synoptic print chapter; for a complete reference list, see ebook)

1. Boyd JD, Hamilton WJ. *The Human Placenta.* Heffer; 1970.
2. Wooding FP, Burton GJ. *Comparative Placentation. Structures, Functions and Evolution.* Springer-Verlag Berlin Heidelberg; 2008.
3. Sadovsky Y, Jansson T. Placenta and placental transport function. In: Plant TM, Zeleznik AJ, eds. *Knobil and Neill's Physiology of Reproduction.* 4th ed. Academic Press; 2015:1741-1782.
4. Mayhew TM, Leach L, McGee R, et al. Proliferation, differentiation and apoptosis in villous trophoblast at 13-41 weeks of gestation (including observations on annulate lamellae and nuclear pore complexes). *Placenta.* 1999;20:407-422.
5. Nelson DM, Johnson RD, Smith SD, et al. Hypoxia limits differentiation and up-regulates expression and activity of prostaglandin H synthase 2 in cultured trophoblast from term human placenta. *Am J Obstet Gynecol.* 1999;180:896-902.
6. Maltepe E, Bakardjiev AI, Fisher SJ. The placenta: transcriptional, epigenetic, and physiological integration during development. *J Clin Invest.* 2010;120:1016-1025.
7. Handwerger S. New insights into the regulation of human cytotrophoblast cell differentiation. *Mol Cell Endocrinol.* 2010;323:94-104.
8. Mi S, Lee X, Li X, et al. Syncytin is a captive retroviral envelope protein involved in human placental morphogenesis. *Nature.* 2000;403:785-789.
9. Benirschke K, Kaufmann P. *Pathology of the Human Placenta.* Springer-Verlag; 2000.
10. Castellucci M, Scheper M, Scheffen I, et al. The development of the human placental villous tree. *Anat Embryol (Berl).* 1990;181:117-128.
11. Getzowa S, Sadowsky A. On the structure of the human placenta with full-time and immature foetus, living or dead. *J Obstet Gynaecol Br Emp.* 1950;57:388-396.
12. Huppertz B. The anatomy of the normal placenta. *J Clin Pathol.* 2008;61:1296-1302.
13. Genbacev O, Zhou Y, Ludlow JW, et al. Regulation of human placental development by oxygen tension. *Science.* 1997;277:1669-1672.

14. Pijnenborg R, Vercruysse L, Hanssens M. The uterine spiral arteries in human pregnancy: facts and controversies. *Placenta*. 2006;27:939-958.

15. Burton GJ, Charnock-Jones DS, Jauniaux E. Regulation of vascular growth and function in the human placenta. *Reproduction*. 2009;138:895-902.

16. Demir R, Seval Y, Huppertz B. Vasculogenesis and angiogenesis in the early human placenta. *Acta Histochem*. 2007;109:257-265.

17. Burton GJ, Jauniaux E, Charnock-Jones DS. The influence of the intra-uterine environment on human placental development. *Int J Dev Biol*. 2010;54:303-312.

18. Red-Horse K, Zhou Y, Genbacev O, et al. Trophoblast differentiation during embryo implantation and formation of the maternal-fetal inter-face. *J Clin Invest*. 2004;114:744-754.

19. Mayhew TM, Charnock-Jones DS, Kaufmann P. Aspects of human feto-placental vasculogenesis and angiogenesis. III. Changes in complicated pregnancies. *Placenta*. 2004;25:127-139.

20. Burton GJ. Oxygen, the Janus gas; its effects on human placental develop-ment and function. *J Anat*. 2009;215:27-35.

21. Schneider H. Oxygenation of the placental-fetal unit in humans. *Respir Physiol Neurobiol*. 2011;178:51-58.

22. Mayhew TM, Jackson MR, Haas JD. Oxygen diffusive conductances of human placentae from term pregnancies at low and high altitudes. *Placenta*. 1990;11:493-503.

37. Costa MA. The endocrine function of human placenta: an overview. *Reprod Biomed Online*. 2016;32:14-43.

38. Smith R. Parturition. *N Engl J Med*. 2007;356:271-283.

39. Fowden AL, Forhead AJ, Sferruzzi-Perri AN, et al. Review: endocrine reg-ulation of placental phenotype. *Placenta*. 2015;36(suppl 1):S50-S59.

40. Smith R, Mesiano S, McGrath S. Hormone trajectories leading to human birth. *Regul Pept*. 2002;108:159-164.

41. Berkane N, Liere P, Oudinet JP, et al. From pregnancy to preeclampsia: a key role for estrogens. *Endocr Rev*. 2017;38:123-144.

42. Mendelson CR, Kamat A. Mechanisms in the regulation of aromatase in developing ovary and placenta. *J Steroid Biochem Mol Biol*. 2007;106:62-70.

43. Fournier T, Guibourdenche J, Evain-Brion D. Review. hCGs: different sources of production, different glycoforms and functions. *Placenta*. 2015;36(suppl 1):S60-S65.

44. Schumacher A. Human chorionic gonadotropin as a pivotal endocrine immune regulator initiating and preserving fetal tolerance. *Int J Mol Sci*. 2017;18(10):2166.

45. Handwerger S, Freemark M. The roles of placental growth hormone and placental lactogen in the regulation of human fetal growth and develop-ment. *J Pediatr Endocrinol Metab*. 2000;13:343-356.

46. Wijayarathna R, de Kretser DM. Activins in reproductive biology and beyond. *Hum Reprod Update*. 2016;22:342-357.

47. Wadhwa PD, Sandman CA, Chicz-DeMet A, et al. Placental CRH modu-lates maternal pituitary adrenal function in human pregnancy. *Ann N Y Acad Sci*. 1997;814:276-281.

48. Gohar J, Mazor M, Leiberman JR. GnRH in pregnancy. *Arch Gynecol Obstet*. 1996;259:1-6.

49. Kim SC, Lee JE, Kang SS, et al. The regulation of oxytocin and oxytocin receptor in human placenta according to gestational age. *J Mol Endocrinol*. 2017;59:235-243.

50. Dewerchin M, Carmeliet P. PlGF: a multitasking cytokine with disease-restricted activity. *Cold Spring Harb Perspect Med*. 2012;2(8):a011056.

51. Schanton M, Maymo JL, Perez-Perez A, et al. Involvement of leptin in the molecular physiology of the placenta. *Reproduction*. 2018;155:R1-R12.

52. Desforges M, Sibley CP. Placental nutrient supply and fetal growth. *Int J Dev Biol*. 2010;54:377-390.

53. Sibley CP, Brownbill P, Glazier JD, et al. Knowledge needed about the exchange physiology of the placenta. *Placenta*. 2018;64(suppl 1):S9-S15.

54. Illsley NP, Baumann MU. Human placental glucose transport in feto-placental growth and metabolism. *Biochim Biophys Acta Mol Basis Dis*. 2020;1866(2):165359.

55. Mayhew TM, Jackson MR, Boyd PA. Changes in oxygen diffusive conduc-tances of human placentae during gestation (10-41 weeks) are commen-surate with the gain in fetal weight. *Placenta*. 1993;14:51-61.

56. Schneider H, Miller RK. Receptor-mediated uptake and transport of mac-romolecules in the human placenta. *Int J Dev Biol*. 2010;54:367-375.

72. Duttaroy AK. Transport of fatty acids across the human placenta: a review. *Prog Lipid Res*. 2009;48:52-61.

74. Scifres CM, Sadovsky Y. Placental fat trafficking. In: Kay HH, Nelson DM, Wang Y, eds. *The Placenta*. Wiley-Blackwell; 2011:75-80.

75. Bildirici I, Schaiff WT, Chen B, et al. PLIN2 is essential for tropho-blastic lipid droplet accumulation and cell survival during hypoxia. *Endocrinology*. 2018;159:3937-3949.

81. Roberts JM, Escudero C. The placenta in preeclampsia. *Pregnancy Hypertens*. 2012;2:72-83.

82. Vaughan OR, Rosario FJ, Powell TL, et al. Regulation of placental amino acid transport and fetal growth. *Prog Mol Biol Transl Sci*. 2017;145:217-251.

83. Burton GJ, Jauniaux E. Placental oxidative stress: from miscarriage to pre-eclampsia. *J Soc Gynecol Investig*. 2004;11:342-352.

84. Jauniaux E, Hempstock J, Greenwold N, et al. Trophoblastic oxidative stress in relation to temporal and regional differences in maternal placen-tal blood flow in normal and abnormal early pregnancies. *Am J Pathol*. 2003;162:115-125.

85. Poston L, Raijmakers MT. Trophoblast oxidative stress, antioxidants and pregnancy outcome – a review. *Placenta*. 2004;25 suppl A:S72-S78.

86. Sultana Z, Maiti K, Aitken J, et al. Oxidative stress, placental ageing-related pathologies and adverse pregnancy outcomes. *Am J Reprod Immunol*. 2017;77(5):e12653.

87. Hempstock J, Jauniaux E, Greenwold N, et al. The contribution of placental oxidative stress to early pregnancy failure. *Hum Pathol*. 2003;34:1265-1275.

88. Chassen S, Jansson T. Complex, coordinated and highly regulated changes in placental signaling and nutrient transport capacity in IUGR. *Biochim Biophys Acta Mol Basis Dis*. 2020;1866(2):165373.

89. Shibata E, Hubel CA, Powers RW, et al. Placental system A amino acid transport is reduced in pregnancies with small for gestational age (SGA) infants but not in preeclampsia with SGA infants. *Placenta*. 2008;29:879-882.

90. Gauster M, Hiden U, Blaschitz A, et al. Dysregulation of placental endo-thelial lipase and lipoprotein lipase in intrauterine growth-restricted preg-nancies. *J Clin Endocrinol Metab*. 2007;92:2256-2263.

91. Cetin I, Giovannini N, Alvino G, et al. Intrauterine growth restriction is associated with changes in polyunsaturated fatty acid fetal-maternal rela-tionships. *Pediatr Res*. 2002;52:750-755.

92. Zamudio S, Torricos T, Fik E, et al. Hypoglycemia and the origin of hypoxia-induced reduction in human fetal growth. *PLoS One*. 2010;5:e8551.

93. Dube E, Gravel A, Martin C, et al. Modulation of fatty acid transport and metabolism by obesity in the human full-term placenta. *Biol Reprod*. 2012;87(1):1-11.

94. Gauster M, Hiden U, van Poppel M, et al. Dysregulation of placental endo-thelial lipase in obese women with gestational diabetes mellitus. *Diabetes*. 2011;60:2457-2464.

95. Scifres CM, Chen B, Nelson DM, et al. Fatty acid binding protein 4 reg-ulates intracellular lipid accumulation in human trophoblasts. *J Clin Endocrinol Metab*. 2011;96:E1083-E1091.

96. Sibley CP, Brownbill P, Dilworth M, et al. Review. Adaptation in placental nutrient supply to meet fetal growth demand: implications for program-ming. *Placenta*. 2010;31 suppl:S70-S74.

97. Constancia M, Angiolini E, Sandovici I, et al. Adaptation of nutri-ent supply to fetal demand in the mouse involves interaction between the Igf2 gene and placental transporter systems. *Proc Natl Acad Sci*. 2005;102:19219-19224.

98. Khong TY, Mooney EE, Ariel I, et al. Sampling and definitions of placental lesions: Amsterdam placental workshop group consensus statement. *Arch Pathol Lab Med*. 2016;140:698-713.

99. Khong TY, Mooney EE, Nikkels PGJ, et al. *Pathology of the Placenta: A Practical Guide*. Springer International Publishing; 2019.

100. Salafia CM, Yampolsky M, Misra DP, et al. Placental surface shape, function, and effects of maternal and fetal vascular pathology. *Placenta*. 2010;31:958-962.

101. Kajantie E, Thornburg KL, Eriksson JG, et al. In preeclampsia, the placenta grows slowly along its minor axis. *Int J Dev Biol*. 2010;54:469-473.

102. Baergen RN. *Manual of Pathology of the Human Placenta*. 2nd ed. Springer US; 2011.

103. Kibel M, Kahn M, Sherman C, et al. Placental abnormalities differ between small for gestational age fetuses in dichorionic twin and singleton pregnancies. *Placenta*. 2017;60:28-35.

104. Sato Y, Benirschke K. Increased prevalence of fetal thrombi in monochorionic-twin placentas. *Pediatrics*. 2006;117:e113-e117.

105. Fitzgerald B. Histopathological examination of the placenta in twin preg-nancies. *APMIS*. 2018;126:626-637.

106. Yampolsky M, Salafia CM, Shlakhter O, et al. Centrality of the umbilical cord insertion in a human placenta influences the placental efficiency. *Placenta*. 2009;30:1058-106

107. Airas U, Heinonen S. Clinical significance of true umbilical knots: a population-based analysis. *Am J Perinatol*. 2002;19:127-132.

108. da Cunha Castro EC, Popek E. Abnormalities of placenta implantation. *APMIS*. 2018;126:613-620.

109. Ernst LM, Linn RL, Minturn L, et al. Placental pathologic associations with morbidly adherent placenta: potential insights into pathogenesis. *Pediatr Dev Pathol*. 2017;20(5):387-393.

110. Brosens I, Pijnenborg R, Vercruysse L, et al. The "Great Obstetrical Syndromes" are associated with disorders of deep placentation. *Am J Obstet Gynecol*. 2011;204:193-201.

111. Catov JM, Scifres CM, Caritis SN, et al. Neonatal outcomes following preterm birth classified according to placental features. *Am J Obstet Gynecol*. 2017;216:411.e411-411.e414.

112. Morgan TK, Tolosa JE, Mele L, et al. Placental villous hypermaturation is associated with idiopathic preterm birth. *J Matern Fetal Neonatal Med*. 2013;26:647-653.

113. Parks WT. Manifestations of hypoxia in the second and third trimester placenta. *Birth Defects Res*. 2017;109:1345-1357.

114. Parks WT. Placental hypoxia: the lesions of maternal malperfusion. *Semin Perinatol*. 2015;39:9-19.

115. Loukeris K, Sela R, Baergen RN. Syncytial knots as a reflection of placental maturity: reference values for 20 to 40 weeks' gestational age. *Pediatr Dev Pathol*. 2010;13:305-309.

116. Veerbeek JH, Nikkels PG, Torrance HL, et al. Placental pathology in early intrauterine growth restriction associated with maternal hypertension. *Placenta*. 2014;35:696-701.

117. Redline RW, Ravishankar S. Fetal vascular malperfusion, an update. *APMIS*. 2018;126:561-569.

118. Chen A, Roberts DJ. Placental pathologic lesions with a significant recurrence risk – what not to miss! *APMIS*. 2018;126:589-601.

119. Kim CJ, Romero R, Chaemsaithong P, et al. Acute chorioamnionitis and funisitis: definition, pathologic features, and clinical significance. *Am J Obstet Gynecol*. 2015;213:S29-S52.

120. Romero R, Miranda J, Chaiworapongsa T, et al. Prevalence and clinical significance of sterile intra-amniotic inflammation in patients with preterm labor and intact membranes. *Am J Reprod Immunol*. 2014;72:458-474.

121. Roberts DJ, Celi AC, Riley LE, et al. Acute histologic chorioamnionitis at term: nearly always noninfectious. *PLoS One*. 2012;7:e31819.

122. Redline RW. Villitis of unknown etiology: noninfectious chronic villitis in the placenta. *Hum Pathol*. 2007;38:1439-1446.

123. Katzman PJ. Chronic inflammatory lesions of the placenta. *Semin Perinatol*. 2015;39:20-26.

131. Barker DJ. The origins of the developmental origins theory. *J Intern Med*. 2007;261:412-417.

132. Burton GJ, Fowden AL, Thornburg KL. Placental origins of chronic disease. *Physiol Rev*. 2016;96:1509-1565.

133. Godfrey KM. The role of the placenta in fetal programming – a review. *Placenta*. 2002;23 suppl A:S20-S27.

134. Barker DJ, Thornburg KL, Osmond C, et al. The prenatal origins of lung cancer. II. The placenta. *Am J Hum Biol*. 2010;22:512-516.

135. Eriksson JG, Kajantie E, Thornburg KL, et al. Mother's body size and placental size predict coronary heart disease in men. *Eur Heart J*. 2011;32:2297-2303.

136. Roseboom TJ, Painter RC, de Rooij SR, et al. Effects of famine on placental size and efficiency. *Placenta*. 2011;32:395-399.

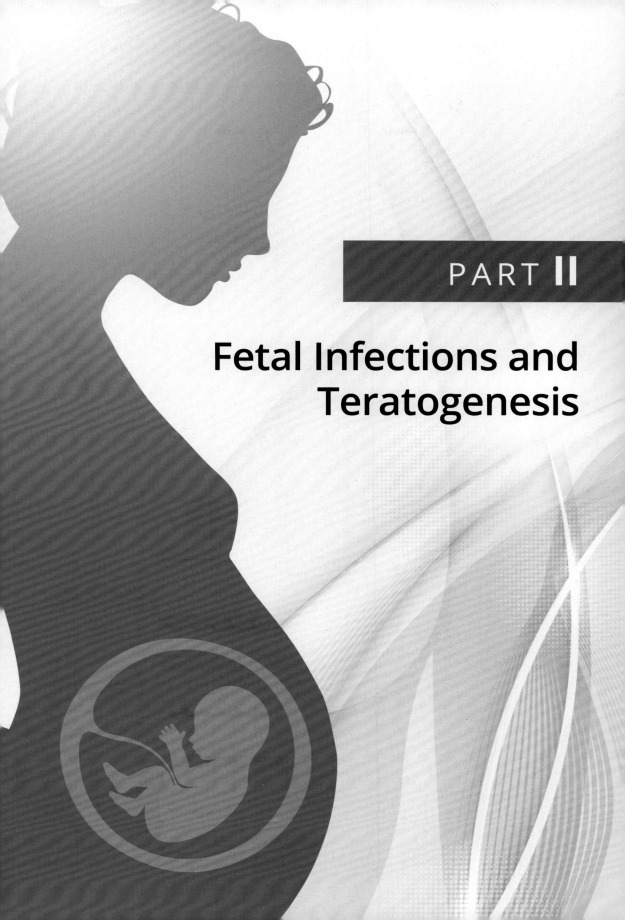

PART II

Fetal Infections and Teratogenesis

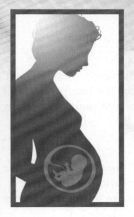

CHAPTER 7

Teratogens

Scott A. Sullivan and Barbara B. Head

Introduction

A teratogen, strictly speaking, is any agent that can contribute or cause a congenital anomaly.

For the purposes of this chapter, we will consider a teratogen to be any nongenetic cause of a malformation.

A number of important factors contribute to the potential risk for an exposure to be a teratogen. These may include:

- the amount or dose of an exposure
- the length and route of the exposure
- the timing in gestation
- pharmacological characteristics, including placental permeability, clearance patterns, solubility, half-life, interactions, and mechanism of action

The foundation for sound patient counseling is quality outcome data. However, limited data are sometimes available on the safety of medications used during pregnancy: a review of prescription medications approved by the U.S. Food and Drug Administration (FDA) from 2000 to 2010 showed that the teratogenic risk was undetermined in 97.7%.[4]

Basic Principles of Teratology

To determine if an agent is teratogenic, it is necessary to characterize the dose, route of exposure, and gestational age of pregnancy when exposure occurred.

Therefore, a list of teratogens indicates only teratogenic *potential*; evaluation of the dose and time of exposure is critical in determining the extent of potential risk. This may not always be precisely known, as patient recall or documentation may at times be incomplete. It is also critically important to determine an accurate gestational

age, if possible, by comparing the menstrual history to the earliest possible ultrasound.

Despite these limitations, physicians and clinicians must be careful to carry out a thorough evaluation of the risks faced by a woman exposed to drugs and chemicals during pregnancy. However, clinicians have a multitude of educational aids to assist them in their evaluations; these include consultations with maternal-fetal medicine subspecialists, geneticists, pharmacists, the medical literature, texts, government and manufacturer websites, and searchable online databases.

The Etiology of Congenital Malformations

The etiology of congenital malformations may be divided into three general categories: unknown, genetic, and environmental (**Table 7.1**).

Factors That Affect Susceptibility to Potential Teratogens

Timing of Exposure

The embryo is most sensitive to the lethal effects of drugs and chemicals during the period of embryonic development, from fertilization through the early postimplantation stage (**Figure 7.1**).[1]

The period of organogenesis (from day 18 through about day 40 post conception in the human) is the period of greatest sensitivity to teratogenic insults and when most anatomic malformations can be induced.[12] Most environmentally produced major malformations occur before the 36th day post conception in humans (**Table 7.2**).

The fetus is most sensitive to the induction of developmental delays and microcephaly at the end of the first and the beginning of the second trimester.[12] Developmental delays or other neurological effects can be induced in the second and third trimesters.[13]

See the eBook for expanded content and a complete reference list.

Table 7.1 Etiology of Human Congenital Malformations Observed During the First Year of Life

Suspected Cause	Percent of Total
Unknown	65-75
Polygenic	
Multifactorial (gene-environment interactions)	
Spontaneous errors of development	
Synergistic interactions of teratogens	
Genetic	15-25
Autosomal and sex-linked inherited genetic disease	
Cytogenetic (chromosomal abnormalities)	
New mutations	
Environmental	10
Maternal conditions: alcoholism, diabetes, endocrinopathies, phenylketonuria, smoking and nicotine, starvation, nutritional deficits	4
Infectious agents: rubella, toxoplasmosis, syphilis, herpes simplex, cytomegalovirus, varicella zoster, Venezuelan equine encephalitis, parvovirus B19	3
Mechanical problems (deformations): amniotic band constrictions, umbilical cord constraint, disparity in uterine size and uterine contents	1-2
Chemicals, prescription drugs, high-dose ionizing radiation, hyperthermia	<1

Modified from Brent RL. Environmental factors: miscellaneous. In: Brent RL, Harris M, eds. *Prevention of Embryonic, Fetal and Perinatal Disease.* John E. Fogarty International Center for Advanced Study in the Health Sciences, NIH; 1976:211.

Dose of the Exposure

The quantitative correlation between the magnitude of the teratogenic effects and the dose of a drug, chemical, or other agent is referred to as the dose-response relationship (**Table 7.3**). For example, a substance given in large enough amounts to cause maternal toxicity is also likely to have deleterious effects on the embryo such as death, growth restriction, or disrupted development. Several considerations affect the interpretation of dose-response relationships and must be carefully reviewed.

Threshold Dose

The threshold dose is the dose below which the incidence of death, malformation, growth restriction, or functional deficit is not statistically greater than that of control subjects (**Table 7.4**).

The incidence and severity of malformations produced by most exogenous teratogenic agents that have been appropriately studied have exhibited threshold phenomena during organogenesis.[1,16]

Genetic Susceptibilities

The genetic constitution of an organism is an important factor in the susceptibility of a species to a drug or chemical. Many disorders of increased sensitivity to drug toxicity or effects in the human may result from an inherited gene or trait.[17]

Environmental Agents Resulting in Toxicity

Table 7.5 lists examples of environmental agents that have resulted in reproductive toxicity and/or congenital malformations in humans. **Table 7.6** lists agents that have had concerns raised about their reproductive effects but after a careful and complete evaluation, have not been found to represent an increased reproductive risk.[18-20]

Interpretation of Animal Study Data

Whole animal teratology studies are helpful in raising concerns about the reproductive effects of drugs and chemicals; however, negative animal studies do not guarantee that these agents are free from reproductive effects in humans.

Well-performed epidemiologic studies still represent a strong methodology for determining the risks and effects of environmental toxicants on humans.

Evaluating Animal Studies to Determine the Potential Risk in Humans

When utilizing animal data to assess the potential risk of a drug or chemical exposure in humans, it is important to critically evaluate the studies using the basic principles of teratology guidelines. One of the

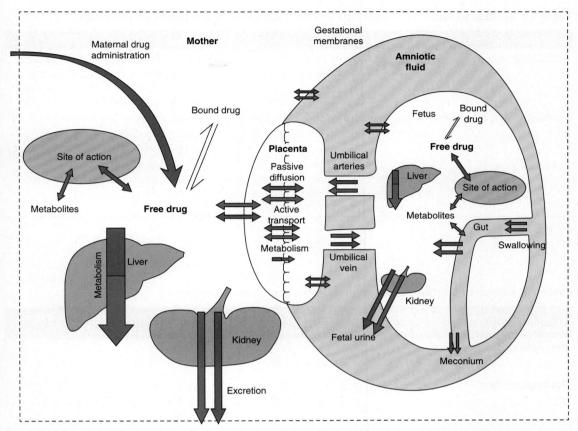

Figure 7.1 Drug disposition in mother and fetus after maternal drug administration. A variety of pharmacokinetic variables, including transplacental transport and metabolism, determine the degree of maternal-to-fetal drug transfer and fetal drug exposure. Red arrows represent parent drug, and blue arrows represent metabolites. The size of the arrows approximates relative importance, although this is drug dependent and will vary during pregnancy with fetal and placental maturation.

(Adapted with permission from Syme MR, Paxton JW, Keelan JA. Drug transfer and metabolism by the human placenta. *Clin Pharmacokinet.* 2004;43(8):487-514, Figure 1.)

most critical factors for consideration is the dose or magnitude of the exposure, and the concept of the threshold-dose effect for reproductive toxicants. A major shortcoming in many studies is the use of weight (mg/kg) as a measure of dose, as dose comparisons based on mg/kg doses are, at best, rough approximations.

One useful aspect of animal studies is in corroborating findings reported in epidemiological studies.

For physicians in practice, reliable and practical sources of information concerning animal testing must be available. This may come from the drug package insert, manufacturer's website, database sites such as REPROTOX, or the Physicians' Desk Reference.[27,28]

The modernized FDA system seeks to give individualized data that are more useful for clinicians. Termed the Pregnancy and Lactation Labelling Final Rule, the new system went into general effect in 2015.[32] Replacing the five categories, the new labeling requires a narrative summarizing the available *in vitro*, animal and human data. The risks are reviewed for pregnancy, lactation, and individuals with reproductive potential.

Table 7.2 Concepts/Factors That Affect the Interpretation of Dose-Response Relationships

Concept	Description	Example
Active metabolites	Metabolites may be the proximate teratogen Rather than the administered drug or chemical	The metabolite phosphoramide mustard and acrolein may produce abnormal development resulting from the metabolism of cyclophosphamide
Duration of exposure	A chronic exposure to a prescribed drug can contribute to an increased teratogenic risk	Anticonvulsant therapy; in contrast an acute exposure to the same drug may present little or no teratogenic risk
Fat solubility	Fat-soluble substances can produce fetal malformations for an extended period after the last ingestion or exposure because they have an unusually long half-life	Polychlorinated biphenyls (PCBs). Etretinate may present a similar risk but the data are not conclusive

Table 7.3 Estimated Outcome of Pregnancy Versus Time From Conception

Time From Conception	Percent Survival to Term[a]	Percent Loss During Interval[a]	Last Time for Induction of Selected Malformations[b]
Preimplantation			
0-6 d	25	54.55	—
Postimplantation			
7-13 d	55	24.66	—
14-20 d	73	8.18	—
3-5 wk	79.5	7.56	22-23 d: cyclopia, sirenomelia, microtia
			26 d: anencephaly
			28 d: meningomyelocele
			34 d: transposition of great vessels
6-9 wk	90	6.52	36 d: cleft lip
			6 wk: diaphragmatic hernia, rectal atresia, ventricular septal defect, syndactyly
			9 wk: cleft palate
10-13 wk	92	4.42	10 wk: omphalocele; 12 wk: hypospadias
14-17 wk	96.26	1.33	—
18-21 wk	97.56	0.85	—
22-25 wk	98.39	0.31	—
26-29 wk	98.69	0.30	—
30-33 wk	98.98	0.30	—
34-37 wk	99.26	0.34	—
38+ wk	99.32	0.68	38+ wk: CNS cell depletion

[a]An estimated 50% to 70% of all human miscarriages occur in the first 3 weeks of gestation.[14,15]
[b]Modified from Schardein J. *Chemically Induced Birth Defects.* 2nd ed. Marcel Dekker; 1993.

Table 7.4 Stochastic and Threshold Dose-Response Relationships of Diseases Produced by Environmental Agents

Relationship	Pathology	Site	Diseases	Risk	Definition
Stochastic phenomena	Damage to a single cell may result in disease	DNA	Cancer, mutation	Some risk exists at all dosages; at low exposures, the risk is below the spontaneous risk	The incidence of the disease increases with the dose, but the severity and nature of the disease remain the same
Threshold phenomena	Multicellular injury	High variation in etiology, affecting many cell and organ processes	Malformation, growth retardation, death, chemical toxicity, *etc.*	No increased risk below the threshold dose	Both the severity and incidence of the disease increase with dose

Modified from Brent RL. Definition of a teratogen and the relationship of teratogenicity to carcinogenicity. *Teratology.* 1986;34:359-360.

Table 7.5 Proven Human Teratogens or Embryotoxins (Drugs, Chemicals, Milieu, and Physical Agents) That Result in Human Congenital Malformations

Reproductive Toxin	Alleged Effects
Aminopterin, methotrexate	Growth retardation, microcephaly, meningomyelocele, mental retardation, hydrocephalus, and cleft palate
Androgens	Along with high doses of some male-derived progestins, can cause masculinization of the developing fetus
Angiotensin-converting enzyme (ACE) inhibitors	Fetal hypotension syndrome in second and third trimester resulting in fetal kidney hypoperfusion and anuria, oligohydramnios, pulmonary hypoplasia, and cranial bone hypoplasia. No effect in the first trimester
Antituberculous therapy	The drugs isoniazid (INH) and para-aminosalicylic (PAS) acid have an increased risk for some CNS abnormalities
Caffeine	Moderate exposure not associated with birth defects; high exposures associated with an increased risk of abortion but data are inconsistent
Chorionic villus sampling (CVS)	Vascular disruptive malformations, ie, limb reduction defects
Cobalt in hematemic multivitamins	Fetal goiter
Cocaine	Very low incidence of vascular disruptive malformations, pregnancy loss
Corticosteroids	High exposures administered systemically have a low risk for cleft palate in some epidemiological studies; however, this is not a consistent finding
Coumarin derivative	Exposure during early pregnancy can result in nasal hypoplasia, stippling of secondary epiphysis, and intrauterine growth retardation. Exposure in late pregnancy can result in CNS malformations as a result of bleeding
Cyclophosphamide and other chemotherapeutic and immunosuppressive agents, eg, cyclosporine, leflunomide	Many chemotherapeutic agents used to treat cancer have a theoretical risk of producing fetal malformations (most are teratogenic in animals); however, clinical data are not consistent. Many have not been shown to be teratogenic, but the numbers of cases in the studies are small; caution is the byword

(Continued)

Table 7.5 Proven Human Teratogens or Embryotoxins (Drugs, Chemicals, Milieu, and Physical Agents) That Result in Human Congenital Malformations (Continued)

Reproductive Toxin	Alleged Effects
Diethylstilbestrol	Genital abnormalities, adenosis, and clear cell adenocarcinoma of the vagina in adolescents. The risk of adenosis can be quite high; the risk of adenocarcinoma is 1:1000-1:10,000
Ethyl alcohol	Fetal alcohol syndrome (microcephaly, mental retardation, growth retardation, typical facial dysmorphogenesis, abnormal ears, and small palpebral fissures)
Ionizing radiation	A threshold greater than 20 rad (0.2 Gy) can increase the risk of some fetal effects such as microcephaly or growth retardation. The threshold for mental retardation is higher
Insulin shock therapy	Microcephaly and mental retardation
Lithium therapy	Chronic use for the treatment of manic depressive illness has an increased risk for Ebstein anomaly and other malformations, but risk appears to be very low
Minoxidil	Hirsutism in newborns (led to the discovery of the hair growth-promoting properties of minoxidil)
Methimazole	Aplasia cutis has been reported[a]
Methylene blue intra-amniotic instillation	Fetal intestinal atresia, hemolytic anemia, and jaundice in the neonatal period. This procedure is no longer utilized to identify one twin
Misoprostol	Low incidence of vascular disruptive phenomena, such as limb reduction defects and Mobius syndrome, has been reported in pregnancies in which this drug was used to induce an abortion
Penicillamine (D-penicillamine)	This drug results in the physical effects referred to as lathyrism, the results of poisoning by the seeds of the genus *Lathyrus*. It causes collagen disruption, cutis laxa, and hyperflexibility of joints. The condition appears to be reversible and risk is low
Progestin therapy	Very high doses of androgen hormone–derived progestins can produce masculinization. Many drugs with progestational activity do not have masculinizing potential. None of these drugs has the potential for producing congenital malformations
Propylthiouracil	Along with other antithyroid medications can result in an infant born with a goiter
Radioactive isotopes	Tissue- and organ-specific damage is dependent on the radioisotope element and distribution, ie, high doses of ^{131}I administered to a pregnant woman can cause fetal thyroid hypoplasia after the eighth week of development
Retinoids, systemic	Systemic retinoic acid, isotretinoin, and etretinate can result in an increased risk of CNS; cardio-aortic, ear, and clefting defects; microtia; anotia; thymic aplasia and other branchial arch and aortic arch abnormalities; and certain congenital heart malformations
Retinoids, topical	This is very unlikely to have teratogenic potential because teratogenic serum levels are not achieved from topical exposure
Streptomycin	Streptomycin and a group of ototoxic drugs can affect the eighth nerve and interfere with hearing; it is a relatively low-risk phenomenon. Children are even less sensitive to the ototoxic effects of these drugs than adults
Sulfa drug and vitamin K	Hemolysis in some subpopulations of fetuses
Tetracycline	Bone and teeth staining
Thalidomide	Increased incidence of deafness, anotia, preaxial limb reduction defects, phocomelia, ventricular septal defects, and GI atresias during susceptible period from the 22nd to the 36th day post conception
Trimethoprim	This drug was frequently used to treat urinary tract infections and has been linked to an increased incidence of neural tube defects. The risk is not high, but it is biologically plausible because of the drug's lowering effect on folic acid levels. This has also resulted in neurological symptoms in adults taking this drug

Table 7.5 Proven Human Teratogens or Embryotoxins (Drugs, Chemicals, Milieu, and Physical Agents) That Result in Human Congenital Malformations   (Continued)

Reproductive Toxin	Alleged Effects
Vitamin A (retinol)	Very high doses of vitamin A have been reported to produce the same malformations as those reported for the retinoids. Dosages sufficient to produce birth defects would have to be in excess of 25,000-50,000 U/d
Vitamin D[a]	Large doses given in vitamin D prophylaxis are possibly involved in the etiology of supravalvular aortic stenosis, elfin facies, and mental retardation
Warfarin (coumarin)	Exposure during early pregnancy can result in nasal hypoplasia, stippling of secondary epiphysis, and intrauterine growth retardation. Exposure in late pregnancy can result in CNS malformations as a result of bleeding
Anticonvulsants	
Carbamazepine	Used in the treatment of convulsive disorders; increases the risk of facial dysmorphology
Diphenylhydantoin	Used in the treatment of convulsive disorders; increases the risk of fetal hydantoin syndrome, consisting of facial dysmorphology, cleft palate, ventricular septal defect (VSD), and growth and mental retardation
Trimethadione and paramethadione	Used in the treatment of convulsive disorders; increases the risk of characteristic facial dysmorphology, mental retardation, V-shaped eyebrows, low-set ears with anteriorly folded helix, high-arched palate, irregular teeth, CNS anomalies, and severe developmental delay
Valproic acid	Used in the treatment of convulsive disorders; increases the risk of spina bifida, facial dysmorphology, and autism
Chemicals	
Carbon monoxide poisoning[a]	CNS damage has been reported with very high exposures, but the risk appears to be low
Gasoline addiction embryopathy	Facial dysmorphology, mental retardation
Lead	Very high exposures can cause pregnancy loss; intrauterine teratogenesis is not established
Methyl mercury	Causes Minamata disease consisting of cerebral palsy, microcephaly, mental retardation, blindness, and cerebellum hypoplasia. Endemics have occurred from adulteration of wheat with mercury-containing chemicals that are used to prevent grain spoilage. Present environmental levels of mercury are unlikely to represent a teratogenic risk, but reducing or limiting the consumption of carnivorous fish has been suggested in order not to exceed the Environmental Protection Agency's (EPA's) maximum permissible exposure (MPE), which is far below the toxic effects of mercury
Polychlorinated biphenyls	Poisoning has occurred from adulteration of food products (cola-colored babies, CNS effects, pigmentation of gums, nails, teeth and groin, hypoplastic deformed nails, intrauterine growth retardation, abnormal skull calcification). The threshold exposure has not been determined, but it is unlikely to be teratogenic at the present environmental exposures
Toluene addiction embryopathy	Facial dysmorphology, mental retardation
Embryonic and Fetal Infections	
Cytomegalovirus	Retinopathy, CNS calcification, microcephaly, mental retardation
Herpes simplex virus	Fetal infection, liver disease, death
Human immunodeficiency virus (HIV)	Perinatal HIV infection

(Continued)

Table 7.5 Proven Human Teratogens or Embryotoxins (Drugs, Chemicals, Milieu, and Physical Agents) That Result in Human Congenital Malformations (Continued)

Reproductive Toxin	Alleged Effects
Parvovirus B19 infection	Stillbirth, hydrops
Rubella virus	Deafness, congenital heart disease, microcephaly, cataracts, mental retardation
Syphilis	Maculopapular rash, hepatosplenomegaly, deformed nails, osteochondritis at joints of extremities, congenital neurosyphilis, abnormal epiphyses, chorioretinitis
Toxoplasmosis	Hydrocephaly, microphthalmia, chorioretinitis, mental retardation
Varicella zoster virus	Skin and muscle defects, intrauterine growth retardation, limb reduction defects, CNS damage (very low increased risk)
Venezuelan equine encephalitis	Hydranencephaly, microphthalmia, CNS destructive lesions, luxation of hip
Maternal Disease States	
Corticosteroid-secreting endocrinopathy	Mothers with Cushing disease can have infants with hyperadrenocortism, but anatomical malformations do not appear to be increased
Iodine deficiency	Iodine deficiency can result in embryonic goiter and mental retardation
Intrauterine problems of constraint and vascular disruption	Defects such as club feet, limb reduction, aplasia cutis, cranial asymmetry, external ear malformations, midline closure defects, cleft palate and muscle aplasia, cleft lip, omphalocele, and encephalocele. More common in multiple-birth pregnancies, pregnancies with anatomical defects of the uterus, placental emboli, and amniotic bands
Maternal androgen endocrinopathy (adrenal tumors)	Masculinization
Maternal diabetes	Caudal and femoral hypoplasia, transposition of great vessels
Folic acid insufficiency in the mother	Increased incidence of neural tube defects (NTDs)
Maternal phenylketonuria	Abortion, microcephaly, and mental retardation. Very high risk in untreated patients
Maternal starvation	Intrauterine growth retardation, abortion, NTDs
Tobacco smoking	Abortion, intrauterine growth retardation, and stillbirth
Zinc deficiency[a]	NTDs

[a]Controversial.

Table 7.6 Agents Erroneously Alleged to Have Caused Human Malformations

Agent	Alleged Effect
Doxylamine succinate (Bendectin)	Alleged to cause numerous types of birth defects including limb reduction defects and heart malformations
Diagnostic ultrasonography	No significant hyperthermia, therefore no reproductive effects
Electromagnetic fields (EMF)	Alleged to cause abortion, cancer, and birth defects
Progestational drugs	Alleged to cause numerous types of congenital birth defects, including limb reduction defects and heart malformations
Trichloroethylene (TCE)	Alleged to cause cardiac defects

Table 7.7 Pregnancy-Related Physiological Alterations in the Mother That Affect Drug Pharmacokinetics

Alteration	Effect on Drug Pharmacokinetics
Decreased gastrointestinal motility; increased intestinal transit time	Results in delayed absorption of drugs in the small intestine owing to increased stomach retention and enhanced absorption of slowly absorbed drugs
Decreased plasma albumin	Alters the kinetics of compounds normally bound to albumin
Renal elimination	Generally increased but is influenced by body position later in pregnancy
Increased plasma and extracellular fluid volumes	Affects concentration-dependent transfer of compounds
Inhibition of metabolic inactivation in the maternal liver	Increases half-life of drug in plasma
Variation in uterine blood flow	May affect transfer across the placenta (although little is known concerning this)

Based on concepts from Jackson M. Drug absorption. In: Fabro S, Scialli A, eds. *Drug and Chemical Action in Pregnancy: Pharmacologic and Toxicologic Principles*. Marcel Dekker; 1986:15, Mattison D. Physiologic variations in pharmacokinetics during pregnancy. In: Fabro S, Scialli A, eds. *Drug and Chemical Action During Pregnancy: Pharmacologic and Toxicologic Principles*. Marcel Dekker; 1986:37-102, and Sonawane B, Yaffe S. Physiologic disposition of drugs in the fetus and newborn. In: Fabro S, Scialli A, eds. *Drug and Chemical Action in Pregnancy: Pharmacologic and Toxicologic Principles*. Marcel Dekker; 1986:103.

Pharmacokinetics and Metabolism of Medications or Chemical

Table 7.7 outlines some examples of pregnancy-related physiological alterations in the mother and fetus, respectively, that can affect the pharmacokinetics of medications.[33,34]

Juchau[37] has defined several experimental criteria to suggest that a suspected metabolite is responsible for the *in vivo* teratogenic effects of a chemical or drug (**Table 7.9**). These criteria may explain why there are marked qualitative and quantitative differences in the species response to a teratogenic agent.

Placental Transport

Most medications and chemicals cross the placenta, and only selected proteins, whose actions are species specific, will cross the placental barrier in one species but not another.

The factors that determine the ability of a drug or chemical to cross the placenta and reach the embryo include molecular weight, lipid affinity or solubility, polarity or degree of ionization, protein binding, and receptor mediation (**Figure 7.2**).

The concentration of an agent in the fetal compartment may also play a role in teratogenesis.

Table 7.9 Criteria to Suggest a Suspected Metabolite Is Responsible for Drug/Chemical Teratogenic Effects *In Vivo*

- The chemical must be convertible to the intermediate
- The intermediate must be found in, or have access to, the tissue(s) affected
- The embryotoxic effect should increase with the concentration of the metabolite
- Inhibiting the conversion should reduce the embryotoxic effect of the agent
- Promoting the conversion should increase the embryotoxicity of the agent
- Inhibiting or promoting conversion should not alter the target tissues
- Inhibiting the conversion should increase the embryotoxicity of the agent

Adapted from Juchau M. Bioactivation in chemical teratogenesis. *Annu Rev Pharmacol Toxicol*. 1989;29:165-187.

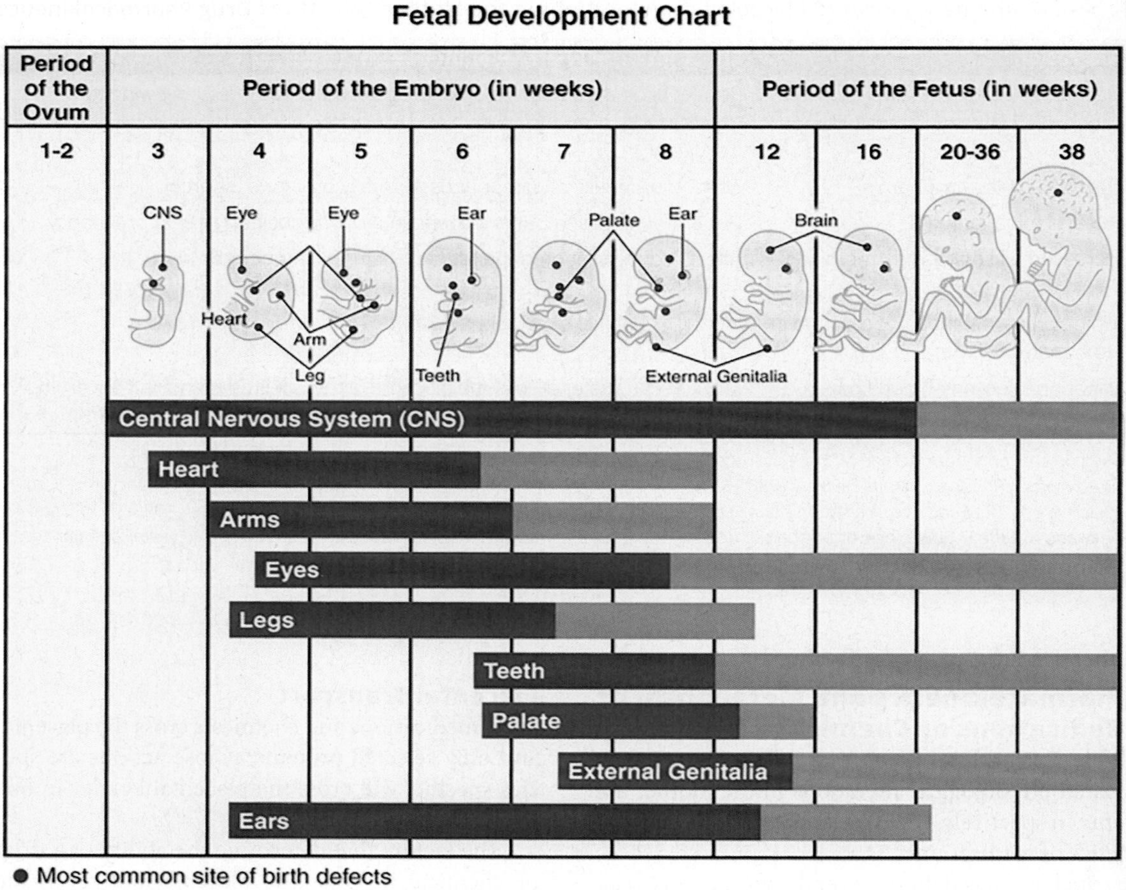

Fetal Development Chart

● Most common site of birth defects

Figure 7.2 Critical period during fetal development when teratogens result in major structural malformation.

The Role of the Physician in Counseling Families

The clinician must be cognizant of the fact that many patients believe that the majority of congenital malformations are caused by a drug or medication taken during pregnancy. Counseling patients about reproductive risks requires a significant degree of knowledge, skill, and sensitivity. Clinicians must also realize that erroneous counseling may result in undue stress, anxiety, and sometimes even legal action.

Only a small percentage of birth defects result from exposure to prescribed medications,[31] chemicals, and physical agents. Even when the drug is listed as a teratogen, to exert a teratogenic effect, it has to be administered during the sensitive period of development for that drug and above the threshold dose. Furthermore, the anomalies in a child should be the same as the malformations in the teratogenic syndrome produced by that particular drug.

Clinical Evaluation

In addition to the usual history and physical evaluation, the physician has to obtain information about the nature, magnitude, and timing of the exposure. The physical examination should include descriptive and quantitative information about the physical characteristics of the child.

KEY POINTS

- Environmental causes account for approximately 10% of human birth malformations, and fewer than 3% of all human malformations are related to prescription drug exposure, chemicals, or radiation.
- Only a small percentage of birth defects are due to prescribed drugs, chemicals, and physical agents. Even when a drug is listed as a teratogen, it has to be administered during the sensitive period of development, and above the threshold dose for producing teratogenesis.
- The etiology of congenital malformations can be divided into three categories: unknown (65%-75%), genetic (15%-25%), and environmental (10%).
- Clinicians should recognize the importance of providing accurate and compassionate counseling about reproductive risks to women exposed to drugs and chemicals during preconception and pregnancy.
- The application of the basic scientific principles of teratology is extremely important in evaluating studies on the reproductive effects of an environmental agent. These principles include the following criteria: the exposure follows a toxicological dose-response curve; the gestational age at which exposure occurs determines what effects (if any) a teratogen has; most teratogens have a consistent group of congenital malformations; and no teratogen can produce every type of malformation.
- The threshold dose for an environmental toxin is the dose below which the incidence of death, malformation, growth restriction, or developmental delays is not greater than that of control subjects.
- Teratogens follow a threshold dose-response curve, whereas mutagens and carcinogens tend to follow a stochastic dose-response curve.
- Physiological alterations in pregnancy and the bioconversion of compounds can significantly influence the teratogenic effects of drugs and chemicals by affecting absorption, body distribution, active form(s), and excretion of the compound.

- Interpretation of dose-response relationships for teratogens must take into account the active metabolites, when metabolites might be the proximate teratogen rather than the administered drug or chemical, the duration of the exposure, and the fat solubility of the agent.
- The role that the placenta plays in drug pharmacokinetics involves transport, the presence of receptors for a number of compounds, and the bioconversion of xenobiotics.
- The genetic variability of an individual is an important factor that affects the susceptibility to a drug or chemical.
- Advances in animal research and epidemiology have enabled scientists to gain a better understanding of the mechanisms and patterns of teratogenesis. Animal teratology studies are helpful in raising concerns about the reproductive effects of drugs and chemicals but are not always generalizable to humans. There are examples of false-positive and false-negative studies in animal populations.
- Well-performed epidemiology studies represent a strong methodology for determining the human risk and the effects of environmental teratogens.
- *In vitro* tests can be used to study the mechanisms of teratogenesis and for preliminary screening studies. However, *in vitro* studies cannot predict human teratogenic risks at particular exposures without the benefit of data obtained from whole animal studies and epidemiological studies.
- The clinician must be able access current, accurate information about the risks for drugs or other exposures taken during pregnancy. Consultation should also be available for complex cases.
- Patients with known exposures should receive detailed counseling about risks/benefits and alternatives when possible. Detailed anatomic ultrasound surveys should be offered as well as serial fetal growth assessments. Multispecialty care is often preferable, potentially involving

Maternal-Fetal Medicine, Genetics, Neonatology, Developmental Pediatrics, and several others.

- The evaluation of the toxicity of drugs and chemicals should (when possible) use data obtained from investigative approaches including (1) epidemiological studies, (2) trend analysis, (3) animal reproductive studies, (4) dose-response relationships, (5) mechanisms of action studies that pertain specifically to the agent, and (6) biological plausibility.

REFERENCES

(only references cited in synoptic print chapter; for a complete reference list, see ebook)

1. Mai CT, Isenburg JL, Canfield MA, et al. National population-based estimates for major birth defects, 2010-2014. *Birth Defects Res.* 2019;111(18):1420-1435. doi:10.1002/bdr2.1589

4. Adam MP, Polifka JE, Friedman JM. Evolving knowledge of the teratogenicity of medications in human pregnancy. *Am J Med Genet C Semin Med Genet.* 2011;157:175-182.

12. Scheuerle A, Aylsworth A. Birth defects and neonatal morbidity caused by teratogen exposure after the embryonic period. *Birth Defects Res A Clin Mol Teratol.* 2016;106:935-939.

13. Hendrix N, Berghella V. Non-placental causes of intrauterine growth restriction. *Semin Perinatol.* 2008;32(3):161-165.

14. Moscovitz J, Alexsunes L. Establishment of metabolism and transport pathways in the rodent and human fetal liver. *Int J Mo Sci.* 2013;14(12):23801-23827.

15. Zhang T, Gao S, Shen Z, et al. Use of selective serotonin-reuptake inhibitors in the first trimester and risk of cardiovascular-related malformations: a meta-analysis of cohort studies. *Sci Rep.* 2017;7:43085.

16. Gilbert-Barness E. Teratogenic causes of malformations. *Ann Clin Lab Sci.* 2010;40(2):99-114.

17. Cassina M, Salviati L, Gianantonio E, Clementi M. Genetic susceptibility to teratogens: state of the art. *Reprod Toxicol.* 2012;34(2):186-191.

18. McKeigue PM, Lamm S, Linn S, Kutcher JS. Bendectin and birth defects: I. A meta-analysis of the epidemiologic studies. *Teratology.* 1994;50(1):27-37.

19. Vedel C, Larsen H, Andreason K, et al. Long-term effects of prenatal progesterone exposure: neurophysiological development and hospital admissions in twins up to 8 years of age. *Ultrasound Obstet Gynecol.* 2016;48(3):382-389.

20. DeSasso J, Coder P, York R, et al. Trichloroethylene in drinking water throughout gestation did not produce congenital heart defects in Sprague Dawley rats. *Birth Defects Res.* 2019;111(16):1217-1233.

27. REPROTOX®. Accessed August 1, 2019. www.reprotox.org

28. *Physician's Desk Reference.* 71st ed. PDR Network, LLC; 2017.

31. Friedman J, Little B, Brent RL, Cordero JF, Hanson JW, Shepard TH. Potential human teratogenicity of frequently prescribed drugs. *Obstet Gynecol.* 1990;75:594-599.

32. Pernia S, DeMaagd G. The new pregnancy and lactation labeling rule. *P T.* 2016;41(11):713-715.

33. Bedson R, Riccoboni A. Physiology of pregnancy: clinical anesthetic implications. *Contin Educ Anaesth Crit Care Pain.* 2014;14(2):69-72.

34. Feghali M, Venkataramanan R, Caritas S. Pharmacokinetics of drugs in pregnancy. *Semin Perinatol.* 2015;39(7):512-519.

37. Juchau M. Bioactivation in chemical teratogenesis. *Annu Rev Pharmacol Toxicol.* 1989;29:165-187.

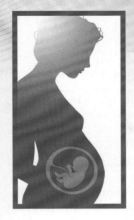

CHAPTER 8

The Effects of Illicit Drug and Alcohol Use in Pregnancy

Katrina Schafer Mark

Introduction

Illicit drug, alcohol, and tobacco use in pregnancy has known risks. As it is the rare exception that a woman will initiate use of these substances during pregnancy, the best strategy to reduce the risk of substance exposure in newborns is to provide comprehensive screening and counseling to women prior to pregnancy.

There is evidence that engagement in prenatal care can significantly improve the outcomes of pregnancies in women who use drugs.[8-11] This may mean that prenatal care is effective in helping women with harm reduction, or it may mean that many of the risks attributed to drug use are actually caused by lack of access to or engagement in care. Notably, punitive action against women who use drugs in pregnancy has not been shown to decrease drug use or improve outcomes, but has been shown to deter women from seeking care.[11,12] This highlights the importance of improving access to compassionate, nonjudgmental care to all women to allow for the best possible maternal and neonatal outcomes.

Women with substance use disorders are more likely to present later for obstetric care. This is likely multifactorial with issues such as late recognition of pregnancy due to irregular menses, lack of access to care, psychosocial issues, and fear of judgment or reprisal from members of the healthcare system. Because one in four people with a substance use disorder also suffer from a mental health disorder, often undiagnosed,[13] increased access to substance use treatment, mental health services, and comprehensive preconception counseling and contraception is paramount.

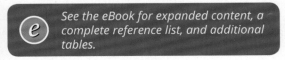

See the eBook for expanded content, a complete reference list, and additional tables.

Alcohol

Alcohol exposure *in utero* is a leading cause of preventable mental disabilities. Pregnant women are advised to avoid alcohol during routine preconception and antenatal care.

The worldwide prevalence of fetal alcohol spectrum disorder (FASD) is estimated to be approximately 7.7 in 1000 births.[16] Estimates of FASD prevalence in the overall US population in 2017 were 15 to 20 per 1000.[16] Although it is difficult to obtain more specific data, it is clear that all cases of full-blown FASD occurred in mothers with chronic alcohol abuse and in mothers who drank heavily throughout pregnancy. It is also clear that binge drinking (≥ 4 drinks during a single occasion) increases the risks of affected children having IQs in the range that is considered intellectual disability.[22]

Work has demonstrated an association between alcohol consumption in pregnancy and increased neurodegeneration via apoptosis (programmed cell death) during synaptogenesis,[26] defects in neuronal migration and decreased numbers of neurons in the mature cortex,[27] and effects on myelination leading to decreases in white matter volume.[28]

Alcohol ingestion by the gravida decreases fetal breathing movements but not gross body movements or fetal heart rate.[35] Alcohol withdrawal effects have been described, even in infants without the stigmata of FASD.[36] The fetal effects of alcohol appear to be multifactorial (**Table 8.1**).

There is no treatment or cure for FASD or alcohol-related birth defects. The best strategy is prevention, and the first component of prevention is educating women of childbearing age of the risks of drinking during pregnancy.

Another critical piece to preventing FASD is identifying mothers at risk. The CAGE (Cut down,

Table 8.1 Effects of Alcohol on the Fetus

Fetal alcohol syndrome—at least one from each of the following categories:

Growth restriction, either prenatal or postnatal in onset

   SGA/IUGR

   Failure to thrive/short stature

Craniofacial abnormalities

   Small eyes

   Epicanthal folds

   Long philtrum

   Midface hypoplasia

Central nervous system abnormalities

   Microcephaly

   Developmental delay

   Mental retardation

   Learning disabilities

Alcohol-related birth defects—any of the preceding problems in the offspring of an alcoholic individual

IUGR, intrauterine growth restriction; SGA, small-for-gestational age.

Annoyed, Guilt, Eye-opener) (**Table 8.3**), T-ACE (Take [number of drinks], Annoyed, Cut down, Eye-opener)[38] (**Table 8.4**), and TWEAK (Tolerance, Worried, Eye-opener, Amnesia, K/Cut down)[39] (**Table 8.5**) questionnaires include basic questions that are effective tools in patient management.

Once an individual at increased risk for having a child with alcohol-related birth defects is identified, attention should be turned to intervention. Counseling programs have proven effective in reducing chronic and binge drinking. Even when a history of alcohol consumption has been identified, interruption of pregnancy is not a recommended intervention because the risks of adverse perinatal outcomes associated with low-level alcohol consumption, or even occasional binges of marked consumption, have not been clearly quantified to date.

Cocaine

Cocaine use among pregnant women varies widely and has been reported in 8% to 24% of pregnant women.[46,47]

Maternal Effects

Medical complications reported with cocaine use include acute myocardial infarction, cardiac arrhythmias, aortic rupture, subarachnoid hemorrhage, strokes, ischemic bowel damage, and

Table 8.3 *CAGE* Questionnaire

1. Have you ever felt the need to **C**ut down drinking?
2. Have you ever felt **A**nnoyed by criticism of your drinking?
3. Have you ever had **G**uilty feelings about drinking?
4. Have you ever taken a morning "**E**ye-opener"?

various other problems in the nonpregnant population.[48] These same complications occur in pregnant women, and a report of intracerebral hemorrhage during the postpartum period confirms that expectation[51] (**Table 8.6**).

Fetal/Neonatal Effects

Withdrawal has been reported in neonates exposed to cocaine. Overall, however, studies have not generally found that cocaine adversely affects mental and motor outcomes.[73,74] Better birth outcomes for cocaine-exposed pregnancies can be achieved by a combination of specialized prenatal care and drug treatment.[8]

Opioids

Opioids are a class of drugs that include morphine, fentanyl, oxycodone, hydrocodone, methadone, and heroin.

Maternal Effects

During pregnancy, much focus is on the effects of opioids on the developing fetus, but these drugs also affect maternal health. Opioids can have direct health consequences, such as opioid-induced constipation, which can be worsened in pregnancy. Many women may also experience hyperalgesia related to chronic opioid use, which makes them experience pain in a more pronounced way.

The most severe health consequence related to opioid use is overdose. Opioid use disorder is associated with a high rate of risk-taking behavior, including risky sexual behavior, needle sharing, and driving while under the influence.[86]

Table 8.4 T-ACE Questionnaire

1. How many drinks can you hold? (**T**olerance)
2. Have you ever felt **A**nnoyed by criticism of your drinking?
3. Have you ever felt the need to **C**ut down drinking?
4. Have you ever taken a morning "**E**ye-opener"?

Table 8.5 TWEAK Questionnaire

Tolerance: How many drinks does it take before you feel the effects of alcohol? (2 points for ≥ 3 drinks)

Worry: Have close friends or family worried or complained about your drinking in the past year? (2 points for yes)

Eye-opener: Do you sometimes take a drink in the morning when you wake up? (1 point for yes)

Amnesia: Are there times when you drink and afterward cannot remember what you said or did? (1 point for yes)

Cut down: Do you sometimes feel the need to cut down on your drinking? (1 point for yes)

Infectious complications of injection drug use are common. The most significant infectious risk facing intravenous drug users and their offspring now is the danger of acquired immunodeficiency syndrome. In addition, women who inject drugs also have an increased risk of abscesses at injection sites, which can lead to systemic infections and sepsis. There is also an increased risk of pneumonia.

Fetal/Neonatal Effects

Opioids cross the placenta and enter the fetal bloodstream. Birth outcomes may also be affected by opioid use; specifically, women with opioid use and use disorders are more likely to deliver low birth weight infants (**Table 8.7**).[91]

Neonatal Abstinence Syndrome

The most striking neonatal effects of perinatal opioid use disorder are neonatal abstinence syndrome (NAS) or neonatal opioid withdrawal syndrome (NOWS).

Table 8.6 Reported Effects of Cocaine on the Fetus and Pregnancy

Placental abruption

Intrauterine growth restriction

Preterm labor

Premature rupture of the membranes with meconium

Spontaneous abortion

Intrauterine cerebral infarctions

Genitourinary tract anomalies

Neurobehavioral disorders

Table 8.7 Reported Effects of Heroin on Pregnancy

Fetal addiction

Intrauterine withdrawal/neonatal abstinence syndrome

Low birth weight

Behavioral teratogenesis

Sudden infant death syndrome

This syndrome includes tremors, restlessness, hyperreflexia, high-pitched cry, sneezing, sleeplessness, tachypnea, yawning, sweating, fever, and, in severe cases, seizures.[98] The onset of symptoms begins anywhere from birth to 5 days of age, depending on the half-life of the opioid to which the neonate was exposed *in utero*, and may persist for a month or more.[99]

Given that NAS/NOWS is caused by withdrawal from opiates, opiate replacement therapy is one of the mainstays of treatment for severe symptoms. Replacement therapy with morphine, methadone, and buprenorphine has been studied, with buprenorphine seemingly having the best short-term outcomes.[100]

NAS/NOW is an expected and manageable outcome of opiate use in pregnancy and should not deter physicians from prescribing medication-assisted therapy for women with opioid use disorder in pregnancy.

Treatment in Pregnancy

Since the 1970s, the standard treatment for opioid use disorder in pregnancy has been methadone. Buprenorphine and methadone were both deemed to be safe and beneficial in pregnancy. However, a woman cannot have recently taken opiates at the initiation of buprenorphine or it may precipitate withdrawal, leading some physicians to continue to prefer methadone due to the ability to prescribe it prior to the experience of withdrawal.

The combination of buprenorphine with naloxone is often used in opioid use disorders. Although there was initially concern for the possible effects of naloxone during pregnancy, subsequent studies have highlighted its efficacy and safety in pregnancy.[108,109]

Naltrexone, a long-acting opioid receptor antagonist that competitively binds and blocks the effects of opioids, has also been shown to be safe in pregnancy.[111]

Hallucinogens, Amphetamines, and Benzodiazapines

Phencyclidine (PCP) use has continued to a greater extent than lysergic acid diethylamide. PCP appears in umbilical cord plasma and amniotic fluid from human pregnancies, and the human placenta is an active site for conversion of PCP to its metabolic products *in vitro*.[114,115]

Case reports describe abnormal neonatal behavior, abnormal brain wave patterns, depressed interactive behaviors, and diminished organizational responses to stimuli in infants exposed to PCP *in utero,* but no epidemiologic studies have quantified the risk.[117-120] Finally, one study demonstrated an increased rate of preterm delivery and meconium-stained amniotic fluid in children exposed to PCP *in utero.*[121]

Adverse pregnancy outcomes, such as preterm birth and low birth weight, have been shown to be increased in women who use methamphetamines, but stopping use improves outcomes and no long-term effects have been noted.[122-124]

Benzodiazepines may be used for psychiatric disorders but are also a commonly misused/abused category of drugs. Although data are limited, there is some suggestion of increased risk of birth defects.[125] Benzodiazepines have a high addiction potential due to their likelihood of physical dependency. Maternal withdrawal from benzodiazepines can be severe and lead to seizures. Due to this, slow weaning is much safer than abrupt cessation.

Tobacco and Nicotine

Maternal smoking is associated with a wide variety of increased obstetric morbidities (**Table 8.8**). Pregnant women who use electronic cigarettes (e-cigarettes) should be counseled that their safety in pregnancy is unknown and their use as a harm reduction or cessation tool should not be overstated.

Attempts to modify smoking behavior during pregnancy have met with mixed success. Smoking during pregnancy continues to be a problem. Behavioral therapies are the first line of intervention. If these therapies fail, then pharmacological

Table 8.8 Obstetric Morbidities Among Pregnant Smokers

Spontaneous abortion
Ectopic pregnancy
Preterm delivery
Placenta previa
IUGR/low birth weight
Placental abruption
PPROM
Sudden infant death syndrome

IUGR, intrauterine growth restriction; PPROM, preterm premature rupture of membranes.

treatment with either bupropion or nicotine replacement treatments (NRTs) can be considered. Bupropion is a U.S. Food and Drug Administration (FDA) class B medication, and all the NRTs are FDA class C medications. A careful assessment of risks and benefits is necessary before starting these therapies in pregnancy.

Caffeine

Caffeine is fat soluble and crosses the placenta. There is no convincing evidence supporting a teratogenic or other adverse role of caffeine in pregnancy when taken in amounts equivalent to less than 10 cups of coffee per day. Pregnant women should be advised to use moderation in their caffeine intake, but it need not be avoided altogether.

Drug Use and Lactation

Many drugs and their metabolites, including alcohol, marijuana, cocaine, hallucinogens, opiates, and caffeine, can be excreted in breast milk. The dose that the infant is exposed to is significantly lower than that consumed by the mother. Some drugs, specifically cocaine, are found in relatively high concentrations in the breast milk and may have a higher potential impact.[181]

As the risk of exposure to drugs through breast milk is largely unknown, the American Academy of Pediatrics recommends that women who breastfeed abstain from consumption of drugs and alcohol. Although many women can achieve abstinence during pregnancy, the rates of relapse postpartum are extremely high.[5]

KEY POINTS

- Drug use in pregnancy is common and most women quit using by the third trimester, but relapse postpartum is high.
- Universal screening for drug use, misuse, and abuse should be performed at the initiation of prenatal care for counseling, treatment, and harm reduction to be maximized; punitive measures are counterproductive.
- Engagement in prenatal care improves many of the adverse prenatal outcomes seen with substance abuse in pregnancy.
- Drug effects on fetal development depend on the dose, the route of administration, physiologic handling of the drug by both the pregnant woman and the fetus, genetic predisposition, and timing of the exposure in the pregnancy.
- Fetal alcohol syndrome (FAS) occurs in 2.5% to 10% of offspring of heavy drinkers and includes growth restriction (either prenatal or postnatal in onset), craniofacial anomalies (small eyes, epicanthal folds, long philtrum, or midface hypoplasia), and central nervous system abnormalities (microcephaly, developmental delay, mental retardation, learning disabilities).
- The categories of alcohol-related birth defects include (1) FAS with confirmed maternal alcohol use; (2) FAS without confirmed maternal alcohol use but with characteristic malformations; (3) partial FAS with confirmed maternal alcohol use and some components of FAS; (4) alcohol-related birth defects with the presence of congenital anomalies resulting from prenatal alcohol exposure; and (5) alcohol-related neurodevelopmental abnormalities.
- Women at risk for problem drinking during pregnancy can be identified using the "CAGE," "T-ACE," or "TWEAK" questionnaires. Interventions in women so identified can decrease problem drinking by more than 50%.
- Drinking cessation before the third trimester of pregnancy will benefit the fetus, so it is never "too late."
- All studies of the impact and effects of a particular illicit drug on developing fetuses are complicated by problems in accurately

quantifying the exposure and the fact that polysubstance abuse is the rule and not the exception.
- Cocaine use during pregnancy is associated with an increased incidence of placental abruption (a side effect of vasoconstriction and hypertension), and this effect persists even if the pregnant cocaine user stops using in the first trimester.
- Maternal medical effects of cocaine use include acute myocardial infarction, cardiac arrhythmias, hypertension, aortic rupture, subarachnoid hemorrhage, and ischemic bowel damage.
- Fetal/neonatal effects of cocaine use in pregnancy include placental abruption, intrauterine growth restriction, preterm labor and delivery, increased incidence of genitourinary birth defects, and withdrawal.
- Medication-assisted therapy with methadone or buprenorphine for women with opioid use disorder significantly improves pregnancy outcomes.
- Structural teratogenicity has not been associated with opioid/narcotic use during pregnancy.
- NAS occurs in 50% to 80% of infants born to mothers chronically using opiates and includes tremors, restlessness, hyperreflexia, high-pitched cry, sneezing, sleeplessness, tachypnea, yawning, sweating, fever, and sometimes seizures.
- NAS is not dose dependent and should not be considered a complication, but rather an expected outcome when medication-assisted therapy is used in pregnancy.
- The major effects of tobacco present in the first trimester are decreased fecundity and increased pregnancy loss and in the second and third trimester as increased growth restriction and preterm labor and delivery.
- The increased incidence of low birth weight and preterm labor and delivery explains the 33% increase in overall perinatal and neonatal morbidity seen in pregnant smokers.
- Cigarette smoking during pregnancy is associated with an increased incidence of orofacial clefts.

(Continued)

- Smoking cessation interventions during pregnancy increase smoking cessation by 30% to 70% in smoking gravidae.
- Caffeine is teratogenic in rodents, but probably only in doses that are exceedingly difficult to achieve in humans (ie, >10 cups of coffee per day).

- Although women who breastfeed should be encouraged to abstain from substance use, in many circumstances, the benefits of breastfeeding outweigh the potential risks of drug exposure through breast milk in women who use illicit substances.

REFERENCES

(only references cited in synoptic print chapter; for a complete reference list, see ebook)

5. Forray A, Merry B, Lin H, Prah Ruger J, Yonkers K. Perinatal substance use: a prospective evaluation of abstinence and relapse. *Drug Alcohol Dep.* 2015;150:147-155.
8. Chazotte C, Youchah J, Freda MC. Cocaine use in pregnancy and low birth weight: the impact of prenatal care and drug treatment. *Semin Perinatol.* 1995;19:293.
9. El-Mohandes A, Herman A, El-Khorazaty M, Katta P, White D, Grylack L. Prenatal care reduces the impact of illicit drug use on perinatal outcomes. *J Perinatol.* 2003;23:354-360.
10. MacGregor SN, Keith LG, Bachicha JA, Chasnoff IJ. Cocaine abuse during pregnancy: correlation between prenatal care and perinatal outcome. *Obstet Gynecol.* 1989;74(6):882-885.
11. Roberts S, Pie C. Complex calculations: how drug use during pregnancy becomes a barrier to prenatal care. *Matern Child Health J.* 2011;15:333-341.
12. Patrick S, Schiff D; Committee on Substance Use and Prevention. A public health response to opioid use in pregnancy. *Pediatrics.* 2017;139(3):e20164070.
13. McCance-Katz E. *The National Survey on Drug Use and Health.* Department of Health and Human Services, Substance Abuse and Mental Health Service Administration; 2017. Accessed May 29, 2019. https://www.samhsa.gov/data/nsduh/reports-detailed-tables-2017-NSDUH
16. Lange S, Probst C, Gmel G, Rehm J, Burd L, Popova S. Global prevalence of fetal alcohol spectrum disorder among children and youth: a systemic review and meta-analysis. *JAMA Pediatr.* 2017;171(10):948-956.
22. Bailey BN, Delaney-Black V, Covington CY, et al. Prenatal exposure to binge drinking and cognitive and behavioral outcomes at age 7 years. *Am J Obstet Gynecol.* 2004;193:1037.
26. Ikonomidou C, Bittigau P, Ishimaru J, et al. Ethanol-induced apoptotic neurodegeneration and fetal alcohol syndrome. *Science.* 2000;287:1056.
27. Miller MW. Effects of alcohol on the generation and migration of cerebral cortical neurons. *Science.* 1986;233:1308.
28. Archibald SL, Gamst A, Riley EP, et al. Brain dysmorphology in individuals with severe prenatal alcohol exposure. *Dev Med Child Neurol.* 2001;43:148.
36. Coles CD, Smith IE, Fernhoff PM, et al. Neonatal ethanol withdrawal: characteristics in clinically normal, nondysmorphic neonates. *J Pediatr.* 1984;105:445.
38. Sokol RJ, Martier SS, Ager JW. The T-ACE questions: practical prenatal detection of risk drinking. *Am J Obstet Gynecol.* 1989;160:863.
39. Russell M, Martier SS, Sokol R, et al. Screening for pregnancy risk-drinking. *Alcohol Clin Exp Res.* 1994;18:1156.
46. Neerhof MG, MacGregor SN, Retzky SS, et al. Cocaine abuse during pregnancy: peripartum prevalence and perinatal outcome. *Am J Obstet Gynecol.* 1989;161:633.
47. Matera C, Warren WB, Moomjy M, et al. Prevalence of use of cocaine and other substances in an obstetric population. *Am J Obstet Gynecol.* 1990;163:797.
48. Creigler LL, Mark H. Special report: medical complications of cocaine abuse. *N Engl J Med.* 1986;315:1495.
51. Mercado A, Johnson G Jr, Calver D, et al. Cocaine, pregnancy, and post-partum intracerebral hemorrhage. *Obstet Gynecol.* 1989;73:467.

73. Coles C, Platzman K, Smith L. Effects of cocaine and alcohol use in pregnancy on neonatal growth and neurobehavioral status. *Neurotoxicol Teratol.* 1992;14:23.
74. Griffith D, Freier C. Methodological issues in the assessment of the mother-child interactions of substance-abusing women and their children. *NIDA Res Monogr.* 1992;117:228.
79. McLeod W, Brien J, Loomis C, et al. Effect of maternal ethanol ingestion on fetal breathing movements, gross body movements, and heart rate at 37 to 40 weeks' gestational age. *Am J Obstet Gynecol.* 1983;145:251.
86. Reece A. Experience of road and other trauma by the opiate dependent patient: a survey report. *Subst Abuse Treat Prev Policy.* 2008;3:1010.
91. Hulse GK, Milne E, English DR, et al. The relationship between maternal use of heroin and methadone and infant birth weight. *Addiction.* 1997;92:1571.
98. Finnegan LP, Connoughton IF, Kron RE, et al. Neonatal abstinence syndrome: assessment and management. In: Harbison RD, ed. *Perinatal Addiction.* Spectrum; 1975:141.
99. Kocherlakota P. Neonatal abstinence syndrome. *Pediatrics.* 2014;134(2):e547.
100. Disher T, Gullickson C, Signh B, et al. Pharmacologic treatments for Neonatal Abstinence Syndrome: a systemic review and network meta-analysis. *JAMA Pediatr.* 2019;173(3):234-243.
108. Juma N, Edwards C, Balfour-Boehm J, et al. Observational study of the safety of buprenorphine+naloxone in pregnancy in a rural and remote population. *BMJ Open.* 2016;6:e011774.
109. Wiegand SL, Stringer EM, Stuebe AM, Jones H, Seashore C, Thorp J. *Obstet Gynecol.* 2015;125(2):363-368.
111. Kelty E, Hulse G. A retrospective cohort study of birth outcomes in neonates exposed to naltrexone in utero: a comparison with methadone, buprenorphine and non-opioid exposed neonates. *Drugs.* 2017;77:1211-1219.
114. Kaufman KR, Petrucha RA, Pitts FN Jr, et al. Phencyclidine in umbilical cord blood: preliminary data. *Am J Psychol.* 1983;140:450.
115. Rayburn WF, Holsztynska EF, Domino EF. Phencyclidine: biotransformation by the human placenta. *Am J Obstet Gynecol.* 1984;148:111.
116. Petrucha RA, Kaufman KR, Pitts FN. Phencyclidine in pregnancy: a case report. *J Reprod Med.* 1982;27:301.
117. Chasnoff D, Burns KA, Burns WJ, et al. Prenatal drug exposure: effects on neonatal and infant growth and development. *Neurotoxicol Teratol.* 1986;8:357.
118. Golden NL, Sokol RI, Rubin IL. Angel dust: possible effects on the fetus. *Pediatrics.* 1980;65:18.
119. Van Dyke DC, Fox AA. Fetal drug exposure and its possible implications for learning in the preschool and school aged population. *J Learn Disabil.* 1990;23:160.
120. Strauss AA, Modanlou HD, Bosu SK. Neonatal manifestations of maternal phencyclidine (PCP) abuse. *Pediatrics.* 1981;68:550.
121. Tabor BL, Smith-Wallace T, Yonekura ML. Perinatal outcome associated with PCP versus cocaine use. *Am J Drug Alcohol Abuse.* 1990;16:337.
122. Smith L, LaGasse L, Derauf C, et al. Motor and cognitive outcomes through three years of age in children exposed to prenatal methamphetamine. *Neurotoxicol Teratol.* 2011;33(1):176-184.
123. Smith L, LaGasse L, Derauf C, et al. The infant development, environment and lifestyle study: effects of prenatal methamphetamine exposure, polydrug exposure, and poverty on intrauterine growth. *Pediatrics.* 2006;118(3):1149.

124. Wright T, Schuetter R, Tellei J, Sauvage L. Methamphetamines and pregnancy outcomes. *J Addict Med*. 2015;9(2):111-117.

125. Tinker SC, Reefhuis J, Bitsko RH, et al; National Birth Defects Prevention Study. Use of benzodiazepine medication during pregnancy and potential risk for birth defects, National birth defects prevention study, 1997-2011. *Birth Defects Res*. 2019;111(10):613-620.

181. Winecker RE, Goldberger BA, Tebbett IR, et al. Detection of cocaine and its metabolites in breast milk. *J Forensic Sci*. 2001;46(5):1221-1223.

CHAPTER 9

Radiation in Pregnancy

Jason K. Molitoris and James W. Snider

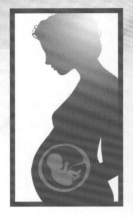

Introduction

Radiation is an important health concern during pregnancy for both the mother and fetus. Exposures are possible in a variety of forms, including in the workplace and at home, along with diagnostic and therapeutic medical interventions. Due to its widespread use, the exquisite sensitivity of the developing embryo, and potential for damaging exposure without knowledge, understanding the potential impacts and methods to safeguard pregnant women against radiation is critical.

Types of Radiation

Radiation is energy emitted as waves or particles and divided into two general types. Nonionizing radiation includes microwave, visible and ultraviolet light, ultrasound, and low frequency radiofrequency. The majority of studies, however, have not found a causal link between nonionizing radiation and undesired fetal effects.[1-3]

Nonionizing radiation is utilized frequently during assessment of *in utero* development. Ultrasound is routinely used in pregnancy, and causal relationships between prenatal ultrasonography and adverse effects have not been observed.[4,5] Magnetic resonance imaging (MRI) is another commonly used imaging modality utilized during pregnancy, especially when ultrasound findings are equivocal, and has also not demonstrated adverse outcomes.[6,7]

Ionizing radiation, on the other hand, has the ability to directly interact with molecules and can either directly or indirectly alter DNA. Actively dividing cells are more sensitive to the effects of radiation and, therefore, cells in the M and G1 cell phases of division are the most radiosensitive, whereas S-phase cells are the least sensitive due to their ability to repair DNA damage. Ionizing radiation causes both single- and double-strand DNA

breaks. Single-strand DNA breaks are typically repairable in an otherwise healthy cell; double-strand DNA breaks can lead to genetic alterations, including chromosomal alterations.[8]

Biological effects of radiation depend on the amount or radiation dose, defined as the energy absorbed per unit mass and measured in gray (Gy). In addition, both the type of radiation and the total amount of absorbed energy exert effects. To account for the role of different radiation types, the biological effect of radiation is expressed through the unit sievert (Sv) and is the product of the radiation dose (Gy) and radiation weighting factor for the type of radiation. For example, alpha particles, which cause a significant amount of damage in small places, have a weighting factor of 20, compared to photons, which are typically used in diagnostic and therapeutic radiation.[8]

Classically, the effects of ionizing radiation are separated into deterministic and stochastic.[9] Stochastic effects of radiation result from insults to the DNA that do not impede the replicative capacity of the cell. These alterations in the DNA can lead to potential consequences, including development of future malignancies. While stochastic effects increase linearly with the radiation dose, there is no minimum absorbed dose. This means that a single radiation-induced DNA change could potentiate a malignant transformation and strongly argues for limiting radiation expose to as low as reasonably achievable. The risk of stochastic effects is the basis for current radiation-related protection practices and standards.[10]

Deterministic effects, on the other hand, are characterized by a threshold dose and begin to occur once the threshold dose is achieved. Deterministic effects are caused by cell death at the time of exposure and in pregnancy can lead to abortion, congenital malformations, growth delay, and neurobehavioral abnormalities. Once the threshold dose is encountered, the likelihood and severity of deterministic effects increases with increased dose, although below the threshold there appears to be no observed effect.[9,11]

Radiation Effects on the Fetus

The majority of our understanding about the effects of radiation during fetal development comes from animal studies, human exposures to diagnostic and therapeutic radiation, and large-scale radiation exposures, including the Chernobyl nuclear power plant exposure and atomic bomb detonations in Hiroshima and Nagasaki during World War II. The majority of published data around radiation dose during pregnancy is from study of these events, and there are limited recent data due to broad implementation of strategies to limit *in utero* radiation exposure. Although these high-dose exposures provide the majority of available data in humans, they may or may not accurately represent findings at lower doses with lower dose rates.[12] It is also often difficult to accurately quantify risks due to the complexity of the fetal developmental process, which remains incompletely understood.

The risks to the fetus associated with radiation exposure are related to the absorbed dose of radiation and the stage of fetal development at which the exposure occurred, and can be carcinogenic, teratogenic, or mutagenic. Because carcinogenic effects are stochastic, these can, theoretically, occur with any amount of exposure. Noncarcinogenic effects, however, are not believed to be observed when the fetus receives a threshold dose below 0.05 Gy. In practice, however, the believed threshold dose increases from 0.1 to 0.2 Gy for an embryo to 0.5 to 0.7 Gy for the fetus at 16 weeks.[13] Due to the significant changes in radiation sensitivity and outcomes, noncarcinogenic radiation effects on the fetus are categorized into preimplantation, organogenesis, and early fetal growth. Significant efforts in animal models during fetal development have subsequently been correlated to human fetal development. Irradiation with 2 Gy of photons delivered through gestation is depicted graphically in **Figure 9.1** along with estimates for the equivalent human embryonic developmental stages.

Prior to implantation, the embryo is exquisitely sensitive to radiation. The primary deleterious effect observed is implantation failure and is felt to occur with doses as low as 0.1 Gy. Failure to implant is believed to represent an "all or nothing" type of event,

and (noncarcinogenic) deleterious effects from radiation are not typically observed if an embryo undergoes successful implantation.[14,15] However, it can be challenging to accurately identify radiation as the causative agent in implantation failure due to the fact that a significant percentage of fertilized embryos do not implant, even in the absence of a known injury.

The period of organogenesis is also highly sensitive to the effects of radiation. The most commonly linked noncarcinogenic effects include mental retardation, microcephaly, and growth restriction.[16-19] Studies from atomic bomb survivors suggest that fetuses between weeks 8 to 15 exposed *in utero* to doses above 1 Gy had a 3% to 4% reduction in height[17] and that there was a threshold dose of 0.3 Gy for an increased risk of mental retardation.[18,19] Microcephaly was observed in fetuses exposed up to 15 weeks' gestation and increased with radiation dose without evidence for a threshold dose.[19] Mental retardation was observed in fetuses exposed from weeks 8 to 25 with the most sensitive period during 8 to 15 weeks. The relationship between absorbed dose and mental retardation appears linear and suggests a probability of 40% chance of mental retardation with a dose of 1 Gy and a

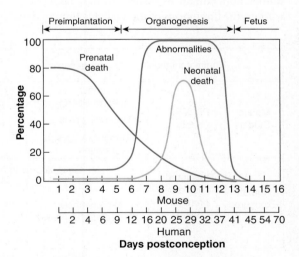

Figure 9.1 Risk of prenatal death, congenital abnormalities, and neonatal death of mice irradiated with 2 Gy during fetal development with estimates of similar human embryo stages included below murine gestational age.

(Reprinted with permission from Hall EJ, Giaccia AJ. *Radiobiology for the Radiologist.* 8th ed. Wolters Kluwer; 2018. Data from Russell LB, Russell WL. An analysis of the changing radiation response of the developing mouse embryo. *J Cell Physiol.* 1954;43[suppl 1]:103-149.)

threshold of at least 0.3 Gy.[20] Based on available data, microcephaly and mental retardation occur with radiation exposure during the critical period of 8 to 15 weeks. Microcephaly also occurs earlier in gestation, while mental retardation can occur later, with significantly higher exposure. However, it can be challenging to determine the specific impact of radiation on early fetal development because 15% of known pregnancies end in spontaneous abortions and 3% of babies have a major congenital malformation in the general population.[21]

Studies have attempted to understand more subtle changes in mental capacity due to radiation exposure using IQ tests. Osei et al evaluated radiation exposure in 50 pregnant women who underwent radiological examinations of the pelvis using risk coefficients and developed a model that suggested that a 30-point IQ decline occurred per 1 Gy of radiation received during weeks 8 to 15 of gestation.[22] It is very challenging to assess these sublethal endpoints, especially when the effects of radiation may not be observable early in life.[12] **Figure 9.2** charts risk of known adverse perinatal and neonatal outcomes after radiation exposure at specific gestational ages, based on data from animal studies and human exposure studies, taking into account the limitations of the available human data.

Unlike noncarcinogenic effects of radiation on the fetus, which are highly dependent on the gestational age, carcinogenic effects of radiation can occur from radiation exposure any time throughout the pregnancy. While initially reported in 1956 that *in utero* exposure to radiation was associated with an increased risk of childhood malignancies, controversy remains regarding whether radiation exposure is the causative agent of childhood cancers due to limited data. Correlation between increased risk of childhood malignancy, especially leukemia, and *in utero* doses of 0.2 Gy has been demonstrated.[23,24] Another estimate places the risk at 1 to 2 cases of childhood malignancies for 3000 *in utero* exposures of 0.1 Gy.[25] A systematic review of 40 years of research suggests *in utero* radiation-induced risk of childhood malignancies with doses as low as 0.1 Gy.[26] Another review did not find an increased risk of childhood cancer after exposure to diagnostic x-rays[27]; however, caution is recommended in interpreting these findings given limited data available. It is also unclear whether exposure at different times of gestation results in different carcinogenic effects, although the prevailing theory is that the risk is constant. Overall, while not conclusive, the International Commission on Radiological Protection (IRCP) suggests a relative risk of 1.4 for

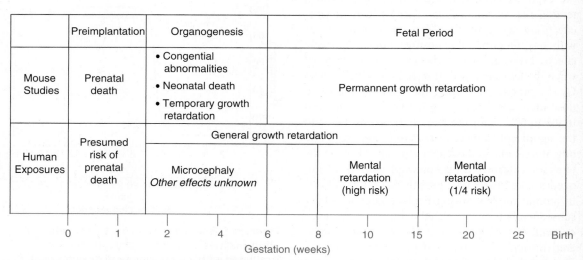

	Preimplantation	Organogenesis	Fetal Period		
Mouse Studies	Prenatal death	• Congential abnormalities • Neonatal death • Temporary growth retardation	Permanent growth retardation		
Human Exposures	Presumed risk of prenatal death	General growth retardation			
		Microcephaly *Other effects unknown*	Mental retardation (high risk)	Mental retardation (1/4 risk)	

Gestation (weeks): 0 1 2 4 6 8 10 15 20 25 Birth

Figure 9.2 Outcomes of mouse studies of fetal radiation exposure experimentation compared with human fetal exposures from survivors of the Japanese atomic bomb. Weeks of gestation for human development are correlated to similar gestation points in mice and both show similarities in increased risk of embryonic death preimplantation. Microcephaly is observed in humans during organogenesis, although other effects are unknown due to limited data. During the fetal period, mice demonstrate growth predominantly and humans display mental retardation, greatest during weeks 8 to 15 of gestation.

development of a radiation-induced malignancy for a 10 mGy fetal exposure, which is felt to be similar to risks of childhood radiation exposure.[13]

Occupational Exposures During Pregnancy

In the United States, the National Council on Radiological Protection and Measurements sets a fetal dose limit of 5 mSv per pregnancy and a corresponding 0.5 mSv per month limit after declaration of a pregnancy for any type of radiation.[28,29] In Europe, the fetal dose limit is 1 mSv/pregnancy.[30] These restrictions are designed to limit the risks of congenital malformations, carcinogenesis, and mental retardation due to radiation exposure. In the United States, there is not a unique dose limit for workers prior to declaration of pregnancy and, once declared, the pregnant worker should meet with the radiation safety officer and/or chair of the radiation safety committee to ensure work-related activities minimize exposure.

In the United States, the American College of Radiology recommends that all women of reproductive age should be screened for pregnancy status prior to radiological examinations using ionizing radiation.[31] In rare circumstances, diagnostic imaging must be performed in an expedited manner that limits the ability to verify the absence of pregnancy. When encountered, it is recommended to utilize practices to minimize dose to the fetus. **Table 9.1** reports the mean and maximum doses of radiation from standard imaging examinations based on the International Commission on Radiological Protection.[13] Alterations in the computed tomography (CT) protocol as well as shielding can be used during diagnostic studies. Despite the known and theorized risks of diagnostic procedures, the risk to the fetus remains low and relatively similar to baseline for probability of malformation and development of childhood malignancies in the ranges of typical diagnostic imaging (**Table 9.2**).[13]

Based on national guidelines in the United States, utilization of radioactive iodine isotopes (I-131) is contraindicated in pregnancy due to the risk of fetal thyroid cancer risk, and Technetium-99m should be used in lieu of I-131 for scintographic thyroid imaging.[32] In contrast, mammography studies have demonstrated minimal fetal exposure and are felt to be safe during pregnancy.[31,33] Based on consensus guidelines from the American College of

Table 9.1 Mean and Maximum Radiation Dose From Imaging Modalities

Procedure	Mean Dose (mGy)	Maximum Dose (mGy)
Conventional radiogram		
Abdomen	1.4	4.2
Chest	<0.01	<0.01
Intravenous urogram	1.7	10
Lumbar spine	1.7	10
Pelvis	1.1	4
Skull	<0.01	<0.01
Thoracic spine	<0.01	<0.01
Fluoroscopic examination		
Barium meal (upper gastrointestinal)	1.1	5.8
Barium enema	6.8	24
Computed tomography		
Abdomen	8.0	49
Chest	0.06	0.96
Head	<0.005	<0.005
Lumbar spine	2.4	8.9
Pelvis	25	79

mGy, milligray.
Reproduced from International Commission on Radiological Protection. Pregnancy and medical radiation. *Ann ICRP.* 2000;30(1):iii-viii, 1-43.

Table 9.2 Probability of Bearing Healthy Children After Radiation Exposure

Absorbed Dose to Fetus Above Background (mGy)	Probability of No Malformation (%)	Probability of Not Developing Childhood Malignancy (%)[a]
0	97	99.7
0.5	97	99.7
1.0	97	99.7
2.5	97	99.7
5	97	99.7
10	97	99.6
50	97	99.4
100	Close to 97[b]	99.1

[a]Rounded values. The risk for fatal cancer is assumed to be 0.6% per 100 mGy fetal dose with a linear relationship, which represents the best estimate from the ICRP, although other published series suggest a lower risk.
[b]Animal studies suggest malformations are unlikely at doses less than 100 to 200 mGy and correlative data corroborate similar expected values in humans.
mGy, milligray.
Reproduced from International Commission on Radiological Protection. Pregnancy and medical radiation. *Ann ICRP.* 2000;30(1):iii-viii, 1-43.

Obstetricians and Gynecologists, solitary diagnostic x-ray imaging tests do not provide enough fetal dose to clearly threaten the growth of the fetus.[31,32]

Pregnancy and Therapeutic Radiotherapy

In most clinical practices, and in general teaching, the avoidance of therapeutic radiotherapy administration during pregnancy remains standard. This principle is driven primarily by a desire to reduce risk to the radiosensitive fetus and by a relative dearth of clear data to guide safe thresholds of exposure during pregnancy.

Fortunately, radiotherapy is most commonly utilized for the treatment of malignancies, and cancer diagnoses either immediately preceding or during pregnancy remain relatively rare. Approximately 1 in 1000 pregnancies will coincide with a cancer diagnosis.[34] The most common malignancies encountered include breast cancer, Hodgkin lymphoma, melanoma, and leukemia.

Of these, only a subset require adjuvant or definitive radiotherapy, and many are candidates for chemotherapeutic, targeted agents or surgical interventions prior to or instead of radiotherapy administration. As such, often in these settings, radiotherapy may be delayed until after delivery. This offers an attractive alternative to the uncertainties that accompany radiotherapy during the pregnancy. In clinical practice, these tactics are often employed. However, as has been pointed out in several important reviews, this approach stems partly from clinical concern and partly from misconceptions of the limited clinical data available to guide radiation oncologists in these scenarios.[35]

To guide decision-making, one must keep in perspective the dose/exposure to both mother and fetus, the stochastic and deterministic effects of radiotherapy exposure, and the risks and benefits to mother and fetus as a result of a course of radiotherapy. Before any such course, a balanced discussion must be had with the pregnant patient regarding each of these factors so that a well-informed decision-making process may ensue.

Scope of Radiotherapy Exposure

As previously mentioned, radiotherapy exposure causes both stochastic and deterministic effects, which are, respectively, independent of and dependent on the extent/dose of exposure. Radiotherapy is most commonly delivered in the modern era by megavoltage energy photon (x-ray) beams or through particle therapies (electron/proton). Radiotherapy doses for therapeutic purposes are generally reported in Gy or Gy radiobiologic effective doses. When referencing older sources, the rad unit, which is equivalent to centigray (cGy = 1/100 Gy), was previously utilized. These units describe absorbed dose, which correlates to the amount of energy deposited into a tissue mass.

For lymphomas and other radiosensitive malignancies, target tissue doses generally range from 20 to 45 Gy. However, for most carcinomas and "solid" tumors, prescription doses extend from 50 to 70 Gy. To provide perspective on this dose in relation to fetal exposure, the Centers for Disease Control and Prevention has generally referenced the National Council on Radiation Protection and Measurements' Report No. 174, "Preconception and Prenatal Radiation Exposure: Health Effects and Protective Guidance," to provide estimates of dose ranges in which negative fetal effects have been encountered.[36] This report generally avoids quantification of stochastic effects (such as secondary malignancy) for which there exists no "threshold" dose beyond which the effect becomes likely. Per this report, with doses less than 0.10 Gy, noncancer health effects have not been detected in higher than normal rates. In the range of 0.10-to-0.50 Gy, failure of implantation or growth restriction are most common depending on the timing of radiotherapy postconception. Above 0.50 Gy, more profound and miscarriage-inducing effects are encountered. It should be noted that the data that inform these estimates come primarily from animal models or from survivors of nuclear explosions/radiation accidents.[13,37]

Therefore, the clinician and patient are faced with the dilemma that approximately 1/100th of the dose needed to treat the malignancy is potentially dangerous to the growing fetus. As such, great caution, thought, and planning from a radiotherapy team of clinicians, physicists, dosimetrists, therapists, and nurses must be undertaken prior to the outset of a radiotherapy course in a pregnant patient. If proceeding with therapy in this setting, the sources of fetal exposure must be understood, modeled, estimated, and measured to appropriately craft the treatment plan as well as to inform the patient of the extent of risk.

Radiotherapy exposure to the fetus comes from several sources during a course of therapeutic radiation.[38] In a megavoltage photon unit, akin to most external beam radiotherapy units worldwide, the dose may primarily come from direct exposure, leakage, collimator/device scatter, and internal scatter. Direct exposure is usually avoided, and any dose near the range of meaningful oncologic effect would be expected to cause fetal demise/miscarriage. Radiotherapy beams may be designed with treatment angles, collimator settings, and jaw apertures to avoid the abdomen and pelvis when the malignancy arises outside of this area. Leakage from the source/target may also be reduced by the use of collimators and distance of the source's position from the patient.

Scatter radiation from the treatment machine head, collimators, and jaws also occurs in low amounts. Exposure to the fetus from leakage and collimator scatter may be further reduced by shielding the pregnant patient's abdomen and/or pelvis. This is most commonly achieved with the application of several half-value (ie, sufficient thickness to attenuate 50% of incident energy) layers of lead shielding, either draped over the patient's abdomen and pelvis (eg, lead aprons) or by external shields placed close to the patient and intervening between the abdomen and the linear accelerator gantry head. Finally, internal scatter to the fetus is unavoidable. Internal scatter represents the energy radiating out from the intentionally exposed area to surrounding tissues within the body. This, of course, depends on the proximity of the target tissue to the fetus/abdomen.

Proton therapy and other particle therapies may be other methods for reducing radiation exposure to the fetus. Due to the Bragg peak effect, these therapies deposit their energy in tissue somewhat through the entrance pathway and primarily at the end of range of the particle within the patient.[39] As a result, there is little to no "exit dose" beyond the target, which may better protect tissues deep within the patient, including the developing fetus. Although there are concerns regarding nuclear interactions and neutron production in these settings, such treatments in pregnant patients have been described.[40]

Brachytherapy, the practice of bringing a radioactive source material close to target tissue for a prescribed period of time, also has very limited range. This technique is often utilized to limit radiation dose to nearby critical structures and limits introduction of scatter radiation from standard external source delivery techniques.

Clinical Use of Radiation Therapy During Pregnancy

There are limited and sparse reports of radiotherapy use during pregnancy in the literature. However, *in vivo* and *in vitro* measurements have seemed to suggest that very low doses to the fetus may be achieved during a course of radiotherapy if careful planning and shielding is utilized. In addition, disease site selection for this technique and distance from the fetus are key.

Breast cancer is the most common malignancy encountered in this setting. Several reports have demonstrated normal births and development in children born to women requiring radiotherapy for breast cancer during pregnancy.[41-43] These efforts have also demonstrated very low measurements for fetal dose with *in vivo* dosimetry. These were all external beam techniques employing doses from 46 to 50 Gy in conventional fractionation. Importantly, it has been demonstrated that normal fetal growth across a standard course of breast radiotherapy (generally delivered with conventional daily fractionation over 5-to-6 weeks) can lead to increasing dose to the fetus across the course of therapy.[44] This happens as the fetus naturally grows closer to the field edge and the irradiated target tissue.

Similar to the experiences treating pregnant patients with breast cancer, several groups have delivered radiotherapy courses to women with Hodgkin lymphoma without significant, documented effects on the fetus or resultant child.[45-48] Phantom dose measurements with thermoluminescent dosimeters have been performed and involve field radiotherapy designed for the management of supradiaphragmatic manifestations of Hodgkin lymphoma.[49] Secondary to distance from the fetus and appropriate field design, doses to the embryo were estimated to be as low as 2.4 to 4.8 cGy and 3.6 to 7.0 cGy for local radiotherapy and 40 Gy to the neck and axilla. With appropriate further shielding, these were reduced to 0.4 to 1.2 and 1.0 to 3.0 cGy, respectively.

In brain tumors, or those of the head and neck, stereotactic and other highly conformal radiotherapy techniques have yielded very low fetal dose measurements, again without any negative impact on the children born of these pregnancies.[50,51] This represents a sampling of the sparse literature, and other disease sites have been addressed.

General Recommendations

Patients diagnosed with a malignancy during pregnancy or those who become pregnant during oncologic care require thoughtful treatment and careful counseling. Multidisciplinary care results in the best and safest outcomes for the pregnant patient and the fetus alike. With regard to radiotherapy, the principle of "as low as reasonably achievable" exposure to nontarget tissues or individuals should still be employed. This may mean avoidance of radiotherapy altogether or delay until after delivery by means of other oncologic or temporizing measures. When delivery during the course is deemed necessary, careful consideration of technique, distance from the fetus, shielding, and dose measurement should be undertaken. The pregnant patient should be made aware of the expected/unavoidable dose to the fetus and associated risks. This should be carefully weighed with the patient, through informed decision-making, against the degree of oncologic benefit of the course of radiotherapy. In general, radiotherapy during pregnancy ideally would be avoided, but when required, it should be done with the utmost attention to detail and caution.

KEY POINTS

- Efforts should be made to limit exposure of pregnant women and women of childbearing age with unknown pregnancy status.
- Effects of radiation are dependent on the type or radiation, developmental stage, and dose.
- *In utero* radiation exposure can lead to carcinogenic, teratogenic, and mutagenic effects.

REFERENCES

1. Brent RL. Reproductive and teratologic effects of low-frequency electromagnetic fields: a review of in vivo and in vitro studies using animal models. *Teratology.* 1999;59(4):261-286.
2. Blaasaas KG, Tynes T, Lie RT. Risk of selected birth defects by maternal residence close to power lines during pregnancy. *Occup Environ Med.* 2004;61(2):174-176. Published correction appears in *Occup Environ Med.* 2004;61(6):559.
3. Li DK, Odouli R, Wi S, et al. A population-based prospective cohort study of personal exposure to magnetic fields during pregnancy and the risk of miscarriage. *Epidemiology.* 2002;13(1):9-20.
4. Salvesen KA. Epidemiological prenatal ultrasound studies. *Prog Biophys Mol Biol.* 2007;93(1-3):295-300.
5. Stålberg K, Haglund B, Axelsson O, et al. Prenatal ultrasound and the risk of childhood brain tumour and its subtypes. *Br J Cancer.* 2008;98(7):1285-1287.
6. Clements H, Duncan KR, Fielding K, et al. Infants exposed to MRI in utero have a normal paediatric assessment at 9 months of age. *Br J Radiol.* 2000;73(866):190-194.
7. Kok RD, de Vries MM, Heerschap A, et al. Absence of harmful effects of magnetic resonance exposure at 1.5 T in utero during the third trimester of pregnancy: a follow-up study. *Magn Reson Imaging.* 2004;22(6):851-854.
8. Walter H. *Review of Radiologic Physics.* 3rd ed. Lippincott Williams & Wilkins; 2010.
9. Fattibene P, Mazzei F, Nuccetelli C, et al. Prenatal exposure to ionizing radiation: sources, effects and regulatory aspects. *Acta Paediatr.* 1999;88(7):693-702.
10. 1990 recommendations of the International Commission on Radiological Protection. *Ann ICRP.* 1991;21(1-3):1-201.
11. Brent RL. Saving lives and changing family histories: appropriate counseling of pregnant women and men and women of reproductive age, concerning the risk of diagnostic radiation exposures during and before pregnancy. *Am J Obstet Gynecol.* 2009;200(1):4-24.
12. Cohen BL. The cancer risk from low level radiation. In: Tack D, Kalra MK, Gevenois PA, eds. *Radiation Dose From Multidetector CT.* Springer Berlin Heidelberg; 2011:61-79.
13. International Commission on Radiological Protection. Pregnancy and medical radiation. *Ann ICRP.* 2000;30(1):1-43.
14. Miller RW. Effects of prenatal exposure to ionizing radiation. *Health Phys.* 1990;59(1):57-61.
15. De Santis M, Cesari E, Nobili E, et al. Radiation effects on development. *Birth Defects Res C Embryo Today.* 2007;81(3):177-182.
16. Lee S, Otake M, Schull WJ. Changes in the pattern of growth in stature related to prenatal exposure to ionizing radiation. *Int J Radiat Biol.* 1999;75(11):1449-1458.
17. Otake M, Fujikoshi Y, Schull WJ, Izumi S. A longitudinal study of growth and development of stature among prenatally exposed atomic bomb survivors. *Radiat Res.* 1993;134(1):94-101.
18. Schull WJ. Brain damage among individuals exposed prenatally to ionizing radiation: a 1993 review. *Stem Cells.* 1997;15(suppl 2):129-133.
19. Otake M, Schull WJ, Lee S. Threshold for radiation-related severe mental retardation in prenatally exposed A-bomb survivors: a re-analysis. *Int J Radiat Biol.* 1996;70(6):755-763.
20. Otake M, Schull WJ. In utero exposure to A-bomb radiation and mental retardation: a reassessment. *Br J Radiol.* 1984;57:409-414.
21. National Council on Radiation Protection and Measurements. *NCRP Report 174. Preconception and Prenatal Radiation Exposure: Health Effects and Protective Guidance. 7910 Woodmont Avenue, Suite 400.* NCRP Publications; 2013.
22. Osei EK, Faulkner K. Fetal doses from radiological examinations. *Br J Radiol.* 1999;72:773-80.
23. Stewart AM, Webb J, Giles D, Hewitt D. Malignant disease in childhood and diagnostic irradiation in utero. *Lancet.* 1956;2:447.
24. Kneale GW, Stewart AM. Mantel-Haenszel analysis of Oxford data. I. Independent effects of several birth factors including fetal irradiation. *J Natl Cancer Inst.* 1976;56:879.
25. Doll R, Wakeford R. Risk of childhood cancer from fetal irradiation. *Br J Radiol.* 1997;70:130-139.
26. Wakeford R, Little MP. Risk coefficients for childhood cancer after intrauterine irradiation: a review. *Int J Radiat Biol.* 2003;79(5):293-309.
27. Schulze-Rath R, Hammer GP, Blettner M. Are pre- or postnatal diagnostic X-rays a risk factor for childhood cancer? A systematic review. *Radiat Environ Biophys.* 2008;47(3):301-312.
28. National Council on Radiation Protection and Measurements. *NCRP Report 116: Limitation of Exposure to Ionizing Radiation.* NCRP Publications; 1993.
29. U.S. Nuclear Regulatory Commission. Standards for Protection Against Radiation. Dose Equivalent to an Embryo/Fetus. 10 CFR Part 20.1208. https://www.nrc.gov/reading-rm/doc-collections/cfr/part020/part020-1208.html.
30. International Commission on Radiological Protection. The 2007 recommendations of the International Commission on Radiological Protection. ICRP Publication 103. *Ann ICRP.* 2007;37(2-4):1-332.
31. *ACR: Practice Guideline for Imaging Pregnant or Potentially Pregnant Adolescents and Women With Ionizing Radiation.* American College of Radiology; 2008.
32. ACOG Committee on Obstetric Practice. ACOG Committee Opinion, number 299, September 2004 (replaces no. 158, September 1995): Guidelines for diagnostic imaging during pregnancy. *Obstet Gynecol.* 2004;104:647-651.

33. Sechopoulos I, Suryanarayanan S, Vedantham S, et al. Radiation dose to organs and tissues from mammography: Monte Carlo and phantom study. *Radiology*. 2008;246:434-443.

34. Pavlidis NA. Coexistence of pregnancy and malignancy. *Oncologist*. 2002;7(4):279-287.

35. Kal HB, Struikmans H. Radiotherapy during pregnancy: fact and fiction. *Lancet Oncol*. 2005;6(5):328-333.

36. [NCRP2013] National Council on Radiation Protection and Measurements. *Preconception and Prenatal Radiation Exposure Health Effects and Protective Guidance*. National Council on Radiation Protection & Measurements; 2013.

37. International Commission on Radiological Protection. Biological effects after prenatal irradiation (embryo and fetus). *Ann ICRP*. 2003;33:205-206.

38. Khan FM. *The Physics of Radiation Therapy*. 5th ed. Lippincott Williams & Wilkins; 2014.

39. Wilson RR. Radiological use of fast protons. *Radiology*. 1946;47(5):487-491.

40. Wang X, Poenisch F, Sahoo N, et al. Spot scanning proton therapy minimizes neutron dose in the setting of radiation therapy administered during pregnancy. *J Appl Clin Med Phys*. 2016;17(5):366-376.

41. Ngu SL, Duval P, Collins C. Foetal radiation dose in radiotherapy for breast cancer. *Australas Radiol*. 1992;36:321-322.

42. Antypas C, Sandilos P, Kouvaris J, et al. Fetal dose evaluation during breast cancer radiotherapy. *Int J Radiat Oncol Biol Phys*. 1998;40:995-999.

43. Van der Giessen PH. Measurement of the peripheral dose for the tangential breast treatment technique with Co-60 gamma radiation and high energy X-rays. *Radiother Oncol*. 1997;42:257-264.

44. Fenig E, Mishaeli M, Kalish Y, et al. Pregnancy and radiation. *Cancer Treat Rev*. 2001;27:1-7.

45. Nisce LZ, Tome MA, He S, et al. Management of coexisting Hodgkin's disease and pregnancy. *Am J Clin Oncol*. 1986;9:146-151.

46. Lishner M, Zemlickis D, Degendorfer P, et al. Maternal and foetal outcome following Hodgkin's disease in pregnancy. *Br J Cancer*. 1992;65(1):114-117.

47. Cygler J, Ding GX, Kendal W, Cross P. Fetal dose for a patient undergoing mantle field irradiation for Hodgkin's disease. *Med Dosim*. 1997;22:135-137.

48. Nuyttens JJ, Prado KL, Jenrette JM, Williams TE. Fetal dose during radiotherapy: clinical implementation and review of the literature. *Cancer Radiother*. 2002;6:352-357.

49. Mazonakis M, Varveris H, Fasoulaki M, Damilakis J. Radiotherapy of Hodgkin's disease in early pregnancy: embryo dose measurements. *Radiother Oncol*. 2003;66:333-339.

50. Yu C, Jozsef G, Apuzzo ML, et al. Fetal radiation doses for model C gamma knife radiosurgery. *Neurosurgery*. 2003;52:687-693.

51. Sharma DS, Jalali R, Tambe CM, et al. Effect of tertiary multileaf collimator (MLC) on foetal dose during three-dimensional conformal radiation therapy (3DCRT) of a brain tumour during pregnancy. *Radiother Oncol*. 2004;70:49-54.

CHAPTER 10

Infectious Disease in Pregnancy

Courtney J. Mitchell and Brenna L. Hughes

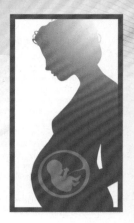

Introduction

Pregnancy is a unique condition with regards to infectious disease. Due to pregnancy-induced changes in the immune system, many diseases that may cause no symptoms or mild illness in nonpregnant subjects trigger much more severe maternal affliction. The advent of antibiotics and vaccines has rendered infectious diseases sometimes a less trendy topic, especially in pregnancy. However, novel organisms continue to emerge and present new challenges to managing these new diseases in pregnancy. Additionally, waning uptake of vaccination in the general population provides opportunities to advocate for recommended immunizations in pregnancy. In this chapter, we will review important infections in the context of pregnancy. Much of this chapter provides a review of enduring science pertinent to infectious disease and pregnancy. However, updates to emerging therapies and changes in guidelines are also provided.

Cytomegalovirus

Cytomegalovirus (CMV), otherwise known as human herpes virus 5, is the most common congenitally acquired infection.[1]

Transmission

In general, the following principles apply to congenital infection with CMV: severe congenital CMV results almost exclusively from primary maternal infection, and clinically evident manifestations in the newborn are more common following primary infection in the mother.

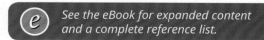
See the eBook for expanded content and a complete reference list.

Clinical Presentation

Patients with CMV may develop fever, pharyngitis, lymphadenopathy, and other generalized symptoms of viral illness, but 90% of adults are asymptomatic.

Characteristics of fetal infection that may aid in prenatal diagnosis include fetal growth restriction, cerebral ventriculomegaly, ascites, microcephaly, hydrocephaly, periventricular calcifications, calcifications of the bowel and liver, hepatosplenomegaly, cardiomegaly, placentomegaly, hyperechogenic bowel, and oligohydramnios or polyhydramnios. CMV may cause nonimmune hydrops. CMV has also been implicated in myocarditis; there have been reports of fetal heart block and of fetal supraventricular tachycardia.[12]

Most infected neonates are asymptomatic at birth, although 10% of these infants present with clinical manifestations at birth. Forty to sixty percent of neonates with symptoms at birth will have permanent sequelae from infection, most commonly, sensorineural hearing loss, followed by cognitive impairment, chorioretinitis, and cerebral palsy[13]; 10% to 15% of neonates asymptomatic at birth will go on to have sensorineural hearing loss.[13] Other common findings in congenital CMV include petechial rash, hepatosplenomegaly, hemolytic anemia, jaundice, interstitial pneumonia, seizures, and microcephaly.

Clinical Assessment

Adult CMV infections usually go unrecognized unless symptoms develop. The presence of CMV-specific immunoglobulin (Ig)G antibodies in the mother confirms a recent or past infection; however, because CMV becomes latent in the mother, previous infection in the mother does not confer immunity against infection in the infant. CMV-specific IgM is detectable in both maternal and neonatal primary infections in 80% of cases.

Shell vial viral culture is the most accurate method of diagnosing CMV infection, although culture positivity cannot distinguish between primary and recurrent infection. Culture sites in the mother include the nasopharynx, cervix, vagina, and urine; in the infant, they include the nasopharynx, conjunctiva, and urine.

When maternal primary infection is suspected or when there are findings on ultrasonography that are suspicious of congenital CMV infection, prenatal diagnosis can be carried out by amniocentesis. Ideally, prenatal diagnosis among women without ultrasound findings including fetal growth restriction, cerebral ventriculomegaly, ascites, microcephaly, hydrocephaly, periventricular calcifications, calcifications of the bowel and liver, hepatosplenomegaly, cardiomegaly, placentomegaly, hyperechogenic bowel, and oligohydramnios or polyhydramnios should occur beyond 21 weeks' gestation, as this optimizes the sensitivity of diagnostic tests.

Fetal blood can be tested for the presence of CMV-specific IgM after 20 weeks' gestation and has a sensitivity of 51% to 58% and a specificity of 100%.[12] The presence of CMV-specific IgM in fetal cord blood, which is detectable in 60% of infants with congenital infection, establishes the diagnosis.[17] On the whole, fetal blood sampling and amniotic fluid analysis have sensitivity, specificity, positive predictive value, and negative predictive value of 80%, 99%, 98%, and 93%, respectively, for CMV.[18] However, as fetal blood sampling adds little additional value to amniotic fluid sampling and is associated with a risk of fetal death, it should not be routinely performed.

Pharmacologic Treatment

The treatment of CMV infection in the mother and infant is directed toward the symptoms, when they are present. Agents that have been used to treat maternal symptoms include adenosine arabinoside, cytosine arabinoside, acyclovir, ganciclovir, and foscarnet (phosphonoformic acid). Unfortunately, these agents have had limited success; adenosine and cytosine arabinoside are toxic, and acyclovir, ganciclovir, and foscarnet have only been used in a very small number of studies.

Currently, there is no proven antenatal treatment of fetal CMV infection recommended outside of research protocols.[12] Because the vast majority of congenital CMV infections occur in instances of maternal primary infection, a reasonable strategy is to vaccinate seronegative women prior to conception. Vaccine development has included investigations into live-attenuated vaccines, recombinant virus vaccines, subunit vaccines, DNA vaccines, and peptide vaccines[20]; however, there is no current CMV vaccine available to prevent maternal CMV infection or decrease vertical transmission. Routine antepartum serologic screening for CMV is not recommended at this time due to no widely available treatment.[2]

Rubella

Rubella, or German measles, is caused by a single-stranded RNA virus that is a member of the Togaviridae family. Out of all the known teratogenic viruses, infection with rubella results in the most severe congenital malformations. The success of vaccination against rubella, and the subsequent decline of congenital rubella syndrome (CRS), stands as one of the major achievements of twentieth-century perinatal and neonatal medicine. Although congenital rubella infections (CRIs) are rare in the United States, it still is prevalent in developing countries. Despite increasing vaccination hesitancy and decreasing rate of measles-mumps-rubella (MMR) immunization, the rate of congenital rubella is still rare in the United States.

Transmission

Rubella virus is spread by respiratory droplets. This requires prolonged close exposure. The virus is present in the nasopharynx and spreads via the lymphatics and then blood. It has an 80% attack rate. Fetal infection requires maternal viremia and placental transmission. Viremia has been thought to occur only with primary infection. Rare cases of reinfection leading to CRS have been reported.[26] Serologic evidence of fetal exposure to rubella has been documented after inadvertent vaccination in pregnancy. To date, no cases of congenital defects secondary to CRS have been reported due to the vaccine.[27] Nevertheless, vaccine administration is contraindicated in pregnancy because the theoretical risk of CRS after vaccination, although low, may not be zero.[28] Although the virus is shed in breast milk, neonatal exposure to rubella during breastfeeding has not been associated with morbidity.[29] Prolonged viral shedding from an infant with CRS may be a source of infection. In addition, virus has been isolated in the urine, cerebrospinal fluid, and even the lens of neonates with CRS.

Clinical Presentation

Maternal

Acquired rubella presents as a mild or asymptomatic infection. The incubation period is 14 to 21 days, with viral shedding beginning 1 week before the onset of a fine "rubelliform" rash which starts on the face and neck and then extends to the trunk and extremities. The rash is macular and lasts 3 days, hence the name 3-day measles. Malaise, fever, and postauricular and suboccipital adenopathy are also common. Arthralgias are common in adult women; arthritis, neuritis, encephalitis, and thrombocytopenia are rare. Because these symptoms are nonspecific, diagnosis should be made on serologic rather than clinical grounds.[32]

Fetal and Neonatal

The pathogenesis of congenital defects due to rubella infection includes impairment in organogenesis due to decreased mitosis and damage secondary to scarring and persistent infection.[33] Abnormalities resulting from impaired organogenesis occur with maternal infection in the first trimester. Other abnormalities, such as progressive hearing loss and pulmonic or aortic stenosis, are due to ongoing damage caused by persistent infection and immune response. Congenital infection may be divided into three categories based on its manifestations: CRS, extended CRS, and delayed CRS. Newborn rubella, or CRS, and extended CRS are apparent at birth. Delayed manifestations of congenital infection may not be apparent for years or decades.

Four major defects in CRS, in order of decreasing frequency, are deafness, cognitive impairment, cardiac lesions, and ophthalmologic abnormalities. Congenital manifestations of rubella are summarized in **Table 10.1** with hearing loss the most common clinical finding in newborns.

Clinical Assessment

Maternal

Clinical diagnosis of postnatal infection is unreliable and must be confirmed by serology. Rubella-specific IgM can be detected 1 week after the onset of the rash and typically persists for up to 8 to 12 weeks; it is detectable by culture of nasopharyngeal swabs, urine, blood, amniotic fluid, placenta, and synovial fluid.[37] Diagnosis of acute rubella infection is also made by the observation

Table 10.1 Clinical Manifestations of Rubella Infection in Newborns and Adults

Birth defects

Congenital rubella syndrome (CRS), which includes any of the following findings:

Neurological: meningoencephalitis, microcephaly, intracranial calcifications, psychomotor retardation, behavioral disorders, autism, chronic progressive panencephalitis, hypotonia, speech defects

Otic: hearing loss

Ophthalmological: cataracts, retinopathy, glaucoma, cloudy cornea, microphthalmia, subretinal neovascularization

Cardiac: patent ductus arteriosus, pulmonary artery stenosis, pulmonary artery hyperplasia, coarctation of the aorta, ventricular septal defect, atrial septal defect, myocarditis, myocardial necrosis

Miscellaneous: thrombocytopenia purpura, chronic rubelliform rash, dermatoglyphic abnormalities, jaundice, hepatosplenomegaly, hepatitis, hemolytic anemia, interstitial pneumonia, bone defects, genitourinary abnormalities (cryptorchidism, polycystic kidneys)

Clinical findings

Mother: macular rubelliform rash, lymphadenopathy (posterior auricular, suboccipital), prodromal symptoms (malaise, fever, headaches), arthralgias, peripheral neuritis; laboratory diagnoses include rubella-specific IgG and IgM, virus isolation from nasopharynx, viral antigen

Infant: CRS (as above); laboratory diagnoses include rubella-specific
IgG and IgM, virus isolation from nasopharynx.

of a fourfold rise in acute and convalescent titers of rubella-specific IgG over a period of 3 to 4 weeks.

Commercially available enzyme immunoassays for rubella IgM and IgG are routinely performed by most laboratories.[38] Indirect antibody assays are more prone to false-positive IgM results, due in part to cross-reactivity with other IgM antibodies or with rheumatoid factor; hence, a second confirmatory test for rubella IgM by a different modality should be performed, especially before 20 weeks' gestation.

Fetal and Neonatal

Prenatal diagnosis of CRI is possible. The presence of rubella-specific IgM in fetal blood confirms infection.[37] Fetal blood sampling to detect IgM must be delayed until 20 to 22 weeks' gestation. There are currently no reverse transcription polymerase chain reaction (RT-PCR) assays approved by the US Food and Drug Administration (FDA) for rubella, but it is available in commercial and public health laboratories.

Rubella-specific IgM is detectable for up to 6 months in infected newborns, and rubella IgG may remain elevated beyond this 6-month period. As in the mother, rubella is detectable by culturing infant blood, stools, cerebrospinal fluid, and urine.

Management of Rubella Infection in Pregnancy

Prevention of *in utero* rubella infection requires the acquisition of immunity by all persons before the childbearing years. Immunity against rubella is considered to be lifelong given the stability of the viral genome and the protective effect of IgG antibody; the humoral-mediated response confers immunity against future reinfection. The American College of Obstetricians and Gynecologists (ACOG) currently recommends all prenatal patients be tested for rubella IgG; and all pregnant women identified as being susceptible to rubella should be advised about the potential risk of CRI and be vaccinated after delivery; however, pregnant women should not be vaccinated.[39] These guidelines also recommend that breastfeeding is not a contraindication to vaccine administration.

There is no specific antiviral therapy for rubella infection. If *in utero* exposure to rubella virus is documented, the woman should be counseled as to the risks and consequences of CRI. With the potentially devastating effects of first trimester infection, a patient may choose to terminate the affected pregnancy if the diagnosis is made in a timely manner.

The treatment of acute rubella in adults and children is based on the symptoms. Most adults have complete recovery from the rash and lymphadenopathy within a week, although one-third may develop late-onset arthralgias. At present, there is no standard method of treating acute CRIs with antiviral therapy.

Varicella Zoster Virus

Varicella zoster virus (VZV) is a DNA virus and a member of the human herpesvirus group that exhibits viral latency. There are two major concerns if VZV infection occurs during pregnancy. The first is the risk that the infection imposes upon the mother; the second is the risk of either teratogenesis or perinatal acquisition by the neonate.

Table 10.2 Clinical Conditions Associated With Congenital Infection With VZV

Manifestation of Congenital Exposure to Varicella	Timing of Maternal Infection
Congenital varicella syndrome	First 20 wk gestation
Neonatal varicella	Between 20 wk gestation and 5 d before delivery
Disseminated varicella	5 d before and up to 2 d after delivery
Neonatal zoster	Reactivation of intrauterine varicella infection or secondary to postnatal exposure to varicella in the neonatal period

Transmission

Varicella Transmission in Pregnancy

Congenital infection with VZV presents as one of the four distinct clinical conditions (**Table 10.2**). The timing of maternal infection determines which clinical syndrome the newborn develops.

Clinical Presentation

Acute VZV infections commonly present with multiple vesicular lesions starting on the head and face and then extending to the truck and, sometimes, the extremities. The skin lesions begin as macules and proceed to a vesicular and then a pustular stage. Approximately 250 to 500 lesions appear during the acute stage and eventually rupture and scab within several days. New vesicles may form as others heal; therefore, the acute phase may involve lesions in different stages of development. The prominent feature of the disease is itching.

The virus is detectable from skin lesions until the scab forms. The attack rate in susceptible individuals after exposure is approximately 90%.[47]

Following inoculation, the incubation period for VZV is approximately 10 to 21 days. Patients are commonly viremic 1 week before and up to 2 days after the onset of clinical symptoms. This period of viremia is accompanied by prodromal symptoms.

Fever and rash commonly occur simultaneously in children after the incubation period. In adults, fever and generalized malaise usually precede the rash by several days. It is recognized that, when adults contract the disease, both constitutional and pulmonary symptoms may be severe. Bacterial infection of the skin with beta-hemolytic strepto-cocci is the common secondary complication of chickenpox.[47] Encephalitis, meningitis, myocarditis, glomerulonephritis, and arthritis are all rare complications in childhood. The most serious complication of varicella infection is pneumonia, which occurs more commonly in adults.

Studies have estimated the risk of varicella pneumonia in pregnancy at 10% to 20% with a higher mortality rate than the general public,[49] although pneumonia does not appear to have an increased prevalence in pregnant women as opposed to other adults.[48]

After the primary infection, VZV remains latent in the dorsal root ganglia and may present later in life as reactivated disease in the form of shingles. In both adults and children, shingles presents as very painful, vesicular lesions that typically follow the dermatomal pattern of the involved dorsal root ganglia. The lesions are almost always unilateral. Peripheral neuralgia, which presents as hypoesthesia on the skin, precedes the lesions by several days. Virus is also recoverable from the lesions of shingles, although the viral load in the vesicular fluid is significantly lower than with primary VZV infection.

Congenital varicella syndrome is a collection of fetal abnormalities, which were first described by Laforet and Lynch[52] in an infant born to a mother who contracted chickenpox at 8 weeks' gestation. The most common findings in congenital varicella syndrome include skin, eye, and limb malformations, such as cicatricial scarring, chorioretinitis, anisocoria, cortical atrophy, limb paresis, and limb hypoplasia ipsilateral to the scarred limb.[52] Ultrasound findings can include limb hypoplasia, ventriculomegaly, microcephaly, gastrointestinal and genitourinary abnormalities, intracranial calcifications, and cortical atrophy.[46] Disseminated varicella presents with generalized vesicular skin lesions, pneumonia, and hepatitis; one-third of these infants die from this severe infection. Neonatal varicella is generally a mild course of chickenpox. Finally, Paryani and Arvin have reported a case of neonatal zoster in a 7-month-old infant without a prior history of chickenpox whose mother developed an acute infection while pregnant.[50]

Clinical Assessment

Most pregnant women have detectable antibodies even if they have a negative history of chickenpox.[53] Pregnant women exposed to chickenpox should have their immune status identified. For the clinician, the main objective is to maintain a high index of suspicion for pneumonia in women who have varicella infection in pregnancy.

Because the clinical presentation—the characteristic rash (lesion) of VZV which presents in multiple stages—is usually characteristic, serology is not usually indicated to confirm the clinical diagnosis. However, serologic testing is indicated in a pregnant woman with exposure to but with a negative or uncertain history of varicella. Virus is recoverable by culture of, and antigen detection in, scrapings of skin lesions. VZV-specific IgM becomes positive within several days of the onset of the rash. VZV-specific IgG confirms previous immunity to VZV and is present in 85% to 95% of adults. Approximately 70% to 90% of patients whose serology status to VZV is uncertain, or whose history of chickenpox in childhood is unknown, demonstrate previous sero-immunity.[54]

Pharmacologic Treatment and Prevention

Women found to be susceptible to VZV should receive varicella zoster immunoglobulin (VZIG) within 96 hours of exposure. Acquisition of maternal antibodies by the fetus is usually protective. However, an infant born after maternal viremia, but before maternal development of antibodies, is at high risk of potentially life-threatening neonatal varicella infection. VZIG has been shown to modify or prevent varicella infection in children and is recommended for use in preventing severe neonatal infections.[47] Accordingly, infants at risk (born to women who develop chickenpox from 5 days before and up to 2 days after delivery) should receive VZIG as passive immunization.

Experts recommend oral acyclovir or valacyclovir for pregnant women with varicella, especially during the second and third trimesters and in cases of with serious complication such as varicella pneumonia.[40,48,56]

Although the Centers for Disease Control and Prevention (CDC) recommends routine vaccination for all children aged 12 to 18 months and vaccination of susceptible persons at older ages, including women of child-bearing ages, the vaccine is contraindicated in pregnancy. Women who receive the vaccine should be advised not to become pregnant for 1 month after administration. The teratogenic potential of the vaccine given inadvertently to pregnant women is not known. In most circumstances, the decision to terminate a pregnancy should not simply be based on vaccine administration during pregnancy. Early studies show no evidence of active VZV in breast milk in postpartum mothers who received the vaccine[57]; therefore, there is no clear evidence that breastfeeding should be discontinued after administration of the vaccine.

Management of VZV in Pregnancy

Women who have varicella infection without complications in pregnancy do not need to be hospitalized. However, women with this infection must be warned to contact their physician immediately in the event of any pulmonary symptoms, including a mild cough. At this point, hospitalization with full respiratory support, if necessary, should be indicated.

Airborne and contact precautions are recommended for neonates born to mothers with varicella until 21 days of age or until 28 days of age if VZIG or intravenous immunoglobulin (IVIG) was administered. To minimize the possibility of infection of the infant, the mother and the infant should be isolated separately until the mother's vesicles have dried, even if the infant has received VZIG.[40] If the infant develops clinical varicella, the mother may care for the infant. If the neonate is born with lesions (eg, congenital varicella), the mother and her newborn should be isolated (they can be isolated together) and discharged home when clinically stable. If the infant is clinically stable for discharge during the incubation period and has not developed varicella, isolation to complete the 21- or 28-day period of viral shedding can be continued at home, as long as relatives and contacts have evidence of immunity to varicella.[2] If the infant needs to see the healthcare provider during that period, the office should be notified of the need for airborne and contact precautions. Infants with varicella embryopathy do not require isolation if they do not have active skin lesions.[2]

Herpes Simplex Virus

Herpes zoster infection is caused by the same virus that causes clinical chickenpox. Zoster occurs rarely in pregnancy, and, because it is a reactivation, maternal antibodies are already present. In healthy women, zoster poses no special threat to the fetus or newborn (1).

Parvovirus B19 Infection

Clinical Presentation

Erythema infectiosum, or fifth disease, is the major clinical presentation of parvovirus B19 infection in children and the classic "slapped cheek" appearance of fifth disease typically presents in children.[64] Adults with parvovirus B19 infection present with a generalized macular rash, anemia, and arthralgias. The rash is macular and reticulate; it typically starts on the face and extends to the trunk and extremities. Constitutional symptoms include fever, coryza, pharyngitis, and malaise; viremia occurs up to a week before the onset of the rash. Adult infections may be accompanied by a transient anemia; immunocompromised patients and patients with hemoglobinopathies may experience transient aplastic crisis.[65]

Fetal parvovirus B19 infection can lead to fetal death, miscarriage, and nonimmune hydrops fetalis; few reports have demonstrated fetal malformations following congenital infections, such as microphthalmia, bilateral cleft lip and palate, micrognathia, and hydrocephalus. Additionally, neonates may have long-term neurodevelopment sequelae after hydrops.[66] The fetal hydrops is thought to result from the transient fetal anemia caused by the infection. A report by Enders and coauthors[67] demonstrated that the rate of development of fetal hydrops following acute infection in pregnancy is 3.9%. This study also revealed a high fetal death rate (6.3%), with the highest rates observed when hydrops developed before 20 weeks' gestation.

Clinical Assessment

The incubation period before the onset of symptoms is usually 4 to 14 days but can be as long as 21 days. Acute infections with parvovirus B19 are diagnosed by the clinical presentation (eg, macular facial rash, arthralgias, anemia). Pregnant women exposed to parvovirus B19 should be screened as soon as possible after exposure. Diagnosis is confirmed by the presence of parvovirus-specific IgM, which is detectable 7 to 10 days after the onset of constitutional symptoms. Parvovirus-specific IgG is produced shortly afterward and persists for years; immunity to parvovirus is permanent. Women who are IgM-negative and IgG-positive and who have had previous exposure are immune.[2] Women who are IgM-positive, no matter their IgG status, should be monitored for possible fetal infection.[2] Women who are IgM-negative and IgG-negative are susceptible to infection; screening should be repeated in 4 weeks. Because IgM does not cross the placenta, parvovirus IgM in cord blood or neonatal blood would indicate congenital infection. Fetal infection can be diagnosed with PCR in amniotic fluid.[2]

Nonpharmacologic Treatment and Prevention

Parvovirus infections in children and adults are self-limited, and treatment is, therefore, supportive based on symptoms. Patients who develop aplastic anemia may require transfusion of blood products. Following diagnosis of acute parvovirus in pregnancy, weekly ultrasonography to detect fetal hydrops and fetal middle cerebral artery Doppler assessment should be performed for 8 to 12 weeks.[2]

Because fetal anemia is the physiological cause of the hydrops, *in utero* transfusion has been shown to significantly improve fetal morbidity and mortality in severe cases. A study by Rodis and coauthors[68] of 5349 cases of fetal hydrops, secondary to acute parvovirus infection in the mother, showed a survival rate of 83%. Most cases of fetal hydrops revert back to normal within 4 weeks. There is clearly no risk of hydrops in mothers who have previous immunity to parvovirus B19. Following intrauterine fetal transfusion, Enders and coauthors[67] reported a survival rate of approximately 85% of hydrops cases. There is a report of spontaneous resolution of 5% of hydrops associated with parvovirus B19.[66]

Options for prevention of infection during an outbreak are limited. The ACOG does not recommend pregnant women be removed from the work environment during an outbreak. Universal precautions and frequent handwashing may decrease the risk of acquisition. Pregnant women who have been exposed to B19 should be counseled on the relative low risk of infection. Serologies should be obtained immediately to assess susceptibility. Of note, suspected or proven intrauterine B19 infections deem amniotic fluid and fetal tissues infectious.

Toxoplasmosis

The organism responsible for toxoplasmosis is *Toxoplasma gondii*, an obligate intracellular protozoan parasite that exhibits a complex life cycle. It exists in three forms: trophozoite (or tachyzoite), cyst, and oocyst. Trophozoites are the proliferative and invasive forms, whereas cysts are the latent forms, persisting in tissue for the lifetime of the host. Oocysts are found in cats that have ingested rodents infected with cysts. Humans become infected if they eat uncooked or undercooked fresh (never frozen) meat from infected animals. Human infection may also occur with hand-to-mouth contact with oocysts excreted in cat feces, most commonly due to poor handling of cat litter of outdoor cats. Inhalation of aerosolized oocysts is another possible mechanism for infection.

Clinical Presentation

Maternal

An immunocompetent adult with acute toxoplasmosis is often only minimally symptomatic or completely asymptomatic. When the disease is clinically apparent, symptoms similar to infectious mononucleosis, including malaise, myalgias, sore throat, and fever, may be present. Painful but nonsuppurative lymph node enlargement, most commonly involving the posterior cervical lymph nodes, is a frequent finding in acute toxoplasmosis. Other associated findings include maculopapular rash, hepatosplenomegaly, and lymphocytosis. Ocular symptoms, such as blurred vision, photophobia, and eye pain, may be present with chronic disease. In the immunocompromised patients, severe disease with pulmonary and central nervous system involvement can be seen.

Fetal

Fetal infection only occurs with acute maternal toxoplasmosis. The likelihood of transmission and the severity of risk to the fetus vary with gestational age. Congenital toxoplasmosis is more frequent, but usually less apparent, when maternal infection occurs later in gestation. Clinical manifestations that may prompt suspicion of infection include intrauterine growth restriction, nonimmune hydrops, hydrocephaly, microcephaly, anencephaly, and hydranencephaly.[69] Ultrasound often fails to identify fetuses affected *in utero*. However, if ultrasound findings are present, they may include scattered intracranial calcifications, ventricular dilation, hepatic enlargement, ascites, and increased placental thickness.[69]

Neonatal

More than half of infants with congenital toxoplasmosis have no signs or symptoms in the newborn period.[69] The classic triad of periventricular calcifications, chorioretinitis, and hydrocephaly is uncommon. Other findings can include growth restriction, low birthweight, hydrocephalus, microcephaly, intracranial calcifications, jaundice, hepatosplenomegaly, cataracts, microphthalmia, strabismus, blindness, epilepsy, psychomotor or mental retardation, petechia secondary to thrombocytopenia, anemia, maculopapular rash, pneumonia, vomiting, and diarrhea.[72] Serious long-term complications include mental disability, severe visual deficits, and seizures. Adverse sequelae have been detected in long-term follow-up of infants with subclinical infection at birth.

Clinical Assessment

Routine screening for toxoplasma infection in pregnancy is not recommended.[2] However, if infection is suspected, detection can be achieved via direct and indirect methods. Indirect techniques should be used in immunocompetent patients, as these methods rely upon serologic analysis, specifically the detection of organism-specific IgG and IgM antibodies. Direct detection with PCR, hybridization, isolation, and histology is largely reserved for diagnosis in immunocompromised individuals.

Detection of IgG and IgM antibodies should be performed in pregnant women who are suspected of having had toxoplasmosis exposure. IgM can appear as early as 1 week after an acute infection, increases rapidly, and then wanes, persisting for several weeks to months; in rare circumstances, IgM may even persist for years. IgG does not appear until several weeks after the levels of IgM increase, but low titers usually persist for years. More recently, enzyme-linked immunosorbent assay, IgG avidity test, and agglutination and differential agglutination tests have been used for the detection of IgG antibodies.[73] Avidity (ie, functional affinity) testing for IgG antibodies is now routinely performed to help to distinguish acute from chronic infection. High-avidity antibodies are not seen in cases of infections acquired in the most recent 3 to 4 months. The differential agglutination (acetone fixed [AC]/formalin fixed [HS]; [AC/HS]) test is useful in distinguishing between a probable acute or chronic infection in pregnant women.

The presence of toxoplasma-specific IgG would indicate protection from further infection. The presence of a high toxoplasma IgG titer with the presence of IgM is suggestive of a recent infection, especially if the IgM titer is high, but it must be remembered that IgM may persist for months or even years following acute infection. A negative IgM test, if found within the first 24 weeks of gestation, especially if associated with low titers of IgG, essentially rules out an acute infection during gestation and points to a chronic infection antedating conception. However, a negative IgM titer in the third trimester does not negate the possibility of an acute infection in the first trimester with a subsequent

decline. In this circumstance, additional testing, such as IgG avidity testing, can be helpful. Finally, women who test positive for IgM antibodies in a nonreference laboratory should always undergo confirmatory testing in a reference laboratory, as 60% of these women are actually found to be previously infected.[74] Maternal diagnosis should only be made after confirmation of serologic findings in a reference laboratory.

Prenatal diagnosis of congenital toxoplasmosis through PCR analysis of amniotic fluid obtained by amniocentesis has essentially eliminated the need for periumbilical fetal blood sampling or serologic testing of amniotic or fetal specimens as this approach has greater sensitivity and is simpler. Sensitivity for PCR analysis of amniotic fluid depends on gestational age but, overall, has a rate of 64% after 18 weeks (and in some studies has been noted to be as high as 98.8%), with a specificity of 100%, a positive predictive value of 100%, and a negative predictive value of 87.8%.[74]

Pharmacologic Treatment and Prevention

In some European countries, large-scale screening and specific therapy are used to prevent congenital toxoplasmosis. The efficacy of medication is approximately 50% in reducing congenital infection. If acute maternal toxoplasmosis is contracted between 2 and 10 weeks' gestation, or if there are major lesions documented by ultrasound, the option of termination should be discussed. The combination of pyrimethamine (a folic acid antagonist) and sulfa drugs (sulfadiazine or triple sulfonamides) is the only effective medication generally available in the United States to reduce the severity of congenital toxoplasmosis. Folic acid should be used with pyrimethamine to minimize its potential side effects of bone marrow suppression and pancytopenia. Spiramycin, a macrolide antibiotic, is used extensively in Europe but is available for use in the United States only through the FDA special drug application. Spiramycin reduces the rate of fetal infection but not the severity of infection. In Western Europe, spiramycin is used from diagnosis to delivery, and pyrimethamine plus sulfadiazine is used to protect against progressive fetopathy. It should be noted, however, that there have been no adequately designed randomized clinical trials demonstrating efficacy of any antenatal therapies to prevent or treat congenital toxoplasmosis.

The primary method of prevention of congenital toxoplasmosis is the application of certain hygienic measures. Pregnant women should be advised to wash their hands thoroughly after contact with raw meat, cats, and materials potentially contaminated by cat feces. Meat should only be eaten when it has been cooked to more than 66 °C (about 151 °F).

Measles

Clinical Presentation

Measles is transmitted via direct contact with infectious droplets, as well as by airborne spread. The incubation of the measles virus is 8 to 10 days. Measles typically presents with 3 to 4 days of prodromal symptoms followed by Koplick spots (small white lesions on an erythematous base) on the buccal mucosa and maculopapular rash that spreads from the head to the trunk to the lower extremities. The prodromal manifestations of the measles include fever, cough, coryza, and conjunctivitis. Complications of measles may include otitis media, bronchopneumonia, croup, and diarrhea. Acute encephalitis occurs in about 1 in 1000 cases of measles and often results in permanent neurologic damage.[40] Subacute sclerosing panencephalitis is a rare complication of measles characterized by degenerative central nervous system diseases manifesting 7-11 years after primary measles infection and leads to neurologic deterioration and seizures.

Women who are pregnant and contract measles are at increased risk for adverse outcomes, including hospitalization, pneumonia, and death,[77] as well as increased risk for elevated liver function tests.[78] Measles in pregnancy is also associated with low birth weight, preterm labor, and neonatal intensive care admission.[79] There has been no definitive link between measles in pregnancy and increased risk of congenital anomalies and fetal loss.

Clinical Assessment

Measles can be diagnosed by detection of viral RNA by RT-PCR, measles-specific IgM, a fourfold increase in measles IgG antibody concentration in paired acute and convalescent serum specimens (collected at least 10 days apart), or isolation of the measles virus in cell culture. Most diagnoses in the United States are now made in conjunction with state health departments and the CDC.

Nonpharmacologic Treatment and Prevention

Supportive care is the treatment for measles; there are no specific antiviral therapy. Pregnant women exposed to measles should receive IVIG (0.5 mL/kg) within 6 days of exposure given the increased risk of measles-related morbidity in pregnancy.[76]

Because the MMR vaccine is a live vaccine, it should not be given in pregnancy. If a woman inadvertently receives the MMR vaccine within 4 weeks of pregnancy, she should be counseled on the theoretical risk of CRS, although no proven cases have occurred. Studies have shown that women who receive the MMR vaccine in pregnancy are not at increased risk of adverse outcomes.[76]

KEY POINTS

- CMV is the most common congenitally acquired infection.
- There is no proven antenatal treatment of fetal CMV infection.
- The most serious complication of varicella infection in pregnancy is pneumonia.
- VZIG should be administered within 96 hours of exposure to pregnant women susceptible to varicella.
- Varicella immunization should be encouraged 1 month prior to pregnancy or in the postpartum period.
- The use of acyclovir or valacyclovir prophylaxis, starting at 36 weeks, effectively reduces the clinical recurrence and asymptomatic shedding of HSV at the time of delivery and the need for cesarean delivery for recurrent disease.
- Following diagnosis of acute parvovirus in pregnancy, weekly ultrasonography to detect fetal hydrops and fetal middle cerebral artery Doppler assessment should be performed for 8 to 12 weeks.
- Routine screening for toxoplasma infection in pregnancy is not recommended.
- There has been no definitive link between measles in pregnancy and increased risk of congenital anomalies and fetal loss.

REFERENCES

(only references cited in synoptic print chapter; for a complete reference list, see ebook)

1. Kimberlin DW, Long SS, Brady MT, Jackson MA. *Red Book 2018: Report of the Committee on Infectious Diseases.* American Academy of Pediatrics; 2018.

2. American College of Obstetricians and Gynecologists. Practice Bulletin No. 151: cytomegalovirus, parvovirus B19, varicella zoster, and toxoplasmosis in pregnancy. *Obstet Gynecol.* 2015;125(6):1510-1525.

12. Revello MG, Gerna G. Diagnosis and management of human cytomegalovirus infection in the mother, fetus, and newborn infant. *Clin Microbiol Rev.* 2002;15(4):680-715.

13. Fowler KB, Boppana SB. Congenital cytomegalovirus infection. *Semin Perinatol.* 2018;42(3):149-154.

17. Stagno S, Pass RF, Dworsky ME, et al. Congenital cytomegalovirus infection: the relative importance of primary and recurrent maternal infection. *N Engl J Med.* 1982;306(16):945-949.

18. Revello MG, Gerna G. Pathogenesis and prenatal diagnosis of human cytomegalovirus infection. *J Clin Virol.* 2004;29(2):71-83.

20. Schleiss MR, Permar SR, Plotkin SA. Progress toward development of a vaccine against congenital cytomegalovirus infection. *Clin Vaccine Immunol.* 2017;24(12):e00268-e00317.

26. Saule H, Enders G, Zeller J, Bernsau U. Congenital rubella infection after previous immunity of the mother. *Eur J Pediatr.* 1988;147(2):195-196.

27. Preblud SR, Williams NM. Fetal risk associated with rubella vaccine: implications for vaccination of susceptible women. *Obstet Gynecol.* 1985;66(1):121-123.

28. Bart SW, Stetler HC, Preblud SR, et al. Fetal risk associated with rubella vaccine: an update. *Rev Infect Dis.* 1985;7(suppl 1):S95-S102.

29. Losonsky GA, Fishaut JM, Strussenberg J, Ogra PL. Effect of immunization against rubella on lactation products. II. Maternal-neonatal interactions. *J Infect Dis.* 1982;145(5):661-666.

32. Freij BJ, South MA, Sever JL. Maternal rubella and the congenital rubella syndrome. *Clin Perinatol.* 1988;15(2):247-257.

33. Hardy JB, McCracken GH Jr, Gilkeson MR, Sever JL. Adverse fetal outcome following maternal rubella after the first trimester of pregnancy. *J Am Med Assoc.* 1969;207(13):2414-2420.

37. Cradock-Watson JE, Miller E, Ridehalgh MK, Terry GM, Ho-Terry L. Detection of rubella virus in fetal and placental tissues and in the throats of neonates after serologically confirmed rubella in pregnancy. *Prenat Diagn.* 1989;9(2):91-96.

38. Banatvala JE, Brown DW. Rubella. *Lancet.* 2004;363(9415):1127-1137.

39. Immunization, Infectious Disease, and Public Health Preparedness Expert Work Group. ACOG Committee Opinion No. 741: maternal immunization. *Obstet Gynecol.* 2018;131(6):e214-e217.

40. American Academy of Pediatrics. Committee on Infectious D, Kimberlin DW, Brady MT, Jackson MA, Long SS. *Red Book: 2018-2021 Report of the Committee on Infectious Diseases.* American Academy of Pediatrics; 2018.

46. Andrews JI. Diagnosis of fetal infections. *Curr Opin Obstet Gynecol.* 2004;16(2):163-166.

47. Wilson CB, Nizet V, Maldonado YA, Remington JS, Klein JO. *Remington and Klein's Infectious Diseases of the Fetus and Newborn Infant.* Elsevier/Saunders; 2016.

48. Harger JH, Ernest JM, Thurnau GR, et al. Frequency of congenital varicella syndrome in a prospective cohort of 347 pregnant women. *Obstet Gynecol.* 2002;100(2):260-265.

49. Lamont RF, Sobel JD, Carrington D, et al. Varicella-zoster virus (chickenpox) infection in pregnancy. *Br J Obstet Gynaecol.* 2011;118(10):1155-1162.

50. Paryani SG, Arvin AM. Intrauterine infection with varicella-zoster virus after maternal varicella. *N Engl J Med.* 1986;314(24):1542-1546.

52. Laforet EG, Lynch CL Jr. Multiple congenital defects following maternal varicella; report of a case. *N Engl J Med.* 1947;236(15):534-537.

53. McGregor JA, Mark S, Crawford GP, Levin MJ. Varicella zoster antibody testing in the care of pregnant women exposed to varicella. *Am J Obstet Gynecol.* 1987;157(2):281-284.

54. Struewing JP, Hyams KC, Tueller JE, Gray GC. The risk of measles, mumps, and varicella among young adults: a serosurvey of US Navy and Marine Corps recruits. *Am J Public Health.* 1993;83(12):1717-1720.

56. Smego RA Jr, Asperilla MO. Use of acyclovir for varicella pneumonia during pregnancy. *Obstet Gynecol.* 1991;78(6):1112-1116.

57. Bohlke K, Galil K, Jackson LA, et al. Postpartum varicella vaccination: is the vaccine virus excreted in breast milk? *Obstet Gynecol.* 2003;102(5 pt 1):970-977.

64. Anderson MJ, Jones SE, Fisher-Hoch SP, et al. Human parvovirus, the cause of erythema infectiosum (fifth disease)? *Lancet.* 1983;1(8338):1378.

65. Serjeant GR, Serjeant BE, Thomas PW, Anderson MJ, Patou G, Pattison JR. Human parvovirus infection in homozygous sickle cell disease. *Lancet.* 1993;341(8855):1237-1240.

66. Bascietto F, Liberati M, Murgano D, et al. Outcome of fetuses with congenital parvovirus B19 infection: systematic review and meta-analysis. *Ultrasound Obstet Gynecol.* 2018;52(5):569-576.

67. Enders M, Weidner A, Zoellner I, Searle K, Enders G. Fetal morbidity and mortality after acute human parvovirus B19 infection in pregnancy: prospective evaluation of 1018 cases. *Prenat Diagn.* 2004;24(7):513-518.

68. Rodis JF, Borgida AF, Wilson M, et al. Management of parvovirus infection in pregnancy and outcomes of hydrops: a survey of members of the Society of Perinatal Obstetricians. *Am J Obstet Gynecol.* 1998;179(4):985-988.

69. Maldonado YA, Read JS. Diagnosis, treatment, and prevention of congenital toxoplasmosis in the United States. *Pediatrics.* 2017;139(2):e20163860.

72. Montoya JG, Remington JS. Management of Toxoplasma gondii infection during pregnancy. *Clin Infect Dis.* 2008;47(4):554-566.

73. Montoya JG, Liesenfeld O. Toxoplasmosis. *Lancet.* 2004;363(9425):1965-1976.

74. Montoya JG. Laboratory diagnosis of Toxoplasma gondii infection and toxoplasmosis. *J Infect Dis.* 2002;185(suppl 1):S73-S82.

76. McLean HQ, Fiebelkorn AP, Temte JL, Wallace GS. Prevention of measles, rubella, congenital rubella syndrome, and mumps, 2013: summary recommendations of the Advisory Committee on Immunization Practices (ACIP). *MMWR Recomm Rep.* 2013;62(RR-04):1-34.

77. Eberhart-Phillips JE, Frederick PD, Baron RC, Mascola L. Measles in pregnancy: a descriptive study of 58 cases. *Obstet Gynecol.* 1993;82(5):797-801.

78. Ali ME, Albar HM. Measles in pregnancy: maternal morbidity and perinatal outcome. *Int J Gynaecol Obstet.* 1997;59(2):109-113.

79. Rasmussen SA, Jamieson DJ. What obstetric health care providers need to know about measles and pregnancy. *Obstet Gynecol.* 2015;126(1):163-170.

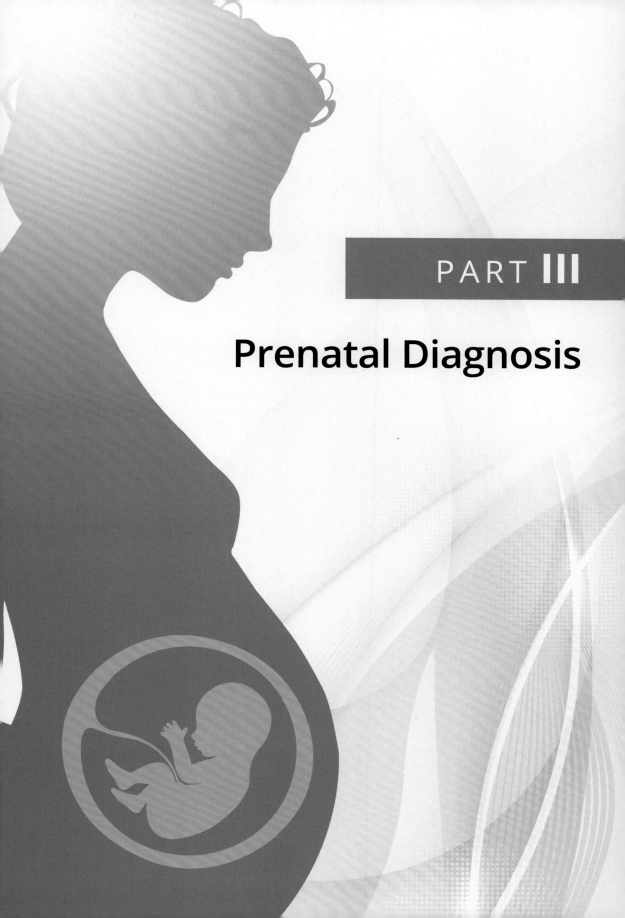

PART III

Prenatal Diagnosis

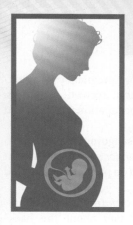

CHAPTER 11

Principles of Genetic Counseling in Prenatal and Perinatal Medicine

Laura Igarzábal and Jeffrey A. Kuller

Introduction

Approximately 2% to 3% of all newborns have a major congenital anomaly, 25% of which have an underlying identifiable *genetic etiology*.[1-3] Some of these defects will be detected in the prenatal period, another percentage at birth or during childhood, and less frequently later in adulthood. In recent decades, there has been an increase in prenatal diagnosis of congenital malformations due to the regular use of ultrasound in pregnancy and improvements of ultrasound equipment. On the other hand, advances in invasive and noninvasive diagnostic tests in pregnancy and molecular studies have contributed to the understanding of the origin of congenital defects and the possibility of carrying out genetic studies. Obstetricians, neonatologists, and other healthcare providers will increasingly encounter fetuses and children with suspected genetic disorders and be asked to order and interpret complex genetic tests.

New screening and diagnostic tests are being introduced regularly in clinical practice. This expanded menu creates a challenge for healthcare providers to keep pace with technologic advances and to effectively provide patients with accurate information related to advantages, disadvantages, limitations, and risks for all testing options.[4] In this scenario, *genetic counseling* has become increasingly important and an integral part of healthcare, to provide a framework to patients for informed decision-making and support.[5] This complex task needs expertise and knowledge, as well as time and resources for adequate counseling.[6,7]

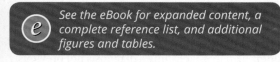

See the eBook for expanded content, a complete reference list, and additional figures and tables.

Principles of Genetic Counseling

The definition of genetic counseling describes a "process of helping people *understand* and *adapt* to the medical, psychological, and familial implications of the genetic contributions to disease."[31]

Genetic counseling is a communication process concerning the occurrence and the risks of recurrence of genetic disorders within a family. Such counseling aims to provide the patient with a clear and comprehensive understanding of all the important *implications* of the disorder in question, as well as the possible *options*. The purpose is also to help families through their *decision making*, and *emotional* adjustments and adaptations, where indicated.[11]

Genetic counseling constitutes an essential component of preconception and prenatal care.[32] All prospective parents need to be told if they have an increased risk of having children with a genetic disorder, or other defects, and what are their options. The physician's duty is to communicate this information *clearly* and in *simple* language (with a translator, if required), to offer specific tests, to offer specific treatments, or to refer couples for expert opinion and to document the consultation and recommendations. Genetic counseling can also provide an otherwise absent opportunity for validation of patient's experiences and concerns about genetic disorders.[7,33]

Prospective parents can seek genetic counseling by themselves or be referred by physicians. No single model of genetic counseling exists with wide variation within and across countries.[34] Genetic counseling should be developed by appropriately *trained professionals* who have the skills to explain genetic concepts and technologies at an appropriate level of complexity, interpret genetic information, communicate uncertainty, and support patient's informed choice.[7,32,35,36] In general, it is best provided by a clinical geneticist or certified genetic counselor under the supervision of a clinical geneticist. In both the United States and Canada, board-certified genetic counselors are available for referral, but this career does not exist in all countries.[34] Genetic counselors are professionals who have specialized education in *genetics* and *counseling* and provide *personalized* help to patients so as they can make *informed decisions* about their genetic health. They are used to interpret genetic disease etiology and clinical consequences, to incorporate new technologic information for pretest counseling, to deal with posttest result interpretation, and to provide an assessment based on patient knowledge, values, and concerns, supporting autonomy.[31,33,37,38]

If an obstetrician or pediatrician or other healthcare provider (midwives, primary care physicians, general practitioners) is well informed, he or she should be able to provide the necessary counseling.[39,40] They should also be able to identify those women or couples with risk factors that should prompt referral to a provider with genetics expertise.[2,4] Referrals for genetic counseling should be initiated in the preconceptional period or early during pregnancy to enable patients with knowledge and guidance to make informed decisions about prevention, testing, and treatment. Caution should guide the primary care physician in avoiding areas outside their expertise. Limited obstetric care provider time and the increasing amount of genomic information for adequate counseling may make it challenging to meet the patient's needs and require an appointment with a clinical geneticist or genetic counselor.[35,37] Documentation of the key elements transmitted during counseling would be regarded as mandatory, regardless of who provides such services.

Reasons for Referral for Genetic Counseling

The primary reasons for referral for genetic counseling, which can be identified both in the prenatal and perinatal period are discussed[3,41,42]:

- Personal history of confirmed or probable *genetic diseases, intellectual disability, or birth defects*.
- Family history of confirmed or probable *genetic disorders, intellectual disability, autism spectrum disorder, or birth defects* (offspring, sibling, parents, grandparents, among others).
- *Maternal medical conditions* associated with an increased risk of congenital anomalies (eg, diabetes mellitus, epilepsy).

- Exposure during or before pregnancy to potential *teratogens* (medication, recreational drugs, alcohol, tobacco, x-ray, occupational agents, and infections).
- Known or suspected consanguinity unions.
- A known or suspected *carrier state* for a particular genetic disorder based on previous or required tests or ethnicity.
- *Recurrent pregnancy* loss or *intrauterine death*.
- The request for *information* about the background risk of birth defects or genetic diseases.
- The request for *information* about the prenatal diagnosis of congenital anomalies.
- *Screening tests* indicating a *high risk* for aneuploidy, congenital disabilities, or pregnancy complications.

The process of genetic counseling in the prenatal and perinatal period integrates the following actions[31]: (1) *interpretation* of family and medical histories to assess the chance of disease occurrence or recurrence; (2) *education* about inheritance, testing, management, prevention, resources, and research; (3) *counseling* to promote informed choices and adaptation to the risk or condition.

Genetic counseling in the prenatal and perinatal period begins with appropriate *risk assessment*. It is essential to determine specific *risk factors* for genetic disorders to provide adequate counseling, selection of tests, and interpretation of results. Comprehensive risk assessment involves the evaluation of a patient's medical, family, pregnancy, and exposure history, as well as other factors such as age and ethnicity. In pregnancy, a family history of the partner should also be obtained.[39,43]

Family information is collected to build a *three-generation pedigree*. The family tree is an easy way to record relevant details (medical conditions, ages of onset, relation to the patient, and appropriate genetic testing results), interpret family relationships, and identify patients with an increased risk for inherited genetic conditions or birth defects.[39,42,44] The family tree can be a handwritten version using standard symbols or an electronic one (**Figure 11.8**). Information is searched on personal and family history of genetic disorders, family's ethnicity, congenital malformations, intellectual disabilities, recurrent pregnancy loss, intrauterine death, childhood death, infertility, primary ovarian insufficiency, and cancer. Examination of previous autopsy reports and x-rays, including those of previous stillborns, is often necessary for confirmation or for help in establishing a diagnosis not previously

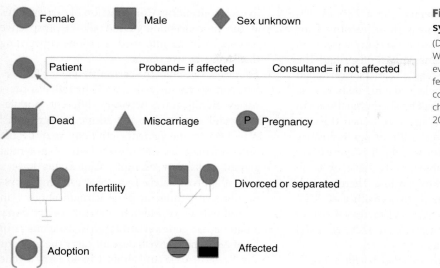

Figure 11.8 Pedigree symbols.

(Data from Wilson RD. Woman's pre-conception evaluation: genetic and fetal risk considerations for counselling and informed choice. *J Obstet Gynaecol Can.* 2018;40(7):935-949.)

made. It is sometimes useful to bring pictures of affected family members who cannot attend the appointment. In the context of congenital malformations, it is important to ask about maternal and paternal age, maternal medical conditions (diabetes mellitus, hypothyroidism, epilepsy), fever, infections (cytomegalovirus, toxoplasmosis, rubella), prenatal exposure to other teratogens (retinoic acid, warfarin, valproic acid), prenatal diagnosis tests, mode of delivery, and childhood development.[38,42,45,46]

At this point, the personal and family history is used to identify genetic disorders or risk factors for genetic disorders, to make a differential diagnosis, to identify and quantify risk for parents and offspring, and to select the right proband and specific tests when considered appropriate.[42,44]

Patients with prolonged infertility of unknown cause or recurrent spontaneous abortion may face a 3% to 8% risk of a parental chromosome abnormality. A history of a previous stillbirth should raise questions about the need for parental chromosome analysis if a karyotype was not performed on the fetus. Between 6% and 11% of stillbirths have a chromosome abnormality.[47]

Certain risk factors increase the risk for *fetal* aneuploidy, single-gene disorders, and structural abnormalities and must also be considered together for individual risk estimation and counseling[2,45,46]:

- *Maternal age*: increasing maternal age increases the risk of aneuploidy.[16,48,49] An arbitrary age of 35 years has long functioned as the age at which maternal age–related risks of chromosome

defects should be discussed and prenatal genetic studies offered, but there is no reason to take this age as a biological cutoff point. Currently, all pregnant women should be informed about available prenatal screening and diagnostic studies to make informed decisions, regardless of age.[50-54]

- *Paternal age*: advancing paternal age has been associated with an increased risk for autosomal dominant single-gene disorder (eg, achondroplasia, Apert syndrome, Crouzon syndrome, Pfeiffer syndrome, multiple endocrine neoplasia type 2A and 2B), epigenetic changes, and chromosomal aneuploidies, but the extent and magnitude of these risks have not been consistently defined.[55-60] The overall risk is low but should be addressed. The best estimate of autosomal dominant disorders in the offspring of fathers who are 40 years of age or older is less than 0.5%.[21] Moreover, there is no consensus for the definition of advanced paternal age. Although most professional societies use a cutoff point of 40 years of age, the optimal definition of advanced paternal age remains to be described.

- *Parental carrier of chromosome rearrangement or aneuploidy*: Patients with prolonged infertility of unknown cause, recurrent pregnancy loss, or intrauterine death may face a 3% to 8% risk of a parental balanced chromosome rearrangement.[11,47,61,62,63] Parental balanced structural chromosomal anomalies increase the risk of unbalanced structural chromosomal anomalies in their offspring. In general, carriers of balanced chromosome translocations, ascertained through the birth of a child with an unbalanced rearrangement, have a 5% to 30% risk of recurrence, whereas those identified for recurrent pregnancy loss or infertility have a 0% to 5% risk of a viable unbalanced offspring.[3] The former risk is higher because carriers ascertained through a liveborn unbalanced child demonstrate the viability for the unbalanced combination. On the contrary, if carriers are ascertained through infertility or miscarriage, without family history of an unbalanced liveborn child, it is most likely that no aneuploid combination is viable, or it will end in spontaneous pregnancy loss. There is much less risk for inversions. Patients with a 47,XXY or 45,X karyotype have a small increased risk of aneuploidy in offspring (47,XXY, 47,XXX, 45,X) although natural fertility is very rare.[3]

- *Parents (or other family members) with a single-gene disorder* (confirmed or possible): if the expectant couple (or other family members) is affected by a single-gene disorder, there should be an in-depth discussion about the disorder and risk to the offspring. Sometimes there may be specific obstetric issues to be evaluated (eg, Marfan syndrome).[32] It is also important to review the diagnosis and natural history of the disease, mode of inheritance, family and individual risk assessment, diagnostic evaluation approach or testing options, management for the condition and treatment recommendations, necessary subspecialty referrals, and to help to make informed reproductive decisions. Molecular diagnosis of the affected proband is usually required for an accurate risk assessment. Sometimes, an obvious pattern of inheritance may emerge without a known disorder. For example, a *maternal* history of nephews, brothers, or uncles with unexplained intellectual disability may point to sex-linked disorder.[21,23,35,46]

- *Carriers of a genetic recessive or X-linked disorder:* Carriers of recessive or X-linked pathogenic variants are usually unaffected by the condition and may be unaware of their carrier status. Their carrier status may be recognized after the birth of an affected child, after the diagnosis of an affected family member, or as the result of a genetic screening program.[32] Two unaffected individuals who are *carriers* of one pathogenic gene variant have a 25% risk of having an affected offspring in each pregnancy (one of four children will be affected; three of four will be phenotypically normal with two of these carriers). Females heterozygous for X-linked disorders have a 50% risk of affected male children

in each conception. Confirmation of carrier status at the preconception period allows prospective parents to make informed decisions concerning their reproductive option.[2,22,23,64,65,66]

- *Ethnic background:* The carrier frequency for specific autosomal recessive or X-linked disorders varies significantly between different populations and is related to the ethnic background.[32] Attention to the patient's ethnicity may be the only warning to the obstetrician of potential genetic risks. For example, Caucasians have a risk of approximately 1 in 25 of carrying a cystic fibrosis pathogenic gene variant; about 1 in 12 individuals of Mediterranean ancestry carry a pathogenic gene variant for β-thalassemia; 1 in 30 of Ashkenazi Jewish descent carry the gene for Tay-Sachs disease, and about 1 in 40 carry a gene pathogenic variant for Canavan disease. Carrier genetic screening is preferably performed in the preconception period to enable prospective parents to make better informed reproductive choices. Carrier genetic screening when the pregnancy is established may limit the options to prenatal diagnosis.[2,22,23,64,65,66] Prenatal diagnosis can be offered only if the parental pathogenic variants are known or if the pregnancy is suspected to be at risk (ie, presence of echogenic fetal bowel increases the risk for cystic fibrosis).

- *Previous fetus or offspring with aneuploidy:* The risk of a future pregnancy being affected by the same or a different trisomy is higher than the maternal age–specific risk. This excess risk is a constant determined by the age at which the first affected pregnancy occurred and is greater for younger women than older women. For example, excess risk at term (above the age-related risk) for a subsequent trisomy 21 was is 0.49% at 20 years and 0.01% at 46 years at the index pregnancy. Excess risk after a previous uncommon trisomy (trisomy 18 and trisomy 13) is 0.37% at 20 years and 0.01% at 50 years[14,16,67,68,69] (**Table 11.5**). In general, though, it is reasonable to counsel patients that the recurrence risk for aneuploidy is 1% to 2% in a patient younger than 35 years. The recurrence risk also appears to be elevated for 47,XXX, and 47,XXY, but not for 45,X.

- *Structural anomalies identified by ultrasonography or at birth:* almost all structural abnormalities increase the likelihood of aneuploidy, copy number variants, and single-gene disorders. These risks are highly dependent on the

Table 11.5 Recurrence Risks for the More Common Chromosome Disorders

Chromosome Disorders	Risk of Recurrence (%)	Notes
Numerical abnormalities		
A previous child born with trisomy 21	1-1.5	Includes risks for all aneuploidy and applies to all women <30 y. Those >30 have maternal age–associated risks of aneuploidy
A previous child born with trisomy 18	<1	
A previous child born with trisomy 13	<1	
A previous child with Turner syndrome (45X)	Population risk	As long as mother is not a Turner syndrome mosaic, risks of recurrence will approximate population risk (1 in 2500 females)
A previous child with XXX syndrome	Population risk	As long as neither parent has sex chromosome mosaicism and mother is <35 y, risks of recurrence will approximate population risk (1 in 1000 females)
A previous child with Klinefelter syndrome (47,XXY)	Population risk	As long as neither parent has sex chromosome mosaicism and mother is <35 y, risk of recurrence will approximate population risk (1 in 1000 males)
A previous child with 47,XYY	Population risk	Population risk approximates 1 in 1000 males
Structural rearrangements		
Robertsonian translocations		
t(13;14) (14;21) maternal		
t(14;21) paternal	Rare	
t(13;21) maternal	11-15	
t(13;21)	1-2	
t(15;21) maternal	11-15	
t(15;21) paternal	1-2	
Reciprocal translocation in general maternal	5-20	Risks depend on how original case was ascertained—if through recurrent miscarriage lower figure applies
In general paternal	3-30	Risks depend on how original case was ascertained—if through recurrent miscarriage lower figure applies
t(11;22) maternal	6	
t(11;22) paternal	S	
Inversions (autosomal)		
Pericentric	5-10	If original case ascertained through a previous child with a structural rearrangement
Pericentric	1-3	If original case ascertained fortuitously and without phenotypic abnormality
Paracentric	<1	

Data from Mc Kinlay Gardner RJ, Amor DJ. *Gardner and Sutherland's Chromosome Abnormalities and Genetic Counseling*. 5th ed. Oxford; 2018, Milunsky A, ed. *Genetic Disorders and the Fetus: Diagnosis, Prevention and Treatment*. Johns Hopkins University Press; 2004, Milunsky A. *Your Genetic Destiny: Know Your Genes, Secure Your Health, Save Your Life*. Perseus Publishing; 2001.

number and type of malformations.[70,71,72,73] Discrepancy between gestational age and fetal growth, disparity in specific measurements (eg, femur length, size of lateral ventricles), or questions of organ presence or normality (eg, large or absent kidneys) will alert the perinatologist to the need for further study, including serial examinations, in order to seek accurate diagnosis.[21] Once a structural anomaly is identified, physicians will try to describe it as accurately as possible, rule out associated anomalies, and classify it as isolated or as part of a syndrome.[74,75,76] The natural history of the malformation should be reviewed, as well as the probable mode of inheritance, prognosis, and risk of recurrence for future pregnancies. The patient should be offered invasive diagnostic testing for fetal karyotype and CMA as the initial investigation.[19,50,74] In the context of a normal cytogenetic result and on a case-by-case basis, it could be appropriate to proceed with molecular sequencing studies for specific genes, genes panels, or whole exome sequencing (WES).[54,77,78,79] Patient decision making requires accurate and detailed counseling.[5,6,7,37] Despite advances in ultrasound and molecular genetics studies, uncertainty may remain regarding the diagnosis until delivery. In these cases, the final assessment should be performed postnatally, or, in cases of pregnancy termination, stillbirth, or neonatal death, an autopsy should be offered.[80]

Screening tests indicating a high risk for congenital abnormalities or pregnancy complications.

Table 11.6 Risk Factors for Genetic Diseases

Genetic Etiology	Risk Factors	
	Preconceptional	Pregnancy
Chromosomal abnormalities	Maternal age Paternal age Previous fetus or offspring with aneuploidy Parental carrier of chromosome rearrangement Parental carrier of aneuploidy History of congenital anomalies Recurrent pregnancy loss: unknown etiology Intrauterine or neonatal death: unknown etiology	Structural anomalies identified by ultrasonography Screening tests indicating a high risk for aneuploidies Increased nuchal translucency Second trimester US soft markers IUGR Oligohydramnios Polyhydramnios
Single-gene disorder		
Autosomal dominant	Paternal age Parents affected by a dominant disorder	Structural anomalies identified by US (eg, skeletal dysplasia)
Autosomal recessive	Ethnic background Parents carrier of a genetic recessive disorder Previous affected offspring with recessive disorder Consanguinity	Structural anomalies identified by US (eg, echogenic bowel)
X-linked	Parents carrier of an X-linked disorder Previous affected offspring with an X-linked disorder Affected males	Structural anomalies identified by US (eg, aqueductal stenosis)
Multifactorial	Previous affected offspring Affected parents Diabetes Epilepsy	Structural anomalies identified by US Polyhydramnios Oligohydramnios

IUGR, intrauterine growth restriction; US, ultrasound.

Data from Harris BS, Bishop KC, Kemeny HR, Walker JS, Rhee E, Kuller JA. Risk factors for birth defects. *Obstet Gynecol Surv.* 2017;72(2):123-135, Committee on Genetics. Committee Opinion No. 643: "identification and referral of maternal genetic conditions in pregnancy". *Obstet Gynecol.* 2015;126(4):913, Wilson RD. Woman's pre-conception evaluation: genetic and fetal risk considerations for counselling and informed choice. *J Obstet Gynaecol Can.* 2018;40(7):935-949.

Couples at risk of affected offspring with specific genetic diseases should be counseled as soon as possible to make informed decisions about reproductive options: prenatal diagnosis for termination of an affected pregnancy or planning for the birth of an affected child, preimplantation genetic testing, use of donor gametes, avoidance of having children or adoption. Psychosocial support for patients and families should be provided[32,81,82,83] (**Table 11.6**).

Counseling About Genetic Tests in the Prenatal and Perinatal Period

For the *low-risk patient*, without identified risk factors for genetic disorders, physicians should counsel about the baseline risk to have a child born with aneuploidy, CNVs, single-gene diseases, and multifactorial disorders, according to maternal and paternal age, and previous genetic tests.[7] Many professional societies consider that all pregnant women, regardless of age, should be offered prenatal assessment for aneuploidy by screening or diagnostic testing in early pregnancy.[51,52,53] Healthcare providers should be aware of the prenatal testing options in their country or institution. At the same time, information about genetic carrier screening should be provided.[7]

Prenatal screening aims to identify pregnancies at increased risk for abnormal outcomes, while simultaneously minimizing the number of normal pregnancies with abnormal test results (the false positive result of the test). Pregnancies identified to be at increased risk are offered diagnostic testing. In addition, negative prenatal screening results may offer the patient reassurance and decreased anxiety.

Prenatal genetic screening tests assess the fetal risk of genetic disorders (eg, trisomy 21) whereas *genetic diagnostic tests* provide a definitive diagnosis of the fetal genetic status. Screening test performance is defined by *detection rate* (DR: the proportion of abnormal pregnancies with positive test results, that is to say the test's ability to correctly detect pregnancies with the condition screened) and *false-positive rate* (FPR). These are measures of the *clinical validity* of the tests.

The *clinical utility* of a test depends on the *prevalence* of the condition in the population being tested and the *impact* on clinical management. The *positive predictive value* (PPV: the chance that a pregnancy is affected with the condition following a positive result) is a measure of clinical utility and depends both on the DR and FPR of the test as well as on the prevalence of the condition being tested. The *negative predictive value* (NPV) is the likelihood that the pregnancy is truly unaffected after a negative test.[39,54,77]

Traditionally, prenatal genetic screening has relied on the identification of pregnancies at increased risk for chromosome abnormalities (trisomy 21, trisomy 18, trisomy 13). Multiple options are available and include serum screening and ultrasound screening (**Table 11.7**). Diagnostic confirmation of fetal chromosomal disorders requires an invasive procedure such as amniocentesis or chorionic villus sampling. For example, women with a positive cell-free fetal DNA in maternal plasma screening test (noninvasive prenatal testing [NIPT]) result for trisomy 21 should be counseled of the increased risk for this trisomy and offered the option of diagnostic testing. When a negative test result is obtained, women should be counseled of the posttest decreased risk for this aneuploidy.[52,77,84,85,86,87]

Patients should always be informed that genetic testing is *optional* and should have the chance for an in-depth discussion of the risks, benefits, and alternatives of the various prenatal diagnostic and screening options, including the option of no testing. Such discussions should allow patients to understand their chance of having a pregnancy or newborn with a specific disorder and empower them to make decisions about whether to proceed with testing or not.[6,7,37] The decision to perform screening or diagnostic testing for aneuploidy will depend on the information provided by the physician and on the patient's understanding, experiences and values, and their desire for informational accuracy.[88]

For the *high-risk patient* for fetal genetic diseases, genetic testing may be offered according to specific risk factors, such as an abnormal ultrasound finding or when parents are both carriers of AR pathogenic variants for the same disorder.[39] Multiple testing methodologies are available for detecting different types of genetic anomalies (**Table 11.8**).

Cytogenetic abnormalities can be detected using standard karyotype and molecular cytogenetic techniques (QF-PCR, MLPA, FISH, CMA). For example, after a positive prenatal screening test for aneuploidy, an invasive prenatal diagnosis for fetal karyotype is offered. Standard karyotype would detect an extra or missing chromosome, and a partial deletion or duplication as small as 5 to 10 Mb (megabases).[3] FISH or

Table 11.7 Prenatal Screening Tests for Aneuploidies

Screening Test	US and Serum Markers	Gestational Age (Weeks)	Detection Rate for Trisomy 21 (%)	False-Positive Rate (%)
First-trimester combined screening	NT PAPP-A Free-BhCG	11-13.6	80-85	5
First-trimester combined screening with additional US markers	Nuchal translucency NB/DV/TV PAPP-A Free-BhCG	11-13.6	90-95	5
Triple test	AFP BhCG Estriol	15-20	65-70	5
Quadruple test	AFP BhCG Estriol Inhibin-A	15-20	75-80	5
Integrated test	NT PAPP-A AFP BhCG Estriol (inhibin-A)	11-13.6 15-20	91-96	5
Sequential test	NT PAPP-A AFP BhCG Estriol (inhibin-A)	11-13.6 15-20	91-95	5
Contingent test	NT PAPP-A AFP BhCG Estriol (inhibin-A)	11-13.6 15-20	90-9	5
Cell-free fetal DNA	Fetal DNA in maternal plasma	9-10	99	0.1

AFP, alpha-fetoprotein; BhCG, beta subunit of human chorionic gonadotropin; DV, ductus venosus Doppler flow pattern; free-BhCG, free beta subunit of human chorionic gonadotropin; NB, nasal bone; NT, nuchal translucency; PAPP-A, pregnancy-associated plasma protein A; TV, Doppler flow through tricuspid valve; US, ultrasound.

Data from Hoskovec JM, Stevens BK. Genetic counseling overview for the obstetrician-gynecologist. *Obstet Gynecol Clin North Am.* 2018;45(1):1-12, Jelin AC, Sagaser KG, Wilkins-Haug L. Prenatal genetic testing options. *Pediatr Clin North Am.* 2019;66(2):281-293, Jelin AC, Vora N. Whole exome sequencing: applications in prenatal genetics. *Obstet Gynecol Clin North Am.* 2018;45(1):69-81.

QF-PCR could be used for rapid cytogenetic results (24-48 hours) for a limited number of chromosomes (eg, FISH for chromosome 21; QF-PCR for chromosomes 21, 18, 13, X, Y). On the other hand, CMA can detect all aneuploidies and other chromosomal anomalies that would be detected by karyotype but with higher-resolution through detection of CNVs. It can be expected to discover a clinically significant CNV in 1% to 2% of structurally normal fetuses and 6% of fetuses with ultrasound anomalies.[5,72,89] CMA does not require cell culture; therefore, it has less turnaround time for results than karyotype, and it will more likely obtain results in cases of fetal demise. CMA is now recommended, when available, as the first-tier test in the postnatal diagnosis of intellectual disability, multiple malformations, and autism spectrum disorder, and in the prenatal diagnosis of birth defects.[90,91,92]

Single-gene disorders are not detectable by CMA and require a sequencing approach, and on

Table 11.8 Test for Prenatal Genetic Diagnosis

Test	Genetic Diagnosis	Turnaround Time
Karyotype	Numerical chromosomal abnormalities Structural chromosomal abnormalities, both balanced and unbalanced 5-10 Mb	7-14 d
FISH	Target aneuploidies (eg, chromosomes 13, 18, 21, X, Y) Target copy number variants	24-48 h (direct testing)
QF-PCR	Target aneuploidies (eg, chromosomes 13, 18, 21, X, Y) Target copy number variants	24-48 h (direct testing)
CMA	Copy number variants Unbalanced 50-200 Kb	3-10 d (culture cells more TAT)
Gene panel	SNPs INDELS Copy number variants (if evaluated)	14 d
WES	SNPs INDELS	14 d

CMA, chromosomal microarray analysis; FISH, fluorescence *in situ* hybridization; INDELS, small insertions and deletions; Kb, kilobases; Mb, megabases; QF-PCR, quantitative fluorescence polymerase chain reaction; SNPs, single-nucleotide polymorphisms; WES, whole exome sequencing.

Data from Mc Kinlay Gardner RJ, Amor DJ. *Gardner and Sutherland's Chromosome Abnormalities and Genetic Counseling*. 5th ed. Oxford; 2018, Post AL, Mottola AT, Kuller JA. What's new in prenatal genetics? A review of current recommendations and guidelines. *Obstet Gynecol Surv*. 2017;72(10):610-617, Wapner RJ, Martin CL, Levy B, et al. Chromosomal microarray versus karyotyping for prenatal diagnosis. *N Engl J Med*. 2012;367(23):2175-2184, American College of Obstetricians and Gynecologists Committee on Genetics. Committee Opinion No. 581: the use of chromosomal microarray analysis in prenatal diagnosis. *Obstet Gynecol*. 2013;122(6):1374-1347, Armour CM, Dougan SD, Brock JA, et al; On-Behalf-Of the Canadian College of Medical Geneticists. Practice guideline: joint CCMG-SOGC recommendations for the use of chromosomal microarray analysis for prenatal diagnosis and assessment of fetal loss in Canada. *J Med Genet*. 2018;55(4):215-221.

a case-by-case basis, the choice of single-gene testing, gene panel, or WES can be considered. For example, in the case of a fetus with normal CMA and a second trimester increased nuchal fold and pleural effusion Noonan syndrome should be suspected, and request a panel of genes associated to RASopathies.[93] On the other hand, if the diagnosis of a specific syndrome is not straightforward and there is suspicion of genetic etiology, WES may be a more useful test.

WES in prenatal diagnosis may be considered in the context of clinical research or in selected cases after normal karyotype and CMA. It has been suggested that WES could be useful in the prenatal genetic diagnosis of fetuses with a single major anomaly or with multiple organ system anomalies that are suggestive of a possible genetic etiology, and in cases of recurrent or lethal fetal anomalies, with expert counseling.[94,95,96] In a prospective cohort of unselected fetuses with structural anomalies, it has been demonstrated that WES identified diagnostic genetic variants in 10% of cases.[95,97]

The joint Position Statement (https://obgyn.onlinelibrary.wiley.com/doi/epdf/10.1002/pd.5195) from the International Society for Prenatal Diagnosis (ISPD), the Society for Maternal Fetal Medicine (SMFM), and the Perinatal Quality Foundation (PQF) on the use of genome-wide sequencing for fetal diagnosis has defined some scenarios where fetal sequencing may be beneficial[94]:

- Fetus with a single major anomaly or with multiple anomalies that are suggestive of a possible genetic etiology after normal CMA.
- Fetus with no available CMA result but with multiple anomalies that strongly suggests a single gene disorder.
- Parental history of a prior undiagnosed fetus or child affected with a major single anomaly or multiple anomalies suggestive of a genetic etiology, and a recurrence of similar anomalies in the current pregnancy after normal karyotype or CMA. If no sample is available from the affected proband, offer sequencing for both parents to

look for carrier status for autosomal recessive diseases that might explain the fetal phenotype.

- In families with a history of recurrent stillbirths of unknown etiology with normal karyotype and/or CMA, where the fetus in the current pregnancy has a recurrent pattern of anomalies.

WES is still expensive, difficult to interpret, and may take several weeks to complete analysis, which limit its utility in prenatal diagnosis. It is also uncertain whether prenatal sequencing should only focus on genes associated with the fetal phenotype or if a full-genome approach would be better. Moving from single gene, to gene panel testing, to WES also increases the potential for VUS and unexpected secondary findings.[98,99,100,101] The trio approach, where fetal and parental samples are analyzed together, benefits interpretation for detected VUS. Ideally, a multidisciplinary team with expertise in clinical genetics and laboratory experience in prenatal diagnosis and fetal sequencing should analyze and categorize the results. The application of prenatal WES is still an evolving field. Although it is increasing rapidly, there is still no evidence on the best way to introduce it into clinical practice.

The purpose of prenatal genetic screening and diagnostic testing is to provide *information* about the fetus to prospective parents so that they can make *informed decisions* about the pregnancy, and to healthcare providers to guide the care or treatment of the pregnant patient and her newborn. Parents should have the option of termination of pregnancy when an abnormality is identified, or be better prepared to receive an affected newborn, depending on personal factors such as attitude toward and previous experience with the disease, ethical and religious principles, level of education, social and legal circumstances.[81,102]

Pretest and *posttest counseling* is essential and must be a part of any screening program and before genetic testing.[6,31,46]

Pretest Counseling

Pretest counseling should be performed by qualified providers who have the skills to communicate the benefits and limitations of tests to patients before testing.[35] Pretest counseling aims to provide *accurate information* about testing options, in a *personalized* (according to patient's culture, education level, language, and values) and *nondirective manner*, and to enable patient *informed decision* making according to personal needs and values.[7,33]

The *informed decision* is one in which the relevant knowledge is high and is consistent with the patient's values, and they are taken into account.[37] Although it is essential to deliver updated information to the patient, based on the best available scientific evidence and not only on personal experience or marketing, which may be biased, it is more than providing data.[35] It is crucial to focus on the patient understanding of the information, preferences, and needs. Pretest counseling would reach informed decision-making if it balances information-giving and psychosocial counseling without overwhelming patients with information.[33,37] Models such as "shared decision-making" better describe the actual counseling process, promoting good communication of best available evidence, patient autonomy, deliberation that includes the process of thinking about and weighing up the pros and cons of the test, and support, to facilitate patient-centered decision-making.[103]

It is essential that physicians have in-depth knowledge of the tests, the conditions for which testing may be offered, and technical issues, in order to answer any questions that may arise during or after the counseling session.[7,33,35,36,37,104]

Each patient will weigh risks and benefits differently and may come to different conclusions about whether to pursue testing.[39,88,105]

Although cost should not preclude offering a medically indicated test to a patient, it could be a barrier to access because many genetic tests are expensive and may not be covered by a patient's insurance.[6] Comprehensive pretest counseling lays the foundation for useful posttest discussion of results.

Posttest Counseling

Posttest counseling can be delivered by any healthcare provider with adequate expertise in the field of medical genetics; if this is not possible, referral to a genetic counselor or medical geneticist is recommended.[6,7] In general, patients with complex findings often benefit from more in-depth time with a physician who can provide specific information and counseling, and who has the skills to translate complex genetic information into informed decision-making.[35] Results should be delivered *promptly*, especially prenatal tests, *clearly* and in a *nondirective* way.[6]

It is important to describe the differences between screening and diagnostic tests. Results from *screening tests* would inform either an *increased risk* for the condition evaluated (positive screening test result or high risk) or a decreased risk (negative screening test result or low risk).

Patients with a positive screening test result should be counseled regarding the higher risk for the screened condition and offered the option of diagnostic testing. It must be emphasized that an abnormal screening test does not mean an affected individual.

On the contrary, when a negative screening result is obtained, patients should be counseled regarding their lower adjusted risk, and not be offered additional screening tests. A low-risk result should prompt a discussion about the NPV and residual risk. Although reassurance should be provided, the patient should understand that a negative result does not eliminate the possibility that the pregnancy has a genetic condition or birth defect.

Diagnostic tests will confirm (or not) the disorder tested, but sometimes an uncertain or noninformative result would be obtained. Information to be shared about abnormal tests includes balanced and up-to-date information on the natural history of the condition, available treatment or therapies, and management options. This situation should also promote a discussion about the scope of the test and residual risk.[6,7,37,104]

A particular challenge in the prenatal period is that information about the fetal phenotype is always incomplete due to limitations inherent to intrauterine development and imaging studies. Moreover, many conditions that are diagnosable *in utero* include a broad spectrum of phenotypes and severity, and for which much of the prognostic information comes from postnatal studies. These issues highlight the limitation in providing accurate prognosis information before delivery in many cases.

When a *noninformative, unexpected,* or *uncertain* diagnosis is obtained, genetic counseling is much more complicated and deserves a physician and/or genetic counselor with extensive experience with these types of results. In the context of prenatal diagnosis, most parents expect reassurance; therefore, this type of diagnosis leads to uncertainty and makes informed decision making difficult.[111]

There could also appear an unexpected diagnosis that may or may not be related to the reason for testing. For example, a microarray study using a platform with single-nucleotide polymorphisms (SNP-microarray), performed for a cardiac malformation, may show a microdeletion in 15q11.2q13.1 demonstrating loss of the maternal allele resulting in Angelman syndrome.[114] Another incidental finding would be a low-penetrance neurosusceptibility loci with unclear significance (VUS).[115] The interpretation of these variants in pregnancy and the clinical implications may be difficult to predict.

If a genetic test reveals a possible pathogenic hereditary gene variant, patients should be encouraged to share the results with other family members at risk of carrying the same disorder.[6] Providing support is imperative, and additional resources may enhance a patient's understanding.

Principles Guiding the Delivery of Genetic Counseling

The principles guiding the delivery of genetic counseling include:

Accurate diagnosis
Nondirective counseling
Confidentiality and trust
Timing
Knowledge, jargon, and empathy
Duty

KEY POINTS

- Approximately 2% to 3% of all newborns have a major congenital anomaly, 25% of which have a known underlying *genetic etiology*.
- The revolutionary breakthrough in molecular diagnostic techniques challenges healthcare providers to keep pace with technologic advances and to effectively provide patients with accurate information related to advantages, disadvantages, limitations, and risks for all testing options.

- *Genetic counseling* has become increasingly important and an integral part of health care, to provide a framework to patients for informed decision-making and support.
- If an obstetrician is well informed, he or she should be able to provide the necessary counseling. Caution should guide the physician in avoiding areas outside expected expertise. If necessary, referral to a provider with genetic expertise should be made.

- Genetic counseling is a communication process to discuss the occurrence and the risks of recurrence of genetic disorders within a family.
- Couples identified at risk of an affected offspring with specific genetic diseases should be counseled as soon as possible to make informed decisions about reproductive options
- *Pretest* and *posttest counseling* is essential and must be a part of any screening program and before genetic testing.

REFERENCES

(only references cited in synoptic print chapter; for a complete reference list, see ebook)

1. Martin JA, Hamilton BE, Osterman MJ, et al. Births: final data for 2015. *Natl Vital Stat Rep.* 2017;66(1):1.
2. Harris BS, Bishop KC, Kemeny HR, Walker JS, Rhee E, Kuller JA. Risk factors for birth defects. *Obstet Gynecol Surv.* 2017;72(2):123-135.
3. Mc Kinlay Gardner RJ, Amor DJ. *Gardner and Sutherland's Chromosome Abnormalities and Genetic Counseling.* 5th ed. Oxford; 2018.
4. McClatchey T, Lay E, Strassberg M, Van den Veyver IB. Missed opportunities: unidentified genetic risk factors in prenatal care. *Prenat Diagn.* 2018;38(1):75-79.
5. Post AL, Mottola AT, Kuller JA. What's new in prenatal genetics? A review of current recommendations and guidelines. *Obstet Gynecol Surv.* 2017;72(10):610-617.
6. Committee on Genetics. Committee Opinion No. 693: counseling about genetic testing and communication of genetic test results. *Obstet Gynecol.* 2017;129(4):e96-e101.
7. Rink BD, Kuller JA. What are the required components of pre- and posttest counseling? *Semin Perinatol.* 2018;42(5):287-289.
11. Milunsky A, ed. *Genetic Disorders and the Fetus: Diagnosis, Prevention and Treatment.* Johns Hopkins University Press; 2004.
14. Hook EB. Chromosomal abnormalities: prevalence, risks and recurrence. In: Brock DJH, Rodeck CH, Ferguson-Smith MA, eds. *Prenatal Diagnosis and Screening.* Churchill Livingstone; 1992:351-392.
16. Snijders RJ, Sundberg K, Holzgreve W, et al. Maternal age-and gestation-specific risk for trisomy 21. *Ultrasound Obstet Gynecol.* 1999;13(3):167-170.
19. Committee on Genetics and the Society for Maternal-Fetal Medicine. Committee Opinion No. 682. Microarrays and next-generation sequencing technology: the use of advanced genetic diagnostic tools in obstetrics and gynecology. *Obstet Gynecol.* 2016;128(6):e262-e268.
21. Milunsky A. *Your Genetic Destiny: Know Your Genes, Secure Your Health, Save Your Life.* Perseus Publishing; 2001.
22. Committee on Genetics. Committee Opinion No. 690: carrier screening in the age of genomic medicine. *Obstet Gynecol.* 2017;129(3):e35-e40.
23. Committee on Genetics. Committee Opinion No. 691. Carrier screening for genetic conditions. *Obstet Gynecol.* 2017;129:e41-e55.
31. National Society of Genetic Counselors' Definition Task Force, Resta R, Biesecker BB, Bennett RL, et al. A new definition of genetic counseling: National Society of Genetic Counselors' Task Force Report. *J Genet Couns.* 2006;15(2):77-83.
32. Ioannides AS. Preconception and prenatal genetic counselling. *Best Pract Res Clin Obstet Gynaecol.* 2017;42:2-10.
33. Brett GR, Wilkins EJ, Creed ET, et al. Genetic counseling in the era of genomics: what's all the fuss about? *J Genet Couns.* 2018;27(5):1010-1021.
35. O'Brien BM, Dugoff L. What education, background, and credentials are required to provide genetic counseling? *Semin Perinatol.* 2018;42(5):290-295.
36. Skirton H. More than an informative service: are counselling skills needed by genetics professionals in the genomic era? *Eur J Hum Genet.* 2018;26(9):1239-1240.
37. Metcalfe SA. Genetic counselling, patient education, and informed decision-making in the genomic era. *Semin Fetal Neonatal Med.* 2018;23(2):142-149.
38. Ormond KE. From genetic counseling to genomic counseling. *Mol Genet Genomic Med.* 2013;1(4):189-193.
39. Hoskovec JM, Stevens BK. Genetic counseling overview for the obstetrician-gynecologist. *Obstet Gynecol Clin North Am.* 2018;45(1):1-12.
40. Mandelberger AH, Robins JC, Buster JE, et al. Preconception counseling: do patients learn about genetics from their obstetrician gynecologists? *J Assist Reprod Genet.* 2015;32(7):1145-1149.
41. ACOG Committee Opinion No. 762: prepregnancy counseling. *Obstet Gynecol.* 2019;133(1):e78-e89.
42. Committee on Genetics. Committee Opinion No. 478: family history as a risk assessment tool. *Obstet Gynecol.* 2011;117(3):747-750.
43. Rashkin MD, Bowes J, Dunaway K, et al. Genetic counseling, 2030: an on-demand service tailored to the needs of a price conscious, genetically literate, and busy world. *J Genet Couns.* 2019;28(2):456-465.
44. Wattendorf DJ, Hadley DW. Family History: the three-generation pedigree. *Am Fam Physician.* 2005;72(3):441-448.
45. Committee on Genetics. Committee Opinion No. 643: "identification and referral of maternal genetic conditions in pregnancy". *Obstet Gynecol.* 2015;126(4):913.
46. Wilson RD. Woman's pre-conception evaluation: genetic and fetal risk considerations for counselling and informed choice. *J Obstet Gynaecol Can.* 2018;40(7):935-949.
47. Page JM, Silver RM. Genetic causes of recurrent pregnancy loss. *Clin Obstet Gynecol.* 2016;59:498-508.
50. American College of Obstetricians and Gynecologists' Committee on Practice Bulletins—Obstetrics, Committee on Genetics; Society for Maternal–Fetal Medicine. Practice Bulletin No. 162: prenatal diagnostic testing for genetic disorders. *Obstet Gynecol.* 2016;127(5):e108-e122.
51. Chitayat D, Langlois S, Wilson RD. No. 261-Prenatal screening for fetal aneuploidy in singleton pregnancies. *J Obstet Gynaecol Can.* 2017;39(9):e380-e394.
52. Committee on Practice Bulletins—Obstetrics, Committee on Genetics, and the Society for Maternal-Fetal Medicine. Practice Bulletin No. 163: screening for fetal aneuploidy. *Obstet Gynecol.* 2016;127(5):e123-37.
53. National Institute for Health and Care Excellence. Antenatal care for uncomplicated pregnancies. Clinical guideline [CG62]. Updated January 2017. Accessed June 25, 2020. https://www.nice.org.uk/guidance/cg62
54. Jelin AC, Sagaser KG, Wilkins-Haug L. Prenatal genetic testing options. *Pediatr Clin North Am.* 2019;66(2):281-293.
55. Sharma R, Agarwal A, Rohra VK, et al. Effects of increased paternal age on sperm quality, reproductive outcome and associated epigenetic risks to offspring. *Reprod Biol Endocrinol.* 2015;13:35-55.
56. Nybo Andersen AM, Urhoj SK. Is advanced paternal age a health risk for the offspring? *Fertil Steril.* 2017;107(2):312-318.
57. Jennings MO, Owen RC, Keefe D, Kim ED. Management and counseling of the male with advanced paternal age. *Fertil Steril.* 2017;107(2):324-328.
58. Brandt JS, Cruz Ithier MA, Rosen T, et al. Advanced paternal age, infertility, and reproductive risks: a review of the literature. *Prenat Diagn.* 2019;39(2):81-87.
59. Hurley EG, De Franco EA. Influence of paternal age on perinatal outcomes. *Am J Obstet Gynecol.* 2017;217(5):566.e1-566.e6.
60. Toriello HV, Meck JM, Professional P, Guidelines C. Statement on guidance for genetic counseling in advanced paternal age. *Genet Med.* 2008;10(6):457-460.
61. Kaser D. The status of genetic screening in recurrent pregnancy loss. *Obstet Gynecol Clin North Am.* 2018;45(1):143-154.
62. Pal AK, Ambulkar PS, Waghmare JE, et al. Chromosomal aberrations in couples with pregnancy loss: a retrospective study. *J Hum Reprod Sci.* 2018;11(3):247-253.
63. Kalotra V, Lall M, Saviour P, Verma IC, Kaur A. Prevalence of cytogenetic anomalies in couples with recurrent miscarriages: a case-control study. *J Hum Reprod Sci.* 2017;10(4):302-309.
64. Edwards JG, Feldman G, Goldberg J, et al. Expanded carrier screening in reproductive medicine—points to consider: a joint statement of the American College of Medical Genetics and Genomics, American College of Obstetricians and Gynecologists, National Society of Genetic Counselors, Perinatal Quality Foundation, and Society for Maternal-Fetal Medicine. *Obstet Gynecol.* 2015;125(3):653-662.

65. Wilson RD, De Bie I, Armour CM, et al. Opinion for Reproductive Genetic Carrier Screening: an update for all Canadian providers of maternity and reproductive healthcare in the era of direct consumer testing. *J Obstet Gynaecol Can*. 2016;38:742-762.

66. Grody WW, Thompson BH, Gregg AR, et al. ACMG position statement on prenatal/preconception expanded carrier screening. *Genet Med*. 2013;15(6):482-483.

67. Grande M, Stergiotou I, Borrell A, et al. Heterotrisomy recurrence risk: a practical maternal age-dependent approach for excess trisomy 21 risk calculation after a previous autosomal trisomy. *J Matern Fetal Neonatal Med*. 2017;30(13):1613-1615.

68. Morris JK, Mutton DE, Alberman E. Recurrences of free trisomy 21: analysis of data from the National Down Syndrome Cytogenetic Register. *Prenat Diagn*. 2005;25(12):1120-1128.

69. Warburton D, Dallaire L, Thangavelu M, et al. Trisomy recurrence: a reconsideration based on North American data. *Am J Hum Genet*. 2004;75(3):376-385.

70. Nicolaides KH, Snijders RJ, Gosden CM, Berry C, Campbell S. Ultrasonographically detectable markers of fetal chromosomal abnormalities. *Lancet*. 1992;340(8821):704-707.

71. Lichtenbelt KD, Knoers NV, Schuring-Blom GH. From karyotyping to array-CGH in prenatal diagnosis. *Cytogenet Genome Res*. 2011;135(3-4):241-250.

72. Wapner RJ, Martin CL, Levy B, et al. Chromosomal microarray versus karyotyping for prenatal diagnosis. *N Engl J Med*. 2012;367(23):2175-2184.

73. Vora NL, Powell B, Brandt A, et al. Prenatal exome sequencing in anomalous fetuses: new opportunities and challenges. *Genet Med*. 2017;19(11):1207-1216.

74. Gagnon A; Genetics Committee. Evaluation of prenatally diagnosed structural congenital anomalies. *J Obstet Gynaecol Can*. 2009;31(9):875-881.

75. Kermorvant-Duchemin E, Ville Y. Prenatal diagnosis of congenital malformations for the better and for the worse. *J Matern Fetal Neonatal Med*. 2017;30(12):1402-1406.

76. Benacerraf BB. The Sherlock Holmes approach to diagnosing fetal syndromes by ultrasound. *Clin Obstet Gynecol*. 2012;55(1):226-248.

77. Jelin AC, Vora N. Whole exome sequencing: applications in prenatal genetics. *Obstet Gynecol Clin North Am*. 2018;45(1):69-81.

78. Hayward J, Chitty LS. Beyond screening for chromosomal abnormalities: advances in non-invasive diagnosis of single gene disorders and fetal exome sequencing. *Semin Fetal Neonatal Med*. 2018;23(2):94-101.

79. de Koning MA, Haak MC, Adama van Scheltema PN, et al. From diagnostic yield to clinical impact: a pilot study on the implementation of prenatal exome sequencing in routine care. *Genet Med*. 2019;21(10):2303-2310. doi:10.1038/s41436-019-0499-9

80. Désilets V, Oligny LL; Genetics Committee of the Society of Obstetricians and Gynaecology Canada; Family Physicians Advisory Committee; Medico-Legal Committee of the SOGC. Fetal and perinatal autopsy in prenatally diagnosed fetal abnormalities with normal karyotype. *J Obstet Gynaecol Can*. 2011;33(10):1047-1057.

81. Paolini CI, Gadow A, Petracchi F, Igarzabal L, Quadrelli R, Gadow EC. Prenatal screening for chromosome abnormalities in a region with no access to termination of pregnancy. *Prenat Diagn*. 2009;29(7):659-663.

82. Chervenak FA, McCullough LB. Ethical issues in perinatal genetics. *Semin Fetal Neonatal Med*. 2011;16(2):70-73.

83. Buccafurni D, Chang PL. Does prenatal diagnosis morally require provision of selective abortion? *Am J Bioeth*. 2009;9(8):65-67.

84. Borrell A. A new comprehensive paradigm for prenatal diagnosis: seeing the forest through the trees. *Ultrasound Obstet Gynecol*. 2018;52(5):563-568.

85. Biggio J. Prenatal screening for fetal aneuploidy: time to examine where we are and where we are going. *Am J Obstet Gynecol*. 2017;21(6):673-675.

86. Committee Opinion No. 640: cell-free DNA screening for fetal aneuploidy. *Obstet Gynecol*. 2015;126(3):e31-e37.

87. Gregg AR, Skotko BG, Benkendorf JL. Noninvasive prenatal screening for fetal aneuploidy, 2016 update: a position statement of the American College of Medical Genetics and Genomics. *Genet Med*. 2016;18(10):1056-1065.

88. Hill M, Johnson JA, Langlois S, et al. Preferences for prenatal tests for Down syndrome: an international comparison of the views of pregnant women and health professionals. *Eur J Hum Genet*. 2016;24:968-975.

89. Oneda B, Rauch A. Microarrays in prenatal diagnosis. *Best Pract Res Clin Obstet Gynaecol*. 2017;23:S1521-S6934.

90. Miller DT, Adam MP, Aradhya S. Consensus statement: chromosomal microarray is a first-tier clinical diagnostic test for individuals with developmental disabilities or congenital anomalies. *Am J Hum Genet*. 2010;86(5):749-764.

91. American College of Obstetricians and Gynecologists Committee on Genetics. Committee Opinion No. 581: the use of chromosomal microarray analysis in prenatal diagnosis. *Obstet Gynecol*. 2013;122(6):1374-1347.

92. Armour CM, Dougan SD, Brock JA, et al; On-Behalf-Of the Canadian College of Medical Geneticists. Practice guideline: joint CCMG-SOGC recommendations for the use of chromosomal microarray analysis for prenatal diagnosis and assessment of fetal loss in Canada. *J Med Genet*. 2018;55(4):215-221.

93. Ali MM, Chasen ST, Norton ME. Testing for Noonan syndrome after increased nuchal translucency. *Prenat Diagn*. 2017;37(8):750-753.

94. International Society for Prenatal Diagnosis; Society for Maternal and Fetal Medicine; Perinatal Quality Foundation. Joint Position Statement from the International Society for Prenatal Diagnosis (ISPD), the Society for Maternal Fetal Medicine (SMFM), and the Perinatal Quality Foundation (PQF) on the use of genome-wide sequencing for fetal diagnosis. *Prenat Diagn*. 2018;38(1):6-9.

95. Mone F, Quinlan-Jones E, Kilby MD. Clinical utility of exome sequencing in the prenatal diagnosis of congenital anomalies: a Review. *Eur J Obstet Gynecol Reprod Biol*. 2018;231:19-24.

96. Drury S, Williams H, Trump N, et al. Exome sequencing for prenatal diagnosis of fetuses with sonographic abnormalities. *Prenat Diagn*. 2015;35(10):1010-1017.

97. Petrovski S, Aggarwal V, Giordano JL, et al. Whole-exome sequencing in the evaluation of fetal structural anomalies: a prospective cohort study. *Lancet*. 2019;393(10173):758-767.

98. Patch C, Middleton A. Point of view: an evolution from genetic counselling to genomic counselling. *Eur J Med Genet*. 2019;62(5):288-289.

99. Ahmad N, Tayoun A, Spinner NB, et al. Prenatal DNA sequencing: clinical, counseling, and diagnostic laboratory considerations. *Prenat Diagn*. 2017;37:1-7.

100. Petersen BS, Fredrich B, Hoeppne MP, et al. Opportunities and challenges of whole-genome and-exome sequencing. *BMC Genet*. 2017;18:14.

101. Carss KJ, Hillman SC, Parthiban V, et al. Exome sequencing improves genetic diagnosis of structural fetal abnormalities revealed by ultrasound. *Hum Mol Genet*. 2014;23(12):3269-3277.

102. Chervenak FA, McCullough LB. Ethical dimensions of the fetus as a patient. *Best Pract Res Clin Obstet Gynaecol*. 2017;43:2-9.

103. Salema D, Townsend A, Austin J. Patient decision-making and the role of the prenatal genetic counselor: an exploratory study. *J Genet Couns*. 2019;28(1):155-163.

104. Fonda Allen J, Stoll K, Bernhardt BA. Pre- and post-test genetic counseling for chromosomal and Mendelian disorders. *Semin Perinatol*. 2016;40:44-55.

105. Kuppermann M, Norton ME, Thao K, et al. Preferences regarding contemporary prenatal genetic tests among women desiring testing: implications for optimal testing strategies. *Prenat Diagn*. 2016;36(5):469-475.

111. Richardson A, Ormond KE. Ethical considerations in prenatal testing: genomic testing and medical uncertainty. *Semin Fetal Neonatl Med*. 2018;23(1):1-6.

114. Srebniak MI, Diderich KE, Joosten M, et al. Prenatal SNP array testing in 1000 fetuses with ultrasound anomalies: causative, unexpected and susceptibility CNVs. *Eur J Hum Genet*. 2016;24(5):645-651.

115. Brabbing-Goldstein D, Reches A, Svirsky R, et al. Dilemmas in genetic counseling for low-penetrance neuro-susceptibility loci detected on prenatal chromosomal microarray analysis. *Am J Obstet Gynecol*. 2018;218(2):247.e1-247.e12.

CHAPTER 12

Basic Principles of Ultrasound

Joanne Stone and Juan A. Peña

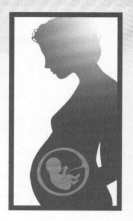

Introduction

Ultrasound has had a profound influence on the practice of medicine, especially in obstetrics. Since its first introduction into medicine, almost half a century ago, ultrasound studies have shown a potential to provide information about the fetus in a noninvasive manner. Most importantly, it does not appear to be associated with any known adverse fetal bioeffects when properly performed. Thus, diagnostic ultrasound gained wide clinical acceptance and became of considerable diagnostic value. The new powerful ultrasound machines, with superb resolution, three-dimensional capabilities, and various Doppler modalities, are convenient to use, comfortable for the patient, and not very expensive. Prenatal ultrasound provides information that allows diagnosis and potential treatment of fetal malformations that otherwise could only be diagnosed postnatally and often in an untimely fashion. However, a major question still remains unequivocally unanswered: Is prenatal diagnostic ultrasound safe? Although no significant adverse outcomes have been identified in children exposed to *in utero* ultrasound, there are some tissue biological effects generated by ultrasound.[1] Even more, the acoustic output of modern equipment constantly changes with the advancement of the technology, whereas investigations into the possibility of subtle or transient fetal adverse ultrasound bioeffects are still at an early stage. Therefore, diagnostic prenatal ultrasound should be used only when indicated and be performed in the shortest time possible with the lowest output.

Basic Physics

Sound consists of waves and is described by frequency, wavelength, amplitude, intensity, and the propagation of speed. An *ultrasound* is a sound with a frequency higher than the human ear can detect. The frequency of ultrasound used in medicine for fetal imaging is in the range of 2 to 12 million cycles per second (megahertz, MHz). Such high-frequency ultrasound is generated by high mechanical deformation of certain materials (eg, crystals or ceramics) caused by electrical stimulation, which produces a generation of waves at ultrasound frequencies. This is described as the *piezoelectric* phenomenon, and it also works in reverse.[2] An ultrasound "receptor" will resonate at certain frequencies, creating electrical impulses when stimulated by reflected ultrasonic waves (echoes).

Materials amenable to the piezoelectric phenomenon make up the core of the ultrasound transducer. These crystals are arrayed at the tip of the ultrasound probe. An ultrasound wave is generated by the electric pulse, transmitted through the tissue, and at some tissue depth is reflected and returned to the transducer. Returned "echoes" are detected and converted by the same transducer into electric impulses of equivalent amplitude that correspond to the depth of the returned ultrasonic wave. The array of the electric impulses is analyzed by the computer software and converted into the image. The arrangement of the crystals and the shape of the transducer alter the image obtained. Depending on the mode of data analysis, we are able to demonstrate tissue structures by: B-mode, two-dimensional real-time sonography; M-mode (eg, used for assessment of heart motion); a pulsed Doppler modality that pictures blood flow in the form of waveforms, which correspond to the systolic and diastolic components of the cardiac cycle; color and power Doppler modes (superimposed blood flow in the form of colored dots/areas over the B-mode picture); and, more recently, three-dimensional sonography that renders analyzed structures in a static three-dimensional image, or four-dimensional ultrasound, which demonstrates a three-dimensional image in real time (**Table 12.1**). All of these advances were possible because of the tremendous advancements in computer technology and software systems that enable quick and accurate analysis of the received ultrasound data.[2]

Ultrasound Image and Resolution

It is imperative to understand that ultrasound images are generated from an ultrasound beam that is three-dimensional in form. The three dimensions are thickness (*azimuthal* resolution), width (*lateral* resolution), and depth (*axial* resolution).

Table 12.1 Basic Ultrasound Modes and Images

Ultrasound Mode	Ultrasound Image	Brief Description	Comment
A-mode (one-dimensional)		Wave spikes occur when a *single* beam passes through objects of different consistency and hardness	Of historical value, now obsolete in medical imaging
B-mode (one-dimensional, 1-D)		Same as A-mode, but wave spikes (upper row) are replaced with *dots* (lower row) where "brightness" corresponds to amplitude of reflected sound	Of historical value, now obsolete in medical imaging
B-mode (two-dimensional in real time)		B-mode generated from multiple crystals (array) in real time (up to 100 images per second)	Today's standard of ultrasound imaging, utilized by almost any ultrasound machine
M-mode		Combination of B-mode one-dimensional (vertical axis) and time (horizontal axis)	Fetal cardiac imaging
Pulsed Doppler		Based on Doppler principle[a] demonstrates blood flow in real time (wave spikes are systolic component of the blood flow)	Used to analyze blood flow characteristics (eg, velocities and resistance to blood flow)
Color Doppler		Codes blood flow (or any motion) by Doppler principle, into two colored dots according to the direction and blood flow velocities; it is superimposed over B-mode image	Used to map blood flow spots within the investigated tissue or organ

Table 12.1 Basic Ultrasound Modes and Images (Continued)

Ultrasound Mode	Ultrasound Image	Brief Description	Comment
Power (color) Doppler		Similar to color Doppler, but codes all blood flow into one color (no directional information)—more sensitive to slow blood flow than color Doppler	Used to enhance blood flow mapping in tissue with slow blood flow states
Three- and four-dimensional (four-dimensional is three-dimensional ultrasound in real time)		Two-dimensional B-mode with a third dimension (depth) analyzed by powerful computer software to render three-dimensional image; three-dimensional image is static, whereas four-dimensional image is the three-dimensional image in real time	Diagnostic value of three- over two-dimensional B-mode real-time ultrasound is controversial, although may significantly reduce scanning time

ªDoppler principle. Source moving toward the receiver has higher frequency than source moving away from receiver, which has lower frequency.

Any transducer that generates an ultrasound beam is capable of focusing that beam at certain depths *via* an electromagnetic lens. Generated ultrasound beams are unevenly thick, with the narrowest part at the level of their focus. If the beam is thick, the reflected echoes from the same plane at a certain depth will be unified in one two-dimensional image that may appear blurry. It is especially true for the images that are closest and farthest away from the probe where the ultrasound beam is the thickest. At the same time, the image is most clear at the focus level where the beam is narrowest.

Axial resolution, or parallel to the direction of the sound waves leaving the transducer, is related to the length of the ultrasound pulse. Shorter ultrasound wavelengths or higher frequencies will produce better axial resolution.

In contrast, *lateral* resolution distinguishes structures that are perpendicular to the acoustic wave. Lateral resolution is equal to the diameter of the ultrasound beam and is significantly affected in curved transducers where the beam diameter increases with depth and becomes equivalent in thickness to the azimuthal resolution. Thus, the image that is away from the probe appears not only blurry but also distorted sometimes. Increasing frequency and a smaller beam diameter may improve lateral resolution.

Although the image quality directly depends on the frequency of the ultrasound probe, resolution has been significantly improved by an increase in the number of transducer crystals (or channels), improvements in transducer crystal technology (creating broadband and high-dynamic-range images), increased array aperture (more crystals firing in a single time frame), faster computational capabilities (faster computer chipsets), improved technical algorithms for focusing on received ultrasound beam (increasing the number of focal zones along the beam), incorporating automatic time-gain controls, and progressively replacing analog portions of the signal path to digital.

The signal path of the beam former (transducer) in the older analog processing data chain ultrasound machines was analyzed based on the axial resolution formed by the use of one focus or multifoci. With the employment of more powerful computers, the whole process became digitized. Super-fast digital beam formers allowed significantly increased numbers of focal points (microfine foci) along the beam to the size of a screen pixel. This technology reduced signal:noise ratio in data processing by several-hundred-fold and created a significantly clearer picture. The most recent advent in use is the so-called *harmonic* imaging (**Figure 12.1**). Tissue harmonic imaging utilizes lower frequency echoes

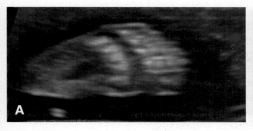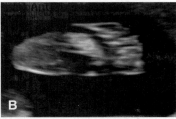

Figure 12.1 Comparison between conventional **(A)** and harmonic ultrasound imaging **(B)**.

for the ultrasound penetration that receives and processes only the higher frequency echoes generated by the body's inherent characteristics. The final product is a dramatically cleaner contrast between adjacent tissue structures that is particularly useful in patients with obesity.

Ultrasound Safety

The diagnostic ultrasound has widespread acceptance due to its clinical utility, convenience, and noninvasiveness. In the United States, approximately 65% of pregnant women have at least one ultrasound examination.[3] We usually reassure any prospective mother that ultrasound is safe and does not have any harmful effects on the baby; therefore, it is of paramount importance to be familiar with ultrasound safety.[4] Some evidence exists that high-energy ultrasound may produce biological effects in exposed tissues. The most studied effects are the local increase in temperature (thermal changes) and oscillatory and potentially catastrophic motions of bubbles, if present, in the tissues (microcavitation).[5]

The nature of ultrasound is such that, during its propagation through the tissue, portions of its energy are absorbed and converted into heat. Although the heat is dissipated by the adjacent tissues and blood flow through the insonated area, tissue temperature may rise a fraction of a degree Celsius.[6] Such temperature aberrations normally occur during the human diurnal cycle, and temperature may increase by 3° to 4°C in febrile states. Hyperthermia is a proven teratogenic agent in various animals (mouse, rat, hamster, monkey, sheep, and others) and is considered so in humans. In addition, certain stages of embryonic and fetal development may be more susceptible to thermal effects.[7] Effects appear to be a threshold phenomenon where temperature increases of 1.5°C or higher are considered necessary for damage to occur. However, the energy output of the diagnostic ultrasound is

of such low intensity that it is unlikely to induce temperature changes of such a degree to produce adverse pregnancy effects.[8] In addition, no recently published study has demonstrated unequivocal adverse effects of diagnostic ultrasound. However, it is a theoretical possibility and should not be completely ignored.

The interaction of sound with microscopic gas bubbles that preexist in tissues may cause a bioeffect termed *microcavitation* or acoustic cavitation.[5] Because of the succession of positive and negative pressures that can cause oscillatory motions of bubbles, stable cavitation or implosion of the bubbles, described as transient cavitation, may result. These can result in cell membrane disruption and even in the release of free radicals that are cytotoxic. Another potential effect is radiation stress, caused by acoustic streaming in liquid media secondary to the pressure gradient generated by the moving sound wave. These biological effects have been produced in plants, insects, and some mammalian tissues. Although there is no direct evidence to suggest that in humans, under clinical conditions, ultrasound-induced microcavitation produces biological effects, the U.S. Food and Drug Administration (FDA), together with the American Institute of Ultrasound in Medicine (AIUM), the American College of Obstetricians and Gynecologists (ACOG), and the National Electrical Manufacturers Association, introduced a method of displaying ultrasonic output that would control and minimize possible bioeffects in insonated fetal tissues.[6,8-11] If an ultrasound machine exceeds predetermined limits for output, either a thermal index or mechanical index must be displayed on the screen. If the thermal index, which is appropriate for Doppler applications, exceeds 1.0, there is a potential for the tissue temperature to rise. If the mechanical index, which is appropriate for scale imaging, exceeds 1.0, there is a potential for cavitational effects.[6,9] It is important to note that although the more recent epidemiologic studies were published in 1998 through 2002, ultrasound examinations consisted exclusively of B-mode, and all machines used predated 1992, ie, the "new" FDA regulations, allowing output to rise to more than 94 mW/cm², the then-accepted upper limit for fetal application. Those acoustic outputs can be considered "low" by today's standards. Still, available published evidence showed no difference in the prevalence of delayed speech or motor development; impaired neurological development, growth, vision, or hearing; low birthweight; dyslexia; or childhood cancer among children exposed to ultrasound *in utero*.[12-14] The only well-designed study showing some effect was a 2013 article that presented a small increase in the frequency of non–right-handedness (ambiguity) in male infants of mothers exposed to diagnostic ultrasound.[15] Nevertheless, in general, it is safe to say that when sonography is performed for a valid medical indication by a well-trained individual who respects the basic rules of time and exposure, the information that can be obtained is of such great value that it clearly overshadows the remote risks that may exist.[16-20]

In contrast with medical indications, performing ultrasound for "keepsake" records of the fetus, especially in the first trimester of the pregnancy, should be discouraged. Embryonic tissue may not have the tensile strength of fetal or adult tissue secondary to underdevelopment of the intercellular matrix to withhold cellular damage due to biological effects caused by ultrasound, especially if the energy output is above recommendations or if it is used for prolonged periods of time.

The risk of thermal bioeffects is increased when imaging is advanced from simple grayscale B-mode (in which the risk may be nonexistent) to pulsed Doppler. Doppler examinations present the highest risk of thermal *bioeffects* owing to their high pulse repetition frequency and longer pulses.[18,19] It also appears that the risks of appreciable harmful *bioeffects* may increase with increasing scanning time, ultrasound frequency (increases thermal risks but decreases cavitation risks), and output power (increasing the gain on the "output" knob, an "energy" trackball, or a "power" cursor) (**Table 12.2**).

Newer technologies, such as harmonic imaging and three-dimensional sonography, may be safer. Both modalities are based on data postprocessing;

Table 12.2 A Summary of the Recommendations Published by Several National and International Organizations, Including the American Institute of Ultrasound in Medicine (AIUM), International Society for Ultrasound in Obstetrics and Gynecology, Australasian Society for Ultrasound in Medicine, British Society for Medical Ultrasound, and World Federation for Ultrasound in Medicine and Biology

- Ultrasound induces biological effects (bioeffects) in the tissues but is generally considered safe if properly used—no epidemiologic studies have shown, so far, harmful effects in humans

- A clear medical indication should be present for performance of diagnostic sonography; when a clear medical indication exists, the benefits outweigh the risks potentially caused by performing sonography

- Ultrasound services should be provided by people with adequate training, including knowledge of safety and bioeffects issues

- An elevation of fetal body temperature above 41°C for 5 min or more is considered hazardous

- Nonthermal bioeffects (microcavitation) may result in capillary bleeding, particularly in the lungs and bowels when gas bubbles are present; fetal lungs and bowels do not contain gas; therefore, a mechanical risk is probably nonexistent

- B- and M-mode sonography appears entirely safe in pregnancy

- Pulsed Doppler and color Doppler sonography with a small region of interest have the greatest potential for bioeffects; these should be carried out with particular care in the first trimester

- New technologies, such as harmonic imaging and three-dimensional sonography, do not present more risk than native B-mode imaging

- Sonographic examination, particularly spectral Doppler sonography, in a pregnant patient with an elevated temperature might pose additional risks to the fetus

- The duration of exposure and output energy levels should be kept at a minimum—ALARA (*as low as reasonably achievable*) principle

- Continuous research and education in ultrasound safety and biological effects are strongly encouraged

Modified from Abramowicz JS. Ultrasound in obstetrics and gynecology: is this hot technology too hot? *J Ultrasound Med.* 2002;21:1327-1333.

therefore, one might speculate that time used for ultrasound scanning may be significantly reduced and, thereby, decrease the potential for adverse ultrasound biological effects. It is important to be cognizant of dwell time, which is the time the ultrasound beam consistently remains in the same tissue proximity. Dwell time is controlled by the individual performing the examination; is related to operator knowledge, experience, and skill; and should be limited to the shortest possible time to minimize potential for tissue heating.[21]

In conclusion, the duration of exposure and output levels should be kept at a minimum, which is the basis of the ALARA (*as low as reasonably achievable*) principle, endorsed, among others, by the AIUM, the National Electrical Manufacturers Association, and the FDA.[6] Nevertheless, continuous research and education on ultrasound safety are strongly encouraged.

Ultrasound Examination

The current ACOG recommendation is that ultrasound in pregnancy should be performed only when there is a valid medical indication. Common indications for a second- or third-trimester ultrasound examination can be found in **Table 12.3**.[22] Clinicians delivering obstetrical care are not obligated to perform ultrasonography in patients who are low risk and with no indications. However, shared decision-making between the patient and clinician can help incorporate ultrasonography in an otherwise low-risk mother's prenatal plan.[16,22]

While there is a small, theoretical risk with ultrasonography,[21] it is our belief that in the era of expanding fetal interventions, the benefits of routine ultrasonography outweigh these risks. The early recognition of fetal anomalies may identify pregnancies that may benefit from *in utero* treatment. At the very minimum, early recognition of fetal anomalies may prepare parents for the emotional ordeal that follows delivery of the fetus with a major malformation. Early recognition of fetal anomalies also provides the opportunity to access early termination, if desired, and, if not, access to additional resources that can prepare a family for a child with an anomaly. Although 90% of infants with congenital anomalies are born to women with no risk factors, a controversy about routine ultrasound use exists.[23] A minimal and inconsistent impact on perinatal morbidity or mortality was observed with the use of routine ultrasound

Table 12.3 Major Indications for Second- and Third-Trimester Ultrasonography[a]

- Screening for fetal anomalies
- Evaluation of fetal anatomy
- Estimation of gestational age
- Evaluation of fetal growth
- Evaluation of vaginal bleeding
- Evaluation of abdominal or pelvic pain
- Evaluation of cervical insufficiency
- Determination of fetal presentation
- Evaluation of suspected multiple gestation
- Adjunct to amniocentesis or other procedure
- Evaluation of a significant discrepancy between uterine size and clinical dates
- Evaluation of a pelvic mass
- Evaluation of a suspected hydatidiform mole
- Adjunct to cervical cerclage placement
- Suspected ectopic pregnancy
- Suspected fetal death
- Suspected uterine abnormalities
- Evaluation of fetal well-being
- Suspected amniotic fluid abnormalities
- Suspected placental abruption
- Adjunct to external cephalic version
- Evaluation of abnormal biochemical markers
- Follow-up evaluation of placental location for suspected placenta previa
- History of previous congenital anomaly
- Evaluation of the fetal condition in late registrants for prenatal care
- Assessment for findings that may increase the risk of aneuploidy

[a]List not exhaustive.
Data from the American College of Radiology (ACR). *ACR-ACOG-AIUM-SRU. Practice parameter for the performance of obstetrical ultrasound. ACR, Diagnostic Radiology: Ultrasonography Practice Parameters and Technical Standards, 2013.* Amended 2014.

screening in the second trimester of pregnancy.[24-26] However, there are data that support its cost-effectiveness when performed in tertiary centers.[27] Moreover, as experience with fetal intervention increases, the literature may bear out additional benefits of routine ultrasonography.

In its most recent clinical management guidelines, the ACOG defined three types of ultrasound examinations performed during the second or third trimesters of pregnancy.[22]

The *standard* second- or third-trimester ultrasound examination includes an evaluation of fetal presentation and number, amniotic fluid volume, cardiac activity, placental position, fetal biometry, and an anatomic survey.[27] Fetal anatomy may be assessed adequately at 16 to 20 weeks of gestation (**Table 12.4**). If technically feasible, the uterus and adnexa should also be examined. A *limited* examination is performed when a specific question requires investigation. For example, it may be employed to verify fetal presentation in a laboring patient, or to confirm heart activity in a patient with absent fetal movements. A *specialized* examination is a detailed or targeted anatomic examination, also known as "76811," that is performed when an anomaly is suspected on the basis of patient history, laboratory abnormalities, results of a limited or standard examination, clinical evaluation, advanced maternal age, maternal complications of pregnancy, or pregnancy after assisted reproductive technology. Other indications include suspected fetal growth restriction or multifetal gestations. Other specialized examinations include fetal Doppler studies,

biophysical profile, fetal echocardiography, additional biometric studies, nuchal translucency (NT), and cervical length.

Updated guidelines that outlined practice parameters for the effective performance and recording of high-quality ultrasound examinations were published in 2018.[28] These guidelines were developed jointly by ACOG, the Society for Maternal-Fetal Medicine, the AIUM, the American College of Radiology, and the Society for Radiologists in Ultrasound. They complement and expand the definitions of the standard first- and second-trimester examination, the limited examination, and the specialized examination. They also provide guidance on the performance of NT in the first trimester, as well as measurement of cervical length.

In addition to indications in the second and third trimesters of pregnancy, **Table 12.5** demonstrates indications for the use of ultrasound in the first trimester of pregnancy. The *standard* first-trimester examination includes an evaluation of the presence, size, location, and number of gestational sacs. The gestational sac is examined for the presence of a yolk sac and embryo/fetus (fetus defined as 10 weeks or greater gestational age). When an embryo/fetus is detected, it should be measured, and the cardiac activity should

Table 12.4 Essential Elements of the Fetal Anatomic Ultrasound Survey

Head and Neck
Cerebellum
Choroid plexus
Cisterna magna
Lateral cerebral ventricles
Midline falx
Cavum septi pellucidi
Upper lip
Chest
Heart
Four-chamber view
Left and right ventricular outflow tracts
Abdomen
Stomach (presence, size, and situs)
Kidneys
Urinary bladder
Umbilical cord insertion site into the fetal abdomen
Umbilical cord vessel number
Spine
Cervical, thoracic, lumbar, and sacral spine
Extremities
Legs and arms (presence or absence)
Gender
In multiple gestations and when medically indicated

Data from AIUM-ACR-ACOG-SMFM-SRU practice parameter for the performance of standard diagnostic obstetric ultrasound examinations. *J Ultrasound Med.* 2018;37(11):E13-E24.

Table 12.5 Indications for Ultrasound in the First Trimester of Pregnancy

To confirm the presence of an intrauterine pregnancy
To evaluate a suspected ectopic pregnancy
To define the cause of vaginal bleeding
To evaluate pelvic pain
To estimate gestational age
To diagnose or evaluate multiple gestations
To confirm cardiac activity
As an adjunct to chorionic villus sampling, embryo transfer, or localization and removal of an intrauterine device
To assess for certain fetal anomalies, such as anencephaly, in patients at high risk
To screen for aneuploidy
To evaluate maternal pelvic masses or uterine abnormalities
To evaluate suspected hydatidiform mole

Data from AIUM-ACR-ACOG-SMFM-SRU practice parameter for the performance of standard diagnostic obstetric ultrasound examinations. *J Ultrasound Med.* 2018;37(11):E13-E24.

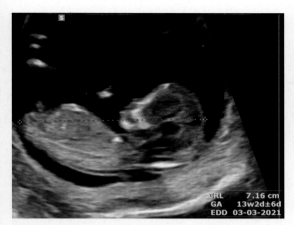

Figure 12.2 Transverse image of the embryo at 13 weeks and 2 days of gestational age depicting a crown-rump length of 71.6 mm.

be recorded by a two-dimensional video clip or M-mode. The routine use of pulsed Doppler ultrasound is discouraged. The uterus, cervix, adnexa, and cul-de-sac region should be examined. The first trimester is a time of rapid embryonic-fetal development. Highly accurate first-trimester dating can be obtained by measuring the crown-rump length (CRL) of the fetus (**Figure 12.2**). A number of studies have demonstrated that fetal CRL is the most accurate measurement for the sonographic dating of pregnancy. It has a high reproducibility and can be used reliably until approximately 12 weeks' gestation. Beyond this period, a variety of sonographic parameters, such as biparietal diameter (BPD), abdominal circumference, and femoral diaphysis length can be used to estimate gestational age. However, the variability of gestational age estimations increases with advancing pregnancy. Guidelines for redating based on ultrasonography can be found in **Table 12.6**.[29] As early as the late first trimester, separate fetal body structures can be examined.

Head

The oval outline of the fetal head should be sought in all examinations. The intracranial anatomy should be examined to ascertain that major midline structures are present, such as thalami, intrahemispheric fissure, and cavum septi pellucidi (**Figure 12.3**). Advanced head evaluation includes the extra- and intraorbital distances, ventricular diameters, occipital frontal distance, and cephalic index,

Table 12.6 Guidelines for Redating Based on Ultrasonography

Gestational Age Range[a]	Method of Measurement	Discrepancy Between Ultrasound Dating and LMP Dating That Supports Redating
8 6/7 wk or less	CRL	More than 5 d
9 0/7 wk to 13 5/7 wk	CRL	More than 7 d
14 0/7 wk to 15 6/7 wk	BPD, HC, AC, FL	More than 7 d
16 0/7 wk to 21 6/7 wk	BPD, HC, AC, FL	More than 10 d
22 0/7 wk to 27 6/7 wk	BPD, HC, AC, FL	More than 14 d
28 0/7 wk and beyond[b]	BPD, HC, AC, FL	More than 21 d

AC, abdominal circumference; BPD, biparietal diameter; CRL, crown-rump length; FL, femur length; HC, head circumference; LMP, last menstrual period.

[a]Based on LMP.

[b]Because of the risk of redating a small fetus that may be growth restricted, management decisions based on third-trimester ultrasonography alone are especially problematic and need to be guided by careful consideration of the entire clinical picture and close surveillance.

Modified from Committee on Obstetric Practice, the American Institute of Ultrasound in Medicine, and the Society for Maternal-Fetal Medicine. Committee Opinion No 700: Methods for Estimating the Due Date. *Obstet Gynecol*. 2017;129(5):e150-e154.

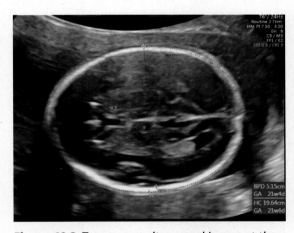

Figure 12.3 Transverse ultrasound image at the level of the biparietal diameters, demonstrating thalami (T) and septum cavum pellucidum (SCP).

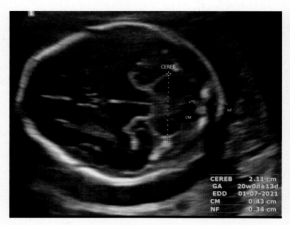

Figure 12.4 Posterior fossa with cerebellar diameter (cereb), cisterna magna (CM), and nuchal fold (NF).

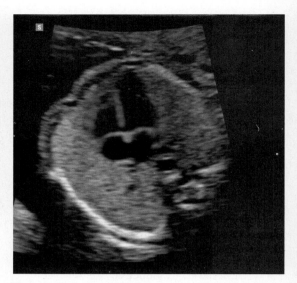

Figure 12.6 Four-chamber view of the fetal heart.

among others. The cephalic index is the ratio of BPD to occipital front distance, which is normally in the range of 0.75 to 0.85. The posterior fossa reveals information about the cerebellar diameter, which correlates with gestational age, presence of the cerebellar vermis, and the size of the cisterna magna (**Figure 12.4**).

Fetal Spine

The fetal spine ossifies as early as 10 weeks and is seen as parallel sets of echoes representing the articulating vertebral facets. It is usually examined in the longitudinal (coronal) plane, although in a targeted examination for neural tube defects, the transverse view of the total spine should be demonstrated (**Figure 12.5**).

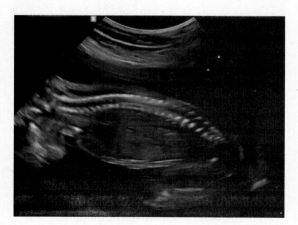

Figure 12.5 Longitudinal image of the fetal spine.

Fetal Heart

Visceral and abdominal situs should be established and correlated with the cardiac apex. A four-chamber heart view (**Figure 12.6**) is a basic part of all examinations after 18 to 20 weeks' gestation. It is fast and easy to perform a screening test for congenital heart disease because the majority of heart structural anomalies may be detected using this single view. The left and right ventricular outflow tracts should also be viewed, and if technically feasible, the three-vessel view and three-vessel tracheal view should also be documented.[28] However, outflow tract anomalies (eg, transposition of the great vessels) can be easily missed if "long-axis" and "short-axis" heart views are not performed (**Figure 12.7**); if possible, these views should be obtained.

Practice parameters have been published to guide clinicians when the need for additional cardiac views is clinically indicated.[30] In addition to the basic cardiac views described above, additional grayscale imaging should include the aortic and ductal arch views and the superior and inferior vena cava views.[30] Color Doppler should also be used to evaluate flow disturbances in the systemic veins, pulmonary veins, foramen ovale, atrioventricular valves, atrial and ventricular septa, semilunar valves, ductal arch, and aortic valve.[30] Additionally, pulsed Doppler sonography

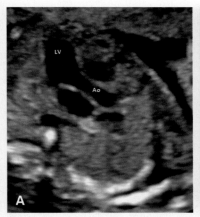

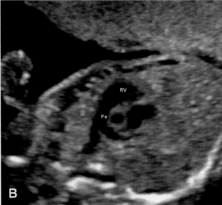

Figure 12.7 Left ventricular outflow tract (**A**) and right ventricular outflow tract (**B**) of the fetal heart. Ao, aorta; LV, left ventricle; Pa, pulmonary artery, RV, right ventricle.

should be used as an adjunct when any structural abnormality is noted or when rhythm abnormalities are suspected.[30] Finally, cardiac biometry and assessment of cardiac function should be considered as clinically indicated.[30]

Abdomen

The fetal abdomen and stomach, as a single cystic area, can be visualized as early as 14 weeks' gestation. Ventral wall defects can be excluded by the demonstration of an intact abdominal umbilical cord insertion (**Figure 12.8**). Fetal kidneys

(**Figure 12.9**) and other upper abdomen organs, such as the gallbladder and liver, can be easily demonstrated. The fetal urinary bladder is usually visible as a fluid-filled structure in the midline of the pelvis.

Extremities

The four fetal limbs are identified routinely during ultrasound examination. Although it is not necessary to measure all six tubular bones in every fetus, measurements of at least one or two segments (femur and humerus) are performed. Both bones of

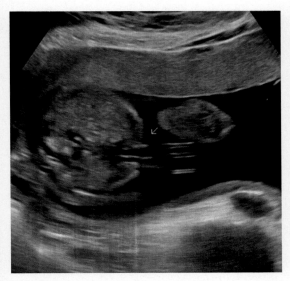

Figure 12.8 Fetal abdominal umbilical cord insertion (arrow).

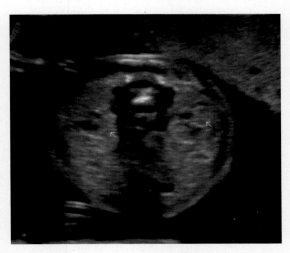

Figure 12.9 Transverse image through the fetal kidneys (arrows).

the normal distal segments should be present. The presence of both fetal hands and feet should be documented (**Figure 12.10**).

Fetal Biometry

Fetal biometry is used to assess the estimated fetal weight and is usually plotted against a growth curve (generated from the large portion of general fetal population) to evaluate fetal growth characteristics. The estimated fetal weight is derived from various combinations of fetal measurements at a certain gestational age, and mainly include BPD, head circumference, abdominal circumference, and femoral diaphysis length, described elsewhere in this text. However, it is important to exercise caution with interpreting the results of the fetal biometry because there is large inter- and intraobserver variation in measurements at extremes of the fetal age (eg, less than 24 or beyond 36 weeks' gestation).

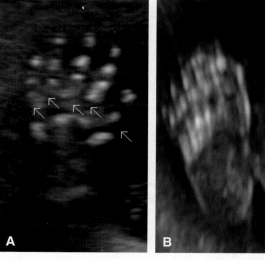

Figure 12.10 Fetal open hand (arrows) **(A)** and a foot **(B)**.

KEY POINTS

- Sonography principles are based on the *piezoelectric phenomenon* and generated ultrasound waves. These ultrasound waves are reflected from tissue boundaries of different density and processed by powerful computer software to generate real-time two- or three-dimensional images.
- Recent advances in ultrasound data processing, such as "harmonic" imaging and super-fast digital beamers, permit significantly improved ultrasound resolution.
- Although three- and four-dimensional (real-time three-dimensional) ultrasounds produce excellent fetal images, their clinical superiority over conventional real-time two-dimensional ultrasound is controversial.
- Ultrasound waves may produce certain biological tissue effects, eg, thermal changes and mechanical effects (microcavitation), if used for prolonged periods of time with extremely high-energy outputs. However, these ultrasound energy output levels are *not* used with diagnostic ultrasound at present time.
- To ensure ultrasound safety, it is the general consensus that the thermal and mechanical indexes are displayed on the screen if the ultrasound machine exceeds predetermined limits for energy output.

- At the present time, diagnostic ultrasound is considered safe for the fetus when used appropriately and prudently. However, casual use of ultrasound, especially during the first trimester of pregnancy, should be avoided, especially implementation of pulsed Doppler ultrasound, which, theoretically, may produce a high thermal index.
- Ultrasound examination in pregnancy is an accurate method of evaluating viability of the pregnancy, fetal number, and placental location, as well as gestational dating, which is most accurately determined in the first trimester of pregnancy.
- Ultrasound is also able to accurately diagnose major fetal anomalies; however, the diagnosis of fetal growth abnormalities is less precise.
- The optimal timing for a single ultrasound examination (if performed in the absence of specific indications) is at 18 to 20 weeks of gestation.
- Appropriate patient counseling before the ultrasound examination regarding its limitations for diagnosis is of paramount importance and should be exercised routinely.

REFERENCES

1. Whitworth M, Bricker L, Mullan C. Ultrasound for fetal assessment in early pregnancy. *Cochrane Database Syst Rev*. 2015;2015(7):CD007058.
2. Kremkau FW. *Diagnostic Ultrasound: Principles and Instruments*. 6th ed. WB Saunders; 2002.
3. Martin JA, Hamilton BE, Sutton PD, et al. Births: final data for 2002. *Natl Vital Stat Rep*. 2003;52:1-113.
4. Reece EA, Assimakopoulos E, Zhen X, Hobbins JC. The safety of obstetrical ultrasound: concerns for the fetus. *Obstet Gynecol*. 1990;76:139-146.
5. Dalecki D. Mechanical bioeffects of ultrasound. *Ann Rev Biomed Eng*. 2004;6:229-248.
6. Fowlkes JB, Holland CK. Mechanical bioeffects from diagnostic ultrasound: AIUM consensus statements. American Institute of Ultrasound in Medicine. *J Ultrasound Med*. 2000;19(2):69-72.
7. Duck FA. Is it safe to use diagnostic ultrasound during the first trimester? (Editorial). *Ultrasound Obstet Gynecol*. 1999;13:385-388.
8. Abramowicz JS, Kossoff G, Marsal K, ter Haar G. International society of ultrasound in obstetrics and gynecology (ISUOG) safety and bioeffects committee: safety statement. *Ultrasound Obstet Gynecol*. 2000;16:594-596.
9. American Institute of Ultrasound in Medicine. *Official Statement: Clinical Safety*. AIUM; 1997.
10. British Medical Ultrasound Society. Guidelines for the safe use of diagnostic ultrasound equipment. *BMUS Bull*. August 2000.
11. Seeds JW. The routine or screening obstetrical ultrasound examination. *Clin Obstet Gynecol*. 1996;39:814-830.
12. Kieler H, Ahlsten G, Haglund B, et al. Routine ultrasound screening in pregnancy and the children's subsequent neurologic development. *Obstet Gynecol*. 1998;91:750-756.
13. Kieler H, Haglund B, Waldenstrom U, Axelsson O. Routine ultrasound screening in pregnancy and the children's subsequent growth, vision and hearing. *Br J Obstet Gynecol*. 1997;104:1267-1272.
14. Kieler H, Cnattingius S, Haglund B, et al. Sinistrality, a side-effect of prenatal sonography: a comparative study of young men. *Epidemiology*. 2001;12:618-623.
15. Kieler H, Axelsson O, Haglund B, et al. Routine ultrasound screening in pregnancy and the children's subsequent handedness. *Early Hum Dev*. 1998;50:233-245.
16. American Institute of Ultrasound in Medicine. AIUM practice guideline for the performance of an antepartum obstetric ultrasound examination. *J Ultrasound Med*. 2003;22:1116-1125.
17. Barnett SB, Kossoff G, Edwards MJ. Is diagnostic ultrasound safe? Current international consensus on the thermal mechanism. *Med J Aust*. 1994;160:33-37.
18. Barnett SB, Maulik D; International Perinatal Doppler Society. Guidelines and recommendations for safe use of Doppler ultrasound in perinatal applications. *J Matern Fetal Med*. 2001;10:75-84.
19. Kurjak A. Are color and pulsed Doppler sonography safe in early pregnancy? *J Perinat Med*. 1999;27:423-430.
20. ter Haar G, Duck F, eds. *The Safe Use of Ultrasound in Medical Diagnosis*. British Medical Ultrasound Society/British Institute of Radiology; 2000.
21. Van den Hof MC, Halifax NS. No. 359-Obstetric ultrasound biological effects and safety. *J Obstet Gynaecol Can*. 2018;40(5):627-632.
22. American College of Obstetricians and Gynecologists. Practice Bulletin No. 175: ultrasound in pregnancy. *Obstet Gynecol*. 2016;128(6):e241-e256.
23. Saari-Kemppainen A, Karjalainen O, Ylostalo P, Heinonen OP. Fetal anomalies in a controlled one-stage ultrasound screening trial. A report from the Helsinki Ultrasound Trial. *J Perinatal Med*. 1994;22:279-289.
24. Long G, Sprigg A. A comparative study of routine versus selective fetal anomaly ultrasound scanning. *J Med Screen*. 1998;5:6-10.
25. Bucher H, Schmidt JG. Does routine ultrasound scanning improve outcome of pregnancy? Meta-analysis of various outcome measures. *Br Med J*. 1993;307:13-17.
26. Vintzileos AM, Ananth CV, Smulian JC, et al. Routine second-trimester ultrasonography in the United States: a cost-benefit analysis. *Am J Obstet Gynecol*. 2000;182:655-660.
27. Leivo T, Tuominen R, Saari-Kemppainen A, et al. Cost-effectiveness of one-stage ultrasound screening in pregnancy: a report from the Helsinki ultrasound trial. *Ultrasound Obstet Gynecol*. 1996;7:309-314.
28. AIUM-ACR-ACOG-SMFM-SRU practice parameter for the performance of standard diagnostic obstetric ultrasound examinations. *J Ultrasound Med*. 2018;37(11):E13-E24.
29. Committee Opinion No 700: Methods for Estimating the Due Date. *Obstet Gynecol*. 2017;129(5):e150-e154.
30. AIUM Practice Parameter for the Performance of Fetal Echocardiography. *J Ultrasound Med*. 2020;39(1):E5-E16.
31. Abramowicz JS. Ultrasound in obstetrics and gynecology: is this hot technology too hot? *J Ultrasound Med*. 2002;21(12):1327-1333.

CHAPTER 13

The First Prenatal Visit— Setting the Stage for Optimal Pregnancy Care

Chloe M. Nielsen, Anna G. Euser, and John C. Hobbins

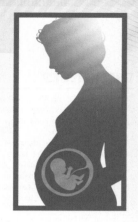

Introduction

The initial prenatal visit can be one of the most important clinician-patient interactions during pregnancy. It may be a time of great anxiety and change for expectant parents and is often the beginning of a long and meaningful relationship with their obstetrician or midwife. Medically, the goal of prenatal care is to prevent complications and to reduce neonatal and maternal morbidity and mortality.[1,2] This initial visit, which generally takes place prior to 12 weeks' gestation, is also a time in which the clinician is tasked with assessing the patient's medical, obstetric, surgical, family, and social histories. There are multiple laboratory tests—from initial prenatal laboratories, to genetic screenings, to patient-specific studies—that must be performed, and with those tests comes a significant counseling responsibility. This obstetrical visit is a pivotal opportunity to assess the patient's overall health and evaluate patient-specific pregnancy risks. The following topics are meant as an overview of the many aspects of prenatal care and are not meant to be an exhaustive review, and many of the introduced topics are covered in more detail elsewhere in this textbook. The arc of obstetrical care will ultimately be guided by the issues and values most important to the patient.[3]

Before going further, we believe that it is important to determine the patient's desires regarding pregnancy continuation. Approximately half of pregnancies in the United States are unintended,[4] and although unintended may not be undesired, it is essential to determine if the patient wishes to continue the pregnancy. Prompt referral for termination services is associated with the ability to use either surgical or medical techniques for evacuation, both of which are associated with low complication rates.[5] Generally speaking, first-trimester abortion is associated with a less than 1% rate of complications.[6] As gestational age increases so do the risks of pregnancy termination—maternal mortality rates increase from 0.1 per 100,000 at 8 weeks to 8.9 deaths per 100,000 at 21 weeks or greater.[7] This is particularly pertinent in women who may have diagnoses (eg, mechanical heart valves or prepregnancy renal failure) or an obstetric history (prior acute fatty liver of pregnancy or decompensated peripartum cardiomyopathy) that would make pregnancy continuation unadvisable.

Laboratory Screening

Prenatal laboratory tests should be obtained for every patient on initiation of obstetrical care. This panel of tests evaluates pregnancy risk associated with maternal alloimmunization, infectious disease, and anemia. The majority of these screening tests are recommended universally for all patients, and other tests should be considered based on individual patient characteristics (**Table 13.1**). There are additional laboratory tests that should be performed based on a woman's obstetric and medical history, and these will be discussed later in this chapter.

Hematologic Screening

An ABO/Rh type and antibody screen evaluates for the presence or absence of the D (Rh) antigen on maternal red blood cells and also detects any other circulating antibodies that may affect pregnancy outcomes and fetal well-being (Chapter 22).[8] A complete blood count is obtained to screen for underlying anemia, hemoglobinopathy, or thrombocytopenia (Chapters 23 and 38).[9]

Table 13.1 Panel of Common Laboratory Tests in Pregnancy

Prenatal Laboratory Testing
Recommended for all patients
Blood type
Blood antibody screen
Complete blood count
Hepatitis B surface antigen
Human immunodeficiency virus
Rubella immunity status
Syphilis screening
Gonorrhea
Chlamydia
Urinalysis
Offer genetic screening/testing and carrier screening
General health screening
Cervical cancer screening
Diabetes mellitus screening
Influenza vaccine
Laboratory tests indicated by patient risk factors
Hepatitis C
Thyroid function testing
Tuberculosis testing
Universal testing is NOT recommended
Bacterial vaginosis
Cytomegalovirus
Toxoplasmosis
Parvovirus
Genital herpes

Infectious Disease Screening

Routine screening for maternal hepatitis B status is recommended using the hepatitis B surface antigen (Chapter 39).[10-12] Although seroprevalence of hepatitis B is relatively low in the United States, vertical transmission can be decreased with third trimester treatment in patients with high viral loads and appropriate neonatal care.[13] Testing for hepatitis C is recommended in women with risk factors, including incarceration, high-risk sexual behavior, or intravenous drug use, and allows for consideration for new curative treatment regimens in the postpartum period (Chapter 39).[14] Human immunodeficiency virus (HIV) testing is recommended for all pregnant patients with each pregnancy confirmation and "opt-out" screening is favored.[15] Appropriate HIV treatment during pregnancy and intrapartum decreases the risk of vertical transmission from 25% to <2% and allows for appropriate care for that woman's future health.[15-18] For patients at high risk of acute infection, it is prudent to obtain an HIV viral load as an additional test. Screening for syphilis by either rapid plasma regain or treponemal testing should performed due to the risk of congenital syphilis and the availability of treatment in pregnancy.[19] Similarly, infectious disease testing should also include gonorrhea and chlamydia assessment, as well as urine evaluation for asymptomatic bacteriuria screening.[20] Rubella immunoglobulin G is tested to determine the risk of maternal rubella infection in pregnancy and allow for immunization postpartum as needed. Consideration of tuberculosis testing in women who have recently emigrated from endemic areas or for women in close proximity to many others (such as those residing in shelters or who are incarcerated) is also prudent.[21]

There are several infectious diseases for which universal prenatal screening is not recommended. This includes cytomegalovirus, toxoplasmosis, parvovirus, genital herpes simplex virus, and bacterial vaginosis (see Chapter 10 for more details regarding congenital infections and testing indications).[22,23,]

General Health Screening

It is important to realize that for many women, pregnancy represents a period of time in which they have more contact with the healthcare system than they do outside of pregnancy. As such, it is prudent to make sure that all appropriate health screenings and interventions that can be safely administered during pregnancy are provided. The Women's Preventative Services Initiative (WPSI) provides guidance that is updated annually with recommendations for well-woman care and includes prevention services recommendations for nonpregnant, pregnant, and postpartum women.[24] Cervical cancer screening with cervical cytology and human papilloma virus testing should be performed if indicated per current guidelines (Chapter 42).[25] All adults, pregnant or not, should be offered an influenza vaccine annually, and this is strongly recommended during pregnancy.[26] Additionally, with increasing rates of obesity and sedentary lifestyles, early screening for pregestational dia-betes mellitus should also be considered based on risk factors (Chapters 30 and 32)[27] Physical activ-ity should be encouraged in all women, pregnant or not, with current recommendations for aerobic activity for at least 150 minutes per week in most women.[28] Thyroid function testing should be per-formed based on personal history of thyroid disease or symptoms and is not universally recommended (Chapter 31).[29]

First-Trimester Ultrasound

Although there are no formal recommendations from professional organizations that all women receive an early ultrasound, first-trimester ultra-sound can be useful to determine fetal viability, pregnancy location, and fetal number; establish dating; and review early fetal anatomy.[30,31] This ultrasound can be either transabdominal or trans-vaginal and should also evaluate the uterus, cervix, and adnexa. In keeping with the ALARA (as low as reasonably achievable) principle, M-mode should be used for demonstration of fetal cardiac activity in the first trimester.[32] These topics are covered in greater detail in Chapters 12, 19, and 20.

At least 10% of clinically recognized preg-nancies result in miscarriage, and 80% of these pregnancy losses occur within the first trimes-ter (Chapter 1).[31,33] Thus, while ascertaining fetal viability is important at every visit, this is partic-ularly important during the first trimester. There are commonly accepted diagnostic criteria for failed pregnancy, and prompt diagnosis allows for expeditious management (Chapter 4).[34] The most accurate manner of establishing pregnancy dating is an ultrasound measurement of the crown-rump length, which can be measured up to 14 weeks.[30,31] In addition, the rate of twin pregnancies (and higher order multiples) has been increasing over time, and first-trimester ultrasound assists diagnosis, chori-onicity assignment, and guiding further prenatal care (see Chapter 5 for full discussion of multifetal pregnancies).

Although first-trimester ultrasound is not meant to replace the later standard anatomic evaluation typically performed in the midsecond trimester, many anatomic abnormalities can be detected sonographically in the first trimester.[31] Early fetal anatomy assessment with a systematic approach can increase the diagnosis of both major struc-tural anomalies and chromosomal aneuploidies in

experienced hands, and this has become an area of expertise in its own right.[35,36] Standardized eval-uations of fetal anatomy in the first trimester may identify severe malformations is 1.0% to 1.4% of low-risk women with detection of 32% to 76% of major structural defects.[36-38] Some anatomic abnor-malities are more reliably detected by ultrasound during the first trimester. For example, acrania and abdominal malformations (omphalocele and gas-troschisis) had a 100% detection rate, while other malformations were not as routinely identified; for example, cardiac defects were only positively iden-tified in 26% of cases and diaphragmatic hernia in 50% of cases.[37]

First-trimester ultrasound has also become a key component of aneuploidy risk assessment, with findings for risk including increased nuchal trans-lucency, cystic hygroma, absent or hypoplastic nasal bone, tricuspid valve regurgitation, and abnormal flow in the ductus venosus (see also Chapter 11 for full discussion). The nuchal translucency measure-ment is also important due to its association with congenital heart disease, even in fetuses with a normal karyotype.[39]

Genetic Testing

Genetic testing options should be addressed early in pregnancy. Chromosomal abnormalities affect approximately 1 in 150 live births, and though the incidence is increased in women of advanced mater-nal age, any pregnancy is at risk.[40] There are multi-ple different screening options available, each with advantages and disadvantages, and these issues are covered in more detail in Chapters 11 and 15. Any testing done, whether screening (cell-free DNA or maternal serum screening) or diagnostic invasive testing (chorionic villus sampling or amniocente-sis), should be focused on the individual patient's risks and preferences.[30,31,40]

Carrier screening is another component of genetic risk assessment and is discussed further in Chapter 15. Current guidelines recommend counseling about carrier screening to all pregnant women.[41] Ideally, carrier screening is completed prior to conception to allow for full risk assess-ment, with testing of both partners as indicated,[3,41] although in practice this may not happen until the initial prenatal visit. Recommended screening for all patients includes the more common auto-somal recessive conditions (cystic fibrosis, spinal muscular atrophy and hemoglobinopathies), with testing for other conditions as part of expanded or ethnic-specific panels (Tay-Sachs disease, phenylketonuria, galactosemia, Gaucher disease) based on patient history and ethnicity.[41] However, expanded carrier screening is also now offered with panels that can test for up to hundreds of recessive conditions. If the mother tests positive for any condition, genetic counseling by certified specialists should be offered as this is an invaluable asset to assist patients as well as the care team to navigate the nuances of the various possible conditions and commensurate diagnostic testing options.

Care Dictated by Maternal History

Central to establishing an appropriate obstetrical care plan is taking a careful medical history. Adverse pregnancy outcomes may be avoided or mitigated by appropriately triaging a patient's concomitant medical conditions and referring to maternal-fetal medicine or other subspecialists as necessary. The obstetric clinician should document any chronic or acute medical problems and should review all medications for teratogenicity or associations with pregnancy complications. For example, patients with chronic hypertension on an angiotensin-converting enzyme inhibitor or an angiotensin receptor blocker should be switched to a different antihypertensive secondary to well-documented teratogenicity.[42] There are a variety of other medications that should be avoided in pregnancy and a much longer list for which a risk-benefit decision must be made regarding continuation or discontinuation of the medication in pregnancy (see Chapter 7 for further discussion). Maternal surgical history, in particular, uterine or cervical procedures, should be reviewed and documented clearly. Certain uterine surgeries, such a large myomectomy or a prior classical cesarean delivery, will affect delivery timing, and prior complex abdominal surgery may influence surgical planning in the event of cesarean delivery.[43]

The obstetric history, often overlooked in other disciplines of medicine, is crucial to determining the patient's risk. Prior adverse outcomes, including prior preterm birth, prior hypertensive disorders of pregnancy, or a prior child affected by aneuploidy or structural abnormality,[31] all increase risk in subsequent pregnancies. As discussed in Chapter 49, patients with a singleton pregnancy that have a prior spontaneous singleton preterm birth should be offered 17-alpha hydroxyprogesterone caproate therapy.[44] History-indicated cervical cerclage, typically placed at the end of the first trimester, may be recommended for those women with a history of prior second trimester pregnancy loss not related to abruption or labor or for women who have had a cerclage in a prior pregnancy (see Chapter 48 for further discussion).[45] For women with a history of preeclampsia, there is a roughly 20% to 50% risk of recurrence depending on risk factors (Chapter 27).[46,47] Initiating low-dose aspirin therapy prior to 16 weeks appears to reduce the rate of recurrent preeclampsia by 10% and for those at risk of preterm preeclampsia reduces that risk by more than half[46] and is now recommended based on assessment of clinical risk factors.[48,49]

Family history, including paternal history, forms an important component of the pregnancy risk assessment and should include questions about congenital anomalies, genetic conditions, and bleeding disorders. There are several hereditary bleeding and clotting disorders that can affect pregnancy management and greatly alter the patient's risk of hemorrhage or thromboembolism, respectively, during pregnancy and are further discussed in Chapters 37 and 38. Bleeding disorders, particularly X-linked bleeding disorders like the hemophilias, may only be evident when taking a family history, as women themselves may be unaffected or affected only mildly. It is also important to assess the paternal medical history for heritable conditions. As well, increased paternal age, generally defined as 40 to 50 years, increases the risk of single-gene disorders such as achondroplasia or Apert syndrome.[50]

All patients should be routinely asked about their use of alcohol, nicotine products, and drugs (both prescription and nonprescribed), including marijuana and opioids, because cessation of drug, tobacco, or alcohol use will improve pregnancy outcomes (see Chapter 8 for a full discussion). In the case of opioid use disorder, use has increased dramatically and universal screening is recommended. Interventions may include opioid agonist medications to support abstinence and decrease at-risk behaviors.[51] With increasing legalization of marijuana, increased use of marijuana in pregnancy has been reported and patients should be counseled on the possible fetal effects.[52] Nicotine replacement can be considered on a patient-by-patient basis to assist with tobacco cessation, and such interventions are commonly used in other countries.[53,54] Environmental exposures should be reviewed, in particular chemicals like diethylstilbestrol, pesticides, mercury, and heavy metals (Chapter 7).[55] Evaluation of the patient's social history also includes evaluation of the patient's support system, their safety in the home, and screening for intimate partner violence.[56]

Care Dictated by Preexisting Maternal Medical Conditions

Although an in-depth discussion of maternal diseases complicating pregnancy is the focus of the chapters (25-43) of Section IV of this text, a brief overview is discussed here.

As the average age at conception rises, it is more common to care for women with one or more chronic medical conditions during pregnancy. Additional evaluation may be indicated based on preexisting maternal health conditions. Although many maternal diseases may dictate adjustments in delivery timing and antenatal surveillance, several maternal conditions require particular attention during a first-trimester visit. Detailed discussion of delivery timing and antenatal surveillance often depends on the disease course and fetal status throughout pregnancy and can be found within the chapters in Section IV.

Depression is one of the most common medical complications during pregnancy and postpartum, and there is a current emphasis to recognize maternal mental health as a vital component of antenatal care.[57] The vital importance of this issue is demonstrated by the statistic that maternal suicide is a greater source of maternal mortality than hemorrhage or hypertensive disorders of pregnancy.[58] The current recommendation is to screen women at least once in the perinatal period for depression and anxiety. To this end, a depression scale instrument that has been validated for use in pregnancy can be administered at this first visit. Either the Edinburgh Postnatal Depression Scale or the Patient Health Questionnaire-9 can be used for this purpose.[57] Screening alone can have clinical benefits that can be further maximized by starting medication and referring for appropriate psychiatric care or counseling when indicated. Many antidepressant medications are safe in pregnancy, and the risks of untreated depression (poor prenatal care, substance use, preterm birth, and low birth weight) need to be balanced against possible

risks of the treatment itself.[59] Evaluation at the first prenatal visit allows the clinician to have a good baseline assessment of the patient's mental health, which is useful in assessing mood at subsequent visits and in the postpartum period. Most importantly, fostering awareness of the importance of maternal mental health, and the stressors imposed by pregnancy and the puerperium, is essential in identifying and promptly treating postpartum depression and psychosis. These topics are further discussed in Chapter 43.

Maternal diabetes type 1, type 2, and other rarer forms (eg, pancreatic diabetes, mature-onset diabetes of the young, latent autoimmune diabetes in adults) may be associated with abnormal fetal growth (either excessive fetal growth or fetal growth restriction), increased rates of hypertensive disorders of pregnancy, and perinatal mortality (further discussion in Chapter 30). Hemoglobin A1c (HbA1c) evaluation can triage patient risk. Ideally, the HbA1c should be less than 6.5%[60] as there is a clear relationship between periconception HbA1c and rates of congenital malformations.[27] For example, in pregnancies with a HbA1c >10%, the risk of fetal anomalies is increased eight-fold, from the baseline risk of 2.5% to approximately 16%.[61] The most common diabetes-associated congenital anomalies are cardiac and neural tube defects. Due to the increased risk of preeclampsia and hypertensive disorders of pregnancy, and possibility of preexisting end-organ dysfunction, baseline laboratory assessment of proteinuria and creatinine is recommended and can prove helpful later in pregnancy.[62] Similar screening is recommended for women with chronic hypertension, with documentation of baseline laboratory assessment and evaluation for preexisting end-organ dysfunction (further discussion in Chapter 27).

The prevalence of obesity in the United States has been well documented, and currently, over one-third of all reproductive age women have overweight (body mass index [BMI] 25 to <30) or obesity (BMI > 30).[63] The National Academy of Medicine has provided guidelines for appropriate gestational weight gain as a function of maternal prepregnancy BMI.[64] These recommendations should be reviewed at the first visit and should be readdressed at each subsequent visit to support appropriate weight gain during pregnancy. Obesity in pregnancy is not without fetal risk with increased rates of miscarriage, congenital anatomic abnormalities, and stillbirth, and patients should be informed of these risks.[65-67] Obesity in pregnancy is further discussed in Chapter 32.

Appropriate and individualized prenatal care sets the stage for a successful pregnancy. It is particularly important for the obstetric clinician to be aware of the all the ways that prenatal care can be optimized for the individual. Many patients will have fetal or maternal complications that will dictate the course of pregnancy care and surveillance, and these adaptations and recommendations are detailed throughout this textbook.

KEY POINTS

- The initial prenatal visit is an essential component of pregnancy care and is an important opportunity to assess the patient's overall health and evaluate patient-specific pregnancy risks.
- A comprehensive health history, physical examination, and laboratory studies are essential components of the first prenatal visit.

- Ultrasound should be performed as early as possible to ensure pregnancy viability, determine fetal number, and establish pregnancy dating.
- Maternal comorbidities may require additional evaluation and monitoring throughout pregnancy, and a plan for this care should be initiated at the first visit.

REFERENCES

1. Rosen MG, Merkatz IR, Hill JG. Caring for our future: a report by the expert panel on the content of prenatal care. *Obstet Gynecol*. 1991;77(5):782-787.
2. Gregory K, Johnson CT, Johnson TR, Entman SS. The content of prenatal care: 2005 update. *Women's Health Issues*. 2006;16:198-215.
3. ACOG Committee Opinion No. 762: prepregnancy counseling. *Obstet Gynecol*. 2019;133(1):e78-e89.
4. Finer L, Zolna M. Declines in unintended pregnancy in the United States, 2008-2011. *N Engl J Med*. 2016;374:843-852.
5. Cunningham G. *Williams Obstetrics*. McGraw-Hill; 2010:363-370.
6. Cleland K, Creinin M. Significant adverse events and outcomes after medical abortion. *Obstet Gynecol*. 2013;121(1):166.
7. Bartlett LA, Berg CJ, Shulman HB, et al. Risk factors for legal induced abortion-related mortality in the United States. *Obstet Gynecol*. 2004;103:729-737.
8. American College of Obstetricians and Gynecologists' Committee on Practice Bulletins—Obstetrics. ACOG Practice Bulletin No. 192: management of alloimmunization during pregnancy. *Obstet Gynecol*. 2018;131(3): e82-e90.
9. ACOG Committee on Obstetrics. ACOG Practice Bulletin No. 78: hemoglobinopathies in pregnancy. *Obstet Gynecol*. 2007;109(1):229-237.
10. U.S. Prevention Services Task Force. Screening for hepatitis B virus infection in pregnancy: reaffirmation recommendation statement. *Ann Intern Med*. 2009;150:869-873.
11. Dionne-Odom J, Tita A, Silverman N. Society for Maternal-Fetal Medicine (SMFM) Consult Series No 38: hepatitis B in pregnancy screening, treatment, and prevention of vertical transmission. *Am J Obstet Gynecol*. 2016;214(1):6-14.
12. ACOG Practice Bulletin No. 86: viral hepatitis in pregnancy. *Obstet Gynecol*. 2007;110(4):941-956.
13. Pan CQ, Duan Z, Dai E, et al. Tenofovir to prevent hepatitis B transmission in mothers with high viral load. *N Engl J Med*. 2016;374:2324-2334.
14. Hughes B, Page CM, Kuller JA; Society for Maternal-Fetal Medicine (SMFM). Consult series No. 43; hepatitis C in pregnancy: screening, treatment, and management. *Am J Obstet Gynecol*. 2017;217(5):B1-B11.
15. ACOG Committee Opinion No. 752: prenatal and perinatal human immunodeficiency virus testing. *Obstet Gynecol*. 2018;132(3):e138-e142.
16. Connor E, Sperling RS, Gelber R, et al. Reduction of maternal infant transmission of human immunodeficiency virus type I with ziduvodine treatment. Pediatric AIDS clinical trials group protocol 076 study group. *N Engl J Med*. 1994;331:1173-1180.

17. Chou R, Cantor AG, Zakher B, et al. Screening for HIV in pregnant women: systematic review to update the 2005 US Preventive Services Task Force recommendation. *Ann Intern Med*. 2012;157:719-728.
18. Fowler M, Qin M, Fiscus CA, et al. Benefits and risks of antiretroviral therapy for perinatal HIV prevention. *N Engl J Med*. 2016;375: 1726-1737.
19. U.S. Preventive Services Task Force. Screening for syphilis infection in pregnancy: reaffirmation recommendation statement. *Ann Intern Med*. 2009;150:705-709.
20. LeFevre ML; U.S. Preventive Services Task Force. Screening for chlamydia and gonorrhea. *Ann Intern Med*. 2014;161:902-910.
21. Lewinsohn G, Leonard MK, LoBue PA, et al. Official American Thoracic Society/Infectious Diseases Society of America/Centers for Disease Control and Prevention Clinical Practice Guidelines: diagnosis of tuberculosis in adults and children. *Clin Infect Dis*. 2017;64(2):111-115.
22. ACOG Practice Bulletin No. 151: cytomegalovirus, parvovirus B19, varicella zoster, and toxoplasmosis in pregnancy. *Obstet Gynecol*. 2015;125(6):1510-1525.
23. U.S. Preventative Services Task Force. Screening for bacterial vaginosis in pregnancy to prevent preterm delivery: USPSTF recommendation statement. *Ann Intern Med*. 2008;148(3):214-219.
24. Women's Preventive Services Initiative. Well-Woman Preventive Visits. Published 2018. Accessed December 4, 2020. https://www.womenspreventivehealth.org/recommendations/well-woman-preventive-visits/
25. Saslow D, Solomon D, Lawson HW, et al. American Cancer Society, American Society for Colposcopy and Cervical Pathology, and American Society for Clinical Pathology screening guidelines for the prevention and early detection of cervical cancer. *J Low Genit Tract Dis*. 2012;16(3): 175-204.
26. ACOG Committee Opinion No. 732: infuenza vaccination during pregnancy. *Obstet Gynecol*. 2018;131(4):e109-e114.
27. American College of Obstetricians and Gynecologists' Committee on Practice Bulletins—Obstetrics. ACOG Practice Bulletin No. 201: pregestational diabetes mellitus. *Obstet Gynecol*. 2018;132(6):e228-e248.
28. ACOG Committee Opinion No. 650: physical activity and exercise during pregnancy and the postpartum period. *Obstet Gynecol*. 2015;126(6): |e135-e142.
29. American College of Obstetricians and Gynecologists. ACOG Practice Bulletin No. 148: thyroid disease in pregnancy. *Obstet Gynecol*. 2015;125:996-1005.
30. AIUM-ACR-ACOG-SMFM-SRU practice parameter for the performance of standard diagnostic obstetric ultrasound examinations. *J Ultrasound Med*. 2018;9999:1-12.

31. Committee on Practice Bulletins—Obstetrics and the American Institute of Ultrasound in Medicine. ACOG Practice Bulletin No. 175: ultrasound in pregnancy. *Obstet Gynecol.* 2018;128(6):e241-256.

32. AIUM practice parameter for the performance of limited obstetric ultrasound examinations by advanced clinical providers. *J Ultrasound Med.* 2018;37:1587-1596.

33. American College of Obstetricians and Gynecologists' Committee on Practice Bulletins—Gynecology. ACOG Practice Bulletin No. 200: early pregnancy loss. *Obstet Gynecol.* 2018;132(5):e197-e207.

34. Doubilet P, Benson CB, Bourne T, et al. Diagnostic criteria for nonviable pregnancy early in the first trimester. *N Engl J Med.* 2013;369:1443-1451.

35. Abuhamad A, Chaoui R. *First Trimester Ultrasound Diagnosis of Fetal Abnormalities.* Wolters Kluwer Health; 2018.

36. Karim JN, Roberts NW, Salomon LJ, Papageorghiou AT. Systematic review of first-trimester ultrasound screening for detection of fetal structural anomalies and factors that affect screening performance. *Ultrasound Obstet Gynecol.* 2017;50(4):429-441.

37. Syngelaki A, Chelemen T, Dagklis T, Allan L, Nicolaides KH. Challenges in the diagnosis of fetal non-chromosomal abnormalities at 11-13 weeks. *Prenat Diagn.* 2011;31:90-102.

38. Iliescu D, Tudorache S, Comanescu A, et al. Improved detection rate of structural abnormalities in the first trimester using an extended examination protocol. *Ultrasound Obstet Gynecol.* 2013;42(3):300-309.

39. Clur S, Ottenkamp J, Bilardo CM. The nuchal translucency and the fetal heart: a literature review. *Prenat Diagn.* 2009;29:739-748.

40. American College of Obstetricians and Gynecologists' Committee on Practice Bulletins—Obstetrics; Committee on Genetics; Society for Maternal–Fetal Medicine. ACOG Practice Bulletin No 163: screening for fetal aneuploidy. *Obstet Gynecol.* 2016;127(5):e123-e137.

41. ACOG Committee Opinion No. 690: carrier screening in the age of genomic medicine. *Obstet Gynecol.* 2017;129:e29-e40.

42. Cooper WO, Hernandez-Diaz S, Arbogast PG, et al. Major congenital malformations after first-trimester exposure to ACE inhibitors. *N Engl J Med.* 2006;354:2443-2451.

43. Landon M, Lynch CD. Optimal timing and mode of delivery after cesarean with previous classical incision or myomectomy: a review of the data. *Semin Perinatol.* 2011;35(5):257-261.

44. Society for Maternal-Fetal Medicine (SMFM) Publications Committee. The choice of progestogen for the prevention of preterm birth in women with singleton pregnancy and prior preterm birth. *Am J Obstet Gynecol.* 2017;216(3):B11-B13.

45. American College of Obstetricians and Gynecologists. ACOG Practice Bulletin No. 142: cerclage for the management of cervical insufficiency. *Obstet Gynecol.* 2014;123:372-379.

46. Rolnik DL, Wright D, Poon LC, et al. Aspirin versus Placebo in Pregnancies at High Risk for Preterm Preeclampsia. *N Engl J Med.* 2017;377(7):613-622.

47. Dildy GA III, Belfort MA, Smulian JC. Preeclampsia recurrence and prevention. *Semin Perinatol.* 2007;31(3):135-141.

48. LeFevre ML; U.S. Preventive Services Task Force. Low-dose aspirin use for the prevention of morbidity and mortality from preeclampsia: U.S. Preventive Services Task Force recommendation statement. *Ann Intern Med.* 2014;161:819-826.

49. World Health Organization. *WHO Recommendations for Prevention and Treatment of Pre-eclampsia and Eclampsia.* WHO; 2011. http://apps.who.int/iris/bitstream/10665/44703/1/978924154833

50. American College of Obstetricians and Gynecologists' Committee on Practice Bulletins—Obstetrics; Committee on Genetics; Society for Maternal–Fetal Medicine. ACOG Practice Bulletin No. 162: prenatal diagnostic testing for genetic disorders. *Obstet Gynecol.* 2016;127(5):e108-e122.

51. ACOG Committee Opinion No. 711: opioid use and opioid use disorder in pregnancy. *Obstet Gynecol.* 2017;127(5):e108-e122.

52. ACOG Committee Opinion No. 722: marijuana use during pregnancy and lactation. *Obstet Gynecol.* 2018;131(1):164.

53. Kapaya M, Tong V, Ding H. Nicotine replacement therapy and other interventions for pregnant smokers: pregnancy Risk Assessment Monitoring System, 2009-2010. *Prev Med.* 2015;78:92-100.

54. ACOG Committee Opinion No. 807: tobacco and nicotine cessation during pregnancy. *Obstet Gynecol.* 2020;135:e221-e229.

55. ACOG Committee Opinion No. 575: exposure to toxic environmental agents. *Fertil Steril.* 2013;100(4):931-934.

56. ACOG Committee Opinion No. 518: intimate partner violence. *Obstet Gynecol.* 2012;119:412-417.

57. ACOG Committee Opinion No. 757: screening for perinatal depression. *Obstet Gynecol.* 2018;132(5):e208-e212.

58. Palladino CL, Singh V, Campbell J, Flynn H, Gold KJ. Homicide and suicide during the perinatal period: findings from the national violent death reporting system. *Obstet Gynecol.* 2011;118(5):1056-1063.

59. Yonkers KA. Diagnosis, pathophysiology, and management of mood disorders in pregnant and postpartum women. *Obstet Gynecol.* 2011;117(4):961-977.

60. American Diabetes Association. 14. Management of diabetes in pregnancy: standards of medical care in diabetes-2021. *Diabetes Care.* 2021;44(Suppl 1):S200-S210.

61. Jensen D, Korsholm L, Ovesen P, et al. Peri-conceptional A1C and risk of serious adverse pregnancy outcome in 933 women with type 1 diabetes. *Diabetes Care.* 2009;32(6):1046-1048.

62. Hypertension in pregnancy. Report of the American College of Obstetricians and Gynecologists' Task Force on Hypertension in Pregnancy. *Obstet Gynecol.* 2013;122(5):1122-1131.

63. Hales CM, Carroll MD, Fryar CD, Ogden CL. Prevalence of obesity among adults and youth: United States, 2015-2016. *NCHS Data Brief.* 2017(288):1-8.

64. ACOG Committee Opinion No. 548: weight gain during pregnancy. *Obstet Gynecol.* 2013;121(1):210-212.

65. ACOG Practice Bulletin No 156 obesity in pregnancy. *Obstet Gynecol.* 2015;126(6):e112-e126.

66. American College of Obstetricians and Gynecologists Committee on Health Care for Underserved Women. ACOG Committee Opinion No. 591: challenges for overweight and obese women. *Obstet Gynecol.* 2014;123(3):726-730.

67. Catalano P. Obesity and pregnancy: mechanisms of short term and long term adverse consequences for mother and child. *Br Med J.* 2017;8:356.

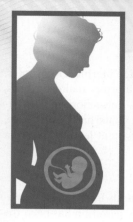

Invasive Diagnostic Procedures

Florencia Petracchi and Silvina Sisterna

Introduction

The prenatal diagnosis gold standard is obtained through the analysis of different fetal or placental tissues: chorionic villus (CVS for chorionic villus sampling), amniotic fluid (for an amniocentesis, AC), or blood (for a cordocentesis, CC).

(see Chapter 11).

Pretest Genetic Counseling
Table 14.3

Prenatal Diagnostic Tests

Chorionic Villus Sampling
Chorionic villus sampling (CVS) consists of obtaining chorionic villi for cytogenetic or molecular test of trophoblastic cells from the placenta.

Technique
Chorionic villi can be obtained by transabdominal or transcervical approaches. The procedure is performed under continuous ultrasound guidance.

- Transabdominal CVS: Local anesthesia can be applied. A 17- to 20-gauge (G) needle, or a needle with 17/19-G outside and 19/20-G inside can be used.[7] Once the needle has reached the target within the placenta, between one and 10 back-and-forth movements are performed, while the vacuum is maintained and the sample is aspirated manually by an assistant or with a vacuum adapter.[5,8]
- Transcervical CVS: A plastic catheter with a metal stylet connected to a syringe is used to make the aspiration. First, a speculum is inserted

into the vagina, and then the vagina and cervix are cleaned with an antiseptic solution. Using ultrasound guidance, the catheter is placed in the cervical canal until it reaches the chorion, from where the sample is suctioned through the tube into the syringe.[9] The number of villi obtained should be verified visually. A minimum amount of 5 mg of villi is required in each sample to achieve a valid result.[9] After the procedure, an ultrasound scanning is recommended to check for fetal heart rate.

Gestational Age
CVS should not be performed before 10 full weeks of gestation, due to the increased risk of fetal loss and complications.[4,10]

Table 14.3 Issues to Discuss During Pretest Counseling Session

Benefits and risks of invasive prenatal tests in comparison with screening tests
Alternative of not carrying out any diagnostic or screening test
Differences between CVS and amniocentesis
Turnaround time of results
Risks of pregnancy loss after the procedure and baseline risks
Precision of the results and limitations of the laboratory techniques that will be used
How the results will be informed
Possibility of inconclusive results and additional tests
Warning guidelines and rest recommendations after the procedure
Indication of anti-D immunization if the patient is Rh negative
Informed content signature

 See the eBook for expanded content, a complete reference list, and additional figures and tables.

Laboratory Aspects

Most prenatal diagnosis clinics in the world have switched to using microarray as the first test whenever a prenatal invasive diagnosis is required.

Errors

The errors reported in CVS results may be due to maternal cell contamination, culture artifacts, or placental and fetal mosaicism.

Mosaicism of placental cells is observed in 1% to 2% of the CVS. As the exact embryo-fetal developmental stage in which the mitotic error occurs cannot be established with certainty with karyotyping, the retrieval of a mosaic in CVS does not necessarily imply a fetal involvement (true fetal mosaicism) as it could be restricted to the placenta (confined placental mosaicism; CPM). For this reason, in this situation, a confirmatory karyotype using amniocentesis is recommended to discriminate a generalized mosaicism (placenta and fetus affected by the abnormal cell line) from a confined mosaicism (only in the placenta affected but not the fetus).

Complications of CVS

Fetal Loss
The risk of fetal loss compared to controls varies between 0.2% and 2%.[4,23]

Vaginal Bleeding
The frequency of vaginal bleeding is around 10%. It seems to be more frequent in the transcervical approach (up to 30% of cases).

Uncommon Complications
Amniotic fluid leakage occurs in less than 0.5% of procedures. The risk of chorioamnionitis and uterine infection are low (1-2/3000) and are probably due to a previous infection.[14] Although an association between CVS and preeclampsia or intrauterine growth restriction has been reported in some studies, a retrospective analysis did not confirm this finding.[33,34]

Risk Factors for Complications
Factors associated with an increased risk of pregnancy loss after CVS include centers that perform less than 100 procedures per year, heavy bleeding during CVS, African-American ethnic background, two or more aspirations/needle insertions, gestational age less than 10 weeks, presence of fetal structural abnormalities, increased nuchal translucency thickness, and low maternal serum PAPP-A levels.[4,37,38] Other factors that may increase the risk of fetal loss after CVS include uterine leiomyomas, advanced maternal age, uterine malformations, chorioamniotic separation, retrochorionic hematoma, previous or current maternal hemorrhage, retroverted uterus, and persistent fetal bradycardia after the procedure.[38,39]

Amniocentesis

Transabdominal amniocentesis used for karyotyping at about 15 to 17 weeks' gestation has been the gold-standard prenatal testing procedure for many years.[40] It has a high degree of safety for both the mother and the fetus, and its cytogenetic results are highly reliable.[16,39]

Technique
An ultrasound is performed to check for gestational age, anatomic scanning, and fetal heart rate. The standard technique aims for choosing an amniotic fluid pocket free of fetal parts and umbilical cord. A 20-22-G spinal needle is inserted transabdominally under continuous ultrasound guidance. Once the needle is in the amniotic cavity, the inner stylet is removed and 20 to 30 mL of fluid is aspirated (as indicated) by the operator, by an assistant, or by using a vacuum.[38] Firm entrance is recommended to avoid pushing the amniotic membrane and not traversing or passing through it, called "tenting" because in ultrasound it can be viewed as a "tent of the membranes".[3,4,9,41,42]

Gestational Age
Amniocentesis for the purpose of genetic diagnosis usually is performed between 15 and 20 weeks of gestation, but it can be performed at any later gestational age.[3] Early amniocentesis (before 14 weeks of gestation) is not recommended.[3,39]

Errors in Amniocentesis
The biological sources of error in amniocentesis include maternal cell contamination, undetected fetal mosaicism, cell mosaicism, and tetraploidy.

Complications of Amniocentesis
Complications of amniocentesis include fetal loss, loss of amniotic fluid, needle injury, chorioamnionitis, and maternal complications.

Fetal loss
Currently, the pregnancy loss rate attributable to the procedure is approximately 0.1% to 0.3% in cases in which the amniocentesis is performed by an experienced physician.[27]

Loss of Amniotic Fluid
The risk varies between 1% and 2%.

Chorioamnionitis
The risk is less than 0.1%.[40]

Needle Injury
Fetal injuries with the needle are extremely rare.

Maternal Complications
Serious maternal complications are very infrequent but can include sepsis or even death[38,66-70] due to an involuntary puncture of the bowel or because of colonization of the gel by microorganisms.[4]

Risk Factors for Complications From Amniocentesis

The main risk factors for complications include centers that perform less than 100 procedures per year, more than three attempts to introduce needles, presence of fetal malformations, and bloody or brownish fluid sample.[4,9,71,72]

Third-Trimester Amniocentesis

Generally, third-trimester amniocentesis is performed to determine fetal karyotype, to rule out fetal compromise after a maternal infection, to diagnose chorioamnionitis, and to, occasionally, determine fetal lung maturity. Third-trimester amniocentesis does not seem to be associated with an increased risk of labor initiation. However, compared to second-trimester procedures, multiple punctures and blood-stained fluid are more frequent. Culture failure rates are higher in third-trimester amniocentesis than in second-trimester amniocentesis (9.7%).[49]

Cordocentesis

Cordocentesis is the ultrasound-guided puncture of the umbilical vein in the umbilical cord, either for diagnostic or therapeutic purposes. In addition, cordocentesis (at the site of insertion of the umbilical cord or in a free portion) or puncture of the intrahepatic portion of the vein through the fetal liver is used to obtain a sample of fetal blood. The risk of fetal loss increases when performed earlier in the pregnancy.[78]

Cordocentesis Technique

First, an ultrasound scan is performed to check for fetal anomalies and localization of the placenta. A 20-22-G needle is inserted transabdominally under continuous ultrasound guidance and inserted into the umbilical vein. There are two techniques: the free-hand technique, which is more frequently used, and the needle-guided technique. If the placenta is anterior, a puncture of the umbilical cord at the placental insertion is suggested. If the placenta is posterior, a sample is taken from the intra-abdominal portion of the umbilical vein or from the placental insertion of the umbilical cord. The sample is taken from a free portion of the umbilical cord in situation where neither hepatic portion or placental insertion approaches are possible.[78]

Once the needle reaches the umbilical vein, a saline wash can be performed to confirm the correct position, and the umbilical arteries should be avoided. An assistant or the same operator performs aspiration with a syringe to obtain a sample of fetal blood.[38]

It is of utmost importance to confirm the fetal origin of the blood. It must be confirmed with an automatic blood analyzer to evaluate the average red blood cells mean corpuscular volume (MCV). The MCV depends on gestational age and is normally above 100 fL. A macrocytosis is characteristic of fetal blood.[78,79]

Complications of Cordocentesis

The risk of fetal loss after a cordocentesis is 1% to 2%. This procedure must be performed by experienced operators. It is expected that the risk of complications or sampling failure decreases as the operator's experience increases. As a cordocentesis carries higher risks than amniocentesis and needs experienced operators, it should be reserved for strict indications.[38]

Indications for an Invasive Prenatal Diagnostic Procedure

Current indications for invasive procedures include an increased risk of fetal chromosomal abnormalities, an increased risk of hereditary genetic or metabolic diseases, suspicion of perinatal infection, and parental request. Before an invasive procedure, a detailed counseling session must be carried out to cover the expected benefits, risks, and technical aspects of the procedure.[3,38]

Checklist for Carrying Out Invasive Diagnostic Procedures

- Signed informed consent should be obtained.
- Before an invasive prenatal procedure, Rhesus status of the mother and the presence of serum alloantibodies should be verified.

- Universal maternal detection of blood-borne viruses (hepatitis B and C virus, HBV and HCV; and human immunodeficiency virus, HIV) is *not recommended*.
- Ultrasound should be performed before and after an invasive diagnostic procedure.
- Asepsis principles should be respected.
- Local anesthesia may be considered, depending on which procedure is performed.
- Patients should be instructed to limit physical activity for 12 to 24 hours post-procedure. No particular pharmacological treatment is recommended.
- Discontinuing thrombotic prophylaxis is not recommended.
- Antibiotic prophylaxis is not recommended.

Multiple Pregnancies

Techniques

Before performing an invasive procedure in multiple pregnancies, chorionicity should be determined as accurately as possible, each twin should be identified and labeled, and sex concordance, or not, should be determined.[39,107,108]

Amniocentesis Technique: Varies According to Chorionicity

Dichorionic twins: It is recommended to take a sample from each sac.

- Two-puncture technique (one for each sac): Low risk (1.8%) of puncture of the same bag.[108] Dye can be instilled in the first bag (eg, indigo carmine) in cases where doubt arises or in a multiple pregnancy of more than 2 fetuses. The use of blue methylene has been abandoned due to the increased risk of congenital anomalies (jejuna atresia).[109,110]
- Single-puncture technique through the intertwin membrane: The first 1 to 2 mL of amniotic fluid sample collected after the passage of the dividing membrane should be discarded to avoid contamination with the first twin.[108] This is a technique not usually used but may be considered when two puncture technique becomes difficult.

Monochorionic, diamniotic twins:

- Sampling from a single bag is sufficient if the chronicity of the pregnancy has been clearly determined by ultrasound prior to 14 weeks and the fetal growth and anatomy are concordant.

- If this is not the case, taking a double sample should be considered. Sampling both sacs should be considered in in vitro fertilization (IVF) pregnancies or in cases where there is structural abnormality or growth discordance because of the remote chance of heterocariotype. When both sacs are sampled, the double-puncture technique is recommended to avoid iatrogenic monoamnionicity.[108]

CVS Technique: Adapted According to Chorionicity

Dichorionic twins: Transabdominally, two separate punctures can be performed, one in each trophoblastic area, or a single sequential puncture technique (double needle with an external 18-19-gauge and two different internal needles of 20 G, one for each placenta). Transcervically, two biopsies are required, one from each placenta. An error occurs in 3% to 4% of cases.[108] Cross contamination with chorionic tissue of different placentas in the same sample may occur in 1% of cases. To reduce this risk, it is recommended to take the sample near the cord insertion site and to avoid the area surrounding the dividing membrane. As an alternative, CVS can be combined transabdominal with transcervical samples.[111]

Monochorionic twins: The recommendation is to take a single sample around the equator. However, amniocentesis should be considered in the two sacs in IVF pregnancies or when there is structural abnormality or growth discordance due to the risk of heterokaryotype.[108]

REFERENCES

(only references cited in synoptic print chapter; for a complete reference list, see ebook)

3. American College of Obstetricians and Gynecologists. Practice Bulletin No. 162 Summary: Prenatal diagnostic testing for genetic disorders. *Obstet Gynecol.* 2016;127(5):976-978.
4. Royal College of Obstetricians and Gynaecologists. *Amniocentesis and Chorionic Villus Sampling.* Green-top Guideline. No. 8; 2010.
5. Young C, von Dadelszen P, Alfirevic Z. Instruments for chorionic villus sampling for prenatal diagnosis. *Cochrane Database Syst Rev.* 2013;(1):CD000114.
7. Carlin AJ, Alfirevic Z. Techniques for chorionic villus sampling and amniocentesis: a survey of practice in specialist UK centres. *Prenat Diagn.* 2008;28:914-919.
8. Battagliarin G, Lanna M, Coviello D, et al. A randomized study to assess two different techniques of aspiration while performing transabdominal chorionic villus sampling. *Ultrasound Obstet Gynecol.* 2009;33: 169-172.
9. Wilson RD, Davies G, Gagnon A, et al; Genetics Committee of the Society of Obstetricians and Gynaecologists of Canada. Amended Canadian guideline for prenatal diagnosis techniques for prenatal diagnosis. *J Obstet Gynaecol Can.* 2005;27:1048-1062.

10. American College of Obstetricians and Gynecologists. Invasive prenatal testing for aneuploidy. *Obstet Gynecol*. 2007;110:1459-1467.

14. Brambati B, Lanzani A, Tului L. Transabdominal and transcervical chorionic villus sampling: efficiency and risk evaluation of 2,411 cases. *Am J Med Genet*. 1990;35:160-164.

16. Gardner RJ, Sutherland GR, Shaffer LG. *Chromosome Abnormalities and Genetic Counseling*. 4th ed. Oxford University Press; 2012.

23. Akolekar R, Beta J, Picciarelli G, et al. Procedure-related risk of miscarriage following amniocentesis and chorionic villus sampling: a systematic review and meta-analysis. *Ultrasound Obstet Gynecol*. 2015;45:16-26.

27. Beta J, Zhang W, Geris S, Kostiv V, Akolekar R. Procedure related risk of miscarriage from chorionic villus sampling and amniocentesis. *Ultrasound Obstet Gynecol*. 2019;54(4):452-457.

33. Basaran A, Basaran M, Topatan B. Chorionic villus sampling and the risk of preeclampsia: a systematic review and meta-analysis. *Arch Gynecol Obstet*. 2011;283:1175-1181.

34. Sotiriadis A, Eleftheriades M, Chatzinikolaou F, et al. Fetal growth impairment after first-trimester chorionic villus sampling: a case-control study. *J Matern Fetal Neonatal Med*. 2015;29:1-5.

37. Odibo AO, Dicke JM, Gray DL, et al. Evaluating the rate and risk factors for fetal loss after chorionic villus sampling. *Obstet Gynecol*. 2008;112:813-819.

38. Ghi T, Sotiriadis A, Calda P, et al. ISUOG Practice Guidelines: invasive procedures for prenatal diagnosis. *Ultrasound Obstet Gynecol*. 2016;48:256-268.

39. Wilson RD, Calgary AB, Gagnon A, et al. Prenatal diagnosis procedures and techniques to obtain a diagnostic fetal specimen or tissue: maternal and fetal risks and benefits. *J Obstet Gynaecol Can*. 2015;37(7):656-668.

40. Sarto GE. Prenatal diagnosis of genetic disorders by amniocentesis. *Wis Med J*. 1970;69:255-260.

41. Tabor A, Alfirevic Z. Update on procedure-related risks for prenatal diagnosis techniques. *Fetal Diagn Ther*. 2010;27:1-7.

42. Cruz-Lemini M, Parra-Saavedra M, Borobio V, et al. How to perform an amniocentesis. *Ultrasound Obstet Gynecol*. 2014;44:727-731.

49. O'Donoghue K, Giorgi L, Pontello V, Pasquini L, Kumar S. Amniocentesis in the third trimester of pregnancy. *Prenat Diagn*. 2007;27:1000-1004.

66. Okyay RE, Gode F, Saatli B, Guclu S. Late-onset maternal mortality after amniocentesis. *Eur J Obstet Gynecol Reprod Biol*. 2011;158:367-368.

67. Bodner K, Wierrani F, Bodner-Adler B. Maternal sepsis due to *Clostridium perfringens* after 2nd-trimester genetic amniocentesis. *J Obstet Gynaecol*. 2011;31:339-340.

68. Pinette MG. Maternal death after second-trimester genetic amniocentesis. *Obstet Gynecol*. 2005;106:409.

69. Elchalal U, Shachar IB, Peleg D, Schenker JG. Maternal mortality following diagnostic 2nd-trimester amniocentesis. *Fetal Diagn Ther*. 2004;19:195-198.

70. Plachouras N, Sotiriadis A, Dalkalitsis N, Kontostolis E, Xiropotamos N, Paraskevaidis E. Fulminant sepsis after invasive prenatal diagnosis. *Obstet Gynecol*. 2004;104:1244-1247.

71. Kahler C, Gembruch U, Heling KS, et al. DEGUM guidelines for amniocentesis and chorionic villus sampling. *Ultraschall Med*. 2013;34:435-440.

72. Hess LW, Anderson RL, Golbus MS. Significance of opaque discolored amniotic fluid at second-trimester amniocentesis. *Obstet Gynecol*. 1986;67:44-46.

78. Berry SM, Stone J, Norton ME, Johnson D, Berghella V. Fetal blood sampling. *Am J Obstet Gynecol*. 2013;209:170-180.

79. Nicolaides KH, Snijders RJM, Thorpe-Beeston JG, Van den Hof MC, Gosden CM, Bellingham AJ. Mean red cell volume in normal, anemic, small, trisomic and triploid fetuses. *Fetal Ther*. 1989;4(1):1-13. doi:10.1159/00026

107. Pergament E, Schulman JD, Copeland K, et al. The risk and efficacy of chorionic villus sampling in multiple gestations. *Prenat Diagn*. 1992;12:377-384.

108. Audibert F, Gagnon A; Genetics Committee of the Society of Obstetricians and Gynaecologists of Canada; Prenatal Diagnosis Committee of the Canadian College of Medical Geneticists. Prenatal screening for and diagnosis of aneuploidy in twin pregnancies. *J Obstet Gynaecol Can*. 2011;33:754-767.

109. Kidd SA, Lancaster PA, Anderson JC, et al. A cohort study of pregnancy outcome after amniocentesis in twin pregnancy. *Paediatr Perinat Epidemiol*. 1997;11:200-213.

110. McFadyen I. The dangers of intra-amniotic methylene blue. *Br J Obstet Gynaecol*. 1992;99:89-90.

111. Weisz B, Rodeck C. Invasive diagnostic procedures in twin pregnancies. *Prenat Diagn*. 2005;25:751-758.

CHAPTER 15

Expanded Mendelian Screening

Mark I. Evans, James D. Goldberg, and Katherine Johansen Taber

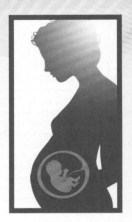

Introduction

The incorporation of new technologies into medical practice has been slower than that of other industries. Medical culture, while aggressively trying to develop new approaches to serious problems, has also simultaneously been notoriously resistant to those changes. The timing of adoption of new techniques is often very variable with some physicians/institutions/countries ranging across a spectrum of "early adopters" to "late adopters." There are many underlying components to such variability, including technological capabilities, resources available to implement new technologies, the cost/benefits of such developments, return on investment, and perceived liability reductions and exposures from such moves.[1,2]

There are two usual requirements for a technology to replace another: the new technology has been reasonably vetted and found to be an improvement or cheaper compared to the existing one, and clinicians become uncomfortable staying with the old approach. With minimal exceptions, there is never universal agreement that a new technology should immediately replace the old one—just as there is usually not universal acceptance that any new paradigm should replace an older one.

Acceptance is affected by a combination of factors that must be in place for the process to move forward. It often depends on perception in the community, resolving practical problems of implementation, and on technical assessments of evidence. Currently debated, disruptive evolutions in obstetrics include the use of cell-free fetal DNA (cffDNA) versus diagnostic procedures such as microarrays, as well as pan-ethnic carrier screening.[3-5] cffDNA utilization has skyrocketed much quicker than any recent technology. It clearly identifies an increased percentage of fetuses with Down syndrome, but it comes at the cost of abandonment of diagnostic procedures from which microarray analysis could detect a far higher number of serious disorders.[4,6] The gap will further increase as whole exome and whole genome sequencing come on line over the next several years.[7] Conversely, there is underutilization of basic, let alone pan-ethnic, carrier screening. Most clinicians are not aware that even in well-defined risk groups, such as the Ashkenazi Jewish population, pan-ethnic screening identifies carriers of more conditions that are not within the typical Ashkenazi panel than those within.[8]

New screening approaches do not always have to include new technologies, per se. Our work on fetal monitoring has shown that the incorporation of other already known variables such as increased uterine contractions and the presence of maternal, fetal, and obstetrical risk factors can significantly increase the performance metrics of screening.[9-11]

Similarly, resistance to change is multifactorial in scope and intensity. For example, it took many years after almost all experts agreed upon the utility of antenatal steroids for lung maturity for the use of these drugs to become the standard of care.[12] More recently, the debate over preeclampsia screening has been intense. National bodies, such as the American College of Obstetricians and Gynecologists (ACOG), are typically late in the game to encourage adoption because, as many critics explain, such recognition could create liability exposure for those late to move to the new technologies.[13]

In the 1990s, ACOG warned its membership that failure to offer low maternal serum alpha-fetoprotein (MSAFP) for Down syndrome screening could create medicolegal exposures. It was intended to protect the membership but had the effect of making such offerings required as a standard of care.[14]

The practice of medicine involves routine use of both diagnostic and screening tests. Obstetrics does

Table 15.1 Characteristics of Screening Tests Versus Diagnostic Tests

Diagnostic Tests
Performed only on at-risk population
Commonly expensive
Commonly have risk
Results give definitive answer

Screening Tests
Offered to general population of patients
Healthy patients
Inexpensive
Easy to perform
Reliable
Rapid return of results
Identify at-risk population
Results do *not* give definitive answer

much more than most specialties. Despite the Pap smear, a screening test that has been standard practice for nearly a century, most patients and, frankly, many physicians do not understand the difference between screening and diagnostic tests[15] (**Table 15.1**). Diagnostic tests are meant to give a definitive answer, may have risks, may be invasive, may be expensive, and are only meant for patients at a risk high enough to warrant them. Conversely, screening tests are meant for everyone, and these tests divide a group with high enough risk to warrant diagnostic testing from those who do not. Screening tests do not give definitive answers.[16] How well a screening test will do its job is defined by the metrics of sensitivity, specificity, positive predictive value (PPV), and negative predictive value.

The principles of evaluation were introduced into medical practice in the 1970s by Galen and Gambino.[16] The performance characteristics establish the boundaries of a playing field and a scoring system within which competitors for better ways to do things can be evaluated.

There are up to 10 criteria generally felt necessary to be considered before deciding (from a public policy perspective) to screen for a condition.[17] We have focused on seven salient, generalizable ones[15] (**Table 15.2**). However, not all screening tests currently being used actually follow these guidelines. Variability in criteria for use can lead to disproportionate expectations, expenditures, and complications from follow-up diagnostic testing that are likely unwarranted. As opposed to the individual patient and physician who are interested in the outcome for a specific person (PPVs and negative predictive values), the goal of a screening program is population based (sensitivity and specificity). The goal is to detect the maximum number of affected individuals for the least number called screen positive. Where to put the cutoff points is arbitrary, but it must be maintained to maximum efficiency. Specifically, a program cannot be judged by whether any particular patient's problem was or was not identified.[16]

Diagnosing patients with disease usually involves tests or procedures performed on persons believed to be at increased risk. Procedures to determine such status may include clinical examinations, laboratory testing, minor invasive procedures (such as obtaining blood), or even major surgical ones. Only a small portion of the overall population generally has enough risk to justify expensive or significant invasive procedures.

Particularly for genetic disorders, there are often population subgroups known to be at disproportionately high risk. Well known subgroups include women at advanced maternal age (AMA) for Down syndrome, Ashkenazi Jewish heritage for Tay-Sachs disease (TSD), African heritage for sickle cell disease, and numerous others.[8] However, for many disorders, although the risk for any given individual in the high-risk category is certainly higher than for anyone in the low-risk category, if the high-risk category is a small proportion of the population, the majority of affected individuals actually come from the low-risk group.[3] Particularly with the advent of increasingly sophisticated molecular technologies, we now have the ability to look for literally thousands of potential disorders in any individual who may be totally asymptomatic.[21]

Screening test results are by definition not pathognomonic for the disease[15]; rather, they delineate who needs further testing. With regard to genetic diseases, for example, asking a patient "how old are you?" is nothing more than a cheap screening test. Historically, using maternal age 35 years as a cutoff, only 30% of chromosomal abnormalities, such as Down syndrome, were detected because that is the percentage that occurred in women older than 35 years compared to those younger than 35 years (before the massive increase in fertility treatments that have increased the number of "older women" having their own children). In the

Table 15.2 Expanded Carrier Screening Panel Criteria

ACOG (2009)[18]	ACMG (2013)[19]	Joint Statement (2015)[20]
Conditions should have a carrier frequency of 1 in 100 or greater	Conditions should be severe enough that at-risk couples would consider having a prenatal diagnosis	Condition should cause cognitive disability, necessitate surgical or medical intervention, and/or have an effect on quality of life
Conditions should have a well-defined phenotype	Conditions with variable expressivity, incomplete penetrance, or mild phenotype should be optional	Prenatal diagnosis can lead to prenatal intervention, delivery management, and/or prenatal education of parents
Conditions should have a detrimental effect on quality of life	Patients should provide consent for any adult-onset disorders tested	Exclude conditions with adult onset, low penetrance, and those that cannot effectively be identified by molecular techniques
Conditions should cause cognitive or physical impairment	Causative gene(s), mutations, and mutation frequencies should be known in the population being tested	—
Conditions should require surgical or medical intervention	Validated clinical association between the mutation(s) detected and the severity of the disorder should exist	—
Conditions should have an onset early in life	—	—
Conditions can be diagnosed prenatally	—	—

ACMG, American College of Medical Genetics and Genomics; ACOG, American College of Obstetricians and Gynecologists.

United States, the AMA group has routinely been offered diagnostic testing. Such targeted group testing can now dramatically increase the detection of certain chromosomal abnormalities from 30% (by age) to about 80% to 90% by combining methodologies,[4] but the principle has been the same for decades: screen widely, routinely, and cheaply (if that it technologically, programmatically, logistically, and fiscally possible), and then perform follow-up tests that are more accurate. Changes in technological capabilities, however, are challenging that approach, specifically for aneuploidy and copy number variants (CNVs).[4,17]

Key Measures of Screening Tests: Sensitivity, Specificity, PPV, and Negative Predictive Value

Four key measures are used in the evaluation of screening tests: sensitivity, specificity, PPV, and negative predictive value[15,16] (**Figure 15.1**). Sensitivity and specificity fundamentally are epidemiologic questions. For example, *sensitivity* is defined by the question, of all the people with a condition, what percentage were identified by the test? Conversely, *specificity* is defined by the question, of all people who do not have the disease process, what

percentage of the patients test negative? Physicians are generally more interested in different questions, however, because only after a positive test does the patient usually receive additional follow-up care. Therefore, the question becomes, of all patients who have a positive test, what percentage of them actually have the disease? This is *PPV*. The *negative*

		Disease	
		Positive	**Negative**
Test	**Positive**	True positive A	False positive B
	Negative	False negative C	True negative D

Test calculations:

Sensitivity = A/A+C

Specificity = D/B+D

Positive predictive value = A/A+B

Negative predictive value = D/C+D

Figure 15.1 Screening metrics.

predictive value is just the opposite—that is, of all the people who have a negative test, what percentage of them are actually negative?

As a principle, sensitivity and specificity do not vary as a function of prevalence, unless there is an influence of other factors on the equation. However, PPVs and negative predictive values do. This has particular relevance, for example, to the mid 1980s when HIV testing first became a subject of public debate. One of the suggestions of the Reagan White House was to have mandatory testing of traditional male/female couples about to marry. In a population in which the prevalence is very low, the proportion of positives that will be false positive will be much higher than in a population in which the prevalence is very high. In the latter population, a large proportion of positives will, in fact, be true positives. In both high and low prevalence areas, the sensitivity and specificity of the tests should be the same, but the positive and negative predictive values will be widely different. If a test is absolutely useless, then the predictive value after the test will be the same as the population risk before the test. Some tests have even been worse than that, that is, the chance of them determining the correct outcome was less than a coin flip.

Newer tests are developed in an effort to refine the sensitivity and specificity of screening, and to reduce the overall costs of the screening programs per se. The goal is to reduce the need for the expenses of invasive testing that follow a positive screening. In addition, although not often mentioned, a good screening prenatal screening test will, in practice, reduce the cost of the care of affected newborns who might, as a result of screening, be detected and terminated during the pregnancy at the wishes of the parents.[21-23] Changing attitudes in society and the lessening paternalistic nature of medicine are bringing new tests onto the market—some, such as ancestry determination, are now available to the public without medical supervision and are aggressively marketed. It remains to be seen how such screening tests will be received, used, and misused.

Use and Misuse of Statistics

The use and misuse of statistical data to justify a particular approach of medical care has been omnipresent for decades. In the 1970s, Galen and Gambino were the first to show that the proper use of statistical principles to interpret laboratory data could significantly improve the quality of clinical care.[16] However, the abuse of such statistics has likewise been used to convince clinicians and patients about less than optimal therapies. For example, with a disorder of low prevalence, even a great test will have a low PPV, and the negative predictive value will be extremely high even before any tests are done. If the population incidence of disease X is 2%, then just saying "hello" to the patient will be associated with a 98% negative predictive value.

Each test must first be judged on its properties. Only if a screen has both good specificity and sensitivity is there a chance that it may be clinically useful. However, there are other criteria that are less specific to the test than to the disease in question and the society or system in which the patients and physicians are embedded.[17] Some screening criteria relate to the disease itself and will change over time along with the development of better screening tests and treatments for those disorders. As the natural history of diseases becomes better understood, treatments will generally become more effective and hopefully available. Additionally, for screening to be appropriate, large populations must be reached, convinced that screening is worthwhile, and confirmatory testing and follow-up must be available. None of these can be taken for granted, but perhaps the most challenging is reaching population segments who could benefit from screening and who, for a variety of reasons, may not be eager to participate.

Screening and testing are powerful public health tools. As specific risk factors are considered, and relevant populations become more constrained, the line between screening and testing can become blurred. This has been most obvious in the poor performance of electronic fetal monitoring for which the difference between screening and testing has been blurred and for which performance metrics have been very poor.[9-11]

History of Screening in Obstetrics

Beyond the Pap smear and blood pressure that have direct relevance to gynecology and in fact all medical specialties, the first obstetric screening test was for Rh status, which, with the development of RhoGAM in the 1970s, was remarkably successful in preventing sensitization and tragic consequences to future pregnancies. While such has been a landmark public health achievement, it is sad to report that its low use in the developing world has left hundreds of thousands of pregnancies at high risk and untreated.[24]

In terms of screening for intrinsic fetal problems, the use of MSAFP in the 1970s (preultrasound) was shown to have about a 90% sensitivity for a 5% false positive rate. The development of the screening test followed the use of amniotic fluid alpha-fetoprotein for diagnosis in couples known to be at high risk. However, because about 95% of all neural tube defects (NTDs) occur to women in the low-risk population and the risk of amniocentesis was felt at the time to be as much as 2%, primarily offering diagnostic procedures to the population at large was neither programmatically nor financially feasible and would likely have led to far more complications from the procedures than the number of abnormalities detected actually warranted.

Next came the discovery that low levels of MSAFP were associated with increased risks of aneuploidy, specifically trisomies 21 and 18. Use of MSAFP screening was much worse for detecting aneuploidies than for detecting NTDs, but it was still an improvement over AMA alone. Given that the risk of a 35-year-old woman carrying a fetus with Down syndrome at midtrimester is about 1/270, the detection of Down syndrome in 1/140 patients following a low MSAFP result was an improvement. Double, triple, and quad screening raised the PPV to about 1/50.[25] In relative terms, such was a big improvement, but there was still much more to be desired. First-trimester combined screening and CffDNA have significantly increased the performance metrics and are discussed in Chapter 11.

The first forays into carrier (Mendelian disorder) screening focused on conditions with simple genetics and simple laboratory requirements. Sickle cell anemia (SSA) is the prototype as every person with SSA on the planet has the same one base pair substitution. Early assessments by "sickle cell prep," hemoglobin electrophoresis, and molecular technologies improved performance metrics.

TSD, a disorder whose consequences were substantial, likewise met the criteria of having a defined population perceived to be at high risk and a laboratory methodology of enzyme analysis that was felt to be sufficiently accurate. Molecular analysis revealed a manageable number of mutations to be investigated. In response, the "Dor Yeshorim" (looking to the future) program was established in the early 1970s for the observant Jewish community in New York. These families by custom and practice had arranged marriages and commonly had large families.[26] TSD carrier status was very common, so disease occurrence was very high. The program featured TSD carrier testing for high school students; however, the patients were not told the results. When parents wanted to have their children marry, the prospective couple and families would meet with the "matchmaker." She would then, in secret, check their carrier statuses. If they were an at-risk couple, she would decide, without explaining why, that they were "not a good match." Hundreds of what would-be carrier couple marriages were prevented, and, because of the large families expected, large numbers of affected children were never conceived.

From a public health perspective, such a method is considered primary prevention. Given that outside of a small number of religious groups, arranged marriages are not common or accepted today in modern society, screening of at-risk patients to identify an affected fetus is considered secondary prevention. Diagnosis after the birth of an affected child is tertiary prevention.

Beginnings of Panels

The identification of the cystic fibrosis (CF) gene in 1989 began the revolution of molecular prenatal diagnosis.[27,28] Identification of risk status became possible for disorders in which there is not a characteristic enzymatic discrimination among affected individuals, carriers, and homozygous normal patients. It also began our understanding of the tremendous genetic heterogeneity of carrier mutations. When the ΔF508 mutation was identified and found to explain about 70% of carriers, it was generally assumed that the "next mutation" might identify 20% of carriers, and that, within a short period, a moderate number of markers would detect almost all the cases. In fact, there are now over 2000 known mutations for CF, which proves the vast superiority of sequencing methods over genotyping methods (discussed later).

As more and more genetic diseases had their DNA structures identified, laboratories began to develop "panels" for determining carrier status. For example, the Ashkenazi Jewish panel went from screening for TSD only; to Canavan, familial dysautonomia, and CF; and then expanding to anywhere from 9 to 40 molecular conditions.[29,30] In the late 2000s, screening for CF, spinal muscular atrophy (SMA), and Fragile X in the Caucasian Christian population was considered by many, but not all, to be the correct approach. It did not help public policy consensus on liability protection that major organizations such as the ACOG and the American College of Medical Genetics and Genomics (ACMG) came to dramatically different conclusions about screening for SMA; ACOG only recently in 2017 added SMA on as a "routine" suggestion, nearly a decade after ACMG and many other countries did.[31,32]

Screening Guidelines

Professional guideline-directed screening for genetic disease has been a long-established part of preconception and prenatal care. Particularly for younger couples, the rate of "at-risk" pregnancies and actual abnormalities that occur is higher for Mendelian disorders than for common chromosome abnormalities such as Down syndrome.[1] As mentioned before, one model for carrier screening has been the community wide screening programs for TSD established in the 1970s.[33] These programs focused on a single severe disease that had an increased carrier frequency in a recognized ethnic group, Eastern European Ashkenazi Jews. Wide implementation of these programs has significantly reduced the incidence of TSD in this ethnic group. This resulted in recommendations from professional organizations to offer prenatal TSD screening to all women of Ashkenazi Jewish descent as discussed below. In fact, the majority of affected infants now come from other ethnic groups because the Ashkenazi Jews were tested and other groups were not.

It has been over a decade since the ACOG and the ACMG initiated guidelines for prenatal and preconception carrier screening of CF.[34] Initial professional guidelines recommended screening Caucasian individuals or those with a family history of CF. In 2011, the ACOG Committee on Genetics updated its CF screening guidelines, stating that it had become increasingly difficult to classify individuals with CF into distinct ethnic categories.[34] The Committee agreed that it was reasonable to offer CF to all couples planning a pregnancy because it allowed expectant parents to consider all reproductive options, including preimplantation genetic diagnosis, prenatal diagnosis, gamete donation, or adoption.

Given the long history of carrier screening, there are still relatively few guidelines available to clinicians, often resulting in inconsistent practices. In addition, there are conflicting recommendations between organizations (ACOG, ACMG) that have published guidelines. Such discrepancies leave the patient and physician at a loss as to the best recommendations and potentially expose the physician to liability if a patient has an affected child who could have been identified.

Outside of the United States, guidelines are even more limited, but there is continuing evolution based upon emerging technologies and public health policies in different countries.

Limitations of Ethnicity-Based Guidelines

Ethnicity-based screening for genetic disorders was for the past four decades the most common and cost-effective means of identifying couples at risk of bearing affected children. Until the past several years, the additive expense of single-gene tests made population-wide screening for recessive diseases cost prohibitive when those diseases largely occurred in specific ethnic groups. Using ethnicity as a screen thus enabled carrier testing to capture individuals most likely to have a mutation.[30] However, mixed ethnicity, adoption, and unknown ancestry compromise the application of the ethnicity-only–based approach.[35] The birth of babies affected with classically "Jewish" disorders to non-Jewish families exemplifies the pitfalls of defining genetic risks based on patients' self-report and increasingly nebulous social constructs of race and ethnicity.[36] In addition, the ACOG statement on CF carrier screening acknowledges the difficulty of assigning a single ethnicity to individuals as a justification for offering pan-ethnic screening.[34] Relying on ethnic categorization implies that most patients have some knowledge of their ancestral heritage, but data indicate that this is limited.[37]

Concerns regarding ethnicity-based screening have been raised in the past.[38] For example, newborn screening (NBS) is not ethnically driven, whereas most carrier screening is, leading Ross to argue that universal NBS is more equitable than ethnicity-based screening because universal screening avoids missed cases of rare disorders where early intervention reduces morbidity and mortality.[38] Similarly, the US Secretary's Advisory

Committee on Heritable Disorders in Newborns and Children (SACHDNC) acknowledges that genetic screening may be appropriate even without the availability of direct medical intervention, particularly if it will inform a family about future reproductive options.[39] A broadened concept of benefit, which includes sparing families from a prolonged diagnostic odyssey and allows for informing relatives of their increased genetic risks, has also been supported.[39] The SACHDNC also stated that an important consideration in the adoption of new screening technologies is the potential for reducing costs involved in the initial workup of a newborn with a rare disease of unknown etiology.[39] These benefits are equally applicable to preconception carrier screening.

Recent developments in laboratory technologies have led to the commercial availability of expanded carrier screening (ECS) panels capable of assessing hundreds of mutations associated with genetic disease without an ethnic predilection or family history. Although many of the disorders on these panels are individually rare, the overall risk of having an affected offspring (approximately 1 in 300 pregnancies)[40] is higher than the risk of having a child with Down syndrome in the average-risk population, or the risk of a child with an NTD, for which screening is essentially universal. Moreover, the cost of ECS is often less than or similar to the cost of currently recommended ethnicity-based panels.

Current Guidelines for Optimal Panel ECS Design

The size and content of ECS panels vary among laboratories, mainly due to the large number of conditions that are possible for inclusion. A 2018 analysis comparing 16 commercially available ECS offerings found that panel size ranged from 41 to 1792 conditions.[19] An ideal ECS panel maximizes the detection of couples at risk for having pregnancies affected with serious conditions without sacrificing the sensitivity of any one condition.

ACOG and ACMG have individually and collectively published their criteria for screening[19,30] (**Table 15.2**). An article authored by five professional societies includes similar suggestions for condition inclusion.[41] There are some subtle differences among the groups, but the central criteria collectively are intended to ensure that conditions

are sufficiently prevalent that couples could reasonably expect to be at risk, are serious enough that couples would want to know that their pregnancy is at risk, and that knowing about such risk would impact pregnancy management or reproductive decision-making.

The design of ECS panels can be approached in different ways.[19] Some panels adopt a more conservative approach by limiting screening only to the most prevalent conditions that have well-understood genotype-phenotype relationships. These panels tend to have high specificity, but they will miss couples at risk for less prevalent conditions or who carry variants with unclear pathogenicity. Panels that screen for a larger number of conditions tend to have higher sensitivity, but some of the conditions may have less well-understood genotype-phenotype relationships and/or are less likely to be serious enough to warrant screening.[19]

A systematic approach for selecting which conditions should be included on ECS panels has been suggested, which prioritizes the principles of severity, actionability, prevalence, and sensitivity, similar to those suggested by ACOG and ACMG.[42]

Severity

The utility of ECS rests on its ability to detect conditions that are severe enough to warrant identification of couples who are at risk. At least two studies have developed frameworks to assist in the classification of disease severity.[43,44] These frameworks rely on traits to describe severity, including the timing of disease onset (infancy/childhood versus adulthood), impact on lifespan (severely shortened versus less so), and disability associated with the disease (intellectual, physical, and sensory impact), with the most severe diseases being those that are early onset, result in reduced lifespan, and cause intellectual or physical impairment.

Actionability

Related to severity, the principle of actionability suggests that panels should only include conditions that would impact reproductive decision-making, pregnancy/perinatal management, or preparation by parents to care for an affected child. For example, "actionability" in the preconception setting may include actions to reduce the risk of having an affected pregnancy, such as *in vitro* fertilization with preimplantation genetic testing for molecular diagnoses to select an unaffected embryo or use of a donor gamete that is not a carrier, whereas "actionability" in the prenatal setting is prenatal diagnostic testing to confirm or rule out a fetal diagnosis, leading to pregnancy management options including termination, and/or preparatory measures for parents for neonatal care.

Prevalence and Carrier Frequency

Inclusion of conditions on ECS panels depends on the prevalence of the condition and the carrier frequency within specific populations (**Figure 15.2**). For example, conditions should not be so rare that pathogenicity of variants cannot be determined and that only a tiny proportion of couples could expect to be at risk. To encourage inclusion of conditions that are sufficiently prevalent, ACOG suggests that the carrier frequency of conditions be 1 in 100 or greater; however, this criterion lacks clarity with regard to which population's carrier frequency should be considered, that is, that of certain ethnicities versus that in any ethnicity.[8,31,45] Others have suggested that the clinical detection rate be used as a threshold, based on the principle that such a threshold would directly measure variant interpretability and indirectly correspond to disease prevalence, whereas a carrier rate threshold alone would not capture variant interpretability.[44] One objection to inclusion of a large number of conditions on a panel is the misconception that the addition of conditions will linearly increase the number of patients screening positive, thus resulting in the need and cost to manage many more patients. However, rarer conditions have lower carrier frequencies, so as rarer conditions are added, the number of positive results will plateau. For example, a panel with the 18 most prevalent conditions typically screened would identify about 84% of at-risk couples. The addition of the 73 next most prevalent conditions increases that identification to approximately 95% of at-risk couples.[45]

The panels offered by several clinical laboratories screen for approximately 150 to 500 conditions and represent a balance between effectively identifying carrier couples and screening for conditions that are reasonably prevalent. A key issue, often misunderstood by nongeneticists, is that the purpose of such screening is to find the maximum number of carrier *couples*, not just heterozygote carriers. As panels increase to include conditions with carrier frequencies much below 1/100, the yield of a nonconsanguineous partner also having the same rare allele is very low. As such, extremely large panels will, with very low prevalence disorders, typically identify very few additional carrier couples.

Timing of ECS

Preconception genetic screening is defined as carrier testing for genetic disorders prior to pregnancy onset, such as at the annual obstetrician-gynecologist well-visit examination, and is not a new concept. Screening for SSA has been routine/mandatory for the African American community for more than 50 years. Likewise, screening for β-thalassemia has been the standard of care for almost as long for Mediterranean populations such as Greeks and Italians. The Jewish community was the first ethnic group to implement multiple disease panels. It started out in the 1970s and a part of the Dor Yeshorim program since the 1980s,[26] significantly reducing the incidence of TSD in Jewish babies. Quickly thereafter, the size of the panel went from one to three to five to now literally dozens of disorders seen disproportionately in the Ashkenazi Jewish population. Multiple Jewish organizations and rabbinical education programs

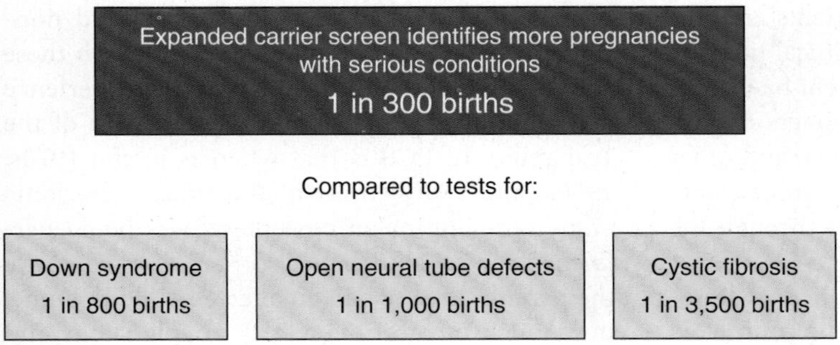

Expanded carrier screen identifies more pregnancies with serious conditions

1 in 300 births

Compared to tests for:

| Down syndrome | Open neural tube defects | Cystic fibrosis |
| 1 in 800 births | 1 in 1,000 births | 1 in 3,500 births |

Figure 15.2 Expanded carrier screen results versus other common diagnostic tests.

have adopted these recommendations, encouraging carrier screening for young Jewish couples during premarital counseling.[46]

Given the low cost of ECS, the preconception screening model in the Jewish community is a model for preconception carrier screening in the general population.[35] Incorporating carrier screening into the well-woman examination, rather than waiting until pregnancy is proximate or underway, improves the standard of care by providing the opportunity for autonomous decision-making and the consideration of modern reproductive technologies. Most women of reproductive age pursue preventive health services annually: 84% of women between the ages of 19 and 39 years have seen a healthcare clinician within the previous year.[47] Healthcare visits during this stage are an ideal time to review family history and discuss carrier screening without the stress of an ongoing pregnancy.[48] The ACOG Committee on Genetics also supports preconception screening over screening in the prenatal period and, since 2005, has released six opinions that recommend preconception genetic screening.[18,28,30,34,47,48] However, only one in six family physicians or obstetrician-gynecologists provides preconception care. This implies the need to improve routine implementation of preconception health and education regarding genetic screening for both physicians and patients.

Genetic Counseling

Patients undergoing carrier screening benefit from informed decision-making, but in-person counseling provided by a genetic counselor is optimal but commonly impractical for large-scale screening because of a shortage of genetics professionals (Chapter 11).[51] Creative and cost-efficient solutions that do not sacrifice quality are needed to carry out informed consent. However, it is outdated and paternalistic to believe that genetic testing requires more patient hand-holding than traditional laboratory testing, particularly when patients are otherwise healthy.[35] This shortage of clinical genetics professionals may actually be of benefit by forcing genetics to become an integral component of general care.[52] Nurses, physician assistants, and other healthcare clinicians will need more professional education in order to guide patients through the screening process.

Given the rapid growth in the number of laboratories providing genetic testing, genetic counselors have been in great demand. Unfortunately, most obstetrician-gynecologists are not well trained to provide up-to-date consultations for their patients, suggesting an educational need for this specialty. Independent telephone and online counseling services have emerged, but it remains to be seen whether this will adequately meet counseling needs as carrier screening is undertaken by more patients. Many laboratories providing carrier screening also provide the option of both pre- and posttest genetic counseling, sometimes at no additional charge to the patient. This solution has the potential to improve genetic counseling access to many more patients than does traditional in-person counseling approaches.[53]

Anxiety and Stigmatization

A more integrated approach to genetics within the field of medicine requires addressing potential anxiety and stigmatization about genetic information that may serve as a barrier to adoption. Concerns about increased anxiety in carriers of recessive diseases appear to be overestimated; a systematic review of 20 studies of the psychological impact of carrier testing for autosomal recessive and X-linked genetic disorders found that several factors influence emotional reactions to carrier testing, including mode of inheritance, existing coping mechanisms, gender, personal connection to a particular disease, and stage of life.[53]

Patients who already had an affected child can experience feelings of guilt and shame associated with their positive carrier status and the birth of the affected child. However, in those who underwent preconception carrier screening as part of routine screening, anxiety largely dissipated within 6 months.[54] For example, carriers of CF who received screening felt no significant difference in anxiety compared to noncarriers. Findings related to feelings of stigmatization and guilt associated with CF screening are similar: no significant difference was noted between carriers and noncarriers in the general population, although these participants did not have any personal experience or family history of CF.[54] A major benefit of the availability of ECS is that whereas in the 1970s, 1980s, and 1990s, most of the time a chorionic villus sampling or amniocentesis was being performed for a Mendelian disorder, it was because the parents already had an affected child at home, now much of the time at-risk couple status and offering prenatal diagnosis comes before the birth of an affected child.[1] The major reaction of couples appears to be relief rather at having options rather than guilt.[1,2,8]

Screening Technology

Today, ECS is typically carried out by either full-exon sequencing or targeted genotyping. In full-exon sequencing, next-generation sequencing (NGS) technologies are used to interrogate nearly all exons and some noncoding regions that are known to affect variant pathogenicity (eg, splice sites). Full-exon sequencing can identify all common and rare novel variants; however, the detection of novel variants necessitates a robust curation process that can determine the clinical impact of each variant.[42] It is important to note that in carrier screening, only pathogenic and likely pathogenic variants are reported; variants of uncertain significance are not.[41]

The other common ECS method is targeted genotyping, in which a set of predefined, known pathogenic or likely pathogenic variants is interrogated using NGS, allele-specific polymerase chain reaction, and/or microarray technology.[42] Because they lack the capability to detect all variants possibly present, targeted genotyping panels often have lower overall detection rates than those performed using full-exon sequencing.[42]

Accurate variant detection and risk prediction for some conditions is technically challenging and requires additional or alternative strategies. For example, an additional NGS step is needed to define the techniques used to detect the risk of a pregnancy affected with Fragile X syndrome. For other conditions, genomic architecture necessitates an alternative strategy. For example, detection of the genetic variants associated with 21-hydroxylase–deficient congenital adrenal hyperplasia is confounded by the presence of a *CYP21A2* pseudogene. Laboratories employ various methods to detect pathogenic variants in such technically challenging genes.[40]

For some conditions, misconceptions that traditional screening methods outperform NGS have persisted. For example, hexosaminidase A (HEXA) enzyme testing has long been the recommended method for TSD carrier screening because it is more sensitive than targeted variant analysis in ethnicities other than Ashkenazi Jewish.[41] However, NGS of HEXA has been employed as an alternative method for TSD carrier screening because it can identify common, rare, and novel variants,[55] and the estimated clinical sensitivity, specificity, and PPV are higher by NGS than by enzyme testing in both Ashkenazi Jewish and non-Ashkenazi Jewish populations.[56] Similarly, for hemoglobinopathies, a complete blood count (CBC) with red blood cell indices, followed by electrophoresis, is recommended to identify carriers.[29] However, this approach cannot provide variant level information or phasing for α-thalassemia; iron deficiency can confound results; and, when CBC and/or electrophoresis results indicate risk, genetic testing is ultimately recommended.[29] This workflow is lengthy and complicated compared to genetic testing as a first-line screening methodology. Furthermore, NGS-based testing for α-thalassemia has higher sensitivity and specificity.[57]

Partner Screening

In order to provide accurate risk based on ECS results, both members of the couple need to be screened. To save money (at the cost of time), couple screening can be accomplished sequentially, in which the female partner is screened by ECS first. Her partner is then only screened for whatever conditions the female was found to carry. Couple screening can also be accomplished concurrently. Sequential screening is more economical, but it takes longer to receive the couple's results as, once the female partner's results are known, the male partner must be contacted, a sample collected, and then the test performed and merged with the female partner's results. With concurrent screening, the couple's results are available more quickly, but the approach is often costlier because both members of the couple are screened with the full ECS panel, rather than only for the conditions that the other partner carries. Some laboratories offer hybrid models in which a sample from both members of the couple is submitted at the same time; the female's sample is tested first, and then the male's sample is tested only if the female is found to be a carrier and only for the conditions the female is found to carry. Deciding which approach is appropriate depends on several factors, including gestational age, availability of the partner for a blood draw or saliva collection, and patient preferences.[41]

Adult-Onset Disorders

The revolution in genetic technologies has resulted in testing that can reveal risk for disorders with an onset in adulthood, rather than during the fetal or childhood periods. There is technically no reason that risk for these adult-onset conditions could not be determined using ECS. Pregnancy is generally considered a time of increased patient receptivity to medical care, so it is an opportunity to provide services that otherwise might be difficult to accomplish—both related to the current pregnancy and for healthcare issues in general. Discussions are ongoing regarding the ethical issues surrounding parental decision-making regarding late-onset conditions that may be present in their offspring.

What Will All This Look Like in 5 to 10 Years?

To paraphrase Winston Churchill, "It is always easier to prophesize after an event has taken place." There has been a parallel development process for both Mendelian and chromosomal/CNV technologies[15,16] (**Table 15.3**). Initially, both could only tackle simple problems, for example, unbanded aneuploidy and simple base pair substitutions

Table 15.3 Parallel Improvements in Mendelian and Chromosomal Testing and Screening

Mendelian	Chromosomal
• Small number of disorders with simple genetics (sickle cell, Tay-Sachs, hemoglobinopathies)	• Low-resolution karyotyping • Whole chromosomes, banding, improved turnaround time
• Expanding, targeted panels (cystic fibrosis, familial dysautonomia, Canavan disease) • How high does the incidence have to be?	• Increased resolution • Molecular vs cytogenetics • Fluorescent *in situ* probes • Quantitative fluorescent polymerase chain reaction for deletions and additions
Expansive by genotype	Expansive by microarrays
Expansive by sequencing	Expansive by sequencing

Extensive improvements in laboratory technology are producing higher quality cheaper panels. The development of sequencing technologies will allow for both many Mendelian and copy number variant disorders to be diagnosable by the same testing platform.

(sickle cell). Parallel advances included banding and simple molecular cytogenetics.

Early Mendelian panels emerged with limited capabilities both for the number of disorders and the sensitivity for each disorder. Next, we moved into a period of more extensive panels using genotyping of increasing number of mutations and microarrays for a "high-resolution" karyotype. Now, both types of disorders are being interrogated by sequencing for even higher clarity of diagnosis for both Mendelian and chromosomal abnormalities. We can predict that over the next several years, capabilities will be further enhanced and progress will occur at a near logarithmic rate. As with all new technological capabilities, we will have our "numerators" of problems before we get the "denominators." Just as the variants of uncertain significance for microarrays and the implications of certain ultrasound findings could be categorized as either pathologic or benign, over time, whole exome sequencing and whole genome sequencing will become routine. However, there will be a period during which uncertain results will need to be clarified.

Our overriding philosophy of practice is to maximize every couple's control over their own lives. More information leads to that. Now, we can expect to identify risk status before a life-changing experience of the birth of a severely impaired child. However, we never tell a patient what they should do. All we seek is to allow them to make such decisions for themselves.

Summary

Several medical professional societies have suggested certain criteria that should be considered in the design of ECS panels. Although some differences in these recommendations exist, there is consensus that conditions screened should be severe, reasonably prevalent, and prenatally diagnosable. We are well beyond the period in which routinely only offering ethnically limited panels can be considered optimal care or even reasonable care. We also believe that genotyping panels are significantly inferior to sequencing ones. These characteristics most effectively support reproductive decision-making and pregnancy management that can reduce the risk of an affected pregnancy and/or lead to improved perinatal care and parental preparation.

KEY POINTS

- The introduction of new medical technologies has often lagged behind other endeavors.
- Most physicians and patients do not have a good understanding of the principles of screening tests and differences versus diagnostic tests.
- Mendelian disorders are far more common than generally recognized, with most couples having a higher incidence than better known conditions such as Down syndrome.
- They are not age dependent so even young couples should be offered such screening.
- Ethnically derived panels miss more than half the carrier couples for most ethnic groups.
- ECS provides a much more comprehensive evaluation than traditional approaches.
- Virtually all national professional organizations of relevance endorse ECS.

REFERENCES

1. Evans MI, Krivchenia EL, Yaron Y. Screening. *Best Pract Res Clin Obstet Gynaecol.* 2002;16(5):645-657.
2. Evans MI, Wapner RJ, Bui TH. Future directions. *Best Pract Res Clin Obstet Gynaecol.* 2002;16(5):757-759.
3. Evans MI, Chik L, O'Brien JE, et al. MOMs (multiples of the median) and DADs (discriminant aneuploidy detection): improved specificity and cost-effectiveness of biochemical screening for aneuploidy with DADs. *Am J Obstet Gynecol.* 1995;172(4 pt 1):1138-1147.
4. Malone FD, Canick JA, Ball RH, et al. First-trimester or second-trimester screening, or both, for Down's syndrome. *N Engl J Med.* 2005;353(19):2001-2011.
5. Orlandi F, Rossi C, Allegra A, et al. First trimester screening with free beta-hCG, PAPP-A and nuchal translucency in pregnancies conceived with assisted reproduction. *Prenat Diagn.* 2002;22(8):718-721.
6. Evans MI, Chick L, O'Brien JE, et al. Logistic regression generated probability estimates for trisomy 21 outcomes from serum alpha fetoprotein and beta human chorionic gonadotrophin: simplification with increased specificity. *J Matern Fetal Med.* 1996;5(1):1-6.
7. Levy B, Wapner R. Prenatal diagnosis by chromosomal microarray analysis. *Fertil Steril.* 2018;109(2):201-212.
8. Guo MH, Gregg AR. Estimating yields of prenatal carrier screening and implications for design of expanded carrier screening panels. *Genet Med.* 2019;21(9):1940-1947.
9. Eden RD, Evans MI, Britt DW, Evans SM, Gallagher P, Schifrin BS. Combined prenatal and postnatal prediction of early neonatal compromise risk. *J Matern Fetal Neonatal Med.* 2019:1-12.
10. Eden RD, Evans MI, Evans SM, Schifrin BS. The "fetal reserve index": re-engineering the interpretation and responses to fetal heart rate patterns. *Fetal Diagn Ther.* 2018;43(2):90-104.
11. Evans MI, Britt DW, Eden RD, Gallagher P, Evans SM, Schifrin BS. The fetal reserve index significantly outperforms ACOG category system in predicting cord blood base excess and pH: a methodological failure of the category system. *Reprod Sci.* 2019;26(6):858-863.
12. American College of Obstetricians and Gynecologists Committee on Obstetric Practice. Committee Opinion No. 713: antenatal corticosteroid therapy for fetal maturation. *Obstet Gynecol.* 2017;130(2):e102-e109.
13. Rolnik DL, Wright D, Poon LC, et al. Aspirin versus placebo in pregnancies at high risk for preterm preeclampsia. *N Engl J Med.* 2017;377(7):613-622.
14. American College of Obstetricians and Gynecologists Committee on Practice Bulletins. Practice Bulletin No. 77: screening for fetal chromosomal abnormalities. *Obstet Gynecol.* 2007;109(1):217-227.
15. Evans MI, Britt DW, Eden RD, Evans SM, Schifrin BS. Re-conceptualizing fetal monitoring. *Eur Gynecol Obstet.* 2019;1:10-17.
16. Galen RS, Gambino SR. *Beyond Normality: The Predictive Value and Efficiency of Medical Diagnoses.* Wiley; 1975.
17. Wilson JMG, Jungner G. *Principles and Practice of Screening for Disease.* World Health Organization; 1968.
18. American College of Obstetricians and Gynecologists Committee on Gynecologic Practice. ACOG Committee Opinion No. 483. primary and preventive care: periodic assessments. *Obstet Gynecol.* 2011;117(4):1008-1015.
19. Chokoshvili D, Vears D, Borry P. Expanded carrier screening for monogenic disorders: where are we now? *Prenat Diagn.* 2018;38(1):59-66.
20. Grody WW, Thompson BH, Gregg AR, et al. ACMG position statement on prenatal/preconception expanded carrier screening. *Genet Med.* 2013;15(6):482-483.
21. Evans MI, Andriole S, Curtis J, Evans SM, Kessler AA, Rubenstein AF. The epidemic of abnormal copy number variant cases missed because of reliance upon noninvasive prenatal screening. *Prenat Diagn.* 2018;38(10):730-734.
22. Evans MI, Evans SM, Bennett TA, Wapner RJ. The price of abandoning diagnostic testing for cell-free fetal DNA screening. *Prenat Diagn.* 2018;38(4):243-245.
23. Evans MI, Wapner RJ, Berkowitz RL. Noninvasive prenatal screening or advanced diagnostic testing: caveat emptor. *Am J Obstet Gynecol.* 2016;215(3):298-305.
24. Neighbor J. *RhoGAM at 50: A Drug Still Saving Lives of Newborns.* Accessed June 17, 2020. http://columbiamedicinemagazine.org/ps-news/spring-2018/rhogam-50-drug-still-saving-lives-newborns
25. Evans MI, Krantz DA, Hallahan TW, Sherwin J. Impact of nuchal translucency credentialing by the FMF, the NTQR or both on screening distributions and performance. *Ultrasound Obstet Gynecol.* 2012;39(2):181-184.
26. Kaback M, Lim-Steele J, Dabholkar D, Brown D, Levy N, Zeiger K. Tay-Sachs disease – carrier screening, prenatal diagnosis, and the molecular era. An international perspective, 1970 to 1993. The International TSD Data Collection Network. *J Am Med Assoc.* 1993;270(19):2307-2315.
27. Casals T, Gimenez J, Ramos MD, Nunes V, Estivill X. Prenatal diagnosis of cystic fibrosis in a highly heterogeneous population. *Prenat Diagn.* 1996;16(3):215-222.
28. Riordan JR, Rommens JM, Kerem B, et al. Identification of the cystic fibrosis gene: cloning and characterization of complementary DNA. *Science.* 1989;245(4922):1066-1073.
29. American College of Obstetricians and Gynecologists Committee on Genetics. Committee opinion No. 691: carrier screening for genetic conditions. *Obstet Gynecol.* 2017;129(3):e41-e55.
30. Gross SJ, Pletcher BA, Monaghan KG; Professional Practice and Guidelines Committee. Carrier screening in individuals of Ashkenazi Jewish descent. *Genet Med.* 2008;10(1):54-56.
31. American College of Obstetricians and Gynecologists Committee on Genetics. Committee opinion No. 690: carrier screening in the age of genomic medicine. *Obstet Gynecol.* 2017;129(3):e35-e40.
32. Prior TW; Professional Practice and Guidelines Committee. Carrier screening for spinal muscular atrophy. *Genet Med.* 2008;10(11):840-842.
33. Kaback MM. Population-based genetic screening for reproductive counseling: the Tay-Sachs disease model. *Eur J Pediatr.* 2000;159(suppl 3):S192-S195.

34. American College of Obstetrics and Gynecology and American College of Medical Genetics. *Preconception and Prenatal Carrier Screening for Cystic Fibrosis: Clinical and Laboratory Guidelines.* American College of Obstetrics and Gynecology; 2001.

35. Nazareth SB, Lazarin GA, Goldberg JD. Changing trends in carrier screening for genetic disease in the United States. *Prenat Diagn.* 2015;35(10):931-935.

36. Park NJ, Morgan C, Sharma R, et al. Improving accuracy of Tay Sachs carrier screening of the non-Jewish population: analysis of 34 carriers and six late-onset patients with HEXA enzyme and DNA sequence analysis. *Pediatr Res.* 2010;67(2):217-220.

37. Shraga R, Yarnall S, Elango S, et al. Evaluating genetic ancestry and self-reported ethnicity in the context of carrier screening. *BMC Genet.* 2017;18(1):99.

38. Ross LF. A re-examination of the use of ethnicity in prenatal carrier testing. *Am J Med Genet A.* 2012;158A(1):19-23.

39. Trotter TL, Fleischman AR, Howell RR, Lloyd-Puryear M; Secretary's Advisory Committee on Heritable Disorders in Newborns and Children. Secretary's Advisory Committee on Heritable Disorders in Newborns and Children response to the president's council on bioethics report: the changing moral focus of newborn screening. *Genet Med.* 2011;13(4):301-304.

40. Hogan GJ, Vysotskaia VS, Beauchamp KA, et al. Validation of an expanded carrier screen that optimizes sensitivity via full-exon sequencing and panel-wide copy number variant identification. *Clin Chem.* 2018;64(7):1063-1073.

41. Edwards JG, Feldman G, Goldberg J, et al. Expanded carrier screening in reproductive medicine-points to consider: a joint statement of the American College of Medical Genetics and Genomics, American College of Obstetricians and Gynecologists, National Society of Genetic Counselors, Perinatal Quality Foundation, and Society for Maternal-Fetal Medicine. *Obstet Gynecol.* 2015;125(3):653-662.

42. Beauchamp KA, Muzzey D, Wong KK, et al. Systematic design and comparison of expanded carrier screening panels. *Genet Med.* 2018;20(1):55-63.

43. Lazarin GA, Hawthorne F, Collins NS, Platt EA, Evans EA, Haque IS. Systematic classification of disease severity for evaluation of expanded carrier screening panels. *PLoS One.* 2014;9(12):e114391.

44. Leo MC, McMullen C, Wilfond BS, et al. Patients' ratings of genetic conditions validate a taxonomy to simplify decisions about preconception carrier screening via genome sequencing. *Am J Med Genet A.* 2016;170(3):574-582.

45. Ben-Shachar R, Svenson A, Goldberg JD, Muzzey D. A data-driven evaluation of the size and content of expanded carrier screening panels. *Genet Med.* 2019;21(9):1931-1939.

46. Jewish Genetic Disease Consortium. *JGDC Launches Rabbi Education Program.* 2019. Accessed November 3, 2019. https://www.jewishgenetic-diseases.org/jgdc-launches-rabbi-education-program-couples-aware/

47. Petterson SM, Bazemore AW, Phillips RL, Rayburn WF. Trends in office-based care for reproductive-aged women according to physician specialty: a ten-year study. *J Womens Health (Larchmt).* 2014;23(12):1021-1026.

48. American College of Obstetricians and Gynecologists Committee on Genetics. Committee Opinion No. 478: family history as a risk assessment tool. *Obstet Gynecol.* 2011;117(3):747-750.

49. American College of Obstetricians and Gynecologists Committee on Genetics. ACOG Committee Opinion No. 486: update on carrier screening for cystic fibrosis. *Obstet Gynecol.* 2011;117(4):1028-1031.

50. American College of Obstetricians and Gynecologists Committee on Genetics. ACOG Committee Opinion No. 442: preconception and prenatal carrier screening for genetic diseases in individuals of Eastern European Jewish descent. *Obstet Gynecol.* 2009;114(4):950-953.

51. Hoskovec JM, Bennett RL, Carey ME, et al. Projecting the supply and demand for certified genetic counselors: a workforce study. *J Genet Couns.* 2018;27(1):16-20.

52. Darcy D, Tian L, Taylor J, Schrijver I. Cystic fibrosis carrier screening in obstetric clinical practice: knowledge, practices, and barriers, a decade after publication of screening guidelines. *Genet Test Mol Biomarkers.* 2011;15(7-8):517-523.

53. Arjunan A, Ben-Shachar R, Kostialik J, et al. Technology-driven noninvasive prenatal screening results disclosure and management. *Telemed J E Health.* 2020;26(1):8-17.

54. Lewis C, Skirton H, Jones R. Can we make assumptions about the psychosocial impact of living as a carrier, based on studies assessing the effects of carrier testing? *J Genet Couns.* 2011;20(1):80-97.

55. Hoffman JD, Greger V, Strovel ET, et al. Next-generation DNA sequencing of HEXA: a step in the right direction for carrier screening. *Mol Genet Genomic Med.* 2013;1(4):260-268.

56. Cecchi AC, Vengoechea ES, Kaseniit KE, et al. Screening for Tay-Sachs disease carriers by full-exon sequencing with novel variant interpretation outperforms enzyme testing in a pan-ethnic cohort. *Mol Genet Genomic Med.* 2019;7(8):1-12.

57. He J, Song W, Yang J, et al. Next-generation sequencing improves thalassemia carrier screening among premarital adults in a high prevalence population: the Dai nationality, China. *Genet Med.* 2017;19(9):1022-1031.

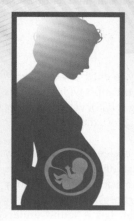

Preimplantation Genetic Diagnosis in Assisted Reproductive Technology

Nanette Santoro, Thanh Ha Luu, and Liesl Nel-Themaat

History of Preimplantation Genetic Testing

Although the first clinical utilization of preimplantation genetic testing (PGT) was published in 1990,[1] the idea was first presented in 1937.[2] It is widely believed that it was Dr John Rock who became known for the first experiments in human *in vitro* fertilization (IVF) during the mid-1940s,[3] who proposed in an unauthored editorial in the *New England Journal of Medicine* that one day parents may have children "according to specification."[2] To grasp how prescient this thinking was, one has to consider that, at the time of this prediction, the structure of DNA was not to be published for another 16 years,[4] DNA sequencing[5] and the first human IVF birth[6] would be reported more than 40 years later, and the polymerase chain reaction (PCR)[7] and fluorescent *in situ* hybridization (FISH)[8] were only to be discovered about 50 years afterward. Both these technologies were instrumental in the evolution of PGT as we know it today.

With significant success in mammalian embryo culture procedures during the second half of the 20th century, ancillary embryo technologies started emerging, including embryo biopsy and fluorescent staining techniques, which were used in the first sexing of preimplantation embryos by Robert Edwards and Richard Gardner in 1967.[9] Rabbit blastocysts produced *in vivo* were biopsied and the trophectoderm assessed for sex chromatin using fluorescent microscopy. The sex of resultant fetuses correlated with the determined sex of the biopsied embryos, confirming the effectiveness of the procedure. A few years later, Whittingham et al reported the first live birth from frozen-thawed embryos in mice,[10] followed by the first human pregnancy from frozen-thawed embryo transfer in 1983.[11] This discovery became especially significant in the 21st century when off-site reference laboratories started doing the majority of genetic testing for clinical laboratories, necessitating cryopreservation of embryos until results became available, after which the appropriate embryos could be thawed and transferred.

Around the same time, Angell et al started analyzing the chromosomes of cleavage-stage human embryos using classic cytology fixation and staining techniques. The authors found evidence of nondisjunction, resulting in an array of chromosomal aberrations in individual blastomeres.[12,13] One of the observations from these experiments was a lack of morphological correlations between euploid and aneuploid embryos, which further highlighted the need for developing an effective selection method based on ploidy. In 1987, an expert meeting held at the Ciba Foundation concluded that collaborative research would be essential to develop PGT as a clinical management alternative to abortion of genetically abnormal fetuses following prenatal testing.[14]

The remainder of the century saw numerous advancements, including the discovery that embryonic genome activation in humans occurs between the 4- and 8-cell stage,[15] the development

See the eBook for case examples.

of cleavage-stage biopsy techniques,[16,17] the first true PGT for a specific mutation in the mouse model,[18] and development of the polar body biopsy technique.[19] The first reported human pregnancies following embryo sex selection were in 1990, when cleavage-stage single blastomeres were sexed using PCR to amplify the DNA of the Y chromosome in patients with X-linked defects.[1] Transfer of embryos deselected for the Y chromosome resulted in female-only pregnancies. Shortly after, normal births following screening of embryos for cystic fibrosis were published[20] using similar techniques. Identification of specific diseases by genetic testing was subsequently coined PGD, for preimplantation diagnosis. Today it is known as preimplantation genetic testing for monogenic gene disorders (PGT-M).

Toward the turn of the millennium, improved embryo culture systems allowed blastocyst culture[21] and trophectoderm biopsy. Human blastocyst biopsy was shown to be a safe alternative to cleavage-stage biopsy, causing IVF programs to switch over.[22] Trophectoderm biopsy allows for a larger sample of cells and is, thus, more representative of the entire embryo, thereby circumventing many concerns raised regarding cleavage-stage biopsy (for review, see references 23-25).

On the molecular genetics side, new technologies continued to provide faster and more accurate diagnoses. In 1994, Munne et al described successful FISH analysis for selection of embryos based on the chromosomes X, Y, 13, 18, and 21.[26,27] Many clinical IVF laboratories thus started routinely performing FISH for what was subsequently called preimplantation genetic screening and today is known as preimplantation genetic testing for aneuploidy (PGT-A). FISH PGT, however, has several key drawbacks: it requires cleavage-stage blastomere biopsy, it is a highly technical procedure, and it can only provide information on a limited number of chromosomes. Whole genome amplification of single blastomeres[28] paired with DNA array–based comparative genomic hybridization[29] and single-nucleotide polymorphism (SNP) microarray[30] soon became the standard testing platforms, each with its unique benefits and drawbacks (see Testing Platforms section and **Table 16.1**). Scientists continued their pursuit of a more accurate, higher resolution platform, and in 2012, Treff et al published development of a quantitative real-time PCR method for identifying aneuploidy in blastocysts.

The most recent technology to enter the PGT market (and quickly becoming the most widely used) is next-generation sequencing (NGS), which provides the highest resolution and most diagnostic power currently available.[31]

The use of PGT in IVF cycles has been steadily increasing to include almost 40% of all IVF cycles reported to the Society for Reproductive Technology (SART) in 2017 (www.sart.org). Therefore, it is imperative that the clinician has a sound understanding of the available options to best serve their patients' genetic testing needs. PGT-A is more broadly utilized to optimize pregnancy outcomes with single-embryo transfers, in cases of advanced maternal age or recurrent implantation failure. PGT-A will also provide sex chromosome information and, thus, can be used for gender selection for disease risk stratification or family balancing goals.

This selection then permits the transfer of a single embryo, a strategy that has contributed to the declining rate of triplet pregnancies due to assisted reproductive technology (ART) in the United States.[32]

Testing Platforms

Most PGT is currently performed on blastocysts using NGS. However, there are still some indications for and some laboratories that utilize older, established technologies. For example, NGS could be used in combination with SNP array to determine parental origin of aneuploidies while also detecting de novo mutations. In addition, the sensitivity and specificity vary, depending on the technology platform used. With NGS, reported sensitivity for detecting aneuploidy is 100% and specificity is 99.98%.[33] Currently, most platforms will report results as euploid, mosaic, or aneuploid. There is no commercially available option to screen for mitochondrial DNA diseases. Follow-up prenatal genetic testing is recommended for all IVF patients because sampling only a few cells within an embryo is never a perfect reflection of the entire embryo (**Figure 16.1**).

Preimplantation Genetic Testing for Monogenic Disorders

Preimplantation genetic diagnosis, now called PGT-M, can be utilized for known single-gene disorders. Specific mutations known to the couple and family for common diseases, such as cystic fibrosis, spinal muscular atrophy, thalassemia, and sickle

Table 16.1 Comparison of Preimplantation Genetic Diagnosis Techniques

Indication	Mostly Cleavage-Stage Biopsy		Blastocyst-Stage Biopsy			
	Single-Cell PCR	FISH	SNP Array	Array CGH	qPCR	NGS
Sex selection		x	x	x	x	x
Monogenic disorders	x		Lab dependent[a]		x	Not developed[a]
De novo mutations						Not developed[a]
Structural abnormalities	Unbalanced only	Unbalanced only		Unbalanced only		Unbalanced only
Aneuploidy		x	x	x	x	x
Triploidy		x	x	Only if XXY or XYY	x	Only if XXY or XYY
Mosaicism			x	x		x
Uniparental disomy			x			
Mitochondria copy number					Lab dependent	x
Parental origin of abnormalities			x			
Main advantages	Detects monogenic diseases from single cells	Detects telomeric or subtelomeric translocation	Allows parental origin of aneuploidy identification	Short turnaround time	Short turnaround time	Parallel sequencing up to 96 samples due to unique barcoding system in single sequencing run
Main limitations	Higher rate of allele dropout than other technologies due to single cell	Only limited chromosomes can be analyzed due to limited probe colors and subjective results depend on analyst	Requires parental support	Labor-intensive, expensive	Very low resolution due to number of probes that are utilized	Unable to detect XXX, UPD, and haploidy
Haploidy			x			

CGH, comparative genomic hybridization; FISH, fluorescent *in situ* hybridization; NGS, next-generation sequencing; PCR, polymerase chain reaction; qPCR, quantitative polymerase chain reaction; SNP, single-nucleotide polymorphism; UPD, uniparental disomy.

[a]It is important to note that different genetics laboratories may use different variations of the same technology platform. In this table, the indicated capabilities are based on what is true in most laboratories. Testing for some of the indications using a specific platform may not have been developed in all laboratories that utilize that technology.

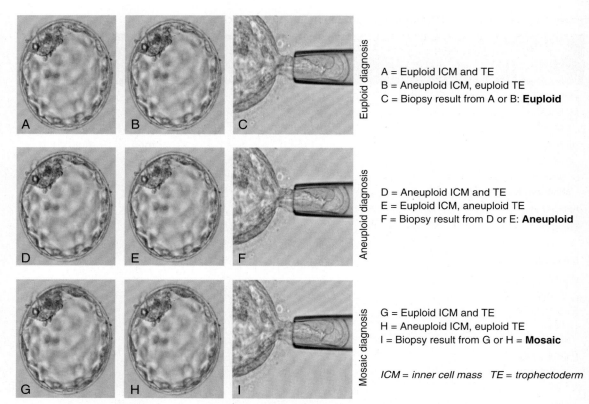

Figure 16.1 Challenges in trophectoderm sampling. Three possible scenarios are shown. Euploid cells within the blastocyst are shown in green and aneuploid cells in red. In panels **A-C**, the embryo would be diagnosed as euploid in both cases, despite the fact that the inner cell mass, destined to become the fetus, is aneuploid in **(B)**. In panels **D-F**, aneuploidy would be diagnosed based on the trophectoderm biopsy, although the inner cell mass is euploid in **(E)**. In panels **G-I**, mosaicism would be diagnosed based on the trophectoderm, although the inner cell mass in case **(G)** is truly mosaic and the inner cell mass in **(H)** is euploid.

cell anemia, can be identified for each embryo, including carrier status. In addition to couples who have already conceived or borne an affected child, more disorders are being detected through widespread antenatal carrier screening, and many couples choose PGT-M to avoid an affected pregnancy.

Testing for adult-onset genetic disease, such as Huntington disease, can also be offered, even in cases when the couple does not want to know their own status but would like to select against an affected embryo.

There are two types of nondisclosure testing, indirect and direct nondisclosure. In indirect nondisclosure, testing is done by linking parental chromosome inheritance patterns rather than probing for the specific mutation of the at-risk individual. Reporting of the results will allow for embryo selection against the inheritance pattern of interest without revealing parental genetic information. In direct nondisclosure testing, the mutation of interest will be sequenced and used to direct embryo transfer recommendations but will not be revealed to the individual. In cases where a couple has a known chromosomal rearrangement, PGT for structural rearrangement can be performed to screen for chromosomal inversions, reciprocal translocations, and Robertsonian translocations to enhance the chance of selecting an unaffected embryo (see Chapter 11).

Clinical Management Issues in Preimplantation Diagnosis

The rapid introduction of preimplantation diagnostic techniques into ART practice has led to a number of areas of uncertainty. Clinical interpretation of results and patient clarity are important goals. It is all the more challenging to have effective dialogues with individuals or couples with infertility because the field and its nomenclature are evolving over time, findings of individual studies are often publicized well before they have achieved an acceptable level of evidence to change practice, and patient expectations of the technology often exceed its ability. What follows are some common clinical scenarios that lead to management dilemmas.

Low Embryo Yields

There is a progressive increase in the proportion of aneuploid embryos with maternal age (**Figure 16.2**)[34]; however, there is large interindividual variation. Therefore, although the a priori odds of embryo aneuploidy can be estimated with reasonable certainty, an individual couple may wind up with unexpected disappointing results. Excess aneuploidy appears to be overwhelmingly related to meiotic errors, especially maternal nondisjunction or failure of chromosomes to separate properly during cell division, which increases with age while aneuploidy due to chromosomal gain or loss occurs in both male and female gametes.[35] Laboratory variation in aneuploidy rates suggests that embryo culture conditions may also contribute to risk of aneuploidy due to mitotic errors after fertilization.[36] Oocyte mitochondrial endowment has been hypothesized to relate to nondisjunction because of the association between reduced oocyte mitochondria, increased aneuploidy, and older reproductive age.[37] Furthermore, couples with a prior history of recurrent miscarriage and those with prior implantation failure are more likely to have a greater than expected proportion of aneuploid embryos.[38] Thus, couples with one or both partners of advanced reproductive age, as well as those with prolonged infertility and/or recurrent miscarriages, are at greater risk of having low embryo yields during an attempted PGT cycle. For such couples, controversy exists about laboratory designation of aneuploidy, and there is uncertainty about what exactly constitutes a good enough embryo suitable for implantation.

Embryo Mosaicism

Chromosomal mosaicism has been known to occur in human embryos for many years.[39] However, the natural history of mosaicism remains poorly understood because there is no noninvasive way of assessing chromosomes in growing embryos.

Mosaic embryos have a lower ongoing pregnancy rate (39.2% vs 63.3%) and higher miscarriage rate (24.3% vs 10.2%).[40] Nonetheless, pregnancy potential remains significant for mosaic embryos. Currently, there are limited data regarding live birth outcomes following mosaic embryo transfers, but standard IVF practice in the era preceding PGT involved the routine transfer of such embryos. Therefore, it appears that mosaic embryos are more likely to result in early miscarriage and not to result in the birth of affected children.

Because aneuploid cells may divide slower than euploid cells or enter apoptosis (programmed cell death), it is also likely that mosaic embryos undergo some degree of "self-correction" over time, thus minimizing the proportion of aneuploid cells and consequently mitigating the phenotype. There is some evidence that this process occurs *in vitro* to a significant degree.[41] There is also the possibility that the trophectoderm undergoing biopsy is chromosomally abnormal but that the inner cellular mass that will give rise to the fetus is normal, leading to a false-positive PGT diagnosis due to the inability to sample all cells (**Figure 16.1**). These two possibilities raise the concern that PGT leads to the disposal of significant numbers of embryos identified as aneuploids that have the potential to result in a healthy child if they were transferred.[42,43] Attention has also recently turned toward transferring embryos with low levels of mosaicism, defined as aneuploidy in 20% to 40% of cells biopsied.[40] However, some programs do not recommend transferring mosaic embryos.[44] High-level mosaic embryos, defined by some platforms as aneuploidy in 40% to 80% of cells biopsied, are generally not recommended for transfer by most IVF programs, but the practice of transferring low-level mosaic embryos is emerging. Additionally, the affected chromosome should be considered. Mosaic embryos with abnormalities involving high-risk chromosomes (ie, 13, 14, 16, 18, 21, X, and Y) should be avoided due to higher rates of uniparental disomy, fetal involvement, miscarriage, and viable aneuploidy.[45] Future improvements in methodology may allow for better selection of mosaic embryos for transfer, as the exact karyotypic anomaly may predict the likelihood of successful implantation.

No Results

Embryos that undergo biopsy but with insufficient DNA content or quality to obtain a result present a

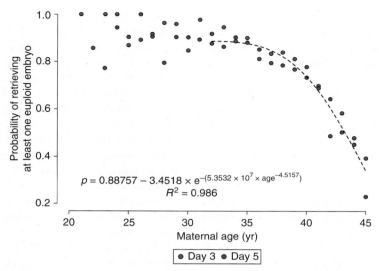

Figure 16.2 Probability of retrieving at least one euploid embryo in a cohort of embryos from women aged 21 to 45 years. For both day 3 and day 5 embryos, the probability of there being at least one euploid embryo was relatively high in women <35 years old, but it decreased rapidly in older women. After the age of 32, this decline is modeled by an exponential curve ($R^2 = 0.986$; dotted black curve). Note that this curve was fit to data from both day 3 and day 5 embryos.

(Reprinted from Demko ZP, Simon AL, McCoy RC, Petrov DA, Rabinowitz M. Effects of maternal age on euploidy rates in a large cohort of embryos analyzed with 24-chromosome single-nucleotide polymorphism-based preimplantation genetic screening. *Fertil Steril*. 2016;105(5):1307-1313.)

particular conundrum for patients. Despite excellent evolution of technique and high rates of embryo survival, embryo biopsy is invasive and exposes the embryo to some degree of compromise, although the exact viability cost of this process is not well quantitated.[46] Subjecting an embryo to a second thaw and biopsy is likely to further reduce its viability regardless of the skill of the laboratory. Reasons for failure to yield an interpretable signal have been linked to DNA amplification failure or poor signal-to-noise ratio preventing accurate interpretation of the results.[47] In addition, due to the high level of technicality, failure of appropriately loading the biopsy into the testing buffer can result in no DNA detection. Embryos with no result can be considered for a rebiopsy, which will usually yield a definitive result.

Costs of PGT

Single-site studies indicate that time to pregnancy is faster with PGT-A in all couples because transfer of noneuploid embryos is avoided.[48] Miscarriage rates also appear to be substantially lower when euploid embryos are selected for transfer.[48] Although this is an overall logical approach, it is not clear whether PGT-A for all is cost-effective.[42,49] The procedure

adds approximately $5000 to $10,000 to the cost of an IVF cycle, depending upon the number of embryos biopsied and local laboratory costs. Therefore, for couples at low risk for aneuploidy, it remains to be determined whether genetic screening of embryos is overall worthwhile, despite its great intellectual appeal. When embryos are scarce, as is the case in women with reduced ovarian reserve, there is evidence that PGT-A can lead to worse outcomes because laboratory diagnosis tends to overestimate the risk of abnormality, thereby eliminating available embryos for transfer that might result in healthy babies.[49] However, the field is evolving very rapidly. Improved technology, use of the trophectoderm biopsy, and the adoption of high-throughput genetic analysis techniques that are less expensive may all bring the costs down to a low enough level to make PGT-A cost-effective for most couples.

Risks to the Fetus and Baby

Because PGT-A involves sampling of trophectoderm, it is reducing the number of placental progenitor cells. Therefore, harm, should it exist, would be expected to occur in placental mass and/or function. When biopsies are carried out on day

5, a relatively small amount of total embryonic tissue (typically between 3 and 10 cells) is removed, and gross outcomes, such as live birth and miscarriage rates, do not appear to be increased.[50] When compared to double-embryo transfer of untested embryos, the reduction of twinning when single-euploid embryos are transferred results in a dramatic reduction in low birth weight, preterm birth, and neonatal intensive care unit admissions.[51] However, more subtle pregnancy outcomes have not been well studied and, as the current standard of care in IVF is evolving to single-embryo transfer for most patients, more data are needed to fully understand the consequences of embryo manipulation and trophectoderm biopsy.

Ethical Conundrums

As with many reproductive technologies, application in certain settings can raise serious ethical concerns. PGT is no exception to this rule. Sex selection of embryos is possible with PGT-A. Sex selection may be used for strictly medical indications, such as to avoid X-linked diseases, and most organizations sanction this use of sex selection. On the other end of the spectrum, couples may request PGT for sex selection for the purpose of family balancing or other nonmedical reasons. The American Society for Reproductive Medicine has evolved in its assessment of this issue, from initially weighing against it to its most recent 2015 Ethics Committee position, which states that "practitioners offering assisted reproductive services are under no ethical obligation to provide or refuse to provide non-medically indicated methods of sex selection" and further recommends that clinics have clear and unambiguous policies and procedures for nonmedical sex selection and that all involved staff are in agreement with these policies.[52] Weighing the costs, risks, and unknown future consequences of PGT, many societies and individual clinics will limit the application of PGT for this use. However, there are numerous scenarios that are intermediate between the two aforementioned ones that require ethical consideration. What if the sex-linked disease is not life-threatening (eg, color blindness)? What if the couple is undergoing PGT-A as part of an IVF cycle and express a preference for a girl or a boy?

Ethical issues are also raised when couples may choose to reproduce to create a child who can be an organ donor for an existing child with a serious illness. Creation of embryos that are human leukocyte antigen–matched to an existing child with a serious illness is a highly controversial issue, colloquially called savior siblings.[53] This issue has captured the public imagination through books and movies such as the novel *Never Let Me Go* or the film *My Sister's Keeper*.

Finally, with the advent of comprehensive genomic screening, couples may wish to select the genetics of their offspring to attempt to create an optimal phenotype. The concept that genotype equals phenotype is widely accepted in the nonmedical community, and this topic has also been adapted into a popular movie, *Gattaca*, named after the genetic code. In the movie, society provides access to power and success only to those who constitute the genetically elite. However, the phenotype of an individual is modified by many factors apart from genetic complement, such as gene penetrance and epigenetic alterations due to environmental factors, and it is generally hazardous to try to forecast the health of the offspring based on the genetics. In addition, thanks to the discovery of precise genome modification by taking advantage of clustered regularly interspaced short palindromic repeats (CRISPR) and CRISPR-associated protein 9, an endonuclease known as Cas9, it is now possible to guide the Cas9 endonuclease to a specific target gene and cause a break in the double-stranded DNA, allowing modifications to the genome. CRISPR/Cas9 technology thereby has the potential to correct genetic errors identified by PGT-M. Use of this technology of course introduces many additional ethical concerns, which are well beyond the scope of this chapter.

Future Directions

PGT as we know it had an incredibly swift invention-to-consumer transition compared to many other services offered in IVF clinics today. For example, it took many years for the majority of laboratories to switch from slow freezing to vitrification, despite the now-obvious advantages of vitrification (for review, see reference 54). The rapid implementation of PGT can be attributed to the highly competitive nature of the field of ART and the strong desire of patients with infertility or recurrent pregnancy loss to have access to any and all potential technological improvements. Unlike most medical practices, IVF clinics generate hard data showing success rates, which are often compared directly across clinics, even though this is not an appropriate practice because it fails to take into account the details of the patient populations at each clinic. Success is usually measured in clinical pregnancy or live birth rates, and these data are heavily used in marketing. In the absence of regulation of newly introduced procedures and technologies, pioneering clinics may initially benefit from increased success rates, but competitors soon follow suit, leveling the playing field. This can make it challenging for clinics to stay "ahead of the crowd." Although such practices often lead to true innovation, they can also introduce costly but ineffective methodologies.

After the first successful PGT reports, several genetic reference laboratories started offering their services to fertility clinics, making it easy to enroll in testing programs. On the IVF laboratory side, most of the equipment already existed for day 3 cleavage-stage embryo biopsies due to the rapid implementation of intracytoplasmic sperm injection in most laboratories after report of the first live human births in 1992.[55] It was thus an easy transition to start offering genetic testing of cleavage-stage embryos. Then, once day 5 blastocyst biopsies were shown to be superior, most laboratories already had the micromanipulation systems as well as the workflow implemented and only needed to add a laser (an optional piece of equipment for blastocyst biopsies) for routine trophectoderm biopsy. This ease of implementation, paired with aggressive marketing by the genetic companies, ensured rapid adoption of routine PGT for all patients in many clinics.

However, the question about the appropriateness of the test-all approach has come under scrutiny with reports of healthy live births from embryos initially diagnosed as mosaic aneuploid.[56] The procedure for blastocyst biopsy is very labor-intensive, requiring increased staff levels in IVF laboratories, and in most cases, PGT requires freezing all embryos until results are available, resulting in an increased need for cryostorage of embryos. There are also risks to the embryos when performing biopsies due to the highly technical nature of the procedure. Therefore, scientists have been exploring alternative modes of assessing the genetic composition of embryos without the need of mechanical disturbance of the embryos.

Palini et al demonstrated that DNA could be isolated from blastocoel fluid and used for whole genome amplification via PCR as well as microarray comparative genomic hybridization.[57] Subsequently, DNA amplified from blastocoel fluid was analyzed by NGS.[58] In addition, the use of spent embryo culture medium for DNA analysis was investigated as an alternative to embryo biopsy for PGT.[59] To date, most data show poor concordance between noninvasive DNA sources and trophectoderm genetic composition, with high amplification failure and low diagnostic accuracy. Thus, the current consensus is that neither spent culture medium nor blastocoel fluid is a reliable source of representative DNA for PGT and should not be offered in a clinical setting.[60] Nongenomic properties that potentially affect viability of embryos after implantation are also under investigation such as modes of cleavage via live imaging; mitochondrial DNA load; and composition, metabolomics, proteomics, and epigenetics. Although the efficiency of most of these technologies is yet to be demonstrated in a clinical setting, they may have the potential to be used complementary to PGT to further aid in selection of the highest potential embryos for transfer in the future.

Ethical debate continues about the wisdom of using PGD and combining it with newer capabilities, such as genome editing, in the evolution of patient care.

Acknowledgment

The authors would like to thank Dr. Cengiz Cinnioglu for critical review of parts of this chapter.

KEY POINTS

- Preimplantation genetic diagnosis has revolutionized the practice of IVF by allowing genetic testing and prescreening of embryos before they ever establish a viable pregnancy.
- Technology has evolved from sampling embryos at the cleavage stage to current methods that involve trophectoderm biopsy to detect common aneuploidies as well as to screen for specific genetic mutations.
- Sampling errors in the detection of embryo abnormalities and sensitivity and specificity of the various PGD modalities in varying patient populations remain the topic of active investigation and are needed to guide its clinical use.

REFERENCES

1. Handyside AH, Kontogianni EH, Hardy K, Winston RML. Pregnancies from biopsied human preimplantation embryos sexed by Y-specific DNA amplification. *Nature.* 1990;344(6268):768-770.
2. Conception in a watch glass. *N Eng J Med.* 1937:678.
3. Rock J, Menkin MF. In vitro fertilization and cleavage of human ovarian eggs. *Science.* 1944;100(2588):105-107.
4. Watson JD, Crick FH. Molecular structure of nucleic acids; a structure for deoxyribose nucleic acid. *Nature.* 1953;171(4356):737-738.
5. Sanger F, Air GM, Barrell BG. Nucleotide sequence of bacteriophage phi X174 DNA. *Nature.* 1977;265(5596):687-695.
6. Steptoe PC, Edwards RG. Birth after the reimplantation of a human embryo. *Lancet.* 1978;2(8085):366.
7. Bartlett JM, Stirling D. A short history of the polymerase chain reaction. *Methods Mol Biol.* 2003;226:3-6.
8. Langer-Safer PR, Levine M, Ward DC. Immunological method for mapping genes on Drosophila polytene chromosomes. *Proc Natl Acad Sci U S A.* 1982;79(14):4381-4385.
9. Edwards RG, Gardner RL. Sexing of live rabbit blastocysts. *Nature.* 1967;214(5088):576-577.
10. Whittingham DG, Leibo SP, Mazur P. Survival of mouse embryos frozen to −196 degrees and −269 degrees C. *Science.* 1972;178(4059):411-414.
11. Trounson A, Mohr L. Human pregnancy following cryopreservation, thawing and transfer of an eight-cell embryo. *Nature.* 1983;305(5936):707-709.
12. Angell RR, Aitken RJ, van Look PFA, Lumsden MA, Templeton AA. Chromosome abnormalities in human embryos after in vitro fertilization. *Nature.* 1983;303(5915):336-338.
13. Angell RR, Templeton AA, Aitken RJ. Chromosome studies in human in vitro fertilization. *Hum Genet.* 1986;72(4):333-339.
14. Whittingham DG, Penketh R. Prenatal diagnosis in the human preimplantation period. Meeting held at the Ciba Foundation on the 13th November 1986. *Hum Reprod.* 1987;2(3):267-270.
15. Braude P, Bolton V, Moore S. Human gene expression first occurs between the four- and eight-cell stages of preimplantation development. *Nature.* 1988;332(6163):459-461.
16. Wilton LJ, Shaw JM, Trounson AO. Successful single-cell biopsy and cryopreservation of preimplantation mouse embryos. *Fertil Steril.* 1989;51(3):513-517.
17. Wilton LJ, Trounson AO. Biopsy of preimplantation mouse embryos: development of micromanipulated embryos and proliferation of single blastomeres in vitro. *Biol Reprod.* 1989;40(1):145-152.
18. Monk M, Hardy K, Handyside A, Whittingham D. Preimplantation diagnosis of deficiency of hypoxanthine phosphoribosyl transferase in a mouse model for Lesch-Nyhan syndrome. *Lancet.* 1987;2(8556):423-425.
19. Verlinsky Y, Ginsberg N, Lifchez A, Valle J, Moise J, Strom CM. Analysis of the first polar body: preconception genetic diagnosis. *Hum Reprod.* 1990;5(7):826-829.
20. Handyside AH, Lesko JG, Tarín JJ, Winston RML, Hughes MR. Birth of a normal girl after in vitro fertilization and preimplantation diagnostic testing for cystic fibrosis. *N Engl J Med.* 1992;327(13):905-909.
21. Huisman GJ, Alberda AT, Leerentveld RA, Verhoeff A, Zeilmaker GH. A comparison of in vitro fertilization results after embryo transfer after 2, 3, and 4 days of embryo culture. *Fertil Steril.* 1994;61(5):970-971.
22. De Boer KA, Catt JW, Jansen RPS, Leigh D, McArthur S. Moving to blastocyst biopsy for preimplantation genetic diagnosis and single embryo transfer at sydney IVF. *Fertil Steril.* 2004;82(2):295-298.
23. De Vos A, Van Steirteghem A. Aspects of biopsy procedures prior to preimplantation genetic diagnosis. *Prenat Diagn.* 2001;21(9):767-780.
24. Scott KL, Hong KH, Scott RT Jr. Selecting the optimal time to perform biopsy for preimplantation genetic testing. *Fertil Steril.* 2013;100(3):608-614.
25. Xu K, Montag M. New perspectives on embryo biopsy: not how, but when and why? *Semin Reprod Med.* 2012;30(4):259-266.
26. Munne S, Lee A, Rosenwaks Z, Grifo J, Cohen J. Diagnosis of major chromosome aneuploidies in human preimplantation embryos. *Hum Reprod.* 1993;8(12):2185-2191.

27. Munne S, Weier HU, Stein J, Grifo J, Cohen J. A fast and efficient method for simultaneous X and Y in situ hybridization of human blastomeres. *J Assist Reprod Genet.* 1993;10(1):82-90.
28. Handyside AH, Robinson MD, Simpson RJ, et al. Isothermal whole genome amplification from single and small numbers of cells: a new era for preimplantation genetic diagnosis of inherited disease. *Mol Hum Reprod.* 2004;10(10):767-772.
29. Hu DG, Webb G, Hussey N. Aneuploidy detection in single cells using DNA array-based comparative genomic hybridization. *Mol Hum Reprod.* 2004;10(4):283-289.
30. Treff NR, Su J, Kasabwala N, Tao X, Miller KA, Scott RT. Robust embryo identification using first polar body single nucleotide polymorphism microarray-based DNA fingerprinting. *Fertil Steril.* 2010;93(7):2453-2455.
31. Zheng H, Jin H, Liu L, Liu J, Wang W-H. Application of next-generation sequencing for 24-chromosome aneuploidy screening of human preimplantation embryos. *Mol Cytogenet.* 2015;8:38.
32. Kulkarni AD, Jamieson DJ, Jones HW, et al. Fertility treatments and multiple births in the United States. *N Engl J Med.* 2013;369(23):2218-2225.
33. Fiorentino F, Biricik A, Bono S, et al. Development and validation of a next-generation sequencing–based protocol for 24-chromosome aneuploidy screening of embryos. *Fertil Steril.* 2014;101(5):1375-1382.e2.
34. Demko ZP, Simon AL, McCoy RC, Petrov DA, Rabinowitz M. Effects of maternal age on euploidy rates in a large cohort of embryos analyzed with 24-chromosome single-nucleotide polymorphism-based preimplantation genetic screening. *Fertil Steril.* 2016;105(5):1307-1313.
35. McCoy RC, Demko ZP, Ryan A, et al. Evidence of selection against complex mitotic-origin aneuploidy during preimplantation development. *PLoS Genet.* 2015;11(10):e1005601.
36. Munne S, Alikani M, Ribustello L, Colls P, Martínez-Ortiz PA, McCulloh DH. Euploidy rates in donor egg cycles significantly differ between fertility centers. *Hum Reprod.* 2017;32(4):743-749.
37. Zhang D, Keilty D, Zhang ZF, Chian RC. Mitochondria in oocyte aging: current understanding. *Facts Views Vis Obgyn.* 2017;9(1):29-38.
38. Kort JD, McCoy RC, Demko Z, Lathi RB. Are blastocyst aneuploidy rates different between fertile and infertile populations? *J Assist Reprod Genet.* 2018;35(3):403-408.
39. Munne S, Weier HUG, Grifo J, Cohen J. Chromosome mosaicism in human embryos. *Biol Reprod.* 1994;51(3):373-379.
40. Kushnir VA, Darmon SK, Barad DH, Gleicher N. Degree of mosaicism in trophectoderm does not predict pregnancy potential: a corrected analysis of pregnancy outcomes following transfer of mosaic embryos. *Reprod Biol Endocrinol.* 2018;16(1):6.
41. Munne S, Velilla E, Colls P, et al. Self-correction of chromosomally abnormal embryos in culture and implications for stem cell production. *Fertil Steril.* 2005;84(5):1328-1334.
42. Paulson RJ. Preimplantation genetic screening: what is the clinical efficiency? *Fertil Steril.* 2017;108(2):228-230.
43. Capalbo A, Ubaldi FM, Rienzi L, Scott R, Treff N. Detecting mosaicism in trophectoderm biopsies: current challenges and future possibilities. *Hum Reprod.* 2017;32(3):492-498.
44. Sachdev NM, Maxwell SM, Besser AG, Grifo JA. Diagnosis and clinical management of embryonic mosaicism. *Fertil Steril.* 2017;107(1):6-11.
45. Grati FR, Gallazzi G, Branca L, Maggi F, Simoni G, Yaron Y. An evidence-based scoring system for prioritizing mosaic aneuploid embryos following preimplantation genetic screening. *Reprod Biomed Online.* 2018;36(4):442-449.
46. Penzias A, Bendikson K, Butts S, et al. The use of preimplantation genetic testing for aneuploidy (PGT-A): a committee opinion. *Fertil Steril.* 2018;109(3):429-436.
47. Cimadomo D, Rienzi L, Romanelli V, et al. Inconclusive chromosomal assessment after blastocyst biopsy: prevalence, causative factors and outcomes after re-biopsy and re-vitrification. A multicenter experience. *Hum Reprod.* 2018;33(10):1839-1846.
48. Rubio C, Bellver J, Rodrigo L, et al. In vitro fertilization with preimplantation genetic diagnosis for aneuploidies in advanced maternal age: a randomized, controlled study. *Fertil Steril.* 2017;107(5):1122-1129.
49. Mastenbroek S, Twisk M, van der Veen F, Repping S. Preimplantation genetic screening: a systematic review and meta-analysis of RCTs. *Hum Reprod Update.* 2011;17(4):454-466.

50. McArthur SJ, Leigh D, Marshall JT, de Boer KA, Jansen RPS. Pregnancies and live births after trophectoderm biopsy and preimplantation genetic testing of human blastocysts. *Fertil Steril*. 2005;84(6):1628-1636.

51. Forman EJ, Hong KH, Franasiak JM, Scott RT Jr. Obstetrical and neonatal outcomes from the BEST Trial: single embryo transfer with aneuploidy screening improves outcomes after in vitro fertilization without compromising delivery rates. *Am J Obstet Gynecol*. 2014;210(2):157.e1-157.e6.

52. Ethics Committee of the American Society for Reproductive Medicine. Use of reproductive technology for sex selection for nonmedical reasons. *Fertil Steril*. 2015;103(6):1418-1422.

53. Wolf SM, Kahn JP, Wagner JE. Using preimplantation genetic diagnosis to create a stem cell donor: issues, guidelines & limits. *J Law Med Ethics*. 2003;31(3):327-339.

54. Nel-Themaat LC, Chang CC, Elliott T, Bernal DP, Wright G, Nagy ZP. Slow freezing of embryos. In: Nagy Z, ed. *In Vitro Fertilization*. Spinger Nature; 2019.

55. Palermo G, Joris H, Devroey P, Van Steirteghem AC, et al. Pregnancies after intracytoplasmic injection of single spermatozoon into an oocyte. *Lancet*. 1992;340(8810):17-18.

56. Greco E, Minasi MG, Fiorentino F. Healthy babies after intrauterine transfer of mosaic aneuploid blastocysts. *N Engl J Med*. 2015;373(21):2089-2090.

57. Palini S, Galluzzi L, De Stefani S, et al. Genomic DNA in human blastocoele fluid. *Reprod Biomed Online*. 2013;26(6):603-610.

58. Zhang Y, Li N, Wang L, et al. Molecular analysis of DNA in blastocoele fluid using next-generation sequencing. *J Assist Reprod Genet*. 2016;33(5):637-645.

59. Xu J, Fang R, Chen L, et al. Noninvasive chromosome screening of human embryos by genome sequencing of embryo culture medium for in vitro fertilization. *Proc Natl Acad Sci U S A*. 2016. 113(42):11907-11912.

60. Capalbo A, Romanelli V, Patassini C, et al. Diagnostic efficacy of blastocoel fluid and spent media as sources of DNA for preimplantation genetic testing in standard clinical conditions. *Fertil Steril*. 2018;110(5):870-879.e5.

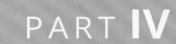

PART IV

Methods of Evaluation of Fetal Development and Well-being

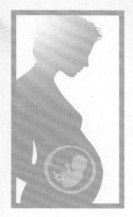

CHAPTER 17

Embryonic Development

Julie A. Rosen and E. Albert Reece

Summary

Please see the ebook chapter for a synopsis of the main events in normal human development, focusing on the embryonic period. The major developmental milestones, structures, and systems depicted in the ebook chapter include embryonic disk folding and formation of the pharyngeal apparatus, face, and palate and development of the respiratory, cardiovascular, urogenital, nervous, and musculoskeletal systems. The reader should consult the following references for a more detailed discussion of individual topics.

 See the ebook for the full chapter content, including animations and interactive images.

REFERENCES

1. Carlson BM. *Human Embryology and Developmental Biology*. 6th ed. Elsevier; 2019.
2. Drews U. *Color Atlas of Embryology*. Thieme Medical Publishers; 2018.
3. Cochard LR. *Netter's Atlas of Human Embryology*. W.B. Saunders; 2012.
4. Bhattacharya N, Stubblefield PG, eds. *Human Fetal Growth and Development: First and Second Trimesters*. Springer; 2016.
5. Schoenwolf GC, Bleyl SB, Brauer PR, Francis-West PH. *Larsen's Human Embryology*. 5th ed. Churchill Livingstone; 2014.
6. Moore KL, Persaud TVN, Torchia MG. *The Developing Human. Clinically Oriented Embryology*. 11th ed. W.B. Saunders; 2019.
7. Steding G. *The Anatomy of the Human Embryo: A Scanning Electron-Microscopic Atlas*. Karger; 2009.
8. Coward K, Wells D, eds. *Textbook of Clinical Embryology*. Cambridge University Press; 2013.
9. Slack JMW. *Essential Developmental Biology*. 3rd ed. Wiley-Blackwell; 2013.
10. Sadler TW. *Langman's Medical Embryology*. 14th ed. Wolters Kluwer; 2019.

CHAPTER 18

Prenatal Diagnosis of Deviant Fetal Growth

Jose R. Duncan and Anthony O. Odibo

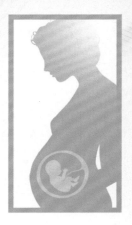

Introduction

This chapter includes discussion of the two extreme types of deviant fetal growth, growth restriction and macrosomia. We review the definition, prenatal diagnosis, associated complications, and antenatal management of both diagnoses, with the aim to provide an updated summary of the most relevant clinical aspects of these conditions.

Fetal Growth Restriction

Definition

Although the term fetal growth restriction (FGR) has been utilized interchangeably with small for gestational age (SGA), the latter refers to birthweight <10th percentile for gestational age (GA) and is not necessarily diagnosed *in utero*.[1] FGR describes a fetus that has failed to meet its growth potential, a criterion that is clinically difficult to establish due to multiple diagnostic criteria utilized to define FGR. Therefore, the true prevalence of FGR is hard to determine.

The American College of Obstetricians and Gynecologists (ACOG) defines FGR as an estimated fetal weight (EFW) less than the 10th percentile for GA. The ACOG also recognizes that utilizing this criterion has flaws, as some constitutionally small fetuses may be misdiagnosed.[2]

Other authors have proposed different diagnostic criteria such as EFW below the 5th percentile or <3rd percentile for the GA, abdominal circumference (AC) <10th percentile, whereas others have utilized some of the criteria mentioned above in addition to abnormal fetal and/or uterine Doppler parameters to decrease the number of false positives.[3-7] The Society for Maternal-Fetal Medicine (SMFM) recommends that FGR be defined as a sonographic EFW or AC below the 10th percentile for GA.[8] Further complicating the definition, most

of the initial studies on intrauterine growth restriction (IUGR) utilized neonatal weight in their criteria instead of fetal weight charts.[9,10]

Other investigators have proposed using the ponderal index, which is a measurement of neonatal nutritional status, a parameter not easily calculated before birth.[11] Studies have shown poor correlation with the ponderal index and FGR diagnosed based on the EFW, as well as with FGR diagnosed by the ponderal index and birthweight.[12] Regardless of the definition, fetuses with FGR are at greater risk for adverse outcomes and increased perinatal mortality.

The adverse perinatal outcomes associated with FGR include neonatal hypoglycemia, hypocalcemia, polycythemia, meconium aspiration, seizures, cerebral palsy, behavioral problems, cardiovascular disease, and perinatal mortality.[13-17] FGR also has long-term effects on these infants, including severe neurodevelopmental deficits and perinatal mortality, depending on GA at delivery, with most of these severe outcomes more common in pregnancies delivered before 32 weeks.[18-20]

Etiologies and Risk Factors

There are several potential causes of FGR. These etiologies can be divided into intrinsic and extrinsic factors (**Table 18.1**). The most common intrinsic causes include genetic disorders (aneuploidy or single-gene disorders),[21,22] structural malformations,[23-26] congenital infections,[27-29] and multiple gestations.[30,31] Placenta abnormalities can be grouped in the intrinsic factors category; however, they may behave similar to extrinsic factors like maternal chronic conditions that cause chronic placenta hypoperfusion.[32-34] Placenta previa and other uncommon placenta locations do not appear to be associated with FGR.[35,36] Extrinsic etiologies include

Table 18.1 Common Etiologies of Fetal Growth Restriction (FGR)

Intrinsic	Extrinsic	Idiopathic
Genetic abnormalities	Hypertensive disorders of pregnancy	Family history of FGR
• Aneuploidies • Trisomies (21,18,13) • Monosomy X • Single-gene disorders	• Chronic hypertension • Preeclampsia • Gestational hypertension	
Structural anomalies	Diabetes mellitus (DM)	
• Congenital heart defects • Gastrointestinal defects • Neural tube defects	• Type 1 DM • Type 2 DM • Gestational DM	
Perinatal infections	Other maternal conditions	
• Cytomegalovirus • Herpes simplex virus • Syphilis • Varicella-zoster virus • AIDS • Malaria	• Systemic lupus erythematosus • Moderate or severe asthma • Obstructive sleep apnea • Renal insufficiency • Inflammatory bowel disease	
Placenta abnormalities	Teratogens	
• Abnormal cord insertions • Chronic abruption • Circumvallate placenta	• Tobacco • Ethanol • Opioids • Cocaine	
Multiple gestations	Medications	
	• Antiepileptics • Warfarin • Chemotherapy drugs	
Metabolic conditions	High altitude	
	Malnourishment or poor maternal weight	

chronic maternal disorders such as hypertensive disorders of pregnancy or diabetes, poor maternal weight gain, and exposure to tobacco, illicit drugs, or teratogens.[37-47]

Despite all the risk factors and etiologies mentioned above, several cases of FGR do not have an identifiable cause and are labeled as idiopathic. However, some of these will be due to a family history of this condition, implying a possible genetic predisposition for this diagnosis.

Classification of IUGR

Historically, the most common classification for FGR included symmetric FGR or asymmetric FGR.[48] Symmetric FGR referred to fetuses with all biometry indices proportionally small. The insult for this group was thought to occur early in gestation and was associated with a worse prognosis. Asymmetric FGR included those fetuses with appropriate head biometry but smaller femur length (FL) and small AC. The insult was thought to occur primarily later in gestation (early third trimester).

Because GA is a critical prognostic factor for neonatal outcomes,[3,6] we favor a more simplistic classification: (1) early-onset FGR, when the diagnosis is made before 32 weeks of gestation; and (2) late-onset FGR, when the diagnosis is made ≥32 weeks of gestation.

Early-Onset FGR

Fetal growth can be restricted as early as in the first trimester as researchers have noted that those pregnancies with smaller-than-expected sized embryos or fetuses in the first trimester were more likely to deliver an SGA neonate.[49] FGR diagnosed during the second trimester (specifically, before 26 weeks) is most commonly associated with chromosomal abnormalities than that diagnosed in the third trimester.[50]

Perinatal infections are also an important etiology for early-onset FGR. Because infections and genetic syndromes may play a role, testing for these etiologies is recommended, especially when there are other clinical indications, such as maternal illness, structural anomalies, or when the diagnosis of FGR is made early in the second trimester. Evidence of placental dysfunction, as illustrated by abnormal umbilical artery (UA) Doppler, also appears more common with early-onset FGR.[51-53] In early-onset FGR, the

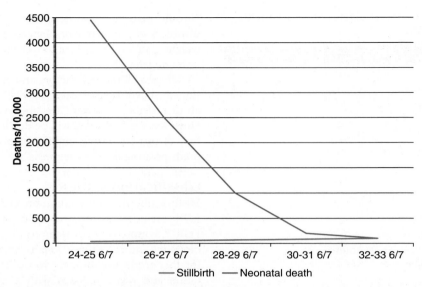

Figure 18.1 Risk of stillbirth and neonatal death for small for gestational age (SGA) pregnancies. The rise in the cumulative risk of stillbirth/10,000 ongoing SGA pregnancies from 24 to 33 6/7 weeks' gestation transposed over the fall in neonatal death/10,000 SGA live births.

(Reprinted with permission from Trudell AS, Tuuli MG, Cahill AG, Macones GA, Odibo AO. Balancing the risks of stillbirth and neonatal death in the early preterm small-for-gestational-age fetus. *Am J Obstet Gynecol.* 2014;211(3):295.e1-295.e7.)

perinatal mortality rate appears better when delivery is accomplished after 29 to 31 weeks[3,20,54,55] (**Figure 18.1**).

Late-Onset FGR
Most of the cases of FGR occur later in gestation, with the great majority (84.9%) being diagnosed at term.[56] A systematic review reported an 8% prevalence of SGA in the third trimester with a mean GA at diagnosis of 35.3 weeks.[57]

In late-onset FGR, the association with smoking is greater than in early-onset FGR. However, the association with preeclampsia, maternal chronic conditions such as hypertension and renal disease, and history of adverse obstetrical outcomes is weaker than in cases of early-onset FGR.[58] Despite these, the same etiologic factors seen more often in early-onset FGR (ie, chromosomal abnormalities, perinatal infections, preeclampsia) could also manifest later in gestation.[51,58,59]

Perhaps the most important difference between the two types of FGR is the different pattern of the vascular Doppler indices. For example, in the early-onset group, UA Doppler abnormalities are more frequent and pronounced, whereas in the late-onset group, most cases have normal UA Doppler waveforms.[51-53]

Diagnosis of FGR
To make an accurate diagnosis of FGR, it is fundamental to have a correct estimation of the GA. Ultrasonography has proven to be superior to the last menstrual period dating, as one-third to one-half of pregnant women cannot recall their last cycle accurately. The accuracy of ultrasound in estimating GA is inversely proportional to GA.[60-62] Although ultrasound is the best method to diagnose FGR, detection rates vary according to the ultrasound parameters and the GA at which the ultrasound is performed.

Once the GA is obtained, the next step is to identify those pregnancies at risk for FGR. Historically, this has been accomplished by measuring the distance (in centimeters) from the pubic symphysis to the fundus (fundal height measurement). However, the accuracy of this method is limited.[63] For the purpose of this chapter, the accuracy of detecting FGR will be defined as those pregnancies evaluated for suspected FGR by ultrasound who give birth to newborns with a birthweight <10th percentile for GA (SGA).

The crown-rump length (CRL) accurately predicts the GA up to 13 weeks and 6 days of gestation.[62] The CRL has been shown to help to identify FGR in the first trimester.[64] In the second and third trimester, FGR is diagnosed by obtaining the EFW, which is usually calculated utilizing multiple fetal biometry parameters, such as the head circumference (HC), biparietal diameter (BPD), the FL, and the AC.[65-68]

There has been some discussion about the best formula or weight chart to estimate the fetal weight. Some authors have proposed using customized EFW charts that adjust for maternal ethnicity and demographic characteristics versus population-based charts.[69-72] The argument for more diverse charts is based on studies where differences in fetal growth have been noted among different races and ethnicities.[73] One of these studies is the INTERGROWTH-21st study that was conducted in eight urban cities from different countries, where the authors developed fetal growth charts, EFW charts, and birthweight charts.[74-76] Despite this, diverse population-based intergrowth charts have failed to perform better than customized charts in detecting neonatal SGA.[77,78] Moreover, neither customized charts nor diverse population-based charts have been shown to be superior in identifying SGA babies with adverse neonatal outcomes compared with traditional methods such as the one reported by Hadlock et al.[79-83] Therefore, in our institution, we utilize the Hadlock method to calculate the EFW.[67,79]

Other Ultrasound Parameters

BPD and HC

The BPD and HC appear to be the best fetal ultrasound parameters to estimate GA in the second trimester and have been utilized to diagnose FGR in the past.[84,85] However, the detection of FGR utilizing a single measurement or serial measurements of the BPD has limited accuracy and should not be encouraged.

Transverse Cerebellar Diameter

Reece and colleagues evaluated the transverse cerebellar diameter (TCD) measurement in FGR.[86] They reported that the TCD measurement was not significantly affected by FGR, and therefore, the TCD could be used as a reliable predictor of GA in pregnancies complicated by FGR. However, Hill and colleagues reported that the TCD was more than two standard deviations below the mean in 60% of cases with FGR,[87] challenging prior results and questioning the utility of this measurement in the evaluation of pregnancies with FGR.

Femur Length

Like the BPD, the FL helps estimate the GA in the early second trimester, and an isolated short femur has been found to be an independent predictor of FGR.[88] However, the FL is inconsistently affected in FGR; therefore, it is an unreliable parameter to detect FGR on its own.

Abdominal Circumference

The AC has been reported to be the best fetal biometric parameter that correlates with fetal weight and is the most sensitive parameter for detecting IUGR.[89-91] Warsof and colleagues found that the AC measurements were more predictive of FGR than BPD or HC.[68] However, the authors used the 25th, rather than the 10th, percentile to increase the sensitivity of the AC as a screening test. Like the EFW, the accuracy in detecting FGR is influenced by the population screened and the GA at which the screening occurs.

AC Versus EFW. Overall the AC and the EFW both appear to have similar detection rates for SGA in the third trimester.[56,92] A study by Chauhan and collaborators found that neonates born from mothers with both EFW and AC <10th percentile had worse outcomes than those with AC <10th and EFW >10th percentile, or those with EFW <10th and AC >10th percentile.[93] However, because the majority of the research on this topic comes from studies that use the EFW, and because assessment of the EFW may be more important in early second trimester, we favor the utilization of the EFW calculation over the AC for the diagnosis of FGR.

Placental Grade

The accuracy of mature placenta grading in detecting FGR is limited, and more accurate methods should be used to identify this condition.[94,95]

Doppler in FGR

The most common fetal vessels used in the evaluation of FGR include the UA, middle cerebral artery (MCA),[6] and the ductus venosus (DV).[75] The uterine artery (UtA) has also been studied in FGR. Doppler resistance can be reported as an S/D ratio (systolic/diastolic ratio), resistance index (RI = systolic velocity − diastolic velocity/systolic velocity), and pulsatility index (PI = systolic velocity − diastolic velocity/mean velocity). In pregnancy, placental resistance declines with advancing

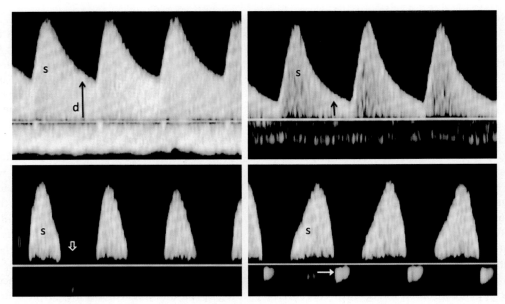

Figure 18.2 Umbilical artery Doppler (UAD) waveform patterns in fetal growth restriction. Long black arrow indicates a normal diastolic flow; short vertical black arrow indicates decreased diastolic flow in the UAD waveforms seen with increased resistance; the thick black arrow indicates absent diastolic flow in the UAD; the horizontal white arrow indicates reverse diastolic flow in the UAD. d, diastolic; s, systolic.

gestation, leading to an increased amount of forward diastolic flow in the UA and the UtA. With progressive uteroplacental insufficiency, there is elevated placental resistance leading to decreased forward diastolic flow, which can progress to absent or even reversed diastolic flow in the UA in severely affected fetuses (**Figure 18.2**).

The fetal MCA is typically a high impedance vessel with low end-diastolic velocity. In cases of progressive FGR, there appears to be preferential shunting of blood toward the brain and heart at the expense of visceral organs, resulting in a lower MCA pulsatility index (PI). This phenomenon is known as the "brain-sparing effect." Finally, evaluation of the fetal venous system is an indirect measure of fetal cardiac compliance. Doppler interrogation of the DV produces a triphasic waveform comprising S, D, and a-waves. The S and D waves occur with ventricular contraction and then passive diastolic filling, respectively. The a-wave is a reflection of ventricular filling, which occurs during atrial systole or "atrial kick." With worsening right ventricular dysfunction, the a-wave will be decreased or even reversed. This reflects decreased or reversed forward flow during atrial systole.

Uterine Artery

Campbell and collaborators were the first to report an increased resistance at the level of the uterine arteries in pregnancies complicated by FGR and preeclampsia.[96] Since then, most of the work has been concentrated on potential prediction or detection rates of the UtA Doppler waveforms for adverse outcomes, including FGR and SGA.

Resistance indices like the PI have been utilized more often; however, the presence of notching in the UtA waveforms have been shown to be an independent predictor of adverse outcomes.[97]

Abnormal UtA Doppler parameters, with or without the addition of biochemical markers, have been shown to be a significant predictor of poor fetal growth in all trimesters of pregnancy.[98-103] However, the clinical utility is limited due to a high false-positive rate (FPR) if performed early in gestation (60% detection rate and 11% FPR)[99] and/or a low detection rate if done in the third trimester (30% with a 10% FPR).[103] A recent survey of international experts recommends UtA Doppler waveform as an additive test to diagnose FGR; however, this parameter has been shown to add limited value to the EFW.[4] Others have promoted the UtA

Doppler assessment as a surveillance tool, as it seems that those with abnormal UtA waveforms are at increased risk to have abnormal MCA and abnormal cerebroplacental ratios (CPRs).[5]

Umbilical Artery

There is good evidence that the presence of abnormal UA Doppler studies in pregnancies with FGR is associated with increased rates of adverse outcomes, such as preeclampsia, respiratory distress syndrome, neonatal acidosis, lower GA at delivery, higher incidence of abnormal fetal surveillance testing, and perinatal mortality.[104-107] A 2013 Cochrane meta-analysis reported a 29% reduction in perinatal mortality in high-risk pregnancies where UA Doppler was included among surveillance options.[108]

An abnormal Doppler interrogation of the UA is described when there are indices suggesting increased resistance (ie, elevated PI, elevated resistive index, elevated systolic/diastolic ratio, absent end-diastolic flow, or reverse diastolic flow). The latter two have been associated with greater rates of acidemia and severe outcomes when compared with elevated indices.[109] However, even in the absence of UA Doppler abnormalities, those with pregnancies with FGR and SGA are at increased risks of adverse neonatal outcomes.[110] The assessment of the UA by Doppler waveforms has become part of the standard of care for the management of pregnancies complicated by FGR.

Middle Cerebral Artery

In normal pregnancies, the MCA follows a parabolic pattern with the resistance as demonstrated by the PI. At the beginning of gestation, the PI is low and then gradually increases followed by a decrease toward the end of gestation. In pregnancies with SGA, a low MCA-PI (<5th percentile for the GA) has been associated with increased incidence of abnormal fetal heart abnormalities, higher neonatal intensive care unit (NICU) admission, and perinatal mortality.[106,111]

Despite these associations, the clinical value of MCA measurement has been questioned because of the lack of evidence showing that this Doppler parameter improves outcomes.

Cerebroplacental Ratio

The CPR is calculated by dividing the MCA PI by the UA PI. A low CPR (less than 1.0 or below the 5th percentile for the GA) in pregnancies complicated by FGR has been associated with increased risks of adverse outcomes such as low Apgar scores, NICU admission, cesarean delivery for fetal distress, metabolic acidosis, and perinatal death.[112,113] There has been a recent international promotion of the MCA and CPR assessment for fetuses with FGR.[4,5] However, their utilization has not been endorsed in the United States due to the limited additive diagnostic value,[114] as well as the lack of clear interventions to reduce the perinatal outcomes associated with brain sparing (low MCA PI or low CPR).[2,115]

Ductus Venosus

Baschat et al[105] showed that growth-restricted fetuses with abnormal venous flow have a higher rate of adverse perinatal outcomes compared to those with Doppler abnormalities in only the UA or MCA. A systematic review and meta-analysis demonstrated a modest predictive ability of abnormal DV Doppler for the prediction of perinatal mortality with a positive likelihood ratio of 4.21 (95% CI 1.98-8.96) and a negative likelihood ratio of 0.43 (95% CI 0.30-0.61).[115] Most recently, the Trial of Umbilical and Fetal Flow in Europe (TRUFFLE)[18] was undertaken to evaluate the role of the DV Doppler assessment as an indication for delivery in preterm FGR. TRUFFLE randomized women with preterm FGR and elevated UA PI to one of three groups as a trigger for delivery: (1) reduced short-term variation on cardiotocography monitoring, (2) early DV changes of elevated PI, or (3) late DV changes of absent or reversed a-wave. They did not find a difference in their primary outcome of survival without neurodevelopmental impairment at the age of 2 years among the groups. There was a significant increase in intact survival for infants randomized to delivery on the basis of late DV changes compared to cardiotocography monitoring; however, this was at the expense of an increased, but nonsignificant, risk of mortality. Based on the available data, the role of the DV Doppler interrogation in the clinical management of the growth-restricted infant remains uncertain.[116,117]

Antenatal Surveillance

UA Doppler assessment is recommended to identify fetuses with FGR at greater risk for adverse outcomes. The nonstress test (NST) or the biophysical profile (BPP) has been used in pregnancies with FGR to further identify those at risk for fetal acidosis or hypoxia and to allow for intervention before deterioration of the fetal status.

Nonstress Test

There is limited evidence supporting NST as a surveillance tool in pregnancies with FGR. McCowan and colleagues[118] conducted a trial comparing a regimen of twice-weekly NST to fortnightly NST in women with SGA fetuses with normal UA Doppler studies. There was no difference in neonatal outcomes between the two groups; however, there was an increased incidence of induction of labor in the twice-weekly NST group. Despite the global utilization of this test, there are no other trials on the efficacy of the NST in reducing adverse outcomes in pregnancies with FGR.

Biophysical Profile and Amniotic Fluid Assessment

The BPP includes the evaluation of the amniotic fluid, fetal movement, fetal tone, and fetal breathing, with or without an NST. When normal, each parameter receives 2 points, for a maximum of 10 points.[119] The NST can be excluded, allowing a maximum score of 8/8.[120]

In a study that included FGR pregnancies, abnormal BPP scores have been associated with fetal acidosis.[121] However, the problem with the BPP, as well as with the NST, is the high FPR and lack of trials demonstrating its efficacy. For example, Kaur and collaborators studied the use of daily BPPs in preterm fetuses with severe FGR (<1000 g with abnormal UA Doppler indices). They reported high false-positive and false-negative rates and concluded that the BPP was not reliable in the evaluation of these pregnancies.[122]

Perhaps one of the most important components of the BPP is the assessment of the amniotic fluid, as investigators have documented that, in cases with FGR, the amniotic fluid index (AFI) progressively decreases.[53,123] In a meta-analysis[92] of pregnancies with FGR, an AFI <5 cm was associated with an increased risk for cesarean deliveries for fetal distress and low 5-minute Apgar scores. However, the authors did not find an association with fetal acidosis. Another retrospective study found that oligohydramnios was an independent risk factor for perinatal mortality in pregnancies with preterm FGR.[124]

Doppler Assessment With Antenatal Surveillance Testing

The optimal strategy of incorporating Doppler studies and tests of fetal well-being is still under investigation. Baschat et al[125] reported that both multivessel Doppler assessments and BPP evaluation can effectively risk-stratify growth-restricted fetuses; however, the Doppler results do not correlate with the BPP results consistently. In another study comparing NST, computerized fetal heart rate analysis, BPP, and arterial and venous Doppler, venous Doppler was found to be the most predictive of fetal acidemia, with a sensitivity of 73% and specificity of 90%.[126] In contrast, a decision analysis evaluated four strategies of antepartum FGR assessment, including Doppler + BPP, BPP only, Doppler only, and no testing. This model demonstrated that BPP was the best strategy to guide physicians on the timing of delivery in preterm growth-restricted fetuses.[127] Perhaps the different conclusions by these studies can be explained by the fact that the alteration in the fetal Doppler assessment in pregnancies with FGR does not follow a pattern, like previously suggested. This is specifically the case in circumstances with pregnancy-related hypertensive disorders and late-onset FGR.[51,128] The SMFM recommends that fetuses with FGR will undergo UA Doppler interrogation every 1 to 2 weeks with NST instead of BPP as the surveillance method.[8]

In conclusion, the optimal way to monitor pregnancies with FGR remains uncertain; therefore, perhaps an accepted approach is to identify those at greater risk (abnormal UA Doppler indices, especially in those with early FGR), followed by a protocol of BPP, NST, or both.

Optimal Time of Delivery in FGR

In pregnancies with FGR, GA is the most important factor determining perinatal survival as the survival rate at 26 weeks exceeds 50% and reaches 90% at 30 weeks of gestation.[3] The Growth Restriction Intervention Trial (GRIT) was a multicenter randomized controlled trial, which compared immediate delivery versus delayed delivery in pregnant women between 24 and 36 weeks' gestation in situations in which the obstetrician was uncertain as to whether to deliver based on current ultrasound and UA Doppler surveillance. There were more intrauterine fetal deaths in the delayed group but fewer neonatal deaths. There was no significant difference in infant survival to the time of hospital discharge between the two groups. On average, patients in the delayed delivery group remained pregnant for an additional 4 days.[129] At 2-year follow-up, the children showed no difference in mortality or severe disability between the two groups; severe disability was limited to the group of patients who were delivered in <31 weeks.[20] Most recently, long-term outcomes for a subset of patients from GRIT were published. These results demonstrated no clinically significant differences between the immediate and delayed delivery group at 9 to 13 years.[130]

In the Disproportionate Intrauterine Growth Intervention Trial at Term (DIGITAT),[20] women with singleton gestations ≥36 weeks with suspected FGR were randomized to undergo delivery or expectant management. The authors found no differences in composite neonatal outcome (death before hospital discharge, 5-minute Apgar score of less than 7, UA pH of less than 7.05, or admission to the intensive care unit) between these two groups, although the study cohort was not large enough to determine a difference in individual outcomes, such as perinatal death.

Based on study results, when there are no clear indications for delivery in the setting of FGR, the current accepted practice is to identify pregnancies with FGR and abnormal UA. Those with a normal UA can be monitored less closely, and if the UA Doppler waveforms remain normal, delivery can be deferred until 38 to 39 weeks (**Figure 18.3**)[131]. In cases where there is elevated UA PI or EFW <3rd percentile for GA, most institutions will increase surveillance with frequent UA Doppler assessment in conjunction of fetal surveillance testing (BPP or NST) and deliver at 37 weeks of gestation. Once the UA end-diastolic flow becomes absent (AEDF) or reversed (REDF), most maternal-fetal medicine services will admit these patients and initiate steroids to promote fetal lung maturity. If the UA Doppler waveforms show persistent REDF and the pregnancy has reached 32 weeks of gestation, some clinicians would suggest delivery in the case of REDF and most will not recommend extending the pregnancy beyond 34 weeks with AEDF, regardless of the BPP or NST result. If the UA PI remains persistently elevated, then delivery will be guided by the antenatal

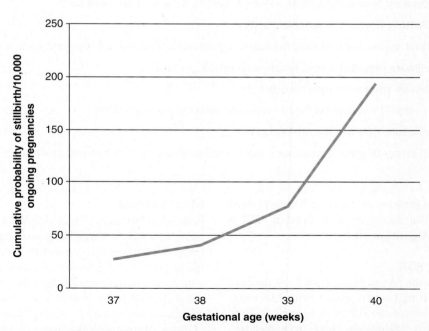

Figure 18.3 Cumulative probability of small for gestational age (SGA) stillbirths over time. This graph displays the rise in the stillbirth risk for the SGA fetus as pregnancy progresses beyond 37 weeks. The risk of stillbirth is reported as SGA stillbirths/10,000 ongoing SGA pregnancies (y-axis).

(Reprinted with permission from Trudell AS, Cahill AG, Tuuli MG, Macones GA, Odibo AO. Risk of stillbirth after 37 weeks in pregnancies complicated by small-for-gestational-age fetuses. *Am J Obstet Gynecol*. 2013;208(5):376.e1-7.)

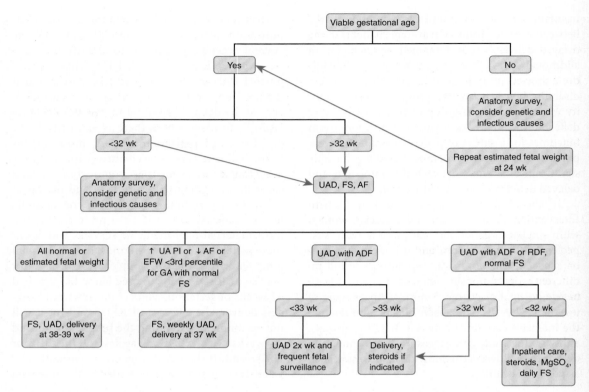

Algorithm 18.1 Management protocol for isolated fetal growth restriction. Fetal growth restriction is defined as estimated fetal weight (EFW) <10th percentile for gestational age (GA).

ADF, absent diastolic flow in the umbilical artery;

AF, amniotic fluid assessment, usually measured by amniotic fluid index or deepest vertical pocket;

FS, fetal surveillance (nonstress test, biophysical profile, or both);

MgSO$_4$, magnesium sulfate for neuroprotection;

PI, pulsatility index (PI = systolic velocity – diastolic velocity/mean velocity);

RDF, reverse diastolic flow in the umbilical artery;

UAD, umbilical artery Doppler assessment, performed primarily at 1 to 2 weeks' gestation.

testing chosen for fetal surveillance. Our proposed protocol for the management of isolated FGR is presented in **Algorithm 18.1**.

Preventing FGR

A 2017 systematic review reported that low doses of aspirin (50-150 mg), when started before 16 weeks of gestation, reduced the risk of developing FGR by more than 40%.[132] However, these were pregnancies considered at high risk based on abnormal UtA Doppler assessment. Because screening for FGR is not currently the standard practice, use of aspirin for the sole purpose of preventing FGR is not recommended.

Macrosomia

Fetal macrosomia has been defined as an EFW of >4500 g at term. Large for gestational age (LGA) refers to birthweight greater than the 90th percentile for GA.[133,134] Earlier in gestation, those fetuses with EFW >90th percentile for their respective GA are suspected to be macrosomic. Similar to FGR and SGA, the etiologies of fetal macrosomia and LGA are commonly unknown.

Risks factors for fetal macrosomia and LGA include preexisting maternal diabetes, uncontrolled gestational diabetes, maternal obesity, excessive gestational weight gain, prior macrosomic infant, postterm pregnancy, and maternal nonsmoking status (**Table 18.2**).[133-138] It has been reported that about 8% of all deliveries in the United States have birthweights ≥4000 g and about 1.1% have birthweights ≥4500 g.[139]

Neonatal and Maternal Outcomes of Macrosomia

Macrosomic infants and their mothers are at increased risk for certain complications. These include cesarean delivery, failed trial of labor, postpartum hemorrhage, and third-degree and fourth-degree lacerations for the mothers.[140-143] Infants are at risk for injuries from shoulder dystocia (brachial plexus injuries, clavicle fracture), admission to NICUs, low Apgar scores, and obesity and diabetes later in life.[143-145] A 2018 retrospective cohort reported an increased risk for fetal demise in pregnancies with suspected LGA.[146]

Diagnosis of Macrosomia

Fundal height measurement is not a good predictor of LGA.[145] However, clinical palpation appears to be as accurate as ultrasound in predicting fetal macrosomia.[147-149] Interestingly, parous women's estimation of fetal weight appears to be comparable to their physicians' clinical estimation of fetal macrosomia once gestation reaches over 41 weeks.[150] A prospective study[151] comparing maternal estimation of fetal weight with clinical estimation of fetal weight by residents, attending physicians, and ultrasound found that ultrasound was the most effective method to detect fetal macrosomia, followed by attending physicians' estimation, and that maternal estimation and resident estimation of fetal weight were identical.

However, ultrasound accuracy for the detection of fetal macrosomia is limited, and it appears that the EFW estimation is less accurate when the EFW is >4500 g.[152] Because the Hadlock et al[80] formula for

Table 18.2 Risk Factors Associated With Fetal Macrosomia

Pregnancy Factors	Maternal Factors
Uncontrolled gestational diabetes	Diabetes mellitus
Prior history of fetal macrosomia	Obesity
Late-term or postterm pregnancies (>41 wk)	Nonsmoking status
Idiopathic	Idiopathic

calculating EFW has been shown to be equal or superior to other formulas or charts,[81-84,153] we utilize this method in our ultrasound unit. However, by using this formula, the mean absolute percent error is significantly greater for fetuses >4500 g than for those <4500 g (12.6% ± 8.4% vs 8.4% ± 6.5, $P = .001$).[154]

The ultrasound measurement of the fetal AC has also been utilized to detect fetal macrosomia with comparable efficacy to ultrasound EFW.[92,155,156] Although the presence of diabetes in pregnancy does not appear to influence the accuracy of ultrasound detecting fetal macrosomia,[157] maternal obesity, another risk factor for macrosomia, may influence the clinical detection rate for fetal macrosomia.[158,159]

Prevention

Prior research evaluating the effect of lifestyle modifications, such as exercise and diet programs, to minimize weight gain during pregnancy reported that these interventions failed to decrease the rates of fetal macrosomia.[160,161] However, a 2016 trial of 1-hour supervised exercise three times a week reduced the rate of birthweights >4000 g from 4.7% in women in the *no exercise group* to 1.8% in the *exercise group*.[162] In contrast, there is good evidence that strict glycemic control decreases the rate of LGA or fetal macrosomia (birthweight >4000 g) in women with mild gestational diabetes from about 14%-21% to 6%-10%.[135,163]

Induction of Labor and Cesarean Delivery for Macrosomia

Scheduled cesarean delivery has been proposed as a measure to decrease the rate of shoulder dystocia and consequences of birth trauma. The ACOG recommends that cesarean delivery should be considered with an EFW >4500 g in mothers with diabetes and when the EFW >5000 g in mothers without diabetes.[133] However, cesarean delivery reduces but does not eliminate the risk of birth trauma complications. Ecker et al[164] calculated that the number of cesarean deliveries needed to prevent one brachial plexus injury was 57 and 19 if the cutoffs utilized are 4000 and 4500 g, respectively. However, the number of cesarean deliveries needed to prevent one permanent brachial plexus injury increases exponentially for each birthweight threshold.[164] The number of cesarean deliveries needed to prevent a permanent injury in infants of mothers without diabetes and with birthweights >4500 g appears to be between 155 and 588 procedures.[165]

Induction of labor when fetal macrosomia is suspected has also been studied. However, the results are conflicting. Retrospective cohorts have found no difference in the rate of shoulder dystocia and neonatal morbidity with an increased cesarean delivery rate.[166,167] Contrary to these findings, a randomized trial in women with EFW >4000 g reported no increased cesarean delivery rate or shoulder dystocia rate in 273 pregnancies randomized to induction of labor or expectant management at 38 weeks.[168] In a larger trial from Europe that randomized women with an EFW >95th percentile for GA into induction of labor or expectant management groups, investigators found a lower rate of composite score that included shoulder dystocia, fracture of the clavicle, brachial plexus injury, intracranial hemorrhage or death, a 68% reduction in shoulder dystocia with induction of labor, and no effect on the rate of cesarean delivery.[169]

Regarding a trial of labor after a cesarean delivery (TOLAC), the diagnosis of fetal macrosomia is not a contraindication for TOLAC, despite the increased rate of cesarean delivery seen in this population.[170,171]

Operative deliveries (vacuum and forceps) appear to be associated with an increased risk for shoulder dystocia in macrosomic fetuses[172]; therefore, the utilization of these procedures should be done with caution.

KEY POINTS

- When the GA is certain, FGR is diagnosed if sonographic biometry reflects an EFW less than the 10th percentile. UA Doppler abnormalities can enhance the prenatal diagnosis of this condition, and serial EFW measurements may be needed when GA is uncertain.
- When the diagnosis of FGR is made early in gestation, genetic syndromes and perinatal infections should be considered.
- The diagnosis of macrosomia is also accomplished by the use of EFW.
- At term, an absolute EFW of 4500 g is utilized to diagnose macrosomia. However, an EFW >90th percentile for GA is preferred before term.

REFERENCES

1. Resnik R. Fetal growth restriction. In: Resnik R, Lockwood C, Moore T, Greene J, Copel J, Silver R, eds. *Creasy and Resnik's Maternal-Fetal Medicine Principles and Practice*. 8th ed. Elsevier; 2018: 798-809.
2. American College of Obstetricians and Gynecologists' Committee on Practice Bulletins—Obstetrics and the Society forMaternal-FetalMedicin. ACOG Practice Bulletin No 204: Fetal growth restriction. *Obstet Gynecol.* 2019;133:e97-e109.
3. Lees C, Marlow N, Arabin B, et al. Perinatal morbidity and mortality in early-onset fetal growth restriction: cohort outcomes of the trial of randomized umbilical and fetal flow in Europe (TRUFFLE). *Ultrasound Obstet Gynecol.* 2013;42:400-408.
4. Gordijn SJ, Beune IM, Thilaganathan B, et al. Consensus definition of fetal growth restriction: a Delphi procedure. *Ultrasound Obstet Gynecol.* 2016;48:333-339.
5. Figueras F, Caradeux J, Crispi F, Eixarch E, Peguero A, Gratacos E. Diagnosis and surveillance of late-onset fetal growth restriction. *Am J Obstet Gynecol.* 2018;218:S790.e1-S802.e1.
6. Unterscheider J, Daly S, Geary MP, et al. Optimizing the definition of intrauterine growth restriction: the multicenter prospective PORTO Study. *Am J Obstet Gynecol.* 2013;208:290.e1-209.e6.
7. Blue NR, Beddow ME, Savabi M, et al. A comparison of methods for the diagnosis of fetal growth restriction between the Royal College of Obstetricians and Gynaecologists and the American College of Obstetricians and Gynecologists. *Obstet Gynecol.* 2018;131: 835-841.
8. Martins JG, Abuhamad A, Biggio JR; Society for Maternal-Fetal Medicine (SMFM) Diagnosis and management of fetal growth restriction. *Am J Obstet Gynecol.* 2020;223(4):B2-B17. doi:10.1016/j.ajog.2020.05.010
9. Lubchenco LO, Hansman C, Dressler M, Boyd E. Intrauterine growth as estimated from liveborn birth-weight data at 24 to 42 weeks of gestation. *Pediatrics.* 1963;32:793-800.
10. Battaglia FC, Lubchenco LO. A practical classification of newborn infants by weight and gestational age. *J Pediatr.* 1967;71:159-163.
11. Walther FJ, Ramaekers LH. The ponderal index as a measure of the nutritional status at birth and its relation to some aspects of neonatal morbidity. *J Perinat Med.* 1982;10:42-47.
12. Ounsted M, Moar V, Scott WA. Perinatal morbidity and mortality in small-for-dates babies: the relative importance of some maternal factors. *Early Hum Dev.* 1981;5:367-375.
13. McIntire DD, Bloom SL, Casey BM, Leveno KJ. Birth weight in relation to morbidity and mortality among newborn infants. *N Engl J Med.* 1999;340:1234-1238.
14. Boulet SL, Alexander GR, Salihu HM, Kirby RS, Carlo WA. Fetal growth risk curves: defining levels of fetal growth restriction by neonatal death risk. *Am J Obstet Gynecol.* 2006;195:1571-1577.
15. Pulver LS, Guest-Warnick G, Stoddard GJ, Byington CL, Young PC. Weight for gestational age affects the mortality of late preterm infants. *Pediatrics.* 2009;123:e1072-e1077.
16. Barker DJ. Fetal growth and adult disease. *Br J Obstet Gynaecol.* 1992;99:275-276.
17. Jarvis S, Glinianaia SV, Torrioli MG, et al. Cerebral palsy and intrauterine growth in single births: European collaborative study. *Lancet.* 2003;362:1106-1111.
18. Lees CC, Marlow N, van Wassenaer-Leemhuis A, et al. 2 year neurodevelopmental and intermediate perinatal outcomes in infants with very preterm fetal growth restriction (TRUFFLE): a randomised trial. *Lancet.* 2015;385:2162-2172.
19. Boers KE, Vijgen SM, Bijlenga D, et al. Induction versus expectant monitoring for intrauterine growth restriction at term: randomised equivalence trial (DIGITAT). *Br Med J.* 2010;341:c7087.
20. Thornton JG, Hornbuckle J, Vail A, Spiegelhalter DJ, Levene M; GRIT Study Group. Infant wellbeing at 2 years of age in the Growth Restriction Intervention Trial (GRIT): multicentred randomised controlled trial. *Lancet.* 2004;364: 513-520.
21. Naeye RL. Prenatal organ and cellular growth with various chromosomal disorders. *Biol Neonat.* 1967;11:248-260.
22. Zhu H, Lin S, Huang L, et al. Application of chromosomal microarray analysis in prenatal diagnosis of fetal growth restriction. *Prenat Diagn.* 2016;36:686-692.

23. Khoury MJ, Erickson JD, Cordero JF, McCarthy BJ. Congenital malformations and intrauterine growth retardation: a population study. *Pediatrics.* 1988;82:83-90.

24. Wallenstein MB, Harper LM, Odibo AO, et al. Fetal congenital heart disease and intrauterine growth restriction: a retrospective cohort study. *J Matern Fetal Neonatal Med.* 2012;25:662-665.

25. Malik S, Cleves MA, Zhao W, et al. National Birth Defects Prevention S. Association between congenital heart defects and small for gestational age. *Pediatrics.* 2007;119:e976-e982.

26. Norman SM, Odibo AO, Longman RE, Roehl KA, Macones GA, Cahill AG. Neural tube defects and associated low birth weight. *Am J Perinatol.* 2012;29:473-476.

27. Hughes BL, Gyamfi-Bannerman C; Society for Maternal-Fetal Medicine. Diagnosis and antenatal management of congenital cytomegalovirus infection. *Am J Obstet Gynecol.* 2016;214:B5-B11.

28. American College of Obstetricians and Gynecologists. Practice Bulletin No. 151: cytomegalovirus, parvovirus B19, varicella zoster, and toxoplasmosis in pregnancy. *Obstet Gynecol.* 2015;125:1510-1525.

29. Desai M, ter Kuile FO, Nosten F, et al. Epidemiology and burden of malaria in pregnancy. *Lancet Infect Dis.* 2007;7:93-104.

30. Grantz KL, Grewal J, Albert PS, et al. Dichorionic twin trajectories: the NICHD fetal growth studies. *Am J Obstet Gynecol.* 2016;215:221.e1-221.e16.

31. Fick AL, Feldstein VA, Norton ME, et al. Unequal placental sharing and birth weight discordance in monochorionic diamniotic twins. *Am J Obstet Gynecol.* 2006;195:178-183.

32. Suzuki S. Clinical significance of pregnancies with circumvallate placenta. *J Obstet Gynaecol Res.* 2008;34:51-54.

33. Esakoff TF, Cheng YW, Snowden JM, Tran SH, Shaffer BL, Caughey AB. Velamentous cord insertion: is it associated with adverse perinatal outcomes? *J Matern Fetal Neonatal Med.* 2015;28:409-412.

34. Hua M, Odibo AO, Macones GA, Roehl KA, Crane JP, Cahill AG. Single umbilical artery and its associated findings. *Obstet Gynecol.* 2010;115:930-934.

35. Harper LM, Odibo AO, Macones GA, et al. Effect of placenta previa on fetal growth. *Am J Obstet Gynecol.* 2010;203:330.e1-330.e5.

36. Salama-Bello R, Duncan JR, Howard SL, et al. Placental location and the development of hypertensive disorders of pregnancy. *J Ultrasound Med.* 2019;38:173-178.

37. Scott A, Moar V, Ounsted M. The relative contributions of different maternal factors in small-for-gestational-age pregnancies. *Eur J Obstet Gynecol Reprod Biol.* 1981;12:157-165.

38. Panaitescu AM, Baschat AA, Akolekar R, et al. Association of chronic hypertension with birth of small-for-gestational-age neonate. *Ultrasound Obstet Gynecol.* 2017;50:361-366.

39. Cunningham FG, Cox SM, Harstad TW, et al. Chronic renal disease and pregnancy outcome. *Am J Obstet Gynecol.* 1990;163:453-459.

40. Kupferminc MJ, Peri H, Zwang E, Yaron Y, Wolman I, Eldor A. High prevalence of the prothrombin gene mutation in women with intrauterine growth retardation, abruptio placentae and second trimester loss. *Acta Obstet Gynecol Scand.* 2000;79:963-967.

41. Said JM, Higgins JR, Moses EK, et al. Inherited thrombophilia polymorphisms and pregnancy outcomes in nulliparous women. *Obstet Gynecol.* 2010;115:5-13.

42. Goetzinger KR, Cahill AG, Macones GA, Odibo AO. The relationship between maternal body mass index and tobacco use on small-for-gestational-age infants. *Am J Perinatol.* 2012;29:153-158.

43. Cliver SP, Goldenberg RL, Cutter GR, et al. The effect of cigarette smoking on neonatal anthropometric measurements. *Obstet Gynecol.* 1995;85:625-630.

44. Tobiasz AM, Duncan JR, Bursac Z, et al. The effect of prenatal alcohol exposure on fetal growth and cardiovascular parameters in a baboon model of pregnancy. *Reprod Sci.* 2018;25:1116-1123.

45. Aviles A, Diaz-Maqueo JC, Talavera A, Guzmán R, García EL. Growth and development of children of mothers treated with chemotherapy during pregnancy: current status of 43 children. *Am J Hematol.* 1991;36:243-248.

46. Unger C, Weiser JK, McCullough RE, Keefer S, Moore LG. Altitude, low birth weight, and infant mortality in Colorado. *J Am Med Assoc.* 1988;259:3427-3432.

47. Ounsted M, Moar VA, Scott A. Risk factors associated with small-for-dates and large-for-dates infants. *Br J Obstet Gynaecol.* 1985;92:226-232.

48. Reece EA, Hagay ZJ. *Prenatal diagnosis of deviant fetal growth.* In: *Reece's Clinical Obstetrics: The Fetus & Mother.* 3rd ed. Wolters Kluwer; 2007:507-520.

49. Bukowski R, Smith GC, Malone FD, et al. Fetal growth in early pregnancy and risk of delivering low birth weight infant: prospective cohort study. *Br Med J.* 2007;334:836.

50. Snijders RJ, Sherrod C, Gosden CM, Nicolaides KH. Fetal growth retardation: associated malformations and chromosomal abnormalities. *Am J Obstet Gynecol.* 1993;168:547-555.

51. Oros D, Figueras F, Cruz-Martinez R, Meler E, Munmany M, Gratacos E. Longitudinal changes in uterine, umbilical and fetal cerebral Doppler indices in late-onset small-for-gestational age fetuses. *Ultrasound Obstet Gynecol.* 2011;37:191-195.

52. Crimmins S, Desai A, Block-Abraham D, Berg C, Gembruch U, Baschat AA. A comparison of Doppler and biophysical findings between liveborn and stillborn growth-restricted fetuses. *Am J Obstet Gynecol.* 2014;211:669.e1-669.e10.

53. Cosmi E, Ambrosini G, D'Antona D, Saccardi C, Mari G. Doppler, cardiotocography, and biophysical profile changes in growth-restricted fetuses. *Obstet Gynecol.* 2005;106:1240-1245.

54. van Wyk L, Boers KE, van der Post JA, et al. Effects on (neuro)developmental and behavioral outcome at 2 years of age of induced labor compared with expectant management in intrauterine growth-restricted infants: long-term outcomes of the DIGITAT trial. *Am J Obstet Gynecol.* 2012;206:406.e1-406.e7.

55. Trudell AS, Tulli MG, Cahill AG, Macones GA, Odibo AO. Balancing the risks of stillbirth and neonatal death in the early preterm small-for-gestational-age fetus. *Am J Obstet Gynecol.* 2014;211:295.e1-295.e7.

56. Ciobanu A, Rouvali A, Syngelaki A, Akolekar R, Nicolaides KH. Prediction of small for gestational age neonates: screening by maternal factors, fetal biometry and biomarkers at 35-37 weeks' gestation. *Am J Obstet Gynecol.* 2019;220(5):486.e1-486.e11.

57. Caradeux J, Martinez-Portilla RJ, Peguero A, Sotiriadis A, Figueras F. Diagnostic performance of third trimester ultrasound for the prediction of late-onset fetal growth restriction: a systematic review and meta-analysis. *Am J Obstet Gynecol.* 2019;220(5):449.e19-459.e19.

58. Crovetto F, Triunfo S, Crispi F, et al. First-trimester screening with specific algorithms for early- and late-onset fetal growth restriction. *Ultrasound Obstet Gynecol.* 2016;48:340-348.

59. Duncan JR, Schenone MH, Argoti PS, Mari G. Middle cerebral artery peak systolic velocity in perinatal cytomegalovirus infection. *J Clin Ultrasound.* 2019;47(6):372-375.

60. Andersen HF, Johnson TR Jr, Flora JD Jr, Barclay ML. Gestational age assessment. II. Prediction from combined clinical observations. *Am J Obstet Gynecol.* 1981;140:770-774.

61. Savitz DA, Terry JW Jr, Dole N, Thorp JM Jr, Siega-Riz AM, Herring AH. Comparison of pregnancy dating by last menstrual period, ultrasound scanning, and their combination. *Am J Obstet Gynecol.* 2002;187:1660-1666.

62. Robinson HP, Fleming JE. A critical evaluation of sonar "crown-rump length" measurements. *Br J Obstet Gynaecol.* 1975;82:702-710.

63. Lindhard A, Nielsen PV, Mouritsen LA, et al. The implications of introducing the symphyseal-fundal height-measurement. A prospective randomized controlled trial. *Br J Obstet Gynaecol.* 1990;97:675-680.

64. Carbone JF, Tuuli MG, Bradshaw R, et al. Efficiency of first-trimester growth restriction and low pregnancy-associated plasma protein-A in predicting small for gestational age at delivery. *Prenat Diagn.* 2012;32:724-729.

65. Shepard MJ, Richards VA, Berkowitz RL, Liebsch J, Odibo AO. An evaluation of two equations for predicting fetal weight by ultrasound. *Am J Obstet Gynecol.* 1982;142:47-54.

66. Deter RL, Hadlock FP, Harrist RB, Carpenter RJ. Evaluation of three methods for obtaining fetal weight estimates using dynamic image ultrasound. *J Clin Ultrasound.* 1981;9:421-425.

67. Hadlock FP, Harrist RB, Sharman RS, Deter RL, Park SK. Estimation of fetal weight with the use of head, body, and femur measurements – A prospective study. *Am J Obstet Gynecol.* 1985;151:333-337.

68. Warsof SL, Gohari P, Berkowitz RL, Hobbins JC. The estimation of fetal weight by computer-assisted analysis. *Am J Obstet Gynecol.* 1977;128:881-892.

69. Gardosi J, Francis A, Turner S, Williams M. Customized growth charts: rationale, validation and clinical benefits. *Am J Obstet Gynecol.* 2018;218:S609-S618.

70. Sovio U, Smith GCS. The effect of customization and use of a fetal growth standard on the association between birthweight percentile and adverse perinatal outcome. *Am J Obstet Gynecol.* 2018;218:S738-S44.

71. Odibo AO, Francis A, Cahill AG, Crane JP, Gardosi J. Association between pregnancy complications and small-for-gestational-age birth weight defined by customized fetal growth standard versus a population-based standard. *J Matern Fetal Neonatal Med.* 2011;24:411-417.

72. Odibo AO, Cahill AG, Odibo L, Macones GA. Prediction of intrauterine fetal death in small-for-gestational-age fetuses: impact of including ultrasound biometry in customized models. *Ultrasound Obstet Gynecol.* 2012;39:288-292.

73. Buck Louis GM, Grewal J, Albert PS, et al. Racial/ethnic standards for fetal growth: the NICHD fetal growth studies. *Am J Obstet Gynecol.* 2015;213:449.e1-449.e41.

74. Papageorghiou AT, Ohuma EO, Altman DG, et al. International standards for fetal growth based on serial ultrasound measurements: the Fetal Growth Longitudinal Study of the INTERGROWTH-21st Project. *Lancet.* 2014;384:869-879.

75. Stirnemann J, Villar J, Salomon LJ, et al. International estimated fetal weight standards of the INTERGROWTH-21st Project. *Ultrasound Obstet Gynecol.* 2017;49:478-486.

76. Villar J, Cheikh Ismail L, Victora CG, et al. International standards for newborn weight, length, and head circumference by gestational age and sex: the Newborn Cross-Sectional Study of the INTERGROWTH-21st Project. *Lancet.* 2014;384:857-868.

77. Anderson NH, Sadler LC, McKinlay CJD, McCowan LME. INTERGROWTH-21st vs customized birthweight standards for identification of perinatal mortality and morbidity. *Am J Obstet Gynecol.* 2016;214:509.e1-509.e7.

78. Odibo AO, Nwabuobi C, Odibo L, Leavitt K, Obican S, Tuuli MG. Customized fetal growth standard compared with the INTERGROWTH-21st century standard at predicting small-for-gestational-age neonates. *Acta Obstet Gynecol Scand.* 2018;97:1381-1387.

79. Hadlock FP, Harrist RB, Martinez-Poyer J. In utero analysis of fetal growth: a sonographic weight standard. *Radiology.* 1991;181:129-133.

80. Hammami A, Mazer Zumaeta A, Syngelaki A, Akolekar R, Nicolaides KH. Ultrasonographic estimation of fetal weight: development of new model and assessment of performance of previous models. *Ultrasound Obstet Gynecol.* 2018;52:35-43.

81. Nwabuobi C, Odibo L, Camisasca-Lopina H, Leavitt K, Tuuli M, Odibo AO. Comparing INTERGROWTH-21st Century and Hadlock growth standards to predict small for gestational age and short-term neonatal outcomes. *J Matern Fetal Neonatal Med.* 2020;33(11):1906-1912.

82. Blue NR, Beddow ME, Savabi M, Katukuri VR, Chao CR. Comparing the Hadlock fetal growth standard to the Eunice Kennedy Shriver National Institute of Child Health and Human Development racial/ethnic standard for the prediction of neonatal morbidity and small for gestational age. *Am J Obstet Gynecol.* 2018;219:474.e1-474.e12.

83. Blue NR, Savabi M, Beddow ME, et al. The Hadlock method is superior to newer methods for the prediction of the birth weight percentile. *J Ultrasound Med.* 2019;38:587-596.

84. Kurtz AB, Wapner RJ, Kurtz RJ, et al. Analysis of biparietal diameter as an accurate indicator of gestational age. *J Clin Ultrasound.* 1980;8:319-326.

85. Hadlock FP, Deter RL, Harrist RB, et al. Fetal biparietal diameter: a critical re-evaluation of the relation to menstrual age by means of real-time ultrasound. *J Ultrasound Med.* 1982;1:97-104.

86. Reece EA, Goldstein I, Pilu G, Hobbins JC. Fetal cerebellar growth unaffected by intrauterine growth retardation: a new parameter for prenatal diagnosis. *Am J Obstet Gynecol.* 1987;157:632-638.

87. Hill LM, Guzick D, Rivello D, Hixson J, Peterson C. The transverse cerebellar diameter cannot be used to assess gestational age in the small for gestational age fetus. *Obstet Gynecol.* 1990;75:329-333.

88. Goetzinger KR, Cahill AG, Macones GA, Odibo AO. Isolated short femur length on second-trimester sonography: a marker for fetal growth restriction and other adverse perinatal outcomes. *J Ultrasound Med.* 2012;31:1935-1941.

89. Campbell S, Wilkin D. Ultrasonic measurement of fetal abdomen circumference in the estimation of fetal weight. *Br J Obstet Gynaecol.* 1975;82:689-697.

90. Kurjak A, Kirkinen P, Latin V. Biometric and dynamic ultrasound assessment of small-for-dates infants: report of 260 cases. *Obstet Gynecol.* 1980;56:281-284.

91. Wittmann BK, Robinson HP, Aitchison T, Fleming JEE. The value of diagnostic ultrasound as a screening test for intrauterine growth retardation: comparison of nine parameters. *Am J Obstet Gynecol.* 1979;134:30-35.

92. Blue NR, Yordan JMP, Holbrook BD, Nirgudkar PA, Mozurkewich EL. Abdominal circumference alone versus estimated fetal weight after 24 weeks to predict small or large for gestational age at birth: a meta-analysis. *Am J Perinatol.* 2017;34:1115-1124.

93. Chauhan SP, Sanderson M, Hendrix NW, Magann EF, Devoe LD. Perinatal outcome and amniotic fluid index in the antepartum and intrapartum periods: a meta-analysis. *Am J Obstet Gynecol.* 1999;181:1473-1478.

94. Grannum PA, Berkowitz RL, Hobbins JC. The ultrasonic changes in the maturing placenta and their relation to fetal pulmonic maturity. *Am J Obstet Gynecol.* 1979;133:915-922.

95. Kazzi GM, Gross TL, Sokol RJ, Kazzi NJ. Detection of intrauterine growth retardation: a new use for sonographic placental grading. *Am J Obstet Gynecol.* 1983;145:733-737.

96. Campbell S, Diaz-Recasens J, Griffin DR, et al. New Doppler technique for assessing uteroplacental blood flow. *Lancet.* 1983;1:675-677.

97. Espinoza J, Kusanovic JP, Bahado-Singh R, et al. Should bilateral uterine artery notching be used in the risk assessment for preeclampsia, small-for-gestational-age, and gestational hypertension? *J Ultrasound Med.* 2010;29:1103-1115.

98. Papageorghiou AT, Yu CK, Nicolaides KH. The role of uterine artery Doppler in predicting adverse pregnancy outcome. *Best Pract Res Clin Obstet Gynaecol.* 2004;18:383-396.

99. Khong SL, Kane SC, Brennecke SP, da Silva Costa F. First-trimester uterine artery Doppler analysis in the prediction of later pregnancy complications. *Dis Markers.* 2015;2015:679730.

100. Garcia B, Llurba E, Valle L, et al. Do knowledge of uterine artery resistance in the second trimester and targeted surveillance improve maternal and perinatal outcome? UTOPIA study: a randomized controlled trial. *Ultrasound Obstet Gynecol.* 2016;47:680-689.

101. Duncan JR, Tobiasz AM, Bursac Z, et al. Uterine artery flow velocity waveforms before and after delivery in hypertensive disorders of pregnancy near term. *Hypertens Pregnancy.* 2018;37:131-136.

102. Obican SG, Odibo L, Tuuli MG, Rodriguez A, Odibo AO. Third trimester uterine artery Doppler indices as predictors of preeclampsia and neonatal small for gestational age. *J Matern Fetal Neonatal Med.* 2020;33(20):3484-3489.

103. Bakalis S, Stoilov B, Akolekar R, Poon LC, Nicolaides KH. Prediction of small-for-gestational-age neonates: screening by uterine artery Doppler and mean arterial pressure at 30-34 weeks. *Ultrasound Obstet Gynecol.* 2015;45:707-714.

104. Kingdom JC, Burrell SJ, Kaufmann P. Pathology and clinical implications of abnormal umbilical artery Doppler waveforms. *Ultrasound Obstet Gynecol.* 1997;9:271-286.

105. Baschat AA, Gembruch U, Reiss I, et al. Relationship between arterial and venous Doppler and perinatal outcome in fetal growth restriction. *Ultrasound Obstet Gynecol.* 2000;16:407-413.

106. Mari G, Hanif F, Treadwell MC, Kruger M. Gestational age at delivery and Doppler waveforms in very preterm intrauterine growth-restricted fetuses as predictors of perinatal mortality. *J Ultrasound Med.* 2007;26:555-559.

107. Gonzalez JM, Stamilio DM, Ural S, Macones GA, Odibo AO. Relationship between abnormal fetal testing and adverse perinatal outcomes in intrauterine growth restriction. *Am J Obstet Gynecol.* 2007;196:e48-e51.

108. Alfirevic Z, Stampalija T, Gyte GM. Fetal and umbilical Doppler ultrasound in high-risk pregnancies. *Cochrane Database Syst Rev.* 2013;(11):CD007529.

109. Kiserud T, Eik-Nes SH, Blaas HG, Hellevik LR, Simensen B. Ductus venosus blood velocity and the umbilical circulation in the seriously growth-retarded fetus. *Ultrasound Obstet Gynecol.* 1994;4:109-114.

110. Triunfo S, Crispi F, Gratacos E, Figueras F. Prediction of delivery of small-for-gestational-age neonates and adverse perinatal outcome by fetoplacental Doppler at 37 weeks' gestation. *Ultrasound Obstet Gynecol.* 2017;49:364-371.

111. Mari G, Deter RL. Middle cerebral artery flow velocity waveforms in normal and small-for-gestational-age fetuses. *Am J Obstet Gynecol.* 1992;166:1262-1270.

112. Bahado-Singh RO, Kovanci E, Jeffres A, et al. The Doppler cerebroplacental ratio and perinatal outcome in intrauterine growth restriction. *Am J Obstet Gynecol.* 1999;180:750-756.

113. Odibo AO, Riddick C, Pare E, Stamilio DM, Macones GA. Cerebroplacental Doppler ratio and adverse perinatal outcomes in intrauterine growth restriction: evaluating the impact of using gestational age-specific reference values. *J Ultrasound Med.* 2005;24:1223-1228.

114. Hernandez-Andrade E, Maymon E, Erez O, et al. A low cerebroplacental ratio at 20-24 Weeks of gestation can predict reduced fetal size later in pregnancy or at birth. *Fetal Diagn Ther.* 2018;44:112-123.

115. Berkley E, Chauhan SP, Abuhamad A; Society for Maternal-Fetal Medicine Publications C. Doppler assessment of the fetus with intrauterine growth restriction. *Am J Obstet Gynecol.* 2012;206:300-308.

116. Morris RK, Selman TJ, Verma M, Robson SC, Kleijnen J, Khan KS. Systematic review and meta-analysis of the test accuracy of ductus venosus Doppler to predict compromise of fetal/neonatal wellbeing in high risk pregnancies with placental insufficiency. *Eur J Obstet Gynecol Reprod Biol.* 2010;152:3-12.

117. Alfirevic Z, Stampalija T, Dowswell T. Fetal and umbilical Doppler ultrasound in high-risk pregnancies. *Cochrane Database Syst Rev.* 2017;6:CD007529.

118. McCowan LM, Harding JE, Roberts AB, Barker SE, Ford C, Stewart AW. A pilot randomized controlled trial of two regimens of fetal surveillance for small-for-gestational-age fetuses with normal results of umbilical artery Doppler velocimetry. *Am J Obstet Gynecol.* 2000;182:81-86.

119. Manning FA, Platt LD, Sipos L. Antepartum fetal evaluation: development of a fetal biophysical profile. *Am J Obstet Gynecol.* 1980;136:787-795.

120. Manning FA, Morrison I, Lange IR, Harman CR, Chamberlain PF. Fetal biophysical profile scoring: selective use of the nonstress test. *Am J Obstet Gynecol.* 1987;156:709-712.

121. Vintzileos AM, Fleming AD, Scorza WE, et al. Relationship between fetal biophysical activities and umbilical cord blood gas values. *Am J Obstet Gynecol.* 1991;165:707-713.

122. Kaur S, Picconi JL, Chadha R, et al. Biophysical profile in the treatment of intrauterine growth-restricted fetuses who weigh <1000 g. *Am J Obstet Gynecol.* 2008;199:264.e1-264.e4.

123. Hecher K, Bilardo CM, Stigter RH, et al. Monitoring of fetuses with intrauterine growth restriction: a longitudinal study. *Ultrasound Obstet Gynecol.* 2001;18:564-570.

124. Scifres CM, Stamilio D, Macones GA, Odibo AO. Predicting perinatal mortality in preterm intrauterine growth restriction. *Am J Perinatol.* 2009;26:723-728.

125. Baschat AA, Galan HL, Bhide A, et al. Doppler and biophysical assessment in growth restricted fetuses: distribution of test results. *Ultrasound Obstet Gynecol.* 2006;27:41-47.

126. Turan S, Turan OM, Berg C, et al. Computerized fetal heart rate analysis, Doppler ultrasound and biophysical profile score in the prediction of acid-base status of growth-restricted fetuses. *Ultrasound Obstet Gynecol.* 2007;30:750-756.

127. Odibo AO, Quinones JN, Lawrence-Cleary K, Stamilio DM, Macones GA. What antepartum fetal test should guide the timing of delivery of the preterm growth-restricted fetus? A decision-analysis. *Am J Obstet Gynecol.* 2004;191:1477-1482.

128. Mari G, Hanif F, Kruger M. Sequence of cardiovascular changes in IUGR in pregnancies with and without preeclampsia. *Prenat Diagn.* 2008;28:377-383.

129. GRIT Study Group. A randomised trial of timed delivery for the compromised preterm fetus: short term outcomes and Bayesian interpretation. *Br J Obstet Gynaecol.* 2003;110:27-32.

130. Walker DM, Marlow N, Upstone L, et al. The Growth Restriction Intervention Trial: long-term outcomes in a randomized trial of timing of delivery in fetal growth restriction. *Am J Obstet Gynecol.* 2011;204:34. e1-34.e9.

131. Trudell AS, Cahill AG, Tuuli MG, Macones GA, Odibo AO. Risk of stillbirth after 37 weeks in pregnancies complicated by small-for-gestational-age fetuses. *Am J Obstet Gynecol.* 2013;278:376.e1-376.e7.

132. Roberge S, Nicolaides K, Demers S, et al. The role of aspirin dose on the prevention of preeclampsia and fetal growth restriction: systematic review and meta-analysis. *Am J Obstet Gynecol.* 2017;216:110.e6-120.e6.

133. American College of Obstetricians and Gynecologists' Committee on Practice Bulletins—Obstetrics. Practice Bulletin No. 173: fetal macrosomia. *Obstet Gynecol.* 2016;128:e195-e209.

134. Kong L, Nilsson IAK, Gissler M, Lavebratt C. Associations of maternal diabetes and body mass index with offspring birth weight and prematurity. *JAMA Pediatr.* 2019;173(4):371-378.

135. Landon MB, Spong CY, Thom E, et al. A multicenter, randomized trial of treatment for mild gestational diabetes. *N Engl J Med.* 2009;361:1339-1348.

136. Ehrenberg HM, Mercer BM, Catalano PM. The influence of obesity and diabetes on the prevalence of macrosomia. *Am J Obstet Gynecol.* 2004;191:964-968.

137. Ferraro ZM, Barrowman N, Prud'homme D, et al. Excessive gestational weight gain predicts large for gestational age neonates independent of maternal body mass index. *J Matern Fetal Neonatal Med.* 2012;25:538-542.

138. Okun N, Verma A, Mitchell BF, et al. Relative importance of maternal constitutional factors and glucose intolerance of pregnancy in the development of newborn macrosomia. *J Matern Fetal Med.* 1997;6:285-290.

139. Hamilton BE, Martin JA, Osterman MJ, Curtin SC, Matthews TJ. Births: final data for 2014. *Natl Vital Stat Rep.* 2015;64:1-64.

140. Jastrow N, Roberge S, Gauthier RJ, et al. Effect of birth weight on adverse obstetric outcomes in vaginal birth after cesarean delivery. *Obstet Gynecol.* 2010;115:338-343.

141. Modanlou HD, Dorchester WL, Thorosian A, Freeman RK. Macrosomia – Maternal, fetal, and neonatal implications. *Obstet Gynecol.* 1980;55:420-424.

142. Stones RW, Paterson CM, Saunders NJ. Risk factors for major obstetric haemorrhage. *Eur J Obstet Gynecol Reprod Biol.* 1993;48:15-18.

143. Esakoff TF, Cheng YW, Sparks TN, Caughey AB. The association between birthweight 4000 g or greater and perinatal outcomes in patients with and without gestational diabetes mellitus. *Am J Obstet Gynecol.* 2009;200:672. e1-672.e4.

144. Perlow JH, Wigton T, Hart J, Strassner HT, Nageotte MP, Wolk BM. Birth trauma. A five-year review of incidence and associated perinatal factors. *J Reprod Med.* 1996;41:754-760.

145. Sparano S, Ahrens W, De Henauw S, et al. Being macrosomic at birth is an independent predictor of overweight in children: results from the IDEFICS study. *Matern Child Health J.* 2013;17:1373-1381.

146. Carter EB, Stockburger J, Tuuli MG, Macones GA, Odibo AO, Trudell AS. Large for gestational age and stillbirth: is there a role for antenatal testing? *Ultrasound Obstet Gynecol.* 2018;54(3):334-337.

147. Sherman DJ, Arieli S, Tovbin J, Siegel G, Caspi E, Bukovsky I. A comparison of clinical and ultrasonic estimation of fetal weight. *Obstet Gynecol.* 1998;91:212-217.

148. Chauhan SP, West DJ, Scardo JA, et al. Antepartum detection of macrosomic fetus: clinical versus sonographic, including soft-tissue measurements. *Obstet Gynecol.* 2000;95:639-642.

149. Chauhan SP, Cowan BD, Magann EF, Bradford TH, Roberts WE, Morrison JC. Intrapartum detection of a macrosomic fetus: clinical versus 8 sonographic models. *Aust N Z J Obstet Gynaecol.* 1995;35:266-270.

150. Chauhan SP, Sullivan CA, Lutton TC, et al. Parous patients' estimate of birth weight in postterm pregnancy. *J Perinatol.* 1995;15:192-194.

151. Harlev A, Walfisch A, Bar-David J, et al. Maternal estimation of fetal weight as a complementary method of fetal weight assessment: a prospective clinical trial. *J Reprod Med.* 2006;51:515-520.

152. O'Reilly-Green CP, Divon MY. Receiver operating characteristic curves of sonographic estimated fetal weight for prediction of macrosomia in prolonged pregnancies. *Ultrasound Obstet Gynecol.* 1997;9:403-408.

153. Shmueli A, Salman L, Hadar E, et al. Sonographic prediction of macrosomia in pregnancies complicated by maternal diabetes: finding the best formula. *Arch Gynecol Obstet.* 2019;299:97-103.

154. Alsulyman OM, Ouzounian JG, Kjos SL. The accuracy of intrapartum ultrasonographic fetal weight estimation in diabetic pregnancies. *Am J Obstet Gynecol.* 1997;177:503-506.

155. Coomarasamy A, Connock M, Thornton J, Khan KS. Accuracy of ultrasound biometry in the prediction of macrosomia: a systematic quantitative review. *Br J Obstet Gynaecol.* 2005;112:1461-1466.

156. Smith GC, Smith MF, McNay MB, Fleming JE. The relation between fetal abdominal circumference and birthweight: findings in 3512 pregnancies. *Br J Obstet Gynaecol.* 1997;104:186-190.

157. Best G, Pressman EK. Ultrasonographic prediction of birth weight in diabetic pregnancies. *Obstet Gynecol.* 2002;99:740-744.

158. Goetzinger KR, Tuuli MG, Odibo AO, Roehl KA, Macones GA, Cahill AG. Screening for fetal growth disorders by clinical exam in the era of obesity. *J Perinatol.* 2013;33:352-357.

159. Drassinower D, Timofeev J, Huang CC, Benson JE, Driggers RW, Landy HJ. Accuracy of clinically estimated fetal weight in pregnancies complicated by diabetes mellitus and obesity. *Am J Perinatol.* 2014;31:31-37.

160. Dodd JM, Turnbull D, McPhee AJ, et al. Antenatal lifestyle advice for women who are overweight or obese: LIMIT randomised trial. *Br Med J.* 2014;348:g1285.

161. de Oliveria Melo AS, Silva JL, Tavares JS, Barros VO, Leite DF, Amorim MM. Effect of a physical exercise program during pregnancy on utero-placental and fetal blood flow and fetal growth: a randomized controlled trial. *Obstet Gynecol.* 2012;120:302-310.

162. Barakat R, Pelaez M, Cordero Y, et al. Exercise during pregnancy protects against hypertension and macrosomia: randomized clinical trial. *Am J Obstet Gynecol.* 2016;214:649.e1-649.e8.

163. Crowther CA, Hiller JE, Moss JR, et al. Effect of treatment of gestational diabetes mellitus on pregnancy outcomes. *N Engl J Med.* 2005;352:2477-2486.

164. Ecker JL, Greenberg JA, Norwitz ER, et al. Birth weight as a predictor of brachial plexus injury. *Obstet Gynecol.* 1997;89:643-647.

165. Bryant DR, Leonardi MR, Landwehr JB, et al. Limited usefulness of fetal weight in predicting neonatal brachial plexus injury. *Am J Obstet Gynecol.* 1998;179:686-689.

166. Combs CA, Singh NB, Khoury JC. Elective induction versus spontaneous labor after sonographic diagnosis of fetal macrosomia. *Obstet Gynecol.* 1993;81:492-496.

167. Leaphart WL, Meyer MC, Capeless EL. Labor induction with a prenatal diagnosis of fetal macrosomia. *J Matern Fetal Med.* 1997;6:99-102.

168. Gonen O, Rosen DJ, Dolfin Z, et al. Induction of labor versus expectant management in macrosomia: a randomized study. *Obstet Gynecol.* 1997;89:913-917.

169. Boulvain M, Senat MV, Perrotin F, et al. Induction of labour versus expectant management for large-for-date fetuses: a randomised controlled trial. *Lancet.* 2015;385:2600-2605.

170. Elkousy MA, Sammel M, Stevens E, et al. The effect of birth weight on vaginal birth after cesarean delivery success rates. *Am J Obstet Gynecol.* 2003;188:824-830.

171. Flamm BL, Goings JR. Vaginal birth after cesarean section: is suspected fetal macrosomia a contraindication? *Obstet Gynecol.* 1989;74:694-697.

172. Kolderup LB, Laros RK Jr, Musci TJ. Incidence of persistent birth injury in macrosomic infants: association with mode of delivery. *Am J Obstet Gynecol.* 1997;177:37-41.

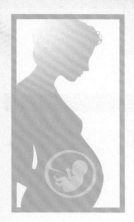

CHAPTER 19

Three- and Four-Dimensional Ultrasound and Magnetic Resonance Imaging in Pregnancy

Shifa Turan and Ozhan M. Turan

Three-dimensional (3D) and four-dimensional (4D) ultrasound

Main Principles of the 3D and 4D Ultrasound

In general, 3D ultrasound consists of four main steps: (1) volume acquisition, (2) three-dimensional (3D) or four-dimensional (4D) visualizations of the volume, (3) optimization of the volume acquisition? with different modes, and (4) storage of volume images, rendered images, or image/volume sequences (**Table 19.1**; **Figure 19.1**).

Volume Acquisition

The main determinants for the ideal volume acquisition are the presence of adequate amniotic fluid in front of the target structure, identifying the area of interest, and using proper angle and time. The region of interest (ROI) box determines the height and width of the acquired volume. The lateral dimensions of the ROI box have the most significant influence on the frame rate; therefore, the narrower the angle, the better the image quality. After identifying the ROI, the volume is acquired symmetrically upwards and downwards toward the targeted image.

See the eBook for expanded content, a complete reference list, and additional figures and tables.

Three- and Four-Dimensional Visualization of the Volume

Multiplanar Display

At the end of the ideal volume acquisition, there will be A, B, and C planes on display. These planes are also called the multiplanar display or orthogonal planes. The image that is displayed in the A plane corresponds to the 2D starting image and, therefore, has the highest image resolution. In contrast, planes B and C are reconstructed images and have lower image resolutions (**Figure 19.2B**). Two main postprocessing applications can be used after obtaining a multiplanar display: tomographic ultrasound imaging (TUI) or virtual organ computer-aided analysis (VOCAL).

TUI is an automated display modality where parallel images in a 3D volume are shown in a multi-image display. TUI allows the examiner to simultaneously display multiple cross-sectional images at specific distances from each other. The number of slices as well as distances between the slices can be adjusted by the position of each plane within the ROI. The advantage of this application is the ability to display sequential parallel planes.

VOCAL utilizes computer technology to provide accurate volume calculations. Manual rotation or constant degree rotation selection, such as 12°, 15°, and 30°, can be selected, and multiple adjacent and sequential planes can manually be measured (**Figure 19.4**).[2]

Table 19.1 Comparisons of Ultrasound and MRI as a Fetal Assessment Method

	Ultrasound	MRI
Advantage	Widely available	No limited views
	Affordable	Able to image whole fetus, uterus
	Allows real-time interpretation	Detection of subtle changes
	Real-time guidance for interventions	Off-line interpretation
Disadvantage	Operator dependent	Operator dependent
	Limited views:	Limited value:
	• Fetal position	• First trimester is not appropriate
	• Oligohydramnios	• Fetal movements
	• Shadowing	• Maternal movements or claustrophobia
	• Maternal obesity	

MRI, magnetic resonance imaging.

Optimization of the 3D Volume With Different Modes

Optimization of the acquired image can be performed using several different display modes (**Table 19.2**). The surface mode is the most common mode to visualize the 3D structures (**Figure 19.5A-C**).

The high-definition (HD)–live mode gives a more realistic visualization of the fetus. In the HD-live mode, the human skin–based color spectrum and movable virtual light source allows almost photographic imaging of the target structure and can show pathological changes that were not detectable with previous 3D surface modes (**Figure 19.5D** and **E**).[3]

Inversion mode inverts the gray scale of the volume voxels. With this mode, anechoic structures, such as the heart chambers, vessel lumen, stomach, gallbladder, renal pelvis, and bladder, appear echogenic in the rendered images, whereas structures that are normally echogenic before grayscale inversion (eg, bones) appear anechoic (**Figure 19.5G** and **H**).[4]

Glass body is another option in which color and power Doppler are used during volume acquisition. This mode allows visualization of the details in blood vessels (**Figure 19.5I**).[5]

Volume contrast imaging (VCI) enhances the appearance of the fetal structures via increasing the balance in contrast (**Figure 19.5F**).

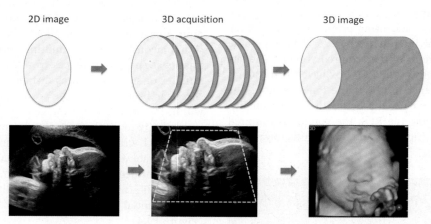

Figure 19.1 Schematic presentation of a three-dimensional (3D) image. During 3D acquisition, multiple two-dimensional (2D) images are obtained to create a 3D image. The single circle represents the 2D image. When the multiple circles are combined, a tridimensional object can be compiled as depicted with a cylinder. The four-dimensional (4D) image can be obtained when the 3D images are captured over time.

Acquisition   Multiplanar display

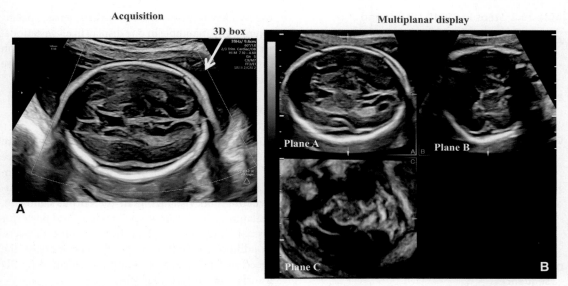

Figure 19.2 Steps of a volume acquisition. The first step is the identification of the area of interest by using the three-dimensional (3D) box **(A)**. Following a volume acquisition, a multiplanar display is obtained **(B)**. Plane A: corresponds to the two-dimensional (2D) starting image and therefore have the highest image resolution; Planes B and C are the transverse and coronal planes, respectively.

Clinical Applications of the 3D and 4D Ultrasound in Pregnancy

The most common mode for visualizing the face is the *surface-rendering mode*. It is usually used to examine the external structures, such as the nose, lips, ears, and profile, and it is an excellent method to show cleft lip, low-set ears, and profile abnormalities such as micrognathia.

The *maximum mode* is the second most common mode used to visualize the fetal face and allows practitioners to assess the bone and sutures of the fetal head and nasal bone. The *reverse rendering mode* is also used in facial evaluations, and the principle of this rendering is to assess the fetal face posteriorly, which allows more precise palate evaluation. *TUI* of the fetal profile at the eye socket view has been

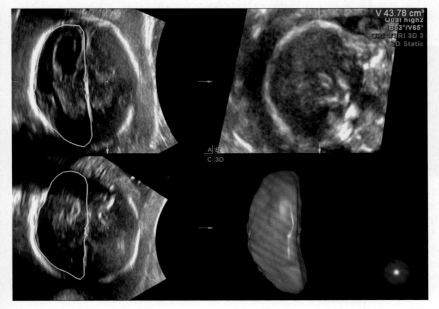

Figure 19.4 Virtual Organ Computer-Aided Analysis (VOCAL). This postprocessing application provides an accurate volume measurement. Manual rotation with 15° selected for measurement of the brain hemisphere.

Table 19.2 Steps in 3D/4D Ultrasound

A. Volume acquisition
- Identifying the 2D image
- Definition of the region of interest
- Volume acquisition

B. 3D and 4D visualization of the volume
- Multiplanar display
- Tomographic ultrasound imaging

C. Optimization of the 3D/4D volume with different modes
- Surface-rendered image with surface mode (light mode/HD Live Mode)
- Transparent display (Maximum mode/x-ray mode)
- Glass body (silhouette, monochrome)
- Inversion mode
- Volume contrast imaging (VCI) mode

D. Storing of the volumes or rendered image sequences

2D, two-dimensional; 3D, three-dimensional; 4D, four-dimensional.

used widely to assess the eye sockets, lenses, palate, tongue, and mandible in one display in all gestational weeks. Postprocessing with the VCI application on top of the TUI improves the appearance of the above structures and helps to delineate the details.

Fetal Central Nervous System

Fetal Brain

Potential benefits of 3D ultrasound in the fetal brain include the ability to identify the location, degree of severity, and extent of central nervous system (CNS) abnormalities; and the possibility of reconstructing and visualizing all the corpus callosum, thalamus, cavum septum pellucidum, and posterior fossa in the sagittal plane from volume datasets. In addition, 3D ultrasonography can increase the speed of fetal neurosonography performed by 2D transvaginal ultrasonography.

Volume acquisition at the level of the transventricular, transcerebellar, and coronal planes allows

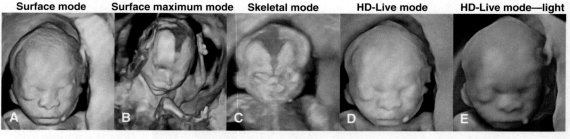

Surface mode   Surface maximum mode   Skeletal mode   HD-Live mode   HD-Live mode—light

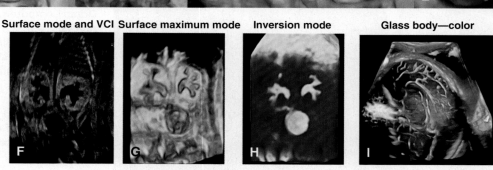

Surface mode and VCI   Surface maximum mode   Inversion mode   Glass body—color

Figure 19.5 Different optimization modes used in three-dimensional (3D) and four-dimensional (4D) ultrasonography. **A,** Surface mode. Using the surface mode, and adjusting threshold and filters, it is possible to display the surface of the fetal face. **B,** Maximum mode of the same volume and with the same region of interest. **C,** Skeletal mode with details of the skeleton of the face. **D,** High-definition live mode. E, High-definition live mode with a light application. **F and G,** Surface mode with volume contrast imaging (VCI) of the kidneys demonstrates renal pelvis size and kidney tissue surround. **H,** Inversion mode of the renal pelvis and bladder. **G,** Demonstration of the pericallosal artery with glass body color.

assessment of the fetal brain by multiplanar and TUI methods. VOCAL can evaluate the hemisphere volumes if asymmetry is suspected (**Figure 19.4**). The color mode by color Doppler or power Doppler allows visualization of brain circulation and abnormalities of the blood vessels in the brain such as vein of Galen malformations.

Fetal Spine

The 3D volume of the spine and application of the multiplanar plane enables assessment of the sagittal, transverse, and coronal view of the spine in one picture. Rendering of the volume will show the spine and ribs very clearly (**Figure 19.10A**). The skeletal mode is the preferred mode for optimization to evaluate fetal spine abnormalities such as hemivertebra and scoliosis (**Figure 19.10B-D**). In addition, it is also helpful to identify the level of the defect in spina bifida cases, which is essential for prognosis and treatment (**Figure 19.10E** and **F**).

OmniView allows interrogation of volume datasets and simultaneous display of up to three independent (nonorthogonal) planes by manually drawing lines from any direction or angle. This modality has a lot of applications in spine and brain assessment. In addition, if volume contrast imaging is applied on top of the initial image, more detail can be seen and definitions of the structures can be more precise.[7]

Fetal Chest and Abdomen

Fetal chest lesions, rib anomalies, intrathoracic masses, abdominal wall defects, and abdominal structures also can be assessed by 3D ultrasound. Minimum mode is constructive to determine cystic structures of the thorax and abdomen. The application of TUI can display thorax and abdominal structures in one picture.

Fetal Heart

Two-dimensional echocardiography is the gold standard for prenatal imaging of the fetal heart and situs. Obtaining the four-chamber view, left and right outflow tract, and the three-vessel and trachea views are the recommended views in obstetric settings.[10] Examining the fetal heart in motion is a critical component of assessing cardiac structure and function.

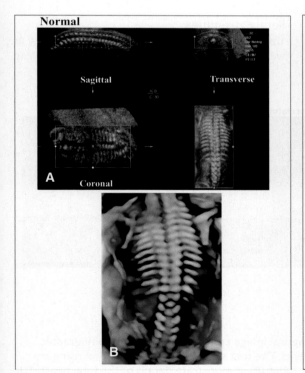
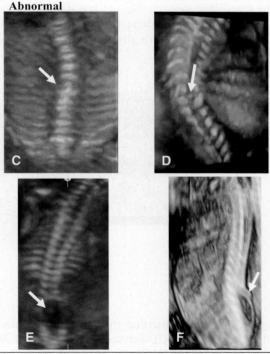

Figure 19.10 The normal spine demonstrated in multiplanar (**A**) and skeletal mode–high-definition (HD) live (**B**). Scoliosis (**C**) and hemivertebra (**D**) were diagnosed in skeletal mode. A spina bifida with skeletal mode was seen in the axial (**E**) and sagittal views (**F**).

Displaying 3D image information as a moving image can be presented as 3D cine-looping and/or 4D real-time imaging. When these modalities are chosen, the spatial and temporal resolution of the image is limited.

Spatiotemporal Image Correlation

Spatiotemporal image correlation (STIC) is an automated volume acquisition that allows synchronization of the imaging data to specific times or phases of the cardiac cycle so that fetal heart motion can be incorporated into the final volume dataset. The transducer array performs single sweep, recording one single 3D dataset over a 7.5- to 15-second time period. The volume of interest is acquired at a sweep angle (approximately 20°-40°) to obtain orthogonal planes, depending on the size of the fetus and gestational age (**Figure 19.13A and B**).

STIC volumes can also be obtained with or without color or power Doppler. The preferred method is obtaining an STIC volume with color or power Doppler. This could be removed by the color off button at the time of postprocessing. Notably, in the first-trimester cardiac evaluation, color or power Doppler is essential and very useful. It allows the practitioner to assess all the cardiac landmarks more precisely and reveals any abnormalities in a precise way.

There are tremendous benefits of applying one of the postprocessing options, such as TUI, in the fetal heart examination. This application allows the examiner to simultaneously display multiple cross-sectional images at specific distances from the four-chamber view, so all the cardiac landmarks can be displayed in one picture (**Figure 19.13C and D**).

Overall, cardiac evaluation performed by 4D ultrasound using STIC and TUI during the first and second trimesters is advantageous in cardiac screening programs as well as in patients with cardiac anomalies (**Figure 19.15**).[11,13]

STIC-M Mode STIC-M mode is another post-processing application that can be used to measure cardiac dimensions, left and right ventricular wall thickness, and interventricular thickness.[14] In addition, STIC-M mode is useful to assess alterations in preload and afterload.

STIC-VOCAL STIC-VOCAL allows a more accurate assessment of the fetal cardiac volumes. After the initial acquisition is obtained with the STIC in traditional or inversion modes, VOCAL is activated to calculate the cardiac ventricular volumes.

Fetal Extremities

Upper and lower extremities, toes, and fingers, as well as the size and shape of the extremities can

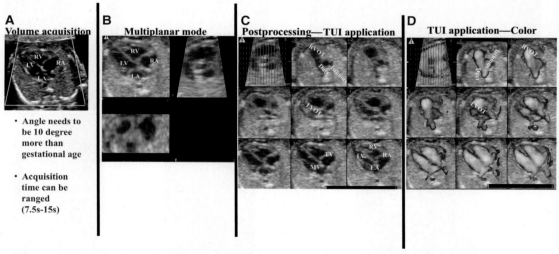

Figure 19.13 Demonstrates the steps for spatiotemporal image correlation (STIC) and tomographic ultrasound imaging (TUI) on the fetal heart at 22 weeks. The first step is volume acquisition using an appropriate setting **(A)**. Multiplanar and rendering modes **(B)** demonstrate details of the fetal heart. TUI allows examining all cardiac structures in a single panel **(C)**, TUI color allows more clear definition of the direction of the blood flow in each vessel and the valve **(D)**. LA, left atrium; LV, left ventricle; LVOT, left ventricular outflow tract; MV, mitral valve; RA, right atrium; RV, right ventricle; RVOT, right ventricular outflow tract; TV, tricuspid valve.

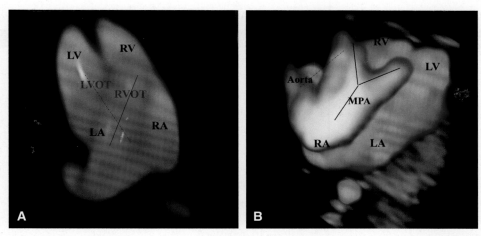

Figure 19.15 Normally connected fetal heart **(A)** at 12 weeks with normal four-chamber and great arteries (crisscross relationship). An abnormal heart **(B)** at first trimester; double outlet right ventricle with parallel relation of the great arteries. LA, left atrium; LV, left ventricle; LVOT, left ventricular outflow tract; MPA, main pulmonary artery; RA, right atrium; RV, right ventricle; RVOT, right ventricular outflow tract.

be evaluated with 3D ultrasound starting from 12 weeks. Surface mode and skeletal mode are the most useful applications to assess all varieties of limb, finger, and toe anomalies in the fetus.

Magnetic Resonance Imaging

Fetal MRI

Procedural Considerations
(**Table 19.3**)
Fetal MRI can be technically challenging due to fetal movements and variable lie and presentation. It is operator dependent and requires appropriate sequences tailored to the organ system and suspected pathology. During MRI data acquisition, the tissue can be characterized by two different relaxation times—T1 (longitudinal relaxation time) and T2 (transverse relaxation time).

The imaging protocol must adapt to fetal movements and to the type of anomaly suspected. The entire fetus should be assessed at the time of MRI examination.

Ideally, three orthogonal planes should be obtained through the fetal head and body in each sequence. The MRI protocol primarily includes T2-weighted sequences. T1-weighted, diffusion-weighted, and additional sequences may be added, if indicated, and ideally should provide documentation of the entire fetus as well as the placenta, uterus, and surrounding maternal structures. Repeated

sequences may be required if the fetus moves during scanning. The field of view should be as small as possible without causing foldover artifacts. Slice thicknesses between 2.5 and 5 mm are used to examine most fetal structures. Thinner slices are possible but increase the signal-to-noise ratio (SNR). At present, the minimum voxel size that may be obtained with fetal MRI is 0.8 × 0.8 × 2.5 mm, with slice thickness.[21] Fetal and maternal movement is usually the limiting factor, and this may lead to a poor resolution in the image capture. Counseling and patient education before the procedure are important to reduce maternal anxiety. The conversation should include the indication for fetal MRI, duration of the procedure, wait time to receive the final results, and any limitations, such as obesity and polyhydramnios, that may affect the image resolution.[24]

Clinical Usage
Generally, fetal MRI is performed using a 1.5 T traditional superconducting magnet with a phased array surface coil allowing a sufficient SNR and an optimal imaging quality. In most cases, the use of ultrafast imaging techniques provides good imaging quality despite fetal motion, even without sedation of the mother-fetus.[25]

The fetal brain is well observed on T2-weighted sequences because of the contrast between cerebrospinal fluid and brain tissue. After 17 weeks, the advantages of MRI in diagnoses of both developmental and acquired intracranial abnormalities

Table 19.3 Primary Diagnostic Tool Based on Fetal Abnormality

Fetal Abnormality	Primary Diagnostic	Adjunct
Face		
Orbits	2D/3D ultrasound	MRI
Ear	2D/3D ultrasound	
Chin	2D/3D ultrasound	MRI
Palate and lips	2D/3D ultrasound	MRI
Brain		
Ventriculomegaly	2D/3D ultrasound	MRI
Hydrocephalus	2D/3D ultrasound	MRI
Midline defects (corpus callosum, cavum septum pellucidum)	2D ultrasound/MRI	3D ultrasound
Posterior fossa	2D/3D ultrasound	MRI
Infection	2D ultrasound/MRI	3D ultrasound
Hemorrhage, ischemia	2D ultrasound/MRI	3D ultrasound
Cortical	2D ultrasound/MRI	3D ultrasound
Spine	2D/3D ultrasound	MRI
Neck	2D/3D ultrasound	MRI
Chest		
Lung	2D/3D ultrasound	MRI
Hernia	2D ultrasound/MRI	3D ultrasound
Heart	2D/4D ultrasound	
Urogenital	2D/3D ultrasound	
Placenta	2D ultrasound/MRI	3D ultrasound

2D, two-dimensional; 3D, three-dimensional; MRI, magnetic resonance imaging.

have been well established; however, determination of some defects may not be possible until after 24 weeks. Additional T1-weighted and diffusion-weighted imaging can provide information about brain development, cell density, myelination, hemorrhage, and ischemic lesions.[21,26]

CNS Anomalies
In general, CNS abnormalities are the most common clinical indication for fetal MRI, representing about 80% of all examinations requested.[27]

Ventriculomegaly When ventriculomegaly is seen on ultrasound, fetal MRI can be a complementary tool to determine if there is any additional abnormality, such as cortical malformations (lissencephaly, schizencephaly, and polymicrogyria), periventricular heterotopia, cerebellar malformations, hemimegalencephaly, periventricular white matter injury, porencephaly, multicystic encephalomalacia,

intraventricular hemorrhage, and germinal matrix hemorrhage.[28] Fetal MRI may also help determine the etiology of the ventriculomegaly or predict any potential poor? neurodevelopmental outcome.

Hydrocephalus Fetal MRI is more useful than ultrasound in diagnosis of congenital hydrocephalus and allows us to investigate brain parenchyma damage secondary to obstruction.[31]

Midline Anomalies Fetal MRI may help to directly visualize the sagittal and coronal planes. In addition, fetal MRI also detects other CNS anomalies associated with agenesis of the corpus callosum such as cortical dysplasia (ie, polymicrogyria) and focal cortical gyration anomalies.[32,33]

Posterior Fossa Abnormalities Fetal MRI allows direct visualization of the cerebellar hemispheres, vermis, and brainstem in three orthogonal planes, although the same views can be obtained by 3D ultrasound if the fetal position is appropriate. Some of the posterior fossa anomalies detected via fetal MRI include those along the Dandy-Walker continuum, cerebellar hypoplasia, cerebellar dysplasia, cerebellar hemorrhage, Joubert syndrome, and Chiari II malformation.

Association between posterior fossa anomalies and supratentorial defects are commonly seen. Therefore, fetal MRI should be used to evaluate the supratentorial brain when an infratentorial defect is identified.

CNS Infection Fetal MRI is useful in detecting CNS anomalies, which may occur after cytomegalovirus (CMV) infection. MRI can identify ischemic-hemorrhagic lesions, clastic lesions, subependymal cysts, intraventricular synechiae, white matter signal alterations, and sulcation and gyral abnormalities associated with CMV infection. Importantly, temporal lobe anomalies, which may be undetectable by prenatal ultrasound, can be more readily visualized by fetal MRI.[36]

Ischemic-Hemorrhagic Lesions When ischemic-hemorrhagic lesions are suspected, MRI can have a crucial role in the diagnosis and localization of the lesion and evaluation of its extension.[37] In case of supratentorial damage, it is essential to evaluate the white matter, potential cerebral cortex involvement, and the continuation of the lesion into the main cerebral areas. If the posterior fossa is involved, imaging must determine if the cerebellar hemispheres and the vermis are damaged. Most of the underlying causes of cerebral/cerebellar hemorrhage can be evaluated on MRI T2-weighted imaging, such as germinal matrix hemorrhage, vascular malformations, and congenital infections. MRI is mandatory for such an assessment because it delineates blood products more precisely.

Fetal MRI can play a dual role in a prenatal diagnostic workup in dural sinus malformations like the vein of Galen aneurysmal malformation. It can confirm the ultrasound diagnosis and may identify prognostically significant secondary findings such as white matter injuries with T2-weighted image sequences.[38]

Cortical Malformations Fetal MRI is an excellent method to identify delayed or absent cerebral sulcation, premature abnormal sulci, thin and irregular

hemispheric parenchyma, wide abnormal overdeveloped gyri, the wide opening of isolated sulci, nodular bulging into the lateral ventricles, cortical clefts, intra-parenchymal echogenic nodules, and cortical thickening.[39] In addition, cortical dysplasia associated with tuberous sclerosis (TS) includes subependymal and cortical nodules, which are difficult to detect by ultrasound but can be easily seen with MRI and appear as a hyperintense signal on T1-weighted image.[40]

Neural Tube Defects Ultrasound is the primary imaging modality used to identify neural tube defects (NTDs). However, MRI has become an important adjuvant tool to confirm and further delineate spinal anomalies and associated cranial and extracranial abnormalities and has become a fundamental study in the presurgical evaluation of fetal patients who are potential candidates for *in utero* repair of myelomeningocele.[41]

Non-CNS Abnormalities
Fetal Oropharynx, Neck, and Face MRI can be used to assess oropharyngeal anatomy if there is a concern of airway patency due to masses or mandibular and other facial malformations.

The exceptional degree of detail in fetal MRI helps determine whether an EXIT (*ex utero* intrapartum treatment) procedure is indicated and, if so, what should be done to secure the airway and manage the tumor during and after the procedure. T2-weighted MRI images in a normal fetus should demonstrate a hyperintense signal throughout the tracheal column, indicating a patent, fluid-filled airway. The absence of such a signal suggests complete high airway obstruction syndrome (CHAOS) as a result of the lesion, indicating that tracheostomy in conjunction with an EXIT procedure may be required. If a tracheostomy is deemed necessary, then the path of a severely deviated trachea may be predicted from the fetal MRI images.[42]

Thoracic Anomalies For malformations such as congenital pulmonary adenomatoid malformation or bronchopulmonary sequestration, MRI can be helpful if the fetal ultrasound cannot provide sufficient information for counseling or management.[43] The other most indicated thoracic anomaly for fetal MRI is a congenital diaphragmatic hernia. MRI can be used to evaluate lung volume and the presence of liver and intra-abdominal organs in the thorax adjunct to fetal ultrasound.

Urogenital Tract Ultrasound is the first-line imaging strategy to detect urogenital tract anomalies; however, MRI could be useful to detect the presence of severe oligohydramnios or anhydramnios. MRI can provide precise information about anatomical localization, borders, and the type of structure that can be helpful in clinical management.[45]

MRI and Placenta Accreta Spectrum

As a research tool, MRI has many applications in the investigation of the placenta. However, its clinical utility is mainly limited to placenta accreta spectrum (PAS) conditions.

The incidence of PAS has increased to 3 in 1000 live births over the last decades because of the inflation of cesarean deliveries.[46,47]

MRI cannot be used as a screening method for PAS. The utility of MRI in PAS has not been clarified yet. Routine use of MRI in PAS remains to be validated by prospective studies. In addition, there is a need for objective standardization and the creation of a reproducible prenatal staging system.[52-54]

The accuracy of MRI in PAS depends on the experience of the individuals who interpret the image and severity of the invasion.[56,57] MRI prediction of the degree of invasion remains challenging (**Figure 19.25**). The timing of imaging also affects

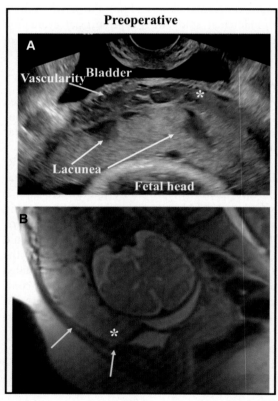
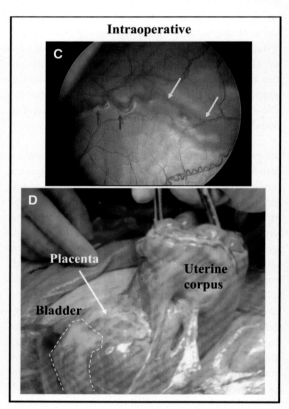

Figure 19.25 Patient with a history of four previous cesarean deliveries with placenta accreta spectrum. The depth of invasion was assessed using preoperative imaging. Two-dimensional (2D) ultrasound **(A)** showed bulge into the bladder, multiple lacunae (white arrows), loss of myometrium (asterisk), and increased vascularity (yellow arrows). The magnetic resonance imaging (MRI) findings **(B)** included a sagittal T2-weighted image in midline showing an anterior placenta without visible myometrium inferiorly (arrows), including adjacent to the urinary bladder with loss of the plane. There is a focal bulging of the placenta adjacent to the urinary bladder (asterisk). The intraoperative assessment via cystoscopy **(C)** showed increased vascularity in the bladder (blue arrows), which communicates with large submucosal blood vessels (yellow arrow). Classical hysterotomy away from the placenta was performed using a linear cutter.[48] After delivery **(D)**, the placenta was bulging out from the lower uterine segment. The bladder was pulled and severely adhered (dashed white line) over the placenta. The pathology report confirmed the bladder invasion.

the accuracy of the MRI. Studies suggest that MRI should be done before 30 weeks because a bulging placenta and thinned myometrium could be challenging to diagnose when the uterus is overstretched later in gestation.[52]

MRI examination for PAS is generally performed using a 1.5 T system. SNR can be maximized by using a phased-array coil.[58] With this protocol, the scanning time is generally 15-30 minutes. The bladder should be comfortably full to assess the degree of placental invasion to the bladder. T2-weighted sequences are more helpful than T1-weighted gradient-echo imaging because T2-weighted sequences give greater tissue contrast. However, T2 sequences have a higher risk of having motion artifacts.[59] The diagnostic MRI features of PAS include uterine bulging, lumpy contour, heterogeneous parenchymal signal intensity, the presence of dark intraplacental bands, and bladder tenting.[59,60]

KEY POINTS

- Prenatal diagnosis expertise requires familiarity with 3D/4D ultrasound and MRI to remain at the cutting edge of technology.
- 3D ultrasound provides data storage that can be accessed to reconstruct any desired image plane.
- Stored volumetric data can be reviewed by multiple examiners long after the examination has ended at any examination location.
- 4D ultrasound is 3D ultrasound with dynamic display of rendered images in real time.
- Postprocessing tools and optimization software in 3D/4D technology improve accuracy of the ultrasound examination.
- 3D ultrasound has been proven useful in the demonstration of complex facial anomalies.
- 3D/4D ultrasound has been promoted as a technique that enhances bonding between the fetus and its parents.
- 4D ultrasound has been proven to enhance accuracy of complex heart defects.
- 3D imaging gives precise information for skeletal abnormalities.
- MRI applications in obstetrics have been proven in the second half of pregnancy, but have limited use in the first trimester.
- Rapid scanning sequences available in modern MRI equipment have obviated the use of paralyzing agents for the fetus.
- Artifacts can be generated on MRI images by both fetal motion and maternal motion.
- The greatest application of MRI in the fetus to date has been in the CNS, with increasing applications in the chest and abdomen.
- The combination of ultrasound and MRI increases the accuracy of fetal diagnosis more than either modality alone.
- The initial evaluation of the placenta should be ultrasound. MRI cannot be used as a screening tool for placenta accreta spectrum
- The accuracy of MRI in the placenta accreta spectrum is strictly related to the experience of the reader.

REFERENCES

(only references cited in synoptic print chapter; for a complete reference list, see ebook)

2. Babucci G, Rosen K, Cappuccini B, Clerici G. 3D evaluation of fetal brain strucutres: reference values and growth curves. *J Matern Fetal Neonatal Med.* 2019;21:1-6. doi:10.1080/14767058.2019.1686477

3. AboEllail MA, Ishimura M, Sajapala S, et al. Three-dimensional color/power Doppler sonography and HD live silhouette mode for diagnosis of molar pregnancy. *J Ultrasound Med.* 2016;35(9):2049-2052.

4. Hata T, Mori N, Tenkumo C, Hanaoka U, Kanenishi K, Tanaka H. Three-dimensional volume-rendered imaging of normal and abnormal fetal fluid-filled structures using inversion mode. *J Obstet Gynaecol Res.* 2011;37(11):1748-1754.

5. Pashaj S, Merz E. Prenatal demonstration of normal variants of the pericallosal artery by 3D ultrasound. *Ultraschall Med.* 2014;35(2):129-136.

7. Araujo Júnior E, Martinez LH, Simioni C, Martins WP, Nardozza LM, Moron AF. Delineation of vertebral area on the coronal plane using three-dimensional ultrasonography advanced volume contrast imaging (VCI) Omni view: intrarater reliability and agreement using standard mouse, high definition mouse, and pen-tablet. *J Matern Fetal Neonatal Med.* 2012; 25(9):1818-1821.

10. American Institute of Ultrasound in Medicine. AIUM practice guideline for the performance of fetal echocardiography. *J Ultrasound Med.* 2013;32(6):1067-1082.

11. Turan S, Turan O, Baschat AA. Three- and four-dimensional fetal echocardiography. *Fetal Diagn Ther.* 2009;25(4):361-372.

13. Turan S, Turan OM, Ty-Torredes K, Harman CR, Baschat AA. Standardization of the first-trimester fetal cardiac examination using spatiotemporal image correlation with tomographic ultrasound and color Doppler imaging. *Ultrasound Obstet Gynecol.* 2009;33(6): 652-656.

14. Turan S, Turan OM, Desai A, Harman CR, Baschat AA. First-trimester fetal cardiac examination using spatiotemporal image correlation, tomographic ultrasound and color Doppler imaging for the diagnosis of complex congenital heart disease in high-risk patients. *Ultrasound Obstet Gynecol.* 2014;44(5):562-567.

21. Patenaude Y, Pugash D, Lim K, et al; Society of Obstetricians and Gynaecologists of Canada. The use of magnetic resonance imaging in the obstetric patient. 2014;36:349-363.

24. Gholipour A, Estroff JA, Barnewolt CE, et al. Fetal MRI: a technical update with educational aspirations. *Concepts Magn Reson Part A Bridg Educ Res.* 2014;43(6):237-266.

25. Manganaro L, Bernardo S, Antonelli A, Vinci V, Saldari M, Catalano C. Fetal MRI of the central nervous system: state-of-the-art. *Eur J Radiol.* 2017;93:273-283.

26. Clouchoux C, Limperopoulos C. Novel applications of quantitative MRI for the fetal brain. *Pediatr Radiol.* 2012;42(suppl 1):S24-S32.

27. Paladini D, Quarantelli M, Sglavo G, et al. Accuracy of neurosonography and MRI in the clinical management of fetuses referred with central nervous system abnormalities, *Ultrasound Obstet Gynecol.* 2014;44(2):188-196.

28. Glen OA. MR imaging of the fetal brain. *Pediatr Radiol.* 2010;40(1):68-81.

31. Ortega E, Muñoz R, Luza N, et al. The value of early and comprehensive diagnoses in a human fetus with hydrocephalus and progressive obliteration of the aqueduct of Sylvius: case report. *BMC Neurol.* 2016;16:45.

32. Manganaro L, Bernardo S, De Vito C, et al. Role of Fetal MRI in the evaluation of isolated and non-isolated corpus callosum dysgenesis: results of a cross-sectional study. *Prenat Diagn.* 2017;37(3):244-252.

33. Alby C, Malan V, Boutaud L, et al. Clinical, genetic and neuropathological findings in a series of 138 fetuses with a corpus callosum malformation. *Birth Defects Res A Clin Mol Teratol.* 2016;106(1):36-46.

36. Doneda C, Parazzini C, Righini A, et al. Early cerebral lesions in cytomegalovirus infection: prenatal MR imaging. *Radiology.* 2010;255(2):613-621.

37. Manganaro L, Bernardo S, La Barbera L, et al. Role of foetal MRI in the evaluation of ischaemic-haemorrhagic lesions of the foetal brain. *J Perinat Med.* 2012;40(4):419-426.

38. Wagner MW, Vaught AJ, Poretti A, Blakemore KJ, Huisman TA. Vein of galen aneurysmal malformation: prognostic markers depicted on fetal MRI. *Neuroradiol J.* 2015;28(1):72-75.

39. Lerman-Sagie T, Leibovitz Z. Malformations of cortical development: from postnatal to fetal imaging. *Can J Neurol Sci.* 2016;43(5):611-618.

40. Goel R, Aggarwal N, Lemmon ME, Bosemani T. Fetal and maternal manifestations of tuberous sclerosis complex: value of fetal MRI. *Neuroradiol J.* 2016;29(1):57-60.

41. Mirsky DM, Schwartz ES, Zarnow DM. Diagnostic features of myelomeningocele: the role of ultrafast fetal MRI. *Fetal Diagn Ther.* 2015;37(3):219-225.

42. Brodsky JR, Irace AL, Didas A, et al. Teratoma of the neonatal head and neck: a 41-year experience. *Int J Pediatr Otorhinolaryngol.* 2017;97:66-71.

43. Pacharn P, Kline-Fath B, Calvo-Garcia M, et al. Congenital lung lesions: prenatal MRI and postnatal findings. *Pediatr Radiol.* 2013; 43(9):1136-1143.

45. Alamo L, Laswad T, Schnyder P, Meuli R, Vial Y, Osterheld MC. Fetal MRI as a complement to the US in the diagnosis and characterization of anomalies of the genito-urinary tract. *Eur J Radiol.* 2010;76:258-264.

46. Silver RM, Landon MB, Rouse DJ, et al. Maternal morbidity associated with multiple repeat cesarean deliveries. *Obstet Gynecol.* 2006;107:1226-1232.

47. Wu S, Kocherginsky M, Hibbard JU. Abnormal placentation: twenty-year analysis. *Am J Obstet Gynecol.* 2005;192:1458-1461.

48. Turan OM, Shannon A, Asoglu MR, Goetzinger KR. A novel approach to reduce blood loss in patients with placenta accreta spectrum disorder. *J Matern Fetal Neonatal Med.* 2019:1-10. doi:10.1080/14767058.2019.16 56194

52. Familiari A, Liberati M, Lim P, et al. Diagnostic accuracy of magnetic resonance imaging in detecting the severity of abnormal invasive placenta: a systematic review and meta-analysis. *Acta Obstet Gynecol Scand.* 2018;97(5):507-520.

53. D'Antonio F, Iacovella C, Palacios-Jaraquemada J, Bruno CH, Manzoli L, Bhide A. Prenatal identification of invasive placentation using magnetic resonance imaging: systematic review and meta-analysis. *Ultrasound Obstet Gynecol.* 2014;44(1):8-16.

54. Finazzo F, D'Antonio F, Masselli G, et al. Interobserver variability in MRI assessment of the severity of placenta accrete spectrum disorders. *Ultrasound Obstet Gynecol.* 2020;55:467-473. doi:10.1002/uog.20381

56. Bhide A, Sebire N, Abuhamad A, Acharya G, Silver R. Morbidly adherent placenta: the need for standardization. *Ultrasound Obstet Gynecol.* 2017;49(5):559-563.

57. Alamo L, Anaye A, Rey J, et al. Detection of suspected placental invasion by MRI: do the results depend on observer' experience? *Eur J Radiol.* 2013;82(2):e51-e57.

58. Masselli G, Gualdi G. MR imaging of the placenta: what a radiologist should know. *Abdom Imaging.* 2013;38:573-587.

59. Kilcoyne A, Shenoy-Bhangle AS, Roberts DJ, Clark Sisodia R, Gervais DA, Lee SI. MRI of placenta accreta, placenta increta, and placenta percreta: pearls and pitfalls. *AJR Am J Roentgenol.* 2017;208:214-221.

60. Baughman WC, Corteville JE, Shah RR. Placenta accreta: spectrum of US and MR imaging findings. *Radiographics.* 2008;28:1905-1916.

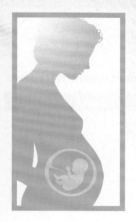

CHAPTER 20

Doppler Ultrasonography and Fetal Well-being

Allison Lankford and Ozhan M. Turan

Introduction

Physics of Doppler

There are several different methods of Doppler sonography used in obstetrics: continuous-wave Doppler, pulsed-wave Doppler, and color and power Doppler. These Doppler techniques differ in a number of ways. Continuous-wave Doppler is sensitive to small vessels and has no upper velocity limit. One drawback is that there is no spatial resolution because the reflected echoes from any moving structure within the ultrasound beam are detected. Continuous-wave Doppler is used in simple fetal heart rate detectors.[4] Pulsed-wave Doppler has the advantage of depth resolution and a variable sample volume. However, there must be sufficient time to characterize the Doppler shift frequency before the next pulse is emitted and, because of this, pulsed-wave Doppler is susceptible to aliasing. Color Doppler is a development of pulsed-wave Dopper where the frequency shift is mapped on the two-dimensional image. The flow toward and away from the transducer is plotted as different colors. Power Doppler is more sensitive than color Doppler for detection and demonstration of blood flow but could not provide information about the direction of the blood flow.[6] Doppler assessment of the maternal and fetal circulation in this chapter primarily focuses on pulsed-wave Doppler.

Doppler Indices

Nondimensional analysis of the flow waveform shape is useful to investigate many vascular beds and can provide information about the proximal (adult peripheral arterial circulation) and distal (fetal circulation) vascular changes.[7] The shape of the waveform can be considered a characteristic of the vascular site. For example, waveforms recorded from arteries supplying low-impedance vascular beds (umbilical and uterine arteries) exhibit relatively high forward velocities throughout diastole. The flow waveform may be described or characterized by the presence or absence of particular features, for example, in the absence of end-diastolic flow and the presence of a post-systolic notch. A triphasic waveform, where there is a period of reverse flow in diastole, is characteristic of vascular sites with high impedance to flow. In addition to the qualitative (shape) assessment of a Doppler waveform, quantitative (absolute velocity and volume flow) and semiquantitative (Doppler indices) measurements can be obtained from each vessel (**Table 20.1**).

Calculation of the absolute flow within a vessel using Doppler ultrasound is extremely challenging, and errors in calculation may arise due to the inaccurate measurement of the vessel cross-sectional area.[7] These errors are further exaggerated when flow calculations are made in small vessels. Therefore, clinicians rely on the semiquantitative Doppler indices in clinical practice. Commonly used semiquantitative Doppler indices include the resistance index (RI), pulsatility index (PI), and systolic/diastolic (S/D) ratio. Among these indices, the PI has a smaller measurement error, narrower reference limit, and is measurable when end-diastolic flow is absent, making it the preferred index. The indices are calculated as ratios between peak systolic velocity (PSV) (A), end-diastolic peak velocity (B), and mean velocity (mean) (**Figure 20.1**).[8]

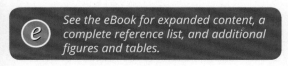

See the eBook for expanded content, a complete reference list, and additional figures and tables.

Table 20.1 Assessment of Maternal and Fetal Doppler Waveforms Using Different Assessment Methods

	Qualitative	Semiquantitative	Quantitative
Maternal			
Uterine artery	Notching Present, absent	Pulsatility index Resistance index	—
Fetal			
Umbilical artery	End-diastolic flow Present, absent, reversed	Pulsatility index Resistance index S/D ratio	—
Middle cerebral artery	—	Pulsatility index	Peak systolic velocity
Ductus venosus	a-wave Present, absent, reversed	Pulsatility index of vein	Velocity ratios S/v, S/D, S/a, v/D, D/a, v/a

a, atrial systole; D, diastolic; S, systolic; v, v-descent.

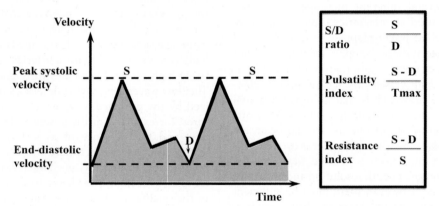

Figure 20.1 This figure depicts the calculation of the semiquantitative Doppler indices on an arterial waveform. The gray-filled area defines time-averaged maximum velocity (T_{max}). D, end diastole; S, peak systole.

Fetal Circulation

An understanding of the fetal circulation is essential to the interpretation and clinical application of Doppler techniques. In the fetus, gas exchange occurs in the placenta. Oxygenated blood from the placenta reaches the systemic fetal systemic circulation through a series of vascular shunts that preferentially divert blood away from the fetal lungs and limit the intermixing of oxygenated and deoxygenated blood that returns to the heart. In circumstances of fetal stress, compensatory mechanisms allow the redistribution of blood flow to critical organs such as the brain.

In the fetal circulation, the umbilical venous blood is the most highly oxygen-saturated blood. The umbilical vein enters the fetal abdomen and is directed to the porta hepatis and into the liver. A portion of the umbilical venous blood flow supplies the liver and the remainder passes through the ductus venosus (DV).[9] At the point where the umbilical vein joins the portal vein to the right, it divides so that a thicker walled DV continues upward and connects the umbilical vein-portal confluence to the inferior vena cava (IVC). In normal fetal development, approximately 50% of the umbilical blood flow passes through the DV and the remaining volume is diverted to the low-resistance hepatic circulation.[10]

Within the thoracic IVC, there are two streams of blood flow: the well-oxygenated blood from the DV and the less oxygenated blood from the abdominal IVC, which drains the lower body. These streams of blood do not mix, and the streaming of blood leads to preferential shunting of well-oxygenated blood from the DV through the foramen ovale toward the left atrium, bypassing the pulmonary circulation. A right-to-left shunt at the level of the foramen ovale allows the oxygenated and nutrient-rich blood to be delivered directly to the cephalic and coronary circulation.

Of the total blood volume that is returned to the right atrium from the thoracic IVC, approximately 40% crosses the foramen ovale to the left atrium and 60% enters the right ventricle across the tricuspid valve.[9] Blood from the hepatic circulation and the superior vena cava is also directed toward the right ventricle. The third vascular shunt, the DA (ductus arteriosus), directs approximately 90% of blood exiting from the right ventricle to the descending aorta. The descending aorta branches into the right and left hypogastric arteries, which distally become the umbilical arteries and return deoxygenated blood to the placenta (**Figure 20.2**).

Arterial Doppler Measurements

Uterine Artery Doppler
Uterine artery (UtA) Doppler assessment provides information about the maternal side of the placenta and acts as surrogate marker for effective trophoblastic invasion and remodeling of the maternal spiral arteries. The UtAs arise from the anterior division of internal iliac arteries and divide into the arcuate, radial, and spiral arteries. Impedance to blood flow in the UtAs decreases as gestational age advances with the development of a low-resistance vascular bed.

The initial fall in vascular resistance during the first and second trimesters is attributed to trophoblastic invasion of spiral arteries. The continued decrease in resistance in the UtAs into the third trimester may be explained by a hormonal effect on the elasticity of the arterial walls.[7] These physiologic changes in spiral arteries result in an increase in the end-diastolic flow of the uterine arteries.[11] Placental ischemic lesions and abnormal development of the spiral arteries may be depicted in the uterine arteries by increased resistance and/or presence of a diastolic notch, which is associated with hypertensive disorders of pregnancy (Chapter 27) and fetal growth restriction (FGR).[11] Color Doppler should be used to locate the UtAs as they cross medial to the external iliac arteries.[12] The region of interest revealed by Doppler should be magnified and a color box should be placed. The Doppler gate is placed within the straight portion of the UtA before it enters the myometrium.

Umbilical Artery Doppler
Umbilical artery (UA) Doppler is a reflection of villous branching in the fetal side of the placenta.

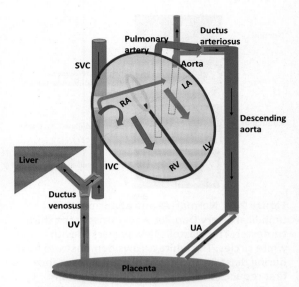

Figure 20.2 Depiction of fetal circulation. The umbilical vein (UV) carries the well-oxygenated blood from the placenta. A portion of the umbilical venous blood flow supplies the liver, and the remainder passes through the ductus venosus (DV) (depicted as green "Y"-shaped organ). Within the thoracic inferior vena cava (IVC), there are two blood flow streams: (1) the well-oxygenated blood from the DV (red arrow) and (2) the less oxygenated blood from the abdominal IVC. These bloodstreams do not mix, and the streaming of blood leads to preferential shunting of well-oxygenated blood from the DV through the foramen ovale (FO) toward the left atrium (LA). The well-oxygenated blood supplies vital organs such as the coronary artery and brain. Blood from the IVC and the superior vena cava (SVC) is directed toward the right ventricle (RV) (blue arrows). RV leads less oxygenated blood to the pulmonary artery (blue arrow). The flow in the pulmonary artery (blue) and aorta (red) mixes at the ductus arteriosus and continues as mixed oxygenated blood (purple) through the descending aorta. The descending aorta branches into the right and left hypogastric arteries, which distally become the umbilical arteries (UA) and return deoxygenated blood to the placenta.

During normal pregnancy, there is a progressive increase in end-diastolic velocity in the UA due to decreasing downstream impedance to flow as the placenta vessels grow. A review of normal ranges for UA measurements illustrates the importance of knowledge of gestational age before an index is

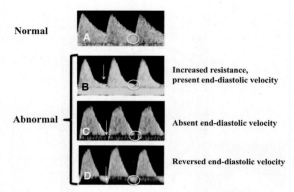

Normal

Abnormal

Increased resistance, present end-diastolic velocity

Absent end-diastolic velocity

Reversed end-diastolic velocity

Figure 20.6 Normal (A) and abnormal (B-D) umbilical artery Doppler waveforms in the third trimester. The diastolic flow is marked with white circles. The white arrows demonstrate flow during diastole. Increased placental resistance first reduces the blood flow during diastole (B). The blood flow stops during diastole (C) or moves backward (D) when the resistance in the placental bed is too high.

considered abnormal. Similar to UtA development, high resistance is seen in the UA in instances of incomplete trophoblastic invasion of maternal spiral arteries. Doppler indices in the UA generally do not start to increase until approximately 60% to 70% of the placental vascular tree is not functioning.[2] This highlights the presence of extensive disease before Doppler detection is possible, and emphasizes the reserve capacity of the placenta.[4] The abnormal UA Doppler waveform is characterized by a pattern of present, absent, or reversed diastolic flow velocities relative to the PSV (**Figure 20.6**).

UA Doppler assessment should be taken in a free-floating midcord segment because the location of the Doppler sampling site in the umbilical cord affects the Doppler waveform. The impedance indices are significantly higher at the fetal end of the cord compared to the placental cord insertion. The color box and magnification should target the area of interest only, and the pulsed Doppler gate should be positioned between the walls of the vessel. External compression of the UA by the transducer has the potential to affect the flow pattern by changing the vascular resistance.

Middle Cerebral Artery

The middle cerebral artery (MCA) arises from the circle of Willis and is the larger terminal branch of the internal carotid artery. Doppler velocimetry of the MCA allows the clinician to assess impedance

to blood flow in the fetal brain circulation. As gestational age advances, normal development leads to an increase in the PSV and average diastolic velocity in the MCA. In abnormal pregnancies, vasodilation of the MCA is considered to be a compensatory mechanism in the fetus to allow increased blood flow to the fetal brain circulation, and this phenomenon is referred to as the "brain-sparing effect." The resistance to blood flow within the vessel can be measured with the PI, which is used in the management of FGR. A reduced PI reflects vasodilation of the MCA. The PSV in the MCA can also be used in assessing fetal anemia and is accurate in any circumstance in which fetal anemia may occur, such as parvovirus infection, hemoglobinopathies, and rhesus alloimmunization.

Utilizing the correct technique to sample the MCA is critical for obtaining accurate measurements. The first step is to obtain a transverse view of the fetal brain at the level of the biparietal diameter. Using color flow imaging, the color box is placed over the region of interest. The MCA runs anterolaterally at the borderline between the anterior and middle cerebral fossae. The pulsed Doppler gate is placed over the vessel, as close as possible to its origin. The point of measurement is critical because the MCA-PSV decreases as the distance from the point of origin increases. The angle of insonation between the ultrasound beam and the direction of blood flow should be kept to 0°. It does not matter whether the near or far side vessel is interrogated. While angle of correction is not necessary when measuring the MCA-PI, PSV measurement should use angle correction and the angle of incidence should be <30°; optimally as close to 0° as possible. Angle correction can be used to measure PSV in the fetal MCA.

The region of interest should be magnified so that the MCA occupies more than 50% of the screen, and the full length of the MCA should be visualized. Fetal breathing and excessive pressure on the fetal head by the transducer may change the MCA waveform. The highest PSV value should be measured, and these steps should be repeated at least three times to improve the accuracy and reproducibility of the measured PSV.[15]

Venous Doppler Assessment

Ductus Venosus

Doppler ultrasonography of the fetal venous circulation has improved our understanding of numerous fetal diseases, and this chapter focuses on the assessment of the DV and the umbilical vein. The DV is different from the hepatic vein and the IVC in that there is a persistence of forward flow throughout the cardiac cycle and retrograde flow during diastole is only seen in pathologic conditions.

The DV is a critical vascular shunt *in utero* that directs oxygenated blood from the umbilical vein to the IVC. Because the DV regulates the amount of umbilical venous return that flows into the heart, it is a direct reflection of cardiac function. As a fetus becomes significantly hypoxemic, myocardial contractility and cardiac output decrease due to increase in right ventricular end-diastolic pressure consequent to an increase in right ventricular afterload. These changes in fetal cardiovascular hemodynamics are reflected in the DV waveform. The DV has a multiphasic blood flow pattern, which depicts cardiac pressure and volume changes in the heart: systolic ventricular ejection (S), declining venous

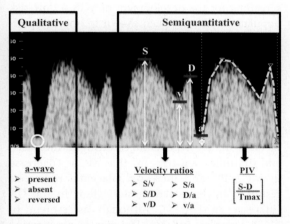

Figure 20.8 Assessment of the ductus venosus waveform. Ventricular systole (S), diastole (D), the opening of atrioventricular valves (v), and atrial contraction (a) were marked on the waveform. Individual velocities can be measured from the maximum velocity of each wave (blue horizontal lines) to baseline. Double-headed white arrows represents individual velocities. A qualitative assessment based on a-wave is demonstrated with the white circle. The a-wave could be present, absent, or reversed. The semiquantitative assessment could be performed tracing a single waveform (yellow dashed line). The ultrasound machine can calculate the pulsatility index of the vein using S, D, and T_{max} (time-averaged maximum velocity). Another semiquantitative assessment is the velocity ratios (S/D, S/v, v/D, S/a, D/a, v/a).

velocities as the ventricles reach the end of systole (v-descent), diastolic velocities (D), and atrial contraction (a-wave) (**Figure 20.8**).

The primary assessment of the DV flow velocity waveform is PI velocity (PIV) that predominantly reflect S/a and to a lesser degree D/a and S/D velocity relationships, or by qualitative analysis focusing on the a-wave. These assessments have limitations in assessing the primary underlying cardiac functional component when the Doppler index is elevated.[16,17] The recognition of distinct venous waveform patterns provides a better understanding of fetal cardiovascular physiology. The a-wave abnormalities are a sensitive marker of impaired venous forward flow but less specific as to the underlying mechanism. In contrast, v-wave abnormalities may be more specific for myocardial relaxation and compliance issues, which would be compromised in FGR. The D-wave abnormalities reflect global diastolic venous dysfunction that is common in right-sided heart defects.[18]

The origin of the DV from the umbilical vein should be identified in a midsagittal view of the upper abdomen or in a cross-sectional plane of the abdomen at the level of the stomach. The color flow box should be applied to the area of the DV, and the portion of the DV with the highest velocity should be identified. This area is identified by looking for an aliasing effect where the blood flow velocity accelerates due to the narrow lumen of the DV. A pulsed-wave Doppler gate of 1 mm in width should be placed over this area, and the waveform should be obtained with the smallest possible angle of insonation. When five constant waveforms with a good signal-to-noise ratios are obtained, the frozen image can be traced, outlining the waveform from the beginning of ventricular systole to the end of atrial systole.[18] The DV waveform is influenced by several intrinsic fetal factors including fetal breathing movements, behavioral states, and cardiac arrhythmias. The DV should be sampled during fetal rest and in the absence of fetal breathing.

Umbilical Vein

The umbilical vein (UV) delivers the oxygenated and nutrient-rich blood from the placenta to the fetus, maintaining a continuous nonpulsatile flow velocity profile throughout the pregnancy. The UV is easy to measure by means of Doppler velocimetry as it courses along with the umbilical arteries. Variations in the UV Doppler waveforms may be demonstrated and will be discussed below in the context of pathologic clinical conditions. The UV should be measured in a free-loop midcord segment with proper magnification. Reduced velocity in the UV typically indicates increased resistance and reduced blood flow through the vein.

Doppler Ultrasound in Normal Pregnancies

First-Trimester Screening for Chromosomal Abnormalities and Congenital Heart Defects

The use of fetal Doppler at the first trimester as a screening tool for certain conditions has shown to be effective.

Multiple authors have suggested that one way to utilize the DV in the first trimester is by using a two-step screening approach. This method may reduce the false-positive rates in fetuses that are considered at increased risk based on nuchal translucency and serum analyte screening and can be used to identify chromosomally normal fetuses that require fetal echocardiogram in the first and second trimesters.[20-24]

The pathophysiologic mechanism explaining abnormal DV waveform patterns in fetuses with increased nuchal translucency and CHD is not completely understood. Several proposed mechanisms include underlying cardiac dysfunction with reduced myocardial compliance and fluid accumulation; impaired neural crest cell migration to the neck and conotruncus secondary to a hypoxic insult; and abnormal innervation or endothelial thickening of the DV.[25-28] In fetuses with normal nuchal translucency measurements, abnormalities in the DV waveform are associated with adverse pregnancy outcomes, including cardiovascular defects, FGR, renal anomalies, and perinatal death.[24] Identification of abnormalities in the DV waveform in the first trimester should be a clue to the clinician that such pregnancies should be monitored closely, and additional surveillance may include fetal echocardiography and third-trimester growth ultrasound in addition to the routine detailed anatomic review at 18 to 20 weeks' gestation.

Early Screening for Preeclampsia and FGR

UtA Doppler has been investigated as screening tool to identify women at risk for developing preeclampsia and/or FGR. Both conditions are thought to be a consequence of impaired trophoblastic invasion of the maternal spiral arteries resulting in an increased vascular resistance in the placental bed. The UtAs provide information regarding the maternal side of the placenta and reflect the effectiveness of trophoblastic invasion. Although the findings of elevated UtA-PI at 22 to 24 weeks may help predict pregnancies at risk for preeclampsia and FGR and result in increased surveillance, it may be too late to implement preventive measures.

A combination of maternal risk factors, mean arterial pressure, UtA Doppler, and maternal serum markers (ie, pregnancy-associated plasma protein A and placental growth factor) identify about 95% of cases of early-onset preeclampsia with a false-positive rate of 10%.[31,32]

Assessment of the uteroplacental circulation by transabdominal ultrasound is feasible starting in the first trimester and may provide a window for early intervention to prevent the most severe forms of preeclampsia and FGR. Although UtA Doppler can be used as a screening tool, routine UA Doppler screening for the development of FGR in low-risk populations has not been shown to improve perinatal outcomes.[13]

Screening for Adverse Perinatal Outcomes Using the Cerebroplacental Ratio

The cerebroplacental ratio (CPR) is a reflection of cerebral vasodilation as a compensatory mechanism for hypoxemia resulting in increased end-diastolic velocity in the MCA (decrease in MCA-PI) and increased placental resistance resulting in decreased diastolic flow in the UA (increase in UA-PI). Although assessment of MCA Doppler and UA Doppler is not routine in low-risk pregnancies in the United States, the CPR may be an important predictor for intrapartum fetal compromise.[34] The CPR is calculated by dividing the Doppler indices of the MCA and umbilical artery UA. A CPR PI <1.08 or less than the 5th percentile for gestational age is considered abnormal.[35-39] In fetuses that were AGA, an abnormal CPR before active labor predicted intrapartum fetal compromise with fetal distress and need for emergency cesarean delivery and academia at birth.[34,40] The clinical application of CPR evaluation during the third trimester of pregnancy for fetuses whose weights are greater than the 10th percentile is uncertain. Several studies have demonstrated that AGA fetuses have a higher incidence of adverse perinatal outcomes when they have a higher CPR. Further studies are needed to determine if late third-trimester evaluation of growth as well as Doppler measurements, including the CPR, should be incorporated into routine antenatal care.

Doppler Ultrasound in Abnormal Pregnancies

Fetal Anemia

Investigation of the MCA-PSV is a powerful and noninvasive technique to assess the presence of fetal anemia.[42] As fetal hemoglobin decreases, the MCA-PSV increases due to increased cardiac output and decreased blood viscosity.[43]

Assessment of MCA-PSV should be considered in any fetal disease associated with anemia. A value of greater than 1.5 multiple of the median (MoM) for the MCA-PSV indicates the need for additional investigation of fetal hemoglobin using cordocentesis and possible intrauterine transfusion. MCA-PSV is a sensitive marker to predict fetal anemia, and it has been shown to decrease to normal reference ranges after fetal anemia has been corrected through intrauterine transfusion.[44,45] Therefore, MCA-PSV can be used both at the time of diagnosis and to monitor the fetal response after intrauterine blood transfusion.

Fetal Growth Restriction

FGR, defined as sonographic estimated fetal weight (EFW) or abdominal circumference (AC) less than the 10th percentile for gestational age, is associated with increased perinatal morbidity and mortality and poor long-term health outcomes.[46,47]

In this chapter, we will focus on uteroplacental origins of FGR because of the critical role of maternal and fetal Doppler assessment to prevent adverse perinatal outcomes.

It is widely accepted that there are two types of FGR: early onset and late onset.

When a fetus is exposed to chronic intrauterine stress and hypoxia, such as in cases of FGR, Doppler ultrasound can be used to assess predictable adaptations in the fetal circulation. The defense and compensatory mechanisms in the fetus include preferential preservation of fetal growth over placental growth, redistribution of blood flow, changes in fetal movement patterns, and eventual deceleration in the fetal heart rate.[50] The characteristics of cardiovascular manifestations (ie, redistribution

of blood flow to the brain, heart, and adrenals) are determined by the gestational age at onset and the severity of placental disease.[51] Doppler abnormalities in these vascular territories display a sequential pattern of disease progression and reflect an initial attempt at compensation for intrauterine hypoxia with eventual decompensation, followed by fetal academia and death. A temporal pattern of disease progression is as follows: decrease in fetal growth, fetal polycythemia, flow redistribution favoring vital organs, decreased amniotic fluid secondary to reduced blood flow to the kidneys, absent end-diastolic flow in the UA, loss of fetal movement, loss of fetal heart rate variability, reversed end-diastolic flow in the UA, reversed a-wave in the DV, fetal circulatory collapse, and fetal death.[50,51]

Early-Onset FGR

Diminished trophoblastic villous vascular area results in increased UA resistance starting in the second trimester.[52] UA velocimetry is one of the most valuable tools for predicting perinatal outcome in the fetus with growth restriction and should be used as part of antepartum surveillance and to help guide timing of delivery.[13] UA Doppler studies should be initiated when FGR is suspected and at a gestational age when the pregnancy is considered viable.[13] Different UA waveform patterns identify worsening degrees of placental insufficiency. With increasing resistance in the fetoplacental circulation, the UA waveform progresses from absent end-diastolic velocities (UA-AEDF) to reversed end-diastolic velocities (UA-REDF). The findings of AEDF or REDF are associated with increased fetal and neonatal mortality and higher incidence of long term neurologic impairment when compared to fetuses with diastolic flow in the UA.[53,54]

The MCA is also an appealing fetal vessel to investigate during intrauterine hypoxia because fetuses divert the oxygenated and nutritionally rich blood to the brain through vasodilation of the cerebral vasculature. This phenomenon is known as "brain sparing" and can be measured with MCA Doppler indices. Alterations from a high-resistance cerebral circulation to a low-resistance state with increased diastolic flow are measured with MCA-PI. Fetuses with FGR that display evidence of brain sparing (MCA-PI < 5th percentile) and have normal UA Doppler studies have a higher risk of poor neurodevelopmental outcomes.[55] Although this compensatory mechanism is commonly seen in early FGR, assessment of MCA Doppler indices has not been evaluated in randomized controlled trials and its relation to the timing of delivery is unclear.

Central venous Doppler defines changes in cardiac loading and contractility, and changes in the DV and UV identify fetuses at an advanced stage of compromise. Absent or reversed flow in the atrial contraction phase of the DV waveform is associated with fetal academia, perinatal morbidity, and perinatal and neonatal mortality.[56] In addition, the duration of absent or reversed flow during atrial systole in the DV is a strong predictor of stillbirth. The time interval between the diagnosis of absent/reversed a-wave and fetal death is approximately 5 days, irrespective of gestational age.[57] When the DV and UA Doppler studies become abnormal, the risk of stillbirth increases dramatically and the combined use of arterial and venous Doppler studies in investigating pregnancies affected by FGR may help identify fetuses with acidemia.[58]

Antepartum fetal surveillance in FGR should be a multimodal approach and include arterial and venous Doppler, the biophysical profile, and computerized cardiotocograph (cCTG) analysis of short-term variability (STV) in the fetal heart rate assessment.[59]

Late-Onset FGR

Late-onset FGR is also associated with increased perinatal morbidity in the form of fetal distress, hypoglycemia, seizures, behavioral problems, cerebral palsy, and cardiovascular disease.[69] Although late-onset FGR is more common than early-onset FGR, it is more challenging to diagnose.[70] The threshold for clinicians to deliver is decreased as neonatal mortality declines significantly after 32 weeks' gestation. The CPR may be used as a marker of failure of a fetus to reach its growth potential at term and may help to identify fetuses at risk for stillbirth.[70] In addition, fetuses with CPR less than the 10th percentile are more likely to be delivered by cesarean delivery for presumed fetal compromise. CPR also is an independent risk factor for neonatal intensive care unit admission.[34,71] Consideration should be given to fetal arterial Doppler assessment in late-onset FGR and may be a valuable tool in detecting fetal hypoxemia secondary to placental insufficiency. Venous Doppler information has not contributed any useful information in assessing late-onset FGR.

Fetal Hydrops

Cardiac Disease–Related Nonimmune Fetal Hydrops

In both structural and functional cardiac causes of NIHF, abnormal venous flow (absent/reversed a-wave in DV and pulsatile flow in the umbilical vein) is strongly associated with mortality.[79] Therefore, detailed venous Doppler evaluation is essential. In cases of structural defects, delivery is the only option in the context of appropriate gestational age. In cases of fetal arrhythmias that are treated with maternal antiarrhythmic therapy, venous Doppler is a useful tool to monitor treatment response. The disappearance of the reversed a-wave in the DV is one of the first signs of successful cardioversion and is often evident before normalization of the heart rate.[77]

Noncardiac Disease–Related Nonimmune Fetal Hydrops

In these cases, MCA-PSV can provide information regarding the degree of fetal anemia, whereas DV and UA Doppler indices will indicate the level of cardiac compromise. Fetal thoracic tumors, congenital pulmonary adenomatoid malformations, and congenital diaphragmatic hernias are all space-occupying lesions that may compress the heart, limit its function, and impair venous return. Evidence of heart failure in these cases will be evident by changes in the DV waveform.

When NIHF is identified in the absence of structural or functional cardiac disease, several additional studies should be considered in conjunction with a detailed Doppler assessment.

Complicated Monochorionic Twins

Twin-to-Twin Transfusion Syndrome

Arterial and venous Doppler assessment has been used in the staging and diagnosis of twin-to-twin transfusion syndrome (TTTS). It is also an important tool to determine monitoring intervals after treatment. The Quintero staging system of TTTS incorporates the use of Doppler and provides prognostic value.[82] Stages I and II are characterized by oligo-polyhydramnios sequence, and in these stages, arterial Doppler and venous Doppler are normal. In stages III and IV, Doppler studies become severely abnormal. Hypervolemia in the recipient results in increased preload and impaired diastolic ventricular filling, and hypovolemia in the donor leads to systemic vasoconstriction. The donor twin will show arterial abnormalities with the absent end-diastolic flow in the UA and/or the recipient will show signs of venous abnormalities such as absent or reversed a-wave in the DV or pulsatile umbilical venous flow.[82,83]

Venous Doppler indices are also useful to monitor response to treatment. Fetoscopic laser coagulation of vascular anastomoses aims to provide definitive therapy for the treatment of TTTS. After successful fetoscopic laser surgery, normalization of a reversed a-wave and noticeable decline in the DV-PIV in the recipient can be seen, and complete recovery from cardiac compromise becomes more apparent by the end of the fourth week after treatment. In contrast, the donor may show signs of impaired cardiac function with abnormal venous flow and tricuspid regurgitation immediately after successful laser treatment.[81] These Doppler changes typically disappear within a couple of weeks and are due to the development of a related state of hypervolemia and abrupt change in cardiac afterload in the donor twin.[84]

Selective Fetal Growth Restriction

Selective fetal growth restriction (sFGR) has been described in three different clinical subtypes, according to UA Doppler findings: type I, UA Doppler with positive end-diastolic flow; type II, persistent absent or reversed end-diastolic flow; and type III, intermittent absent or reversed end-diastolic flow[87] (**Figure 20.11**). Type I pregnancies represented the lower end of the spectrum of severity with a relatively favorable prognosis. However, close follow-up with UA Doppler assessment is essential to exclude progression to type II or III. Type II pregnancies are characterized by a more severe form of placental discordance, which may explain the early onset of UA-AEDF. The progression of Doppler patterns in type II sFGR

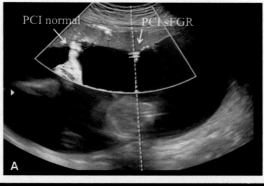

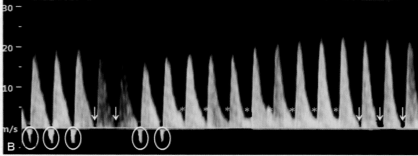

Figure 20.11 Diagnosis of type III selective fetal growth restriction (sFGR) using umbilical artery Doppler at the placental cord insertion (PCI) of the growth restricted fetus. A, PCIs of normal and growth-restricted fetuses are labeled. The Doppler gate (green box) and gate (dashed yellow line) placed over the PCI. In the presence of arterial-to-arterial anastomoses, the blood flow shifts from one side to another for a short period. B, Reduced speed of the waveform allows documenting this blood flow shift in one step, as reversed (white circles), absent (white arrows), and present (white asterisks) end-diastolic flow at the same time.

is similar to what is seen in singletons with early-onset FGR, and the presence of abnormal DV Doppler (reversed a-wave) is critically important for allowing timely intervention or delivery. Type III is a unique condition in that there is an atypical, unpredictable evolution of Doppler changes that presents significant challenges in identifying fetal deterioration.[88] Intermittent absent end-diastolic flow occurs due to bidirectional flow in large artery-to-artery anastomoses.[87] Management of type III is always more challenging than with types I and II due to an increased risk of unexpected fetal death, which is about 15%. None of the other arterial or venous Doppler techniques have been shown to provide useful prognostic information in managing type III sFGR.

Twin Anemia-Polycythemia Sequence

MCA-PSV is the key Doppler assessment for diagnosing twin anemia-polycythemia sequence (TAPS). Suggested antenatal diagnostic criteria for TAPS include an MCA-PSV > 1.5 MoM in the donor consistent with fetal anemia and MCA-PSV < 1.0 MoM for the recipient, which is consistent with polycythemia. Routine assessment of MCA-PSVs in monochorionic twin pregnancies should begin early and occur on regular bases (at least every 2 weeks).[89] Due to the heterogeneity of the disease, predicting perinatal outcomes is challenging. Several management strategies have been proposed and include expectant management, delivery, intrauterine fetal transfusion, selective reduction, and fetoscopic laser coagulation.

KEY POINTS

- Continuous-wave Doppler is sensitive to small vessels and has no upper velocity limit, which is a significant advantage. However, it cannot provide spatial resolution.
- Color Doppler is a development of pulsed-wave Dopper where the frequency shift is mapped on the two-dimensional image. The flow toward and away from the transducer is plotted as different colors.
- Power Doppler is more sensitive than color Doppler for detection and demonstration of blood flow but could not provide information about the direction of the blood flow.
- Doppler ultrasound measurements may be used to determine the presence of flow and the direction of flow, identify time-varying velocity characteristics, and detect velocity disturbances.
- Commonly used semiquantitative Doppler indices include the RI, PI, and S/D ratio. The PI has a smaller measurement error, has narrower reference limit, and is measurable when the end-diastolic flow is absent.
- In the fetal circulation, two blood flow streams run without mixing in the thoracic IVC: (1) well-oxygenated blood from the DV and (2) less oxygenated blood from the abdominal IVC, which drains the lower body. The well-oxygenated blood from the DV passes through the foramen ovale toward the left atrium.

- UtA Doppler assessment provides information about the maternal side of the placenta and acts as a surrogate marker for effective trophoblastic invasion and remodeling of the maternal spiral arteries.
- UA Doppler is a reflection of villous branching in the fetal side of the placenta.
- UA Doppler assessment should be taken in a free-floating midcord segment. This is because the impedance indices are significantly higher at the fetal end of the cord compared to the placental cord insertion.
- An angle correction is not necessary when measuring the MCA-PI. However, the angle correction should be used and the angle should optimally be as close to 0° as possible (<30°) during the measurement of the PSV.
- The DV directly reflects cardiac function.
- The DV a-wave abnormalities are a sensitive marker of impaired venous forward flow but less specific as to the underlying mechanism. In contrast, v-wave abnormalities may be more specific for myocardial relaxation and compliance issues, which would be compromised in FGR. The D-wave abnormalities reflect global diastolic venous dysfunction that is common in right-sided heart defects.
- In fetuses with normal nuchal translucency measurements, abnormalities in the DV waveform are associated with adverse

pregnancy outcomes, including cardiovascular defects, FGR, renal anomalies, and perinatal death.

- Assessment of the uteroplacental circulation by transabdominal ultrasound is feasible, starting in the first trimester, and may provide a window for early intervention to prevent the most severe forms of preeclampsia and FGR.
- The clinical application of CPR evaluation during the third trimester of pregnancy for fetuses whose weights are greater than the 10th percentile is uncertain.
- Investigation of the MCA-PSV is a powerful and noninvasive technique to assess the presence of fetal anemia.
- Umbilical Doppler studies should be initiated when FGR is suspected and at a gestational age when the pregnancy is considered viable.
- DV absent or reversed flow is a strong predictor of stillbirth in early-onset FGR. The time interval between the diagnosis

of absent/reversed a-wave and fetal death is approximately 5 days, irrespective of gestational age.

- Antepartum fetal surveillance in FGR should be a multimodal approach and include arterial and venous Doppler, the biophysical profile, and cCTG analysis of STV in the fetal heart rate assessment.
- After 32 weeks' gestation, UA Doppler plays a critical role in determining the delivery timing in early-onset FGR.
- Although late-onset FGR is more common than early-onset FGR, it is more challenging to diagnose.
- In nonimmune hydrops, an abnormal venous flow (in DV or umbilical vein) is strongly associated with mortality.
- Arterial and venous Doppler assessment has been used in the staging and diagnosis of TTTS. It is also an important tool to determine monitoring intervals after treatment.

REFERENCES

(only references cited in synoptic print chapter; for a complete reference list, see ebook)

2. Alfirevic Z, Stampalija T, Gyte GM. Fetal and umbilical Doppler ultrasound in high-risk pregnancies. In: The Cochrane Collaboration , ed. *Cochrane Database of Systematic Reviews*. John Wiley & Sons, Ltd; 2010. doi:10.1002/14651858.CD007529.pub2

4. Trudinger BJ. *Doppler ultrasonography and fetal well-being*. In: *Clinical Obstetrics*. John Wiley & Sons, Ltd; 2008:561-585. https://onlinelibrary.wiley.com/doi/abs/10.1002/9780470753293.ch31. Accessed May 25, 2019.

6. Nelson T, Pretorius D. The Doppler signal: where does it come from and what does it mean? *Am J Roentgenol*. 1988;151(3):439-447. doi:10.2214/ajr.151.3.439

7. Nicolaides K, Rizzo G, Hecher K, Ximenes R. *Doppler in Obstetrics*. The Fetal Medicine Foundation & ISUOG; 2002. Accessed February 11, 2020. https://fetalmedicine.org/var/uploads/Doppler-in-Obstetrics.pdf.

8. Burns PN. Principles of Doppler and color flow. *Radiol Med*. 1993;85(5 suppl 1):3-16.

9. Creasy RK, Resnik R, Iams JD, Lockwood CJ, Moore T, Greene MF. *Creasy and Resnik's Maternal-Fetal Medicine: Principles and Practice E-Book*. Elsevier Health Sciences; 2013..

10. Edelstone DI, Rudolph AM, Heymann MA. Liver and ductus venosus blood flows in fetal lambs in utero. *Circ Res*. 1978;42(3):426-433.

11. Ferrazzi E, Bulfamante G, Mezzopane R, Barbera A, Ghidini A, Pardi G. Uterine Doppler velocimetry and placental hypoxic-ischemic lesion in pregnancies with fetal intrauterine growth restriction. *Placenta*. 1999;20(5-6):389-394. doi:10.1053/plac.1999.0395

12. Arduini D, Rizzo G, Boccolini MR, Romanini C, Mancuso S. Functional assessment of uteroplacental and fetal circulations by means of color Doppler ultrasonography. *J Ultrasound Med*. 1990;9(5):249-253.

13. Berkley E, Chauhan SP, Abuhamad A. Doppler assessment of the fetus with intrauterine growth restriction. *Am J Obstet Gynecol*. 2012;206(4):300-308. doi:10.1016/j.ajog.2012.01.022

15. Detti L, Mari G. Noninvasive diagnosis of fetal anemia. *Clin Obstet Gynecol*. 2003;46(4):923-930.

16. Baschat AA, Turan OM, Turan S. Ductus venosus blood-flow patterns: more than meets the eye? *Ultrasound Obstet Gynecol*. 2012;39(5):598-599. doi:10.1002/uog.10151

17. Sanapo L, Turan OM, Turan S, Ton J, Atlas M, Baschat AA. Correlation analysis of ductus venosus velocity indices and fetal cardiac function: ductus venosus waveform and fetal cardiac function. *Ultrasound Obstet Gynecol*. 2014;43(5):515-519. doi:10.1002/uog.13242

18. Turan OM, Turan S, Sanapo L, Rosenbloom JI, Baschat AA. Semiquantitative classification of ductus venosus blood flow patterns: ductus venosus waveform patterns. *Ultrasound Obstet Gynecol*. 2014;43(5):508-514. doi:10.1002/uog.13207

20. Antolín E, Comas C, Torrents M, et al. The role of ductus venosus blood flow assessment in screening for chromosomal abnormalities at 10-16 weeks of gestation: ductus venosus blood flow and chromosomal abnormalities. *Ultrasound Obstet Gynecol*. 2001;17(4):295-300. doi:10.1046/j.1469-0705.2001.00395.x

21. Timmerman E, Clur SA, Pajkrt E, Bilardo CM. First-trimester measurement of the ductus venosus pulsatility index and the prediction of congenital heart defects. *Ultrasound Obstet Gynecol*. 2010;36(6):668-675. doi:10.1002/uog.7742

22. Bilardo CM, Müller MA, Zikulnig L, Schipper M, Hecher K. Ductus venosus studies in fetuses at high risk for chromosomal or heart abnormalities: relationship with nuchal translucency measurement and fetal outcome. *Ultrasound Obstet Gynecol*. 2001;17(4):288-294.

23. Maiz N, Valencia C, Emmanuel EE, Staboulidou I, Nicolaides KH. Screening for adverse pregnancy outcome by ductus venosus Doppler at 11–13+6 Weeks of gestation. *Obstet Gynecol*. 2008;112(3):598-605. doi:10.1097/AOG.0b013e3181834608

24. Oh C, Harman C, Baschat AA. Abnormal first-trimester ductus venosus blood flow: a risk factor for adverse outcome in fetuses with normal nuchal translucency. *Ultrasound Obstet Gynecol*. 2007;30(2):192-196. doi:10.1002/uog.4034

25. Bekker MN, Arkesteijn JB, van den Akker NM, et al. Increased NCAM expression and vascular development in trisomy 16 mouse embryos: relationship with nuchal translucency. *Pediatr Res*. 2005;58(6):1222. doi:10.1203/01.pdr.0000187795.82497.31

26. Clur SAB, Oude Rengerink K, Mol BWJ, Ottenkamp J, Bilardo CM. Fetal cardiac function between 11 and 35 weeks' gestation and nuchal translucency thickness. *Ultrasound Obstet Gynecol.* 2011;37(1):48-56. doi:10.1002/uog.8807

27. Coceani F, Adeagbo AS, Cutz E, Olley PM. Autonomic mechanisms in the ductus venosus of the lamb. *Am J Physiol.* 1984;247(1):H17-H24. doi:10.1152/ajpheart.1984.247.1.H17

28. Nakamura T, Gulick J, Colbert MC, Robbins J. Protein tyrosine phosphatase activity in the neural crest is essential for normal heart and skull development. *Proc Natl Acad Sci USA.* 2009;106(27):11270-11275. doi:10.1073/pnas.0902230106

31. Poon LC, Nicolaides KH. Early prediction of preeclampsia. *Obstet Gynecol Int.* 2014;2014:1-11. doi:10.1155/2014/297397

32. Poon LC, Shennan A, Hyett JA, et al. The International Federation of Gynecology and Obstetrics (FIGO) initiative on pre-eclampsia: a pragmatic guide for first-trimester screening and prevention. *Int J Gynecol Obstet.* 2019;145(suppl 1):1-33. doi:10.1002/ijgo.12802

34. Prior T, Mullins E, Bennett P, Kumar S. Prediction of intrapartum fetal compromise using the cerebroumbilical ratio: a prospective observational study. *Am J Obstet Gynecol.* 2013;208(2):124.e1-124.e6. doi:10.1016/j.ajog.2012.11.016

35. Arbeille P, Body G, Saliba E, et al. Fetal cerebral circulation assessment by Doppler ultrasound in normal and pathological pregnancies. *Eur J Obstet Gynecol Reprod Biol.* 1988;29(4):261-273. doi:10.1016/0028-2243(88)90066-4

36. Arias F. Accuracy of the middle-cerebral-to-umbilical-artery resistance index ratio in the prediction of neonatal outcome in patients at high risk for fetal and neonatal complications. *Am J Obstet Gynecol.* 1994;171(6):1541-1545. doi:10.5555/uri:pii:0002937894903980

37. Baschat AA, Gembruch U. The cerebroplacental Doppler ratio revisited. *Ultrasound Obstet Gynecol.* 2003;21(2):124-127. doi:10.1002/uog.20

38. Gramellini D, Folli MC, Raboni S, Vadora E, Merialdi A. Cerebral-umbilical Doppler ratio as a predictor of adverse perinatal outcome. *Obstet Gynecol.* 1992;79(3):416-420. doi:10.1097/00006250-199203000-00018

39. Odibo AO, Riddick C, Pare E, Stamilio DM, Macones GA. Cerebroplacental Doppler ratio and adverse perinatal outcomes in intrauterine growth restriction. *J Ultrasound Med.* 2005;24(9):1223-1228. doi:10.7863/jum.2005.24.9.1223

40. Morales-Roselló J, Khalil A, Morlando M, Bhide A, Papageorghiou A, Thilaganathan B. Poor neonatal acid-base status in term fetuses with low cerebroplacental ratio. *Ultrasound Obstet Gynecol.* 2015;45(2):156-161. doi:10.1002/uog.14647

42. Mari G, Deter RL, Carpenter RL. Noninvasive diagnosis by Doppler ultrasonography of fetal anemia due to maternal red-cell alloimmunization. Collaborative Group for Doppler Assessment of the Blood Velocity in Anemic Fetuses. *N Engl J Med.* 2000;342(1):9-14.

43. Fan FC, Chen RY, Schuessler GB, Chien S. Effects of hematocrit variations on regional hemodynamics and oxygen transport in the dog. *Am J Physiol.* 1980;238(4):H545-H522.

44. Pretlove S, Fox C, Khan K, Kilby M. Noninvasive methods of detecting fetal anaemia: a systematic review and meta-analysis. Noninvasive methods of detecting fetal anaemia. *Br J Obstet Gynaecol.* 2009;116(12):1558-1567. doi:10.1111/j.1471-0528.2009.02255.x

45. Stefos T, Cosmi E, Detti L, Mari G. Correction of fetal anemia on the middle cerebral artery peak systolic velocity. *Obstet Gynecol.* 2002;99(2):211-215. doi:10.1016/S0029-7844(01)01724-0

46. American College of Obstetricians and Gynecologists' Committee on Practice Bulletins—Obstetrics and the Society for Maternal-FetalMedicin. ACOG Practice Bulletin No. 204: Fetal growth restriction. *Obstet Gynecol.* 2019;133:e97-109.

47. Garite TJ, Clark R, Thorp JA. Intrauterine growth restriction increases morbidity and mortality among premature neonates. *Am J Obstet Gynecol.* 2004;191(2):481-487. doi:10.1016/j.ajog.2004.01.036

50. Maulik D, Mundy D, Heitmann E, Maulik D. Evidence-based approach to umbilical artery Doppler fetal surveillance in high-risk pregnancies: an update. *Clin Obstet Gynecol.* 2010;53(4):869-878. doi:10.1097/GRF.0b013e3181fbb5f5

51. Turan OM, Turan S, Gungor S, et al. Progression of Doppler abnormalities in intrauterine growth restriction. *Ultrasound Obstet Gynecol.* 2008;32(2):160-167. doi:10.1002/uog.5386

52. Arabin B, Jimenez E, Vogel M, Weitzel HK. Relationship of utero- and fetoplacental blood flow velocity wave forms with Pathomorphological placental findings. *Fetal Diagn Ther.* 1992;7(3-4):173-179. doi:10.1159/000263695

53. Baschat AA, Gembruch U, Harman CR. The sequence of changes in Doppler and biophysical parameters as severe fetal growth restriction worsens: Doppler and biophysical profile in IUGR. *Ultrasound Obstet Gynecol.* 2001;18(6):571-577. doi:10.1046/j.0960-7692.2001.00591.x

54. Valcamonico A, Danti L, Frusca T, et al. Absent end-diastolic velocity in umbilical artery: risk of neonatal morbidity and brain damage. *Am J Obstet Gynecol.* 1994;170(3):796-801. doi:10.1016/S0002-9378(94)70285-3

55. Eixarch E, Meler E, Iraola A, et al. Neurodevelopmental outcome in 2-year-old infants who were small-for-gestational age term fetuses with cerebral blood flow redistribution. *Ultrasound Obstet Gynecol.* 2008;32(7):894-899. doi:10.1002/uog.6249

56. Baschat AA, Gembruch U, Weiner CP, Harman CR. Qualitative venous Doppler waveform analysis improves prediction of critical perinatal outcomes in premature growth-restricted fetuses. *Ultrasound Obstet Gynecol.* 2003;22(3):240-245. doi:10.1002/uog.149

57. Turan OM, Turan S, Berg C, et al. Duration of persistent abnormal ductus venosus flow and its impact on perinatal outcome in fetal growth restriction. *Ultrasound Obstet Gynecol.* 2011;38(3):295-302. doi:10.1002/uog.9011

58. Baschat AA, Güclü S, Kush ML, Gembruch U, Weiner CP, Harman CR. Venous Doppler in the prediction of acid-base status of growth-restricted fetuses with elevated placental blood flow resistance. *Am J Obstet Gynecol.* 2004;191(1):277-284. doi:10.1016/j.ajog.2003.11.028

59. Turan S, Turan OM, Berg C, et al. Computerized fetal heart rate analysis, Doppler ultrasound and biophysical profile score in the prediction of acid-base status of growth-restricted fetuses. *Ultrasound Obstet Gynecol.* 2007;30(5):750-756. doi:10.1002/uog.4101

69. Boers KE, Vijgen SMC, Bijlenga D, et al. Induction versus expectant monitoring for intrauterine growth restriction at term: randomised equivalence trial (DIGITAT). *Br Med J.* 2010;341:c7087. doi:10.1136/bmj.c7087

70. Khalil A, Thilaganathan B. Role of uteroplacental and fetal Doppler in identifying fetal growth restriction at term. *Best Pract Res Clin Obstet Gynaecol.* 2017;38:38-47. doi:10.1016/j.bpobgyn.2016.09.003

71. Khalil AA, Morales-Rosello J, Elsaddig M, et al. The association between fetal Doppler and admission to neonatal unit at term. *Am J Obstet Gynecol.* 2015;213(1):57.e1-57.e7. doi:10.1016/j.ajog.2014.10.013

77. Krapp M, Baschat AA, Gembruch U, Geipel A, Germer U. Flecainide in the intrauterine treatment of fetal supraventricular tachycardia: flecainide in fetuses with SVT. *Ultrasound Obstet Gynecol.* 2002;19(2):158-164. doi:10.1046/j.0960-7692.2001.00562.x

79. Hofstaetter C, Gudmundsson S. Venous Doppler in the evaluation of fetal hydrops. *Obstet Gynecol Int.* 2010;2010:1-7. doi:10.1155/2010/430157

81. Van Mieghem T, Klaritsch P, Doné E, et al. Assessment of fetal cardiac function before and after therapy for twin-to-twin transfusion syndrome. *Am J Obstet Gynecol.* 2009;200(4):400.e1-400.e7. doi:10.1016/j.ajog.2009.01.051

82. Quintero RA, Morales WJ, Allen MH, Bornick PW, Johnson PK, Kruger M. Staging of twin-twin transfusion syndrome. *J Perinatol.* 1999;19(8):550-555. doi:10.1038/sj.jp.7200292

83. Rychik J, Tian Z, Bebbington M, et al. The twin-twin transfusion syndrome: spectrum of cardiovascular abnormality and development of a cardiovascular score to assess severity of disease. *Am J Obstet Gynecol.* 2007;197(4):392.e1-392.e8. doi:10.1016/j.ajog.2007.06.055

84. Gratacós E, Van Schoubroeck D, Carreras E, et al. Transient hydropic signs in the donor fetus after fetoscopic laser coagulation in severe twin-twin transfusion syndrome: incidence and clinical relevance. *Ultrasound Obstet Gynecol.* 2002;19(5):449-453.

87. Gratacós E, Lewi L, Muñoz B, et al. A classification system for selective intrauterine growth restriction in monochorionic pregnancies according to umbilical artery Doppler flow in the smaller twin. *Ultrasound Obstet Gynecol.* 2007;30(1):28-34. doi:10.1002/uog.4046

88. Gratacós E, Carreras E, Becker J, et al. Prevalence of neurological damage in monochorionic twins with selective intrauterine growth restriction and intermittent absent or reversed end-diastolic umbilical artery flow: brain damage in twins. *Ultrasound Obstet Gynecol.* 2004;24(2):159-163. doi:10.1002/uog.1105

89. Slaghekke F, Kist WJ, Oepkes D, et al. Twin anemia-polycythemia sequence: diagnostic criteria, classification, perinatal management and outcome. *Fetal Diagn Ther.* 2010;27(4):181-190. doi:10.1159/000304512

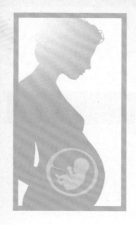

Antepartum and Intrapartum Surveillance of the Fetus and the Amniotic Fluid

Maria Andrikopoulou, Michael G. Ross, and Anthony M. Vintzileos

ANTEPARTUM SURVEILLANCE TECHNIQUES (FETUS AND AMNIOTIC FLUID)

There are multiple maternal and fetal indications to perform antepartum surveillance. Although the mechanisms controlling sleep and activity cycles in the fetus are not well understood, knowledge of these behaviors is imperative to appropriately interpret fetal heart rate (FHR) monitoring and fetal biophysical profile (BPP) activities.

In the near-term fetus, there are four behavioral states (occurring repeatedly and stable over time) that have been described: quiet sleep, active sleep, quiet awake, and active awake.[1] The fetus predominantly spends its time in either a quiet or an active sleep state.[2]

Table 21.2 shows the various pathophysiologic processes, examples of maternal/fetal conditions, and the specific surveillance tests that may be the most appropriate.

Fetal Movement Monitoring

This method of surveillance (also known as "fetal kick counts") by the mother is simple, inexpensive, noninvasive, and understandable to patients. In general, the presence of good fetal movement is a sign of fetal well-being and an indirect measure of normal fetal acid-base status. Awareness of fetal movements will vary from patient to patient and is also affected by other maternal, fetal, and uterine factors.

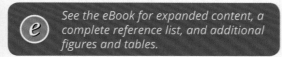

See the eBook for expanded content, a complete reference list, and additional figures and tables.

A popular approach is to have the patient lie on her left side and count distinct fetal movements.[7] Counting 10 movements in a period of up to 2 hours is felt to be reassuring. In another approach, women were advised to count fetal movements for 1 hour, three times per week.[8] If the count is nonreassuring or decreased, further assessment is recommended (such as nonstress test [NST] with amniotic fluid volume [AFV] assessment or BPP), and the physician should be contacted immediately.

Contraction Stress Test

Historically, a contraction stress test (CST) was the first antepartum fetal heart test used to detect uteroplacental insufficiency. This test is based on the response of the FHR to uterine contractions and relies on the premise that fetal oxygenation will be transiently worsened by contractions, which primarily occurs intrapartum. Therefore, in a suboptimally oxygenated fetus, the resultant intermittent worsening in oxygenation will, in turn, lead to the FHR pattern of late decelerations.[20] This test is rarely used today because it is cumbersome, is costly, has a high false-positive rate, and has been replaced by noninvasive tools such as the NST and Doppler velocimetry. However, the CST may be of particular value in preterm fetuses who demonstrate intermittent, "spontaneous" heart rate decelerations to assess the potential for uteroplacental insufficiency.

Nonstress Test

The purpose of the NST is to identify healthy fetuses and prolong preterm pregnancies, as well as identify those in jeopardy so that timely intervention can

Table 21.2 Condition-Specific Antepartum Fetal Testing

Pathophysiologic Condition	Maternal/Fetal Condition	ªAppropriate Test(s)
Metabolic abnormalities	Type 1 diabetes	NST, CST, BPP, Doppler in class F-R diabetes, maternal blood glucose (goal is normal)
Decreased uteroplacental blood flow	Hypertensive disorders Collagen, renal, vascular disease Most cases IUGR (<32-34 wk)	NST, CST, BPP, AF assessment, Doppler, EFW by US (growth rate)
Decreased gas exchange	Postdate pregnancy Some cases IUGR (>32-34 wk)	NST, CST, BPP, AF assessment, first-trimester US (accurate dating), EFW by US
Fetal sepsis	PROM Intra-amniotic infection Maternal fever, primary subclinical intra-amniotic infection	NST, BPP, AF assessment, amniocentesis (rule out infection)
Fetal anemia	Fetomaternal hemorrhage Erythroblastosis fetalis Parvovirus B19 infection	NST (if hydrops present), CST (if hydrops present), BPP (if hydrops present), MCA peak systolic velocity, US to rule out hydrops, fetal liver length, cordocentesis, amniocentesis (>28 wk)
Fetal heart failure	Cardiac arrhythmia Nonimmune hydrops Chorioangioma placenta	Doppler (venous circulation), US to rule out hydrops, continuous FHR monitoring (determine time spent in sinus rhythm), M-mode echo (rule out arrhythmias)
Umbilical cord accident	Umbilical cord entanglement (monoamniotic twins) Velamentous cord insertion/funic presentation Noncoiled umbilical cord	Frequent NST, umbilical artery Doppler, color Doppler on US (verify diagnosis)
Fetal stroke	Oligohydramnios	NST, BPP, AF assessment

AF, amniotic fluid; BPP, biophysical profile; CST, contraction stress test; EFW, estimated fetal weight; FHR, fetal heart rate; IUGR, intrauterine growth restriction; MCA, middle cerebral artery; NST, nonstress test; PROM, premature rupture of membranes; US, ultrasound.
ªSpecific surveillance tests that may be the most appropriate and are suggested guidelines.

improve outcomes. This testing modality is based on the premise that the heart rate of the fetus that is not acidemic or neurologically depressed will temporarily accelerate with fetal movement. FHR reactivity is speculated to be a good indicator of normal fetal autonomic function and well-being.

Technique

FHR is monitored using a Doppler ultrasound transducer, while a tocodynamometer may be used to record any uterine contractions. Fetal activity is also recorded on the strip; however, the patient does not need to document fetal movement for the test to be interpreted. Less than 1% of NSTs provide unsatisfactory results owing to inadequate recording of the FHR tracing.[37] Technical difficulties that may be encountered include obesity, fetal hiccups, excessive fetal activity, and polyhydramnios.[29]

Possible Results

The FHR tracing can be categorized as reactive or nonreactive. Although various definitions of reactivity have been used, the most common is ≥2 FHR accelerations (which peak, but do not necessarily remain, at least 15 beats per minute [bpm] in amplitude above the baseline, and last 15 seconds from baseline to baseline) within a 10- or 20-minutes period, with or without fetal movement.[38] In preterm fetuses <32 weeks, FHR acceleration is defined as 10 bpm above baseline for at least 10 seconds. It may be necessary to continue the NST for 40 minutes to account for variations in the fetal sleep-wake cycle because it may take longer for a healthy term fetus to display two FHR accelerations.[39] If, after 40 minutes, the criteria are still not met, fetal movement may be induced by acoustic stimulation (see below).[37] Other factors besides fetal compromise that can lead to a nonreactive NST include depressants (narcotics, phenobarbital), beta-blockers (propranolol), and smoking.[40-42]

NST interpretation should take gestational age into account; this is an important consideration, as preterm fetuses are less likely to have FHR accelerations in association with fetal movements.

Studies also have evaluated the predictive value of NSTs in pregnancies <32 weeks of gestation based on a lower threshold for accelerations (ie, at least 10 bpm above the baseline and at least 10 seconds from baseline-to-baseline) and have shown that there is no appreciable difference between the 10-beat criteria and 15-beat criteria in predicting outcomes.[49,50] This concept should be kept in mind, as many fetuses may undergo antepartum surveillance at <32 weeks. Preterm fetuses may also normally exhibit decelerations between 20 and 30 weeks.[51] They become less common as gestation advances and are more frequent at <30 weeks. However, although gestational age should always be considered when interpreting NSTs, nonreassuring FHR patterns in the preterm fetus should not be automatically—and perhaps improperly—attributed to prematurity.

The American College of Obstetricians and Gynecologists (ACOG) states that NSTs and antenatal testing are typically repeated if the clinical condition that prompted testing persists. Even though the ideal interval has not been established, they are typically repeated at weekly intervals or in more frequent intervals in high-risk conditions.[20]

Whereas a reactive NST has excellent specificity, the predictive value of a positive test has been reported to be <40%.[58] Concomitantly, the false-positive rate of a nonreactive NST has been found to be 57% to 100% for perinatal mortality, and 44% to 92% for perinatal morbidity.[29] Therefore, when an NST is nonreactive, either prolongation of the time of the NST or use of other forms of testing (such as the BPP and/or Doppler velocimetry) is recommended. Even after prolongation of monitoring, a nonreactive NST may still be consistent with good fetal outcomes. However, persistent absence of reactivity without an identified underlying cause, such as medication, prematurity, or congenital anomalies, may be associated with fetal compromise.[59] Those fetuses that remained nonreactive after 90 minutes had 67% and 93.3% perinatal mortality and morbidity rates, respectively.

In summary, while a reactive NST is usually associated with good outcomes, absence of accelerations is not necessarily linked to fetal compromise.

Vibroacoustic Stimulation

Because the majority of nonreactive NSTs occur in healthy fetuses secondary to a physiologically normal sleep state, fetal stimulation has been used as a way to distinguish normal fetal sleep from fetal compromise. VAS is an effective technique to improve the efficiency of antepartum FHR testing because it safely reduces the time needed to perform an NST without compromising detection of the sick fetus.[60]

Technique

To perform a VAS, an artificial larynx is positioned on the maternal abdomen over the fetal vertex with a stimulus of 1 to 2 seconds. This procedure may be repeated up to three times (at 1-minute intervals) for progressively longer durations of up to 3 seconds to elicit FHR accelerations. The increases in intrauterine sound decibels created by VAS are thought to be safe and harmless to the fetus.

Possible Results

The normal fetal response to VAS includes not only FHR accelerations, but also increases in variability and gross body movements. Utilizing this approach on a normal fetus may elicit accelerations that appear to be suggestive of fetal well-being. Studies have demonstrated the advantages of using VAS in conjunction with the NST. Trudinger and Boylan reported that using VAS with NST versus NST alone had higher sensitivity in detecting abnormal fetal outcomes (66% vs 39%).[61] Those fetuses with an abnormal response, who remained nonreactive after VAS, demonstrated increased rates of intrapartum fetal distress, fetal growth restriction, and lower Apgar scores.[62]

Biophysical Profile

The BPP is unique in that it assesses both acute (ie, FHR reactivity, fetal breathing movements, fetal movements, fetal tone) and chronic (ie, AFV) markers of fetal condition. It is a noninvasive modality with a high negative predictive value for adverse perinatal outcomes.[34,64] When used in conjunction with other surveillance and testing measures, the BPP helps to assess fetal hypoxia and acidemia, presence of infection in patients with premature rupture of membranes, placental dysfunction, and stillbirth.

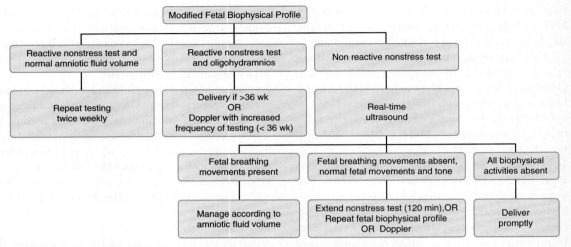

Algorithm 21.1 Suggested protocol for the modified fetal biophysical profile.

The BPP is based on the premise that the biophysical activities developed last *in utero* are the first to become abnormal in the presence of fetal acidemia or infection.[65]

Technique

The BPP is performed using real-time ultrasonography to assess multiple fetal biophysical activities as well as AFV. Sonographic observation is continued until either normal activity is seen or after 30 consecutive minutes of scanning have elapsed. The interval of BPP testing frequency (1-2 per week) is arbitrary; however, it is often a matter of individual clinical judgment, training, preferences, and experience.

The modified BPP is composed of the NST (an acute indicator of fetal acid-base status) and AFV (indicator of chronic uteroplacental function). **Algorithm 21.1** shows our suggested protocol for the modified BPP.

Possible Results

Current scoring systems assign a numeric value (usually 0 or 2) to each of the biophysical

Table 21.5 Biophysical Profile Scoring: Technique and Interpretation

Biophysical Variable	Normal (Score = 2)	Abnormal (Score = 0)
Fetal breathing movements	≥1 episode of ≥30 s in 30 min	Absent or no episode of ≥30 s in 30 min
Gross body movements	≥3 discrete body limb movements in 30 min (episodes of active continuous movement considered)	≤2 episodes of body limb movements in 30 min as single movement
Fetal tone	≥1 episode of active extension with return to flexion of fetal limb(s) or trunk Opening and closing of hand considered normal tone	Either slow extension with return to partial flexion movement of limb in full extension or absent fetal movement
Reactive fetal heart rate	≥2 episodes of acceleration of ≥15 bpm and of ≥15 s associated with fetal movement in 20 min	<2 episodes of acceleration of fetal heart rate or acceleration of <15 bpm in 20 min
Qualitative amniotic fluid volume	≥1 pocket of fluid measuring 2 cm in vertical axis	Either no pockets or largest pocket <2 cm in vertical axis

bpm, beats per minute.

components (**Table 21.5**). A normal modified BPP exists when the NST is reactive and the AFI is >5 cm.[20] An abnormal test occurs if either the NST is nonreactive or the AFI is 5 cm or less.

A BPP score of 8 or more is considered reassuring. In fact, if all four sonographic components are normal, the NST may be omitted without compromising the validity of the BPP test results.[73] When the score is <8, however, analyzing which individual components of the BPP are abnormal can assist in determining true fetal status and minimize false-positive examinations. The BPP score should also be interpreted within the overall clinical context. In general, a score of 6 is considered equivocal, and a score of ≤4 is abnormal. In the mature fetus, a BPP of 6/10 may indicate compromise and may be an indication for delivery; however, in the immature fetus, repeat testing or use of Doppler velocimetry may be in order before intervention is recommended.

Regardless of the total score, in the presence of oligohydramnios (largest vertical pocket of AFV ≤2 cm), further evaluation is warranted.[74]

A normal BPP conveys a low risk of stillbirth; however, the false-negative rate of the BPP (fetal death within 1 week of a last normal test result) ranges from 0.645 to 7 per 1000.[75,77,79] There is also a strong relationship between the last BPP score and perinatal morbidity variables.[74,78] Combinations of these variables (fetal distress, admission to neonatal intensive care unit, intrauterine growth restriction, 5-minutes Apgar score ≤ 7, and cord pH < 7.20) also showed the same highly significant inverse linear correlation with BPP score.

Amniotic Fluid Volume Assessment

Amniotic fluid is essential to pregnancy, providing an environment for normal development, growth, and movement of the fetus. AFV is a chronic marker of fetal well-being, and a normal AFV also protects the fetus from cord compression during fetal activity or uterine contractions. This volume changes during pregnancy: at 22 weeks, the average AFV is 630 mL, and this increases to 770 mL at 28 weeks.[87] Between 29 and 37 weeks, there is little change in volume, which averages 800 mL. Beyond 39 weeks, AFV decreases sharply (average 515 mL at 41 weeks).

It is only under pathologic conditions where fetal modulation of fluid secretion (urine and lung liquid) and resorption (swallowing and intramembranous flow) contribute to marked changes in AFV.

Technique

Although a variety of techniques have been developed to assess AFV, the two predominant approaches in use today are measurement of a single vertical (largest) AF pocket and use of the AFI, the sum of measurements (cm) of the deepest cord-free amniotic fluid pocket in each of the maternal abdominal quadrants.[89]

Controversy remains as to the superiority of the AFI or the single vertical pocket and studies have reported varying advantages and disadvantages of both modalities.[75,90]

Possible Results

An AFI > 5 cm is generally considered to be an adequate volume.[83] In low-risk pregnancies, the mean AFI is 16.2 ± 5.3 cm and remains relatively stable from 24 weeks through term. Polyhydramnios is defined as an AFI >25 cm, and oligohydramnios is defined as an AFI ≤5 cm.[90,93]

Intrapartum Fetal Surveillance Techniques

Fetal Heart Rate Monitoring

The main surveillance technique for intrapartum fetal evaluation is FHR monitoring, which can be performed either intermittently or continuously. Intermittent FHR monitoring can be performed by either intermittent auscultation of FHR (using a hand-held Doppler ultrasound on the abdomen or DeLee stethoscope) or using a continuous electronic FHR monitor intermittently (recorded on a tracing).

Continuous electronic FHR monitoring (EFM) determines the FHR on a beat-to-beat basis and displays data continuously. It can be performed either externally or internally.

An essential adjunctive component to FHR monitoring is uterine contraction monitoring, which can be accomplished via an external tocodynamometer (most commonly) on the maternal abdomen. Although uterine frequency and duration of contractions are measured with reasonable accuracy, the strength/amplitude of the contractions cannot be determined using this modality. In contrast, insertion of an intrauterine pressure catheter, which requires cervical dilation and ruptured membranes, can assess the strength, amplitude, duration, and frequency of contractions.

EFM is now the main screening method for intrapartum fetal assessment in most developed countries, but has been disappointing on account of its subjective nature, frequency of falsely nonreassuring patterns, and persistent questions regarding efficacy.[102] In addition, the widespread use of EFM does not appear to have reduced cerebral palsy,[103] as nonreassuring patterns occur in about 15% of labors,[104] and the positive predictive value is not as good as its accuracy in confirming fetal well-being.

Technique

The FHR is generally recorded during a contraction, and for 30 seconds afterward. Although there are no studies providing data on the optimal intervals for monitoring in low-risk patients, it is generally recommended that the FHR should be determined at every hour in the latent phase, every 30 minutes in the active phase, and every 15 minutes in the second stage of labor. In high-risk patients, it is recommended that the FHR be determined every 30 minutes during the latent phase, every 15 minutes during the active phase, and every 5 minutes during the second stage of labor.

Possible Results

The interpretation of FHR patterns should incorporate knowledge of gestational age, maternal condition, medications, and other factors that could influence FHR components. Standard definitions for the components of EFM have been recommended by several organizations, and a three-tiered classification system for interpretation of FHR patterns, Categories I, II and III, is shown in **Table 21.9**.

A clinical rule-of-thumb is that FHR decelerations reflect the nature of the insult to the fetus, whereas FHR variability reflects the fetus' ability to tolerate the insult. If decreased variability is associated with baseline FHR changes, or is seen with recurrent decelerations, the likelihood of fetal compromise increases.[115-117] Four types of decelerations are seen intrapartum—early, variable, late, or prolonged—based on their temporal relationship with contractions, as well as their configuration. Any deceleration is quantitated by the depth of the nadir (in bpm) below the baseline (excluding transient spikes or electronic artifacts), and the duration is quantitated in minutes and seconds from the beginning to the end of the deceleration.[119] Decelerations are defined as recurrent if they occur with ≥50% of uterine contractions in any 20-minutes segment. Early decelerations are thought to be secondary to an increase in vagal tone due to fetal head compression

Table 21.9 Categories of FHR Patterns According to the 2008 NICHD Classification System

Category I (normal)
It should include *all* of the following:
• Baseline rate: 110-160 bpm • Variability: Moderate • Accelerations: Present or absent • Decelerations: No late, variable, or prolonged decelerations
Category II (indeterminate)
Includes all FHR patterns not classified as Category I or Category III
Category III (abnormal)

• Absent variability with any of the following:
  • Recurrent late decelerations
  • Recurrent variable decelerations
  • Bradycardia
Or
• Sinusoidal pattern

FHR, fetal heart rate; NICHD, *Eunice Kennedy Shriver* National Institute of Child Health and Human Development.
Data from National Institute of Child Health and Human Development Research Planning Workshop. Electronic fetal heart rate monitoring: research guidelines for interpretation. *Am J Obstet Gynecol.* 1997;17:1385.

during the contraction. These decelerations are innocuous, are not associated with fetal hypoxemia or acidemia,[115,123] can be observed throughout labor (but are seen most often at cervical dilations of 4-8 cm),[124] and do not require corrective measures.

Variable decelerations are the most common decelerations seen in labor, are most often seen during the second stage, and indicate umbilical cord compression. Variable decelerations have been graded by some as mild, moderate, and severe based on the duration of the deceleration and the level to which the FHR drops.[123]

Late decelerations are caused by fetal hypoxia, which is often due to decreased intervillous exchange between mother and fetus secondary to decreased placental perfusion.

A sinusoidal FHR differs from variability in that it has a smooth, sine wave–like pattern of regular frequency and amplitude[127] (**Figure 21.5**). This pattern has been associated with severe fetal anemia and/or hypovolemia. A transient "sinusoid-like" pattern may also be seen after maternal administration of some narcotic analgesics.[128] However, in this setting, it does not indicate fetal compromise.

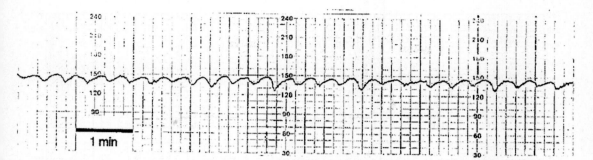

Figure 21.5 Varying degrees of fetal heart rate variability showing the sinusoidal pattern. Original scaling, 30 bpm/cm vertical axis, and paper speed 3 cm/min horizontal axis.

(Reprinted from Electronic fetal heart rate monitoring: research guidelines for interpretation. National Institute of Child Health and Human Development Research Planning Workshop. *Am J Obstet Gynecol.* 1997;177(6):1385-1390.)

A sawtooth FHR pattern has been associated with fetal CNS injury *in utero* of ischemic or hemorrhagic etiology[129] (**Figure 21.6**). This FHR pattern has unstable or indeterminate baseline, periods of sawtooth-like oscillations with a frequency of 3 to 5 per minute and amplitude greater than 20 bpm. Three cases have been reported with this FHR pattern, all linked to cases with evidence of *in utero* fetal CNS injury.[129]

A Category I fetal heart rate tracing generally implies that the fetus has normal fetal acid-base status.[119,121] On the other hand, Category III fetal heart rate tracing, with absent variability and recurrent late or variable decelerations, fetal bradycardia, or sinusoidal pattern, is predictive of abnormal fetal acid-base status.[119,121] These situations are associated with a significant likelihood of fetal compromise with strong possibility for adverse outcomes. A Category II FHR is one that does not fit into Category I or III and accounts for the overwhelming majority of FHR patterns in labor. Given great variation of FHR patterns that are included in this category, the standardization of management of these FHR patterns is challenging and at times controversial. **Algorithm 21.2** shows a suggested protocol for managing Category II FHR tracings in labor.[130]

This clinical application of the algorithm becomes extremely important to prevent progression to Category III FHR (**Algorithm 21.3**).

Fetal Acid-Base Evaluation

During labor, fetal acidemia may be secondary to impaired maternal-fetal exchange in the intervillous space. In acute umbilical cord compression, rapid CO_2 accumulation leads to a respiratory acidemia. Metabolic acidemia can occur secondary to lactic acid accumulation when the anaerobic pathway of energy production is used. If enough hypoxemia and acidemia develop and persist, significant fetal morbidity/mortality may result. Therefore, fetal scalp capillary blood sampling was developed to evaluate fetal acid-base status during labor and has been used to improve the positive predictive value of FHR tracings.

Given the cost, patient discomfort, invasive nature of the test, high failure rate, and unavailability of equipment, intermittent fetal scalp blood sampling is not routinely used in the United States and is only used in Europe.[135]

Technique

Umbilical cord acid-base values are often obtained at the time of delivery and are used to establish an objective measure of fetal status at the time of birth. Although umbilical artery blood gases are preferable to venous blood, sampling of both provides information on the fetal and uteroplacental circulations respectively. The ACOG recommends that cord gases should be obtained in cases where labor and delivery or the pregnancy has been complicated,[136] or when the 5-minutes Apgar score is 5 or less.[137]

Possible Results

Both fetal cord pH and lactate can be measured. A fetal scalp pH $\geq$ 7.25 is considered normal,[112] pH 7.20 to 7.24 indicates preacidemia, and a pH $\leq$ 7.19 indicates fetal acidemia. However, it is understood that pH values associated with pathologic fetal acidemia may be significantly lower. Significant neonatal morbidity is usually associated with umbilical artery pH < 7.10, and this cutoff may be as low as 7.00.[139,140]

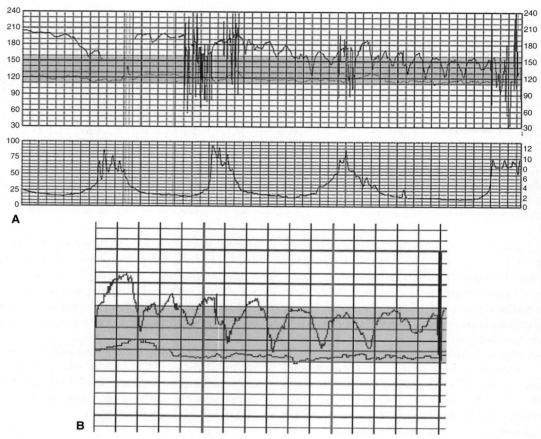

Figure 21.6 Sawtooth fetal heart rate patterns. **A,** Sudden onset of fetal tachycardia with sawtooth pattern. **B,** Sawtooth pattern with unstable baseline.

(Reprinted from Andrikopoulou M, Vintzileos AM. Sawtooth fetal heart rate pattern due to in utero fetal central nervous system injury. *Am J Obstet Gynecol.* 2016;214:403.e1-403.e4.)

Normal values for arterial and venous blood samples have been described.[141,142] However, it is important to note that fetal pH values normally fall during labor, and fetal acidemia in the presence of labor has been defined as a cord artery pH < 7.15 or cord vein pH < 7.20.[143]

Fetal Stimulation Techniques

Fetal scalp stimulation and VAS have been proposed to further evaluate a nonreassuring FHR pattern during intrapartum FHR management. These fetal stimulation techniques have many advantages; they are noninvasive, are not technically difficult, can be performed earlier in labor, and can be used when scalp pH sampling is not feasible. Many of the commonly used stimulation tests—VAS, digital scalp stimulation, fetal scalp puncture, and Allis clamp

scalp stimulation—have shown similar effectiveness in predicting the absence of fetal acidemia.[149] In our opinion, if the fetus has a normal response to either VAS or scalp stimulation, significant acute fetal acidemia can be ruled out, and thus a scalp pH may be unnecessary, even in the presence of equivocal or nonreassuring FHR tracings. However, absence of acceleration after simulation was not necessarily associated with fetal acidemia.[149]

Fetal Pulse Oximetry

Fetal pulse oximetry (FPO) emerged in the late 1980s as a tool to continuously and directly measure fetal arterial O_2 saturation during labor thereby improving the evaluation of fetal well-being. It is generally reserved for use when a nonreassuring FHR has been recorded, to assist in identifying

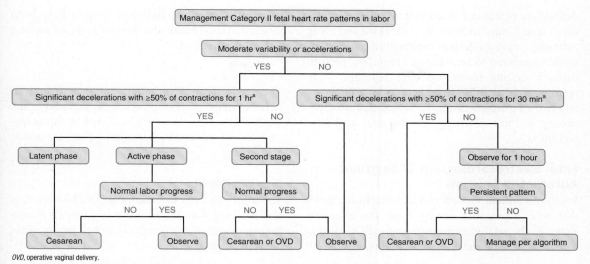

OVD, operative vaginal delivery.

ªThat have not resolved with appropriate conservative corrective measures, which may include supplemental oxygen, maternal position changes, intravenous fluid administration, correction of hypotension, reduction or discontinuation of uterine stimulation, administration of uterine relaxant, amnioinfusion, and/or changes in second stage breathing and pushing techniques.

Algorithm 21.2 Algorithm for managing Category II fetal heart rate (FHR) patterns in labor.

(Modified from Clark SL, Nageotte MP, Garite TJ, et al. Intrapartum management of category II fetal heart rate tracings: towards standardization of care. *Am J Obstet Gynecol*. 2013;209(2):89-97.)

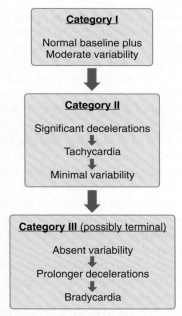

Algorithm 21.3 Gradual progression of Category I to Category III fetal heart rate (FHR) pattern due to primary uteroplacental insufficiency or excessive uterine activity.

(Adapted from Vintzileos AM, Smulian JC. Decelerations, tachycardia, and decreased variability: have we overlooked the significance of longitudinal fetal heart rate changes for detecting intrapartum fetal hypoxia? *Am J Obstet Gynecol*. 2016;215(3):261-264.)

hypoxemic fetuses who may benefit from further intervention, and as an adjunct to FHR monitoring. The initial hope was to decrease the cesarean rate for fetal distress when fetal O_2 saturation is normal. However, studies have proven inconclusive as to the utility and benefit of FPO as a standard practice, and the ACOG has not endorsed its use.[164]

Technique

A variety of FPO sensors have been studied. Some are placed during a vaginal examination to attach to the top of the fetal head by suction,[165] and others lie against the fetal temple or cheek.[166] The sensor remains *in situ*, and FPO values are recorded for approximately 81% of the monitoring time.

Possible Results

Fetal acidemia is rare when the fetal arterial O_2 saturation is continually >30% (critical threshold). Thus, FPO values ≥30% are considered reassuring (even when the EFM is nonreassuring), whereas values <30% warrant consideration of interventions such as maternal position change or urgent cesarean delivery.[167] FHR abnormalities associated with normal scalp blood analysis and normal Apgar scores at delivery have been demonstrated in association with stable arterial O_2 saturation patterns.[168] An ominous EFM pattern has been defined as prolonged deceleration below 70 bpm for at least 7 min. In 2003, the U.S. Food and Drug Administration guidelines expanded the EFM patterns considered to be ominous, requiring prompt delivery despite reassuring FPO readings. They reemphasized that FPO is meant as an adjunct to, and not a replacement for, EFM and that no technology is 100% predictive of the fetal acid-base condition.

Fetal Electrocardiogram ST Segment Automated Analysis

Studies in animal models and humans have shown that fetal hypoxemia during labor can alter the shape of the fetal electrocardiogram (ECG) waveform (notably the elevation or depression of the ST segment). Therefore, technical systems have been developed to monitor the fetal ECG as an adjunct to continuous EFM.[177]

Technique

The fetal ECG ST segment automated analysis (STAN) analyzes the repolarization segment of the ECG (ST) waveform, which is altered by intramyocardial potassium release, resulting from metabolic acidemia.[178]

Possible Results

The utility of ECG as an adjunct to EFM remains unclear. Larger studies have not consistently shown improvement of perinatal outcomes or decrease operative-delivery rates.

KEY POINTS

- Both antepartum and intrapartum surveillance of the fetus have the intent of detecting fetal compromise so that appropriate and timely interventions can be accomplished. As fetal compromise has a diverse etiology, modalities of testing must be able to survey both acute fetal status and chronic disease states as well as application of condition-specific fetal testing.
- Fetal movement monitoring ("fetal kick counts") by the mother is an advantageous form of surveillance because it lacks contraindications, is simple, inexpensive, noninvasive, and understandable to patients. The relationship between decreased fetal activity and poor perinatal outcome has been well established.
- A negative contraction stress test indicates fetal ability to tolerate uterine contractions. In general, however, a positive test implies potential uteroplacental insufficiency and has been associated with adverse perinatal outcome and an increased incidence of intrauterine demise. However, the test is cumbersome, time consuming, costly, and has a high false-positive rates.
- FHR reactivity is a good indicator of normal fetal autonomic function and well-being; it relies on normal neurologic development and normal integration of the central nervous system control of FHR.

- Preterm fetuses are less likely to have FHR accelerations in association with fetal movements.
- The predictive value of a negative NST (normal outcome associated with a reactive NST) is very high. The reactive NST predicts good perinatal outcome in about 95% of cases. The false-positive rate of a nonreactive NST is also very high.
- The normal fetal response to VAS includes not only FHR accelerations, but also increases in long-term FHR variability and gross body movements.
- VAS has been conclusively demonstrated to be effective in achieving fetal arousal, is reasonably safe, and improves the efficiency of antepartum FHR testing. Utilizing VAS on the nonacidemic fetus may elicit accelerations that appear to be valid in predicting fetal well-being. It also offers the advantage of safely reducing testing time, without compromising detection of the acidemic fetus.
- The BPP is unique in that it assesses both acute (FHR reactivity, fetal breathing movements, fetal movements, fetal tone) and chronic (amniotic fluid volume) markers of fetal condition.
- The "gradual hypoxia concept" implies that the biophysical activities developed last *in utero* are also the first to become abnormal in the presence of fetal acidemia or infection. In

accordance with this concept, early stages of fetal compromise are manifested by abnormalities in FHR reactivity and breathing, while movement and tone are generally not abolished until much later stages of compromise.

- In the second half of pregnancy, the main sources of amniotic fluid include fetal urine excretion (especially) and fluid secreted by the fetal lung. However, unlike the role of the kidneys, the fetal lung does not play a role in regulating fetal body fluid homeostasis.

- Polyhydramnios (pathologic accumulation of amniotic fluid), which is defined as an amniotic fluid index >25 cm, occurs in 0.2% to 1.6% of the general population. When the cause of polyhydramnios can be found, the diagnosis usually falls into the following categories: fetal malformations and genetic disorders, diabetes, Rh sensitization, and congenital infections. Fetal swallowing impairment may also result in excess amniotic fluid volume.

- Oligohydramnios (reduced amniotic fluid volume) occurs in 5.5% to 37.8% of pregnancies and is significant because of its known association with adverse pregnancy outcome, such as umbilical cord occlusion, fetal distress in labor, meconium aspiration, operative deliveries, and stillbirth.

- The pathophysiologic processes that can lead to fetal death/damage include decreased uteroplacental blood flow, decreased gas exchange at the trophoblastic membrane level, metabolic processes, fetal sepsis, fetal anemia, fetal heart failure, umbilical cord accidents, or fetal strokes (ischemic or hemorrhagic). Multiple parameter assessment or combinations of different tests may often be the optimal fetal strategy, depending on the testing indication. In order to improve accuracy, condition-specific fetal testing should be utilized.

- The interpretation of FHR patterns should incorporate knowledge of gestational age, maternal condition, medications, and other factors that could influence FHR components.

- In 2008, the National Institute of Child Health and Human Development Research Planning Workshop developed standardized definitions for electronic FHR patterns, developed FHRT categories (I, II, III) and recommendations for interpreting them.

- The diagnostic accuracy of electronic FHR monitoring in predicting fetal compromise (positive predictive value) is not as good as its accuracy in confirming fetal well-being.

- In order to determine the appropriate timing of delivery during labor, progression of Category I or II to Category III FHR pattern should be avoided, by considering the characteristic longitudinal sequential FHR changes.

- Other methods of evaluating a nonreassuring FHR pattern have been proposed, such as fetal scalp stimulation and VAS intrapartum. FHR acceleration as a response to fetal stimulation indicates a nonacidemic fetus, and thus scalp blood sampling may be omitted. Using VAS or scalp stimulation intrapartum may reduce the need for scalp pH when FHR tracings are equivocal/nonreassuring.

- Fetal pulse oximetry has not proven to be of clinical value for reduction in cesarean rate for nonreassuring electronic FHR monitoring patterns and is not currently used.

- Technical systems have been developed to monitor the fetal ECG during labor, as an adjunct to continuous electronic FHR monitoring, with the aim of improving fetal outcome and minimizing unnecessary obstetric interference. However, large studies demonstrated that this technology did not consistently improve perinatal outcomes or decrease operative-delivery rates.

REFERENCES

(only references cited in synoptic print chapter; for a complete reference list, see ebook)

1. Nijhuis JG, Prechtl HF, Martin CB Jr, Bots RS. Are there behavioral states in the human fetus? *Early Hum Dev.* 1982;6:177.

2. van Woerdan EE, van Geijn HP. Heart-rate patterns and fetal movements. In: Nijhuis JG, ed. *Fetal Behavior: Developmental and Perinatal Aspects.* Oxford University Press; 1992:41.

7. Moore TR, Piacquadio K. A prospective evaluation of fetal movement screening to reduce the incidence of antepartum fetal death. *Am J Obstet Gynecol.* 1989;160:1075.

8. Neldam S. Fetal movements as an indicator of fetal well-being. *Dan Med Bull.* 1983;30(4):274.

20. *ACOG Practice Bulletin No 9.* In: *Antepartum Fetal Surveillance.* American College of Obstetricians and Gynecologists; 1999:911.

29. Thacker SB, Berkelman RL. Assessing the diagnostic accuracy and efficacy of selected antepartum fetal surveillance techniques. *Obstet Gynecol Surv.* 1986;41:121.

34. Devoe LD. Antenatal fetal assessment: contraction stress test, nonstress test, vibroacoustic stimulation, amniotic fluid volume, biophysical profile, and modified biophysical profile – an overview. *Semin Perinatol.* 2008;32(4):247-252.

37. Phelan JP. The nonstress test: a review of 3000 tests. *Am J Obstet Gynecol.* 1981;139:7.

38. Evertson LR, Gauthier RJ, Schifrin BS, Paul RH. Antepartum fetal heart rate testing. I. Evolution of the nonstress test. *Am J Obstet Gynecol.* 1979;133:29.

39. Patrick J, Carmichael L, Chess L, Staples C. Accelerations of the human fetal heart rate at 38 to 40 weeks' gestational age. *Am J Obstet Gynecol.* 1984;148:35.

40. Phelan JP. Diminished fetal reactivity with smoking. *Am J Obstet Gynecol.* 1980;136:230.

41. Margulis E, Binder D, Cohen AW. The effect of propanolol on the non-stress test. *Am J Obstet Gynecol.* 1984;148:340.

42. Keegan KA, Paul RH, Broussard PM, et al. Antepartum fetal heart testing. III: the effect of phenobarbital on the nonstress test. *Am J Obstet Gynecol.* 1979;133:579.

49. Cousins LM, Poeltler DM, Faron S, Catanzarite V, Daneshmand S, CaselFe H. Nonstress testing at ≤32.0 weeks' gestation: a randomized trial comparing different assessment criteria. *Am J Obstet Gynecol.* 2012;207(4):311.e1-311.e7.

50. Glantz JC, Bertoia N. Preterm nonstress testing: 10-beat compared with 15-beat criteria. *Obstet Gynecol.* 2011;118(1):87-93.

51. Sorokin Y, Dierker LJ, Pillay SK, et al. The association between fetal heart rate patterns and fetal movements in pregnancies between 20 and 30 weeks' gestation. *Am J Obstet Gynecol.* 1982;143:243.

58. Devoe LD. The nonstress test. *Obstet Gynecol Clin North Am.* 1990;17:111.

59. Devoe LD, McKenzie J, Searle NS, Sherline DM. Clinical sequelae of the extended nonstress test. *Am J Obstet Gynecol.* 1985;151:1074.

60. Smith CV, Phelan JP, Platt LD, et al. Fetal acoustic stimulation testing. II. A randomized clinical comparison with the nonstress test. *Am J Obstet Gynecol.* 1986;155:131.

61. Trudinger BJ, Boylan P. Antepartum fetal heart rate monitoring: value of sound stimulation. *Obstet Gynecol* 1980;55:265.

64. Liston R, Sawchuck D, Young D. No. 197a-Fetal Health surveillance: ante-partum consensus guideline. *J Obstet Gynaecol Can.* 2018;40(4):e251-e271.

65. Vintzileos AM, Campbell WA, Ingardia CJ, Nochimson DJ. The fetal bio-physical profile and its predictive value. *Obstet Gynecol.* 1983;62:271.

73. Manning FA, Morrison I, Lange IR, et al. Fetal biophysical profile scoring: selective use of the nonstress test. *Am J Obstet Gynecol.* 1987;156:709.

74. Manning FA, Harman CR, Morrison I, et al. Fetal assessment based on fetal biophysical profile scoring. IV. An analysis of perinatal morbidity and mortality. *Am J Obstet Gynecol.* 1990;162:703.

75. Chamberlain PF, Manning FA, Morrison I, et al. Ultrasound evaluation of amniotic fluid volume. I. The relationship of marginal and decreased amni-otic fluid volumes to perinatal outcome. *Am J Obstet Gynecol.* 1984;150:245.

77. Manning FA, Morrison I, Lange IR, et al. Fetal assessment based upon fetal biophysical profile scoring: experience in 12620 referred high risk pregnancies. I. Perinatal mortality by frequency and etiology. *Am J Obstet Gynecol.* 1985;151:343.

78. Baskett TF, Allen AC, Gray JH, et al. Fetal biophysical profile and perinatal death. *Obstet Gynecol.* 1987;70:357.

79. Platt LD, Eglinton GS, Sipos L, et al. Further experience with the fetal bio-physical profile. *Obstet Gynecol.* 1983;61:480.

83. Vintzileos AM, Feinstein SJ, Lodeiro JG, Campbell WA, Weinbaum PJ, Nochimson DJ. Fetal biophysical profile and the effect of premature rup-ture of the membranes. *Obstet Gynecol.* 1986;67(6):818-823.

87. Brace RA, Wolf EJ. Normal amniotic fluid volume changes throughout pregnancy. *Am J Obstet Gynecol.* 1989;161:382.

89. Phelan JP, Smith CV, Broussard P, Small M. Amniotic fluid volume assess-ment with the four quadrant technique at 36-42 weeks' gestation. *J Reprod Med.* 1987;32:540.

90. Rutherford SE, Phelan JP, Smith CV, Jacobs N. The four-quadrant assess-ment of amniotic fluid volume: an adjunct to antepartum fetal heart rate testing. *Obstet Gynecol.* 1987;70:353.

93. Phelan JP, Martin GI. Polyhydramnios: Fetal and Neonatal Implications. *Clin Perinatol.* 1989;16(4):987-994.

102. Freeman RK. Problems with intrapartum fetal heart rate monitoring interpretation and patient management. *Obstet Gynecol.* 2002;100:813.

103. Clark SL, Hankins GD. Temporal and demographic trends in cerebral palsy – fact and fiction. *Am J Obstet Gynecol.* 2003;188:628.

104. Umstad MP. The predictive value of abnormal fetal heart rate patterns in early labour. *Aust N Z J Obstet Gynaecol.* 1993;33:145.

112. Alfirevic Z, Devane D, Gyte GM, Cuthbert A. Continuous cardiotocogra-phy (CTG) as a form of electronic fetal monitoring (EFM) for fetal assess-ment during labour. *Cochrane Database Syst Rev.* 2017;2(2):Cd006066.

115. Beard RW, Filshie GM, Knight CA, Roberts GM. The significance of the changes in the continuous fetal heart rate in the first stage of labour. *J Obstet Gynaecol Br Commonw.* 1971;78(10):865-881.

116. Paul RH, Suidan AK, Yeh SY, et al. Clinical fetal monitoring. VII. The evaluation and significance of intrapartum baseline FHR variability. *Am J Obstet Gynecol.* 1975;123:206.

117. Martin CB. Physiology and clinical use of fetal heart rate variability. *Clin Perinatol.* 1982;9:339.

119. Macones GA, Hankins GD, Spong CY, Hauth J, Moore T. The 2008 National Institute of Child Health and Human Development workshop report on electronic fetal monitoring: update on definitions, inter-pretation, and research guidelines. *J Obstet Gynecol Neonatal Nurs.* 2008;37(5):510-515.

121. American College of Obstetricians and Gynecologists. ACOG Practice Bulletin No. 106: Intraparturn fetal heart rate monitoring. Nomenclature, interpretation, and general management principles. *Obstet Gynecol.* 2009;114:192-202.

123. Kubli FW, Hon EH, Khazin AF, Takemura H. Observations on heart rate and pH in the human fetus during labor. *Am J Obstet Gynecol.* 1969;104:1190.

124. Sheiner E, Levy A, Ofir K, et al. Changes in fetal heart rate and uterine pat-terns associated with uterine rupture. *J Reprod Med.* 2004;49(5):373-378.

127. National Institute of Child Health and Human Development Research Planning Workshop. Electronic fetal heart rate monitoring: research guidelines for interpretation. *Am J Obstet Gynecol.* 1997;17:1385.

128. Angel JL, Knuppel R, Lake M. Sinusoidal fetal heart rate patterns asso-ciated with intravenous butorphanol administration: a case report. *Am J Obstet Gynecol.* 1984;149:465.

129. Andrikopoulou M, Vintzileos AM. Sawtooth fetal heart rate pattern due to in utero fetal central nervous system injury. *Am J Obstet Gynecol.* 2016;214(3):403.e1-403.e4.

130. Clark SL, Nageotte MP, Garite TJ, et al. Intrapartum management of cat-egory II fetal heart rate tracings: towards standardization of care. *Am J Obstet Gynecol.* 2013;209(2):89-97.

135. Chandraharan E. Should national guidelines continue to recommend fetal scalp blood sampling during labor? *J Matern Fetal Neonatal Med.* 2016;29(22):3682-3685.

136. *ACOG Technical Bulletin No. 216.* In: *Umbilical Artery Blood Acid-Base Analysis.* American College of Obstetricians and Gynecologists; 1995.

137. Committee on Obstetric Practice American Academy of Pediatrics-Committee on Fetus and Newborn. ACOG Committee Opinion No. 64, October 2015: the Apgar score. *Obstet Gynecol.* 2015;126:e52-e55.

139. Winkler CL, Hauth JC, Tucker M, et al. Neonatal complications at term as related to the degrees of umbilical artery acidemia. *Am J Obstet Gynecol.* 1991;164:637.

140. Goldaber KG, Gilstrap LC, Leveno KJ, et al. Pathologic fetal acidemia. *Obstet Gynecol.* 1991;78:1103.

141. Helwig JT, Parer JT, Kilpatrick SJ, Laros RK Jr. Umbilical cord blood acid-base state: what is normal? *Am J Obstet Gynecol.* 1996;174(6):1807-1814.

142. Goodwin TM, Milner-Masterson L, Paul RH. Elimination of fetal scalp blood sampling on a large clinical service. *Obstet Gynecol.* 1994;83:971.

143. Vintzileos AM, Egan JFX, Campbell WA, et al. Asphyxia at birth as deter-mined by cord blood pH measurements in preterm and term gestations: correlation with neonatal outcomes. *J Matern Fetal Med* 1992;1:7.

149. Skupski DW, Rosenberg CR, Eglinton GS. Intrapartum fetal stimulation tests: a meta-analysis. *Obstet Gynecol.* 2002;99(1):129-134.

164. American College of Obstetricians and Gynecologists Committee on Obstetric Practice. ACOG Committee Opinion, no. 258. Fetal pulse oxim-etry. *Obstet Gynecol.* 2001;98:523.

165. Arikan GM, Scholz HS, Haeusler MCH, et al. Low fetal oxygen saturation at birth and acidosis. *Obstet Gynecol* 2000;95:565.

166. Mallinckrodt Inc. *OxiFirst™ fetal oxygen saturation monitoring system. Operator's Manual. N-400 Fetal Pulse Oximeter.* Mallinckrodt Inc.; 2000.

167. Seelbach-Gobel B, Heupel M, Kuhnert M, Butterwegge M. The prediction of fetal acidoses by means of intrapartum fetal pulse oximetry. *Am J Obstet Gynecol.* 1999;180:73.

168. Dildy GA, Clark SL, Loucks CA. Intrapartum fetal pulse oximetry: past, present, and future. *Am J Obstet Gynecol.* 1996;175:1.

177. East CE, Begg L, Colditz PB, Lau R. Fetal pulse oximetry for fetal assess-ment in labour. *Cochrane Database Syst Rev.* 2014;2014(10):CD004075.

178. Luttkus AK, Stupin JH, Callsen TA, Dudenhausen JW. Feasibility of simul-taneous application of fetal electrocardiography and fetal pulse oximetry. *Acta Obstet Gynecol Scand.* 2003;82:443.

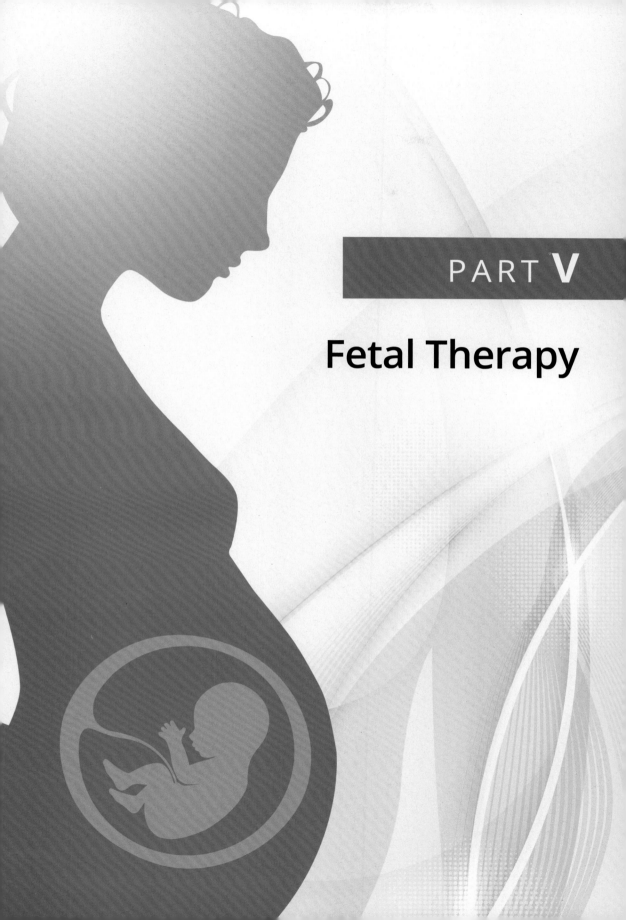

PART V

Fetal Therapy

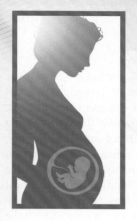

CHAPTER **22**

Maternal Alloimmunization and Fetal Hemolytic Disease

Mae-Lan Winchester and Carl P. Weiner

Introduction

Red Blood Cell Antigens
There are two main blood group antigens, ABO (with blood types A, AB, AB, and O) and RhD (either positive or negative). The most common system causing serious alloimmunization is the Rh antigen system.

Rh Antigen System Nomenclature
The Fisher-Race system, first proposed in the 1940s, presumes the presence of three genetic loci, each with two major alleles—Dd, Cc, Ee.[6] An Rh gene complex is described by three letters: Cde, cde, cDE, cDe, Cde, cdE, CDE, CdE. The first three complexes, Cde, cde, and cDE, are the most common, and the last one, CdE, is yet to be demonstrated.

The presence or absence of the D antigen determines the Rh status. Approximately 45% of D-positive individuals are homozygous for D antigen. For example, offspring conceived by a man who is homozygous D-positive (Rh-positive) and a woman who is homozygous D-negative (Rh-negative) will be D positive; if he is heterozygous, there is an equal chance that the offspring will be D negative or D positive in each pregnancy.

Immunology
The Rh antigen system is highly immunogenic. Ten different antigenic epitopes have been identified to date. One theory suggests the different epitopes are

variably expressed within the erythrocyte membrane, and that this immunologic variation accounts for the spectrum of fetal hemolytic disease.

Rh Functionality
Rh antigens are transmembrane proteins thought to maintain appropriate erythrocyte shape and are expressed on the fetal erythrocytes by day 38 of gestation. Expression of these antigens may have a role in maintaining erythrocyte integrity, and contributing to electrolyte and volume flux across the erythrocyte membrane.

PATHOGENESIS OF MATERNAL ALLOIMMUNIZATION

For Rh alloimmunization to occur:

1. The woman must be Rh negative and the fetus Rh positive.
2. Fetal erythrocytes must enter the maternal circulation in sufficient quantity.
3. The mother must be immune competent.

Transplacental Hemorrhage
A major cause of maternal alloimmunization is transplacental hemorrhage (TPH), which was shown to cause Rh immunization by Chown. Seventy-five percent of women have a fetal TPH at some time during pregnancy or at delivery.[20] The hemorrhage volume is usually small, but exceeds 5 mL in 1% and 30 mL in 0.25% of pregnancies. The prevalence and volume of TPH rises with advancing gestation, from 3% (0.03 mL) in the first trimester, to 12% (usually < 0.1 mL) in the second trimester, to 45% (occasionally up to 25 mL) in the

See the eBook for expanded content, a complete reference list, and additional figures.

third trimester.[20] Antenatal invasive procedures, such as chorionic villus sampling or amniocentesis, increase the risk of TPH, although hemorrhage volume remains small.[21] Antepartum hemorrhage, cesarean section, manual removal of the placenta, and external cephalic version each increase both the rate and volume of TPH. Spontaneous abortion has a low risk of TPH (typically < 0.1 mL). However, the risk may be as high as 25% after therapeutic abortion, with volumes exceeding 0.2 mL in 4% of pregnancies.[22] Women who become Rh immunized after spontaneous abortion are considered "good responders," and frequently have very severely affected fetuses in subsequent pregnancies.

In 1957, the Kleihauer acid elution test was developed, which provided a sensitive, but only semiquantitative, method of detecting TPH.[23] Currently, more sensitive testing can be accomplished using flow cytometry, which measures directly the concentration of either the Rh antigen or hemoglobin F in maternal circulation. Flow cytometry can detect total blood volumes of <2.0 mL and is especially useful in mothers with hemoglobinopathies, such as sickle cell disease, where the maternal fetal hemoglobin level is higher than that of unaffected women.[24] However, flow cytometry is not yet available in all hospitals, perhaps due to equipment and staffing requirements, and many centers only provide the Kleihauer-Betke.

Maternal Response

At least two factors affect whether alloimmunization occurs. First, 30% of Rh-negative individuals behave as immunologic nonresponders and do not become sensitized, regardless of the Rh-antigen load. Second, ABO incompatibility has a protective effect. ABO incompatibility decreases the risk of alloimmunization to 1.5% to 2% after the delivery of an Rh-positive neonate. However, ABO incompatibility provides no protection once Rh immunization has developed.[27]

Antibody Detection and Measurement Methods

3. Indirect antiglobulin test (IAT)[30]—Antihuman globulin (AHG) antibody (Coombs serum) is produced by the injection of human serum (or specific human IgG) into an animal. IgG anti-D antibodies, if present, adhere to Rh-positive erythrocytes after incubation with the serum being screened for Rh antibodies. The erythrocytes are then washed with isotonic saline and suspended in the AHG antibody serum. The erythrocytes agglutinate if coated with antibody (a positive IAT or indirect Coombs test). The reciprocal of the highest dilution causing agglutination is the indirect antiglobulin titer. IAT screening is more sensitive than albumin screening. IAT titers are usually one to three dilutions higher than albumin titers. A critical titer is defined as the titer associated with a significant risk of fetal hydrops. This varies with the institution and methodology. Most centers have a critical titer between 8 and 32.

4. Enzyme—The incubation of erythrocytes with various enzymes (ie, papain, trypsin, or bromelin) reduces the negative electrical potential of the cells. As a result, the erythrocytes lie closer together in saline and are agglutinated by IgG anti-D antibodies.

5. Autoanalyzer (AA)—AA methods (bromelin[31] and low ionic[32]) are the most sensitive for the detection of Rh antibodies. In this technique, erythrocytes are mixed with agents to enhance agglutination by the anti-D antibodies. Agglutinated cells are separated from nonagglutinated cells and lysed. The amount of released hemoglobin is then compared to an international standard. A modification of the bromelin method is used to measure accurately (µg/mL) the amount of serum anti-D antibodies.[33]

PATHOGENESIS OF FETAL HEMOLYTIC DISEASE

Degrees of Rh Hemolytic Disease

The severity of hemolytic disease reflects the amount of maternal IgG anti-D antibodies (the titer) produced, the antibodies' particular affinity or avidity for the fetal red cell membrane D antigen, and the ability of the fetus to tolerate hypoxemia before developing hydrops secondary to myocardial pump failure.

Mild Disease

Approximately 50% of affected fetuses do not require treatment postnatally. Their umbilical cord blood hemoglobin is above 12 g/dL, and their umbilical cord serum bilirubin is less than 68 µmol/L (<4 mg/100 mL). In the nursery, their hemoglobin does not drop below 11 g/dL, and their serum indirect bilirubin remains below 340 µmol/L (20 mg/dL) or 260 to 300 µmol/L (15-17.5 mg/dL) if preterm. Postdischarge hemoglobin remains above 7.5 g/dL.

Intermediate Disease

Approximately 25% to 30% of affected fetuses have intermediate disease. They are born at or near term in good condition, with an umbilical cord blood hemoglobin between 9 g/dL and 12 g/dL. Extramedullary erythropoiesis is modest and liver function normal.

Some of these infants develop severe hyperbilirubinemia; those with kernicterus are deeply jaundiced. Thankfully, the current incidence of this potentially devastating condition is 1 in 650 to 1000 infants born above 35 weeks' gestation.[39] They become lethargic by day 3 to 5 and then hypertonic. They assume an opisthotonic position with their necks hyperextended; backs arched; and knees, wrists, and elbows flexed. Their vegetative reflexes disappear, and apneic spells develop. The mortality rate approaches 90%. In the remaining 10%, the jaundice fades and spasticity lessens. However, they show severe central nervous system dysfunction over time with profound neurosensory deafness and choreoathetoid spastic cerebral palsy. Developmental delay may be relatively mild, but learning and functioning are hindered by deafness and spastic choreoathetosis.

Severe Disease

The remaining 25% are the most severely affected fetuses, who, despite maximal red blood cell production, become progressively more anemic. Ascites with anasarca (generalized edema) occurs. Half these fetuses become hydropic between 18 and 34 weeks' gestation; the other half between 34 weeks and term.

The mechanism underlying hydrops has become clearer over time. There is always a large hemoglobin deficit.[40] Because hemoglobin concentration rises with advancing gestational age, hydrops occurs at higher absolute hemoglobin levels in late compared to early gestation and is rare before 20 weeks' gestation. Cardiac dysfunction secondary to severe fetal anemia and the resultant inadequate oxygen-carrying capacity is evident in at least 90% of hydropic fetuses. Fetal cardiac dysfunction is characterized by an increase in the biventricular cardiac diameter, systolic atrial-ventricular valve regurgitation, abnormal peak velocity index for veins in the ductus venosus and an elevated umbilical pressure for gestational age.[41] Cardiac dysfunction is detectable prior to the development of hydrops and within 48 hours of transfusion (well before the hydrops resolves), the umbilical venous pressure decreases into the normal range for gestation.[42,43] Although hepatomegaly was once thought to cause portal hypertension and decrease cardiac return, it is clear this is not the typical mechanism. Additionally, whereas hypoalbuminemia (secondary to fetal liver failure) was once thought to be a contributing factor, fetal studies have revealed that the albumin concentration is normal in all but premoribund, hydropic fetuses.[41,44]

Monitoring the Mother and Fetus at Risk

A blood sample is obtained from every woman during her first prenatal visit for blood type and antibody screening. Ideally, all women should have two blood type determinations on record that are in agreement.

The American College of Obstetricians and Gynecologists recommends routine repeat testing of all women at 28 weeks to detect RhD sensitization due to early fetomaternal hemorrhage.[45]

The fetal risk is determined once the mother is found to have a clinically significant alloantibody.

Historically, amniocentesis was the preferred method of evaluating fetal antigen status. Furthermore, fetal cells obtained by chorionic villus sampling may also be used. Currently, other methods to determine Rh status include cloning complementary DNA to detect the fetal Rh D genotype and using probes for other known Rh antigens.

Advances in plasma cell-free fetal DNA (cffDNA) processing have allowed for the accurate determination of fetal antigen status from maternal blood across all three trimesters.[48-50]

At delivery, umbilical cord and maternal blood are tested: umbilical cord blood for ABO, Rh type, and direct Coombs status; and maternal blood for the presence of Rh antibody and fetal red cells.

PREDICTING THE SEVERITY OF RH HEMOLYTIC DISEASE

Medical History

The severity of hemolytic disease may remain similar from pregnancy to pregnancy (mild, moderate, or severe), but is more likely to progress in severity with each Rh-positive pregnancy. The risk of hydrops is 8% to 10% in a first sensitized pregnancy. If a woman has had a hydropic fetus, there is a 90% chance that the next affected fetus will also develop hydrops without intervention, typically at the same or an earlier time in gestation.

Rh Antibody Titers

If Rh antibody titers are measured in the same laboratory by the same experienced personnel using the same methods, the results are reproducible and of some value in predicting the risk of severe hemolytic disease. Because the binding constant of the Rh antibody varies from fetus to fetus, as may the density of Rh antigen on the red blood cell membrane and the ability of the fetus to compensate for RBC hemolysis, the titer indicates only which fetus is at risk. The maternal antibody titer that puts the fetus at risk must be determined by each laboratory. However, in general, an albumin titer of 16 or an indirect antiglobulin titer of 32 to 64 carries a 10% risk that the fetus will become hydropic without intervention. The exact titer threshold that is deemed critical will vary by lab. Titers of at-risk women should be repeated monthly after the first prenatal visit.

Fetal Blood Sampling

Maternal history and antibody titer alone are inadequate for the proper management of the Rh-immunized pregnancy, and fetal blood sampling by cordocentesis may be necessary. Fetal blood sampling is by far the most accurate means of determining the degree of severity of hemolytic disease.

Ultrasound

Ultrasound has a central role in the management of the alloimmunized pregnancy because it establishes gestational age, can predict moderate and severe anemia, and can detect hydrops fetalis.[55-60]

Doppler Ultrasonography

A number of investigators found that decreasing fetal hemoglobin levels, which would be associated with a lower blood viscosity and increased cardiac output, also produce higher blood velocities.[61-63] Vessels studied include the descending aorta, the umbilical vein, the splenic artery, the common carotid artery, and the middle cerebral artery (MCA). The most commonly interrogated vessel is the MCA.

The Society for Maternal-Fetal Medicine recommends that MCA-PSV be used as the primary technique to detect fetal anemia, with MCA-PSV greater than 1.5 MoM (multiples of median) as the threshold for cordocentesis to confirm that a fetal intravascular transfusion is needed.[65] More than 70% of invasive tests can be avoided using this threshold. (See Amniotic Fluid Analysis in eBook online.)

Cell-Mediated Maternal Antibody Functional Assays

Because of the relatively poor correlation between blood group antibody and severity of hemolytic disease, various functional assays were developed to reflect the antibody-binding avidity for the red blood cell membrane antigen. These assays include the monocyte monolayer assay,[58] antibody-dependent cellular cytotoxicity (ADCC) using lymphocytes,[59] ADCC using monocytes,[67] and monocyte chemiluminescence.[68] However, all tests are incapable of differentiating the unaffected antigen-negative fetus from the affected antigen-positive fetus and appear to have modest clinical value as currently formulated.

MANAGEMENT OF THE RH-IMMUNIZED WOMAN AND HER FETUS

Nonsensitized Women (First Affected Pregnancy)

Management of the newly sensitized woman begins upon identification of an antibody against a clinically significant antigen. The care team must be familiar with their laboratory's maternal indirect Coombs antibody titers (assuming the results are reproducible) and threshold.

When the maternal indirect Coombs antibody titers are below the threshold (below which severe fetal hemolytic disease does not occur), they should be repeated monthly. Once the critical titer is exceeded, the fetus is followed with serial measurements of the MCA-PSV. An MCA-PSV greater than 1.5 MoM indicates the need for invasive fetal testing. A determination of the fetal PCR Rh genotype should be standard in any at-risk women undergoing chorionic villus sampling or second-trimester amniocentesis because a negative result eliminates the need for further testing.

Cordocentesis is indicated when the peak MCA Doppler velocity exceeds 1.5 MoM. With the declining incidence of maternal isoimmunization, these patients should be referred to maternal-fetal medicine specialists with experience in the field. Approximately 50% of isoimmunized women will require only one cordocentesis and, with the use of Doppler ultrasound, delivery may be safely deferred until term.[69]

Laboratory tests performed on the first fetal specimen include type and Rh status, direct Coombs test, complete blood count (CBC), manual reticulocyte count, and total bilirubin. Laboratory tests sent on subsequent fetal specimens include CBC, manual reticulocyte count, and total bilirubin. If the fetus is not anemic when first sampled, a strongly positive direct Coombs test or a manual reticulocyte count outside the 95% confidence interval are strong risk factors for the development of anemia *in utero*.

Rh-Immunized Women With a Previously Affected Fetus or Infant

Patients should be referred to a tertiary care center if they have documented isoimmunization. Maternal titers are not predictive of the degree of fetal anemia. If the paternal phenotype is heterozygous or the father is unknown, either a maternal plasma sample or an amniocentesis is performed at 15 weeks to determine fetal RhD status. If the fetus is antigen positive, initiating serial MCA Doppler measurements by 18 weeks to monitor the pregnancy is recommended. Testing is repeated every 1 to 2 weeks as long as results are normal. If a rising value for peak MCA Doppler velocity greater than 1.5 MoM is found, a cordocentesis is performed and the fetus transfused if the hematocrit is <30%.

Treatment

Intrauterine Fetal Transfusion

Fetal transfusion therapy should never be undertaken in the absence of hydrops without first confirming that the fetus has significant anemia. These procedures should only be performed by individuals with considerable experience.

Intraperitoneal Fetal Transfusions

Intraperitoneal fetal transfusion is the original method of fetal transfusion and is now considered a rarely needed backup to intravascular transfusion.

Direct Intravascular Fetal Transfusion

IVT should be performed using blood from a fresh donor whenever possible, group O, and negative for the antigen (or antigens) to which the mother is sensitized (D negative if the mother is Rh negative with anti-D antibodies). It should also be negative for hepatitis B surface antigen, human immunodeficiency virus, hepatitis C virus, and cytomegalovirus. The blood unit is centrifuged, and the supernatant plasma with its buffy coat is discarded. Gamma irradiation of the donor red cells

is recommended. Sterile isotonic saline is added to the packed red cells immediately before the intrauterine transfusion (IUT) raising the hematocrit to between 70% and 75%. Transfused blood with a higher hematocrit mixes much more slowly.

The mother is made comfortable with pillows placed under her knees (to take pressure off the lower spine) and a pillow positioned on the left to displace the uterus to avoid supine hypotension. Diazepam (5-10 mg) administered orally or intravenously is used to foster relaxation during the procedure. There is no reason to administer indomethacin or a neuraxial anesthetic. The maternal abdomen is surgically prepared. Prophylactic antibiotic administration is neither effective nor cost-efficient. The unit of blood at room temperature is attached to a blood filter and then a three-way valve. A length of extension tubing is attached to the stopcock end and filled with donor red cells, taking great care to ensure that no air bubbles are in the tubing, stopcock, or syringe.

Once prepared, the operator selects the easiest approach to the umbilical vein and, under real-time ultrasound guidance (the transducer being enclosed in a sterile drape), directs a 10-cm, 20 to 22-gauge spinal puncture needle into the umbilical vein. The selected skin site is infiltrated with 1% lidocaine, although some women may decline use of a local anesthetic as the burning sensation is often greater than the discomfort from the needle puncture.

If the artery is inadvertently punctured, the needle should be removed and redirected to the vein unless there is no other option. When the needle appears within the vessel, the stylet is withdrawn and, upon return of blood, the fetus is paralyzed with pancuronium (0.2-0.3 mg/kg estimated fetal weight [EFW]) intravenously, to ensure fetal quiet, as any fetal movement may cause catastrophic events such as vessel laceration or cord hematoma. Pancuronium is also advantageous for IVT specifically because its sympathomimetic effect helps maintain cardiac output as the fetus is volume loaded. After fetal paralysis, the umbilical venous pressure is measured. It provides definitive identification of the vessel punctured and allows for the monitoring of the fetal response to volume loading. Furosemide (3 mg/kg EFW) may also be administered to ameliorate volume loading; however, research has failed to show a clear benefit.[75]

The donor blood is injected in 20-mL aliquots over 2 to 3 minutes. The transfusion is monitored continuously by ultrasound (streaming turbulence is seen as the donor red cells pass down the vein). Meanwhile, the assistant must be ready to halt the infusion if there is any abrupt change in the resistance to flow. Because only 2 to 3 mm of needle is in the fetal vessel, there is a significant risk of dislodgement, either into the amniotic cavity (easily recognized and not hazardous) or into the cord substance producing a cord hematoma with risk of umbilical venous compression and vasospasm-induced bradycardia. Excluding the first transfusion of a hydropic fetus, the target for the posttransfusion fetal hematocrit is 48% to 55%. Consequently, the volume infused depends on the gestational age and the initial hematocrit.

Intrahepatic IVT

The intrahepatic portion of the umbilical vein has been used as a transfusion site, especially for severely affected fetuses who require transfusion in the early second trimester. This technique was first described by Nicolini in 1990.[77] Claimed benefits of this approach include needle stabilization by the surrounding tissue. This technique is considered a safe alternative to umbilical vein transfusion, especially in cases of a posterior placenta when the practitioner is uncomfortable with a free loop transfusion.

Fetal Monitoring During Transfusion

A variety of options exist to monitor the fetus during the transfusion. First, obtaining images of the fetal heart to rule out bradycardias, but this is of limited value. A second option is to periodically measure the umbilical venous pressure.[43] If the fetus does not tolerate the transfusion, the umbilical venous pressure will increase (fetal bradycardias also increase the umbilical venous pressure); an increase of >10 mm Hg is associated with increased perinatal mortality, and the transfusion should be stopped and, if needed, blood volume should be removed to reduce the fetal preload. Another option is Doppler ultrasound to evaluate fetal well-being during the transfusion.

Intrauterine Transfusion in the Presence of Hydrops Fetalis

Most hydropic fetuses have myocardial dysfunction. As a result, they frequently fail to tolerate the typical transfusion volume load.[41] Thus, the target hematocrit after the first transfusion should be no more than 25%. A day later, the hematocrit can safely be brought up to the target 48% to 55% with a second transfusion.

Umbilical vein pH (UVpH) maintenance is especially important in the hydropic fetus.

The blood volume transfused depends on gestational age and the starting hematocrit. Several formulae exist to calculate the volume needed; however, none is reliable enough to terminate the procedure without first checking the hematocrit. Donor blood with a hematocrit <75% equilibrates rapidly (likely because of the rapid fluid exchange across the placenta) whereas donor blood with a hematocrit > 80% does not equilibrate as rapidly (likely because of increased viscosity).

The last transfusion is done between 34 and 35 weeks' gestation, and delivery is planned at 38 to 39 weeks. Transfusion therapy is not an indication for cesarean delivery.

Fetal Hematologic Response to Transfusion

One goal of transfusion therapy is the complete suppression of fetal erythropoiesis, and the average fetal reticulocyte count is usually <1% by the third transfusion. Complications of hyperbilirubinemia are less if at least two transfusions have been performed 3 weeks apart. The longer fetal erythropoiesis is suppressed, the longer it takes to resume postnatally. It is common after initiating therapy before 24 weeks to have to support the neonate with small transfusions to maintain the hematocrit between 25% and 30% until erythropoiesis resumes after a month.

Timing of Repeat Transfusion

The traditional method to determine the timing of repeat transfusion involves estimating the rate of red blood cell destruction by a reduction in either fetal hemoglobin (or hematocrit) in between transfusions. This estimation commonly assumes a decrease in fetal hemoglobin of 0.3 g/dL/d or hematocrit 1%/d between IUTs. It does not take into account the impact of the percent remaining fetal red blood cells and gestational age.

MCA Doppler velocimetry can also be used to time IVT. Improvement in fetal anemia after IVT is associated with the normalization of the MCA-PSV.

Procedure-Related Complications

Possible complications related to cordocentesis and IUT include bleeding, umbilical vessel thrombosis, preterm premature rupture of membranes, emergent delivery due to bradycardia, and fetal death.

Survival After Fetal Transfusion

Survival after IUT varies with center experience and with the presence or absence of hydrops. Practitioners should refer patients to experienced units.

The presence or absence of hydrops impacts survival even when appropriate alterations in technique are made.

Gestational age at time of IUT has large effect on fetal mortality. Fetuses requiring early second trimester transfusion have increased disease severity. This plus the technical challenges of early procedures increase the risk of perinatal death as much as fourfold compared to fetuses in whom the transfusion can be delayed.[83] Given the increased risks of early transfusion, several strategies to decrease disease severity and therefore the need for early transfusion have been proposed. These include differing puncture sites as discussed previously (intrahepatic, intraperitoneal), but also methods of decreasing the maternal immune response to the fetal antigen (discussed later in this chapter).

Delivery of the Fetus After IUT

There is no justification for preterm induction of labor if a transfusion can be performed.

Infants who have received *in utero* transfusion therapy do well after birth. Generally, the neonatal capillary hematocrit increases about 15% within the first few hours of life (likely secondary to fluid shifts) and then decreases slowly to a level at or below the umbilical cord hematocrit level at delivery over the next few days to weeks. As these infants are now delivered at term, they have a higher tolerance to bilirubin levels and can usually be managed with phototherapy alone. The infant may develop anemia by 5 weeks after delivery; this is expected as the transfused blood is nearing the end of its lifespan. This neonatal anemia is also likely associated with a low reticulocyte count. These neonates should have their hematocrit and reticulocyte count monitored weekly. The therapeutic goal is to maintain them with a modest anemia; small transfusions will keep the infant asymptomatic but leave the erythropoietic stimulus unblunted. Once reticulocytosis is observed, the neonate will no longer need further transfusion therapy.

Maternal Effects of IUT

Alloimmunized Rh-negative women are functional hyperresponders and frequently develop other blood group antibodies, such as M, S, s, Jk[a], Fy[a], and so on. A second antibody may manifest after one or two IUTs, jeopardizing the lifespan of the donor red cells transfused next if not corrected. The second antibody can be derived from either the fetus or the transfused (donor) blood. Antibodies to C and E are thought to be most commonly the result of fetal exposure, whereas those to Duffy and S are often due to the transfused unit.

Suppression of Rh Immunization
Plasma Exchange

Large amounts of maternal antibody-containing plasma (3 L/d, 5 days per week) are removed and replaced with saline, 5% albumin, and intravenous gamma globulin to reduce the circulating maternal blood group antibody levels by 75% to 80%. Such reductions are transient and at best, delay the need for IUT by 2 to 3 weeks. With the advent of fetal blood sampling and IVT as early as 18 to 20 weeks' gestation, intensive plasmapheresis is only rarely indicated.

Intravenous Immune Serum Globulin

Intravenous immunoglobulin (IVIG) has been reported to reduce the severity of hemolytic disease.[88] The recommended dose is 1 g/kg maternal body weight administered weekly. IVIG may exert a beneficial effect by negative feedback, reducing maternal antibody levels by 50%; by saturating the trophoblastic Fc receptor sites to impede placental transfer of antibody to the fetus; or by saturating fetal splenic Fc receptor sites, preventing the destruction of antibody-coated fetal red blood cells. The combination of IVIG and plasmapheresis in severely affected fetuses has demonstrated fetal safety and tolerability in several case reports.[89-91] However, technical challenges of each component limit its use.

PREVENTION OF RH IMMUNIZATION

Primary prevention aims to reduce the incidence of Rh isoimmunization by reducing the exposure to foreign antigens.

The goal of secondary prevention is to slow down or even reverse the progression of disease. This is accomplished using prophylactic Rh immunoglobulin (RhIG). RhIG has reduced the prevalence of fetal hemolytic disease secondary to Rh isoimmunization from 16% to <1%.[9]

IUT is a form of tertiary prevention, aimed at ameliorating the disease severity.

Rh Immunoglobulin

The standard dose in the United States is 300 µg given intramuscularly (i.m.). Smaller doses of 100 to 125 µg i.m. are used in Canada, Europe, and Australia. All these doses appear to be effective.

RhIG prevents Rh immunization with two provisos: it must be given in an adequate amount, and it must be given before Rh immunization has begun. RhIG administration does not suppress Rh immunization once it has begun, no matter how weak the immunization.[92]

Because the half-life of RhIG is approximately 1623 days, 15% to 20% of patients receiving it at 28 weeks have a very low anti-D titer at term. In the United States, it is recommended that 300 µg of RhIG be administered within 72 hours of delivery of an Rh-positive infant. This dose will protect against sensitization from a fetal-maternal hemorrhage (FMH) of 30 mL of fetal whole blood. Approximately 1 in 1000 deliveries exceed this volume, and recognized risk factors will identify only 50%. Therefore, routine screening at delivery for excessive FMH is indicated. The rosette test, a qualitative yet sensitive test for FMH, is performed first. A negative test result implies that the patient can receive the standard dose of RhIG. A Kleihauer-Betke stain is performed if the rosette test is positive. The percentage of fetal blood cells is multiplied by 50 to estimate the FMH volume, and additional vials of RhIG are administered to prevent maternal sensitization. No more than five units of RhIG should be administered intramuscularly in a 24-hour period. Should a large dose of RhIG be required, the entire calculated dose may be given using an intravenous preparation.

Antenatal Rh Prophylaxis

Antenatal Rh prophylaxis is widely accepted, although many centers give a single injection of 300 µg of RhIG at or as close to 28 weeks' gestation as possible. The single dose at 28 weeks' gestation has been highly successful.[98]

The administration of RhIG during pregnancy does not harm the fetus.

Postpartum Rh Prophylaxis

One prophylactic dose unit of RhIG should be administered to the Rh-negative nonimmune woman as soon as her infant is determined to be Rh positive and no later than 72 hours postpartum. If the Rh status of the baby remains unknown at 72 hours, the woman should be given RhIG regardless. It is better to treat unnecessarily than to fail to treat an at-risk woman.

Rh Prophylaxis Problems

Residual problems still exist[104,105] and include the following:

1. Failure of compliance after delivery.
2. Failure to give prophylaxis after abortion.
3. Failure to give prophylaxis after amniocentesis.
4. Failure to protect after massive fetal TPH.
5. Failure to protect against Rh immunization during pregnancy.
6. The question of augmentation of the risk of Rh immunization.
7. The question of Rh immunization during infancy.
8. The question of the "weak D" or D^u mother.
9. The question of suppression of weak Rh immunization.
10. Reactions to intramuscular RhIG-ion exchange and RhIG-monoclonal RhIG.
11. Challenges of obesity in RhIG dosing and administration

If massive TPH is diagnosed after delivery of an Rh-positive baby, 600 µg (two vials) of RhIG should be administered if the TPH is greater than 25 mL but less than 50 mL; 900 µg (three vials) of RhIG administered if the TPH is greater than 50 mL but less than 75 mL; and. up to 1200 µg (four vials) of RhIG can be given i.m. every 12 hours until the appropriate dose has been administered.

It is prudent to consider delivery after the TPH exceeds 50 mL if the fetus is 33 weeks or greater and there is evidence of pulmonary maturity.

If a fetal TPH greater than 50 mL is diagnosed early in pregnancy before evidence of fetal lung maturity, cordocentesis should be performed, and a transfusion carried out if a significant anemia is discovered. RhIG (600 µg) should be given to the mother if the fetus is Rh positive.

Reactions to Intramuscular RhIG— Newer Forms of RhIG

Ion-Exchange RhIG

RhIG prepared using ion-exchange chromatography produces a very pure product with greater efficiency of yield, low total protein, no demonstrable IgM, and an IgA content only 0.3% of that in the Cohn-prepared RhIG.[110] It also has very low anticomplement activity and can be given safely intravenously (i.v.). It is twice as effective when given i.v.; thus, only half the dose is needed after delivery (120 μg). However, the antenatal prophylaxis dose must be the same (300 μg) because its half-life is the same.

SUMMARY OF RECOMMENDATIONS FOR RH PROPHYLAXIS

1. Every Rh-negative unimmunized woman who delivers an Rh-positive baby must be given one prophylactic dose of RhIG as soon as possible after delivery.
2. Every Rh-negative unimmunized woman who aborts or threatens to abort must be given RhIG, unless her husband (or father of the baby) is known to be Rh negative.
3. Every Rh-negative unimmunized woman who undergoes amniocentesis or chorionic villus sampling, unless the father of the baby is known to be Rh negative, must be given 300 μg of RhIG at the time of the procedure, with subsequent doses at 12-week intervals until delivery.
4. Every Rh-negative unimmunized woman should be given 300 μg of RhIG at 28 weeks' gestation if the father of the baby is Rh positive or Rh unknown. A second dose should be given 12 weeks later if delivery has not taken place, but does not need to be repeated postpartum if delivery occurs within 3 weeks.
5. If massive TPH is diagnosed, 300 μg of RhIG should be given i.m. for every 25 mL of fetal blood or fraction thereof in the maternal circulation. The dose may be reduced by one-third if RhIG is given i.v.
6. One prophylactic dose of RhIG should be given antepartum to the mother who has an Rh antibody detectable only by AA methods and again after delivery, if she delivers a Rh-positive baby. If the antibody is detectable by a manual enzyme method, administration of RhIG will not prevent progressive immunization. However, it should be given if there is any question about the specificity of the enzyme reactions.

NON-RHD BLOOD GROUP IMMUNIZATION

ABO Hemolytic Disease

Although ABO-incompatible hemolytic transfusion reactions are intravascular and much more serious than extravascular Rh-incompatible hemolytic transfusion reactions, ABO hemolytic disease is much milder than Rh hemolytic disease. Kernicterus due to ABO hemolytic disease is reported, but hydrops caused by ABO hemolytic disease is extremely rare.[116,117]

The management of ABO erythroblastosis is entirely a pediatric concern. Amniocentesis and other fetal investigative measures are not required in the ABO-incompatible pregnancy.

Hemolytic Disease Caused by Atypical Blood Group Antibodies

Non-D alloantibodies, therefore, have assumed greater significance in the etiology of hemolytic disease and are numerous.[118] However, the only antibodies implicated in moderate-to-severe disease are all those in the Rh blood group system plus anti-K, -Jk^a, -Js^a, -Js^b, -Ku, -Fy^a, -M, -N, -s, -U, -PP$_1$p^k, -Di^b, -Lan, -LW, -Far, -Good, -Wr^a, and -Zd (**Table 22.1**). Pregnant women with atypical antibodies should be managed in the same manner as if they were Rh negative and RhD immunized.

Anti-Kell alloimmunization is a special case. There are several reports of severe Kell alloimmune

Table 22.1 Association of Hemolytic Disease With Maternal Blood Group Antibodies

Common	c(cE)—incidence high, disease common, may be severe
	Kell—incidence high, disease uncommon but, if present, may be severe
	E—incidence high, disease uncommon, usually mild, rarely severe
	C(Ce, C^w)—incidence moderate, disease common, usually mild
Uncommon	K—rarely present but, when present, may be very severe
	Kp^a(Kp^b) —rare, disease may require treatment, very rarely severe
	Jk^a—uncommon, may require treatment, rarely severe
	Fy^a—uncommon, usually mild, may require treatment, rarely severe
	S—uncommon, usually mild, may require treatment, rarely severe
Rare	s, U, M, Fy^b, N, Do^a, Di^a, Di^b, Lu^a, Yt^a, Jk^b—rarely cause hemolytic disease
Never	Le^a, Le^b, P—never cause hemolytic disease

disease with low, misleading ΔOD 450 values.[119,120] It has been hypothesized that the expression of the Kell antigen on early fetal red blood cell precursors plays an important role in direct suppression of erythropoiesis evidenced by *in vitro* experiments with anti-Kell antibodies. However, phagocytosis of red blood cell precursors expressing the Kell antigen has also been observed *in vitro*, making it plausible that the lack of hyperbilirubinemia observed in fetuses affected by maternal anti-Kell antibodies is due in part to immune-mediated clearance of very early red blood cell precursors, which do not contain hemoglobin. Anti-Kell antibodies have been postulated to cause destruction of poorly hemoglobinized marrow erythroid precursors,[121] which may explain the reports of more severe Kell hemolytic disease of the newborn than was predicted from the ΔOD 450 readings.[115,116] The management of Kell isoimmunization is the same as for Rh disease and is based on serial MCA Doppler peak velocity measurements and cordocentesis when abnormal.

KEY POINTS

- For Rh alloimmunization to occur:
  - The woman must be Rh negative and the fetus Rh positive.
  - Fetal erythrocytes must enter the maternal circulation in sufficient quantity.
  - The mother must be immune competent.
- The primary maternal Rh immune response is slow (typically over 6-12 weeks)—it is usually weak and predominantly IgM (which does not cross the placenta). The second TPH in an immunized woman produces a rapid (within days) secondary immune response (IgG anti-D antibodies), which can readily cross the placenta, coat fetal erythrocytes, and trigger hemolysis.
- ABO incompatibility between an Rh-positive fetus and an Rh-negative mother reduces the risk of immunization to 1.5% to 2%. This protection is in part because of rapid intravascular hemolysis of the fetal ABO-incompatible cells and their sequestration in the liver. Remember ABO incompatibility confers no protection once Rh immunization has developed.
- Fetal blood is produced as early as the third week in the yolk sac, but moves to the liver and, finally, to the bone marrow by 16 weeks' gestation. The Rh antigen is detectable on the red cell membrane by the sixth week.
- Pathogenesis—maternal IgG anti-D antibodies cross the placenta (TPH) and coat the D-positive fetal red cells. These fetal red cells are destroyed extravascularly, resulting in anemia, which stimulates the synthesis of fetal erythropoietin. Reticulocytosis occurs when fetal hemoglobin deficit exceeds 2 g/dL (compared with gestational age-appropriate norms). Nucleated red cell precursors from normoblasts to primitive erythroblasts are released into the circulation (erythroblastosis fetalis). During hemolysis, the globin chain is split from hemoglobin. The remaining heme pigment is converted by hemeoxygenase to biliverdin, and then by biliverdin reductase to neurotoxic indirect bilirubin. The fetal and newborn liver is deficient in glucuronyl transferase and Y transport protein; therefore, the increased indirect bilirubin is deposited in the extravascular fluid. Indirect bilirubin is water insoluble and, when the albumin-binding capacity is exceeded, the excess indirect bilirubin diffuses into fatty tissues (ie, the neuron), where it interferes with cellular metabolism causing the mitochondria to swell, balloon, and then the neuron dies.
- Doppler velocimetry to assess the peak MCA systolic velocity is the primary screening technique for fetal anemia, using a threshold of 1.5 MoM. Cordocentesis should be performed when this threshold is exceeded.
- Cordocentesis is the most accurate means of determining degree of severity of hemolytic disease, in the absence of hydrops fetalis—it allows the measurement of all blood parameters that can be measured after birth (hemoglobin, hematocrit, serum bilirubin, direct and indirect platelet count, leukocyte count, serum proteins, and blood gases).

- Management of the newly sensitized woman begins with identification. If titers are below the threshold (below which severe fetal hemolytic disease does not occur), they should be repeated monthly. Once the critical titer is exceeded, the fetus is followed with serial measurements of the peak MCA velocity. The timing of invasive fetal testing (cordocentesis) is determined by ultrasound evidence of fetal anemia (when the peak MCA velocity becomes elevated).

- Management of the woman with a previously sensitized fetus again begins with identification. If the fetus is deemed to be at risk, initiate serial MCA Doppler measurements by 18 weeks to monitor these pregnancies. Testing should be repeated every 1 to 2 weeks as long as the MCA Doppler measurements are normal. If a rising value for peak MCA Doppler velocity of more than 1.5 MoM is found, a cordocentesis should be performed and the fetus transfused if the hematocrit is <30%.

- Transfusion therapy is initiated when the fetal hematocrit is <30%, a value less than the 2.5th per centile at all gestational ages above 20 weeks.

- The blood used for fetal transfusion should be from a fresh donor, group O, and negative for the antigen (or antigens) to which the mother is sensitized. It should also be negative for infectious diseases.

- Transfusion therapy suppresses fetal erythropoiesis, and the average reticulocyte count is usually <1% by the third transfusion. The complications of hyperbilirubinemia are less if at least two transfusions are performed 3 weeks apart. The last transfusion can be done between 34 and 35 weeks' gestation and delivery planned at 38 to 39 weeks. Transfusion therapy is not an indication for cesarean delivery.

- RhIG prevents Rh immunization with two provisos: it must be given in adequate amounts, and it must be given before Rh immunization has begun. RhIG administration does not suppress Rh immunization once it has begun, no matter how weak the immunization.

- In the United States, it is recommended that 300 µg of RhIG be administered within 72 hours of delivery of an Rh-positive infant. This dose will protect against sensitization from TPH of 30 mL of fetal whole blood. Approximately 1 in 1000 deliveries will exceed this volume. Therefore, routine screening at delivery for excessive TPH is indicated. The rosette test is performed first; if negative, the patient needs to receive only the standard dose of RhIG and, if positive, a Kleihauer-Betke stain is performed to determine the number of additional vials of RhIG that are needed to prevent maternal sensitization.

- RhIG administration is also recommended for all invasive diagnostic procedures, external cephalic version, and abortion.

REFERENCES

(only references cited in synoptic print chapter; for a complete reference list, see ebook)

6. Race RR. The Rh genotype and Fisher's theory. *Blood.* 1948;3:27.

9. Issitt PD. The Rh blood group system, 1988: eight new antigens in nine years and some observation on the biochemistry and genetics of the system. *Transfus Med Rev.* 1989;3:1.

20. Bowman JM, Pollock JM, Penton LE. Fetomaternal transplacental hemorrhage during pregnancy and after delivery. *Vox Sang.* 1986;51:117.

21. Bowman JM, Pollock JM. Transplacental fetal hemorrhage after amniocentesis. *Obstet Gynecol.* 1985;66:749.

22. Goldman JA, Eckerling B. Transplacental hemorrhage during spontaneous and therapeutic artificial abortion. *Obstet Gynecol.* 1970;35(6):903-908.

23. Kleihauer E, Braun H, Betke K. Demonstration von fetalem Haemoglobin in den Erythrozyten eines Blutausstriches. *Klin Wochenschr.* 1957;35:637.

24. Farias MG, Dal Bó S, Castro SM, et al. Flow cytometry in detection of fetal red blood cells and maternal F cells to identify fetomaternal hemorrhage. *Fetal Pediatr Pathol.* 2016;35(6):385-391.

27. Bowman JM. Fetomaternal ABO incompatibility and erythroblastosis fetalis. *Vox Sang.* 1986;50:104.

30. Zipursky A, Israels LG. The pathogenesis and prevention of Rh immunization. *Can Med Assoc J.* 1967;97:1245.

31. Rosenfield RE, Haber GV. *Detection and measurement of homologous human hemagglutinins.* In: *Automation in Analytical Chemistry-Technicon Symposia.* Mediad, Inc.; 1965:503.

32. Lalezari P. A polybrene method for the detection of red cell antibodies. *Fed Proc.* 1967;26:756.

33. Moore BPL. Automation in the blood transfusion laboratory. I. Antibody detection and quantitation in the Technicon Auto Analyzer. *Can Med Assoc J.* 1969;100:381.

39. Bhutani VK, Johnson L. Kernicterus in the 21st century: frequently asked questions. *J Perinatol.* 2009;29 Suppl 1:S20-S24. doi:10.1038/jp.2008.212

40. Nicolaides KH, Warenski JC, Rodeck CH. The relationship of fetal protein concentration and haemoglobin level to the development of hydrops in rhesus isoimmunization. *Am J Obstet Gynecol.* 1985;152:341.

41. Weiner CP, Williamson RA, Wenstrom KD, et al. Management of fetal hemolytic disease by cordocentesis: I. Prediction of fetal anemia. *Am J Obstet Gynecol.* 1991;165:546.

42. Weiner CP, Williamson RA, Wenstrom KD, et al. Management of fetal hemolytic disease by cordocentesis: II. Outcome of treatment. *Am J Obstet Gynecol.* 1991;165:1302.

43. Weiner CP, Pelzer GD, Heilskov J, Wenstrom KD, Williamson RA. The effect of intravascular transfusion on umbilical venous pressure in anemic fetuses with and without hydrops. *Am J Obstet Gynecol.* 1989;161(6 Pt 1): 1498-1501. doi:10.1016/0002-9378(89)90912-5.

44. Weiner CP. Human fetal bilirubin and fetal hemolytic disease. *Am J Obstet Gynecol.* 1992;116:1449.

45. American College of Obstetrics and Gynecology. Practice bulletin No. 181: prevention of Rh D alloimmunization. *Obstet Gynecol.* 2017;130(2):e57-e70.

48. Scheffer PG, van der Schoot CE, Page-Christiaens GC, de Haas M. Noninvasive fetal blood group genotyping of rhesus D, c, E and of K in alloimmunised pregnant women: evaluation of a 7-year clinical experience. *Br J Obstet Gynecol.* 2011;118:340-1348.

49. Manzanares S, Entrala C, Sánchez-Gila M, et al. Noninvasive fetal RhD status determination in early pregnancy. *Fetal Diag Ther.* 2014;35:7-12.

50. Boggione CT, LujánBrajovich ME, Mattaloni SM, et al. Genotyping approach for non-invasive foetal RHD detection in an admixed population. *Blood Transfus.* 2017;15:66-73.

55. Nicolaides KH, Fontanarosa M, Gabbe SG, Rodeck CH. Failure of ultrasonographic parameters to predict the severity of fetal anemia in rhesus isoimmunization. *Am J Obstet Gynecol.* 1988;158:920.

56. Mari G, Adrignolo A, Abuhamad AZ, et al. Diagnosis of feta anemia with Doppler ultrasound in pregnancy complicated by maternal blood group immunization. *Ultrasound Obstet Gynecol.* 1995;5:400.

57. Detti L, Mari G, Akiyama M, et al. Longitudinal assessment of the middle cerebral artery peak systolic velocity in healthy fetuses and in fetuses at risk for anemia. *Am J Obstet Gynecol.* 2002;187:937.

58. Zupanska B, Brojer E, Richards Y, et al. Serological and immunological characteristics of maternal anti-Rh(D) antibodies in predicting the severity of haemolytic disease of the newborn. *Vox Sang.* 1989;56:247.

59. Urbaniak SI, Greiss MA, Crawford RJ, et al. Prediction of the outcome of Rhesus haemolytic disease of the newborn: additional information using an ADCC assay. *Vox Sang.* 1984;46:323.

60. Bahado-Singh R, Oz U, Mari G, et al. Fetal splenic size in anemia due to Rh-alloimmunization. *J Ultrasound Med.* 2005;24:697.

61. Mari G. Doppler ultrasonography in obstetrics: from the diagnosis of fetal anemia to the treatment of intrauterine growth-restricted fetuses. *Am J Obstet Gynecol.* 2009;200(6):613.e1-613.e6139. doi:10.1016/j.ajog. 2008.10.054

62. Moise KJ Jr. The usefulness of middle cerebral artery Doppler assessment in the treatment of the fetus at risk for anemia. *Am J Obstet Gynecol.* 2008;198(2):161.e1-161.e1614. doi:10.1016/j.ajog.2007.10.788

63. Pretlove SJ, Fox CE, Khan KS, Kilby MD. Noninvasive methods of detecting fetal anaemia: a systematic review and meta-analysis. *BJOG.* 2009;116(12):1558-1567. doi:10.1111/j.1471-0528.2009.02255.x

65. Society for Maternal-Fetal Medicine (SMFM); Mari G, Norton ME, et al. Society for Maternal-fetal Medicine (SMFM) Clinical Guideline #8: the fetus at risk for anemia – diagnosis and management. *Am J Obstet Gynecol.* 2015;212:697-710.

67. Engelfriet CP, Brouwers HAA, Huiskes E, et al. Prognostic value of the ADCC with monocytes and maternal antibodies for haemolytic disease of the newborn. Abstract presented at: XXIst Congress ISH and XIXth Congress ISBT; 1986; Sydney, Australia. 162(abst).

68. Hadley AB, Kumpel BM, Leader KA, et al. Correlation of serological, quantitative and cell-mediated functional assays of maternal alloantibodies with the severity of haemolytic disease of the newborn. *Br J Haematol.* 1991;77:221.

69. Sánchez-Durán MÁ, Higueras MT, Halajdian-Madrid C, et al. Management and outcome of pregnancies in women with red cell isoimmunization: a 15-year observational study from a tertiary care university hospital. *BMC Pregnancy Childbirth.* 2019;19(1):356. doi:10.1186/s12884-019-2525-y

75. Chestnut DH, Pollack KL, Weiner CP, et al. Does furosemide alter the hemodynamic response to rapid intravascular transfusion of the anemic fetal lamb. *Am J Obstet Gynecol.* 1989;161:1571.

77. Nicolini U, Santolaya J, Ojo OE, et al. The fetal intrahepatic umbilical vein as an alternative to cord needling for prenatal diagnosis and therapy. *Prenat Diag.* 1998;9:665-671.

83. Lindenburg IT, van Kamp IL, van Zwet EW, et al. Increased perinatal loss after intrauterine transfusion for alloimmuneanaemia before 20 weeks of gestation. *Br J Obstet Gynecol.* 2013;120:847-852.

88. Bartsch F, Sandberg L. Incidence of anti-D at delivery in previously non-immunized Rh-negative mothers with Rh-positive babies. *Vox Sang.* 1979;36:50. Presented at McMaster Conference on Prevention of Rh Immunization, 28-30 September, 1977.

89. Nwogu LC, MoiseJr KJ, Klein KI, Tint H, Castillo B, Bai Y. Successful management of severe red blood cell alloimmunization in pregnancy with a combination of therapeutic plasma exchange, intravenous immune globulin, and intrauterine transfusion. *Transfusion.* 2018;58:677-684.

90. Fernandez Alba JJ, Leon R, Gonzalez-Macias C, et al. Treatment of D alloimmunization in pregnancy with plasmapheresis, intravenous immune globulin, and intrauterine transfusion: case report. *Transfus Apher Sci.* 2014;51:70-72.

91. Houston BL, Govia R, Abov-Setta AM, et al. Severe alloimmunization and hemolytic disease of the fetus managed with plasmapheresis, intravenous immunoglobulin, and intrauterine transfusion: a case report. *Transfus Apher Sci.* 2015;53:399-402.

92. Bowman JM, Pollock JM. Reversal of Rh alloimmunization. Fact or fancy? *Vox Sang.* 1984;47:209.

98. Bowman JM, Pollock JM. Antenatal Rh prophylaxis: 28-week gestation service program. *Can Med Assoc J.* 1978;118:627.

104. Bowman JM. Controversies in Rh prophylaxis: who needs Rh immune globulin and when should it be given? *Am J Obstet Gynecol.* 1985;151:289.

105. Bowman JM. The prevention of Rh immunization. *Transfus Med Rev.* 1988;2:129.

110. Hoppe HH, Mester T, Hennig W, Krebs HJ. Prevention of Rh-immunization: modified production of IgG anti Rh for intravenous application by ion exchange chromatography (IEC). *Vox Sang.* 1973;25:308.

115. MacDonald G, Primrose S, Biggins K, et al. Production and characterizationofhuman-humanandhuman-mousetohybridomassecretingRh(D)-specific monoclonal antibodies. *Scand J Immunol.* 1987;25:477.

116. Miller DF, Petrie SJ. Fatal erythroblastosisfetalis secondary to ABO incompatibility: report of a case. *Obstet Gynecol.* 1963;22:773.

117. Gilja BK, Shah VP. Hydropsfetalis due to ABO incompatibility. *Clin Pediatr.* 1988;27:210.

118. Mollison PL, Engelfriet CP, Contreras M. Hemolytic disease of the newborn. In: Mollison PL, ed. *Blood Transfusion in Clinical Medicine.* 8th ed. Blackwell Scientific Publications; 1987:639.

119. Caine ME, Mueller-Heubach E. Kell sensitization in pregnancy. *Am J Obstet Gynecol.* 1986;154:85.

120. Hadi HA, Robertson A. Kell sensitization, hydrops, and low delta OD$_{450}$. *J Matern Fetal Med.* 1992;1:293.

121. Vaughan JI, Warwick R, Letsky E, et al. Erythropoietic suppression in fetal anemia because of Kellalloimmunization. *Am J Obstet Gynecol.* 1994;171:247.

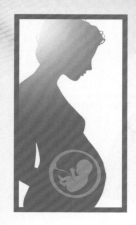

CHAPTER 23

Fetal Neonatal Alloimmune Thrombocytopenia

Victoria Lindstrom Chase and Michael J. Paidas

Introduction

Fetal and neonatal thrombocytopenia is defined by a platelet count less than 150,000/μL. Thrombocytopenia can be the result of a variety of different etiologies ranging from immunologic disorders, to antenatal infections, to genetic conditions. Platelet counts above 50,000/μL are unlikely to cause significant sequelae. However, when the fetal platelet count drops below this threshold, significant sequela may arise, with the most serious being spontaneous intracranial bleeding. Of fetuses and neonates with severe thrombocytopenia, defined by a platelet count less than 50,000/μL, fetal and neonatal alloimmune thrombocytopenia (FNAIT) is the most common cause.

Etiology

FNAIT is a pregnancy complication that affects a fetus or baby's platelets and can lead to serious fetal or neonatal morbidity and mortality. Platelets have protein on their surface called human platelet antigens (HPAs) that are both maternally and paternally inherited in an autosomal codominant fashion. In pregnancy and at the time of delivery, fetal platelets enter maternal circulation. If the maternal immune system identifies foreign, paternally inherited HPAs, maternal alloantibodies against the fetal HPAs may occur. The maternal immunoglobulin (Ig) G antibodies produced then cross the placenta and invoke fetal platelet destruction (**Figure 23.1**).

FNAIT is considered the platelet equivalent of hemolytic disease of the fetus and newborn (HDFN; and see Chapter 22). However, there are important differences between the two diseases. Approximately 2% of women are HPA-1-negative, as compared to approximately 10% of Rh-negative women. FNAIT frequently occurs in the first pregnancy, in contrast to HDFN, in which clinically affected fetuses and newborns rarely occur in the first pregnancy, but disease is manifested in the second and subsequent pregnancies. Sensitization following an incompatible transfusion rarely occurs with the HPA-1a antigen, whereas anti-D is the most common antibody response during incompatible transfusions. Routine antenatal screening for FNAIT does not exist but does for Rh phenotyping. Prevention does not exist for FNAIT but does for HDFN related to anti-D, namely antenatal and postnatal RhIG (anti-D).

The incidence of FNAIT is 1 in 1000 to 1 in 2000 live births.[1,2] Severity of thrombocytopenia ranges from clinically asymptomatic neonates to fetuses or neonates with intracranial hemorrhage (ICH) and/or death.[3] Death or long-term neurological damage resulting from ICH that occurs at or soon after delivery is historically quoted at 25%[4] with *in utero* spontaneous ICH occurring in 5% to 10% of pregnancies.[5] In more contemporary literature of pregnancies affected by FNAIT, the rate of ICH has been reported as 8.9% and mortality approximately as 1%.[6]

As mentioned, FNAIT may occur in the first pregnancy of an at-risk couple. The fetal bleeding risk is a result of thrombocytopenia and, in mouse studies, maternal alloantibody mediated damage to vascular integrity and angiogenesis.[7-9] The severity of thrombocytopenia differs depending on the platelet antigen involved,[10] may worsen with increasing gestation,[3] and is more severe if prior pregnancies have been affected.

Biologic Activity of Human Platelet Antigens

Over 30 HPAs have been identified (**Table 23.1**). They are carried on platelet membrane glycoproteins (GP) 1a-V-IX, more commonly known as the

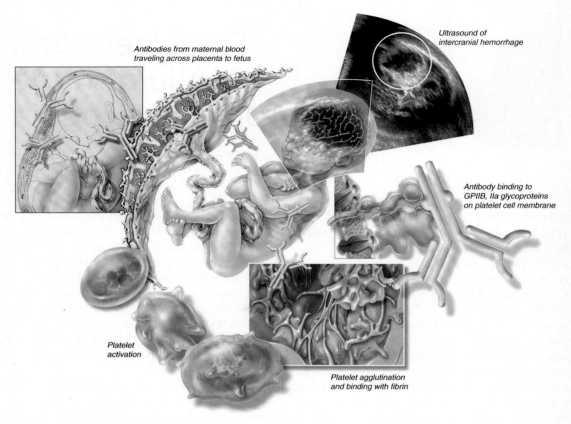

Antibodies from maternal blood
traveling across placenta to fetus

Ultrasound of
intercranial hemorrhage

Antibody binding to
GPIIB, IIa glycoproteins
on platelet cell membrane

Platelet
activation

Platelet agglutination
and binding with fibrin

Figure 23.1 Pathophysiology of fetal neonatal alloimmune thrombocytopenia.

(Reprinted from Paidas MJ, Thung S, Beardsley DS. Unmasking the many faces of maternal and fetal thrombocytopenia. *Contemp Ob Gyn*. 2006;51(9):42-52.)

von Willebrand receptor; GPIIb/IIIa, an αIIb/β3 integrin and fibrinogen receptor; heparin platelet (HP) Ia/IIa, a collagen receptor; and cluster of differentiation (CD) 109, a glycosylphosphatidylinositol-anchored protein. Platelet glycoproteins function by interacting with extracellular matrix protein and coagulation factors to achieve hemostasis. Glycoprotein IV, a class B scavenger receptor, can elicit a FNAIT-like clinical picture. Deficiency in this glycoprotein is more common in those with African or Asian descent (**Figure 23.2**).[11]

Many HPAs are biallelic and codominant. The most commonly implicated platelet antibody in FNAIT is due to anti-HPA-1a alloimmunization in mothers who are HPA-1b homozygous, which is responsible for approximately 80% of cases of FNAIT in non-Hispanic white women.[3] The HPA-1a and HPA-1b alleles are variants of the β3 integrin molecule on glycoprotein IIIa

which are a result of a substitution of a proline for leucine base at amino acid 33.[12] The next most common antibodies implicated in FNAIT in non-Hispanic whites are against HPA-5a and HPA-15. In contrast, in Asian women, HPA-4a, HPA-6a, and HPA-21b incompatibility is more frequently causative.[11,13]

Additionally, an increased immunologic susceptibility to alloimmunization has been associated with certain human leukocyte antigens (HLAs). HLA-DRB3*0101 is an example of one of these HLAs studied due to its association with alloimmunization in women who are HPA-1a-negative. Women who carry one or two copies of HLA-DBR3*0101 and are delivering a HLA-1a-positive child have a 12.7% risk of alloimmunization versus a 0.5% risk in those negative for the allele.[12] An increased risk of alloimmunization is also seen in women with Dw52a, DQB1*0201, and DR6 alleles.[14]

Table 23.1 Human Platelet Antigen (HPA) System

HPA System Name	Antigen	Familiar Name
Polymorphisms of GpIIIa		
HPA-1	HPA-1a	P1[A1], Zw[a]
	HPA-1b	P1[A1], Zw[b]
HPA-4	HPA-4a	Pen[a], Yuk[b]
	HPA-4b	Pen[b], Yuk[a]
HPA-6	HPA-6bw	Ca, Tu
HPA-7	HPA-7bw	Mo
HPA-8	HPA-8w	Sr-a
HPA-10	HPA-10bw	La(a)
HPA-11	HPA-11bw	Gro(a)
HPA-14	HPA-14bw	Oe(a)
HPA-16	HPA-16bw	Duv(a)
Polymorphisms of GpIIb		
HPA-3	HPA-3a	Bak[a], Lek
	HPA-3b	Bak[b]
HPA-9	HPA-9bw	Max[a]
Polymorphisms of GpIa		
HPA-5	HPA-5a	Br[b], Zavb
	HPA-5b	Br[a], Zava
HPA-13	HPA-13bw	Sit(a)
Polymorphisms of GpIb		
HPA-2	HPA-2b	Ko[a], Sib-a
HPA-12	HPA-12bw	Ly(a)
Other Probable Platelet Alloantigen Specificities		
HPA-15	HPA-15a	Gov a
	HPA-15b	Gov b

Adapted from Kamphuis MM, Tiller H, van den Akker ES, Westgren M, Tiblad E, Oepkes D. Fetal and neonatal alloimmune thrombocytopenia: management and outcome of a large international retrospective cohort. *Fetal Diagn Ther*. 2017;41(4):251-257.

Diagnosis

FNAIT should be suspected in all the cases of fetal ICH identified sonographically or when neonatal thrombocytopenia is identified. Scenarios that warrant a parental evaluation for FNAIT include a history of an affected child, direct relation to an affected child, previous child with unexplained thrombocytopenia, and a woman incidentally found to lack the HPA-1a antigen (**Algorithm 23.1**). The diagnosis is typically made following maternal and paternal HPA genotyping identifying platelet antigen incompatibility and maternal antibodies to the foreign paternal antigen. Murphy et al used platelet immunofluorescence tests and monoclonal antibody immobilization of platelet antigen assays for platelet typing and detection of HPA antibodies (**Table 23.2**).[15] In the setting of paternal platelet antigen heterozygosity, fetal platelet antigen typing may be evaluated by polymerase chain reaction. Fetal DNA may be obtained via chorionic villus sampling or amniocentesis. However, chorionic villus sampling is typically avoided due to theoretical risk of increased sensitization with the procedure. Fetal HPA-1a genotyping via cell-free DNA testing in the early second trimester produces reliable results but is not widely available as a routine clinical test.[16]

Antenatal Management and Screening

High-quality evidence for screening and management of FNAIT is limited. The most robust data regarding treatment modalities evaluated are focused on preventative management in future pregnancies. Platelet transfusion, maternal steroid administration, and intravenous immunoglobulin (IVIG) are the most commonly studied management approaches. However, evidence supporting these interventions is limited due to the lack of standardized treatment dosing and timing of interventions.

Universal Screening

Universal screening for FNAIT would enable detection of the condition in a mother's first affected pregnancy. The goal would be to prevent ICH and its associated morbidity and mortality. However, this would require balancing the risk and benefits of screening and treatment.

In a Scottish observational prospective study of 26,503 women, they identified 546 women who were HPA-1a-negative giving a prevalence of approximately 2%.[17] Of this population, 7.9% were then identified to have anti-HPA-1a antibodies. Of women with antibodies, 32% had neonates that had thrombocytopenia at birth. There were no cases of ICH. Women who were HPA-1a-negative were screened for anti-HPA-1a antibodies during pregnancy, at delivery, and 10 to 14 days following delivery. The overall incidence of NAIT and severe NAIT was 43 per 100,000 and 27 per 100,000 live births, respectively.[17]

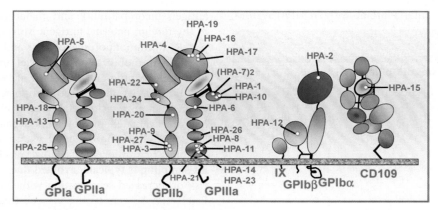

Figure 23.2 Structure of the human platelet antigen (HPA). Antigens known to trigger maternal sensitization in fetal neonatal alloimmune thrombocytopenia are located on four different platelet membrane glycoproteins and glycoprotein complexes.

(Reprinted with permission from Peterson JA, McFarland JG, Curtis BR, Aster RH. Neonatal alloimmune thrombocytopenia: pathogenesis, diagnosis and management. *Br J Haematol*. 2013;161(1):3-14.)

A Norwegian study of 100,448 women performed universal HPA-1 allotyping at the time of RhD typing.[2] Two percent of women were HPA-1a-negative, and of those, 10.6% had anti-HPA-1a antibodies. In women with HPA-1a antibodies, cesarean delivery was recommended and occurred at a median gestational age of 37 1/7 weeks. ICH occurred in two HPA-1a-positive infants.[2]

Table 23.2 FNAIT Laboratory Workup[a]

- Flow cytometry is a rapid method of detecting platelet reactive antibodies. It is used to test maternal serum against washed paternal and maternal platelets and a panel of platelets from normal O donors typed for HPA ag.
- Screen for class I HLA antibodies. Maternal and paternal red cells are typed for ABO.
- Solid phase assay is used to detect the specific glycoprotein the maternal ab is targeting.
  - MACE (modified antigen capture ELISA), used for GPIIb/IIIa, GP Ia/IIa.
  - ACE ELISA (antigen capture ELISA) screen for antibodies GPIb/IX.
  - MAIPA monoclonal ab immobilization of platelet antigen (alternative method).
  - Platelet typing: Type paternal and maternal DNA.

ab, antibody; ag, antigen; DNA, deoxyribonucleic acid; ELISA, enzyme-linked immunosorbent assay; FNAIT, fetal neonatal alloimmune thrombocytopenia; GP, glycoprotein; HLA, human leukocyte antigen; HPA, human platelet antigen.
[a]Use an experienced reference lab.
Data from Peterson JA, McFarland JG, Curtis BR, Aster RH. Neonatal alloimmune thrombocytopenia: pathogenesis, diagnosis and management. *Br J Haematol*. 2013;161(1):3-14. PMID: 23384054.

Williamson et al[1] performed an observational study that evaluated the HPAs of 24,417 women, umbilical cord platelet counts, and infant morbidity. Following HPA genotyping, 2.5% were HPA-1a-negative and 12.5% of those had HPA-1a antibodies. Nine infants were born with severe thrombocytopenia, and one infant was born with evidence of a large occipitoparietal porencephalic cyst with encephalomalacia, consistent with prior hemorrhage.

These universal screening studies identify a low prevalence of FNAIT and an inability to predict the severity of cases. They are also limited to screening for HPA-1a incompatibility and antibodies which are most common in the non-Hispanic white population and responsible for approximately 80% of FNAIT cases.[3] However, HPA-1a screening would not be adequate for women of other racial descents. At this time population-wide screening for platelet antigens or antiplatelet antibodies is not currently performed in the United States. Consequently, FNAIT is diagnosed following diagnosis of *in utero* ICH, neonatal thrombocytopenia, or neonatal ICH.

Screening by Antibody Titers

Both retrospective and prospective studies have examined antibody titers to better stratify women for risk of severe FNAIT. In the individual studies evaluating the association of antibody titers and FNAIT, results are mixed. However, in a meta-analysis evaluating a total of 256 HPA-1a

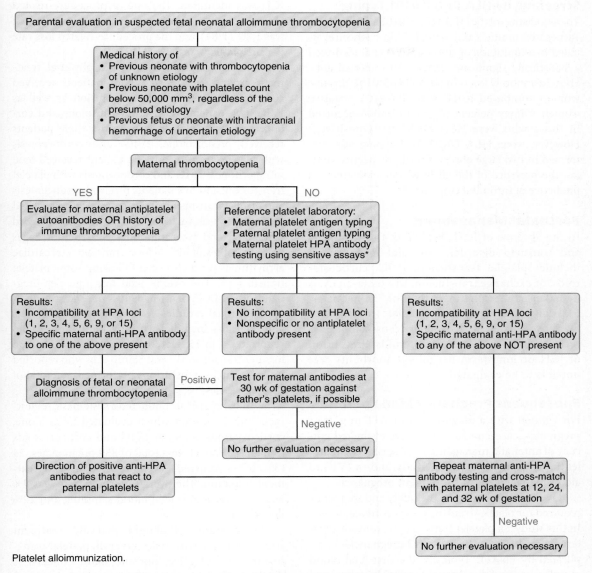

Platelet alloimmunization.

ELISA, enzyme-linked immunosorbent assay; HPA, human platelet antigen; MACE, modified antigen capture enzyme-linked immunosorbent assay; MAIPA, monoclonal antibody immobilization of platelet antigens; NAIT, neonatal alloimmune thrombocytopenia.

*Examples of sensitive assays include MACE and MAIPA.

Algorithm 23.1 Parental evaluation for suspected fetal neonatal alloimmune thrombocytopenia.

(From Pacheco LD, Berkowitz RL, Moise KJ Jr, Bussel JB, McFarland JG, Saade GR. Fetal and neonatal alloimmune thrombocytopenia: a management algorithm based on risk stratification. *Obstet Gynecol.* 2011;118(5):1157-1163.)

immunized pregnancies, HPA-1a antibody levels drawn in the third trimester or at delivery were correlated with the newborn platelet count.[18] For severe FNAIT, the positive and negative predictive values were low.[18] Of those studies evaluating the primiparous population, antibody titers were first detected at 17 and 21 weeks' gestation.[1,17]

Screening by HLA DRB3*0101 Typing

The association of the HLA DRB3*0101 allele in HPA-1a-negative mothers and risk of FNAIT has been evaluated in a multitude of studies. Killie et al identified a statistically significant increase in maternal anti-HPA-1a antibody levels in HLA DRB3*0101-positive women compared to HLA DRB3*0101-negative women. Ninety percent of immunization occurred in those who were HLA DRB3*0101-positive.[19] However, when HLA DRB3*0101 typing was performed in two large observational prospective studies, the presence of the allele was not identified as predictive of thrombocytopenia.[1,12]

Postnatal Management

In the absence of ICH, FNAIT is a self-limiting and transient disorder. Postnatal management includes platelet transfusion, IVIG, corticosteroids, or exchange transfusion. In a meta-analysis by Baker et al evaluating a total of 754 neonates, 51% of infants required platelet transfusions. Of those treated with platelet transfusion, 37% received IVIG and/or corticosteroids. Prevention of ICH or long-term neurologic morbidity was not able to be evaluated.[6]

Subsequent Pregnancy Management

For women with a diagnosis of FNAIT in a prior pregnancy, case-control series have evaluated efficacy of antenatal management via serial fetal platelet transfusions, maternal steroids, and/or IVIG to aid in management of subsequent pregnancies.

Overton et al evaluated the safety and frequency required for platelet transfusion via cordocentesis.[20] In this study, 84 platelet transfusions were administered over a 10-year period in 12 pregnancies complicated by FNAIT. Typically, the first fetal blood sampling occurred at 22 to 24 weeks' gestation and was repeated at weekly intervals until delivery. Early in the study period, the transfusions continued until 35 to 36 weeks, at which time delivery was enacted. In the latter portion of the study, the investigators performed platelet transfusions until 32 weeks' gestation with delivery occurring 1 to 2 days following the final transfusion. In addition to platelet transfusions, three mothers received IVIG at 1 g/kg/d and 1 fetus directly received IVIG at 1 g/kg of estimated fetal weight. The outcomes included 10 pregnancies that resulted in healthy infants who did not require platelet transfusions in the neonatal period. No

ICH was identified. The rate of procedure-related losses, defined as those occurring within 48 hours, was 1.2% (1/84), and the procedure-related loss rate per pregnancy was 8.3% (1/12).[20]

In a study of 15 patients by Murphy et al, treatment groups overlapped.[15] Four patients received cordocentesis with platelet transfusion as well as IVIG; two patients received prednisolone and cordocentesis with platelet transfusion; three patients received prednisolone, IVIG, and cordocentesis with platelet transfusion; one patient received fetal intraperitoneal IVIG and cordocentesis with platelet transfusion; and five patients received cordocentesis and platelet transfusion alone. Complications related to cordocentesis included a fetal loss due to cord hematoma and two additional cord hemorrhages that did not result in fetal loss. Transient fetal cardiac arrhythmias were also seen following some platelet transfusions. The overall fetal loss rate per pregnancy was 1 in 15 or a 1 in 69 loss per transfusion.[15]

Additional studies examining cordocentesis and fetal loss included work by Kahnai et al who reported a 1 in 15 fetal loss per pregnancy (1 in 36 loss per transfusion)[21] and Sainio et al who reported no losses in 34 transfusions performed in a total of 13 pregnancies.[22]

Winkelhorst et al conducted a systematic review[7] including 26 studies which evaluated IVIG alone, corticosteroids alone, or IVIG and corticosteroids to manage FNAIT. In a total of 839 pregnancies, 24 (3%) ICHs occurred. Seven occurred prior to treatment initiation. The overall mortality rate was 4% with 53% related to fetal blood sampling and 22% due to ICH.

These studies highlight that all treatment strategies come with risks. Overall, platelet transfusions are effective, but the main concern is the high fetal loss rate. Fetal bradycardia, cord tamponade, and exsanguination have all been reported. The overall pooled loss rate is 1.3% per transfusion and 5.5% per pregnancy. Due to the required weekly platelet transfusions for 10 or more weeks, risk of increased maternal sensitization, and the fetal loss rate, a noninvasive treatment approach with IVIG with or without steroids has become the cornerstone of management. However, IVIG serious adverse effects can include hemolytic anemia, renal failure, aseptic meningitis, and thrombotic complications. Corticosteroids increase the risk of hypertension and diabetes.[23] Therefore, some groups advocate different treatment regimens depending on the level of risk for severe FNAIT which in most cases appears to be directly proportional to the severity in the prior pregnancy.[24-26]

Paidas et al provided a detailed study describing the risks of exsanguination associated with fetal blood sampling in the setting of FNAIT and highlighted the distinguishing features among pregnancies whose fetuses fatally exsanguinated and those that survived the cordocentesis.[27] Since that publication, an *in utero* platelet transfusion is typically performed prior to needle removal when a fetal platelet count of <50 × 10⁹/l is encountered. Post cordocentesis, observation for streaming, bradycardia, and clot formation are recommended, as well as fetal heart rate tracing monitoring when appropriate. **See Table 23.3 for details regarding *in utero* platelet transfusion.**

It is known that fetuses with platelet counts less than 20,000/mL³ have lower response rates to IVIG alone at the standard dose of 1 g/kg/wk. Therefore,

Table 23.3 *In Utero* Platelet Transfusion

- Aim for concentration >2000 × 106/µL (avg. 5-15 mL platelet concentrate).
- Leukoreduced and irradiated platelets to prevent graft-versus-host disease.
- If maternally derived platelets, wash platelets to remove alloantibody.
- Administer rho(d) immune globulin (human) if indicated:

Volume of platelet concentrate transfused (mL) = (volume of fetoplacental unit in mL) × (final – initial platelet count) × 2 divided by (platelet count of the transfused concentrate)

Fetoplacental volume: multiply estimated fetal weight (grams) by 0.14

Data from Paidas MJ, Berkowitz RL, Lynch L, et al. Alloimmune thrombocytopenia: fetal and neonatal losses related to cordocentesis. *Am J Obstet Gynecol*. 1995;172(2 pt 1):475-479. PMID: 7856672, Mandelbrot L, Daffos F, Forestier F, MacAleese J, Descombey D. Assessment of fetal blood volume for computer-assisted management of *in utero* transfusion. *Fetal Ther*. 1988;3(1-2):60-66. PMID: 3257068, Leduc L, Moise KJ Jr, Carpenter RJ Jr, Cano LE. Fetoplacental blood volume estimation in pregnancies with Rh alloimmunization. *Fetal Diagn Ther*. 1990;5(3-4):138-146, and Murphy MF, Waters AH, Doughty HA, et al. Antenatal management of fetomaternal alloimmune thrombocytopenia – Report of 15 affected pregnancies. *Transfus Med*. 1994;4(4):281-292. PMID: 7889140.

some recommend cordocentesis to evaluate the initial platelet count and/or response to treatment. To address this concern, a multicenter, randomized controlled trial evaluated the effectiveness of two antenatal treatment regimens for standard-risk women who were defined as those with documented alloimmune thrombocytopenia but no prior child with ICH.[26] Study groups received IVIG 2 g/kg/wk or IVIG 1 g/kg/wk plus prednisone (0.5 mg/kg/d) beginning around 20 weeks' gestation. Cordocentesis was performed at 32 weeks' gestation to assess response. For those with fetal platelets less than 30,000/mL³ in the IVIG 2 g/kg/wk group, prednisone was added, and in the IVIG 1 g/kg/wk group, the dose was increased to 2 g/kg/wk. A total of 73 women were randomized to the two groups. There were no differences in the average platelet counts at the time of cordocentesis or delivery or need for salvage therapy. One ICH occurred in each group, but neither was attributed to treatment failure. Cordocentesis complications occurred in 6% of cases and resulted in emergent delivery or intrauterine fetal death of 14% of infants.[26]

In contrast to standard-risk women, women with a history of ICH in a fetus or neonate have a documented recurrence risk of nearly 100%. Given this high risk for recurrence, Bussel et al evaluated a cohort of 33 women with 37 pregnancies risk-stratified by prior timing of ICH.[25] Women received IVIG 1 g/kg/wk or 2 g/kg/wk with or without prednisone beginning at 12 weeks' gestation. Cordocentesis with platelet transfusion was performed in these pregnancies. Following treatment, ICH occurred in five infants, two of which were confirmed due to treatment failure, and both of whom had received 1 g/kg/wk with prednisone 1 mg/kg/wk.[25]

Because of serious fetal and neonatal morbidity associated with cordocentesis, there is clearly a need for noninvasive therapy. However, without invasive platelet monitoring, the optimal treatment that maximizes fetal platelet response but minimizes maternal complications is not clearly defined. Treatment algorithms have been proposed based on best evidence available but are not backed by randomized controlled trials. One risk-stratified treatment algorithm by Pacheco et al[24] is illustrated in **Algorithm 23.2**. For women with a history of a fetus or newborn with thrombocytopenia or unexplained ICH, paternal incompatibility for

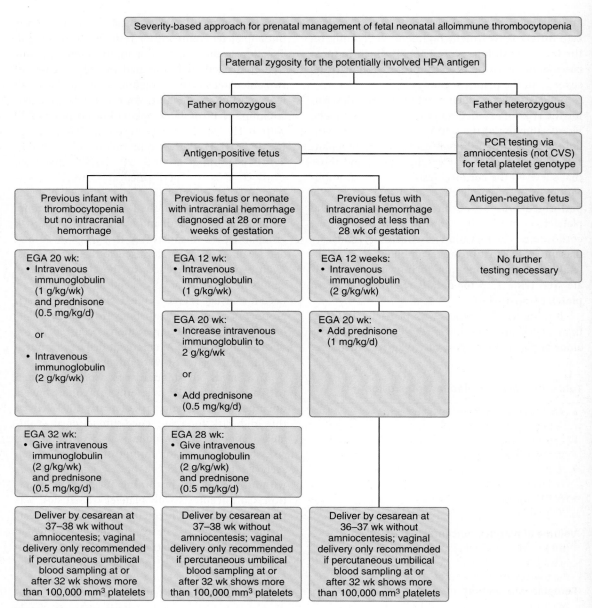

Platelet alloimmunization.

CVS, chorionic villus sampling; EGA, estimated gestational age; HPA, human platelet antigen; NAIT, neonatal alloimmune thrombocytopenia; PCR, polymerase chain reaction.

Algorithm 23.2 **Severity-based approach for prenatal management of neonatal alloimmune thrombocytopenia.**

(From Pacheco LD, Berkowitz RL, Moise KJ Jr, Bussel JB, McFarland JG, Saade GR. Fetal and neonatal alloimmune thrombocytopenia: a management algorithm based on risk stratification. *Obstet Gynecol.* 2011;118(5):1157-1163.)

HPA antigens, but no anti-HPA antibodies identified, serial anti-HPA antibody screening is recommended. If antibodies are present, treatment would be initiated. If no antibodies develop by 30 weeks' gestation, no further evaluation is required. For women with a history of confirmed FNAIT, the predominant management strategy is based upon the severity of FNAIT in prior pregnancy.[23]

KEY POINTS

- The pathophysiology of FNAIT is well described at this point in time, but continuing advances are required to refine immune aspects of this disease.
- Progress has been made over the past 30 years in tailoring management strategies for pregnancies at risk for FNAIT.
- Universal screening as well as robust prevention and safer diagnostic and treatment modalities represent urgent unmet needs in this disorder.

- More research is needed to develop treatment approaches which maximize fetal platelet response but minimize maternal complications.
- For women with a diagnosis of FNAIT in a prior pregnancy, a risk-stratified approach to antenatal management is the preferred management strategy currently, with therapeutic options consisting of IVIG, maternal steroids, and serial fetal platelet transfusions.

REFERENCES

1. Williamson LM, Hackett G, Rennie J, et al. The natural history of feto-maternal alloimmunization to the platelet-specific antigen HPA-1a (PlA1, Zwa) as determined by antenatal screening. *Blood*. 1998;92(7):2280-2287.
2. Kjeldsen-Kragh J, Killie MK, Tomter G, et al. A screening and intervention program aimed to reduce mortality and serious morbidity associated with severe neonatal alloimmune thrombocytopenia. *Blood*. 2007;110(3):833-839.
3. Mueller-Eckhardt C, Kiefel V, Grubert A, et al. 348 cases of suspected neonatal alloimmune thrombocytopenia. *Lancet*. 1989;1(8634):363-366.
4. Kaplan C, Morel-Kopp MC, Kroll H, et al. HPA-5b (Br(a)) neonatal alloimmune thrombocytopenia: clinical and immunological analysis of 39 cases. *Br J Haematol*. 1991;78(3):425-429.
5. Reznikoff-Etievant MF. Management of alloimmune neonatal and antenatal thrombocytopenia. *Vox Sang*. 1988;55(4):193-201.
6. Baker JM, Shehata N, Bussel J, et al. Postnatal intervention for the treatment of FNAIT: a systematic review. *J Perinatol*. 2019;39(10):1329-1339.
7. Winkelhorst D, Murphy MF, Greinacher A, et al. Antenatal management in fetal and neonatal alloimmune thrombocytopenia: a systematic review. *Blood*. 2017;129(11):1538-1547.
8. Liu ZJ, Bussel JB, Lakkaraja M, et al. Suppression of in vitro megakaryopoiesis by maternal sera containing anti-HPA-1a antibodies. *Blood*. 2015;126(10):1234-1236.
9. Yougbare I, Lang S, Yang H, et al. Maternal anti-platelet beta3 integrins impair angiogenesis and cause intracranial hemorrhage. *J Clin Invest*. 2015;125(4):1545-1556.
10. Bussel JB, Zabusky MR, Berkowitz RL, McFarland JG. Fetal alloimmune thrombocytopenia. *N Engl J Med*. 1997;337(1):22-26.
11. Peterson JA, McFarland JG, Curtis BR, Aster RH. Neonatal alloimmune thrombocytopenia: pathogenesis, diagnosis and management. *Br J Haematol*. 2013;161(1):3-14.
12. Kjeldsen-Kragh J, Titze TL, Lie BA, Vaage JT, Kjær M. HLA-DRB3*01:01 exhibits a dose-dependent impact on HPA-1a antibody levels in HPA-1a-immunized women. *Blood Adv*. 2019;3(7):945-951.
13. Arnold DM, Smith JW, Kelton JG. Diagnosis and management of neonatal alloimmune thrombocytopenia. *Transfus Med Rev*. 2008;22(4):255-267.
14. L'Abbe D, Tremblay L, Filion M, et al. Alloimmunization to platelet antigen HPA-1a (PlA1) is strongly associated with both HLA-DRB3*0101 and HLA-DQB1*0201. *Hum Immunol*. 1992;34(2):107-114.
15. Murphy MF, Waters AH, Doughty HA, et al. Antenatal management of fetomaternal alloimmune thrombocytopenia – Report of 15 affected pregnancies. *Transfus Med*. 1994;4(4):281-292.

16. Scheffer PG, Ait Soussan A, Verhagen OJ, et al. Noninvasive fetal genotyping of human platelet antigen-1a. *Br J Obstet Gynaecol*. 2011;118(11):1392-1395.
17. Turner ML, Bessos H, Fagge T, et al. Prospective epidemiologic study of the outcome and cost-effectiveness of antenatal screening to detect neonatal alloimmune thrombocytopenia due to anti-HPA-1a. *Transfusion*. 2005;45(12):1945-1956.
18. Kjaer M, Bertrand G, Bakchoul T, et al. Maternal HPA-1a antibody level and its role in predicting the severity of fetal/neonatal alloimmune thrombocytopenia: a systematic review. *Vox Sang*. 2019;114(1):79-94.
19. Killie MK, Husebekk A, Kjeldsen-Kragh J, Skogen B. A prospective study of maternal anti-HPA 1a antibody level as a potential predictor of alloimmune thrombocytopenia in the newborn. *Haematologica*. 2008;93(6):870-877.
20. Overton TG, Duncan KR, Jolly M, Letsky E, Fisk NM. Serial aggressive platelet transfusion for fetal alloimmune thrombocytopenia: platelet dynamics and perinatal outcome. *Am J Obstet Gynecol*. 2002;186(4):826-831.
21. Kanhai HH, Porcelijn L, Engelfriet CP, et al. Management of alloimmune thrombocytopenia. *Vox Sang*. 2007;93(4):370-385.
22. Sainio S, Teramo K, Kekomaki R. Prenatal treatment of severe fetomaternal alloimmune thrombocytopenia. *Transfus Med*. 1999;9(4):321-330.
23. Rossi KQ, Lehman KJ, O'Shaughnessy RW. Effects of antepartum therapy for fetal alloimmune thrombocytopenia on maternal lifestyle. *J Matern Fetal Neonatal Med*. 2016;29(11):1783-1788.
24. Pacheco LD, Berkowitz RL, Moise KJ Jr, Bussel JB, McFarland JG, Saade GR. Fetal and neonatal alloimmune thrombocytopenia: a management algorithm based on risk stratification. *Obstet Gynecol*. 2011;118(5):1157-1163.
25. Bussel JB, Berkowitz RL, Hung C, et al. Intracranial hemorrhage in alloimmune thrombocytopenia: stratified management to prevent recurrence in the subsequent affected fetus. *Am J Obstet Gynecol*. 2010;203(2):135. e1-135.e14.
26. Berkowitz RL, Lesser ML, McFarland JG, et al. Antepartum treatment without early cordocentesis for standard-risk alloimmune thrombocytopenia: a randomized controlled trial. *Obstet Gynecol*. 2007;110(2 pt 1):249-255.
27. Paidas MJ, Berkowitz RL, Lynch L, et al. Alloimmune thrombocytopenia: fetal and neonatal losses related to cordocentesis. *Am J Obstet Gynecol*. 1995;172(2 pt 1):475-479. PMID: 7856672.
28. Mandelbrot L, Daffos F, Forestier F, MacAleese J, Descombey D. Assessment of fetal blood volume for computer-assisted management of in utero transfusion. *Fetal Ther*. 1988;3(1-2):60-66. PMID: 3257068.

29. Leduc L, Moise KJ Jr, Carpenter RJ Jr, Cano LE. Fetoplacental blood volume estimation in pregnancies with Rh alloimmunization. *Fetal Diagn Ther*. 1990;5(3-4):138-146.

30. Murphy MF, Waters AH, Doughty HA, et al. Antenatal management of fetomaternal alloimmune thrombocytopenia – Report of 15 affected pregnancies. *Transfus Med*. 1994;4(4):281-292. PMID: 7889140.

31. Paidas MJ, Thung S, Beardsley DS. Unmasking maternal and fetal thrombocytopenia. *Contemp Ob Gyn*. 2006;51(9):42-52.

32. Paidas MJ. *Fetal and Neonatal Alloimmune Thrombocytopenia: Parental Evaluation and Pregnancy Management*. UpToDate. 2020. Accessed September 21, 2020. https://www.uptodate.com/contents/fetal-and-neonatal-alloimmune-thrombocytopenia-parental-evaluation-and-pregnancy-management

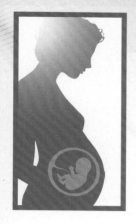

CHAPTER 24

Fetal Surgical Interventions

Eftichia Kontopoulos, Ruben Quintero, Ramen H. Chmait, Andrew H. Chon, and Denise Araujo Lapa

FETAL INTERVENTIONS FOR MONOCHORIONIC TWIN PREGNANCY COMPLICATIONS

Table 24.1 presents a summary and comparison of the most common surgical approaches to treat monochorionic twin pregnancy complications, which include twin-twin transfusion syndrome (TTTS), twin anemia-polycythemia sequence (TAPS), selective intrauterine growth restriction (sIUGR), and twin reverse arterial perfusion (TRAP) sequence.

Treatment of TTTS

Unless delivery of the fetuses can be considered, TTTS needs to be treated as soon as logistically feasible, mainly since the progression of the condition is unpredictable. Treatment of TTTS has included expectant medical management,[9] *sectio parva*,[10] serial amniocenteses,[11-13] and laser photocoagulation of the placental vascular anastomoses.[14-19] However, the perinatal mortality rate of expectantly managed TTTS is as high as 95%,[11] and selective reduction via umbilical cord occlusion (UCO) (*sectio parva*) of one of the fetuses is an extreme measure that should only be entertained in extraordinary circumstances. Therefore, serial amniocentesis and laser therapy are the two approaches more commonly used, with laser photocoagulation being the treatment modality of choice.

Serial Amniocentesis

Serial amniocentesis, also called serial amniodrainage or amnioreduction, consists of removing the

See the eBook for expanded content, a complete reference list, and additional figures and tables.

excessive amount of amniotic fluid from the recipient twin's sac as often as necessary. Typically, an 18- to 20-gauge spinal needle is used.[20] The volume of amniotic fluid that should be withdrawn has not been standardized, although some authors suggest removing enough fluid to bring the MVP to approximately 6 cm.[21] The purpose of reducing the amount of amniotic fluid volume in the recipient's sac is to diminish the overall uterine distention and the risk of miscarriage or prematurity. Serial amniodrainage should be viewed as a contemporizing treatment measure, for it serves only to ameliorate the polyhydramnios, but does not treat the underlying etiology.

Laser Therapy

Unlike serial amniocentesis, laser therapy addresses the primary pathogenic cause of TTTS by ablating all vascular communications.[18] This surgery is performed using fetal endoscopes, which are used to directly visualize the vessels on the placental surface. Once mapping of the vascular communications has been performed, the vessels are photocoagulated using a special type of laser energy that is delivered into the amniotic cavity by quartz fibers through the operating channel of the endoscope. Quintero et al developed the selective technique (selective laser photocoagulation of communicating vessels, or SLPCV), which selectively ablates only the vascular communications and does not require location of the dividing membrane.[18] Ablation of all vascular anastomoses after SLPCV essentially transforms a monochorionic twin pregnancy into a "functional" dichorionic twin pregnancy, with no further exchange of blood between the fetuses.[31]

A third-generation laser technique has been reported[41] which involves lasering the arteriovenous anastomoses in a specific sequence (sequential

Table 24.1 Comparison of Twin-Twin Transfusion Syndrome (TTTS), Selective Intrauterine Growth Restriction (sIUGR), and Twin Anemia-Polycythemia Sequence (TAPS)

Condition	Diagnostic Criteria	Amniotic Fluid Discordance	Growth Restriction	Growth Discordance >20%-25%	Role of Placental Vascular Anastomoses	Staging	Optimal Treatment
TTTS	MVP >8 cm in one twin, <2 cm in the other twin	Yes	May be present, but not part of the diagnosis	May be present, but not part of the definition	Causal	I-V, based on visualization of bladder, arterial and venous Dopplers, hydrops.	Laser photocoagulation of placental vascular anastomoses, regardless of stage.
sIUGR	EFW <10th percentile in one twin	May be present, but not >8 <2 cm.	Integral to the definition	May be present, but not essential to the definition	Causal, contributing, or only means of survival	Types I-III, based on diastolic flow in the umbilical artery	Laser ablation of placental vascular anastomoses, type II.
TAPS	MCA-PSV >1.5 MoM in one twin, <1.0 MoM in the other twin	May be present, but not >8 <2 cm.			Causal	I-V, based on MCA-PSV values, arterial and venous Dopplers, hydrops.	Laser ablation of placental vascular anastomoses

EFW, estimated fetal weight; MCA-PSV, peak systolic velocity of the middle cerebral artery; MoM, multiples of the median.

laser photocoagulation of communicating vessels, or SQLPCV), such that the AV anastomoses from the donor to the recipient are lasered first, followed by the remaining communications.[33] Although a sequential technique may not be required in all cases, it could be indicated in patients where the condition of the donor twin would be most compromised.

Complications of Laser Therapy

Residual patent vascular anastomoses (RPVAS) may result in persistent TTTS (the condition continues) or reverse TTTS (the roles of the twins are reversed, such that the original donor becomes the new recipient, and the original recipient becomes the new donor). Persistent TTTS results from remaining AVDR anastomoses, whereas reverse TTTS results from remaining AVRDs. If both AVDRs and AVRDs remain patent, persistent or reverse TTTS may occur depending on the direction of the net exchange of blood between the fetuses.

Incomplete or inadequate laser therapy may also result in another condition, twin anemia-polycythemia sequence (TAPS), defined below and described in Chapter 5.

Failed laser surgery is defined as persistent or reverse TTTS or TAPS. Suspected anemia of a surviving twin after demise of the co-twin, by assessment of the peak systolic velocity of the middle cerebral artery (MCA-PSV), may also be due to RPAVs, although it may reflect the sequence of how the anastomoses were lasered. Dual fetal demise with postmortem demonstration of RPVASs is considered failed laser therapy.

In view of the relatively high incidence of RPVAS seen by some groups, some authors proposed "connecting the dots" between photocoagulated areas on the surface of the placenta.[49] The resulting surgical technique of lasering healthy interanastomotic areas of the placenta has been called the "the Solomon technique."[49]

However, the superiority of the Solomon technique to the SLPCV technique has not been proven.

Accuracy of Laser Therapy

Theoretically, one could combine the rate of adequate placental assessment and of selective laser surgery with the rate of either residual patent placental vascular anastomoses (when available) and the rate of persistent or reverse TTTS to determine how accurate the laser surgery is being performed at a given center or by a given surgeon. Accuracy of SLPCV could thus be defined as:

$$AccSLPCV = QSI \times (1 - RPPVA) \times (1 - PRTTTS)$$

where, AccSLPCV is the accuracy in performing SLPCV, QSI is the rate of Quintero selectively performed surgeries, RPPVA is the rate of residual patent placental vascular anastomoses (when available), and PRTTTS is the rate of persistent or reverse TTTS. **Table 24.6** shows such a theoretical calculation and its use to compare outcomes of different reports.

Twin Anemia-Polycythemia Sequence

Treatment of TAPS and Outcomes

The treatment options that have been proposed for patients with TAPS include expectant management, intrauterine transfusion (IUT) of the anemic twin, and partial exchange transfusion (PET) of the polycythemic twin, laser therapy, or cord occlusion of one of the fetuses.

Intrauterine transfusions and partial exchange transfusions may result in postnatal morbidity to either twin. The recipient twin may develop polycythemia hyperviscosity syndrome, including skin necrosis and limb ischemia and thrombocytopenia.[45,68-70] Neurological damage of the donor or the recipient twin has also been reported either

Table 24.6 Accuracy of Laser Surgery for Twin-Twin Transfusion Syndrome (TTTS)

Author	Rate of Selectively Performed Surgeries	1 - Rate of Residual Patent Placental Vascular Anastomoses	1 - Rate of Persistent/ Reverse TTTS	Accuracy of SLPCV
USFetus group[34,44]	98.7%	0.95	0.99	92%
Solomon[41-43]	87%	0.81	0.99	69.7%
Solomon[41-43] "standard"	89%	0.66	0.93	54%

SLPCV, selective laser photocoagulation of communicating vessels.
1 - rate of adverse outcome = rate of success.

spontaneously or with IUT and PET.[71] Long-term neurodevelopmental morbidity after laser therapy has also been reported.[41-43,65]

Selective Intrauterine Growth Restriction

Management
Current counseling of patients with sIUGR involves consideration of the following management options: expectant management, UCO, termination of pregnancy, or laser therapy.

Expectant Management
Expectant management of patients with sIUGR may be associated with an increased risk of adverse perinatal outcomes, including prematurity and its attendant complications.[88]

The risk of adverse outcomes may be higher depending on the umbilical artery Doppler waveform of the sIUGR fetus, such that fetuses with persistent AEDV (sIUGR type II) are thought to be at a higher risk than sIUGR fetuses with umbilical artery forward diastolic flow (sIUGR type I).[88,108] Fetuses with intermittent AEDV (sIUGR type III) are believed to have an unpredictable prognosis.[87] To avoid the potential complications associated with expectant management, patients with sIUGR are often asked to consider either termination of pregnancy or cord occlusion of the sIUGR twin.[109]

Umbilical Cord Occlusion
Selective feticide of the sIUGR twin in monochorionic pregnancies is aimed at sparing the surviving AGA twin from the risks of the spontaneous demise of the sIUGR twin. Several methods have been described, including intravascular injection of fibrin glue,[110] metal coils,[111-114] or alcohol-embedded suture material[115]; induction of cardiac tamponade[116]; and utilization of clips.[117]

Other approaches include fetoscopic and ultrasound-guided UCO,[1] which results in instantaneous, complete interruption of the blood flow; bipolar coagulation; and radiofrequency ablation.[118]

Laser Therapy
The rationale for laser therapy to treat sIUGR stems from the fact that placental vascular anastomoses mediate the adverse effects on the AGA twin which occur as the result of the spontaneous demise of the sIUGR twin. Thus, occlusion of the anastomoses interrupts the blood exchange between fetuses, rendering them functionally as dichorionic twins.

Twin Reverse Arterial Perfusion Sequence

Treatment
Fetoscopic UCO can be performed using a variety of surgical techniques, each of which is particularly suited to a given clinical presentation. The most important preoperative consideration is surgical access.[123] Entering the sac of the perfused twin offers all of the possible occlusion alternatives. In addition, if rupture of the sac of the perfused twin occurs, it may not necessarily affect the pump twin. Disruption of the dividing membrane should be avoided at all times.[123]

The choice of surgical technique depends on the specific characteristics of the cord and of the vascular anastomoses. Umbilical cord laser photocoagulation or laser of the vascular communications are possible options, if the cord is not amenable to ligation. Bipolar electrocautery is also an alternative, although this technique can be limited by the size of the umbilical cord and may result in bleeding from the cord itself.[124] One of the limitations of intrafetal radiofrequency ablation is that the extent of the thermal damage is not entirely under the control of the operator, and intraoperative exsanguination of the pump twin may occur, which may result in intrafetal hemorrhage and death.[125,126]

Discordant (Obligate Lethal) Anomalous Twins
Patients with monochorionic twins discordant for the presence of an obligate lethal condition other than TRAP, such as anencephaly or other severe congenital anomaly in which the affected twin has a significant risk of *in utero* demise and, thus, poses a risk to the co-twin, can be offered the option of UCO. The presence of discordance itself is not an indication for UCO. UCO is utilized in a similar fashion as described for TRAP sequence.

DEVELOPMENTAL STRUCTURAL ABNORMALITIES

Fetal Lung Masses

Thoracic Space-Occupying Lesions
Pulmonary hypoplasia and subsequent neonatal death may result from various space-occupying lesions, including congenital diaphragmatic

hernia (CDH), cystic adenomatoid malformation (CCAM) (also known as congenital pulmonary airway malformation [CPAM]), lobar or extralobar bronchopulmonary sequestration (BPS), pulmonary emphysema, bronchial atresia, and hydrothorax, among others (**Table 24.8**).[127-129]

Fetal therapy may be considered in select cases to counter the effect of the lesion and avoid the development of pulmonary hypoplasia.[127,130-132] The fundamental steps required to offer fetal therapy include an as accurate as possible prenatal differential diagnosis, knowledge of the natural history of each condition, development of antenatal criteria for intervention, and appropriate form of treatment. Prenatal differential diagnosis can be undertaken using ultrasound, color and pulsed Doppler, as well as fetal magnetic resonance imaging (MRI).

Congenital Diaphragmatic Hernia (CDH)

Congenital diaphragmatic hernia (CDH) remains one of the most challenging conditions in fetal therapy. Approximately 10% of cases are associated with a chromosomal anomaly, the most prevalent of which is trisomy-18 (accounting for 37%), a genetic syndrome or a microdeletion.[137] Most cases are left-sided (85%). Nonisolated cases include congenital heart disease (14%) and central nervous system (4.8%), limb, and urinary system anomalies (5%).[137] Overall survival rates for isolated cases are approximately 72% at the first week of life and approximately 65% at 1 year of age.[137] The challenges in the antenatal management of fetuses with CDH stem both from the definition

of high-risk groups, as well as from the antenatal surgical techniques used.

Definition of High-Risk Groups

Neonatal morbidity and mortality from CDH is the result of pulmonary hypoplasia, pulmonary hypertension, or both. The identification of fetuses at risk for neonatal death is based on the prediction of pulmonary hypoplasia and less on pulmonary hypertension.[138,139]

Treatment of CDH

A palliative measure to promote lung growth via tracheal occlusion (TO) would achieve the goal of averting the development of pulmonary hypoplasia with subsequent postnatal repair of the hernia and improved neonatal survival.[154-156]

Intraluminal tracheal occlusion methods, in contrast to the previous extraluminal fetal neck dissection approach, were developed.[159-161]

While most groups use a similar TO surgical approach, there are differences in choice of occluding device. Some groups have favored the use of detachable balloons that can be deployed percutaneously under fetoscopic guidance.[162-165] Others use self-expanding covered stents with an attached suture for removal.[159,160,166]

Cystic Adenomatoid Malformation/Congenital Pulmonary Airway Malformation

Incidence and Clinical Presentation

Congenital cystic adenomatoid malformation (CCAM), more recently called congenital pulmonary

Table 24.8 Thoracic Space–Occupying Lesions

Condition	Diagnostic Criteria	Classification	Criteria for Antenatal Treatment	Ideal Treatment
CDH	Ultrasound demonstration of abdominal contents in the fetal chest	Left, right	Small contralateral lung, defined as a QLI <0.6 (left-CDH), <0.5 (right-CDH)	Tracheal occlusion with expandable stent
CPAM/CCAM	Cystic or hyperechogenic lung mass	Types I, II, III depending on cyst size	Hydrops or small contralateral lung	Percutaneous fetal sclerosis
BPS	Cystic or hyperechogenic mass with systemic or pulmonary feeding vessel.	Intralobar, extralobar	Hydrops or small contralateral lung	Ablation of feeding vessel

BPS, bronchopulmonary sequestration; CCAM, cystic adenomatoid malformation; CDH, congenital diaphragmatic hernia; CLE, congenital lobar emphysema; CPAM, congenital pulmonary airway malformation; QLI, quantitative lung index.

airway malformation (CPAM), consists of increased cell proliferation in the bronchial structures with lack of differentiation of the alveoli and decreased apoptosis.[171] These lesions usually occur in the first 6 weeks of gestation.[172]

CCAM/CPAM has been classified into three major types.[175,176] Type I, macrocystic, accounts for 50% to 70% of cases, contain one or more large cysts >2 cm with ciliated pseudostratified columnar epithelium. Type III, microcystic, is the most rare type and consists of several noncystic masses <0.5 cm with cuboidal epithelium. Type II is a mixture of type I and III and presents with several cysts, each <1 cm in size.[171] CCAM/CPAM communicates in a normal fashion with the bronchial tree.[177]

Treatment

Selection of patients for antenatal therapy for CCAM/CPAM is based on the prediction of pulmonary hypoplasia, hydrops, and neonatal death using an ultrasound index. Crombleholme et al proposed a CCAM/CPAM volume ratio (CVR)[180] calculated by dividing the volume of prolate ellipsoid (L × W × H × 0.52) by head circumference, where L, W, and H are the length, width, and height of the CCAM/CPAM, and 0.52 is a constant. Using this formula, they found that the mean CVR in fetuses that did not develop hydrops was 0.74, ±0.48.[180] The authors proposed that a value two standard deviations above the mean (0.74 + [0.48 × 2], or 1.7) would serve as a cut-off to predict the development of hydrops or neonatal death.

Several forms of antenatal therapy have been proposed for CCAM/CPAM, including thoracoamniotic shunting,[183] intralesional laser,[184] and lobectomy via open fetal surgery for fetuses with hydrops.[185,186] Antenatal corticosteroids have also been proposed, but outcomes have been unpredictable.[187] Complicated type I CCAM/CPAM may lend itself to thoracoamniotic shunting. However, shunting is not possible for types II and III CCAM/CPAM, and antenatal resection of the CCAM/CPAM via open fetal surgery has been proposed.[185,186]

Bermudez et al reported on the use percutaneous intralesional injection of sclersoing agents in patients with types II-III CCAM/CPAM with hydrops (fetal sclerotherapy, or FST).[131] Intralesional injection resulted in resolution of hydrops and of the mass effect in all cases without any complications.

Bronchopulmonary Sequestration

Bronchopulmonary sequestration (BPS) is a rare developmental anomaly of the lung characterized by nonfunctional pulmonary tissue without communication with the tracheobronchial tree and with an aberrant systemic arterial blood supply.[177] Extra- and intralobar types have been described, with the extralobar type usually located within the abdominal cavity, and the intralobar type typically located within the pleural cavity with an arterial feeding vessel generally arising from the thoracic aorta and with venous drainage into the left atrium.[189,190] Pulmonary hypoplasia in patients with BPS may result from atelectasis from compression of the normal lung, rather solely by the size of the mass.[146,147] The prognosis is poor in cases diagnosed before 26 weeks and is associated with mediastinal shift, polyhydramnios, and fetal hydrops.[130,191]

Therapeutic options for patients with complicated BPS include immediate delivery, medical therapy with diuretics and inotropic drugs, palliative serial amniodrainage, thoracoamniotic shunting of fetal pleural effusions, percutaneous sclerosis[132,192] or laser[191,193] of the vascular pedicle, and open fetal surgery.[132-134] Fetal bronchoscopy, with intraoperative lavage of the bronchial tree and immediate expansion of the normal lung parenchyma, has also been reported in one patient with BPS.[146,147]

Lower Urinary Tract Obstruction

Fetal lower urinary tract obstruction (LUTO) is due to a congenital obstruction at the level of the bladder or urethra. Male fetuses are more commonly affected, while the diagnosis of LUTO in a female fetus is often associated with more complex pathology (ie, cloacal malformations, megacystis-microcolon-intestinal hypoperistalsis syndrome). Long-standing LUTO can lead to abnormal renal development, and concurrent oligohydramnios is associated with pulmonary hypoplasia and skeletal abnormalities.[198-202]

The obstruction of the lower urinary tract may be partial or complete. The most common cause of LUTO is a posterior urethral valve (PUV), followed by urethral atresia/stenosis and congenital megalourethra.[195,204,205] The severity, duration, and timing of the obstruction impact renal growth and development as well as long-term survival. However, this is not a linear relationship and is difficult to predict prenatally.[206]

Various biomarkers have also been investigated as surrogate indicators for *in utero* renal function and postnatal prognosis.[196]

Clinical Assessment

LUTO can be prenatally diagnosed by ultrasound as early as in the first trimester; however, most cases are diagnosed in the second trimester during routine anatomy assessment.[197,229,230] In some patients, megacystis diagnosed in the first trimester spontaneously resolves and may represent a transient physiologic state.[231,232] In the cases where spontaneous resolution does not occur, serial ultrasound examinations are necessary. Characteristic ultrasound findings include a megacystis with oligohydramnios/anhydramnios present in severe cases (**Figure 24.2**). A visually enlarged bladder failing to empty during an extended ultrasound examination (ie, greater than 45 minutes) is commonly used in clinical practice.[234,235] Additional findings may include a dilated proximal urethra ("keyhole" sign), bladder wall thickening, bilateral hydroureteronephrosis, and hyperechogenic cystic kidneys.[209,229,230] Of note, the reliability of using the keyhole sign to predict the postnatal diagnosis of PUV is limited, with 35% of fetuses having underlying pathologies, such as vesicoureteral reflux, other than PUV identified after birth.[236]

The differential diagnosis of LUTO includes obstructive uropathies, such as PUV and other types of urethral obstruction, ureteroceles, megaureter, prune belly syndrome, megacystismicrocolon-hypoperistalsis syndrome, neurogenic bladder, primary vesicoureteral reflux, or a cloacal malformation.[197,229,230,232,233,240,241]

Treatment

Given the significant morbidity of untreated LUTO, *in utero* interventions have been developed, with the most common minimally invasive technique being VAS placement[38,39,196,244-249](**Figure 24.3**).

The main rationale for VAS placement is to restore the amniotic fluid volume and prevent lethal pulmonary hypoplasia. VAS-related complications include shunt dislodgement or obstruction,[219,244,247,250] urinary ascites,[237] iatrogenic gastroschisis,[251] and preterm premature rupture of membranes.[219,250,252]

Other *in utero* interventions include guide-wire passage or hydroablation of the PUV,[260] balloon catheter urethroplasty,[261] transurethral stenting,[262] urethral vesicoamniotic shunting,[263,264] and fetoscopic transvesical laser ablation of posterior urethral valves.[205,263,264]

Depending on the severity, postnatal survivors often have to deal with a spectrum of long-term morbidities, including bladder dysfunction, chronic renal impairment necessitating dialysis or transplantation, pulmonary insufficiency, poor growth, sexual dysfunction, and neurodevelopmental impairment.[202,258,266]

Amniotic Band Syndrome

Amniotic band syndrome (ABS) is a congenital anomaly complex that occurs in association with *in utero* entrapment of fetal parts by fibrous bands of amnion.[268-270]

The pathophysiology of ABS is not clearly understood and is likely multifactorial. A widely accepted theory is disruption of the amnion early in pregnancy leading to entanglement of fetal structures by amniochorionic mesoblastic fibrous strands.[272,275] The strands of amnion can lead to congenital malformations, deformations, and/or disruptions.[276] The cause of amnion rupture is unknown in most cases, but possible risk factors include connective tissue disorders and invasive *in-utero* procedures.[277-282] Other proposed etiologies of ABS include intrinsic defect of the germinal disc development, vascular compromise, and genetic mutations.[269,272,283] Risk factors for ABS may include prior uterine surgery, cigarette smoking, and high altitude.[272,284,285] Pseudoamniotic band syndrome (PABS) is a rare iatrogenic complication after invasive *in utero* procedures in which free floating amniotic bands are subsequently formed from fibrous strands extending from the surface of the denuded chorion.[277] PABS has been reported after amniocentesis, fetoscopy, thoracoamniotic shunt placement, fetal tracheal occlusion for CDH, and open fetal surgery.[277-279] The diagnosis of PABS requires a high degree of suspicion because, at most, only 27% are diagnosed prenatally by ultrasound.[277-279,286,287] Similar to spontaneous ABS, the amniotic bands from PABS can lead to constriction of fetal body parts and the umbilical cord.[280,288,289]

Clinical Assessment

ABS can be diagnosed early as the first trimester in the setting of characteristic fetal malformations.[290,291] The visualization of amniotic bands themselves is not required for diagnosis; however, a careful

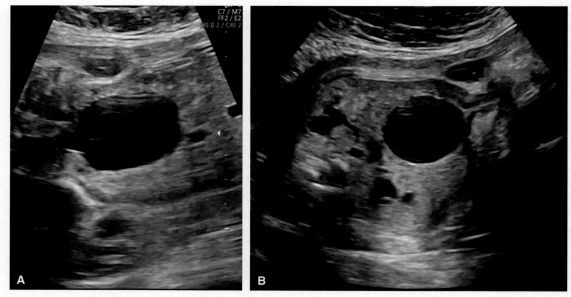

Figure 24.2 Ultrasound images at 30 weeks' gestation of a male fetus with lower urinary tract obstruction and oligohydramnios. **A,** Megacystis with "keyhole sign." **B,** Axial view of bilateral hydronephrosis and megacystis.

search of thin membrane-like strands should be performed using ultrasound. Importantly, the visualization of free-floating membranes alone in the absence of fetal malformations or restricted movement does not establish the diagnosis of ABS.[292]

The differential diagnosis of intrauterine linear echogenicities includes synechiae, uterine duplication anomalies, circumvallate placenta, or physiologic chorioamniotic membrane nonfusion.[293] Although ultrasound remains the mainstay of prenatal diagnosis, fetal MRI may be a complementary imaging modality that can assist in visualizing amniotic bands and their secondary manifestations when ultrasound findings are equivocal.[294]

Clinical Presentation

The clinical spectrum of ABS is heterogeneous and includes limb, craniofacial, central nervous system, body wall, and umbilical cord abnormalities.[268-270,276,292,295,296] The organ systems involved may be singular or multiple, and defects can be symmetric or asymmetric.[297] The most common abnormalities observed involve the fetal extremities (ie, constrictions, amputations, talipes equinovarus).[269,284] In cases of limb constriction, the extremity demonstrates circumferential constriction with distal edema[295,298] (**Figure 24.4**).

Treatment

There is a subset of patients who are candidates for *in utero* lysis of amniotic bands under fetoscopic and/or ultrasound guidance.[305,306] In the setting of limb involvement, the release of the constriction is considered to reduce the risk of irreversible loss of function and/or amputation.[295,296,299,306,307] The ideal time to intervene or the point in which amniotic band lysis would be futile is unknown. Of note, the fetus may potentially possess unique plasticity in fetal limb recovery. Depending on the degree of band adherence, release of the bands can be achieved using blunt dissection, endoshears, diathermy, or laser[295,296,299,307] (**Figure 24.5**).

Spina Bifida Repair

Open spina bifida (OSB) is characterized by the nonclosure of the elements that protect the medulla, leaving it exposed to the amniotic fluid throughout pregnancy. The primary postnatal consequences of OSB are related to a lifelong impairment of the control of sphincters and motor function at or below the level of the lesion, sometimes leading to paralysis.[310,311] The lesion is associated with Chiari II malformation, characterized by herniation of the cerebellum through the foramen magnum into the spinal canal.[312]

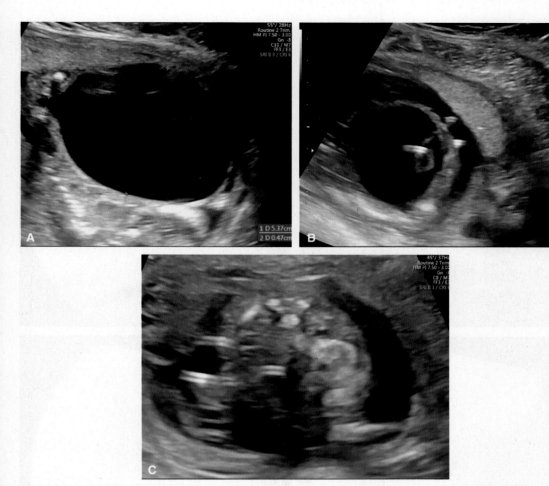

Figure 24.3 Ultrasound images at 17 weeks' gestation of a male fetus with lower urinary tract obstruction and oligohydramnios. **A,** Preoperative image with megacystis and "keyhole sign." **B,** Intraoperative image during vesicoamniotic shunt placement. **C,** Postoperative day 1 with the vescioamniotic shunt in place and decompressed fetal bladder. Normal amniotic fluid volume.

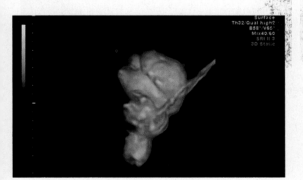

Figure 24.4 A three-dimensional (3D) ultrasound demonstrating amniotic band constriction of the fetal wrist with distal edema of the hand.

Postnatal Treatment of OSB

The primary goal of postnatal treatment of OSB is to stop the leakage of cerebral spinal fluid (CSF) from the lesion and to prevent infection of the exposed nervous tissue. To accomplish this, the neural placode is released and reshaped, the dura mater is closed in a watertight fashion, the paravertebral muscles are approximated, and the skin is closed. Approximately 52% to 91% of babies will require a ventriculoperitoneal (VP) shunt to treat an ensuing hydrocephalus.[313]

Two types of complications can arise from the postnatal surgical repair and VP shunting: problems with the VP shunt (eg, obstruction or infection) and

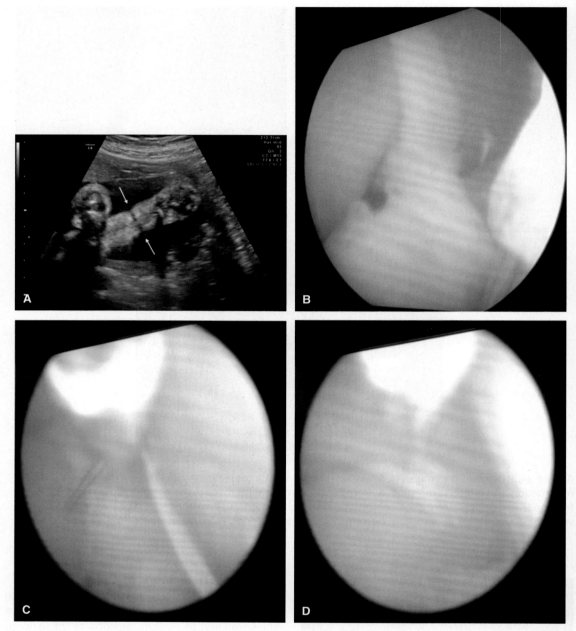

Figure 24.5 Amniotic band around lower extremity. **A,** Circumferential constriction by amniotic band (arrows) with mild distal swelling of right lower extremity. **B-D,** Fetoscopic release of the amniotic band around the lower extremity using endoshears.

tethered cord syndrome. Both complications require subsequent neurosurgical operations, which can cause further loss of neurological function.[311]

Prenatal Repair of OSB

As of this publication, there are two main fetoscopic techniques used for prenatal repair of OSB: the entirely percutaneous skin-over-biocellulose for antenatal fetoscopic repair (SAFER) technique and the laparotomy-assisted approach. Of note, fetal OSB repair provides *in utero* watertight sealing of placode lesions, the primary objective of postnatal repair approaches, thereby promoting reversal of the hindbrain herniation. Both the SAFER

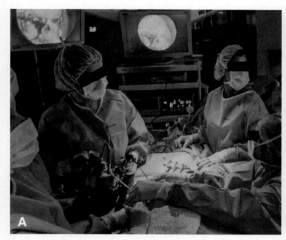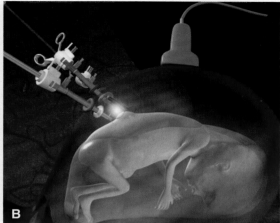

Figure 24.6 A, External view of the operating room during surgery. **B,** Schematics of the fetal repair.

technique and the laparotomy-assisted approach achieve similar neurological outcomes, but utilize very different neurosurgical approaches.

Fetoscopic Techniques

The SAFER technique (**Figure 24.6**) comprises an approach where the skin is sutured above a biocellulose patch (one patch) or, if there is not enough skin to be sutured in the midline, an artificial skin is used (two patches). This approach relies on the induction of fetal self-repair to close the lesion.

The laparotomy-assisted approach uses a primary watertight suture to repair the dura mater.

As of this writing, there has not been a prospective randomized, controlled trial comparing the open versus fetoscopic approach to repair OSB due to ethical concerns and because the open surgical approach has undergone modifications that would not be possible to directly parallel fetoscopically. However, comparison between long-term outcomes after any fetoscopic and the open fetal surgery approach have not shown any differences.[332,333]

KEY POINTS

Twin-Twin Transfusion Syndrome

- Standardization of diagnostic criteria for TTTS using ultrasound, recognition of the heterogeneous presentation of the condition with the Quintero staging system, and successful treatment of the disorder with laser therapy have made TTTS a success story in fetal therapy.
- Definitive treatment is achieved with complete laser obliteration of all placental vascular anastomoses.
- Benchmark outcomes include >90% survival of at least twin, 65% to 75% survival of both twins, <5% incidence of patent placental vascular anastomoses, <5% of persistent or reverse TTTS, <5% of

postlaser TAPS, <5% neurodevelopmental impairment, and 34 weeks' mean gestational age at delivery.
- Further research is still aimed at decreasing complications and improving surgical outcomes.

Twin Anemia-Polycythemia Sequence

- TAPS is the latest entity in the list of complications of monochorionic twins.
- The pathophysiology of TAPS is poorly understood, with small arteriovenous anastomoses playing a permissive role. Initial diagnostic criteria are being revised.
- Laser treatment appears to offer advantages over any of the other treatment modalities.

(Continued)

Selective Intrauterine Growth Restriction

- Monochorionic pregnancies complicated by sIUGR that do not meet sonographic criteria for TTTS represent a separate clinical entity.
- sIUGR pregnancies manifest higher rates of morbidity and mortality compared to dichorionic and uncomplicated monochorionic gestations and, therefore, need close monitoring and proper management.
- The classification of sIUGR into types I, II, and III, while useful in differentiating the various presentations, should not be interpreted as type III having the worse prognosis. Type II sIUGR is associated with the highest risk of an adverse perinatal outcome.
- SLPCV is indicated in type II sIUGR and should be associated with >90% survival of the AGA twin and 40% or greater chance of survival of the IUGR twin.
- Cord occlusion of the sIUGR twin should be considered only as a last resort, if SLPCV is not deemed feasible.

TRAP Sequence and Other Discordant Anomalous Twins

- TRAP sequence and other discordant anomalies of monochorionic twins may pose a risk to the healthy co-twin.
- The diagnosis of TRAP sequence requires the demonstration of reverse arterial flow into the anomalous twin with the combined use of color and pulsed Doppler.
- Criteria for antenatal intervention in TRAP sequence include large TRAP/pump ratio (>100%), polyhydramnios, abnormal Doppler studies (typically venous), hydrops of the pump twin, shortened cervix, and gestational age <26 weeks.
- Criteria for intervention in discordant anomalous twins depends on whether the anomalous twin is likely to die spontaneously in utero, or whether it poses any other risk (eg, polyhydramnios) to the healthy co-twin.
- Suture ligation is the preferred method for cord occlusion, compared to thermal methods (laser photocoagulation, bipolar electrocautery or radiofrequency ablation [RFA]).

- Disruption of the dividing membrane should be avoided while performing cord occlusion, to avoid development of a pseudoamniotic twin pregnancy and its attendant complications (cord entanglement, demise of the healthy co-twin).
- Ligation and transection of the umbilical cord is the preferred surgical method for the treatment of complicated monoamniotic discordant anomalous twins.

Congenital Diaphragmatic Hernia

- CDH remains an unsolved dilemma in fetal therapy.
- Differences in the sonographic criteria for the identification of high-risk groups as well as in which medical device is ideal to achieve the best palliative in utero treatment for the condition summarize the state of affairs in CDH.
- Successful antenatal management of patients with CDH is undoubtedly the holy grail in fetal therapy.

Fetal Lung Masses

- Fetal lung lesions, while rare, may be associated with significant fetal and perinatal mortality.
- Antenatal sonographic classifications have changed, and so have the criteria to predict fetuses at risk for the development of hydrops, pulmonary hypoplasia, and neonatal death.
- Depending on the type of lesion, different therapeutic modalities have been proposed, with less emphasis on open fetal surgery techniques.

Lower Urinary Tract Obstruction

- Fetal LUTO is a relatively common fetal therapy condition.
- Untreated, LUTO may result in neonatal death from pulmonary hypoplasia or chronic renal damage.
- Appropriate selection of LUTO patients involves detailed ultrasound evaluation and assessment of karyotype, microarray, and fetal renal function.

- Treatment of LUTO with standard double pigtail catheters is fraught with substantial catheter malfunction.
- Treatment of LUTO with the Q-shunt is associated with less risk for shunt dislodgement and improved neonatal outcomes.

Amniotic Band Syndrome

- ABS is a rare nonlethal entity that may be associated with limb amputations.
- Criteria for antenatal intervention have not been established, but include evidence of significant limb constriction with distal edema and possibly distal arterial Doppler abnormalities.
- Lysis of amniotic bands, which represented the treatment of the first nonlethal fetal condition in utero, may avoid spontaneous limb amputation and improved postnatal limb function.

Spina Bifida Repair

- Prenatal repair of open spina bifida reduces shunt rates and may improve postnatal motor and neurodevelopmental outcomes.
- The hysterotomy required for the open fetal surgery leaves subsequent pregnancies at risk of uterine rupture.
- Fetoscopic repair is feasible and seems to achieve the same, postnatal neurological outcomes as the open repair.
- Fetoscopy can be accomplished by a laparotomy-based approach, or it can be entirely percutaneous.
- Surgical techniques for the repair of the defect are not yet standardized, and the type of defect repair may affect long term outcomes, especially regarding walking, neurogenic bladder, and cord tethering.
- The role of open fetal surgery for the management of spina bifida may be restricted to selected cases in the very near future.

REFERENCES

(only references cited in synoptic print chapter; for a complete reference list, see ebook)

1. Quintero R, Reich H, Puder K, et al. Brief report: umbilical-cord ligation of an acardiac twin by fetoscopy at 19 weeks of gestation. *N Eng J Med.* 1994;330:469-471.
9. Jones J, Sbarra A, Dilillo L, et al. Indomethacin in severe twin-to-twin transfusion syndrome. *Am J Perinatol.* 1993;10:24-26.
10. Urig MA, Simpson GF, Elliott JP, Clewell WH. Twin-twin transfusion syndrome: the surgical removal of one twin as a treatment option. *Fetal Ther.* 1988;3(4):185-188.
11. Saunders NJ, Snijders RJ, Nicolaides KH. Therapeutic amniocentesis in twin-twin transfusion syndrome appearing in the second trimester of pregnancy. *Am J Obstet Gynecol.* 1992;166(3):820-824.
12. Wax JR, Blakemore KJ, Blohm P, Callan NA. Stuck twin with cotwin nonimmune hydrops: successful treatment by amniocentesis. *Fetal Diagn Ther.* 1991;6(3-4):126-131.
13. Dennis LG, Winkler CL. Twin-to-twin transfusion syndrome: aggressive therapeutic amniocentesis. *Am J Obstet Gynecol.* 1997;177(2):342-347; discussion 7-9.
14. De Lia JE, Cruikshank DP, Keye WR Jr. Fetoscopic neodymium:YAG laser occlusion of placental vessels in severe twin-twin transfusion syndrome. *Obstet Gynecol.* 1990;75(6):1046-1053.
15. Ville Y, Hecher K, Ogg D, Warren R, Nicolaides K. Successful outcome after Nd: YAG laser separation of chorioangiopagus-twins under sonoendoscopic control. *Ultrasound Obstet Gynecol.* 1992;2(6):429-431.
16. De Lia JE, Kuhlmann RS, Harstad TW, Cruikshank DP. Fetoscopic laser ablation of placental vessels in severe previable twin-twin transfusion syndrome. *Am J Obstet Gynecol.* 1995;172(4 pt 1):1202-1208; discussion 8-11.
17. Ville Y, Hyett J, Hecher K, Nicolaides K. Preliminary experience with endoscopic laser surgery for severe twin-twin transfusion syndrome. *N Engl J Med.* 1995;332:224-227.
18. Quintero R, Morales W, Mendoza G, et al. Selective photocoagulation of placental vessels in twin-twin transfusion syndrome: evolution of a surgical technique. *Obstet Gynecol Surv.* 1998;53(12):S97-S103.
19. Hecher K, Diehl W, Zikulnig L, Vetter M, Hackeloer BJ. Endoscopic laser coagulation of placental anastomoses in 200 pregnancies with severe mid-trimester twin-to-twin transfusion syndrome. *Eur J Obstet Gynecol Reprod Biol.* 2000;92(1):135-139.
20. Dickinson JE. Severe twin-twin transfusion syndrome: current management concepts. *Aust N Z J Obstet Gynaecol.* 1995;35(1):16-21.
21. Jauniaux E, Holmes A, Hyett J, Yates R, Rodeck C. Rapid and radical amniodrainage in the treatment of severe twin-twin transfusion syndrome. *Prenat Diagn.* 2001;21(6):471-476.
31. Lenclen R, Paupe A, Ciarlo G, et al. Neonatal outcome in preterm monochorionic twins with twin-to-twin transfusion syndrome after intrauterine treatment with amnioreduction or fetoscopic laser surgery: comparison with dichorionic twins. *Am J Obstet Gynecol.* 2007;196(5):450.e1-450.e7.
33. Quintero RA. *Twin-Twin Transfusion Syndrome.* InformaHealth; 2007.
34. Crisan LS, Kontopoulos EV, Quintero RA. Appraisal of the selectivity index in a cohort of patients treated with laser surgery for twin-twin transfusion syndrome. *Am J Obstet Gynecol.* 2010;202(2):157.e1-157.e5.
38. Quintero RA, Chmait RH, Bornick PW, Kontopoulos EV. Trocar-assisted selective laser photocoagulation of communicating vessels: a technique for the laser treatment of patients with twin-twin transfusion syndrome with inaccessible anterior placentas. *J Matern Fetal Neonatal Med.* 2010;23(4):330-334.
39. Quintero RA, Gomez Castro LA, Bermudez C, Chmait RH, Kontopoulos EV. In utero management of fetal lower urinary tract obstruction with a novel shunt: a landmark development in fetal therapy. *J Matern Fetal Neonatal Med.* 2010;23(8):806-812.
41. Slaghekke F, Lopriore E, Lewi L, et al. Fetoscopic laser coagulation of the vascular equator versus selective coagulation for twin-to-twin transfusion syndrome: an open-label randomised controlled trial. *Lancet.* 2014;383(9935):2144-2151.
42. Slaghekke F, Lewi L, Middeldorp JM, et al. Residual anastomoses in twin-twin transfusion syndrome after laser: the Solomon randomized trial. *Am J Obstet Gynecol.* 2014;211(3):285.e1-285.e7.
43. Slaghekke F, van Klink JM, Koopman HM, Middeldorp JM, Oepkes D, Lopriore E. Neurodevelopmental outcome in twin anemia-polycythemia sequence after laser surgery for twin-twin transfusion syndrome. *Ultrasound Obstet Gynecol.* 2014;44(3):316-321.

44. Kontopoulos E, Chmait R, Baker B, Llanes A, Quintero R. USFetus surgical benchmarks of selective laser therapy for twin-twin transfusion syndrome. *Am J Obstet Gynecol.* 2015;212(1):S91-S92.

45. Robyr R, Lewi L, Salomon LJ, et al. Prevalence and management of late fetal complications following successful selective laser coagulation of chorionic plate anastomoses in twin-to-twin transfusion syndrome. *Am J Obstet Gynecol.* 2006;194(3):796-803.

49. Chalouhi GE, Essaoui M, Stirnemann J, et al. Laser therapy for twin-to-twin transfusion syndrome (TTTS). *Prenat Diagn.* 2011;31(7):637-646.

65. Taniguchi K, Sumie M, Sugibayashi R, Wada S, Matsuoka K, Sago H. Twin anemia-polycythemia sequence after laser surgery for twin-twin transfusion syndrome and maternal morbidity. *Fetal Diagn Ther.* 2015;37(2):148-153.

68. Stranak Z, Korcek P, Hympanova L, Kyncl M, Krofta L. Prenatally acquired multiple limb ischemia in a very low birth weight monochorionic twin. *Fetal Diagn Ther.* 2017;41(3):237-238.

69. Lopriore E, Slaghekke F, Oepkes D, Middeldorp JM, Vandenbussche FP, Walther FJ. Hematological characteristics in neonates with twin anemia-polycythemia sequence (TAPS). *Prenat Diagn.* 2010;30(3):251-255.

70. Sarkar S, Rosenkrantz TS. Neonatal polycythemia and hyperviscosity. *Semin Fetal Neonatal Med.* 2008;13(4):248-255.

72. Genova L, Slaghekke F, Klumper FJ, et al. Management of twin anemia-polycythemia sequence using intrauterine blood transfusion for the donor and partial exchange transfusion for the recipient. *Fetal Diagn Ther.* 2013;34(2):121-126.

87. Gratacos E, Lewi L, Munoz B, et al. A classification system for selective intrauterine growth restriction in monochorionic pregnancies according to umbilical artery Doppler flow in the smaller twin. *Ultrasound Obstet Gynecol.* 2007;30(1):28-34.

88. Ishii K, Murakoshi T, Takahashi Y, et al. Perinatal outcome of monochorionic twins with selective intrauterine growth restriction and different types of umbilical artery Doppler under expectant management. *Fetal Diagn Ther.* 2009;26(3):157-161.

108. Buca D, Pagani G, Rizzo G, et al. Outcome of monochorionic twin pregnancy with selective intrauterine growth restriction according to umbilical artery Doppler flow pattern of smaller twin: systematic review and meta-analysis. *Ultrasound Obstet Gynecol.* 2017;50(5):559-568.

109. Parra-Cordero M, Bennasar M, Martinez JM, Eixarch E, Torres X, Gratacos E. Cord occlusion in monochorionic twins with early selective intrauterine growth restriction and abnormal umbilical artery Doppler: a consecutive series of 90 cases. *Fetal Diagn Ther.* 2016;39(3):186-191.

110. Grab D, Schneider V, Keckstein J, et al. Twin, acardiac, outcome. *Fetus.* 1992;2(7615):11-13.

111. Hamada H, Okane M, Koresawa M, Iwasaki H. Fetal therapy in utero by blockage of the umbilical blood flow of acardiac monster in twin pregnancy. *Nihon Sanka Fujinka Gakkai Zasshi.* 1989;41:1803.

112. Bebbington MW, Wilson RD, Machan L, Wittmann BK. Selective feticide in twin transfusion syndrome using ultrasound-guided insertion of thrombogenic coils. *Fetal Diagn Ther.* 1995;10(1):32-36.

113. Porreco R, Barton S, Haverkamp A. Occlusion of umbilical artery in acardiac, acephalic twin. *Lancet.* 1991;337:326-327.

114. Roberts R, Shah D, Jeanty P, Beattie J. Twin, acardiac, ultrasound-guided embolization. *Fetus.* 1991;1(7615):5-10.

115. Holzgreve W, Tercanli S, Krings W, Schuierer G. A simpler technique for umbilical-cord blockade of an acardiac twin. *N Eng J Med.* 1994;331(1):56-57.

116. Seeds JW, Herbert WN, Richards DS. Prenatal sonographic diagnosis and management of a twin pregnancy with placenta previa and hemicardia. *Am J Perinatol.* 1987;4(4):313-316.

117. Donnenfeld AE, van de Woestijne J, Craparo F, Smith CS, Ludomirsky A, Weiner S. The normal fetus of an acardiac twin pregnancy: perinatal management based on echocardiographic and sonographic evaluation. *Prenat Diagn.* 1991;11(4):235-244.

118. Bebbington MW, Danzer E, Moldenhauer J, Khalek N, Johnson MP. Radiofrequency ablation vs bipolar umbilical cord coagulation in the management of complicated monochorionic pregnancies. *Ultrasound Obstet Gynecol.* 2012;40(3):319-324.

123. Quintero RA, Chmait RH, Murakoshi T, et al. Surgical management of twin reversed arterial perfusion sequence. *Am J Obstet Gynecol.* 2006;194(4):982-991.

124. Nicolini U, Poblete A, Boschetto C, Bonati F, Roberts A. Complicated monochorionic twin pregnancies: experience with bipolar cord coagulation. *Am J Obstet Gynecol.* 2001;185(3):703-707.

125. Livingston JC, Lim FY, Polzin W, Mason J, Crombleholme TM. Intrafetal radiofrequency ablation for twin reversed arterial perfusion (TRAP): a single-center experience. *Am J Obstet Gynecol.* 2007;197(4):399.e1-399.e3.

126. Morel O, Malartic C, Barranger E. Radiofrequency ablation for twin-reversed arterial perfusion sequence: the unknown cord occlusion delay calls for long term neonatal follow-up of the surviving twins. *Am J Obstet Gynecol.* 2007;197(5):557-558; author reply 8.

127. Cavoretto P, Molina F, Poggi S, Davenport M, Nicolaides KH. Prenatal diagnosis and outcome of echogenic fetal lung lesions. *Ultrasound Obstet Gynecol.* 2008;32(6):769-783.

128. Stanton M, Njere I, Ade-Ajayi N, Patel S, Davenport M. Systematic review and meta-analysis of the postnatal management of congenital cystic lung lesions. *J Pediatr Surg.* 2009;44(5):1027-1033.

129. Laje P, Wilson RD, Guttenberg M, Liechty KW. Survival in primary congenital pulmonary lymphangiectasia with hydrops fetalis. *Fetal Diagn Ther.* 2008;24(3):225-229.

130. Witlox RS, Lopriore E, Oepkes D. Prenatal interventions for fetal lung lesions. *Prenat Diagn.* 2011;31(7):628-636.

131. Bermudez C, Perez-Wulff J, Arcadipane M, et al. Percutaneous fetal sclerotherapy for congenital cystic adenomatoid malformation of the lung. *Fetal Diagn Ther.* 2008;24(3):237-240.

132. Bermudez C, Perez-Wulff J, Bufalino G, Sosa C, Gomez L, Quintero RA. Percutaneous ultrasound-guided sclerotherapy for complicated fetal intralobar bronchopulmonary sequestration. *Ultrasound Obstet Gynecol.* 2007;29(5):586-589.

133. Biyyam DR, Chapman T, Ferguson MR, Deutsch G, Dighe MK. Congenital lung abnormalities: embryologic features, prenatal diagnosis, and postnatal radiologic-pathologic correlation. *Radiographics.* 2010;30(6):1721-1738.

134. Murotsuki J, Uehara S, Okamura K, Yajima A, Murakami K. Prenatal diagnosis of congenital cystic adenomatoid malformation of the lung by fetal lung biopsy. *Prenat Diagn.* 1994;14(7):637-639.

137. McGivern MR, Best KE, Rankin J, et al. Epidemiology of congenital diaphragmatic hernia in Europe: a register-based study. *Arch Dis Child Fetal Neonatal Ed.* 2015;100(2):F137-F144.

138. Achiron R, Heggesh J, Mashiach S, Lipitz S, Rotstein Z. Peripheral right pulmonary artery blood flow velocimetry: Doppler sonographic study of normal and abnormal fetuses. *J Ultrasound Med.* 1998;17(11):687-692.

139. Chaoui R, Kalache K, Tennstedt C, Lenz F, Vogel M. Pulmonary arterial Doppler velocimetry in fetuses with lung hypoplasia. *Eur J Obstet Gynecol Reprod Biol.* 1999;84(2):179-185.

146. Quintero RA, Kontopoulos EV, Quintero LF, Landy DC, Gonzalez R, Chmait RH. The observed vs. expected lung-to-head ratio does not correct for the effect of gestational age on the lung-to-head ratio. *J Matern Fetal Neonatal Med.* 2012;26:552-557.

147. Quintero RA, Kontopoulos E, Reiter J, Pedreira WL, Colin AA. Fetal bronchoscopy: its successful use in a case of extralobar pulmonary sequestration. *J Matern Fetal Neonatal Med.* 2012;25(11):2354-2358.

154. Bealer JF, Skarsgard ED, Hedrick MH, et al. The 'PLUG' odyssey: adventures in experimental fetal tracheal occlusion. *J Pediatr Surg.* 1995;30(2):361-364; discussion 4-5.

155. Hedrick MH, Estes JM, Sullivan KM, et al. Plug the lung until it grows (PLUG): a new method to treat congenital diaphragmatic hernia in utero. *J Pediatr Surg.* 1994;29:612.

156. Skarsgard ED, Meuli M, VanderWall KJ, Bealer JF, Adzick NS, Harrison MR. Fetal endoscopic tracheal occlusion ('Fetendo-PLUG') for congenital diaphragmatic hernia. *J Pediatr Surg.* 1996;31(10):1335-1338.

159. Quintero R, Quintero L, Pivatelli A, Bornick P, Allen M, Johnson P. The donor-recipient (D-R) score: in vivo endoscopic evidence to support the hypothesis of a net transfer of blood from donor to recipient in twin-twin transfusion syndrome. *Prenat Neonat Med.* 2000;5:84-91.

160. Quintero R, Morales W, Bornick P, Allen M, Johnson P. Minimally-invasive intraluminal tracheal occlusion in a human fetus with left congenital diaphragmatic hernia at 27 weeks' gestation via direct fetal laryngoscopy. *Prenat Neonat Med.* 2000;5:134-140.

161. Deprest J. Towards an endoscopic intra-uterine treatment for congenital diaphragmatic hernia. *Verh K Acad Geneeskd Belg.* 2002;64(1):55-70.

162. Harrison MR, Albanese CT, Hawgood SB, et al. Fetoscopic temporary tracheal occlusion by means of detachable balloon for congenital diaphragmatic hernia. *Am J Obstet Gynecol.* 2001;185(3):730-733.

163. Deprest J, Gratacos E, Nicolaides KH. Fetoscopic tracheal occlusion (FETO) for severe congenital diaphragmatic hernia: evolution of a technique and preliminary results. *Ultrasound Obstet Gynecol.* 2004;24(2):121-126.

164. Jani J, Gratacos E, Greenough A, et al. Percutaneous fetal endoscopic tracheal occlusion (FETO) for severe left-sided congenital diaphragmatic hernia. *Clin Obstet Gynecol.* 2005;48(4):910-922.

165. Kohl T, Gembruch U, Filsinger B, et al. Encouraging early clinical experience with deliberately delayed temporary fetoscopic tracheal occlusion for the prenatal treatment of life-threatening right and left congenital diaphragmatic hernias. *Fetal Diagn Ther.* 2006;21(3):314-318.

166. Sosa-Sosa C, Bermudez C, Chmait RH, et al. Intraluminal tracheal occlusion using a modified 8-mm Z-stent in a sheep model of left-sided congenital diaphragmatic hernia. *J Matern Fetal Neonatal Med.* 2012;25(11):2346-2353.

171. Evrard V, Ceulemans J, Coosemans W, et al. Congenital parenchymatous malformations of the lung. *World J Surg.* 1999;23(11):1123-1132.

172. Sanders R. *Cystic adenomatoid malformation of the lung.* In: *Structural Fetal Abnormalities: Total Picture.* Mosby; 1996:180-183.

175. Stocker JT, Madewell JE, Drake RM. Congenital cystic adenomatoid malformation of the lung. Classification and morphologic spectrum. *Hum Pathol.* 1977;8(2):155-171.

176. Askin FB, Gilbert-Barness E. Respiratory system. In: Gilbert-Barness E, ed. *Potter's Pathology of the Fetus, Infant and Child.* Vol 2. 2nd ed. Mosby Elsevier; 2007:1108-1109.

177. Barnes NA, Pilling DW. Bronchopulmonary foregut malformations: embryology, radiology and quandary. *Eur Radiol.* 2003;13(12):2659-2673.

180. Crombleholme TM, Coleman B, Hedrick H, et al. Cystic adenomatoid malformation volume ratio predicts outcome in prenatally diagnosed cystic adenomatoid malformation of the lung. *J Pediatr Surg.* 2002;37(3):331-338.

183. Wilson RD, Baxter JK, Johnson MP, et al. Thoracoamniotic shunts: fetal treatment of pleural effusions and congenital cystic adenomatoid malformations. *Fetal Diagn Ther.* 2004;19(5):413-420.

184. Bruner JP, Jarnagin BK, Reinisch L. Percutaneous laser ablation of fetal congenital cystic adenomatoid malformation: too little, too late? *Fetal Diagn Ther.* 2000;15(6):359-363.

185. Adzick NS, Flake AW, Crombleholme TM. Management of congenital lung lesions. *Semin Pediatr Surg.* 2003;12(1):10-16.

186. Harrison MR, Adzick NS, Jennings RW, et al. Antenatal intervention for congenital cystic adenomatoid malformation. *Lancet.* 1990;336:965-967.

187. Derderian SC, Coleman AM, Jeanty C, et al. Favorable outcomes in high-risk congenital pulmonary airway malformations treated with multiple courses of maternal betamethasone. *J Pediatr Surg.* 2015;50(4):515-518.

189. Romero R, Chervenak FA, Kotzen J, Berkowitz RL, Hobbins JC. Antenatal sonographic findings of extralobar pulmonary sequestration. *J Ultrasound Med.* 1982;1(3):131-132.

190. Reece EA, Lockwood CJ, Rizzo N, Pilu G, Bovicelli L, Hobbins JC. Intrinsic intrathoracic malformations of the fetus: sonographic detection and clinical presentation. *Obstet Gynecol.* 1987;70(4):627-632.

191. Witlox RS, Lopriore E, Walther FJ, Rikkers-Mutsaerts ER, Klumper FJ, Oepkes D. Single-needle laser treatment with drainage of hydrothorax in fetal bronchopulmonary sequestration with hydrops. *Ultrasound Obstet Gynecol.* 2009;34(3):355-357.

192. Nicolini U, Cerri V, Groli C, Poblete A, Mauro F. A new approach to prenatal treatment of extralobar pulmonary sequestration. *Prenat Diagn.* 2000;20(9):758-760.

193. Oepkes D, Devlieger R, Lopriore E, Klumper FJ. Successful ultrasound-guided laser treatment of fetal hydrops caused by pulmonary sequestration. *Ultrasound Obstet Gynecol.* 2007;29(4):457-459.

195. Malin G, Tonks AM, Morris RK, Gardosi J, Kilby MD. Congenital lower urinary tract obstruction: a population-based epidemiological study. *Br J Obstet Gynecol.* 2012;119(12):1455-1464.

196. Cheung KW, Morris RK, Kilby MD. Congenital urinary tract obstruction. *Best Pract Res Clin Obstet Gynaecol.* 2019;58:78-92.

197. Osborne NG, Bonilla-Musoles F, Machado LE, et al. Fetal megacystis: differential diagnosis. *J Ultrasound Med.* 2011;30(6):833-841.

198. Freedman AL, Johnson MP, Gonzalez R. Fetal therapy for obstructive uropathy: past, present.future? *Pediatr Nephrol.* 2000;14(2):167-176.

199. Nakayama DK, Harrison MR, de Lorimier AA. Prognosis of posterior urethral valves presenting at birth. *J Pediatr Surg.* 1986;21(1):43-45.

201. Matsell DG, Yu S, Morrison SJ. Antenatal determinants of long-term kidney outcome in boys with posterior urethral valves. *Fetal Diagn Ther.* 2016;39(3):214-221.

202. Morris RK, Ruano R, Kilby MD. Effectiveness of fetal cystoscopy as a diagnostic and therapeutic intervention for lower urinary tract obstruction: a systematic review. *Ultrasound Obstet Gynecol.* 2011;37(6):629-637.

204. Bornes M, Spaggiari E, Schmitz T, et al. Outcome and etiologies of fetal megacystis according to the gestational age at diagnosis. *Prenat Diagn.* 2013;33(12):1162-1166.

205. Sananes N, Cruz-Martinez R, Favre R, et al. Two-year outcomes after diagnostic and therapeutic fetal cystoscopy for lower urinary tract obstruction. *Prenat Diagn.* 2016;36(4):297-303.

206. Chevalier RL. Congenital urinary tract obstruction: the long view. *Adv Chronic Kidney Dis.* 2015;22(4):312-319.

209. Robyr R, Benachi A, Daikha-Dahmane F, Martinovich J, Dumez Y, Ville Y. Correlation between ultrasound and anatomical findings in fetuses with lower urinary tract obstruction in the first half of pregnancy. *Ultrasound Obstet Gynecol.* 2005;25(5):478-482.

219. Chon AH, de Oliveira GH, Lemley KV, Korst LM, Assaf RD, Chmait RH. Fetal serum beta2-microglobulin and postnatal renal function in lower urinary tract obstruction treated with vesicoamniotic shunt. *Fetal Diagn Ther.* 2017;42(1):17-27.

229. Ibirogba ER, Haeri S, Ruano R. Fetal lower urinary tract obstruction: what should we tell the prospective parents? *Prenat Diagn.* 2020.

230. Dias T, Sairam S, Kumarasiri S. Ultrasound diagnosis of fetal renal abnormalities. *Best Pract Res Clin Obstet Gynaecol.* 2014;28(3):403-415.

231. Sebire NJ, Von Kaisenberg C, Rubio C, Snijders RJ, Nicolaides KH. Fetal megacystis at 10-14 weeks of gestation. *Ultrasound Obstet Gynecol.* 1996;8(6):387-390.

232. Liao AW, Sebire NJ, Geerts L, Cicero S, Nicolaides KH. Megacystis at 10-14 weeks of gestation: chromosomal defects and outcome according to bladder length. *Ultrasound Obstet Gynecol.* 2003;21(4):338-341.

233. Taghavi K, Sharpe C, Stringer MD. Fetal megacystis: a systematic review. *J Pediatr Urol.* 2017;13(1):7-15.

234. Fontanella F, Duin LK, Adama van Scheltema PN, et al. Prenatal diagnosis of LUTO: improving diagnostic accuracy. *Ultrasound Obstet Gynecol.* 2018;52(6):739-743.

235. Montemarano H, Bulas DI, Rushton HG, Selby D. Bladder distention and pyelectasis in the male fetus: causes, comparisons, and contrasts. *J Ultrasound Med.* 1998;17(12):743-749.

236. Bernardes LS, Aksnes G, Saada J, et al. Keyhole sign: how specific is it for the diagnosis of posterior urethral valves? *Ultrasound Obstet Gynecol.* 2009;34(4):419-423.

237. Ruano R. Fetal surgery for severe lower urinary tract obstruction. *Prenat Diagn.* 2011;31(7):667-674.

240. Biard JM, Johnson MP, Carr MC, et al. Long-term outcomes in children treated by prenatal vesicoamniotic shunting for lower urinary tract obstruction. *Obstet Gynecol.* 2005;106(3):503-508.

241. Banuelos Marco B, Gonzalez R, Ludwikowski B, Lingnau A. Effectiveness of prenatal intervention on the outcome of diseases that have a postnatal urological impact. *Front Pediatr.* 2019;7:118.

244. Jeong BD, Won HS, Lee MY. Perinatal outcomes of fetal lower urinary tract obstruction after vesicoamniotic shunting using a double-basket catheter. *J Ultrasound Med.* 2018;37(9):2147-2156.

245. McLorie G, Farhat W, Khoury A, Geary D, Ryan G. Outcome analysis of vesicoamniotic shunting in a comprehensive population. *J Urol.* 2001;166(3):1036-1040.

246. Clark TJ, Martin WL, Divakaran TG, Whittle MJ, Kilby MD, Khan KS. Prenatal bladder drainage in the management of fetal lower urinary tract obstruction: a systematic review and meta-analysis. *Obstet Gynecol.* 2003;102(2):367-382.

247. Saccone G, D'Alessandro P, Escolino M, et al. Antenatal intervention for congenital fetal lower urinary tract obstruction (LUTO): a systematic review and meta-analysis. *J Matern Fetal Neonatal Med.* 2018;33:1-161.

248. Kilby MD, Morris RK. Fetal therapy for the treatment of congenital bladder neck obstruction. *Nat Rev Urol.* 2014;11(7):412-419.

249. Manning FA, Harrison MR, Rodeck C. Catheter shunts for fetal hydronephrosis and hydrocephalus. Report of the International Fetal Surgery Registry. *N Engl J Med.* 1986;315(5):336-340.

250. Ethun CG, Zamora IJ, Roth DR, et al. Outcomes of fetuses with lower urinary tract obstruction treated with vesicoamniotic shunt: a single-institution experience. *J Pediatr Surg.* 2013;48(5):956-962.

251. Debska M, Kretowicz P, Oledzka A, et al. Early vesico-amniotic shunting – does it change the prognosis in fetal lower urinary tract obstruction diagnosed in the first trimester? *Ginekol Pol.* 2017;88(9):486-491.

252. Morris RK, Malin GL, Khan KS, Kilby MD. Systematic review of the effectiveness of antenatal intervention for the treatment of congenital lower urinary tract obstruction. *Br J Obstet Gynecol.* 2010;117(4):382-390.

258. Freedman AL, Johnson MP, Smith CA, Gonzalez R, Evans MI. Long-term outcome in children after antenatal intervention for obstructive uropathies. *Lancet*. 1999;354(9176):374-377.

260. Welsh A, Agarwal S, Kumar S, Smith RP, Fisk NM. Fetal cystoscopy in the management of fetal obstructive uropathy: experience in a single European centre. *Prenat Diagn*. 2003;23(13):1033-1041.

262. Ruano R, Yoshizaki CT, Giron AM, Srougi M, Zugaib M. Cystoscopic placement of transurethral stent in a fetus with urethral stenosis. *Ultrasound Obstet Gynecol*. 2014;44(2):238-240.

263. Quintero RA, Johnson MP, Romero R, et al. In-utero percutaneous cystoscopy in the management of fetal lower obstructive uropathy. *Lancet*. 1995;346(8974):537-540.

264. Quintero RA, Hume R, Smith C, et al. Percutaneous fetal cystoscopy and endoscopic fulguration of posterior urethral valves. *Am J Obstet Gynecol*. 1995;172(1 pt 1):206-209.

266. Monteiro S, Nassr AA, Yun PS, et al. Neurodevelopmental outcome in infants with lower urinary tract obstruction based on different degrees of severity. *Fetal Diagn Ther*. 2020;47:1-10.

268. Society for Maternal-Fetal Medicine, Gandhi M, Rac MWF, McKinney J. Amniotic band sequence. *Am J Obstet Gynecol*. 2019;221:B5-B6.

269. Seeds JW, Cefalo RC, Herbert WN. Amniotic band syndrome. *Am J Obstet Gynecol*. 1982;144:243-248.

271. Barros M, Gorgal G, Machado AP, Ramalho C, Matias A, Montenegro N. Revisiting amniotic band sequence: a wide spectrum of manifestations. *Fetal Diagn Ther*. 2014;35:51-56.

272. Cignini P, Giorlandino C, Padula F, Dugo N, Cafa EV, Spata A. Epidemiology and risk factors of amniotic band syndrome, or ADAM sequence. *J Prenat Med*. 2012;6:59-63.

275. Torpin R. Amniochorionic mesoblastic fibrous strings and amnionic bands: associated constricting fetal malformations or fetal death. *Am J Obstet Gynecol*. 1965;91:65-75.

276. Higginbottom MC, Jones KL, Hall BD, Smith DW. The amniotic band disruption complex: timing of amniotic rupture and variable spectra of consequent defects. *J Pediatr*. 1979;95:544-549.

277. Ting YH, Lao TT, Law KM, Cheng YK, Lau TK, Leung TY. Pseudoamniotic band syndrome after in utero intervention for twin-to-twin transfusion syndrome: case reports and literature review. *Fetal Diagn Ther*. 2016;40:67-72.

278. Cruz-Martinez R, Van Mieghem T, Lewi L, et al. Incidence and clinical implications of early inadvertent septostomy after laser therapy for twin-twin transfusion syndrome. *Ultrasound Obstet Gynecol*. 2011;37:458-462.

279. Graf JL, Bealer JF, Gibbs DL, Adzick NS, Harrison MR. Chorioamniotic membrane separation: a potentially lethal finding. *Fetal Diagn Ther*. 1997;12:81-84.

280. Han M, Afshar Y, Chon AH, et al. Pseudoamniotic band syndrome post fetal thoracoamniotic shunting for bilateral hydrothorax. *Fetal Pediatr Pathol*. 2017;36:311-318.

281. Young ID, Lindenbaum RH, Thompson EM, Pembrey ME. Amniotic bands in connective tissue disorders. *Arch Dis Child*. 1985;60:1061-1063.

282. Sakiyama T, Umegaki-Arao N, Sasaki T, Kosaki K, Amagai M, Kubo A. Case of dominant dystrophic epidermolysis bullosa with amniotic band syndrome. *J Dermatol*. 2017;44:102-103.

283. Halder A. Amniotic band syndrome and/or limb body wall complex: split or lump. *Appl Clin Genet*. 2010;3:7-15.

284. Barzilay E, Harel Y, Haas J, et al. Prenatal diagnosis of amniotic band syndrome – risk factors and ultrasonic signs. *J Matern Fetal Neonatal Med*. 2015;28:281-283.

285. Castilla EE, Lopez-Camelo JS, Campana H. Altitude as a risk factor for congenital anomalies. *Am J Med Genet*. 1999;86:9-14.

286. Shamshirsaz AA, Shamshirsaz AA, Nayeri UA, Bahtiyar MO, Belfort MA, Campbell WA. Pseudoamniotic band syndrome: a rare complication of monochorionic triplets with twin-to-twin transfusion syndrome. *Prenat Diagn*. 2012;32:97-98.

287. Winer N, Salomon LJ, Essaoui M, Nasr B, Bernard JP, Ville Y. Pseudoamniotic band syndrome: a rare complication of monochorionic twins with fetofetal transfusion syndrome treated by laser coagulation. *Am J Obstet Gynecol*. 2008;198:393.e1-393.e5.

288. Rodrigues A, Araujo C, Carvalho R, Melo MA, Pinto L, da Graca LM. Limb constriction secondary to pseudoamniotic band syndrome after selective fetoscopic laser surgery: report of a case with a favorable outcome. *Fetal Diagn Ther*. 2012;32:288-291.

289. Heifetz SA. Strangulation of the umbilical cord by amniotic bands: report of 6 cases and literature review. *Pediatr Pathol*. 1984;2:285-304.

290. Proffitt E, Phillips M, DeMauro C, Conde K, Powell J. Ultrasonographic diagnosis of intrauterine fetal decapitation secondary to amniotic band sequence: a case report. *J Emerg Med*. 2016;50:e129-e131.

291. Niu Z, Meng H, Zhang X, Ouyang Y, Zhang Y, Wu X. Two case reports: early detection of amniotic band syndrome by adhesion between hand and umbilical cord at 11 to 14 weeks' gestation. *Medicine (Baltimore)*. 2019;98:e18302.

292. Burton DJ, Filly RA. Sonographic diagnosis of the amniotic band syndrome. *AJR Am J Roentgenol*. 1991;156:555-558.

293. Jensen KK, Oh KY, Kennedy AM, Sohaey R. Intrauterine linear echogenicities in the gravid uterus: what radiologists should know. *Radiographics*. 2018;38:642-657.

294. Neuman J, Calvo-Garcia MA, Kline-Fath BM, et al. Prenatal imaging of amniotic band sequence: utility and role of fetal MRI as an adjunct to prenatal US. *Pediatr Radiol*. 2012;42:544-551.

295. Abdel-Sattar M, Chon A, Chen B, Burkhalter W, Chmait RH. Salvage of necrotic-appearing limb after in utero endoscopic lysis of constriction bands. *AJP Rep*. 2017;7:e74-e78.

296. Derderian SC, Iqbal CW, Goldstein R, Lee H, Hirose S. Fetoscopic approach to amniotic band syndrome. *J Pediatr Surg*. 2014;49:359-362.

297. Hata T, Tanaka H, Noguchi J. 3D/4D sonographic evaluation of amniotic band syndrome in early pregnancy: a supplement to 2D ultrasound. *J Obstet Gynaecol Res*. 2011;37:656-660.

298. Javadian P, Shamshirsaz AA, Haeri S, et al. Perinatal outcome after fetoscopic release of amniotic bands: a single-center experience and review of the literature. *Ultrasound Obstet Gynecol*. 2013;42:449-455.

299. Quintero RA, Morales WJ, Phillips J, Kalter CS, Angel JL. In utero lysis of amniotic bands. *Ultrasound Obstet Gynecol*. 1997;10:316-320.

305. Husler MR, Wilson RD, Horii SC, Bebbington MW, Adzick NS, Johnson MP. When is fetoscopic release of amniotic bands indicated? Review of outcome of cases treated in utero and selection criteria for fetal surgery. *Prenat Diagn*. 2009;29:457-463.

306. Gueneuc A, Chalouhi GE, Borali D, Mediouni I, Stirnemann J, Ville Y. Fetoscopic release of amniotic bands causing limb constriction: case series and review of the literature. *Fetal Diagn Ther*. 2019;46:246-256.

307. Assaf R, Llanes A, Chmait R. In utero release of constriction amniotic bands via blunt dissection. *Fetal Pediatr Pathol*. 2012;31:25-29.

310. Oakeshott P, Hunt GM. Long-term outcome in open spina bifida. *Br J Gen Pract*. 2003;53(493):632-636.

311. Oakeshott P, Hunt GM, Poulton A, Reid F. Open spina bifida: birth findings predict long-term outcome. *Arch Dis Child*. 2012;97(5):474-476.

312. Stevenson KL. Chiari Type II malformation: past, present, and future. *Neurosurg Focus*. 2004;16(2):E5.

313. Chakraborty A, Crimmins D, Hayward R, Thompson D. Toward reducing shunt placement rates in patients with myelomeningocele. *J Neurosurg Pediatr*. 2008;1(5):361-365.

332. Sanz Cortes MS, Torres P, Yepez M, et al. Comparison of brain microstructure after prenatal spina bifida repair by either laparotomy assisted fetoscopic or open approach. *Ultrasound Obstet Gynecol*. 2020;55:87-95.

333. Sanz Cortes MS, Lapa DA, Acacio G, et al. Proceedings of the First Annual Meeting of the International Fetoscopic Myelomeningocele Repair Consortium. *Ultrasound Obstet Gynecol*. 2019;53:855-863.

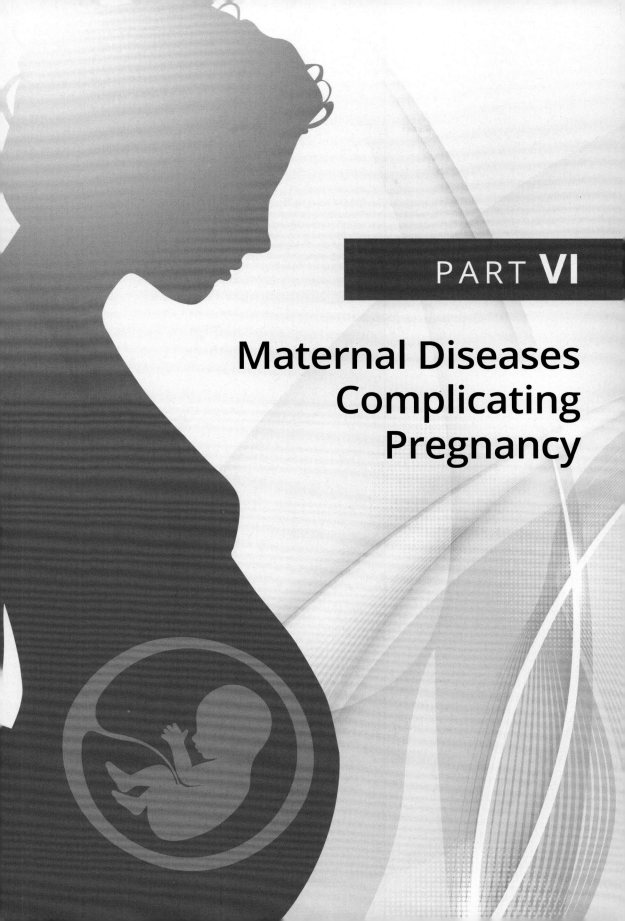

PART **VI**

Maternal Diseases Complicating Pregnancy

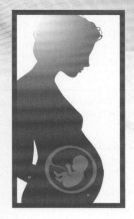

CHAPTER 25

Critical Care Obstetrics

Luis D. Pacheco, Antonio F. Saad, and
Mohamed Ibrahim

Shock is a condition in which circulation fails to meet the nutritional needs of the cell and remove metabolic wastes.[1] Shock may be further divided into four types: hypovolemic, distributive, cardiogenic, and obstructive. **Table 25.1** summarizes the characteristics of the most common forms of shock.

Hypovolemic shock, the most common form seen in obstetrics, is due to excessive blood loss. When the circulating blood volume is less than the capacity of its vascular bed, hypotension with diminished tissue perfusion results, leading to cellular hypoxia, acidosis, and cell death.[2] Depending on the duration and severity of the insult, irreversible organ damage or even death may occur.

Initial General Management of Shock in Pregnancy

Algorithm 25.1 summarizes the initial basic management of patients in shock. Several important initial steps should be performed when the diagnosis of shock is made in the obstetric patient. First, two large-bore intravenous (IV) lines, preferably 16-gauge, are placed for rapid expansion of intravascular volume.

An indwelling bladder catheter is placed for hourly determination of urine output. An arterial line allows continuous measurement of systemic blood pressure, as well as easy access for laboratory investigations. Oxygen may be administered via a face mask at 8 to 10 L/min, and the inspired oxygen concentration adjusted according to arterial blood gas results. Inability to protect the airway, poor arterial oxygenation, and airway obstruction may require early endotracheal intubation and mechanical ventilation. In viable pregnancies, electronic

See the eBook for expanded content, a complete reference list, and additional tables.

fetal monitoring and ultrasound examination are recommended. Importantly, during the initial phase of shock resuscitation, maternal care should not be interrupted or delayed due to fetal concerns.

Screening

Initial laboratory investigation usually includes blood type and cross-match, complete blood count, platelets, fibrinogen, electrolytes, blood urea nitrogen, creatinine, and arterial blood gas. Urine should be sent for analysis and microscopic evaluation as indicated. In cases of suspected sepsis, early cultures (blood, urine, respiratory, genital tract) and serum lactate levels should be obtained without delay.[4]

Nonpharmacologic Treatment

Volume Replacement Therapy

Volume replacement is commonly the first intervention in the management of hypovolemic and distributive shock. Fluids may be divided into colloids and crystalloids.

The three most commonly used crystalloids are normal saline, Lactated Ringer's, and PlasmaLyte.

We recommend the use of balanced crystalloids as opposed to normal saline for shock resuscitation. Current guidelines recommend 30 mL/kg of crystalloids in cases of suspected septic shock.[7]

Overzealous fluid resuscitation should be avoided since there is a linear correlation between positive fluid balance and mortality among critically ill patients.[8] The use of passive measurements of preload, such as central venous pressure and pulmonary artery occlusion pressure, to guide fluid resuscitation is discouraged because they do not predict fluid responsiveness.[9] We recommend that fluid therapy in shock resuscitation be guided by dynamic measures of preload such as pulse pressure variation (PPV) and/or passive leg raising (PLR).

Table 25.1 Clinical Characteristics of Shock

Hemorrhagic	Most common cause of shock in obstetrics. Decreased preload results in decreased cardiac output and compensatory increase in systemic vascular resistances. Transthoracic echocardiography reveals a hyperdynamic "empty" left ventricle.
Distributive	Characterized by peripheral vasodilation with low systemic vascular resistances. The decreased afterload commonly results in an increased cardiac output. Sepsis and anaphylaxis are typical forms of distributive shock.
Obstructive	Shock secondary to acute obstruction of blood flow with decreased preload to the heart. Commonly seen with massive pulmonary embolism, cardiac tamponade, and tension pneumothorax.
Cardiogenic	"Pump" failure resulting in decreased heart contractility as seen in acute systolic dysfunction from peripartum cardiomyopathy or myocardial, myocardial infarction, or viral myocarditis.

PPV is a dynamic measure of volume responsiveness. PPV only predicts fluid responsiveness in patients on mechanical ventilation not triggering the ventilator and on sinus rhythm. Briefly, during inspiration, when the ventilator delivers a preset tidal volume, the intrathoracic pressure increases with a concomitant decrease in preload. The opposite occurs during expiration. This variability in preload will result in different amounts of preload to the left ventricle, with resultant variability in stroke volume (and consequently in pulse pressure) only among individuals who are in fact fluid responsive (stroke volume increases with increased preload and vice versa).

During PLR, the clinician raises the patient's legs to 30° to 45° for 2 to 3 minutes. This maneuver results in an acute increase in preload to the heart of 300 mL. If the patient is volume responsive, an increase in stroke volume will be present. The latter may be documented with the concomitant use of a noninvasive cardiac output monitor.[11] If baseline cardiac output increases after performing the PLR maneuver, the patient is considered fluid responsive, and fluid should be administered. During late pregnancy, the uterus may compress the inferior vena cava (IVC). A small fluid bolus (250-500 mL) may be administered through an IV access in an upper extremity. If the cardiac output increases, then the patient will respond to further fluid.

The use of sodium bicarbonate is not recommended. Although bicarbonate by itself does not cross the placenta, its administration in a pregnant patient may result in fetal respiratory acidosis because it increases CO_2 levels, which can diffuse transplacentally toward the fetus after buffering hydrogen ions.

Blood Component Therapy

Hypovolemic shock frequently requires blood product transfusion. Resuscitation based on crystalloids and packed red cells is strongly discouraged as it results in dilutional coagulopathy and increased mortality. Many massive transfusion protocols now incorporate the concept of hemostatic resuscitation, in which similar ratios of packed red cells, fresh frozen plasma, and platelets are given regardless of laboratory values.

Transfusion of multiple blood products may result in transfusion-related acute lung injury (TRALI). The management of TRALI is supportive care with mechanical ventilation when indicated.[15]

Packed red blood cells (PRBCs) are administered to increase oxygen-carrying capacity to the tissues. Each unit of PRBCs (volume of 200-250 mL) will increase the hemoglobin by 1 g/dL and the hematocrit by 3%. Each unit of fresh frozen plasma (FFP; 200-250 mL) contains all clotting factors. On average, each unit contains 500 mg of fibrinogen and will raise the serum fibrinogen by 10 mg/dL. Ideally, FFP should be ABO compatible, although it does not require cross-matching. If no ABO compatible units are available, the "universal donor type" of FFP is AB because there are no naturally occurring anti-A or anti-B antibodies in these donors. However, due to the rarity of the AB blood type, the use of type A FFP is a safe alternative. In the actively bleeding patient, the platelet count should ideally be maintained above 50,000/mm^3. Each unit of platelets (20-40 mL) will increase the platelet count by 5000 to 10,000/mm^3. Commonly, platelets are administered as "six-packs"; each six-pack will consequently increase the platelet count by 30,000 to 60,000/mm^3.

In the setting of severe obstetrical hemorrhage, we recommend early administration of FFP together with PRBCs and platelets to avoid dilutional coagulopathy.[16]

Patient with suspected shock of unknown etiology

- Perform focused physical exam and history
- Oxygen administration and secure airway if indicated
- Obtain peripheral venous access (consider intraosseous if unable to obtain)
- Administer 1-2 L of crystalloid if suspect distributive or hypovolemic shock
- Send laboratory exams as indicated (cultures, serum lactate, complete blood count, liver/kidney function, electrolytes, coagulation studies)
- Bedside transthoracic echocardiography
- If viable, consider electronic fetal monitoring

Obstructive:
- If cardiac tamponade, immediate pericardial drainage indicated
- If tension pneumothorax, immediate needle decompression indicated
- If pulmonary embolism, start systemic thrombolysis with tissue plasminogen activated (t-PA)

Hemorrhagic:
- Early control of bleeding sources (surgically or with radiologic embolization when indicated)
- Avoid massive replacement of crystalloid and or colloid
- Consider 1:1:1 replacement of packed red cells, fresh frozen plasma, and platelets in setting of massive hemorrhage
- Maintain fibrinogen above 150-200 mg/dL with administration of cryoprecipitate
- Tranexamic acid in postpartum hemorrhage or trauma within 3 hours of onset

Distributive (septic):
- Start early broad-spectrum antibiotics
- Perform early source control as indicated (eg, drain collections, appendectomy, soft tissue debridement)
- Guide fluid resuscitation based on dynamic measures of preload, such as pulse pressure variation or passive leg raising
- If no fluid responsive and mean arterial blood pressure below 65 mm Hg, start norepinephrine through central line*

Distributive (anaphylactic):
- Secure airway as indicated
- Epinephrine
- Fluid resuscitation
- Albuterol for bronchospasm/racemic epinephrine for upper airway edema
- Adjunctive treatments include antihistamine agents (H1 and H2) and steroids

Cardiogenic:
- Noninvasive or invasive mechanical ventilation may be needed depending on severity of pulmonary edema
- Avoid excessive fluids
- Furosemide to decrease preload
- If hypertensive, vasodilators indicated (eg, hydralazine, nicardipine) to decrease afterload
- Maintain blood pressure with use of norepinephrine and inotropic support if needed (dobutamine or milrinone)
- Severe cases may need mechanical support with left ventricular assist devices or veno-arterial ECMO

*Pregnant women in the midtrimester may have lower blood pressures due to physiological vasodilation. Initiation of norepinephrine may not be required arbitrarily to keep mean arterial blood pressure above the threshold of 65 mm Hg, as long as there is no evidence of hypoperfusion (normal mentation, normal urine output, normal distal extremities, adequate capillary refill, normal lactate). ECMO, extracorporeal membrane oxygenation.

Algorithm 25.1 Initial management of pregnant patients with most common forms of shock.

In addition, although most massive transfusion protocols do not include cryoprecipitate, during obstetrical hemorrhage we recommend that early administration of cryoprecipitate be strongly considered as early severe fibrinogen consumption is common.

Recently, the use of fibrinogen concentrates has been used to raise serum fibrinogen in actively bleeding patients. It is currently recommended that serum fibrinogen be maintained above 150 to 200 mg/dL with the use of cryoprecipitate or fibrinogen concentrates.[17] Cryoprecipitate contains fibronectin and factors I, VIII, von Willebrand, and XIII. Each unit is approximately 20 to 40 mL and contains 150 to 350 mg of fibrinogen. One unit will raise serum fibrinogen by 10 mg/dL and is effective without the need to administer large amounts of volume.

Vasopressor and Inotrope Therapy

Vasopressors are mainly used in the setting of distributive shock.

Norepinephrine is the vasopressor of choice in most clinical situations, including septic shock complicating pregnancy.[4] It should be administered through a central line to avoid extravasation. The usual starting dose is 0.05 µg/kg/min, which is then titrated until the patient reaches a desired MAP (usually above 65 mm Hg).

Phenylephrine increases blood pressure mainly by increasing SVR. The usual starting dose is 0.5 µg/kg/min. Phenylephrine may result in decreases in cardiac output as it does not provide any inotropic support, and low cardiac output may be worsened by an isolated increase in afterload. Bradycardia is a common side effect.

Vasopressin is a stress hormone secreted by the posterior pituitary. In the setting of sepsis, vasopressin is a second-line pressor with a recommended dose of 0.03 U/min. Importantly, the dose is fixed and should not be titrated as higher doses may result in ischemia to different organs, including the heart, kidneys, bowel, and skin. The use of vasopressin in pregnancy is not recommended as it may activate oxytocin receptors, resulting in uterine contractions.

Pure inotropes (dobutamine, milrinone) act mainly by increasing cardiac output. Dobutamine is indicated when increases in cardiac output are required. The starting dose is 2.5 µg/kg/min and may be titrated to the desired effect (improved cardiac output as evidenced by improved blood pressure, urine output, resolution of hyperlactatemia, and improved mental status). The most common side effects are tachycardia and hypotension. Milrinone, another pure inotrope, inhibits cellular processes, which, in turn, allow calcium to enter the myocardial cells. The starting dose is 0.125 µg/kg/min. Main side effects are similar to those of dobutamine: hypotension and tachycardia.

Epinephrine is both a powerful vasoconstrictor and inotrope. The usual starting dose is 0.03 µg/kg/min. Common side effects from epinephrine include a higher rate of tachyarrhythmias (as compared to norepinephrine and vasopressin) and mild elevations in lactate.

Hemodynamic Monitoring

The use of transthoracic echocardiography by noncardiologist physicians has dramatically changed the management of patients with shock.[23]

Hemorrhagic (Hypovolemic) Shock

Hemorrhagic shock is the most common form of shock in obstetrics. Most cases occur secondary to postpartum hemorrhage due to uterine atony and abnormal placentation.

Management of Hemorrhagic Shock in Pregnancy

Medical and surgical treatments usually involve administration of uterotonics; repair of genital lacerations as indicated; and a variety of surgical procedures, including uterine artery ligation, B-Lynch stitches, placement of intrauterine balloons, and hysterectomy. From a critical care point of view, the most important intervention is to maintain hemodynamic stability until the bleeding is controlled (usually surgically).

Nonpharmacologic and Pharmacologic Treatments

Early administration of blood products (PRBCs at a ratio of 1:1:1 with platelets and FFP) results in improved outcomes.[14] Certain adjuvant pharmacological products may be used in the management of severe hemorrhage.

Where available, fibrinogen concentrates may be used to maintain the serum fibrinogen above 150 to 200 mg/dL in the actively bleeding patient.

Among patients with postpartum hemorrhage, the antifibrinolytic agent tranexamic acid within 3 hours of birth is currently recommended to treat established postpartum hemorrhage that is unresponsive to first-line measures such as uterotonics.

Distributive Shock

Anaphylactic Shock

Anaphylaxis is a series of events that occur in a sensitized individual on subsequent exposure to a specific antigen.

Clinical Assessment and Management of Anaphylactic Shock in Pregnancy

Early recognition and management of anaphylactic reactions is essential. Risk factors, including a prior history of anaphylaxis, should be noted carefully at admission. Anaphylaxis usually presents with acute onset of urticaria, hypotension, bronchospasm, angioedema, and cardiovascular collapse. Acute management of anaphylaxis in the obstetrical patient should not differ from that in the nonpregnant patient.

Pharmacologic Treatment

Epinephrine is the cornerstone of treatment; 0.3 to 0.5 mg (0.3-0.5 mL of a 1:1000 [1 mg/mL] solution) of intramuscular epinephrine should be administered as soon as possible (usually apply in the mid-lateral thigh).

Adjuvant therapies include the use of antihistamines (50 mg IV diphenhydramine or 20 mg IV famotidine) and steroids (eg, 125 mg IV methylprednisolone or 100 mg IV hydrocortisone). However, use of these adjunctive interventions should never delay the administration of epinephrine.[31]

Nonpharmacologic Treatment

Delivery is rarely necessary because the fetal condition usually improves with maternal stabilization.

Septic Shock

The incidence of septic shock among maternal critical care admissions has been reported to be around 10%.[40] In addition, the maternal fatality rate from severe sepsis or septic shock has been reported to be lower in pregnant women compared to nonpregnant individuals (9.6% vs 16.8%, respectively).[41]

Clinical Assessment

The three most common sources of infection among pregnant and postpartum women requiring intensive care unit admission due to severe sepsis or septic shock are respiratory (39%), genital tract (24%), and urinary tract (9%).[40]

Management of Septic Shock in Pregnancy

Management should be individualized depending on gestational age and maternal and fetal conditions. A multidisciplinary approach is critical for the management of the obstetric patient with septic shock and should involve maternal-fetal, critical care, anesthesia, and neonatology specialists. In 2019, the Society of Maternal-Fetal Medicine updated guidelines regarding the management of sepsis in the obstetrical population.[4] In this publication, the committee recommended that, as soon as sepsis is suspected in healthy woman with organ dysfunction, cultures (blood, urine, sputum) and serum lactate should be obtained, and empiric broad-spectrum antibiotics administered within 1 hour of diagnosis.[7] The next step of management should be dedicated to searching for a focus of infection through imaging. After identifying the focus of infection, the least invasive method to achieve source control is recommended, such as percutaneous drainage.[7] One exception is cases of necrotizing soft tissue infections that usually require extensive and repetitive debridement procedures to attain adequate source control.

Nonpharmacologic and Pharmacologic Treatment

Simultaneously with source control, initial interventions include fluid resuscitation with 1 to 2 L of crystalloid.[7] Due to concerns of pulmonary edema, third-spacing, cerebral edema, bowel edema, and higher mortality, aggressive fluid resuscitation should be avoided, emphasizing the importance of using dynamic rather than static measures of preload to guide fluid therapy.[51,52] Fluid responsiveness can be assessed by either PLR or PPV. The former is achieved by raising legs 30° to 45° for 2 to 3 minutes, leading to autotransfusion of ~300 mL of blood to the chest. Fluid responders will have an increase in stroke volume or cardiac output measured by noninvasive cardiac output monitors.[53] PLR is not reliable in the third trimester due to uterine aortocaval compression and should be replaced with a 250 to 500-mL small fluid bolus.[12] PPV consists of analyzing the arterial line wave form; if it varies by more than 13% with the respiratory cycle, the patient is considered fluid responsive. This technique requires patients to be in sinus rhythm, sedated, and receiving positive pressure mechanical ventilation.[54]

Another method to assess fluid responsiveness is by measuring the diameter of the IVC with respiration using bedside ultrasound. An IVC diameter <1.5 cm with significant variation with respiratory cycle indicates that the patient is a fluid responder.

Vasopressors should be administered in patients with suspected hypoperfusion or hypotension refractory to initial fluid resuscitation. Norepinephrine has been shown to be safe in pregnant women and should be considered as the first-line therapy to achieve a MAP ≥65 mm Hg with signs of hypoperfusion.[7,55]

For adrenergic refractory patients, hydrocortisone of 200 mg/day should be considered.[7] If cardiac dysfunction is present, an ionotropic agent, such as dobutamine, should be administered.[7] Indication for delivery should be based on obstetrical indications after maternal stabilization. Regardless of prior or concomitant steroid use, steroids for fetal lung maturity are not contraindicated.

Cardiogenic Shock

Clinical Presentation
Cardiogenic shock should be considered in patients with persistent hypotension (systolic blood pressure <90 mm Hg or MAP 30 mm Hg lower than baseline) with cardiac index <2.2 L/min/m² and adequate or elevated left-sided filling pressures.[59] In the obstetric population, possible etiologies of cardiogenic shock include myocardial infarction, viral myocarditis, arrhythmias, peripartum cardiomyopathy, pulmonary hypertension, and valvular heart disease.

Management of Cardiogenic Shock in Pregnancy
Overall management of cardiogenic shock should not differ from the nonpregnant population. Initial management should focus on maintenance of ventilation and oxygenation with the use of mechanical ventilation (invasive or noninvasive) as needed.

Nonpharmacologic and Pharmacologic Treatment
Blood pressure is usually raised with the use of vasopressors (norepinephrine) as fluid is commonly contraindicated in the setting of severe pulmonary edema. Cardiac output may be improved with the use of inotropes, such as milrinone or dobutamine. Pulmonary edema and peripheral organ congestion improve with the use of furosemide. If the etiology is ischemic, immediate coronary revascularization (either percutaneously or surgically) is mandatory. Mechanical assist devices are indicated in patients with refractory poor tissue perfusion with no improvement in hemodynamic parameters. Available devices include percutaneous ventricular assist devices (eg, Tandemheart, Impella), venoarterial extracorporeal membrane oxygenation (ECMO), and intra-aortic balloon counterpulsation pumps.

Acute Respiratory Distress Syndrome

Clinical Presentation
The acute respiratory distress syndrome (ARDS) is a form of noncardiogenic pulmonary edema that leads to hypoxic respiratory failure. ARDS may be classified by severity based on the ratio between the partial pressure of oxygen (Pao_2) and the inspired fraction of oxygen (Fio_2), known as the Pao_2/Fio_2 ratio. Mild ARDS has a Pao_2/Fio_2 ratio of 200 to 300, moderate ARDS has a ratio of 100 to 199, and severe cases have a ratio <100. Importantly, the ratio should be measured while receiving at least 5 cmH_2O of positive end expiratory pressure (PEEP).

ARDS occurs due to an inflammatory insult to the lung, resulting in endothelial injury and fluid/protein leakage into the alveolar space.

Management of ARDS in Pregnancy
The management of ARDS may be divided into ventilatory and nonventilatory. Ventilatory management includes the use of lung-protective mechanical ventilation with the use of low tidal volumes to avoid high injurious transpulmonary pressures.[63]

Similarly, during pregnancy, a higher plateau pressure up to 35 cmH_2O may be tolerated (due to increased abdominal pressures and chest wall/breast edema), allowing tidal volumes close to 8 mL/kg (ideal body weight). The latter two strategies will ameliorate CO_2 retention. During pregnancy, the normal partial pressure of CO_2 is 30 mm Hg. To avoid fetal acidosis from CO_2 retention, we recommend targeting a $Paco_2$ lower than 50 to 60 mm Hg, if possible. Together with low tidal volume ventilation, adequate PEEP should be used to recruit alveolar units.[64]

Nonpharmacologic and Pharmacologic Treatment

Prone ventilation has recently been proven beneficial in ARDS with a Pao_2/Fio_2 ratio below 150.[65] When applied, ventilation in the prone position should occur at least 16 hours every day.

The use of high-frequency oscillatory ventilation is not beneficial and not currently recommended.[66]

Nonventilatory treatment includes the use of a restrictive fluid management approach and neuromuscular paralysis for 48 hours with cisatracurium.[67,68]

The use of low-dose steroids as an attempt to decrease pulmonary inflammation in ARDS has been controversial. Steroids should not be used in ARDS secondary to influenza pneumonia as mortality is increased with their use.[70]

Severe refractory cases may require venous-venous ECMO as a rescue therapy.

Trauma

Clinical Presentation

An increased incidence of minor trauma has been observed as pregnancy progresses.[73] In most cases, injury is minimal and not associated with a significant increase in perinatal mortality.[74,75] Major trauma, however, may place the mother and infant at severe risk.

Physiological changes occurring in pregnancy may affect management of trauma victims. The circulatory changes in pregnancy are the most significant. Due to blood volume expansion, blood loss of up to 1 L may occur without any hemodynamic changes. The gravid uterus may decrease cardiac output (up to 30%) in the supine position, thus necessitating the left uterine displacement during management of the traumatic patient to facilitate adequate preload. The cephalic displacement of the diaphragm during the second half of pregnancy mandates placement of chest tubes at a higher than usual level, usually in the third or fourth intercostal spaces (as opposed to fourth or fifth spaces). Significant ventilatory changes include an elevated pH with a $Paco_2$ of 30 mm Hg and HCO_3 between 18 and 22 mEq/L (limited buffering capacity due to lower bicarbonate levels). A 20% decrease in the functional residual capacity, together with increased oxygen consumption, results in faster oxygen desaturation at the time of tracheal intubation and impacts airway management.

Management of Trauma in Pregnancy

Overall, trauma management during pregnancy should follow the same principles as in nonpregnant individuals. Most of the landmark studies in the topic while be quoted as we believe they provide invaluable information despite being published decades ago.

Initial resuscitation efforts should focus on maternal resuscitation, as the latter usually will improve fetal status. Resuscitation efforts should be based on a systematic approach based on the principles of advanced trauma life support (ATLS). The primary survey includes the "ABCDE approach": evaluation of **a**dequate airway protection, **b**reathing, **c**irculation, **d**isability, and **e**xposure.[76,77]

A quick focused neurological exam and exposure of the patient are pivotal. Absent chest movements and/or air entry on chest auscultation requires immediate intervention to open the airway (ie, chin lift, head tilt, jaw thrust maneuver; placement of an oropharyngeal airway). If cervical spine injury is suspected, excessive head tilt should be avoided; however, even in this situation, opening the airway takes precedence. Neck stabilization while maintaining an in-line neutral position of the neck protects against a possible spinal cord injury. Nasopharyngeal airways should be avoided if a base skull fracture is suspected (the latter may be suspected by the presence of periocular and/or retroauricular equimosis together with leakage of cerebrospinal fluid through the nose and/or ears). Airway management should be performed by the most skilled clinician as airway edema during pregnancy may limit visualization of the glottis.[78]

Rapid sequence induction (RSI) is recommended to facilitate tracheal intubation. RSI involves the administration of an induction agent (ie, propofol, ketamine, etomidate) followed immediately by a paralytic (ie, succinylcholine, rocuronium).

Once the airway is secured, proper oxygenation and ventilation are essential for the mother's and fetus' well-being. If adequate oxygenation cannot be achieved (usually together with an increased effort to deliver a tidal volume manually with a bag mask device), a tension pneumothorax should be suspected and treated accordingly with immediate needle decompression, followed by placement of a chest tube. As previously discussed, the thoracostomy tube needs to be placed one or two intercostal spaces above the normal fifth intercostal space to avoid risk of intra-abdominal injury.[79]

Once initial maternal stabilization is ensured, fetal care should be started. If the fetus is viable, continuous fetal electronic monitoring is recommended.[80] If stable, a bedside ultrasound targeting the placental location, amniotic fluid volume, presentation, number of fetuses, and estimated fetal weight may be performed.

Nonpharmacologic and Pharmacologic Treatment

Classically, it has been recommended that 2 L of crystalloid be administered to trauma victims who are hypotensive; however, this practice may result in worsening of coagulopathy, and many argue that this practice should be abandoned.[81] Instead, in nonpregnant patients with blunt or penetrating torso injuries (prior to definite surgical control), hypotensive resuscitation aiming at systolic blood pressures between 80 and 90 mm Hg, with the use of no fluid or only small boluses, is advocated in an attempt to avoid massive fluid resuscitation and resultant dilutional coagulopathy.[81]

There are no data on the safety of hypotensive resuscitation during pregnancy. We recommend that a systolic blood pressure >90 mm Hg be targeted in the pregnant trauma victim. If massive transfusion is initiated, as previously discussed, maintaining a 1:1:1 ratio of packed red cells, plasma, and platelets is recommended.

Similar to nonpregnant patients, a basic blood workup, including a complete blood count, coagulation profile, electrolytes, arterial blood gas, toxicology screen, urine analysis, and type and screen, is usually obtained. The Kleihauer-Betke (KB) elution test is used to detect fetal red blood cells in maternal blood.

In RH-negative women it is necessary to calculate the required dose of RhoGAM. Each vial of RhoGAM (300 μg) neutralizes 30 mL of fetal blood (15 mL of red cells). The number of vials needed may be calculated by the following formula:

$$\text{\# of vials required} = \frac{50 \times \% \text{ positive KB stain}}{30}.$$

If the result ends in a decimal ≥0.5, rounding to the higher number is recommended (eg, if the result of the equation is 3.54, round to 4 vials). One extra vial should always be added to the result of the prior equation.[82] The maximum number of vials that may be administered per day IM is 5. If a higher dose is indicated, IV administration may be required (ie, 600 μg every 8 hours until the total dose is completed).

Most trauma victims will require some form of body imaging. Clinicians should not refrain from ordering imaging studies as needed due to concerns of fetal exposure to ionizing radiation. If the study is indicated, it should be performed. If possible, abdominal shielding should be used.

Abdominal ultrasound is useful in detecting intra-abdominal fluid collections; the FAST (focused assessment sonography in trauma) scan includes a four-quadrant screen (pericardium, perihepatic, perisplenic, and pelvic) looking for free fluid (likely blood) following blunt trauma.

Blunt Trauma

Blunt trauma is more common than penetrating during pregnancy[83] and is often the result of automotive accidents and deployment of safety air bags and strain against 3-point restraint seatbelts. During motor vehicle accidents, the forward displacement of the uterus followed by counter movement can generate enough force to cause placental shearing and abruption. About 40% of patients following severe motor vehicle accidents may present with placental abruption.[84,85]

Simple falls are also a common cause of blunt trauma during pregnancy. Placental abruption may occur in 4% to 5% of cases, and direct abdominal trauma is not necessary for abruption to develop. In viable pregnancies, a 4-hour period of fetal monitoring usually suffices, as long as there is no evidence of placental abruption (ie, vaginal bleeding, abdominal pain, contractions more often than 1 every 10 minutes). If the latter develops, longer periods of observation are usually indicated (24 hours of continuous fetal monitoring).

Uterine rupture is an infrequent complication of blunt traumatic injury during pregnancy. The incidence increases with advancing gestation and severity of force. Most traumatic uterine ruptures involve the uterine fundus or the posterior aspect of the uterus.[86] Patients with a history of cesarean delivery may be at increased risk.

Penetrating Trauma

Similar to nonpregnant patients, stab wounds and gunshots are the most common types of penetrating traumas. The cephalic displacement of intra-abdominal organs by the gravid uterus decreases the incidence of maternal visceral injury but results in a high rate of direct fetal injuries with a high rate of fetal mortality.[87,88]

The traditional management of gunshot wounds to the abdomen has included exploratory laparotomy to determine the extent of visceral injury. Patients in whom the projectile or object enters anteriorly and below the level of the uterine fundus often do not have maternal visceral involvement and may be considered for expectant management if otherwise stable.[89] However, most recommend abdominal exploration for all extrauterine intra-abdominal gunshot wounds and most intrauterine wounds.

Abdominal stab wounds require surgical repair in approximately one-half of reported cases.[90] Small bowel involvement is more frequent with upper abdominal stab wounds in pregnancy due to upper displacement of the small bowel by the gravid uterus.[89,91] Because of the propensity of small intestinal injury and the potentially lethal effect of diaphragmatic rupture with herniation of intra-abdominal organs, exploration of upper abdominal stab wounds during pregnancy is recommended. As with gunshot wounds, if the wound is confined to the lower abdomen, the uterus usually sustains most injuries, whereas other viscera are spared. The use of bedside ultrasound (FAST) may aid in the decision to proceed with an exploratory laparotomy.

If direct uterine injury is encountered during exploration, the extent of the injury will determine the surgical intervention, ranging from observation to hysterectomy. Cesarean delivery is indicated for fetal distress at a viable gestational age. Exploratory laparotomy is not a reason to perform a cesarean delivery if another indication does not exist.

Cardiopulmonary Resuscitation

Cardiac arrest during pregnancy should be managed with the use of conventional cardiopulmonary resuscitation (CPR). **Algorithm 25.2** summarizes the basic steps of CPR during pregnancy.

Similar to nonpregnant individuals, the hands should be placed on the lower half of the sternum.

A defibrillator should be used as soon as possible if the patient shows a shockable rhythm (pulseless ventricular tachycardia or ventricular fibrillation). Defibrillation is not harmful for the fetus and can be safely used in any trimester. Together with defibrillation and CPR, patients with these two rhythms may require epinephrine (IV or IO) and amiodarone.

If the initial rhythm is nonshockable (asystole or pulseless electrical activity), then CPR along with epinephrine are the mainstay of treatment. If the pregnancy is estimated to be 20 weeks or further (fundal height above the umbilicus), then manual left lateral displacement of the uterus by an assistant is fundamental to prevent compression of the IVC and the aorta.

It is of paramount importance that during the arrest, clinicians think about potential reversible causes to the arrest (ie, hypovolemia, hypoxia, acidosis, hypothermia, hyperkalemia, tension pneumothorax, tamponade, and thrombosis: either myocardial infarction or pulmonary embolism).

Electronic Fetal Heart Rate Monitoring During Maternal Resuscitation

During the development of shock in the pregnant patient, redistribution of maternal cardiac output to vital organs, such as the brain and heart, may occur at the expense of the uteroplacental fetal unit. In most cases, delivery is not indicated in the underresuscitated patient; on the contrary, adequate hemodynamic resuscitation with the use of fluids, blood products, vasopressors, or inotropes as indicated usually improves the fetal status.

The appropriate duration of electronic fetal monitoring after trauma is unclear. It is commonly suggested that a period of continuous fetal monitoring is prudent in most cases of trauma during pregnancy of more than 23 to 24 weeks' gestation.[95] In cases of hemodynamic instability, the maternal condition should be stabilized before delivery is considered for persistent evidence of fetal distress. The fetus may recover as maternal hypoxia, acidosis, and hypotension are corrected. Serial evaluations of fetal status and *in utero* resuscitation are generally preferable to the emergency delivery of a depressed infant from a hemodynamically unstable mother.

Maternal cardiac arrest

- Start immediate high-quality CPR at a 30:2 ratio if no advanced airway in place.
- If airway in place, provide 100-120 chest compressions/minute together with one ventilation every 6 seconds.
- If > 20 weeks, manually displace uterus leftward.
- Avoid hyperventilation.
- Provide CPR as uninterrupted cycles of 2 minutes.
- After each cycle, a pause shorter than 10 seconds is used to analyze the baseline rhythm and to check for a carotid pulse.

Place defibrillator pads as soon as available and analyze initial rhythm during the following pulse check pause

Shockable rhythm (ventricular fibrillation or pulseless ventricular tachycardia):

- Early defibrillation and repeat as needed every 2 minutes of CPR (if > 20 weeks, prepare for perimortem cesarean delivery)
- If persistent after two shocks, start IV/IO epinephrine 1 mg every 3-5 minutes
- If persistent after three shocks, administer amiodarone 300 mg IV/IO

Nonshockable rhythm (asystole or pulseless electrical activity):

- Continue CPR with pulse checks every 2 minutes (if > 20 weeks, prepare for perimortem cesarean delivery)
- Administer epinephrine 1 mg IV/IO every 3-5 minutes

In all cases, consider potentially reversible causes, such as hypovolemia, hypoxemia, acidosis, hypothermia, hyper/hypokalemia, tension pneumothorax, cardiac tamponade, myocardial infarction, or pulmonary embolism.

CPR, cardiopulmonary resuscitation; IV, intravenous; IO, intraosseous.

Algorithm 25.2 Initial cardiopulmonary resuscitation during pregnancy.

KEY POINTS

- The use of targeted ultrasound in the early management of shock is recommended to guide initial treatment decisions.
- Fluid resuscitation should be started with the use of balanced crystalloids as opposed to normal saline or colloids.
- Fluid responsiveness should be assessed with dynamic measures of preload as opposed to static measures.
- In the setting of massive hemorrhage, early hemostatic resuscitation and activation

of massive transfusion protocols is recommended.
- For distributive shock during pregnancy, norepinephrine is the vasopressor of choice.
- In patients with ARDS, lung protective mechanical ventilation and a conservative fluid strategy result in improved outcomes.
- Overall, in pregnant women with trauma and in cardiac arrest, similar guidelines applied to nonpregnant individuals should be followed.

REFERENCES

(only references cited in synoptic print chapter; for a complete reference list, see ebook)

1. Holcroft JW, Blaisdell FW. Shock: causes and management of circulatory collapse. In: Sabiston DC, ed. *Textbook of Surgery*. 13th ed. W.B. Saunders; 1986:38.
2. Cavanagh D, Knuppel RA, Shepherd JH, Anderson R, Rao PS. Septic shock and the obstetrician/gynecologist. *South Med J*. 1982;75(7):809-813.
3. Plante LA, Pacheco LD, Louis JM. SMFM Consult Series #47: sepsis during pregnancy and the puerperium. *Am J Obstet Gynecol*. 2019;220:B2-B10.
7. Rhodes A, Evans LE, Alhazzani W, et al. Surviving Sepsis Campaign. International guidelines for management of sepsis and septic shock: 2016. *Intensive Care Med*. 2017;43(3):304-377.
8. Sadaka F, Juarez M, Naydenov S, O'Brien J. Fluid resuscitation in septic shock: the effect of increasing fluid balance on mortality. *J Intensive Care Med*. 2014;29(4):213-217.
9. Marik PE, Baram M, Vahid B. Does central venous pressure predict fluid responsiveness? A systematic review of the literature and the tale of seven mares. *Chest*. 2008;134(1):172-178.
11. Gidwani H, Gomez H. The crashing patient: hemodynamic collapse. *Curr Opin Crit Care*. 2017;23(6):533-540.
12. Marques NR, Martinello C, Kramer GC, et al. Passive leg raising during pregnancy. *Am J Perinatol*. 2015;32(4):393-398.
14. Holcomb JB, Tilley BC, Baraniuk S, et al. Transfusion of plasma, platelets, and red blood cells in a 1:1:1 vs a 1:1:2 ratio and mortality in patients with severe trauma: the PROPPR randomized clinical trial. *J Am Med Assoc*. 2015;313(5):471-482.
15. Looney MR, Gropper MA, Matthay MA. Transfusion-related acute lung injury: a review. *Chest*. 2004;126(1):249-258.
16. Pacheco LD, Saade GR, Costantine MM, Clark SL, Hankins GDV. The role of massive transfusion protocols in obstetrics. *Am J Perinatol*. 2013;30(1):1-4.
17. Pacheco LD, Saade GR, Hankins GDV. Medical management of postpartum hemorrhage: an update. *Semin Perinatol*. 2019;43(1):22-26.
23. Orme RM, Oram MP, McKinstry CE. Impact of echocardiography on patient management in the intensive care unit: an audit of district general hospital practice. *Br J Anaesth*. 2009;102(3):340-344.
31. Muraro A, Roberts G, Worm M, et al; EAACI Food Allergy and Anaphylaxis Guidelines Group. Anaphylaxis: guidelines from the European academy of allergy and clinical immunology. *Allergy*. 2014;69(8):1026-1045.
40. Acosta CD, Harrison DA, Rowan K, Lucas DN, Kurinczuk JJ, Knight M. Maternal morbidity and mortality from severe sepsis: a national cohort study. *BMJ Open*. 2016;6(8):e012323.
41. Kidson KM, Henderson WR, Hutcheon JA. Case fatality and adverse outcomes are reduced in pregnant women with severe sepsis or septic shock compared with age-matched comorbid-matched nonpregnant women. *Crit Care Med*. 2018;46(11):1775-1782.
51. Marik P, Bellomo R. A rational approach to fluid therapy in sepsis. *Br J Anaesth*. 2016;116(3):339-349.
52. Osman D, Ridel C, Ray P, et al. Cardiac filling pressures are not appropriate to predict hemodynamic response to volume challenge. *Crit Care Med*. 2007;35(1):64-68.
53. Monnet X, Marik P, Teboul JL. Passive leg raising for predicting fluid responsiveness: a systematic review and meta-analysis. *Intensive Care Med*. 2016;42(12):1935-1947.
54. Enomoto TM, Harder L. Dynamic indices of preload. *Crit Care Clin*. 2010;26(2):307-321, table of contents.
55. Ngan Kee WD, Lee SW, Ng FF, et al. Randomized double-blinded comparison of norepinephrine and phenylephrine for maintenance of blood pressure during spinal anesthesia for cesarean delivery. *Anesthesiology*. 2015;122(4):736-745.
59. Reynolds HR, Hochman JS. Cardiogenic shock: current concepts and improving outcomes. *Circulation*. 2008;117(5):686-697.
63. Brower RG, Matthay MA, Morris A, et al. Ventilation with lower tidal volumes as compared with traditional tidal volumes for acute lung injury and the acute respiratory distress syndrome. *N Engl J Med*. 2000;342(18):1301-1308.
64. Phoenix SI, Paravastu S, Columb M, et al. Does a higher positive end expiratory pressure decrease mortality in acute respiratory distress syndrome? A systematic review and meta-analysis. *Anesthesiology*. 2009;110(5):1098-1105.
65. Guerin C, Reignier J, Richard JC, et al. Prone positioning in severe acute respiratory distress syndrome. *N Engl J Med*. 2013;368(23):2159-2168.
66. Frat JP, Thille AW, Mercat A, et al. High-flow oxygen through nasal cannula in acute hypoxemic respiratory failure. *N Engl J Med*. 2015;372(23):2185-2196.
67. Wiedemann HP, Wheeler AP, Bernard GR, et al. Comparison of two fluid-management strategies in acute lung injury. *N Engl J Med*. 2006;354(24):2564-2575.
68. Papazian L, Forel JM, Gacouin A, et al. Neuromuscular blockers in early acute respiratory distress syndrome. *N Engl J Med*. 2010;363(12):1107-1116.
70. Brun-Buisson C, Richard JC, Mercat A, et al. Early corticosteroids in severe influenza A/H1N1 pneumonia and acute respiratory distress syndrome. *Am J Respir Crit Care Med*. 2011;183(9):1200-1206.
73. Fort AT, Harlin RS. Pregnancy outcome after noncatastrophic maternal trauma during pregnancy. *Obstet Gynecol*. 1970;35(6):912-915.
74. Plauche WC, Von Almen W, Muller R. Catastrophic uterine rupture. *Obstet Gynecol*. 1984;64(6):792-797.
75. Rothenberger DA, Quattlebaum FW, Zabel J, et al. Diagnostic peritoneal lavage for blunt trauma in pregnant women. *Am J Obstet Gynecol*. 1977;129(5):479-481.
76. Mohammad A, Branicki F, Abu-Zidan FM. Educational and clinical impact of Advanced Trauma Life Support (ATLS) courses: a systematic review. *World J Surg*. 2014;38(2):322-329.
77. American College of Surgeons. *Advanced Trauma Life Support*. 7th ed. First Impressions; 2004.
78. Kuhlmann RS, Cruikshank DP. Maternal trauma during pregnancy. *Clin Obstet Gynecol*. 1994;37(2):274-293.
79. Brown HL. Trauma in pregnancy. *Obstet Gynecol*. 2009;114(1):147-160.
80. Dahmus MA, Sibai BM. Blunt abdominal trauma: are there any predictive factors for abruptio placentae or maternal-fetal distress? *Am J Obstet Gynecol*. 1993;169(4):1054-1059.
81. King DR. Initial care of the severely injured patient. *N Engl J Med*. 2019;380(8):763-770.
82. Moise KJ Jr, Argoti PS. Management and prevention of red cell alloimmunization in pregnancy: a systematic review. *Obstet Gynecol*. 2012;120(5):1132-1139.
83. Petrone P, Jimenez-Morillas P, Axelrad A, Marini CP. Traumatic injuries to the pregnant patient: a critical literature review. *Eur J Trauma Emerg Surg*. 2019;45:383-392. doi:10.1007/s00068-017-0839-x
84. Metz TD, Abbott JT. Uterine trauma in pregnancy after motor vehicle crashes with airbag deployment: a 30-case series. *J Trauma*. 2006;61(3):658-661.
85. Pearlman MD, Viano D. Automobile crash simulation with the first pregnant crash test dummy. *Am J Obstet Gynecol*. 1996;175(4 pt 1):977-981.
86. Maull KI. Maternal-fetal trauma. *Semin Pediatr Surg*. 2001;10(1):32-34.
87. Sakala EP, Kort DD. Management of stab wounds to the pregnant uterus: a case report and a review of the literature. *Obstet Gynecol Surv*. 1988;43(6):319-324.
88. Sandy EA II, Koerner M. Self-inflicted gunshot wound to the pregnant abdomen: report of a case and review of the literature. *Am J Perinatol*. 1989;6(1):30-31.
89. Stone IK. Trauma in the obstetric patient. *Obstet Gynecol Clin North Am*. 1999;26(3):459-467, viii.
90. Buchsbaum HJ. Penetrating injury of the abdomen. In: Buchsbaum HJ, ed. *Trauma in Pregnancy*. W.B. Saunders; 1979:82.
91. Cunningham FG, Gant NF, Leveno KJ, et al. *Maternal adaptations to pregnancy*. In: *Williams Obstetrics*. 21st ed. Appleton and Lange; 2001:167.
95. Mendez-Figueroa H, Dahlke JD, Vrees RA, et al. Trauma in pregnancy: an updated systematic review. *Am J Obstet Gynecol*. 2013;209(1):1-10.

CHAPTER 26

Anesthesia in the Normal and High-Risk Patient

Bhavani Shankar Kodali and
Andrew M. Malinow

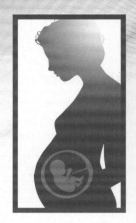

Introduction
(**Figure 26.1**)

Anesthesia for Labor and Delivery in a Patient With a Routine Pregnancy

The most effective labor analgesia is provided by neuraxial spinal, continuous labor epidural (CLE), combined spinal epidural (CSE), or continuous spinal anesthesia (CSA) injection.

(**Figure 26.2A-C**)

With all but single-injection spinal analgesia, an epidural catheter is routinely sited at the vertebral L2 to L4 level.

CLE infusions contain low-concentration local anesthetics, such as bupivacaine (0.0625%-0.125%) or ropivacaine (0.1%),[2,3] routinely augmented by the addition of fentanyl (2 µg/mL).

In CSE, a 25- to 27-gauge spinal needle is introduced through an epidural needle into the intrathecal space (**Figure 26.2C**). Bupivacaine (1.5-2 mg) with fentanyl (25 µg) is injected to provide quicker onset of pain relief, and then it is immediately followed by the insertion of epidural catheter through the epidural needle.

CSA involves puncture of the dura to facilitate placement of a catheter to allow titration of small injections of local anesthetic or opioid, a technique employed mainly (and rarely) in the management of high-risk delivery (vide infra).

Analgesia is provided via a patient-controlled electromechanical pump in either continuous, patient-controlled epidural analgesia (PCEA)[4], or programmed intermittent epidural bolus (PIEB) analgesia.

The choice of anesthetic technique for cesarean delivery depends on several factors, including: experience of anesthesiologist and obstetrician; indication for and urgency of cesarean delivery; presence of an *in situ* functioning epidural catheter placed for labor analgesia; and patient factors (such as patient cooperation, maternal preference, obesity, and presence of coagulation disorders, spine deformities, and anticipated difficult airway). Neuraxial anesthesia is almost always preferred to general anesthesia as it is safer for the parturient.

However, the need for general anesthesia cannot be eliminated entirely; it is required for emergent cesarean delivery and in the case when neuraxial anesthesia has failed or is contraindicated.

Spinal anesthesia for cesarean delivery is achieved by subarachnoid injection of bupivacaine (10-15 mg) through a 25- to 27-gauge needle inserted at vertebral level L3 to L4. This dose yields surgical anesthesia for up to 120 minutes. Both Whitacre and Sprotte spinal needles are designed with a noncutting leading edge and are associated with a decreased incidence of post–dural puncture headache. Fentanyl (10-20 µg) is routinely added to the local anesthetic to enhance the quality of sensory blockade. Further addition of preservative-free morphine (150-200 µg), especially when combined with postoperative administration of nonopioid adjuvants (eg, acetaminophen or nonsteroidal anti-inflammatory drugs [NSAIDs]), provides excellent postoperative pain relief for about 18 to 24 hours.[1] If prolonged duration of surgery is anticipated, CSE allows additional epidural catheter injections to supplement the required level of

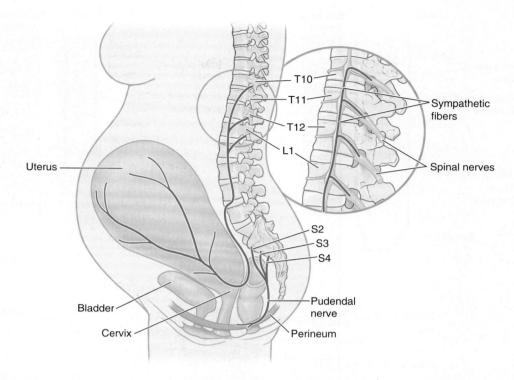

Figure 26.1 Parturition pain pathways. Afferent pain impulses from the cervix and uterus are carried by nerves that accompany sympathetic fibers and enter the neuraxis at T10, T11, T12, and L1 spinal levels. Pain pathways from the perineum travel to S2, S3, and S4 via the pudendal nerve.

anesthesia. The epidural catheter can also be injected with preservative-containing morphine (2-3 mg) to provide postoperative pain relief as an alternative to intrathecal morphine.[1] If a parturient in labor with an *in situ* epidural catheter requires cesarean delivery, the T4 rostral level of surgical anesthesia can be achieved in approximately 10 to 15 minutes after injection of 2% lidocaine with 1:200,000 epinephrine (usually 18-24 mL injected in intermittent 3- to 5-mL bolus doses). If immediate cesarean delivery is required, injection of 3% chloroprocaine is often used to expeditiously achieve surgical anesthesia (approximately 7-10 minutes) and thus avoid general anesthesia.[1] Prophylactic administration of intravenous metoclopramide and ondansetron minimizes the incidence of intraoperative and immediate postoperative nausea and vomiting.

Anesthesia for Labor and Delivery in a Patient With a High-Risk Pregnancy

General Principles

Management of the high-risk pregnancy involves meticulous antenatal care given by the obstetrician and consultant subspecialists to achieve maternal physiologic stability in the face of maternal comorbidity. In labor, the goal is to maintain fetal well-being (in general, meaning maintaining uteroplacental blood flow) while providing maternal cardiorespiratory stability.

Therefore, any well-communicated delivery plan should include not only an analgesia/anesthesia plan for labor/vaginal delivery (ie, "Plan A") but also for induction of surgical anesthesia for an unplanned nonemergent ("Plan B") or immediate, emergent abdominal delivery ("Plan C").

Obesity

Placing the patient supine, in lithotomy, or on the bed in Trendelenburg position all accentuate the reduction in lung volume. Together with the decrease in FRC and ERV, all exacerbate ventilation/perfusion mismatch, maternal arterial hypoxemia, and atelectasis. Left uterine displacement (LUD) and supplemental oxygen by mask are standard.

Due to the risk of respiratory compromise, caution should be used if prescribing parenteral narcotics or self-administered inhaled nitrous oxide

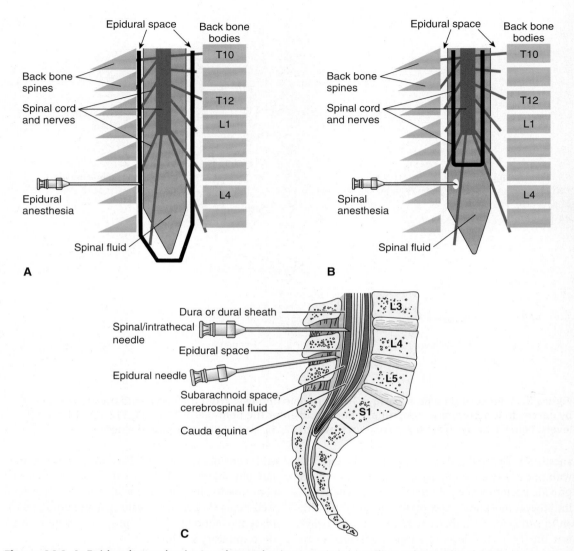

Figure 26.2 A, Epidural anesthesia: Local anesthetic agent is injected into the epidural space via epidural catheter. Epidural space is in the vertebral canal outside of dural sac containing cerebrospinal fluid and the spinal cord. The transmission of impulses are blocked in the nerve roots as they traverse the epidural space. **B,** Spinal anesthesia: Local anesthetic agent is injected into cerebrospinal fluid. The transmission of impulses is blocked as nerve roots traverse from the spinal cord through the subarachnoid space containing cerebrospinal fluid. Subarachnoid space surrounds the spinal cord and within the dural sac. **C,** Needle placement for spinal and epidural anesthesia.

(Adapted with permission from Taylor C, Lillis CA, LeMone P. *Fundamentals of Nursing.* 2nd ed. JB Lippincott; 1993.)

in the laboring patient with obesity. Analgesia after single injection of subarachnoid local anesthetic/opioid solution lasts less than 120 minutes.

More importantly, it does not provide a catheter for injection of successive doses of local anesthetic, later necessary for prolonged labor or for abdominal delivery. Siting a neuraxial catheter (as part of epidural, CSE, or CSA analgesia) and injecting dilute solutions of local anesthetic/opioid is

the preferred technique for labor analgesia. In the patient with morbid obesity, successful siting of a neuraxial catheter is often technically difficult and requires a prolonged duration period, necessitating ultrasound imaging and/or retrieval of long-length (eg, 5-, 6- or 7-inch) epidural needles required to pass through superficial adipose layers to reach the epidural/subarachnoid space. As for parturients without obesity, a T8 to T10 sensory dermatomal level is adequate for labor analgesia. In parturients with super-morbid obesity (body mass index [BMI] > 40), we have induced CSA for labor analgesia. Unlike an epidural catheter, the withdrawal of cerebrospinal fluid (CSF) before injection of local anesthetic is reassuring that the catheter tip is correctly placed, predictive that injected drug will be effective, and a surgical level of anesthesia can easily be obtained.

For cesarean delivery, neuraxial anesthesia at the rostral T4 sensory dermatomal level is preferred to general. In patients with obesity, due to the (often) prolonged duration of surgery, many anesthesiologists prefer siting a neuraxial catheter (eg, CLE, CSE, CSA) to single-injection spinal anesthesia.

Cardiac Disease

To maintain cardiovascular stability, the anesthesiologist will focus on the cardiovascular stress of labor and expected vaginal or unplanned abdominal delivery.[13] Central to any plan is the maintenance of forward flow, based on providing/maintain homeostasis of four basic cardiac parameters—preload, afterload, contractility, and heart rate—throughout delivery until immediate bedside responsibilities are transferred back to the cardiologist.

The induction of neuraxial anesthesia is associated with sympathetic-mediated vasodilation, and this coupled with unanticipated obstetric hemorrhage can decrease circulating volume returning to the heart (preload). Right ventricular preload is maintained with a combination of metered bolus infusions of intravenous fluid and/or low doses of vasopressor drugs, mitigating maternal tachycardia. Maternal tachycardia can result in decreased ventricular filling time and decreased forward flow and increased myocardial oxygen demand.

Most drugs currently used to induce or maintain general anesthesia have little or no effect on cardiac contractility. However, the induction of anesthesia in a patient with cardiac disease is much different in dose and time sequence of administration as compared to routine induction of general anesthesia for immediate abdominal delivery.

In addition to pulse oximetry (measuring both maternal peripheral arterial saturation and heart rate), routine monitoring of a patient with cardiac disease is often expanded to include continuous electrocardiography; siting an intra-arterial catheter to measure maternal systemic arterial pressure; siting a central venous catheter in anticipation of infusion of vasoactive drugs; and intermittent "point-of-care" (bedside) ultrasound to intermittently image inferior caval diameter, biventricular and septal motion, and interstitial lung water.

Neuraxial analgesia/anesthesia for labor can be modified for selected patients undergoing assisted vaginal delivery indicated to shorten the expulsive phase of delivery. For expected vaginal delivery, the patient is usually placed in a low lithotomy (with tilt or manual uterine displacement) or modified Sims position.

Neuraxial anesthesia for cesarean delivery can be induced using epidural anesthesia or spinal anesthesia knowing that the relative ("slow" or "fast," respectively) onset of upper thoracic sympathectomy will increase peripheral capacitance, decreasing central circulating volume, and often, increase maternal heart rate. The anesthesiologist may induce a two-step CSE anesthetic injecting subarachnoid opioid and then may inject a local anesthetic via the catheter to achieve surgical anesthesia while titrating intravenous crystalloid boluses to maintain normovolemia.

Cardiac output is routinely increased after delivery of the placenta, most likely due to an increase in central circulating volume.

Temporary amelioration is often observed in the immediate postpartum, allowing further assessment of maternal condition and a window of time if transfer back to a cardiac nursing unit is desired.

Specific Cardiac Conditions

Left-to-right shunts occur with congenital lesions such as patent ductus arteriosus (PDA), ventricular septal defect (VSD), and atrial septal defect (ASD). With pregnancy-associated vasodilation, these patients usually tolerate pregnancy well. Anesthesiologists will often site a neuraxial catheter early in active labor using saline for loss of resistance (LOR) instead of air in the syringe while advancing the epidural needle and will connect in-line air traps to all intravenous infusion sets to help prevent paradoxical air emboli.

Eisenmenger syndrome, caused by a left-to-right shunt, results in an increase in pulmonary artery pressure if left untreated.

Labor analgesia can be accomplished with a lumbar epidural, intrathecal opioids, or a pudendal block early in the second stage of labor.

The most common cyanotic heart lesion is tetralogy of Fallot.

Care should be taken to avoid a decrease in SVR, as with single-shot spinal anesthesia, which may cause insufficient venous return, increase in shunt, and worsening hypoxemia.

Maintaining SVR and euvolemia analgesia for labor and expected vaginal delivery can be managed with neuraxial (epidural, CSE, spinal or continuous spinal) injection of opioids with dilute local anesthetic or as an alternative systemic medication (eg, PCA remifentanil) with pudendal[15] or low-spinal anesthetic for assisted delivery.[16]

Parturients with *antepartum dilated, hypokinetic ventricle cardiac failure* often present for delivery already on digoxin-like inotropes; low-dose, beta-adrenergic blockers; diuretics; peripheral arterial vasodilators; and anticoagulants.[17,18] Unless the patient has contraindication to regional anesthesia, vaginal or cesarean delivery may be facilitated by neuraxial anesthesia. The aim of the anesthesiologist is to attenuate wide swings in cardiac demand, maintain preload (adequate central circulating volume) with warmed intravenous fluids, and obviate an increase in afterload and heart rate due to pain-associated circulating catecholamines.

The use of CLE, CSE, CSA, and single-injection spinal anesthetic for induction of cesarean delivery have all been reported in patients with severe peripartum cardiomyopathy.[19] At induction, metered volumes of intravenous fluids are given with injection of vasopressor to support cardiac return without reflex change to cardiac rate or even arrhythmia. If general anesthesia is required, then the obstetric anesthesiologist will alter the routine induction and maintenance to avoid profound myocardial depression.[20] If immediate delivery is required, then induction of "cardiac" anesthesia may delay skin incision.

With general anesthesia for nonimmediate delivery, invasive monitoring of maternal central venous (also allowing infusion of vasoactive drugs) and systemic intra-arterial pressures and, more recently, transesophageal echocardiography can prove invaluable, if not for preoperative, for postoperative management.

Patients with *aortic insufficiency* (AI) and *mitral regurgitation* usually tolerate labor and delivery without major issue. Induction of neuraxial analgesia/anesthesia is routine (**Table 26.1**). Anesthetic management of patients with *stenotic valvular disease* focuses on the concept of a "fixed" maximum CO in a patient challenged by routine fluctuations in CO seen in labor and delivery.[21,22]

To avoid any hypotension, neuraxial injection of intrathecal narcotics (single-injection spinal, CSE, CSA) have been used, followed by a pudendal block or neuraxial injection (especially via a continuous spinal catheter) of extremely dilute local anesthetic for assisted delivery. Although neuraxial anesthesia has been reported,[23] many obstetric anesthesiologists have, especially in the past, chosen general anesthesia for cesarean delivery.

With *pulmonary hypertension*, the increase in pulmonary artery afterload not only induces right ventricular but, indirectly, left ventricular dysfunction.

Right ventricular failure is associated with ischemia and dysrhythmia (**Table 26.2**).

In a seeming contradiction, some of these patients require diuresis to decrease the size of a dilated right ventricle, increasing the efficiency

Table 26.1 Cardiac Valvular Disease—Desired Hemodynamics to Maintain Forward Flow

	Aortic Insufficiency	Mitral Regurgitation	Mitral Stenosis	Aortic Stenosis
Preload	Normovolemia	Normovolemia	May tolerate slight increase	May tolerate slight increase
Afterload	Decrease SVR	Maintain or decrease SVR	Maintain SVR Right ventricle may not tolerate increase in PVR	Maintain or increase for coronary perfusion
Heart Rate (sinus)	Normocardia to slight tachycardia	Normocardia to slight tachycardia	Decrease or maintain—will not tolerate tachycardia	Decrease or maintain—will not tolerate tachycardia
Contractility	Maintain or increase	Maintain	Right ventricle may need support	Maintain

PVR, pulmonary vascular resistance; SVR, systemic vascular resistance.

Table 26.2 Anesthetic Implications of Pulmonary Hypertension and Its Pathophysiology

	Right Ventricle (RV)	Left Ventricle (LV)	Useful Medications
Pathology	• Hypertrophy • Dilation • Fibrosis • Impaired RCA flow (during diastole and systole) • Ischemia/arrhythmia	Impingement from RV → Impaired LV filling Impaired wall motion Ventricular uncoupling	
Preload	Normovolemia hypovolemia will inadequately fill RV hypervolemia will further RV impingement on LV function	Normovolemia May not tolerate hypervolemia	To increase: bolus of IV volume; phenylephrine infusion To decrease: diuretic
Afterload	Decrease PVR	Maintain SVR to ensure circulating volume return central circulation	To decrease PVR: iNO; iPGI$_2$; milrinone; dobutamine; isoproterenol
Heart Rate (sinus)	Maintain sinus normocardia (ensure RV filling)	Maintain sinus normocardia (ensure LV filling)	
Contractility	? Hypercontractile with hypertrophy (response to chronic increased PAP) ±Hypocontractile with dilation/fibrosis (response to acute increase in PAP)		If hypocontractile: milrinone; low-dose epi/nepi; dobutamine

iNO, inhaled nitric oxide; iPGI2, inhaled epoprostenol; IV, intravenous; low-dose epi, epinephrine (<0.06 µg/kg/min); LV, left ventricle; nepi, norepinephrine; PAP, pulmonary artery pressure; PVR, pulmonary vascular resistance; RCA, right coronary artery; RV, right ventricle; SVR, systemic vascular resistance.

of the left ventricle. Rapid increases or decreases in central circulating volume are not well tolerated; euvolemia must be maintained. Although inhaled nitric oxide (iNO) is often indicated in afflicted adults, iNO is routinely administered via tracheal tube (titrating the dose by vaporizer in parts per million changes) mitigating its use in an awake patient during labor or at cesarean delivery.[24]

An alternative to iNO, inhaled nebulized epoprostenol, is routinely administered via tight-fitting facemask[25] and does not have toxicity (NO$_2$) for caregivers. Prostacyclin does possess platelet inhibitory effects but has been reported in conjunction with neuraxial anesthesia.

Preeclampsia

Often, maternal risks of neuraxial analgesia/anesthesia center around the possibility of epidural hematoma after neuraxial anesthesia in a patient with preeclampsia, with or without changes in the laboratory test results compatible with coagulopathy. Monitoring platelet count is the laboratory test most routinely obtained. Most anesthesiologists feel confident that neuraxial insertion of a needle in a patient with at least 70,000 platelets per mm^3 (without any overt signs of coagulopathy) is not contraindicated[27]; insertion with less than 50,000 per mm^3 presents a relative contraindication. Reassuring results from other tests of coagulation (eg, TEG/ROTEM) are reason to reassure the anesthesiologist that it is relatively safe to proceed with neuraxial anesthesia in a patient whose platelet count is below 70,000 per mm^3.[28]

Neuraxial analgesia provides excellent maternal pain relief and is demonstrated to increase uteroplacental perfusion in the preeclamptic pregnancy.[1] In most cases, neuraxial analgesia can be converted to surgical anesthesia obviating general anesthesia. Therefore, anesthesia for labor and delivery in the patient with preeclampsia is desirable and often necessary.[26]

Another risk often discussed is neuraxial anesthesia-induced, untreated maternal hypotension and its effects on placental perfusion to an often fragile, and perhaps premature, fetus.

In multiple studies of neuraxial anesthesia for cesarean delivery in patients with severe preeclampsia, little (ie, latency to hypotension, amount of vasopressor used, nadir of decrease in blood pressure) or no differences (ie, incidence of hypotension, amount of intravenous fluid volume) in hemodynamic effects occur between those receiving spinal and those receiving epidural anesthesia.[29]

Although less desirable than neuraxial anesthesia, general anesthesia may still be indicated due to maternal contraindication or obstetric emergency.

Severe hypertension can be observed at induction/tracheal intubation and emergence from general anesthesia. As with a patient suffering from cardiac disease, this pressor response can be blunted with intravenous injection of adjuvant antihypertensive drugs (eg, labetalol or esmolol) or rapid-onset short-acting opioids (eg, remifentanil or alfentanil) prior to the more routine rapid sequence of injection of intravenous propofol (or barbiturate) and succinylcholine.

Neurologic Disease

Cesarean delivery is often urgently indicated; the aim of surgical anesthesia is to mitigate an increase in ICP. Maternal monitoring should include an intra-arterial catheter (eg, radial) to monitor beat-to-beat systemic arterial pressure and a (eg, subclavian) central venous catheter, inserted primarily for infusion of vasoactive drugs but also used to monitor central vascular pressures. Maternal infusion of intravenous (low-dose) mannitol and steroids to pharmacologically ameliorate increased ICP may be indicated (**Figure 26.3**).

General anesthetics have been most often reported for these patients.

The pressor response associated with the induction of general anesthesia and intubation will increase intracranial blood volume, possibly enough to cause cerebral herniation or stroke. To attenuate this hypertensive response, the anesthesiologist will often inject rapid-acting, short- to medium-duration opioids (eg, fentanyl, remifentanil) or antihypertensives (eg, esmolol) at both induction and (with the patient still with increased ICP/intracranial mass) at emergence from general anesthesia at the end of surgery.

Neuraxial anesthesia is generally considered safe in other *intracranial* conditions without evidence of intracranial hypertension such as *Moyamoya*, arteriovenous malformation (*AVM*), *aneurysm*, *pseudotumor cerebri*, asymptomatic *Arnold-Chiari I* (with no evidence of tethering, minimal tonsillar descent and unobstructed CSF flow), and *cerebral venous thrombosis* (if the patient is not anticoagulated).

A diagnosis of *multiple sclerosis* does not contraindicate induction of neuraxial analgesia/anesthesia for labor and vaginal or abdominal delivery.

CLE using an injectate of dilute solution of local anesthetic (with or without opioid) is accepted as safe for labor analgesia in these patients.[32]

Myasthenia gravis is characterized by episodes of weakness affecting muscles of respiration, laryngeal muscles, and facial and ocular muscles.

Pain-induced increase in respiratory work indicates early labor analgesia. Parenteral opioids should be used cautiously to avoid any residual respiratory compromise. Neuraxial analgesia is a preferred method of pain relief and can be modified to provide anesthesia for an assisted vaginal delivery to shorten the duration of maternal expulsive efforts phase or obstetric-indicated abdominal delivery.[34]

Although neuraxial anesthesia is preferred over general anesthesia for cesarean delivery, a patient with adequate neuraxial surgical anesthesia whose degree of respiratory compromise precludes spontaneous ventilation while supine may require mechanical ventilation (ie, general anesthesia) when positioned on the operating room table. Unless severely debilitated, the menu of drugs chosen and conduct of routine *induction* of general anesthesia for obstetrics are unchanged.

Use of neuraxial opioids for postoperative analgesia spares the systemic effects of large doses of parenteral opioids; however, many anesthesiologists wish to avoid any opioids. Protocols for non-opioid postoperative analgesia should be employed, including combinations of oral and intravenous acetaminophen and NSAIDs, and intravenous ketamine and dexmedetomidine. Consideration should be given to placing transversus abdominis plane nerve blocks or continuous infusion of low-volume, dilute local anesthetic injectate via a lower thoracic neuraxial catheter.

Although patients with previous mid–thoracic cord (or higher) injury may retain some vague sensation (usually not discerned as typical labor pain), they sometimes present to the labor and delivery suite unaware they are in advanced labor. Neuraxial injection of local anesthetic (and not solely an

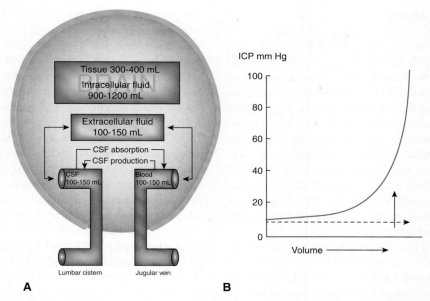

Figure 26.3 A and B, Intracranial compliance in a patient with an intracranial mass: **(A)** Applying a three-compartment (tissue, cerebrospinal fluid [CSF], blood) model in a patient with already increased intracranial compliance, **(B)** small increases in intracranial or neuraxial volume will greatly increase intracranial pressure (ICP). Such increases are seen with: uterine contraction (~2-3 mm Hg) epidural bolus injection with 5 mL or 10 mL (5 and 21 mm Hg, respectively); increasing noncommunicating hydrocephalus, acute increase in systemic hypertension (untreated pressor response to tracheal intubation and extubation); and enlarging mass (eg, tumor, blood clot).

(Adapted with permission from Leffert LR, Schwamm LH. Neuraxial anesthesia in parturients with intracranial pathology. *Anesthesiology.* 2013;119:703-718.)

opioid) is required to interrupt the afferent and efferent arcs of the intact (but disinhibited) reflex.

In a patient with para- or quadriplegia, sensory and motor testing of the block is obviously difficult. However, in a laboring patient for expected vaginal delivery, injection of routine volumes of epidural bupivacaine (8-12 mL of 0.25% or 0.375%) should interrupt neural reflexes while eliminating muscle reflexes at the ankle and patella; sensory testing above the level of cord transection should be routine. Because sensation of uterine contractions is attenuated or eliminated, use of a patient-controlled infusion of dilute local anesthetic/opioid injectate may not be optimal. Intermittent bolus injection of the catheter is indicated on a regular time-based schedule, as well as a bolus delivery dose of local anesthetic to reinforce attenuation of the neural reflex at the time of intense abdomino pelvic stimulation (eg, digital vaginal examination, assisted delivery, manual extraction of the placenta). In a laboring patient with a transection level below T10, neuraxial analgesia is induced to eliminate the pain of labor or produce required surgical anesthesia.

Patients with mid- to high thoracic transection will often "feel" surgical stimulation. It is our experience to routinely dose (concentration and volumes) neuraxial anesthesia for cesarean delivery. Optimal monitoring of these patients includes an intra-arterial catheter for beat-to-beat monitoring of maternal systemic blood pressure, a central venous catheter for infusion of vasoactive medications (eg, nicardipine, sodium nitroprusside, labetalol, esmolol), and a continuous five-lead electrocardiograph (ECG).

In these patients, instead of succinylcholine (associated with a massive hyperkalemic response), anesthesiologists intravenously inject a rapid-sequence intubating dose of a nondepolarizing paralytic (eg, rocuronium [1.2 mg/kg]), hastening the onset of "intubating conditions" to facilitate tracheal intubation.

Substance Abuse

Polysubstance abuse in pregnancy is not uncommon.[36] A parturient may present in opioid withdrawal, acutely opioid intoxicated, or even in opioid overdose. In the face of required immediate cesarean delivery, induction of anesthesia is often complicated by limited intravenous access; plans should be in place to obtain central or even intraosseous access. Unless there is a more routine contraindication, neuraxial anesthetic techniques are preferred for labor and vaginal or cesarean delivery.[36] Intravenous drug abusers are prone to an increased incidence of epidural abscesses; therefore, a neurological assessment should be carried out before induction of neuraxial anesthesia.[36]

A required induction and maintenance of general anesthesia is accomplished with routinely used agents (eg, propofol, paralytics, opioids, benzodiazepines, inhalational gases). Cross-tolerance is not a routine problem while anesthetized. Postoperative analgesic regimens often include bilateral transverse abdominus plane regional block (with bupivacaine or ropivacaine) or low-rate, dilute local anesthetic (with or without supplemental fentanyl) via PCEA, as well as a menu of intravenous and oral NSAIDs, acetaminophen, and gabapentin.[37] The patient's daily narcotic dose should be met. Opioid agonist-antagonists should be avoided.

Induction of neuraxial analgesia/anesthesia in cocaine abusers, who are both volume and catecholamine depleted, may lead to an unexpected degree of hypotension; ephedrine (which releases catecholamines) may be ineffective. Therefore, intravenous volume repletion and phenylephrine are routinely used to treat hypotension. If induction of general anesthesia is required for immediate delivery, then the anesthesiologist should be prepared to prevent and aggressively treat (eg, labetalol, esmolol, nicardipine) an exaggerated pressor response to tracheal intubation.

KEY POINTS

- Pregnancy is associated with physiological changes such as increased ventilation and cardiac out.
- Neuraxial labor analgesia is the most desirable method during labor.
- Pregnancy is associated with pregnancy-related complications or superimposed on a preexisting morbidity such as obesity, diabetes, hypertension, etc.

- Due to tremendous progress in the management of congenital heart diseases, many women with congenital heart diseases are reaching childbearing age.
- Multidisciplinary team approach is the pathway to success in the management of pregnant women with complex pregnancies and complex comorbidities.

REFERENCES

(only references cited in synoptic print chapter; for a complete reference list, see ebook)

1. Datta S, Kodali BS, Segal S. *Obstetric Anesthesia Handbook.* Springer-Verlag; 2010. doi:10.1007/978-0-387-88602-2
2. Epsztein Kanczuk M, Barrett NM, Arzola C, et al. Programmed intermittent epidural bolus for labor analgesia during first stage of labor: a biased-coin up-and-down sequential allocation trial to determine the optimum interval time between boluses of a fixed volume of 10 mL of bupivacaine 0.0625% with fentanyl 2 μg/mL. *Anesth Analg.* 2017;124:537-541.
3. Carvalho B, George RB, Cobb B, McKenzie C, Riley ET. Implementation of programmed intermittent epidural bolus for the maintenance of labor analgesia. *Anesth Analg.* 2016;123:965-971.
4. Ojo OA, Mehdiratta JE, Gamez BH, Hunting J, Habib AS. Comparison of programmed intermittent epidural boluses with continuous epidural infusion for the maintenance of labor analgesia: a randomized, controlled, double-blind study. *Anesth Analg.* 2020;130(2):426-435. doi:10.1213/ANE.0000000000004104
13. Cohen KM, Minehart RD, Leffert LR. Anesthetic treatment of cardiac disease during pregnancy. *Curr Treat Options Cardiovasc Med.* 2018;20:66.

15. Kuczkowski KM. Labor analgesia for the parturient with cardiac disease: what does an obstetrician need to know? *Acta Obstet Gynecol Scand.* 2004;83:223-233.
16. Ghai B, Mohan V, Khetarpal M. Epidural anesthesia for cesarean section in a patient with Eisenmenger's syndrome. *Int J Obstet Anesth.* 2002;11:44-47.
17. Billebeau G, Etienne M, Cheikh-Khelifa R, et al. Pregnancy in women with a cardiomyopathy: outcomes and predictors from a retrospective cohort. *Arch Cardiovasc Dis.* 2018;111:199-209.
18. Stergiopoulos K, Shiang E, Bench T. Pregnancy in patients with pre-existing cardiomyopathies. *J Am Coll Cardiol.* 2011;58:337-350.
19. Velickovic IA, Leicht CH. Continuous spinal anesthesia for cesarean section in a parturient with severe recurrent peripartum cardiomyopathy. *Int J Obstet Anesth.* 2004;13:40-43.
20. Breen TW, Janzen JA. Pulmonary hypertension and cardiomyopathy: anaesthetic management for caesarean section. *Can J Anaesth.* 1991;38:895-899.
21. Dennis A. Valvular heart disease in pregnancy. *Int J Obstet Anesth.* 2016;25:4-8.
22. Windram JD, Colman JM, Wald RM, Udell JA, Siu SC, Silversides CK. Valvular heart disease in pregnancy. *Best Pract Res Clin Obstet Gynaecol.* 2014;28:507-518.

23. Ioscovich AM, Goldszmidt E, Fadeev AV, Grisaru-Granovsky S, Halpern SH. Peripartum anesthetic management of patients with aortic valve stenosis: a retrospective study and literature review. *Int J Obstet Anesth.* 2009;18(4):379-386. doi:10.1016/j.ijoa.2009.02.019

24. Kawabe A, Nakano K, Aiko Y, et al. Successful management of pregnancy in a patient with systemic lupus erythematosus-associated pulmonary arterial hypertension. *Intern Med.* 2018;57:1655-1659.

25. Hill LL, De Wet CJ, Jacobsohn E, Leighton BL, Tymkew H. Peripartum substitution of inhaled for intravenous prostacyclin in a patient with primary pulmonary hypertension. *Anesthesiology.* 2004;100:1603-1605.

26. Dennis AT. Management of pre-eclampsia: issues for anaesthetists. *Anaesthesia.* 2012;67:1009-1020.

27. Lee LO, Bateman BT, Kheterpal S, et al. Risk of epidural hematoma after neuraxial techniques in thrombocytopenic parturients: a report from the multicenter perioperative outcomes group. *Anesthesiology.* 2017;126:1053-1063.

28. Levy N, Goren O, Cattan A, Weiniger CF, Matot I. Neuraxial block for delivery among women with low platelet counts: a retrospective analysis. *Int J Obstet Anesth.* 2018;35:4-9.

29. Henke VG, Bateman BT, Leffert LR. Focused review: spinal anesthesia in severe preeclampsia. *Anesth Analg.* 2013;117:686-693.

32. Ferrero S, Pretta S, Ragni N. Multiple sclerosis: management issues during pregnancy. *Eur J Obstet Gynecol Reprod Biol.* 2004;115:3-9.

34. Almeida C, Coutinho E, Moreira D, et al. Myasthenia gravis and pregnancy: anaesthetic management – A series of cases. *Acta Anaesthesiol Scand.* 2010;27:985-990.

36. Kuczkowski KM. The cocaine abusing parturient: a review of anesthetic considerations. *Can J Anaesth.* 2004;51:145-154.

37. Raymond BL, Kook BT, Richardson MG. The opioid epidemic and pregnancy: implications for anesthetic care. *Curr Opin Anesthesiol.* 2018;31:243-250.

CHAPTER 27

Hypertensive Diseases in Pregnancy

Conisha M. Holloman and Baha M. Sibai

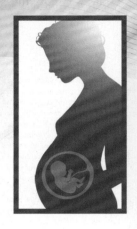

The incidence of hypertensive disorders vary according to the population studied and the criteria used for diagnosis but is still one of the leading causes of maternal and perinatal mortality worldwide. In Latin America and the Caribbean, they are responsible for almost 26% of maternal deaths, which contrasts to the 9% of deaths in Africa and Asia. Despite maternal mortality being higher in lower to middle-income countries when compared to high-income counties, 16% of maternal deaths are attributed to hypertensive disorders in countries like the United States. Between 1987 and 2004, preeclampsia increased by 25% in the United States.[1-4]

Preeclampsia

Clinical Assessment

Preeclampsia is a syndrome primarily defined as new-onset hypertension that develops in the second half of pregnancy (after 20 weeks of gestation). Diagnostic criteria require the development of hypertension defined as a persistent systolic blood pressure (BP) of 140 mm Hg or greater or diastolic BP of 90 mm Hg or higher on two occasions at least 4 hours apart after 20 weeks gestation in a woman with previously normal blood pressure. The optimal measurement of BP is with the patient seated comfortably, with legs uncrossed, and arm and back supported so that the middle of the cuff on the upper arm is at the level of the atrium. Ideally, 5 to 10 minutes should pass before taking the blood pressure.[12]

Proteinuria is defined as the excretion of 300 mg or more of protein in a 24-hour urine collection or protein/creatinine ratio of at least 0.3 mg/dL. A urine dipstick protein of 2+ is also used as a surrogate marker when quantitative methods are unavailable (due to increased false-positive and false-negative results). Prior to 2013, proteinuria was a requirement for the diagnosis of preeclampsia, but it was later recognized that some patients have advanced disease before protein is detected in the urine. This criterion was removed in the 2013 ACOG Task Force and instead features of end-organ dysfunction were highlighted such as thrombocytopenia, liver or renal impairment, pulmonary edema, and neurologic or visual dysfunction.[13] Although it is often accompanied with an acute development of proteinuria, preeclampsia can be associated with other signs and symptoms such as persistent headache, visual changes, right upper quadrant pain, epigastric pain, nausea, and vomiting. However, maternal symptoms, such as headache and right upper quadrant pain, may not always correlate with laboratory-confirmed abnormalities or have multiple etiologies.[14,15]

Preeclampsia is also classified in the presence or absence of severe features (**Tables 27.1** and **27.2**): blood pressure greater than 160 mm Hg systolic or 110 mm Hg diastolic, acute kidney injury with creatinine greater than 1.1 or an increase greater than twofold above the baseline, doubling of liver function tests, persistent or severe central nervous system symptoms, platelet count less than 100×10^9/L, and the presence of pulmonary edema. Severe proteinuria ($\geq$5 g in a 24-hour urine collection) is no longer used because it does not correlate to outcomes.[16,17]

In normal pregnancy, invasion of uterine arteries transforms cytotrophoblasts from an epithelial to an endothelial phenotype. This process is called pseudovasculogenesis (**Figure 27.1**). The remodeling is meant to increase the supply of oxygen

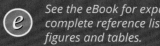

See the eBook for expanded content, a complete reference list, and additional figures and tables.

Table 27.1 Criteria for the Diagnosis of Preeclampsia Without Severe Features

- Systolic BP ≥ 140 mm Hg or diastolic BP ≥ 90 mm Hg on two occasions 4 h apart after 20 wk of gestation in a woman known not to have chronic hypertension prior to the pregnancy
- Systolic BP ≥ 160 mm Hg or diastolic BP ≥ 110 mm Hg, hypertension can be confirmed within a short interval (minutes) to allow the administration of antihypertensive medication on two separate occasions

BP, blood pressure.

Table 27.2 Criteria for the Diagnosis of Preeclampsia With Severe Features

- Systolic BP ≥ 160 mm Hg or diastolic BP ≥ 110 mm Hg on two occasions 4 h apart
- Thrombocytopenia (platelet count less than 100,000/μL)
- Pulmonary edema
- Cerebral or visual disturbances
- Epigastric pain/right upper quadrant pain
- Pulmonary edema
- Abnormal liver function tests: aspartate aminotransferase (AST) or alanine aminotransferase (ALT) more than twice the upper limit for the laboratory
- Serum creatinine concentration of 1.1 mg/dL or doubling of baseline serum creatinine with no other renal pathology

BP, blood pressure.

and nutrients to the fetus. This is achieved by the cytotrophoblasts' upregulated expression of molecules that are important to uterine inversion such as those from the vascular endothelial growth factor (VEGF) family (eg, VEGF-A, VEGF-C, and placental growth factor [PlGF]). The end result is cytotrophoblastic invasion of the uterine wall and replacement of the highly resistant uterine spiral arteries and arterioles with a low resistance vascular system. In preeclampsia, this process is thought to be defective (probably secondary to altered immunologic response at the fetal-maternal interface) and leads to ischemia. As a result, there is an excessive production of soluble Flt1 (sFlt-1) that binds in the blood to both the VEGF and PlGF. The state of high sFlt-1 and low VEGF/PlGF contributes to the development of hypertension.[18-22]

Clear racial differences can be noted in the United States in regard to the incidence and level of severity of preeclampsia. African American women have a higher incidence of preeclampsia than Caucasian women and a threefold higher rate of maternal fatality. Disparities in access to health care combined with differences in comorbid conditions may be to blame for this stark difference.[24]

Eclampsia

Factors determining the degree of dysfunction include a delay in the treatment of preeclampsia and the presence of complicating obstetric and medical factors.

In one study, there were no preceding symptoms in 25% of women with eclampsia. Out of 20,000 patients, 21% experienced postpartum eclampsia.[26] The seizures are usually generalized tonic-clonic in nature, lasting 60 to 90 seconds and followed by a postictal phase.[10,27] Laboratory

findings also vary. Serum uric acid and creatinine are usually elevated, and creatinine clearance is reduced. Hemoconcentration, reflected by an increased hematocrit and reduced plasma volume, is common as liver enzymes are found in 11% to 74% of eclamptic patients. HELLP (**h**emolysis, **e**levated **l**iver enzymes, and **l**ow **p**latelets) syndrome complicates approximately 10% of eclampsia and usually occurs in longstanding disease and in patients with medical complications.[24]

According to the World Health Organization, there is a reported increase in eclampsia from 0.1% to 0.8% in developed countries. This contrasts from the incidence of eclampsia in Western countries of 4 to 5 per 10,000 pregnancies.[28]

Several mechanisms have been suggested as predisposing factors to the development of eclampsia:

- Cerebral vasospasm;
- Cerebral hemorrhage;
- Cerebral ischemia;
- Cerebral edema;
- Hypertensive encephalopathy; and
- Metabolic encephalopathy.

Clinical Assessment

Most women with eclamptic seizures have an abnormal electroencephalogram. However, electroencephalographic changes are almost always transient and resolve completely. The neurologic and cerebrovascular changes of eclampsia serve as a model for hypertensive encephalopathy, with

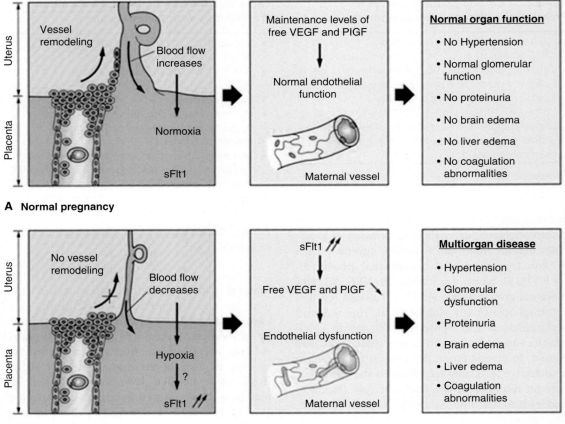

Figure 27.1 Hypothesis on the role of soluble Flt1 (sFlt1) in preeclampsia. A, During normal pregnancy, the uterine spiral arteries are infiltrated and remodeled by endovascular invasive trophoblasts, thereby increasing blood flow significantly in order to meet the oxygen and nutrient demands of the fetus. B, In the placenta of preeclamptic women, trophoblast invasion does not occur and blood flow is reduced, resulting in placental hypoxia. In addition, increased amounts of sFlt1 are produced by the placenta and scavenge vascular endothelial growth factor (VEGF) and placental growth factor (PlGF), thereby lowering circulating levels of unbound VEGF and PlGF. This altered balance causes generalized endothelial dysfunction, resulting in multiorgan disease. It remains unknown whether hypoxia is the trigger for stimulating sFlt1 secretion in the placenta of preeclamptic mothers and whether the higher sFlt1 levels interfere with trophoblast invasion and spiral artery remodeling.

the occipital and parietal zones most vulnerable. The similar pathogenetic events of forced vasodilation and altered cerebral autoregulation seen in hypertensive encephalopathy may be operative in eclampsia. However, an additional factor, such as endothelial cell dysfunction, seems to be present in eclampsia. Although routine neuroimaging studies are not advocated for all women with eclampsia, focal neurologic deficits or prolonged coma (atypical eclampsia) require prompt investigation.[31]

HELLP Syndrome

Most experts consider HELLP syndrome to be a manifestation of preeclampsia rather than a distinct hypertensive pathology of pregnancy.

In the series reported by Sibai, women with HELLP syndrome may present with a variety of signs and symptoms, none of which is diagnostic and all of which may be found in women with severe preeclampsia or eclampsia without HELLP syndrome.[35] Nausea, vomiting, and epigastric pain are the most common symptoms.

About 15% to 50% of HELLP cases have mild hypertension, about 12% to 18% have no hypertension, and 13% of cases have no proteinuria.[38] As a result, patients are often misdiagnosed as having various medical and surgical disorders, including appendicitis, gastroenteritis, glomerulonephritis, pyelonephritis, viral hepatitis, or even acute fatty liver of pregnancy (AFLP).

Microangiopathic hemolytic anemia develops in response to destructive forces that act on red blood cells in small blood vessels, resulting in the formation of schistocytes. The exact mechanism for the cause of underlying liver hematoma with HELLP syndrome is not known. The speculated mechanism involves ischemic lesions of the liver secondary to the preeclampsia-associated micro-angiopathy, further progressing to hepatic necrosis and hemorrhage. The process of neovascularization in the affected parenchyma and newly formed vessels are more prone to bleeding with hypertensive episodes. The subcapsular hematoma is formed from intrahepatic hemorrhage that can rupture into the peritoneal cavity with hematoma expansion after hypertension or trauma.[39]

The criteria for the diagnosis of HELLP syndrome: (1) hemolysis (abnormal peripheral blood smear, total bilirubin exceeding 1.2 mg/dL, and lactic dehydrogenase [LDH] > 600 U/L), (2) elevated liver enzymes (serum aspartate aminotransferase [AST] > 70 U/L, elevated alanine aminotransferase [ALT] and LDH > 600 U/L), and (3) low platelet count (<100,000/μL).[40]

Chronic Hypertension

Other factors that may suggest the presence of chronic hypertension (CHTN) include

- Retinal changes on fundoscopic examination;
- Radiologic and electrocardiographic evidence of cardiac enlargement;
- Compromised renal function or associated renal disease; and
- Multiparity with a previous history of hypertensive pregnancies.

The most common etiology of CHTN is essential or primary hypertension, contributing 90% of CHTN cases, while secondary hypertension accounts for the remaining 10%.

They include renal diseases (glomerulonephritis, polycystic kidneys, renal artery stenosis, or reno-vascular disease), systemic lupus erythematosus,

polyarteritis nodosa, endocrine disorders (hyper-aldosteronism, pheochromocytoma, diabetes mellitus), and coarctation of the aorta.[47] Most of the secondary causes require specific treatment in addition to antihypertensive therapy. Early diagnosis is important because, if untreated, many of these disorders are associated with significant maternal/fetal morbidity and mortality.

CHTN in pregnancy may be subclassified into mild hypertension (diastolic BP ≥ 90 to < 110 mm Hg or systolic BP ≥ 140 to < 160 mm Hg) or severe hypertension (diastolic BP > 110 mm Hg or systolic BP ≥ 160 mm Hg). For the purpose of clinical management, CHTN in pregnancy may also be divided into a low-risk group (hypertension with no end-organ damage or associated significant comorbidities) or a high-risk CHTN group (hypertension with end-organ damage or associated morbidities). These subdivisions are discussed in detail under the management of CHTN in pregnancy. Between 13% and 40% of pregnant women with CHTN will develop superimposed preeclampsia.[48]

Gestational Hypertension

Gestational hypertension, previously called pregnancy-induced hypertension, is the development of new-onset hypertension after 20 weeks of gestation in the absence of diagnostic criteria for preeclampsia. Gestational hypertension develops in 6% to 17% or healthy nulliparous women and 2% to 4% of multiparous women.[50] Of those women who are initially diagnosed with gestational hypertension, 15% to 46% will develop preeclampsia.[51]

Clinical Presentation

The diagnosis can be changed to CHTN if elevated beyond 12 weeks postpartum. If the blood pressure normalizes after 12 weeks, then the diagnosis is changed to transient hypertension of pregnancy.[2,13] If proteinuria occurs before 12 weeks postpartum, then the diagnosis will be gestational hypertension with progression to postpartum preeclampsia. If high blood pressure alone persists beyond 12 weeks of the postpartum period, then the patient has CHTN.

Gestational hypertension can be further divided into two categories, mild and severe. Mild gestational hypertension is defined as systolic BP ≥ 140 mm Hg or diastolic BP ≥ 90 mm Hg (without proteinuria) measured on two occasions at least 4 hours apart and no more than 7 days apart after 20 weeks of gestation.

It often occurs close to term and intrapartum, or within 24 hours of delivery. Mild gestational hypertension often resolves within 10 days of the postpartum period without treatment.

Severe gestational hypertension is defined as sustained systolic BP ≥ 160 mm Hg and/or diastolic BP ≥ 110 mm Hg measured at least 4 hours apart with no proteinuria. The diagnosis may need to be confirmed within a shorter interval than 4 hours to facilitate timely antihypertensive therapy. Women with severe gestational hypertension have higher maternal and perinatal morbidities than those with mild gestational hypertension, with disease progression reaching 50% when gestational hypertension develops before 30 weeks of gestation.[2,52]

Management of Hypertension in Pregnancy

The Hypertension Task Force states that the first consideration in the management of women with gestational hypertension or preeclampsia without severe features is the safety of the mother and her fetus. Second is delivery of a mature newborn that will not require neonatal intensive care. When the diagnosis has been confirmed, subsequent management will depend on the results of maternal and fetal evaluation, gestational age, presence of labor or ruptured membranes, vaginal bleeding, and maternal wishes.[53]

Antepartum Management

All women diagnosed with hypertension in pregnancy should have a complete blood count, serum creatine, liver enzymes, 24-hour urine collection or urine protein to creatinine ratio, and symptom inventory. Fetal evaluation should include ultrasound evaluation for estimated fetal weight (EFW) and amniotic fluid index (AFI) (in centimeters), nonstress test (NST), and biophysical profile (BPP) if the NST is nonreactive.

Continued observation is appropriate for a woman with a gestational age less than 37 weeks if she has gestational hypertension or preeclampsia without severe features. Fetal monitoring includes fetal testing with daily kick counts, ultrasounds for fetal growth evaluation every 3 weeks, as well as NST once weekly for patients with gestational hypertension and twice weekly for patients with preeclampsia without severe features. Maternal evaluation includes complete blood count and checking liver enzymes and serum creatinine levels at least once

a week. For women with gestational hypertension, the assessment for proteinuria should occur at least once a week in the office. Symptoms and serial blood pressure checks should be monitored at least once a week for gestational hypertension and twice weekly for those with preeclampsia without severe features. Patient education is also imperative and should stress the importance of accessing care if severe symptoms develop. Symptoms considered concerning include severe headaches, visual changes, epigastric pain, shortness of breath and persistent symptoms of abdominal pain, contractions, vaginal spotting, ruptured membranes, or decreased fetal movement. Women with mild gestational hypertension or preeclampsia with a persistent blood pressure less than 160 mm Hg systolic or 110 mm Hg diastolic should not be started on antihypertensive therapy.[2,7,53]

Intrapartum Management

There are currently no randomized controlled trials that indicate expectant management will either improve perinatal outcomes or increase maternal or fetal risks in women who are 34 0/7 to 37 0/7 weeks of gestation. The risk associated with expectant management include the development of severe hypertension (10%-15%), eclampsia (0.2%-0.5%), HELLP syndrome (1%-2%), placental abruption (0.5%-2%), fetal growth restriction (10%-12%), and fetal death (0.2%-0.5%). However, immediate preterm delivery is associated with increased rates of admission to the neonatal intensive care unit, neonatal respiratory complications, and a slight increase in neonatal death when compared to infants born at 37 weeks or more gestational age. Taking this into consideration, the risk-benefit ratio between expectant management and immediate delivery is in favor or the former until 37 weeks' gestation in the absence of any other severe condition (eg, premature rupture of membranes, preterm labor, or vaginal bleeding).[6,54] Conservative management of mild or severe preeclampsia beyond term is not beneficial to the fetus because uteroplacental blood flow may be suboptimal. After 37 weeks' gestation, labor should be induced as soon as the cervix is favorable.

Indications favoring against expectant management include some of the following conditions[2]:

- Uncontrolled severe-range blood pressures (persistent systolic of 160 mm Hg or greater OR diastolic of 110 mm Hg or greater not responsive to antihypertensive medications)

- Persistent headaches unresponsive to treatment
- Epigastric pain or right upper pain unresponsive to treatment
- Visual disturbances, motor deficits or altered mental status
- HELLP syndrome
- Eclampsia
- Suspected placental abruption
- Abnormal fetal testing
- Fetal death
- Persistent reverse end-diastolic flow in umbilical artery

Condition-Specific Management

Preeclampsia With Severe Features

Preeclampsia with severe features can cause acute and long-term complications for both mother and newborn. Maternal complications of severe preeclampsia include pulmonary edema, myocardial infarction, stroke, acute respiratory distress syndrome, coagulopathy, severe renal failure, and retinal injury. These complications are more likely to occur in the presence of preexisting medical conditions and with acute maternal organ dysfunction related to preeclampsia.[55,56]

The clinical course of severe preeclampsia is often plagued with progressive deterioration of maternal and fetal conditions if delivery is not imminent. Therefore, the ACOG recommends when gestational age is at or beyond 34 0/7 weeks, and in those with unstable maternal-fetal conditions irrespective of gestational age, delivery should be initiated after maternal stabilization.[2,7,53]

Severe preeclampsia warrants hospitalization, administration of magnesium sulfate for seizure prophylaxis while antihypertensive medication is instituted for diastolic BP ≥ 110 mm Hg or systolic BP ≥ 160 mm Hg, and delivery of the fetus (except where conservative management is indicated as discussed above). The therapeutic goals include reduction of blood pressure to prevent maternal cerebrovascular accidents and congestive heart failure without compromising cerebral perfusion or jeopardizing uteroplacental blood flow. Profound and rapid reduction in blood pressure may compromise the uteroplacental circulation; therefore, continuous fetal monitoring should be employed. Thus, the goal of initial antihypertensive therapy is to limit the reduction in mean arterial pressure to 20% to 25% or to a diastolic blood pressure of 100 mm Hg.[57,58]

Parenteral or oral antihypertensive agents (ie, labetalol, hydralazine, nifedipine, sodium nitroprusside, etc) are used for acute reduction of blood pressure in women with severe features of preeclampsia or eclampsia. Oral medications are also used for maintenance or chronic therapy (**Table 27.7**). The choice of agents is dependent on the stage in pregnancy (antepartum, intrapartum, or postpartum), the side effect profile of the agent in question, the presence of other medical problems (renal insufficiency, diabetes mellitus, pulmonary edema, myocardial ischemia, etc), and, if postpartum, whether the woman is breastfeeding or not. The different agents used are discussed later under antihypertensive agents.

Eclampsia

The protocol used to manage eclampsia is outlined in **Table 27.8**. Preventing maternal injury and supporting respiratory and cardiovascular functions is the first priority in the management of eclampsia. Supportive care should be given during and immediately after an acute convulsive episode. To ensure adequate maternal oxygenation, the airway potency must be assessed and established. Supplemental oxygen can be administered via a face mask with or without oxygen reservoir at 8 to 10 L/min. Transcutaneous pulse oximetry should be used to monitor oxygenation in all eclamptic patients. If the acute event is occurring in an inpatient setting, the bed's side rails should be elevated and padded, a padded tongue blade should be inserted between the teeth, and physical restraints may be needed. To minimize aspiration, the patient should lie in the lateral decubitus position and vomitus and oral secretions suctioned as needed. Once convulsions have been abolished, arterial blood gas measurements and a chest radiograph should be obtained to insure adequate maternal oxygenation and exclude aspiration. Hypoxemia and acidemia should be corrected and maternal hypertension treated.

The fetal heart rate and uterine activity must be closely monitored. Fetal bradycardia is a common finding during an eclamptic seizure, but the rate usually returns to normal once convulsions cease.[59] If bradycardia persists or the uterus is hypertonic, placental abruption should be suspected and evaluated as appropriate. After stabilization of the maternal condition, steps should be taken to deliver the fetus, which is the definitive treatment for eclampsia. The mode of delivery is dependent on the usual obstetric indications.

Table 27.7 Antihypertensive Medication in Pregnancy

Class	Medication	Dose Starting Dose	Dose Maximum Dose
Common drugs for chronic therapy of hypertension			
Calcium channel blocker	Nifedipine (extended release)	30 mg orally, once a day	120 mg/d orally, four times a day
Alpha- and beta-blocker	Labetalol	100 mg orally, twice a day	2400 mg/d
Thiazide diuretic	HCTZ	12.5 mg orally, once a day	50 mg/d
Loop diuretic	Furosemide	20-120 mg orally, once a day	40 mg/d
Common drugs for acute therapy of severe hypertension			
Arteriolar dilator	Hydralazine		5-10 mg IV or IM every 20-40 min to a maximum cumulative dose of 20 mg
Calcium channel blocker	Nifedipine (immediate release)		10-20 mg orally, repeat in 20 min if needed; then 10-20 mg every 2-6 h; maximum dose of 180 mg
Alpha- and beta-blocker	Labetalol		20 mg IV per dose, then 20-80 mg every 10 min (maximum dose is 140 mg) or constant infusion 1-2 mg/min IV
Arterial and venous dilator	Nitroprusside		0.2-0.5 µg/kg/min

HCTZ, hydrochlorothiazide; IM, intramuscular; IV, intravenous.

HELLP Syndrome

Delivery is the definitive therapy for HELLP syndrome beyond 34 weeks' gestation or fetal or maternal jeopardy. For women with HELLP syndrome before fetal viability, it is recommended that delivery occur shortly after initial maternal stabilization. Without laboratory evidence of DIC, steroid therapy may be given to promote fetal lung maturity at gestational ages under 34 weeks for 24 to 48 hours if maternal and fetal conditions remain stable to complete the course. During this period of conservative management, maternal and fetal conditions must be continuously assessed.

HELLP syndrome is not an indication for immediate cesarean delivery. Guidelines similar to those described above for women with severe preeclampsia should be followed. The use of pudendal block or epidural anesthesia is contraindicated because of the bleeding risk. General anesthesia is the method of choice for cesarean delivery.

After delivery, the woman with HELLP syndrome should be monitored closely in an intensive care facility (labor and delivery recovery unit or medical/surgical intensive care unit) for at least 48 hours. Most women show evidence of resolution of the disease process within 48 hours postpartum. Some (especially those with DIC) may demonstrate delayed resolution or even deterioration. These

Table 27.8 Protocol for the Management of Eclampsia

- Convulsions are controlled or prevented with a loading dose of 6 g magnesium sulfate in 100 mL of 5% dextrose in Ringer lactated solution, given over 15 min, followed by a maintenance dose of 2 g/h. The dose is adjusted according to patellar reflexes and urine output in the previous 4-h period
  - Induction or delivery is initiated within 4 h after maternal stabilization
  - Magnesium sulfate is continued for 24 h after delivery or, if postpartum, 24 h after the last convulsion. In some cases, the infusion may be continued for a longer period
  - Diuretics, plasma volume expanders, and invasive hemodynamic monitoring used only if clinically indicated

women are at risk for the development of pulmonary edema from transfusion of blood products, fluid mobilization, and compromised renal function and should be closely monitored.

HELLP syndrome may also develop in the postpartum period. The time of onset in the postpartum group ranges from a few hours to 6 days, with the majority developing HELLP syndrome within 48 hours postpartum. Postpartum management is similar to that in the antepartum woman with HELLP syndrome, including the need for antiseizure prophylaxis. Steroids (dexamethasone or betamethasone) have been suggested in a few studies to improve the hematological parameters and, possibly, the clinical outcome of HELLP syndrome.[60,61] However, the use of steroids in HELLP syndrome is considered experimental.

Women presenting with shoulder pain, shock, or evidence of massive ascites or pleural effusions should have imaging studies of the liver to rule out the presence of subcapsular hematoma of the liver. A ruptured subcapsular liver hematoma resulting in shock is a surgical emergency requiring an acute multidisciplinary approach. Resuscitation should consist of massive transfusion of blood products, correction of coagulopathy with fresh frozen plasma (FFP) and platelets, and immediate laparotomy. Options at laparotomy include any combination of the following: packing, drainage, surgical ligation of the hepatic artery, embolization of the hepatic artery to the involved liver segment, resection of the involved hepatic segment, and liver transplantation, if indicated.[39] (**Table 27.9**).

CHTN and CHTN With Superimposed Preeclampsia

Uncomplicated CHTN in pregnancy is labeled low-risk CHTN, whereas the high-risk group (**Table 27.10**) includes patients with renal disease, diabetes mellitus, and other comorbidities. The discussion of management focuses on the control of blood pressure and the assessment of fetal and maternal well-being. Women should be seen by a nutritionist and given dietary advice. Daily sodium intake should be restricted to 2 g. The harmful effects of smoking, stress, and caffeine on maternal blood pressure and fetal well-being are emphasized, and frequent rest periods are encouraged.

Women with severe CHTN in early pregnancy or underlying renal disease require early referral for

Table 27.9 Evaluation of Pregnancy Complicated by Chronic Hypertension

Name:	Date of birth:
Parity: G. . . P. . .:	LMP:
Gestational age:	EDD or EDC:

Ultrasound:
  First-trimester ultrasound (for correct dating and nuchal translucence [NT] measurement)
  Fetal biometry/anatomy ultrasound (at 18-20 wk)
  Follow-up growth ultrasound at 3-weekly intervals starting in late second trimester

Fetal testing starting in late second or early third trimester (for patients with renal insufficiency):
  Twice-weekly testing or BPP
  Nonstress test (NST) if there is poor growth
  NST and Doppler studies if IUGR (<10%)

Renal evaluation: 24-h urine protein and creatinine clearance
electrolytes, urea, and creatinine levels
OR urine protein creatinine ratio
ECG: (cardiology consultation if ECG is abnormal)
Cardiac echocardiography:
Comments/comorbid conditions:

BPP, biophysical profile; ECG, electrocardiogram; EDC, estimated date of conception; EDD, estimated delivery date; IUGR, intrauterine growth restriction; LMP, last menstrual period.

antenatal care, intensive fetal and maternal monitoring as described earlier, and delivery in a tertiary care center. Antihypertensive therapy is indicated and should maintain systolic blood pressure between 140 and 150 mm Hg and diastolic pressure between 90 and 100 mm Hg. Persistent blood pressure levels below these ranges in women who have previously been very hypertensive may jeopardize placental perfusion.

Pharmacologic Treatment

Antiseizure Medications in Preeclampsia

Magnesium causes relaxation of smooth muscle by competing with calcium for entry into cells at the time of cellular depolarization, but its exact mechanism of action in the control of eclamptic seizures is unknown. Central nervous system depression and suppression of neuronal activity are postulated as mechanisms. The antiseizure benefit of magnesium may be the result of antagonism at the N-methyl-D-aspartate receptors.[65] Additional theories about the efficacy of magnesium sulfate therapy for seizure prophylaxis include its role as a cerebral

Table 27.10 High-Risk Factors of Chronic Hypertension in Pregnancy

Maternal age older than 40 y (may consider age ≥ 35 y)
Duration of hypertension more than 15 y
Blood pressure exceeding 160 over 110 mm Hg early in pregnancy
Diabetes mellitus (classes B-F)
Cardiomyopathy
Renal disease
Connective tissue disorders
Consider morbid obesity (weight ≥ 300 lb)

vasodilator (particularly acting on the smaller diameter vessels). The potential for magnesium to relieve cerebral ischemia through its antagonism of calcium-dependent arterial constriction may explain its antiseizure activity. Conversely, once widespread cerebral vasoconstriction has occurred in severe preeclampsia, the resultant cerebral ischemia could lower the threshold for seizure activity in those affected areas.[66]

The first sign of magnesium toxicity is loss of patellar reflexes (10-12 mg/dL). Other early signs and symptoms of magnesium toxicity include nausea, feeling of warmth, flushing, slurred speech, and somnolence (9-12 mg/dL). Magnesium toxicity should also be considered in women who do not regain consciousness after an eclamptic seizure.

Serum magnesium levels may also be used for monitoring evidence of drug toxicity. Magnesium is excreted by the kidneys; renal dysfunction may result in toxicity. The following guidelines may help to prevent magnesium toxicity:

- Monitor hourly urine output;
- Evaluate deep tendon reflexes hourly;
- Monitor respiratory rate; and
- Monitor serum magnesium levels regularly.

Antihypertensive Therapy

Treatment of severe hypertension is associated with a reduction in maternal morbidity and mortality. Severe elevations in blood pressure are associated with acute maternal cerebrovascular and coronary events; however, the blood pressure level at which adverse events are increase is not precisely known and is likely to vary depending on comorbidities. Importantly, antihypertensive therapy does not prevent preeclampsia or abruptio placentae, nor does it improve perinatal outcome.[53] First-line long-term pharmacologic treatment of pregnancy women with hypertension includes labetalol and nifedipine.

Alpha- and Beta-Blocking Agents

Labetalol is a nonselective, combined alpha- and beta-adrenoceptor blocker and the most commonly used antihypertensive agent in pregnancy. Parenteral labetalol has a rapid onset of action. It can be used for immediate and long-term control of blood pressure. The initial intravenous dose is 20 mg with subsequent escalating doses every 20 minutes (40 mg and then 80 mg) until either a desired effect or a maximum dose of 300 mg is reached. Oral labetalol may also be used for long-term therapy: an initial oral dose of 200 mg twice daily may be increased to a maximum daily dose of 2400 mg. Side effects of labetalol therapy include scalp tingling, tremulousness, and headache. Another maternal side effect is bronchoconstriction; therefore, labetalol should be avoided in patients with asthma as well as those with bradycardia.[12] Avoid the use of labetalol in women with second-degree heart block.

Other beta blockers (metoprolol, atenolol, oxprenolol) have been studied in pregnancy. Use of atenolol in the first trimester has been reported to be associated with intrauterine growth restriction, but the evidence is inconclusive.[67] Metoprolol is sometimes used as a last resort in the management of hypertension not responding to other common antihypertensive agents.

Calcium Channel Blockers

Calcium channel blockers (CCBs) have a very good safety profile in pregnancy and have been used successfully to manage hypertension in pregnancy. They may have a renoprotective effect that might be useful in patients with renal insufficiency. Nifedipine is a dihydropyridine CCB that can be associated with fusing, peripheral edema, reflex tachycardia, and headache. Nifedipine is used extensively in obstetric practice for both blood pressure control and preterm labor with no obvious teratogenic effects documented. The maximum daily dose for nifedipine is 120 mg. Common side effects include headache, flushing, tachycardia, and fatigue. Caution is advised when administering nifedipine with magnesium due to reports of hypotension and neuromuscular blockade.[68]

Nifedipine is available orally in both short-acting and extended-release forms. It may improve uteroplacental blood flow and has a tocolytic effect on the uterus. In addition to oral therapy for CHTN in pregnancy, nifedipine may be used for emergent reduction of severe hypertension. The use of sublingual nifedipine in the past for rapid reduction in blood pressure posed significant risks to the mother and fetus; hence, the sublingual route is contraindicated in pregnancy.

Although less often used, other CCBs (verapamil and diltiazem) may be used for blood pressure control in patients with cardiac disease. Additional experience with verapamil use in pregnancy is available because of its use in treating arrhythmias in pregnancy.

Hydralazine

Hydralazine is a potent vasodilator that acts directly on smooth muscle. It is administered as an intravenous bolus injection. After intravenous administration, the hypotensive effects develop gradually over 15 to 30 minutes. The usual bolus dose is 5 to 10 mg to be repeated every 20 to 40 minutes as needed. Maternal side effects include maternal hypotension, reflex tachycardia, headache, facial flushing, palpitations, nausea, and vomiting. Fetal distress secondary to hypotension has been reported from overtreatment in two of six cases.[69] Chronic administration may be associated with a maternal lupus syndrome and neonatal thrombocytopenia. Oral hydralazine is a weak antihypertensive when used alone and is usually combined with another first-line medication or diuretic.

Sodium Nitroprusside

Sodium nitroprusside is a potent arterial and venous dilator used for emergency therapy of patients with hypertensive crisis. It is given as a continuous intravenous infusion because of its immediate onset of action and short duration of action (1-10 minutes). It is metabolized by the liver and excreted by the kidneys. The initial infusion dose in gravid women should be 0.2 µg/kg/min rather than the usual dose of 0.5 µg/kg/min, as is standard in nonpregnant patients. This drug should be reserved for hypertensive emergencies because of concerns about thiocyanate toxicity in the neonate if used longer than 4 hours. Thus, nitroprusside is generally viewed as an agent used if other first- and second-line agents have failed to achieve adequate blood pressure control.[70]

Diuretics

Thiazide diuretics are commonly used to treat hypertension in the nonpregnant population, but their role in pregnancy is highly controversial. Although patients with preeclampsia and eclampsia may have edema and appear to be fluid overloaded, they are very frequently intravascularly depleted and may have a marked reduction in volume if treated with diuretics.[45] Plasma volume depletion is associated with poor perinatal outcomes. However, there is no reason not to use a diuretic in the postpartum period when there is pooling of fluid from the periphery and the uterus into the circulation, thus increasing the intravascular fluid volume. We recommend that more physicians start using diuretics as first-line antihypertensive agents in the postpartum period.

Thiazide diuretics may cause hyperglycemia, thus adversely affecting the control of hyperglycemia in patients with diabetes, but this side effect is unlikely to have a huge impact on outcome because these medications are only used for a short period. Other side effects include hyponatremia, hyperuricemia, acute pancreatitis, and fetal thrombocytopenia.

Loop diuretics are useful in patients with signs of fluid overload or pulmonary edema. Prolonged use of loop diuretics may lead to hypokalemia. Therefore, the serum potassium level should be checked if the woman is receiving a loop diuretic for more than a couple of days.

Angiotensin-Converting Enzyme Inhibitors

The chronic use of angiotensin-converting enzyme (ACE) inhibitors in pregnancy is associated with fetal renal insufficiency/renal failure, fetal growth retardation, oligohydramnios, cranial anomalies, severe fetal hypotension, and death, especially in the second and third trimesters. Therefore, ACE inhibitors are contraindicated in pregnancy but may be useful in the postpartum period.[45] Postpartum use of ACE inhibitors is indicated for women with diabetic kidney disease and peripartum cardiomyopathy. Women are advised to stop ACE inhibitors prior to conception; however, if exposed to ACE inhibitors in the first trimester, the medication may be stopped without significant damage to the fetus.

Aspirin

Evidence has shown that an imbalance in prostacyclin and thromboxane A_2 metabolism is involved in the development of preeclampsia, which has prompted interest in the study of aspirin for preeclampsia prevention.[71] There is a preferential inhibition of thromboxane at lower doses of aspirin as well as platelet aggregation. In 2014, the ACOG recommended that women at high risk of preeclampsia should start aspirin treatment with 81 mg daily between 12 and 28 weeks and should continue until delivery.[72] Initiating after 28 weeks is unlikely to be beneficial and should not be used in women with risk factors for gastrointestinal hemorrhage (eg, bleeding disorders or peptic ulcer disease).

KEY POINTS

- Hypertensive disorders or pregnancy are one of the most common medical complications of pregnancy, being present in 10% of pregnancies.
- Preeclampsia without severe features is systolic blood pressure (BP) ≥ 140 mm Hg or diastolic BP ≥ 90 mm Hg observed on two occasions at least 4 hours apart with proteinuria, OR new onset thrombocytopenia, renal insufficiency, or impaired renal insufficiency.
- Preeclampsia with severe features is systolic BP ≥ 160 mm Hg or diastolic BP ≥ 110 mm Hg or the presence of cerebral or visual disturbances. Other features of severe preeclampsia include persistent headache, persistent visual changes (scotomata), right upper quadrant pain, epigastric pain, nausea, and vomiting.
- The pathophysiology of preeclampsia is thought to be related to abnormal placentation and placental ischemia.
- Preeclampsia and eclampsia may be associated with the development of posterior reversible encephalopathy syndrome (PRES).
- The outcome in women with chronic hypertension (CHTN) is closely related to the development of superimposed preeclampsia and abruptio placentae.
- Patients with hypertension in pregnancy have an increased incidence of eclampsia, abruptio placentae, preterm delivery (mainly iatrogenic preterm delivery due to obstetric intervention secondary to hypertension or its complications), disseminated intravascular coagulation (DIC), hemorrhage, renal insufficiency, pulmonary edema, stroke, and death.
- Hypertension in pregnancy increases perinatal morbidity and mortality including preterm delivery/prematurity and intrauterine growth retardation.
- Treatment of severe hypertension is associated with a reduction in maternal morbidity and mortality, but does not prevent preeclampsia or abruptio placentae, nor does it improve perinatal outcomes.
- The most effective therapy for preeclampsia is delivery of the fetus and placenta.
- No clinically useful and universally accepted predictive or screening test has been identified for preeclampsia.
- Preconception counseling is very important in the management of patients with CHTN. It is important to establish the etiology and severity of hypertension, to identify end-organ damage, and to achieve adequate blood pressure control prior to conception.
- Because of their renoprotective effects, calcium channel blockers (i.e., nifedipine) are helpful in patients with CHTN and diabetes mellitus.
- Angiotensin-converting enzyme inhibitors may cause fetal renal insufficiency, oligohydramnios, growth restriction, cranial anomalies, and severe fetal hypotension especially in the second and third trimesters.
- ACOG's 2014 recommendations for women at high risk of preeclampsia are to start aspirin treatment with 81 mg daily between 12 and 28 weeks and to continue until delivery.

REFERENCES

(only references cited in synoptic print chapter; for a complete reference list, see ebook)

1. Steegers EA, von Dadelszen P, Duvekot JJ, et al. Pre-eclampsia. *Lancet.* 2010;376:631-644.
2. Gestational Hypertension and Preeclampsia. ACOG Practice Bulletin No. 202. American College of Obstetricians and Gynecologists. *Obstet Gynecol.* 2019;133:e1-e25.
3. Nissaisorakarn P, Sharif S, Belinda J. Hypertension in pregnancy: defining blood pressure goals and the value of biomarkers for preeclampsia. *Curr Cardiol Rep.* 2016;18(12):131. doi:0.1007/s11886-016-0782-1
4. Ankumah NE, Sibai BM. Chronic hypertension in pregnancy: diagnosis, management, and outcomes. *Clin Obstet Gynecol.* 2017;60(1):206-214. doi:10.1097/grf.0000000000000255
6. Sibai BM. Management of late preterm and early-term pregnancies complicated by mild gestational hypertension/pre-eclampsia. *Semin Perinatol.* 2011;35(5):292-296. doi:10.1053/j.semperi.2011.05.010
7. Chronic Hypertension in Pregnancy. ACOG Practice Bulletin No. 203. American College of Obstetricians and Gynecologists. *Obstet Gynecol.* 2019;133:e26-e50.
10. Leeman L, Dresano LT, Fontaine P. Hypertensive disorders of pregnancy. *Am Fam Physician.* 2016;93:121-127.
12. Garovic VD. Hypertension in pregnancy: diagnosis and treatment. *Mayo Clin Proc.* 2000;75:1071-1076.
13. Wilkerson RG, Ogunbodede AC. Hypertensive disorders of pregnancy. *Emerg Med Clin North Am.* 2019;37(2):301-316. doi:10.1016/j.emc.2019.01.008
14. Sperling JD, Dahlke JD, Huber WJ, et al. The role of headache in the classification and management of hypertensive disorders in pregnancy. *Obstet Gynecol.* 2015;126:297-302.
15. Thangaratinam S, Gallos ID, Meah N, et al; TIPPS (Tests in Prediction of Preeclampsia's Severity) Review Group. How accurate are maternal symptoms in predicting impending complications in women with preeclampsia? A systematic review and meta-analysis. *Acta Obstet Gynecol Scand.* 2011;90:564-573.
16. Phipps E, Prasanna D, Brima W, Jim B. Preeclampsia: updates in pathogenesis, definitions, and guidelines. *Clin J Am Soc Nephrol.* 2016;11(6):1102-1113. doi:10.2215/cjn.12081115
17. Newman MG, Robichaux AG, Stedman CM, et al. Perinatal outcomes in preeclampsia that is complicated by massive proteinuria. *Am J Obstet Gynecol.* 2003;188(1):264-268.
18. Bokslag A, van Weissenbruch M, Mol BW, de Groot CJ. Preeclampsia: short and long-term consequences for mother and neonate. *Early Hum Dev.* 2016;102:47-50.
19. Mayrink J, Costa ML, Cecatti JG. Preeclampsia in 2018: revisiting concepts, physiopathology, and prediction. *Sci World J.* 2018;2018:6268276. doi:10.1155/2018/6268276
20. Jim B, Karumanchi SA. Preeclampsia: pathogenesis, prevention, and long-term complications. *Semin Nephrol.* 2017;37:386-397. doi:10.1016/j.semnephrol.2017.05.011
21. El-Sayed AAF. Preeclampsia: a review of the pathogenesis and possible management strategies based on its pathophysiological derangements. *Taiwan J Obstet Gynecol.* 2017;56(5):593-598. doi:10.1016/j.tjog.2017.08.004
22. Roberts JM, Hubel CA. The two stage model of preeclampsia: variations on the theme. *Placenta.* 2009;30(suppl A):S32-S37.
24. Sibai BM. Best practices for diagnosis and management of preeclampsia. Part 1 of 3. Preeclampsia: 3 preemptive tactics. *Obstet Gynecol Manage.* 2005;17(2):20-32.
26. Vigil-De Gracia P, Ramirez R, Duran Y, et al. Magnesium sulfate for 6 vs 24 hours post delivery in patients who received magnesium sulfate for less than 8 hours before birth: a randomized clinical trial. *BMC Pregnancy Childbirth.* 2017;17(1):241. doi:10.1186/s12884-017-1424-3
27. Berhan Y, Berhan A. Should magnesium sulfate be administered to women with mild pre-eclampsia? A systematic review of published reports on eclampsia. *J Obstet Gynaecol Res.* 2015;41(6):831-842.
28. Hart LA, Sibai BM. Seizures in pregnancy: epilepsy, eclampsia, and stroke. *Semin Perinatol.* 2013;37(4):207-224. doi:10.1053/j.semperi.2013.04.001
31. Sibai BM, Spinnato JA, Watson DL, et al. Eclampsia IV. Neurological findings and future outcome. *Am J Obstet Gynecol.* 1985;152:184.

35. Sibai BM, Taslimi MM, El-Nazer A, et al. Maternal-perinatal outcome associated with the syndrome of hemolysis, elevated liver enzymes, and low platelets in severe preeclampsia-eclampsia. *Am J Obstet Gynecol.* 1986;155:501.
38. Sibai BM. Diagnosis, controversies, and management of the syndrome of hemolysis, elevated liver enzymes, and low platelet count. *Obstet Gynecol.* 2004;103(5 pt 1):981-991.
39. Haram K, Svendsen E, Abildgaard U. The HELLP syndrome: clinical issues and management. A review. *BMC Pregnancy Childbirth.* 2009;9:8.
40. Ditisheim A, Sibai BM. Diagnosis and management of HELLP syndrome complicated by liver hematoma. *Clin Obstet Gynecol.* 2017;60:190-197.
45. Sibai BM, Abdella TN, Anderson GD. Pregnancy outcome in 211 patients with mild chronic hypertension. *Obstet Gynecol.* 1983;61:571.
47. Moussa HN, Arian SE, Sibai BM. Management of hypertensive disorders in pregnancy. *Womens Health.* 2014;10(4):385-404.
48. Khosravi S, Dabiran S, Lotfi M, et al. Study of the prevalence of hypertension and complications of hypertensive disorders in pregnancy. *Open J Prev Med.* 2014;4(11):860-867.
50. Sibai BM, Stella CL. Diagnosis and management of atypical preeclampsia-eclampsia. *Am J Obstet Gynecol.* 2009;200:481.e1-481.e7.
51. Sibai BM. Diagnosis and management of gestational hypertension and preeclampsia. *Obstet Gynecol.* 2003;102(1):181-192.
52. Bernstein PS, Martin JN Jr, Barton JR, et al. National Partnership for Maternal Safety: consensus bundle on severe hypertension during pregnancy and the postpartum period. *Obstet Gynecol.* 2017;130:347-357.
53. Roberts JM, August PA, Bakris G, et al. Hypertension in pregnancy report of the American College of Obstetricians and Gynecologists' Task Force on hypertension in pregnancy. *Obstet Gynecol.* 2013;122(5):1122-1131.
54. Barton JR, O'Brien JM, Bergauer NK, et al. Mild gestational hypertension remote from term: progression and outcome. *Am J Obstet Gynecol.* 2001;184(5):979-983.
55. Ganzevoort W, Sibai BM. Temporising versus interventionist management (preterm and at term). *Best Pract Res Clin Obstet Gynaecol.* 2011;25:463-476.
56. Sibai BM; Publications Committee, Society for Maternal-Fetal Medicine. Evaluation and management of severe preeclampsia before 34 weeks' gestation. *Am J Obstet Gynecol.* 2011;205:191-198.
57. Calhoun DA, Oparil S. Treatment of hypertensive crisis. *N Engl J Med.* 1990;323:1177-1183.
58. Sibai BM, Mercer BM, Schiff E, et al. Aggressive versus expectant management of severe preeclampsia at 28 to 32 weeks gestation: a randomized controlled trial. *Am J Obstet Gynecol.* 1994;174:818-822.
59. Paul RH, Koh KS, Bernstein SG. Changes in fetal heart rate—uterine contraction patterns associated with eclampsia. *Am J Obstet Gynecol.* 1978;130:165.
60. Isler CM, Magann EF, Rinehart BK, et al. Dexamethasone compared with betamethasone for glucocorticoid treatment of postpartum HELLP syndrome. *Int J Gynecol Obstet.* 2003;80:291-297.
61. Mao M, Chen C. Corticosteroid therapy for management of hemolysis, elevated liver enzymes, and low platelet count (HELLP) syndrome: a meta-analysis. *Med Sci Monit.* 2015;21:3777-3783.
65. Lambert G, Brichant JF, Hartstein G, et al. Preeclampsia: an update. *Acta Anaesthesiol Belg.* 2014;65(4):137-149.
66. Belfort MA, Moise KJ. Effect of magnesium sulfate on maternal brain blood flow in preeclampsia: a randomized, placebo-controlled study. *Am J Obstet Gynecol.* 1992;167:661-666.
67. Chahine KM, Sibai BM. Chronic hypertension in pregnancy: new concepts for classification and management. *Am J Perinatol.* 2018;36(2):161-168. doi:10.1055/s0038-1666976
68. Ben-Ami M, Giladi Y, Shalev E. The combination of magnesium sulphate and nifedipine: a cause of neuromuscular blockade. *Br J Obstet Gynaecol.* 1994;101(3):262-263.
69. ElFarra J, Bean C, Martin JN. Management of hypertensive crisis for the obstetrician/gynecologist. *Obstet Gynecol Clin North Am.* 2016;43(4):623-637.
70. Magee LA, Abalos E, Dadelszen von P, et al. How to manage hypertension in pregnancy effectively. *Br J Clin Pharmacol.* 2011;72(3):394-401.
71. Masotti G, Galanti G, Poggesi L, et al. Differential inhibition of prostacyclin production and platelet aggregation by aspirin. *Lancet.* 1979;2:1213-1217.
72. LeFevre ML. Low-dose aspirin use for the prevention of morbidity and mortality from preeclampsia: U.S. Preventive Services Task Force recommendation statement. U.S. Preventive Services Task Force. *Ann Intern Med.* 2014;161:819-826.

CHAPTER 28

Cardiac Diseases in Pregnancy

Ji Eun Park, Charles C. Hong, and
Susie N. Hong

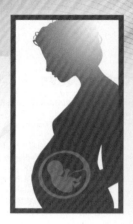

Introduction

Advances in cardiovascular medicine and cardiothoracic surgery have improved long-term outcomes in patients with congenital heart disease (CHD), and as such, most patients with CHD reach childbearing age. Given an observed increasing prevalence of pregnancies among women with cardiovascular disease, estimated to range between 0.1% and 4%, the need for obstetricians to be well-versed in proper counseling and management of these conditions is paramount.[1] Despite advances in the diagnosis and management of maternal cardiovascular disease, such conditions continue to account for 15% of maternal deaths in pregnancy.[2] This chapter focuses on the interaction between structural cardiovascular disease and pregnancy, with an emphasis on the means of achieving optimal maternal and perinatal outcomes.

Clinical Assessment of the Cardiac Patient During Pregnancy

Prepregnancy counseling in women with cardiac disease is ideal to individualize peripartum cardiac risk. The World Health Organization (WHO) classification of maternal cardiovascular risk (**Table 28.1**) provides a lesion-based maternal risk assessment that is widely utilized.[3,4]

The WHO classification takes into account the New York Heart Association (NYHA) classification of heart failure (HF) based on clinical function (classes I-IV, **Table 28.2**).

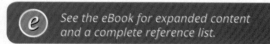

See the eBook for expanded content and a complete reference list.

The Cardiac Disease in Pregnancy (CARPREG) study identified four predictors of maternal cardiac events: prior cardiac event or arrhythmias, poor functional status (NYHA class III or IV) or cyanosis, high-risk left-sided valvular lesion or obstruction, and left ventricular (LV) systolic dysfunction (ejection fraction [EF] < 40%).[7] The predictors were further evaluated in CARPREG II, with the addition of lesion-specific variables (mechanical prosthesis, coronary artery disease, high-risk aortopathy, and pulmonary hypertension [PH]) and late pregnancy assessment into a risk score.[8]

The Boston Adult Congenital Heart group found reduced right ventricular (RV) function and severe pulmonic regurgitation (PR) were predictors of adverse cardiac outcomes in pregnancy.[9] Additionally, the ZAHARA (Zwangerschap bij Aangeboren HARtAfwijking) study investigated outcomes with particular interest in women with CHD, finding that moderate to severe aortic or pulmonic valve regurgitation, presence of a mechanical valve prosthesis, and cyanotic heart disease were independent predictors of adverse outcomes.[10] The WHO classification, incorporating these predictors from the above studies, has been validated in pregnant women with heart disease, both in resource-rich and resource-limited settings.[11,12]

These studies have shown that, although women with cardiac disease have significant morbidity, maternal mortality is rare at <1%.[7,8,11,13,14] However, maternal mortality is higher in women with heart disease compared to the general population.[13,15,16]

However, not all clinical variables can be captured through risk predictors or indices and individual patient risk assessment based on clinical judgment remains crucial to providing the best possible pre-, peri-, and antenatal patient care.

Table 28.1 Modified WHO Classification of Maternal Cardiovascular Risk

	WHO I	WHO II	WHO II-III	WHO III	WHO IV
Diagnosis	Small or mild • pulmonary stenosis • patent ductus arteriosus • mitral valve prolapse Successfully repaired simple lesions (atrial or ventricular septal defect, patent ductus arteriosus, anomalous pulmonary venous drainage)	Unoperated atrial or ventricular septal defect Repaired tetralogy of Fallot Supraventricular tachycardias Turner syndrome without aortic dilatation	Mild left ventricular impairment (EF > 45%) Hypertrophic cardiomyopathy Native or tissue valve disease not considered WHO I or IV (mild mitral stenosis, moderate aortic stenosis) Marfan syndrome without aortic dilatation Repaired coarctation	Moderate left ventricular impairment (EF 30%-45%) Previous peripartum cardiomyopathy without any residual left ventricular impairment Mechanical valve Unrepaired cyanotic heart disease Other complex heart disease Moderate mitral stenosis Severe asymptomatic aortic stenosis Moderate aortic dilatation Ventricular tachycardia	Pulmonary arterial hypertension Severe systemic ventricular dysfunction (EF < 30% or NYHA class III-IV) Previous peripartum cardiomyopathy with any residual left ventricular impairment Severe mitral stenosis Severe symptomatic aortic stenosis Systemic right ventricle with moderate or severely decreased ventricular function Severe aortic dilatation Vascular Ehlers-Danlos Severe (re)coarctation
Risk	No detectable increased risk of maternal mortality and no/mild increased risk in morbidity	Small increased risk of maternal mortality or moderate increase in morbidity	Intermediate increased risk of maternal mortality or moderate to severe increase in morbidity	Significantly increased risk of maternal mortality or severe morbidity	Extremely high risk of maternal mortality or severe morbidity
Maternal cardiac event rate	2.5%-5%	5.7%-10.5%	10%-19%	19%-27%	40%-100%

EF, ejection fraction; NYHA, New York Heart Association; WHO, World Health Organization classification.
Modified from Regitz-Zagrosek V, Roos-Hesselink JW, Bauersachs J, et al. 2018 ESC Guidelines for the management of cardiovascular diseases during pregnancy. *Eur Heart J.* 2018;39(34):3165-3241 by permission of Oxford University Press.

Specific Maternal Cardiac Diseases Affecting Pregnancy

Arrhythmias

Clinical Presentation

Pregnancy, especially in the setting of cardiac disease, may increase the risk of arrhythmias and arrhythmia exacerbation. Supraventricular tachycardias (SVTs), as well as atrial fibrillation and atrial flutter, are more common in pregnancies in women with CHD than in women without CHD. Importantly, although generally well tolerated (WHO risk class II), adverse maternal and fetal outcomes have been described with SVT in pregnancy, emphasizing the need for treatment.[3,19]

Table 28.2 New York Heart Association (NYHA) Functional Classification for Heart Failure

Functional Class	Symptoms
I	No limitation of physical activity. Ordinary physical activity does not cause undue fatigue, palpitation, or dyspnea.
II	Slight limitation of physical activity. Comfortable at rest. Ordinary physical activity results in fatigue, palpitation, or dyspnea.
III	Marked limitation of physical activity. Comfortable at rest. Less than ordinary activity causes fatigue, palpitation, or dyspnea.
IV	Unable to carry on any physical activity without discomfort. Symptoms of heart failure at rest. If any physical activity is undertaken, discomfort increases.

Adapted from Regitz-Zagrosek V, Roos-Hesselink JW, Bauersachs J, et al. 2018 ESC Guidelines for the management of cardiovascular diseases during pregnancy. *Eur Heart J.* 2018;39(34):3165-3241.

Pharmacologic Treatment

Beta blockers, such as metoprolol and propranolol, although effective, must be used through joint decision-making with the mother given the risk of intrauterine growth restriction. Verapamil or digoxin may be used, as well as, less commonly, flecainide, propafenone, or sotalol.[3,20] In cases of supraventricular arrhythmias refractory to pharmacologic therapy, catheter ablation or cardioversion may be necessary.

Congenital Cardiac Diseases

Advances in cardiovascular intervention and cardiothoracic surgery have enabled the surgical correction of many previously fatal congenital cardiac lesions. Thus, patients with CHD now account for the vast majority of pregnant women with heart disease.

We preface our discussion regarding congenital cardiac lesions with the acknowledgment that patients at risk of developing right-to-left shunts with increased PH are at highest risk for unacceptably high maternal and fetal morbidity and mortality; surgical correction prior to the development of increased pulmonary vascular resistance and PH

(Eisenmenger syndrome) is the greatest single contributor to improved outcomes observed over the preceding 4 decades.

Atrial Sepal Defects
Clinical Presentation

Atrial septal defects (ASDs) are the most common congenital lesions seen during pregnancy and are generally asymptomatic.[25,26]

The two significant potential complications seen with ASDs are arrhythmias and right atrial and/or ventricular enlargement.

As a result of pregnancy-associated increases in atrial volume, biatrial enlargement and resultant supraventricular dysrhythmias are occasionally encountered. In general, although atrial arrhythmias are not uncommon in patients with ASDs, their onset generally occurs after the fourth decade of life. Thus, such arrhythmias are unlikely to be encountered in the majority of pregnant women. That said, in patients with ASDs, atrial fibrillation is the most common arrhythmia encountered; however, SVT and atrial flutter also may occur.[28]

ASDs are characterized by high pulmonary blood flow associated with normal pulmonary artery pressures. Because pulmonary artery pressures are low, PH is unusual.

Clinical Assessment

The hypervolemia and increased cardiac output associated with pregnancy accentuates the left-to-right shunt through the ASD, increasing the burden on the right ventricle. Those with impaired functional capacity, right atrial or RV enlargement, or a left-to-right shunt large enough to cause physiologic sequelae (pulmonary to systemic blood flow ratio Qp:Qs ≥ 1.5:1) should be evaluated for surgical or transcatheter closure prior to conception.[1]

Management of ASDs in Pregnancy

ASD closure is recommended postpartum for most patients who present initially during pregnancy.[1,3] Although ASDs are tolerated well by most patients, congestive failure and death have been reported.[29-31] Thus, peripartum management focuses on avoiding vascular resistance changes that increase the degree of the shunt.

The majority of patients with ASDs tolerate pregnancy, labor, and delivery without complication (WHO risk class II, with successfully repaired simple ASDs classified as WHO I).[3]

During labor, placement of the patient in the lateral recumbent position, avoidance of fluid overload, oxygen administration, and pain relief with epidural anesthesia to avoid increased cardiac output can be helpful.

Ventricular Septal Defects
Clinical Presentation
Ventricular septal defects (VSDs) may occur as an isolated lesion or in conjunction with other congenital cardiac anomalies, including tetralogy of Fallot, transposition of the great vessels, and coarctation of the aorta. The size of the septal defect is the most important determinant of clinical prognosis during pregnancy. Small defects are tolerated well, whereas larger defects in the high-pressure/high-flow, left-to-right shunt are associated more frequently with congestive heart failure (CHF), arrhythmias, and the development of PH.

Management of VSDs in Pregnancy
Management considerations for patients with uncomplicated VSDs are similar to those outlined for ASDs. Pregnancy, labor, and delivery are tolerated well by patients with uncomplicated VSD (WHO risk class II, with successfully repaired simple lesions classified as WHO risk I).[3] Schaefer and colleagues compiled a series of 141 pregnancies in 56 women with VSD.[29] The only two maternal deaths were in women whose VSD was complicated by PH (Eisenmenger syndrome).

Nonpharmacologic Treatment
Those with evidence of LV volume overload and hemodynamically significant shunts (Qp:Qs ≥ 1.5:1) should undergo VSD closure prior to pregnancy, as long as severe PH is not present.[1] Although very rarely indicated, successful primary closure of a large VSD during pregnancy has been reported.[30,32] Right heart catheterization with measurement of pulmonary pressures may be helpful to assist in determining appropriate treatments. In general, invasive hemodynamic monitoring is unnecessary.

Patent Ductus Arteriosus
Clinical Presentation
As with uncomplicated ASD and VSD, most patients are asymptomatic and pregnancy, labor, and delivery are generally well tolerated in patients with PDA (WHO risk class I).[3] As with a large VSD,

however, the high-pressure/high-flow, left-to-right shunt associated with a large, uncorrected PDA can lead to PH.

Management of PDA in Pregnancy
Management considerations for patients with uncomplicated PDA without PH are similar to those for patients with ASDs.

Nonpharmacologic Treatment
Those with evidence of left atrial or LV enlargement in the absence of severe PH should have transcatheter or surgical PDA closure performed prior to conception.[1]

PH and Eisenmenger Syndrome
Clinical Presentation
PH is defined as a mean pulmonary arterial pressure (PAP) ≥25 mm Hg at rest, diagnosed by right heart catheterization. PH is classified into five broad categories: idiopathic pulmonary arterial hypertension (PAH, WHO Group I); PH due to left heart disease (WHO Group II); PH due to lung disease (WHO Group III); PH due to thromboembolic disease (WHO Group IV); and PH due to unclear or multifactorial etiologies (WHO Group V).

PAH carries a high mortality risk during pregnancy, although this risk is decreasing,[34] because the pulmonary circulation is not able to adapt to increased cardiac output seen in pregnancy, leading to further increased PAP and RV failure.[34] PH is further exacerbated by the prothrombotic state of pregnancy.

Eisenmenger syndrome develops when, in the presence of left-to-right shunt, progressive PH leads to shunt reversal or bidirectional shunting as a result of chronically increased pulmonary vascular blood flow with accompanying pulmonary vascular resistance exceeding systemic vascular resistance. Although this syndrome may rarely occur with ASD, VSD, or PDA, the low-pressure/high-flow shunt seen in ASD is far less likely to result in PH and shunt reversal than is the condition of high-pressure/high-flow symptoms seen with VSD and PDA.

In Eisenmenger syndrome, during the antepartum period, decreased systemic vascular resistance in the setting of fixed, high pulmonary resistance increases both the likelihood and the degree of right-to-left shunting. Pulmonary perfusion decreases, with systemic hypotension resulting in hypoxemia with subsequent maternal, then fetal deterioration. The peripartum development of systemic hypotension leads to decreased RV filling pressures; in the concomitant presence of a fixed cardiac output state (eg, PH), such decreased right heart pressures may be insufficient to perfuse the pulmonary arterial bed, leading to a sudden and profound hypoxemia and death.

Eisenmenger syndrome associated with VSDs appears to carry a higher mortality risk than that associated with PDA or ASDs.

Thromboembolic phenomena have been associated with up to 43% of all maternal deaths in Eisenmenger syndrome.[37]

Sudden delayed postpartum death, occurring 4 to 6 weeks after delivery, has also been reported.[37,40] Such deaths may involve a rebound worsening of PH associated with the loss of pregnancy-associated hormones, causing RV failure, arrhythmias, or thromboembolic events.

Management of PH and Eisenmenger Syndrome in Pregnancy

The current American College of Cardiology (ACC) and European Society of Cardiology (ESC) guidelines advise against pregnancy in women with PAH and recommend termination for those who become pregnant due to the high mortality associated with continuing pregnancy (WHO risk class IV).[3,35]

Management centers on decreasing pulmonary vascular resistance, maintaining RV preload, LV afterload, and RV contractility. Thus, factors that increase pulmonary vascular resistance ought to be avoided, and patients should be routinely monitored for occurrence of symptoms, signs of HF, worsening RV function, and increased levels of brain natriuretic peptide.

The mainstays of therapy and management for hypoxia continue to be inpatient care in a tertiary care center with experienced clinicians, with continuous administration of oxygen, use of pulmonary vasodilators, avoidance of hypotension and anemia, judicious diuretic use as necessary, and limited use of operative deliveries requiring general anesthesia, as these have been associated with worse outcomes.[39,43,44]

Inhaled nitric oxide has been used to decrease pulmonary vascular resistance and improved pulmonary blood flow and oxygenation, in conjunction with supplemental oxygen.[35]

Evidence suggests early planned delivery around 32 to 34 weeks for women with moderate to severe PH and 35 to 37 weeks for women with mild PH may be reasonable.[34,41,42,45] Prophylaxis for endocarditis with antibiotics should be considered as described in **Table 28.3**.[22] Given the elevated mortality risk postpartum, immediately postdelivery patients should be monitored in an intensive care setting, where careful monitoring of hemodynamics can take place.[35] Additionally, current recommendations include at least 1 week of in-hospital monitoring for RV failure and PH medication titration.[35]

Table 28.3 Antibiotic Prophylaxis for Cardiac Lesions With Highest Risk of Bacterial Endocarditis

Cardiac lesion
Prosthetic cardiac valves or prosthetic material used for cardiac valve repair
Previous infective endocarditis
CHD:
Unrepaired cyanotic heart disease, including palliative shunts and conduits
Completely repaired CHD using prosthetic material or device, whether replaced by surgery or by transcatheter intervention, during the first 6 mo after procedure
Repaired CHD with residual defects at the site or adjacent to the site of a prosthetic patch or device
Patients who underwent cardiac transplantation with valvular regurgitation due to a structurally abnormal valve

CHD, congenital heart disease.

These recommendations are based on American College of Cardiology/American Heart Association guidelines, which specifically discourage endocarditis prophylaxis for "routine" vaginal or cesarean delivery. Specifically, the guidelines comment on prophylaxis as reasonable for patients *at the highest risk of adverse outcomes from infective endocarditis,* as listed above. Given a possible increased risk of endocarditis with complicated deliveries such as retained placenta, alongside recommendations to give antibiotics before or within 30 minutes of starting a "complicated" procedure, the decision to hold or administer bacterial endocarditis prophylaxis is not necessarily straightforward.[22] Thus, many obstetricians may elect to administer prophylactic antibiotics to cover unpredictable complicated deliveries.

Adapted from Nishimura RA, Otto CM, Bonow RO, et al. 2017 AHA/ACC focused update of the 2014 AHA/ACC Guideline for the management of patients with valvular heart disease: a report of the American College of Cardiology/American Heart Association Task Force on Clinical Practice Guidelines. *Circulation.* 2017;135(25):e1159-e1195.

Table 28.4 Reference Values With Central Hemodynamic Assessment

Parameter	Nonpregnant	Pregnant
Cardiac output (L/min)	4.3	6.2
Heart rate (bpm)	71	83
Pulmonary vascular resistance (dyne/cm/s⁵)	119	78
Systemic vascular resistance (dyne/cm/s⁵)	1530	1210
Mean arterial pressure (mm Hg)	86	90
Pulmonary capillary wedge pressure (mmHg)	6.3	7.5
Central venous pressure (mm Hg)	3.7	3.6

Bpm, beats per minute. Values are derived from 10 selected patients at 36 to 38 weeks' gestation and again at 11 to 13 weeks postpartum with arterial lines and Swan-Ganz catheters to characterize central hemodynamic values of pregnancy. From Clark SL, Cotton DB, Lee W, et al. Central hemodynamic assessment of normal term pregnancy. *Am J Obstet Gynecol.* 1989;161(6):1439-1442.

Invasive monitoring with an arterial line and central venous catheter is indicated for close monitoring for hypotension and volume status of the decompensating patient. A pulmonary artery catheter will provide useful information among some patients with moderate to severe PH from interatrial shunts.[6,44,47] Reference values are provided in **Table 28.4**.

However, among patients with interventricular shunts, catheter placement is associated with a high rate of complications, including arrhythmias, embolization, and pulmonary artery rupture.[34] In instances in which pulmonary artery catheterization may be of benefit, simultaneous cardiovascular imaging may be helpful in catheter placement. If the possibility of right-to-left shunting exists, balloon inflation with carbon dioxide is preferable to that with air in an effort to avoid systemic air embolus associated with the rare occurrence of balloon rupture.

In consideration of catheter placement, it is of note that, during labor, uterine contractions are associated with a decrease in the ratio of pulmonary to systemic blood flow.[48,49] Pulmonary artery catheterization and serial arterial blood gas determinations thus theoretically allow the clinician to detect and treat early changes in cardiac output, pulmonary artery pressure, and shunt fraction. Because the primary concern in such patients is the avoidance of hypotension, any attempt at preload reduction (ie, diuresis) must be undertaken with caution, even in the face of initial fluid overload. Some clinicians prefer to manage such patients on the "wet" side (wedge pressure range of 16-18 mm Hg), maintaining a preload margin of safety against unexpected blood loss with an a priori acknowledged risk of pulmonary edema. Because of the increased risk of significant blood loss and hypotension associated with operative delivery, cesarean delivery should be reserved for standard obstetric indications, although many patients have elected to schedule cesarean deliveries in an attempt to avoid overt hemodynamic fluctuations.[35] Similarly, midforceps delivery is not warranted to shorten the second stage but should be reserved for obstetric indications only. Likewise, large volume boluses should be avoided, as these can alter the peripartum hemodynamics.

The issue of pulmonary artery catheterization is controversial in Eisenmenger and specifically advised against in patients with this disorder the most recent ACC Scientific Statement.[35]

If operative delivery is necessary, meticulous attention to hemostasis and surgical technique with an experienced surgical team minimizes the risk of blood loss, hypotension, and death in these patients. Despite expert management, a substantial risk of maternal mortality remains during labor and delivery. Laparoscopic tubal ligation under local anesthesia has also been described in a group of women with various types of cyanotic cardiac disease.[50]

Anesthesia for patients with PH is controversial. Theoretically, general and single-dose spinal anesthesia, with its accompanying risk of hypotension, should be avoided. Regional techniques for both vaginal (epidural) and cesarean (spinal) delivery have been described and successfully used.[34,51]

Eisenmenger syndrome most frequently results from hemorrhage or complications of spinal anesthesia.[38] Thus, avoidance of systemic hypotension is the principal clinical concern in the intrapartum management of patients with PH of any etiology. This fact is underscored by the longstanding knowledge that the greatest maternal risk occurs in the peripartum period, and most deaths occur between

2 and 9 days' postpartum.[34] The precise pathophysiology of such decompensation is unclear, and it is uncertain what, if any, therapeutic maneuvers prevent or ameliorate such deterioration.

Pharmacologic Treatment

The therapies for PAH are specific to the disease; the therapies for other forms of PH are usually consistent of treating the underlying etiology, such as HF (WHO Group II), obstructive lung disease (WHO Group III), obstructive sleep apnea (WHO Group III), or chronic pulmonary embolism (WHO Group IV). Therapies for PAH include calcium channel blockers for those who have been shown to respond to vasoreactivity testing. Women with vasoreactive PH and on stable dosages of medications have been shown to have improved pregnancy outcomes as compared to those with nonvasoreactive PH, which makes up the majority of PH cases.[34] Phosphodiesterase inhibitors, such as sildenafil and tadalafil, and prostacyclin analogues, such as epoprostenol and treprostenil, have not been associated with increased fetal risk and are likely beneficial in women with PAH.[34] Endothelin receptor antagonists, such as bosentan and ambrisentan, as well as guanylate cyclase agonists, such as riociguat, have been shown to be teratogenic in animal studies, making them Federal Drug Administration category X.

Studies suggest that earlier institution of therapies is beneficial for PAH, and, thus, it is recommended to start therapies at least 3 months prior to delivery.[34]

In general, after Eisenmenger pathophysiology is established, PH is permanent, and surgical correction of the defect is unhelpful and increases mortality.[1,3,35,40]

Coarctation of the Aorta
Clinical Presentation

The most common site of coarctation is the origin of the left subclavian artery. Associated anomalies of the aorta and left heart, including VSDs and PDA, are common, as are intracranial aneurysms in the circle of Willis.[55] Coarctation is usually asymptomatic. Its presence is suggested by hypertension confined to the upper extremities.

Resting cardiac output may be increased, but increased left atrial pressure with exercise suggests occult LV dysfunction. Aneurysms may also develop below the coarctation, or involve the intercostal arteries, and may lead to rupture. In addition, ruptures without prior aneurysm formation have been reported.[54,55]

Tetralogy of Fallot
Clinical Presentation

Tetralogy of Fallot is a conotruncal defect that encompasses the cyanotic complex of VSD, overriding aorta, RV hypertrophy, and pulmonic valve stenosis.

Management of Tetralogy of Fallot in Pregnancy

Most cases of tetralogy of Fallot are corrected during infancy or childhood; the vast majority of women may be assumed to have undergone repair in order to survive to reproductive age. Several published reports attest to the relatively good outcome of pregnancy in patients with corrected tetralogy of Fallot, with cardiac complications in 8%, due to arrhythmias and HF (WHO risk class II).[3,58]

However, in patients with unrepaired Tetralogy, maternal mortality ranged from 4% to 15%, with 30% fetal mortality as a result of hypoxia.[5,59] In patients with uncorrected VSD, the decline in systematic vascular resistance that accompanies pregnancy can lead to worsening of the right-to-left shunt.[5] This condition can be aggravated further by systemic hypotension as a result of peripartum blood loss. A poor prognosis has been associated with RV dysfunction and severe PR.[3]

Pulmonic Stenosis
Clinical Presentation

Pulmonic stenosis is a common congenital defect. Although obstruction can be valvular, supravalvular, or subvalvular, the degree of obstruction, rather than its site, is the principal determinant of clinical performance. A transvalvular pressure gradient exceeding 60 mm Hg is considered severe and can result in right HF and arrhythmias. Pulmonic stenosis in association with cyanotic congenital lesions has a worse prognosis.

Management of Pulmonic Stenosis in Pregnancy

Pregnancy in women with mild (classified as WHO risk class I) and moderate pulmonic stenosis is generally well tolerated.[3]

Most patients can be managed medically, but percutaneous balloon valvuloplasty is an option if resistant to medical therapy. Severe pulmonic stenosis mandates surgical correction.[6]

Ebstein Anomaly
Clinical Presentation
Ebstein anomaly consists of apical displacement of the tricuspid valve with secondary tricuspid regurgitation (TR) and enlargement of both the right atrium and ventricle, resulting in variable clinical presentation, including asymptomatic patients to those with cyanosis and HF. Ebstein anomaly has also been associated with an increased risk of SVT, including atrioventricular reentrant tachycardia.[63]

Management of Ebstein Anomaly in Pregnancy
Pregnancy in women with uncomplicated Ebstein is usually tolerated well (WHO risk class II), but those with severe, symptomatic cyanosis, or HF should be advised against pregnancy.[3] Usually symptomatic patients can be managed medically but should be monitored for worsening cyanosis and paradoxical emboli from patent foramen ovale/ASD.

Acquired Valvular Disease
It is helpful to keep a few commonly accepted considerations regarding acquired valvular lesions in mind. First, regurgitant lesions are generally better tolerated in pregnancy than stenotic lesions due to pregnancy-associated systemic vascular resistance improving forward flow and thus limiting the effects of regurgitation (assuming an absence of LV dysfunction).

Second, maternal and fetal risks of acquired cardiac lesions in pregnancy generally vary with the functional classification at pregnancy onset and term.

Women with NYHA functional class I or II heart disease have a favorable prognosis in pregnancy (with the notable exception of mitral stenosis [MS], **Table 28.2**).[3,22] Moreover, patients who reach term as class I or II usually tolerate properly managed labor without invasive monitoring. Third, because of increasing cardiovascular demand in the high-output state, functional status will deteriorate during pregnancy among functional class III and IV patients.[5,13,15,19,47]

Clinical Presentation
Acquired valvular lesions are commonly rheumatic in origin, although endocarditis secondary to intravenous drug use is becoming more prevalent. During pregnancy, maternal morbidity and mortality with rheumatic lesions results from CHF or arrhythmias with a final common sequela of pulmonary edema, embolic event, or fatal dysrhythmia, with pulmonary edema being the leading cause of death in patients with rheumatic heart disease during pregnancy.[15,17,47]

The onset of atrial fibrillation during pregnancy carries with it a higher risk of RV and LV failure (63%) than atrial fibrillation with onset before gestation. In addition, the risk of systemic embolization after the onset of atrial fibrillation during pregnancy may exceed that associated with onset in the nonpregnant state.[15] In the presence of prosthetic valve replacement or repair, endocarditis prophylaxis is reasonable (**Table 28.3**).[22]

Right-Sided Valvular Disease: Pulmonic and Tricuspid Lesions
Clinical Presentation
Physiologic valvular regurgitation is common during pregnancy, especially with right-sided valves, and the degree of regurgitation progresses as pregnancy advances.[64] Isolated right-sided valvular lesions of rheumatic origin are uncommon; however, such lesions are seen with increased frequency in intravenous drug abusers, in whom the lesions are secondary to valvular endocarditis. TR may also occur in patients with CHDs such as Ebstein anomaly. PR is seen commonly in patients after tetralogy of Fallot repair and less commonly in patients after valvuloplasty for pulmonic stenosis.

Management of Right-Sided Valvular Disease in Pregnancy
A successful pregnancy has been reported after Fontan repair of congenital tricuspid atresia.[66] Even after complete tricuspid valvectomy for endocarditis, subsequent pregnancy, labor, and delivery are generally well tolerated. However, PR is a predictor of adverse outcomes during pregnancy, including HF and arrhythmias, which appear to be related to the degree of RV dysfunction.[9,10] Given the propensity toward pulmonary edema peripartum, cautious fluid administration is the mainstay of labor and delivery management in patients with right-sided lesions.[64-67] In general, invasive hemodynamic monitoring during labor and delivery is not necessary.

Left-Sided Valvular Disease
Mitral Stenosis
Clinical Presentation MS is the most common rheumatic valvular lesion encountered during pregnancy.[59] It can occur as an isolated lesion or

in conjunction with aortic or right-sided lesions. Maternal mortality in severe MS has decreased (severe MS, WHO risk class IV; moderate MS, WHO risk class II-III).

Rates of cardiac morbidity, such as pulmonary edema, are high, and careful attention to hemodynamics can help decrease cardiac morbidity. Secondary to severe stenosis, impaired ventricular diastolic filling yields elevated left atrial pressure with a relatively fixed cardiac output. Marked increases in heart rate, cardiac output, and plasma volume accompany normal pregnancy, labor, and delivery (**Table 28.4**). During pregnancy, women with MS are unable to accommodate volume fluctuations, resulting in atrial arrhythmias and pulmonary edema. Complications, occurring most commonly in the third trimester and in the first week postpartum, are associated with NYHA class and severity of MS.[68,70]

Management of MS in Pregnancy The ability to accommodate an increased cardiac output in patients with MS depends largely on two factors.[40] First, these patients depend on adequate diastolic filling time.

A second important consideration in patients with MS centers on LV preload.

Any preload manipulation (ie, diuresis) must be undertaken with caution and attention to the maintenance of cardiac output.

The most hazardous time for these women appears to be the immediate postpartum period. Such patients often enter the postpartum period already operating at their maximum cardiac output and cannot accommodate the volume shifts that follow delivery. In one series of patients with severe MS, a postpartum rise in wedge pressure of up to 16 mm Hg could be expected in the immediate postpartum period.[6] Because frank pulmonary edema generally does not occur with wedge pressures of less than 28 to 30 mm Hg,[73] it follows that the optimal pre-delivery wedge pressure for such patients is 14 mm Hg or less, as indicated by pulmonary artery catheterization.[6] Such a preload may be approached by cautious intrapartum diuresis with careful attention to the maintenance of adequate cardiac output. Active diuresis is not always necessary in patients who enter with evidence of only mild fluid overload. In such patients, simple fluid restriction alongside sensible and insensible fluid losses endogenous to labor can result in a significant fall in wedge pressure before delivery.

In symptomatic patients with moderate to severe MS, many of the same management considerations apply as those previously discussed under the section dealing with Eisenmenger syndrome and PH. Bed rest with the administration of oxygen to maintain the therapeutic goal of a Pao_2 of greater than 70 mm Hg is essential. As previously discussed, pulmonary artery catheterization can allow the hemodynamics to be optimized before the stress of labor.

Previous recommendations for delivery in patients with cardiac disease have included an assisted second stage to shorten its duration. In cases of severe disease, cesarean delivery with general anesthesia has also been advocated as the preferred mode of delivery. With the aggressive and attentive management scheme presented, spontaneous vaginal delivery is generally safe and preferable, even in patients with severe disease and PH.

Pharmacologic and Nonpharmacologic Treatment Given that an increase in heart rate of approximately 10 beats per minute (bpm) is common in normal pregnancy, labor, and delivery, oral beta blocker therapy should be considered for any patient with moderate to severe MS who enters labor with even a mild tachycardia. Because pulmonary edema is the major concern in these patients, we recommend incremental diuresis be carried out to approach a wedge pressure of 12 to 14 mm Hg. Such manipulation, however, must be performed with careful attention to maintaining cardiac output; patients with MS cannot necessarily tolerate a normal wedge pressure. Thus, wedge pressures of 20 mm Hg or more may be necessary to maintain cardiac output and blood pressure.[6,44] If the heart rate rises to more than 100 bpm, we recommend the administration of a beta blocker to avoid tachycardia and subsequent falls in cardiac output. Women with refractory symptoms despite medical therapy may be considered for percutaneous mitral valve balloon valvuloplasty. Surgical valve replacement is rare given the high rate of fetal mortality and only considered when other methods have failed.[68,74-76] Atrial fibrillation should be treated with prompt anticoagulation and restoration of sinus rhythm when necessary.

Mitral Regurgitation
Clinical Presentation Hemodynamically significant mitral regurgitation (MR) is usually rheumatic in

origin in young women or due to mitral valve prolapse (MVP). Rheumatic MR usually occurs with other valvular lesions. Fortunately, MR, especially with normal LV size and function, is tolerated well during pregnancy, due to the decrease in systemic vascular resistance and blood pressure during pregnancy. However, these patients are at risk for the development of HF and arrhythmias in the setting of increased cardiac output and plasma volume, especially when LV dilation and/or systolic dysfunction is present.

Congenital MVP is much more common during pregnancy than rheumatic MR and can occur in up to 17% of young healthy women. This condition is generally asymptomatic (mild MVP stratified as WHO risk class I).[5,44,47,77] The midsystolic click and murmur associated with congenital MVP are characteristic. However, the intensity of this murmur, as well as that associated with rheumatic mitral insufficiency, may decrease during pregnancy because of decreased systemic vascular resistance.[78]

Pharmacologic Treatment Patients with MR may develop atrial enlargement and subsequent atrial fibrillation, which should be treated with beta blockers and anticoagulation.

Aortic Stenosis
Clinical Presentation Aortic stenosis (AS) is commonly congenital in origin secondary to a bicuspid aortic valve, less commonly from rheumatic disease, and thus represents 5% of all congenital cardiac anomalies.[80] The most contemporary studies in patients with congenital AS indicate low maternal mortality.[70,81] The increase in cardiac output and plasma volume may be poorly tolerated in the setting of fixed obstruction. Women with mild to moderate AS often do well (WHO risk class II-III).[3,22] With severe disease, however, a fixed cardiac output limits adequate coronary artery or cerebral perfusion under conditions of physical exertion (WHO risk class III in the setting of severe, asymptomatic AS; WHO risk class IV if severe, symptomatic AS).[3] Inadequate cardiac perfusion subsequently results in angina, syncope, arrhythmias, or sudden death.

Management of AS in Pregnancy In patients with severe AS, limitation of physical activity may be necessary. Pulmonary edema should be treated with diuretics; however, hypovolemia should be avoided, as preload is of the utmost importance.

Of note, because hypovolemia is of greater concern than pulmonary edema, the wedge pressure should be maintained in the range 14 to 18 mm Hg in order to provide a margin of safety against unexpected peripartum blood loss. Hypotension resulting from blood loss, ganglionic blockade from epidural anesthesia, or supine vena cava occlusion by the gravid uterus may result in sudden death. Similarly, during labor and delivery, hypervolemia from relief of inferior cava compressions, autotransfusions from a contracting uterus, and aggressive intravenous fluid administration may not be tolerated either.

Nonpharmacologic Treatment Women who have severe stenosis or symptoms are advised to undergo repair prior to attempting pregnancy in an effort to substantially reduce pregnancy-associated morbidity and mortality.[80-82] That said, there are reports of women with severe AS having undergone successful balloon valvuloplasty in pregnancy in the setting of refractory disease.[83] Percutaneous aortic valve implantation during pregnancy has not yet been reported. Open valve replacement is associated with a 30% fetal mortality risk.[84] Pregnancy termination in the mid-trimester may be especially hazardous due to blood loss and has been reported to carry a mortality of up to 40%.[85]

Aortic Regurgitation
Clinical Presentation Aortic regurgitation is most commonly associated with bicuspid aortic valve disease and less commonly with aortopathy with dilated aorta or endocarditis.

Management and Pharmacologic Treatment of Aortic Regurgitation in Pregnancy The increase in cardiac output and plasma volume can cause worsen HF in patients with LV dysfunction, and these patients should be treated with medical therapy for HF.

If symptomatic, patients respond favorably to diuretics and vasodilators; epidural anesthesia is thus appropriate and reduces the risk of LV failure at delivery.[24,86]

Peripartum Cardiomyopathy

Clinical Presentation
Peripartum cardiomyopathy (PPCM) is defined as cardiomyopathy occurring during pregnancy or the first 6 months' postpartum in women without

previous cardiac disease and after exclusion of other causes of cardiac failure, as shown in **Table 28.5**.[87-90]

PPCM is characterized by the development of HF in the setting of systolic dysfunction, with or without LV dilation, and is a diagnosis of exclusion that should not be made without a concerted effort to identify valvular, metabolic, infectious, or toxic causes of cardiomyopathy.[91] Other peripartum complications, such as amniotic fluid embolism, severe preeclampsia, and corticosteroid- or sympathomimetic-induced pulmonary edema, must also be considered before making the diagnosis of PPCM.[91] However, prior to concluding a definitive etiologic role for beta agonists, it must be considered that sympathomimetic agents may unmask rather than induce an underlying PPCM.[92] To date, there remains no definitive proven association between tocolytic therapy and PPCM.

Epidemiology and Risk Factors

The incidence of PPCM is estimated at between 1 in 3000 live births in the United States.[93-97]

An incidence as high as 1% has been suggested in women from certain African tribes.[95]

Risk factors for PPCM include African American descent, older maternal age, multifetal gestations, and hypertensive disorders during pregnancy.[93,95,98]

Some cases of PPCM may occur in a familial pattern, suggesting a genetic contribution.[99,100] The overall mortality from PPCM in the United States ranges from 0% to 19%.[93-96] Risk factors for death include older age, multiparity, severe LV systolic dysfunction, African American descent, and delayed diagnosis.[101-103]

The clinical course of PPCM can be variable, with spontaneous recovery within days to months in some patients to persistent, severe LV dysfunction in other patients.

Due to the low prevalence of pre-existing dilated cardiomyopathy (DCM) prior to pregnancy in young females, little data are available on pregnancy in women with pre-existing DCM.

Moderate to severe LV dysfunction and NYHA class III to IV are risk factors for cardiovascular morbidity (WHO risk class III-IV).[3,106]

Clinical Assessment

PPCM manifests clinically by increasing fatigue, dyspnea, and peripheral and/or pulmonary edema. As most women in the last trimester of pregnancy manifest these conditions, high clinical suspicion for a cardiomyopathy should arise with paroxysmal nocturnal dyspnea, chest pain, nocturnal cough, new regurgitant murmurs, pulmonary crackles, and hepatomegaly.[107]

Delayed diagnosis >1 week has been associated with worse cardiovascular outcomes.[104] Physical examination reveals classic evidence of CHF, including elevated jugular venous pressure, rales, and an S3 gallop. Serum n-terminal pro–b-type natriuretic peptide may be elevated. Cardiomegaly and pulmonary edema are found on chest radiograph, and the electrocardiogram often demonstrates LV and atrial dilation, with the nonspecific ST and T wave changes. In addition, up to 50% of patients with PPCM may manifest evidence of pulmonary or systemic embolic phenomena. The diagnosis rests on the echocardiographic finding of new LV systolic dysfunction (LVEF < 45%) during or after pregnancy (**Table 28.5**).[87]

Etiology

The etiology of PPCM remains unclear, with suggestions of low selenium levels, viral infections, cytokine-induced pathways, inflammation, and autoimmune pathways contributing to its development. There is some evidence that PPCM may result

Table 28.5 Clinical Parameters Defining Peripartum Cardiomyopathy

Parameter	Echocardiographic Parameters
Heart failure presenting toward the end of pregnancy or following delivery	—
No prior history of cardiac disease	—
Absence of clearly identifiable etiology	—
Echocardiographic findings of left ventricular dysfunction	EF < 45% and/or M-mode fractional shortening of <30%
—	End-diastolic dimension/body surface area >2.72 cm/m²

EF, ejection fraction.
Echocardiographic parameters as described by Hibbard et al.[87,98]
Adapted from Hibbard JU, Lindheimer M, Lang RM. A modified definition for peripartum cardiomyopathy and prognosis based on echocardiography. *Obstet Gynecol.* 1999;94(2):311-316 and Sliwa K, Hilfiker-Kleiner D, Petrie MC, et al. Current state of knowledge on aetiology, diagnosis, management, and therapy of peripartum cardiomyopathy: a position statement from the Heart Failure Association of the European Society of Cardiology Working Group on peripartum cardiomyopathy. *Eur J Heart Fail.* 2010;12(8):767-778.

from vascular disease caused by hormonal changes in pregnancy.

Data suggest the contribution of oxidative stress, angiogenic imbalance, and impaired cardiomyocyte protection to PPCM and the potential for prolactin inhibition by bromocriptine as a therapeutic option, for which studies are underway.[95,111]

Pharmacologic and Nonpharmacologic Treatment

Medical therapy for PPCM includes guideline-directed medical therapy for HF, including beta blockers (preferably beta-1 selective, metoprolol tartrate) and diuretics (furosemide 20-40 mg oral daily), and fluid and sodium restriction (1 L/d and 2000 mg/d, maximum, respectively).[3,98,112] Because angiotensin-converting enzyme (ACE) inhibitors and angiotensin receptor blockers are contraindicated in pregnancy, afterload reduction with vasodilators (25-100 mg of oral hydralazine three times a day being the drug of choice peripartum, with 10-40 mg oral isosorbide dinitrate three times a day postpartum) should be used. Digoxin can be used once optimized on beta blockers and vasodilators. Spironolactone is relatively contraindicated during pregnancy due to antiandrogenic effects and limited safety data but may be considered postpartum, as the active metabolite of spironolactone is found in breast milk at insignificant doses.

In general, because of the adverse effects of negative ionotropic agents, nondihydropyridine calcium channel blockers should be avoided during pregnancy. In recent years, ACE inhibitors (2.5-20 mg oral enalapril twice daily and 6.25-50 mg oral captopril three times a day) have been the mainstay of treatment postpartum; breastfeeding women should be counseled accordingly.

Patients with poor cardiac function (EF < 40%) are at increased risk of thromboembolism; therefore, we recommend prophylaxis with unfractionated heparin (UFH) (5000-7500 units subcutaneously) or low-molecular-weight enoxaparin (40 mg subcutaneously) during pregnancy.[34]

Given recent reports of ventricular fibrillation in women with PPCM and severely low EF, it may be reasonable to consider a wearable cardioverter-defibrillator with appropriate shock for particularly high-risk patients.[113]

Management of PPCM in Pregnancy

Women with stable disease on appropriate medical therapy can be monitored to determine the optimal timing and mode of delivery. Women with severe LV dysfunction and uncontrolled symptoms, particularly NYHA class III to IV (WHO risk class IV), on optimal medical therapy, should be offered the option of termination of pregnancy or early delivery, as this may result in clinical improvement.[3,34]

When PPCM occurs in the last trimester of pregnancy, delivery is indicated. The mode of delivery should be based on obstetric indications.

Regional epidural analgesia has the distinct advantage of reducing both preload and afterload, as well as minimizing fluctuations in cardiac output associated with labor.[107] In instances of obstetrically indicated cesarean delivery, we and others recommend careful monitoring of fluid balance with central monitoring in an effort to clearly define and monitor the central venous pressure.[107]

Maternal Outcomes

Although PPCM is associated with a more favorable prognosis than other cardiomyopathies, it is associated with significant morbidity and mortality.

Most studies suggest recovery within 6 months of diagnosis, although recovery of LV function may be further delayed.[93,104,114-116] Lower EF (LVEF ≤ 30%), larger LV end-diastolic diameter (≥ 60 mm), and African American descent predict worse prognosis for recovery.[103,117] Additionally, women with PPCM in one pregnancy are more likely to have recurrent PPCM in subsequent pregnancies.

Even women with recovered LV function are at higher risk of deterioration of LV function in a subsequent pregnancy.

Hypertrophic Cardiomyopathy

Clinical Presentation

Hypertrophic cardiomyopathy (HCM) is an autosomal-dominant condition with variable penetrance, generally characterized by LV hypertrophy with reduced LV size and compliance.

HCM includes heterogeneous morphologies of the LV, but the most problematic for pregnancy is LV hypertrophy involving the septum to a greater extent than the free wall, resulting in obstruction to LV outflow tract (LVOT) and secondary MR, the two principal hemodynamic concerns for the clinician.[120-123]

Although the increased blood volume associated with normal pregnancy should enhance LV filling and improve hemodynamic performance, this positive effect of pregnancy is countered by the fall in arterial pressure and vena cava obstruction common in the last trimester of pregnancy. In addition, tachycardia resulting from pain in labor and Valsalva maneuver with active maternal efforts in the second stage of labor diminish LV filling and aggravate the relative outflow obstruction. Thus, it may be generally surmised that reduction of preload and afterload in patients with HCM results in an increase in the outflow gradient with a concomitant reduction in LV filling.

Maternal morbidity is increased with severe LVOT obstruction, diastolic dysfunction, and arrhythmias.[120]

Management of HCM in Pregnancy

The keys to successful management of the peripartum period in patients with HCM involve avoidance of hypotension, control of tachycardia, conduction of labor in the left lateral recumbent position, and avoidance of maternal Valsalva maneuver with the use of an assisted second stage of labor. Intravenous fluids should be used judiciously. The use of regional anesthesia, with its accompanying hemodynamic alterations, should be carefully monitored and single-dose spinal anesthesia should be avoided. Cesarean delivery of patients with HCM should be reserved for obstetric indications and those with severe LVOT obstruction.

Maternal outcomes in patients with HCM are generally good (WHO risk class II-III), and HCM is rarely an indication for pregnancy termination.[3,124]

Pharmacologic Treatment

Beta blockers should be continued if already being taken and started when symptoms occur.[3,125]

Marfan Syndrome

Clinical Assessment

Pregnancy is associated with an increased risk of aortic dissection.

The risk of aortic dissection in pregnancy in women with Marfan syndrome is about 3%, with increased risk in those with prior pregnancy, larger aortic diameter, and greater rate of aortic growth during pregnancy.[128,129] Aortic dissection usually occurs during the third trimester or postpartum but can occur throughout gestation.[130] Thus, patients are followed up prior to and during pregnancy for aortic root diameter, as it predicts the risk of aortic dissection or rupture.

Prognosis is best individualized and should be based on echocardiographic (both transthoracic

and transesophageal), computed tomography, and/ or cardiac magnetic resonance imaging assessment of proximal and distal aortic diameter, valvular function, and global cardiac function.[131-134] It is important to note that enlargement of the aortic root is not demonstrable by chest radiograph until dilation has become pronounced.[134] Mortality is correlated with size of the aortic root, but even women with aortic root <40 mm have 1% risk of dissection (WHO risk class II-III).[3,128,135]

Nonpharmacologic Treatment

Generally, replacement of the ascending aorta in asymptomatic patients is recommended when the aortic root diameter exceeds 4.5 cm.[3,34] Elective prepregnancy surgery should be considered in women with Marfan with aortic root dilation >45 mm (WHO risk class IV if not repaired).[3]

In women with aortic root of 40 to 45 mm (WHO risk class III), surgical repair should be considered during pregnancy if there is >5-mm increase in diameter and/or with family history of premature aortic dissection.[3] Even with repair, there is risk of distal aortic dissection.

Pharmacologic Treatment

Aggressive control of hypertension with beta blocker therapy has been shown to decrease the rate of aortic growth in patients with Marfan syndrome.[129,138,139] Utilization of labetalol (an alpha and beta antagonist) has the added advantage of controlling mean arterial blood pressure in a rapid fashion, alongside its ability to decrease pulsatile pressure on the aorta.[136]

Management of Marfan Syndrome in Pregnancy

In instances of aortic root dilation approximating 4.5 cm, cesarean delivery is recommended to minimize episodic hypertension that may precipitate aortic root dissection.[3] In counseling women with Marfan syndrome, the high risk of transmission, risk of maternal aortic dissection, and high rate of obstetric complications with increased risk of neonatal mortality should be discussed.[140,141]

Vascular Ehlers-Danlos Syndrome

Vascular Ehlers-Danlos syndrome (EDS), formerly known as type IV EDS, is an inherited disorder of collagen severely affecting the vasculature. Vascular EDS bears a high risk of vascular complications with high maternal mortality (WHO risk class IV) and ACC/ESC guidelines do not recommend pregnancy in women with this disease.[3,142]

Pregnancy-Associated Myocardial Infarction

Clinical Presentation

Acute myocardial infarction (MI) is three times more common in pregnancy and postpartum, as compared to nonpregnant women of the same age, and appears to be more common in pregnant women who are older than 30 years.[144]

Pharmacologic and Nonpharmacologic Treatment

Nitrates have been used in pregnant women with angina with careful monitoring for maternal hypotension without adverse fetal effects.[34] Aspirin at low doses has been used extensively without significant maternal and fetal bleeding risk. Cardiac catheterization when necessary should minimize the use of radiation if possible, aiming to result in <1 rad in fetal exposure.[34] Percutaneous coronary intervention should be utilized for standard indications of ST elevation MI and unstable non-ST elevation MI (NSTEMI), with particular attention to avoiding iatrogenic coronary dissection as a result of coronary contrast injections or interventions. A noninvasive approach to stabilize women with NSTEMI is preferred.

Management of MI in Pregnancy

Studies report that most patients have spontaneous healing in spontaneous coronary artery dissection, and thus, conservative management in stable patients has been advised.[146,147] In contrast, those who are unstable or with left main disease should be referred for bypass surgery.

Use of Anticoagulation Therapy in Pregnancy

Use of anticoagulation therapy in the patient with a mechanical prosthetic heart valve or atrial fibrillation during pregnancy is critical to avoid thromboembolism but is associated with increased rate of maternal and fetal complications associated with the anticoagulation agent (WHO risk class III).[3,22] Treatment regimens are outlined in **Table 28.6**.

Warfarin (Coumadin) is effective in reducing the risk of thromboembolism in pregnant women

Table 28.6 Treatment Approaches for Women With Mechanical Heart Valves[a]

Approach	Therapeutic Parameters
Unfractionated heparin (UFH) throughout pregnancy	Maintain midinterval aPTT at a minimum of twice control
Low-molecular-weight heparin (LMWH) until 36 wk, then UFH	Maintain peak antifactor Xa heparin levels (4-6 h post injection) 0.8-1.2 U/mL
UFH or LMWH in adjusted dose (as above) through the 12th week of gestation, then warfarin until 36 wk, followed by reinitiation of UFH (as above)	Target INR 2.5-3.5 with warfarin therapy
Warfarin during first trimester if dose required to reach therapeutic level ≤5 mg, then UFH or LMWH (as above), followed by UFH after 36 wk	Target INR 2.5-3.5 with warfarin therapy

aPTT, activated partial thromboplastin time; INR, international normalized ratio.
[a]All regimens should include aspirin 81 mg daily.

with mechanical valves. However, its use in the first 6 to 12 weeks of gestation has been associated with fetal warfarin syndrome (warfarin embryopathy, characterized by nasal hypoplasia and stippled epiphyses), miscarriage, and fetal intracranial hemorrhage.

Balancing the fetal risks with warfarin therapy are the maternal risks with UFH and low-molecular-weight heparin (LMWH) therapy.

LMWH has been shown to be superior to UFH, with stable and more predictable dose response, less bleeding, and lower risk of heparin-induced thrombocytopenia.[155]

ACC/American Heart Association guidelines suggest continuation of warfarin during the first trimester is reasonable if the daily dose of warfarin required to achieve a therapeutic dose is ≤5 mg, with the recommendation that twice daily subcutaneous LMWH with dose-adjusted anti-Xa levels be used in the first trimester if the warfarin dose is >5 mg.[22] After the first trimester, warfarin is continued until 35 to 36 weeks, followed by use of intravenous UFH until delivery.

Alternatively, other programs have used LMWH in lower risk women in the first 35 to 36 weeks of gestation with good results.[34]

Patients with bioprosthetic or xenograft valves are not usually treated with anticoagulants during pregnancy. Patients with a bioprosthetic valve who are in atrial fibrillation or have evidence of thromboembolism, however, should receive anticoagulant therapy with doses controlled accordingly.[156]

KEY POINTS

- Normal physiologic changes of pregnancy may mimic cardiac disease.
- Despite the first key point, suspected cardiovascular abnormalities must be worked up aggressively in pregnancy.
- Most maternal deaths in developed countries due to cardiac disease are secondary to cardiomyopathy, ischemic heart disease, endocarditis, PH, and arrhythmia.
- Women with cardiac disease should seek preconception counseling.
- Women with PH, severe aortic or mitral valve stenosis, and severe right or LV dysfunction are at the highest risk of maternal morbidity and mortality and should be counseled prior to pregnancy. Interventions should be planned prior to conception if possible.
- Women with PPCM are at risk of morbidity and should be closely monitored throughout their pregnancy.
- No method of anticoagulation is ideal or risk free in patients with mechanical valves during pregnancy.
- Any woman with suspected PH must have a definitive diagnosis as soon as possible, usually via right heart catheterization.
- Modified WHO classification of maternal cardiovascular risk can be used to guide pregnancy risk and prepregnancy counseling.
- In women with cyanotic heart disease, fetal deterioration is a common cause of early delivery.

- Most valvular regurgitation is tolerated well during pregnancy.
- In patients with significant MS, the risks of pulmonary edema due to peripartum volume shifts must be weighed against the risks of falling cardiac output if active diuresis is considered during labor.
- The postpartum period is the time of greatest risk of pulmonary edema in women with MS.
- The major hemodynamic considerations complicating pregnancy in women with heart disease are increased intravascular volume, decreased systemic vascular resistance, increased tendency for pathologic clot formation, and hemodynamic fluctuations during the peripartum period.
- The need for endocarditis prophylaxis during uncomplicated vaginal delivery in women with structural heart disease is not recommended and should be reserved for those with the highest risk of bacterial endocarditis.
- Even in most forms of severe cardiac disease, forceps or vacuum delivery should be reserved for standard obstetric indications.
- With proper management, many women with cardiac disease can expect successful pregnancy.
- Management of significant cardiac disease in pregnancy should be a team effort, involving obstetrics, cardiology, maternal-fetal medicine, and anesthesia specialists.

REFERENCES

(only references cited in synoptic print chapter; for a complete reference list, see ebook)

1. Stout Karen K, Daniels Curt J, Aboulhosn Jamil A, et al. 2018 AHA/ACC guideline for the management of adults with congenital heart disease: a report of the American College of Cardiology/American Heart Association Task Force on Clinical Practice Guidelines. *Circulation.* 2019;139(14):e698-e800. doi:10.1161/CIR.0000000000000603

2. Center for Disease Control. Pregnancy Mortality Surveillance System. Maternal and Infant Health. Accessed April 8, 2019. https://www.cdc.gov/reproductivehealth/maternalinfanthealth/pregnancy-mortality-surveillance-system.htm

3. Regitz-Zagrosek V, Blomstrom Lundqvist C, Borghi C, et al. ESC Guidelines on the management of cardiovascular diseases during pregnancy: the Task Force on the Management of Cardiovascular Diseases during pregnancy of the European Society of Cardiology (ESC). *Eur Heart J.* 2011;32(24):3147-3197. doi:10.1093/eurheartj/ehr218

4. Thorne S, MacGregor A, Nelson-Piercy C. Risks of contraception and pregnancy in heart disease. *Heart.* 2006;92(10):1520-1525. doi:10.1136/hrt.2006.095240

5. Shime J, Mocarski EJM, Hastings D, Webb GD, McLaughlin PR. Congenital heart disease in pregnancy: short-and long-term implications. *Am J Obstet Gynecol.* 1987;156(2):313-322.

6. Clark SL, Phelan JP, Greenspoon J, Aldahl D, Horenstein J. Labor and delivery in the presence of mitral stenosis: central hemodynamic observations. *Am J Obstet Gynecol.* 1985;152(8):984-988.

7. Siu SC, Sermer M, Colman JM, et al. Prospective multicenter study of pregnancy outcomes in women with heart disease. *Circulation.* 2001;104(5):515-521.

8. Silversides CK, Grewal J, Mason J, et al. Pregnancy outcomes in women with heart disease: the CARPREG II study. *J Am Coll Cardiol.* 2018;71(21):2419-2430. doi:10.1016/j.jacc.2018.02.076

9. Khairy P, Ouyang DW, Fernandes SM, Lee-Parritz A, Economy KE, Landzberg MJ. Pregnancy outcomes in women with congenital heart disease. *Circulation.* 2006;113(4):517-524.

10. Drenthen W, Boersma E, Balci A, et al; ZAHARA Investigators. Predictors of pregnancy complications in women with congenital heart disease. *Eur Heart J.* 2010;31(17):2124-2132. doi:10.1093/eurheartj/ehq200

11. Balci A, Sollie-Szarynska KM, van der Bijl AG, et al. Prospective validation and assessment of cardiovascular and offspring risk models for pregnant women with congenital heart disease. *Heart.* 2014;100(17):1373-1381.

12. van Hagen IM, Boersma E, Johnson MR, et al. Global cardiac risk assessment in the Registry of Pregnancy and Cardiac disease: results of a registry from the European Society of Cardiology. *Eur J Heart Fail.* 2016;18(5):523-533.

13. Roos-Hesselink JW, Ruys TP, Stein JI, et al. Outcome of pregnancy in patients with structural or ischaemic heart disease: results of a registry of the European Society of Cardiology. *Eur Heart J.* 2012;34(9):657-665.

14. Schlichting LE, Insaf TZ, Zaidi AN, Lui GK, Van Zutphen AR. Maternal comorbidities and complications of delivery in pregnant women with congenital heart disease. *J Am Coll Cardiol.* 2019;73(17):2181-2191. doi:10.1016/j.jacc.2019.01.069

15. Szekely P, Turner R, Snaith L. Pregnancy and the changing pattern of rheumatic heart disease. *Br Heart J.* 1973;35(12):1293-1303.

16. Jacob S, Bloebaum L, Varner MW. Maternal mortality in Utah. *Obstet Gynecol.* 1998;91(2):187-191.

17. De Swiet M. *Cardiac disease.* In: *Why Mothers Die 1997-1999: The Confidential Enquiries Into Maternal Deaths in the United Kingdom.* RCOG Press; 2001:153.

19. Drenthen W, Pieper PG, Roos-Hesselink JW, et al. Outcome of pregnancy in women with congenital heart disease: a literature review. *J Am Coll Cardiol.* 2007;49(24):2303-2311.

20. Page RL, Joglar JA, Caldwell MA, et al. 2015 ACC/AHA/HRS Guideline for the management of adult patients with supraventricular tachycardia: a report of the American College of Cardiology/American Heart Association Task Force on Clinical Practice Guidelines and the Heart Rhythm Society. *J Am Coll Cardiol.* 2016;67(13):e27-e115.

22. Nishimura Rick A, Otto Catherine M, Bonow Robert O, et al. 2014 AHA/ACC Guideline for the management of patients with valvular heart disease: executive summary. A report of the American College of Cardiology/American Heart Association Task Force on Practice Guidelines. *Circulation.* 2014;129(23):2440-2492. doi:10.1161/CIR.0000000000000029

24. Reimold SC, Rutherford JD. Valvular heart disease in pregnancy. *N Engl J Med.* 2003;349(1):52-59.

25. Ullery JC. The management of pregnancy complicated by heart disease. *Am J Obstet Gynecol.* 1954;67(4):834-866.

26. Perloff JK. Congenital heart disease and pregnancy. *Clin Cardiol.* 1994;17(11):579-587.

28. Ellison RC, Sloss LJ. Electrocardiographic features of congenital heart disease in the adult. *Cardiovasc Clin.* 1979;10(1):119.

29. Schaefer G, Arditi LI, Solomon HA, Ringland JE. Congenital heart disease and pregnancy. *Clin Obstet Gynecol.* 1968;11(4):1048-1063.

30. Hibbard LT. Maternal mortality due to cardiac disease. *Clin Obstet Gynecol.* 1975;18(3):27-36.

31. Neilson G, Galea EG, Blunt A. Congenital heart disease and pregnancy. *Med J Aust.* 1970;1(22):1086-1088.

32. Zitnik RS, Brandenburg RO, Sheldon R, Wallace RB. Pregnancy and open-heart surgery. *Circulation.* 1969;39(5S1):I-257-I-262.

34. Elkayam U, Goland S, Pieper PG, Silversides CK. High-risk cardiac disease in pregnancy: Part II. *J Am Coll Cardiol.* 2016;68(5):502-516. doi:10.1016/j.jacc.2016.05.050

35. Canobbio MM, Warnes CA, Aboulhosn J, et al. Management of pregnancy in patients with complex congenital heart disease: a scientific statement for healthcare professionals from the American Heart Association. *Circulation.* 2017;135(8):e50-e87. doi:10.1161/CIR.0000000000000458

36. Gleicher N, Midwall J, Hochberger D, Jaffin H. Eisenmenger's syndrome and pregnancy. *Obstet Gynecol Surv.* 1979;34(10):721-741.

38. Weiss BM, Zemp L, Seifert B, Hess OM. Outcome of pulmonary vascular disease in pregnancy: a systematic overview from 1978 through 1996. *J Am Coll Cardiol.* 1998;31(7):1650. doi:10.1016/S0735-1097(98)00162-4

39. Bédard E, Dimopoulos K, Gatzoulis MA. Has there been any progress made on pregnancy outcomes among women with pulmonary arterial hypertension? *Eur Heart J.* 2009;30(3):256-265. doi:10.1093/eurheartj/ehn597

40. Avila WS, Grinberg M, Snitcowsky R, et al. Maternal and fetal outcome in pregnant women with Eisenmenger's syndrome. *Eur Heart J.* 1995;16(4):460-464.

41. Katsuragi S, Yamanaka K, Neki R, et al. Maternal outcome in pregnancy complicated with pulmonary arterial hypertension. *Circ J.* 2012;76(9):2249-2254. doi:10.1253/circj.CJ-12-0235

42. Subbaiah M, Kumar S, Roy KK, Sharma JB, Singh N. Pregnancy outcome in women with pulmonary arterial hypertension: single-center experience from India. *Arch Gynecol Obstet.* 2013;288(2):305-309. doi:10.1007/s00404-013-2761-8

43. Pieper PG, Lameijer H, Hoendermis ES. Pregnancy and pulmonary hypertension. *Best Pract Res Clin Obstet Gynaecol.* 2014;28(4):579-591. doi:10.1016/j.bpobgyn.2014.03.003

44. Clark SL, Cotton DB, Hankins GD, Phelan JP. *Critical Care Obstetrics.* Blackwell Science Malden; 1997.

45. Kiely DG, Condliffe R, Webster V, et al. Improved survival in pregnancy and pulmonary hypertension using a multiprofessional approach. *Br J Obstet Gynaecol.* 2010;117(5):565-574. doi:10.1111/j.1471-0528.2009.02492.x

46. Committee on Practice Bulletins-Obstetrics. ACOG Practice Bulletin No. 199: use of prophylactic antibiotics in labor and delivery. *Obstet Gynecol.* 2018;132(3):e103-e119. doi:10.1097/AOG.0000000000002833

47. Clark SL, Cotton DB, Lee W, et al. Central hemodynamic assessment of normal term pregnancy. *Am J Obstet Gynecol.* 1989;161(6):1439-1442.

48. Penning S, Robinson KD, Major CA, Garite TJ. A comparison of echocardiography and pulmonary artery catheterization for evaluation of pulmonary artery pressures in pregnant patients with suspected pulmonary hypertension. *Am J Obstet Gynecol.* 2001;184(7):1568-1570. doi:10.1067/mob.2001.114857

49. Midwall J, Jaffin H, Herman MV, Kupersmith J. Shunt flow and pulmonary hemodynamics during labor and delivery in the Eisenmenger syndrome. *Am J Cardiol.* 1978;42(2):299-303. doi:10.1016/0002-9149(78)90915-3

50. Snabes MC, Poindexter AN. Laparoscopic tubal sterilization under local anesthesia in women with cyanotic heart disease. *Obstet Gynecol.* 1991;78(3):437-440.

51. Rout CC. Anaesthesia and analgesia for the critically ill parturient. *Best Pract Res Clin Obstet Gynaecol.* 2001;15(4):507-522.

54. Deal K, Wooley CF. Coarctation of the aorta and pregnancy. *Ann Intern Med.* 1973;78(5):706-710.

55. Goodwin JF. Pregnancy and coarctation of the aorta. *Clin Obstet Gynecol.* 1961;4(3):645-664.

58. Balci A, Drenthen W, Mulder BJM, et al. Pregnancy in women with corrected tetralogy of Fallot: occurrence and predictors of adverse events. *Am Heart J.* 2011;161(2):307-313. doi:10.1016/j.ahj.2010.10.027

59. Meyer EC, Tulsky AS, Sigmann P, Silber EN. Pregnancy in the presence of tetralogy of Fallot: observations on two patients. *Am J Cardiol.* 1964;14(6):874-879.

63. Lima FV, Koutrolou-Sotiropoulou P, Yen TY, Stergiopoulos K. Clinical characteristics and outcomes in pregnant women with Ebstein anomaly at the time of delivery in the USA: 2003-2012. *Arch Cardiovasc Dis.* 2016;109(6-7):390-398.

64. Gei AF, Hankins GD. Cardiac disease and pregnancy. *Obstet Gynecol Clin North Am.* 2001;28(3):465-512.

65. Chesley LC. Severe rheumatic cardiac disease and pregnancy: the ultimate prognosis. *Am J Obstet Gynecol.* 1980;136(5):552-558.

66. Campos O, Andrade JL, Bocanegra J, et al. Physiologic multivalvular regurgitation during pregnancy: a longitudinal Doppler echocardiographic study. *Int J Cardiol.* 1993;40(3):265-272.

67. Robson SC, Hunter S, Boys RJ, Dunlop W. Serial study of factors influencing changes in cardiac output during human pregnancy. *Am J Physiol.* 1989;256(4):H1060-H1065.

68. Silversides CK, Colman JM, Sermer M, Siu SC. Cardiac risk in pregnant women with rheumatic mitral stenosis. *Am J Cardiol.* 2003;91(11):1382-1385. doi:10.1016/S0002-9149(03)00339-4

70. Hameed A, Karaalp IS, Tummala PP, et al. The effect of valvular heart disease on maternal and fetal outcome of pregnancy. *J Am Coll Cardiol.* 2001;37(3):893-899. doi:10.1016/S0735-1097(00)01198-0

73. Forrester JS, Swan HJ. Acute myocardial infarction: a physiological basis of therapy. *Crit Care Med.* 1974;2(6):283-292.

74. Weiss BM, von Segesser LK, Alon E, Seifert B, Turina MI. Outcome of cardiovascular surgery and pregnancy: a systematic review of the period 1984-1996. *Am J Obstet Gynecol.* 1998;179(6):1643-1653.

75. Parry AJ, Westaby S. Cardiopulmonary bypass during pregnancy. *Ann Thorac Surg.* 1996;61(6):1865-1869.

76. John AS, Gurley F, Schaff HV, et al. Cardiopulmonary bypass during pregnancy. *Ann Thorac Surg.* 2011;91(4):1191-1196. doi:10.1016/j.athoracsur.2010.11.037

77. Avila WS, Rossi EG, Ramires JAF, et al. Pregnancy in patients with heart disease: experience with 1,000 cases. *Clin Cardiol.* 2003;26(3):135-142.

78. Hass JM. The effect of pregnancy on the midsystolic click and murmur of the prolapsing posterior leaflet of the mitral valve. *Am Heart J.* 1976;92(3):407-408.

79. Rayburn WF, Fontana ME. Mitral valve prolapse and pregnancy. *Am J Obstet Gynecol.* 1981;141(1):9-11.

80. Sullivan HJ. Valvular heart surgery during pregnancy. *Surg Clin North Am.* 1995;75(1):59-75.

81. Silversides CK, Colman JM, Sermer M, Farine D, Siu SC. Early and intermediate-term outcomes of pregnancy with congenital aortic stenosis. *Am J Cardiol.* 2003;91(11):1386-1389. doi:10.1016/S0002-9149(03)00340-0

82. Carabello BA. Evaluation and management of patients with aortic stenosis. *Circulation.* 2002;105(15):1746-1750.

83. Presbitero P, Prever SB, Brusca A. Interventional cardiology in pregnancy. *Eur Heart J.* 1996;17(2):182-188. doi:10.1093/oxfordjournals.eurheartj.a014833

84. Chambers CE, Clark SL. Cardiac surgery during pregnancy. *Clin Obstet Gynecol.* 1994;37(2):316-323.

85. Arias F, Pineda J. Aortic stenosis and pregnancy. *J Reprod Med.* 1978;20(4):229-232.

86. Klein LL, Galan HL. Cardiac disease in pregnancy. *Obstet Gynecol Clin North Am.* 2004;31(2):429-459.

87. Hibbard JU, Lindheimer M, Lang RM. A modified definition for peripartum cardiomyopathy and prognosis based on echocardiography. *Obstet Gynecol.* 1999;94(2):311-316.

88. Demakis JG, Rahimtoola SH, Sutton GC, et al. Natural course of peripartum cardiomyopathy. *Circulation.* 1971;44(6):1053-1061.

89. Brown CS, Bertolet BD. Peripartum cardiomyopathy: a comprehensive review. *Am J Obstet Gynecol.* 1998;178(2):409-414.

90. De Souza JL Jr, de Carvalho Frimm C, Nastari L, Mady C. Left ventricular function after a new pregnancy in patients with peripartum cardiomyopathy. *J Card Fail.* 2001;7(1):30-35.

91. Felker GM, Thompson RE, Hare JM, et al. Underlying causes and long-term survival in patients with initially unexplained cardiomyopathy. *N Engl J Med.* 2000;342(15):1077-1084.

92. Blickstein I, Zazel Y, Katz Z, Lancet M. Ritodrine-induced pulmonary edema unmasking underlying peripartum cardiomyopathy. *Am J Obstet Gynecol.* 1988;159(2):332-333.

93. Elkayam U. Clinical characteristics of peripartum cardiomyopathy in the United States: diagnosis, prognosis, and management. *J Am Coll Cardiol.* 2011;58(7):659-670.

94. Fett JD, Christie LG, Carraway RD, Murphy JG. *Five-year prospective study of the incidence and prognosis of peripartum cardiomyopathy at a single institution.* In: *Mayo Clinic Proceedings.* Vol 80. Elsevier; 2005:1602-1606.

95. Sliwa K, Fett J, Elkayam U. Peripartum cardiomyopathy. *Lancet.* 2006;368(9536):687-693.

96. Brar SS, Khan SS, Sandhu GK, et al. Incidence, mortality, and racial differences in peripartum cardiomyopathy. *Am J Cardiol.* 2007;100(2):302-304.

97. Kolte D, Khera S, Aronow WS, et al. Temporal trends in incidence and outcomes of peripartum cardiomyopathy in the United States: a nationwide population-based study. *J Am Heart Assoc.* 2014;3(3):e001056.

98. Sliwa K, Hilfiker-Kleiner D, Petrie MC, et al. Current state of knowledge on aetiology, diagnosis, management, and therapy of peripartum cardiomyopathy: a position statement from the Heart Failure Association of the European Society of Cardiology Working Group on peripartum cardiomyopathy. *Eur J Heart Fail.* 2010;12(8):767-778. doi:10.1093/eurjhf/hfq120

99. Morales A, Painter T, Li R, et al. Rare variant mutations in pregnancy-associated or peripartum cardiomyopathy. *Circulation.* 2010;121(20):2176-2182.

100. van Spaendonck-Zwarts KY, van Tintelen JP, van Veldhuisen DJ, et al. Peripartum cardiomyopathy as a part of familial dilated cardiomyopathy. *Circulation.* 2010;121(20):2169-2175. doi:10.1161/CIRCULATIONAHA.109.929646

101. Pearson GD, Veille JC, Rahimtoola S, et al. Peripartum cardiomyopathy: National Heart, Lung, and Blood Institute and Office of Rare Diseases (National Institutes of Health) workshop recommendations and review. *J Am Med Assoc.* 2000;283(9):1183-1188.

102. Whitehead SJ, Berg CJ, Chang J. Pregnancy-related mortality due to cardiomyopathy: United States, 1991-1997. *Obstet Gynecol.* 2003;102(6):1326-1331.

103. McNamara DM, Elkayam U, Alharethi R, et al. Clinical outcomes for peripartum cardiomyopathy in North America: results of the IPAC study (Investigations of Pregnancy-Associated Cardiomyopathy). *J Am Coll Cardiol.* 2015;66(8):905-914.

104. Goland S, Modi K, Bitar F, et al. Clinical profile and predictors of complications in peripartum cardiomyopathy. *J Card Fail.* 2009;15(8):645-650.

106. Grewal J, Siu SC, Ross HJ, et al. Pregnancy outcomes in women with dilated cardiomyopathy. *J Am Coll Cardiol.* 2009;55(1):45-52.

107. Ray P, Murphy GJ, Shutt LE. Recognition and management of maternal cardiac disease in pregnancy. *Br J Anaesth.* 2004;93(3):428-439.

111. Haghikia A, Podewski E, Libhaber E, et al. Phenotyping and outcome on contemporary management in a German cohort of patients with peripartum cardiomyopathy. *Basic Res Cardiol.* 2013;108(4):366.

112. Yancy CW, Jessup M, Bozkurt B, et al. 2017 ACC/AHA/HFSA focused update of the 2013 ACCF/AHA Guideline for the management of heart failure: a report of the American College of Cardiology/American Heart Association Task Force on Clinical Practice Guidelines and the Heart Failure Society of America. *Circulation.* 2017;136(6):e137-e161. doi:10.1161/CIR.0000000000000509

113. Duncker D, Haghikia A, König T, et al. Risk for ventricular fibrillation in peripartum cardiomyopathy with severely reduced left ventricular function – Value of the wearable cardioverter/defibrillator. *Eur J Heart Fail.* 2014;16(12):1331-1336. doi:10.1002/ejhf.188

114. Blauwet LA, Libhaber E, Forster O, et al. Predictors of outcome in 176 South African patients with peripartum cardiomyopathy. *Heart.* 2013;99(5):308-313.

115. Amos AM, Jaber WA, Russell SD. Improved outcomes in peripartum cardiomyopathy with contemporary. *Am Heart J.* 2006;152(3):509-513.

116. Fett JD, Sannon H, Thélisma E, Sprunger T, Suresh V. Recovery from severe heart failure following peripartum cardiomyopathy. *Int J Gynecol Obstet.* 2009;104(2):125-127.

117. Goland S, Bitar F, Modi K, et al. Evaluation of the clinical relevance of baseline left ventricular ejection fraction as a predictor of recovery or persistence of severe dysfunction in women in the United States with peripartum cardiomyopathy. *J Card Fail.* 2011;17(5):426-430.

120. Autore C, Conte MR, Piccininno M, et al. Risk associated with pregnancy in hypertrophic cardiomyopathy. *J Am Coll Cardiol.* 2002;40(10):1864-1869. doi:10.1016/S0735-1097(02)02495-6

121. Autore C, Brauneis S, Apponi F, Commisso C, Pinto G, Fedele F. Epidural anesthesia for cesarean section in patients with hypertrophic cardiomyopathy: a report of three cases. *Anesthesiology.* 1999;90(4):1205-1207.

122. Kolibash AJ, Ruiz DE, Lewis RP. Idiopathic hypertrophic subaortic stenosis in pregnancy. *Ann Intern Med.* 1975;82(6):791-794.

123. Oakley GD, McGarry K, Limb DG, Oakley CM. Management of pregnancy in patients with hypertrophic cardiomyopathy. *Br Med J.* 1979;1(6180):1749-1750.

124. Schinkel AFL. Pregnancy in women with hypertrophic cardiomyopathy. *Cardiol Rev.* 2014;22(5).

125. Elliott PM, Anastasakis A, Borger MA, et al; Authors/Task Force members. 2014 ESC guidelines on diagnosis and management of hypertrophic cardiomyopathy: the Task Force for the Diagnosis and Management of Hypertrophic Cardiomyopathy of the European Society of Cardiology (ESC). *Eur Heart J.* 2014;35(39):2733-2779. doi:10.1093/eurheartj/ehu284

128. Smith K, Gros B. Pregnancy-related acute aortic dissection in Marfan syndrome: a review of the literature. *Congenit Heart Dis.* 2017;12(3):251-260. doi:10.1111/chd.12465

129. Donnelly RT, Pinto NM, Kocolas I, Yetman AT. The immediate and long-term impact of pregnancy on aortic growth rate and mortality in women with Marfan syndrome. *J Am Coll Cardiol.* 2012;60(3):224-229. doi:10.1016/j.jacc.2012.03.051

130. Goland S, Elkayam U. Cardiovascular problems in pregnant women with Marfan syndrome. *Circulation.* 2009;119(4):619-623. doi:10.1161/CIRCULATIONAHA.104.493569

131. Rossiter JP, Repke JT, Morales AJ, Murphy EA, Pyeritz RE. A prospective longitudinal evaluation of pregnancy in the Marfan syndrome. *Am J Obstet Gynecol.* 1995;173(5):1599-1606.

132. Lipscomb KJ, Clayton Smith J, Clarke B, Donnai P, Harris R. Outcome of pregnancy in women with Marfan's syndrome. *Br J Obstet Gynaecol.* 1997;104(2):201-206.

133. Murdoch JL, Walker BA, Halpern BL, Kuzma JW, McKusick VA. Life expectancy and causes of death in the Marfan syndrome. *N Engl J Med.* 1972;286(15):804-808.

134. Pyeritz RE, McKusick VA. The Marfan syndrome: diagnosis and management. *N Engl J Med.* 1979;300(14):772-777.

135. Pyeritz RE. Maternal and fetal complications of pregnancy in the Marfan syndrome. *Am J Med.* 1981;71(5):784-790. doi:10.1016/0002-9343(81)90365-X

136. Slater EE, DeSanctis RW. Dissection of the aorta. *Med Clin North Am.* 1979;63(1):141-154.

138. Koo H, Lawrence KA, Musini VM. Beta-blockers for preventing aortic dissection in Marfan syndrome. *Cochrane Database Syst Rev.* 2017;11(11). doi:10.1002/14651858.CD011103.pub2

139. Shores J, Berger KR, Murphy EA, Pyeritz RE. Progression of aortic dilatation and the benefit of long-term β-adrenergic blockade in Marfan's syndrome. *N Engl J Med.* 1994;330(19):1335-1341. doi:10.1056/NEJM199405123301902

140. Meijboom LJ, Drenthen W, Pieper PG, et al. Obstetric complications in Marfan syndrome. *Int J Cardiol.* 2006;110(1):53-59. doi:10.1016/j.ijcard.2005.07.017

141. Goland S, Barakat M, Khatri N, Elkayam U. Pregnancy in Marfan syndrome: maternal and fetal risk and recommendations for patient assessment and management. *Cardiol Rev.* 2009;17(6):253-262.

142. Murray ML, Pepin M, Peterson S, Byers PH. Pregnancy-related deaths and complications in women with vascular Ehlers-Danlos syndrome. *Genet Med.* 2014;16:874-880.

144. Roth A, Elkayam U. Acute myocardial infarction associated with pregnancy. *J Am Coll Cardiol.* 2008;52(3):171-180. doi:10.1016/j.jacc.2008.03.049

146. Jacqueline S, Aymong E, Sedlak T, et al. Spontaneous coronary artery dissection: association with predisposing arteriopathies and precipitating stressors and cardiovascular outcomes. *Circ Cardiovasc Interv.* 2014;7(5):645-655. doi:10.1161/CIRCINTERVENTIONS.114.001760

147. Hassan S, Prakash R, Starovoytov A, Saw J. Natural history of spontaneous coronary artery dissection with spontaneous angiographic healing. *JACC Cardiovasc Interv.* 2019;12(6):518-527. doi:10.1016/j.jcin.2018.12.011

155. Goland S, Elkayam U. Anticoagulation in pregnancy. *Cardiol Clin.* 2012;30(3):395-405. doi:10.1016/j.ccl.2012.05.003

156. Wyse DG, Waldo AL, DiMarco JP, et al. A comparison of rate control and rhythm control in patients with atrial fibrillation. *N Engl J Med.* 2002;347(23):1825-1833. doi:10.1056/NEJMoa021328

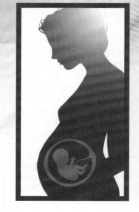

CHAPTER 29

Maternal Pulmonary Disorders Complicating Pregnancy

Steven James Cassady, Janaki Deepak, Neal Dodia, Jeffrey D. Hasday, William Brian Karkowsky, and Kathryn S. Robinett

Introduction

Pregnant women can be afflicted by the same respiratory illnesses as nonpregnant women, but these conditions may be complicated by the physiologic changes that occur during pregnancy. In this chapter, we will review the evaluation and diagnosis of lung disease in the pregnant patient, discuss the pertinent physiologic changes of the respiratory system that occur during pregnancy, and discuss specific respiratory illnesses with regard to the pregnant population.

Clinical Assessment of the Pregnant Pulmonary Patient

Pregnant patients should be evaluated for pulmonary disease in a similar manner to those who are nonpregnant. The core evaluation should stem from a thorough history, which can guide the need for serum blood testing, pulmonary function testing, and advanced imaging. Documenting baseline symptoms and function prior to pregnancy can be helpful to quantify change during pregnancy. Dyspnea is a common complaint during pregnancy and affects approximately 60% to 70% of pregnant women during both rest and exertion.[1] It is thought to be related largely to elevated circulating progesterone causing larger tidal volume breaths and increased perception of respiratory discomfort from these larger breaths. To a lesser degree, mechanical forces external to the lungs contribute to dyspnea as well.[2,3]

Differentiating a physiologic change from a pathologic change requires an understanding of the normal physiologic changes that occur during pregnancy and a careful history taking. For example, despite the common complaint of dyspnea, most pregnant patients should not experience a change in exercise tolerance and should not have abnormalities on physical examination. If these findings are present, further workup and potentially pulmonary consultation may be warranted.[4,5]

Pulmonary Physiology in Pregnancy
Normal Respiratory Physiology

To understand the mechanical changes that occur in pregnancy, we must first review the respiratory physiology of healthy nonpregnant patients. Lung volume is determined by the balance between the force exerted by the chest wall and the elastic recoil of the lung. In forced exhalation, contraction of the respiratory muscles (eg, the rectus abdominis, transverse abdominis, internal and external obliques, and intercostals) reduces lung volumes until compression of the noncartilagenous segments of the bronchial tree terminates further exhalation (**Figure 29.1**). The volume remaining in the lung at this point is the residual volume (RV). The lung volume at maximal inspiration, including the RV, is the total lung capacity (TLC). The total volume that can be exhaled from a full inspiration is the vital capacity (VC). The forced VC (FVC) is measured with a forced expiration and is usually the same as when measured during an unforced or slow VC (SVC). Maintaining RV or TLC requires active work by the respiratory muscles. The volume remaining in the lungs at the end of a normal effortless exhalation when the outward recoil of the relaxed respiratory muscles is balanced by the inward force of elastic recoil is the functional residual capacity (FRC). Abnormal lung volumes may be caused by

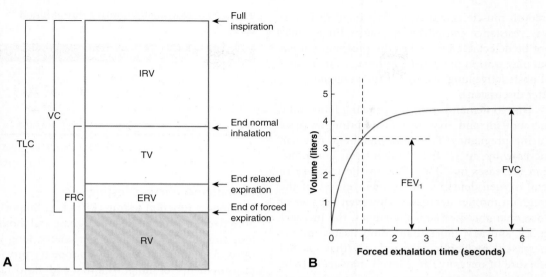

Figure 29.1 Lung volumes and capacities. Lung volumes and lung capacities, comprising two or more lung volumes, are shown schematically in panel A. ERV, expiratory reserve volume; FRC, functional residual capacity; IRV, inspiratory reserve volume; RV, residual volume; TLC, total lung capacity; TV, tidal volume; VC, vital capacity. A representation of a spirogram is shown in panel B with forced expiratory volume in 1 second (FEV_1) and forced vital capacity (FVC) indicated.

changes in the shape or compliance of the chest wall or abdomen, changes in respiratory muscle function, reduced pleural compliance or accumulation of pleural fluid, or reduced compliance of lung parenchyma. The flow rates in the airways are determined by airway luminal diameter. Air flow limitation occurs when airway lumens are narrowed by airway wall thickening, bronchoconstriction, or the presence of intraluminal mucus.

Respiratory Physiology Changes During Pregnancy
During pregnancy, FRC decreases by 9.5% to 25% as the gravid uterus gradually displaces the diaphragm upwards.[6] However, expansion of the chest wall compensates for loss of volume due to this diaphragmatic displacement so that TLC remains unchanged, and inspiratory capacity and tidal volume usually increase during pregnancy.[7,8] Respiratory muscle strength is not affected by the mechanical changes of pregnancy, which may be the result of changes in the curvature of the diaphragm due to uterine enlargement that leads to increased muscle fiber stretch. Measurements of maximal inspiratory and expiratory force also remain preserved. While respiratory muscle strength is preserved, increases in pleural and intra-abdominal pressures increase the respiratory muscle work required to achieve the same level of lung expansion.[7,9]

Hormonal and Metabolic Changes During Pregnancy
The increases in progesterone and estrogen levels that occur during normal pregnancy modify respiratory drive. Total respiration, often quantified as the minute ventilation (MV), the product of the respiratory rate (RR), and tidal volume (TV or V_T), is managed both consciously and unconsciously. Unconscious regulation is controlled by central respiratory centers in the medulla that primarily respond to blood levels of carbon dioxide (CO_2). Progesterone acts on receptors present in the central respiratory centers to increase sensitivity to CO_2, thereby increasing TV and MV and reducing blood partial pressure of CO_2 (Pco_2). Estrogen can augment the effect of progesterone on respiratory drive by increasing the sensitivity and number of progesterone receptors. In addition to its effects on MV, progesterone can cause mucosal edema of the upper airways, which can contribute to upper airway obstruction.[6,8,10]

Prostaglandins circulate throughout pregnancy and can have various effects on the respiratory system. Prostaglandins E_1 and E_2 have a dilatory effect on the bronchial smooth muscle, whereas prostaglandin $F_{2\alpha}$, a uterine smooth muscle stimulant during labor, causes bronchial smooth muscle constriction. The increase in airway resistance caused by prostaglandin $F_{2\alpha}$ may not be detectable by the healthy pregnant patient but may worsen preexisting asthma or other types of obstructive lung disease during pregnancy (see later discussion).[8]

Due to demand from the growing fetus, total metabolism and oxygen consumption increase during pregnancy. The basal metabolic rate can increase by up to 15%, and oxygen consumption increases by 20%.[11] Due to the increase in fetal oxygen demand, the oxygen reserve of the pregnant mother decreases. However, because of hormonal and mechanical changes, the increase in TV and MV more than compensates for the increased metabolic demand so that partial pressure of oxygen (Pao_2) levels may actually be higher in pregnant women than nonpregnant women.[6]

Screening

Blood Gas Evaluation

Measuring serum venous or arterial blood can be a useful determinant of acid-base status, and the latter can provide detailed information about maternal oxygenation. Venous blood gases (VBG) can provide a close estimate of arterial pH but do not evaluate oxygenation. VBGs have the benefit of being easier and less painful to obtain than arterial blood gases (ABGs) and carry less risk of vessel injury.[12,13]

If a precise measurement of the pH and arterial Pco_2 ($Paco_2$) or an evaluation of the Pao_2 is required, then an ABG may be indicated. ABG values can be useful in determining an underlying diagnosis of respiratory failure and triaging patients. Normal values for blood gas measurements differ between nonpregnant and pregnant patients (**Table 29.1**).[11] Overall, respiratory changes during pregnancy result in a respiratory alkalosis with slightly increased Pao_2 or arterial oxygen tension. Both are normal physiologic changes that result from the increase in ventilation that occurs primarily due to circulating progesterone; this mechanism is further described in the physiology section of the chapter.[13] It is important to understand that results from the blood gas tests may be reported as abnormal because most testing laboratories do not change normal values for pregnant patients.

Table 29.1 Normal Values of Arterial Blood Gases[11]

Measurement	Nonpregnant	Pregnant
pH	7.35-7.45	7.40-7.47
$Paco_2$ (mm Hg)	35-40	27-32
HCO_3 (mmol/L)	22-24	18-22
Pao_2 (mm Hg)	80-100	100-108

HCO_3, bicarbonate; $Paco_2$, arterial Pco_2; Pao_2, partial pressure of oxygen.

Pulmonary Function Testing

Pulmonary function testing (PFT) is an important objective test to diagnose lung disease and monitor lung function. PFTs include spirometry, lung volumes, and diffusion capacity. Spirometry provides measurements of lung volumes and flow rates, including FVC and the exhaled volume in the first second of a forced expiration, known as the forced expiratory volume in 1 second (FEV_1), which can help identify and distinguish between obstructive and restrictive disease.

A ratio of the FEV_1/FVC ratio of less than 0.70 is generally considered diagnostic for obstruction or the presence of airflow limitation, although subtler findings on spirometry, such as "scooping" of the expiratory limb of the flow volume loop, may suggest obstruction with borderline values for FEV_1/FVC ratio. Once obstruction is established, its severity can then be determined based on the patient's FEV_1 result as it compares to normal values.[14] Restrictive lung disease is suggested by a decrease in the FVC below 80% of predicted without evidence of obstruction (ie, FEV_1/FVC ratio > 0.70).

Because spirometry can only measure exhaled volume, lung volume testing is required for measurement of RV and the volume measures that incorporate the RV, including the FRC and TLC. Values for TLC less than 80% of predicted confirm the presence of a restrictive defect. In some cases, spirometry and lung volumes may indicate the presence of both obstructive and restrictive defects.[15]

Imaging

Radiographic imaging is frequently obtained to assist with the evaluation and diagnosis of pulmonary disease. A justified concern for many pregnant patients is whether radiation exposure is safe for the fetus. Fortunately, in most circumstances, radiation exposure from chest imaging does not pose a significant risk to the mother or fetus. The risk for radiation-associated fetal abnormalities is greatest in the first trimester and early second trimester, but the doses of radiation used for standard x-ray or computed tomography (CT) imaging are well below the threshold level for causing fetal abnormalities. For example, conservative estimates place 50 mGy as a potential threshold of radiation exposure to cause embryonic death, whereas a complete chest CT scan exposes a fetus to only 0.01 to 0.66 mGy. Overall, the consensus is that chest imaging should not be withheld in the pregnant patient if it is clinically indicated.[16] See Chapter 9 for detailed discussion on radiation in pregnancy.

Chest x-rays remain an effective modality for diagnosing a myriad of pulmonary conditions, including pneumonia, pulmonary edema, and pneumothorax. However, a CT of the chest may be required for higher resolution imaging of the lung parenchyma. CT angiography of the chest using intravenous contrast can be performed safely in pregnancy to evaluate vascular structures and diagnose pulmonary embolism.[17] Animal studies and observational reports have not shown any negative impacts of intravenous contrast on fetal development.[16]

Effects of Pulmonary Disorders on Pregnancy

Asthma

Clinical Presentation
Asthma is a common lung disorder characterized by the classic clinical manifestations of bronchospasm, such as wheezing, shortness of breath, chest tightness, and cough in response to triggers. Because airway resistance is often variable in asthma, patients with asthma may have normal expiratory airflow on PFT. If suspicion of asthma is high and PFTs fail to show an obstructive pattern, repeated home measurements of peak flow rates may identify asthma by demonstrating peak flow rate variability.

Epidemiology
Asthma is the most common chronic disease in women during their childbearing years and is the most common chronic disease affecting pregnant women.[18] The prevalence of asthma in pregnant woman is between 8% and 13%.[18] Asthma has a significant impact on

1% to 4% of pregnancies with life-threatening exacerbations occurring in between 0.5% and 5% of pregnancies.[18] Women often experience changes in their asthma control during pregnancy, and there is a general "rule of thirds" that one-third of women experience improved asthma control, one-third of women experience worsening control, and one-third of women have unchanged control.[19] The burden of asthma-related complications in pregnancy is greater for African-American women, who have higher rates of morbidity and mortality associated with asthma.[18,20] Fortunately, if asthma is well controlled during pregnancy, there is almost no increased risk of complication for the mother or fetus.[20]

Maternal Risk From Asthma
There are a variety of reasons why asthma may worsen symptomatically during pregnancy, including the effects of the normal physiological changes that during pregnancy. Pregnant women have significant hormonal changes that affect respiratory drive and gravidae are more susceptible to viral respiratory infections, such as influenza, both of which can lead to increased frequency of asthma exacerbations, especially in the second trimester.[23,24] An important cause of pregnancy-related asthma exacerbations is inadequate treatment of underlying asthma due to unwarranted concerns of adverse medication effects by patients and/or their healthcare clinicians. However, undertreatment of asthma poses a greater risk for mother and fetus and can result in asthma exacerbations, preeclampsia, preterm delivery, low birth weight, and increased perinatal mortality, as discussed in the section on fetal risk below.[18,23]

Fetal Complications of Maternal Asthma
Concerns regarding the risks to the fetus associated with maternal asthma include the impact of suboptimal asthma control and the potential adverse effects of asthma treatments. With regard to the former, several large cohort studies clearly demonstrate a consistent association between poor asthma control and numerous obstetric and neonatal complications. The largest of these studies, which evaluated pregnancy outcomes in 37,585 pregnant women with asthma and 243,434 pregnant women without asthma, demonstrated a small but statistically significant increase in the incidence of miscarriage, antepartum hemorrhage, postpartum hemorrhage, anemia, depression, and need for

cesarean delivery in patients with asthma.[22] A large retrospective US-based cohort study evaluated the effect of asthma in 223,512 singleton pregnancies on multiple pregnancy-related complications and found that, after adjustment for multiple variables, pregnant women with asthma have higher odds of preeclampsia, pulmonary embolism, and preterm labor compared to those without asthma.[21] A meta-analysis of 21 studies comparing pregnancies in women with and without asthma found that the risk of congenital malformations was slightly increased in women with asthma, although this increased risk was not seen when controlling for women receiving active asthma management, suggesting that control of underlying asthma mitigated this risk.[25]

The underlying mechanisms driving the risk of obstetrical complications in pregnant women with poorly controlled asthma have not been conclusively defined, but may include maternal hypoxia, disruptions of uteroplacental blood flow, or increased administration of systemic oral corticosteroids. A large analysis of pregnant women with asthma found that poorly controlled asthma increased the risk of spontaneous abortion by 26%.[26] Interestingly, no association was found between asthma severity and spontaneous or induced abortion.[26] Similarly, maternal asthma exacerbations and oral corticosteroid use were associated with low birth weight and preterm delivery. Moderate to severe asthma during pregnancy was associated with an increased risk of small for gestational age and low birth weight infants.[26]

Management of Asthma Exacerbations in Pregnancy

Management of asthma exacerbations in pregnant women does not differ substantially from that of the nonpregnant patient. Treatment plans should emphasize appropriate maternal and fetal monitoring, identification of triggers (including infections and medication nonadherence), appropriate supportive care, and prompt initiation of severity-dependent pharmacologic therapies. As mentioned previously, because the risks associated with asthma exacerbations far exceed maternal or fetal risks from the adverse effects of pharmacologic therapies, prompt treatment of exacerbations is crucial.

Definitions of asthma exacerbation are neither uniform nor comprehensive, but broadly include worsening respiratory symptoms of breathlessness, wheezing, chest tightness, or cough, along with evidence of airflow obstruction by peak flow monitoring. Once a reasonable suspicion for asthma exacerbation exists, rapid assessment of severity should ensue with a focused evaluation for evidence of labored breathing, respiratory distress, and inadequate oxygenation or ventilation. In urgent care and emergency settings, appropriate monitoring of mother and fetus, including pulse oximetry and fetal heart monitoring, should be initiated.

Pharmacologic and Nonpharmacologic Treatment of Stable Asthma

Fortunately, treatment of asthma with nonpharmacologic and pharmacologic therapies effectively mitigates the risks of obstetrical complications with a favorable safety profile. The mainstay of nonpharmacologic therapies includes appropriate patient education on respiratory trigger avoidance and smoking cessation. In terms of pharmacologic management, the cornerstone for rapid reversal of acute asthma symptoms remains short-acting beta-agonists (SABAs) such as albuterol. Some case-controlled studies have shown a small increase in the risk of some congenital malformations, including gastroschisis, cleft palate, and cardiac defects, associated with SABA use, but the general consensus is that this class of drugs is safe to use during pregnancy.[27-29] The risk of these associated defects appears to be small, and these studies are difficult to interpret because SABA use itself is an indicator of suboptimal asthma control. Long-acting beta-agonist (LABA) bronchodilators also appear to be quite safe for use in pregnancy, with most of the safety data generated for salmeterol and formoterol.[30]

In general, oral corticosteroids are best reserved for salvage therapy or for patients experiencing a severe respiratory exacerbation. Systemic corticosteroids have been associated with distinct congenital malformations, specifically cleft palate, preterm birth, and low birth weights.[27] Inhaled corticosteroids as a stand-alone therapy or in combination with an LABA are associated with a much lower risk of fetal abnormalities than systemic corticosteroids. Use of inhaled budesonide was found not to be associated with an increased rate of congenital malformations in a Swedish registry of nearly 3000 pregnant women.[31] Similar to the results with budesonide, the use of fluticasone did not affect rates of low birth weight, small for gestational age births, and preterm delivery.[30]

Studies of leukotriene modifiers, including leukotriene receptor antagonists such as montelukast and zafirlukast, have shown no increase in major birth defects or other adverse outcomes in women taking these medications during pregnancy.[32-34] In the last decade, treatment of asthma has expanded to include an array of monoclonal antibodies, including anti-immunoglobulin (Ig) E, anti-interleukin (IL)-5, and anti-IL-4 therapies. To date, no significant teratogenicity has been observed with the use of these medications, but it remains too early to assure the safety of these medications during pregnancy as these antibodies likely cross the placenta and are not approved for use in pregnancy by the U.S. Food and Drug Administration (FDA). However, omalizumab is categorized as pregnancy category B by the FDA based on the publication of an omalizumab pregnancy registry.[35]

Supplemental oxygen may be beneficial in individuals who are unable to maintain oxygen saturations above 95% or a Pao_2 of greater than 80 mm Hg. It is worth emphasizing that a near-"normal" $Paco_2$ on an ABG measurement based on nonpregnant normal values may fail to identify relative decompensation and impaired ventilatory reserve when superimposed on the typical alkalosis that occurs during pregnancy.

Medications typically used for acute asthma include systemic corticosteroids, short-acting bronchodilator agents, and intravenous magnesium sulfate. Doses and routes of systemic corticosteroids need not differ substantially from that used in non-pregnant females, but optimal doses during pregnancy have not been conclusively identified. Standard doses of systemic corticosteroids range between 40 and 60 mg for prednisone or the equivalent dose of methylprednisolone (32-48 mg). Higher doses of corticosteroids are often used in patients with particularly severe asthma exacerbations or for those who are critically ill. Short-acting bronchodilators, such as albuterol and ipratropium, are used similarly in pregnant and nonpregnant patients and are typically administered as a nebulized form during acute exacerbations. Given its well-studied safety profile, intravenous magnesium sulfate is often given for its bronchodilator effects. Use of the intravenous beta-agonist epinephrine is generally avoided during pregnancy due to concerns for potential circulatory effects on uteroplacental blood flow.

Aspiration in Pregnancy

Clinical Presentation

Aspiration of low pH gastric contents into the tracheobronchial tree can lead to a chemical pneumonitis and bacterial pneumonia. A number of physiological factors predispose pregnant women to aspiration, including elevated intragastric pressure due to the gravid uterus and increased prevalence of gastroesophageal reflux disease (GERD) due to the negative effects of circulating estradiol and progesterone on lower esophageal sphincter tone.[36] The risks of aspiration are highest during and immediately following labor and are further increased by the use of sedation and analgesic medications, repositioning during labor, and by tracheal intubation if general anesthesia is required.

Chemical pneumonitis due to aspiration of gastric contents with a pH 2.5 or lower is characterized by early alveolar injury, hemorrhage, and edema followed by acute inflammation and formation of hyaline membranes. Patients may develop fever, abrupt-onset dyspnea, diffuse crackles on lung examination, and potentially marked hypoxemia. Chest x-ray or CT chest imaging may demonstrate consolidation in the region portion of the lung. Severe cases of aspiration pneumonitis may progress to respiratory failure or acute respiratory distress syndrome (ARDS).

Aspiration pneumonia, which may develop as a superimposed infection of the injured lung, usually presents with a similar symptom profile as other forms of bacterial pneumonia (see below), including fever, dyspnea, and cough productive of purulent sputum. However, because the causative pathogens in aspiration pneumonia are usually anaerobic bacteria and other oral flora that are more indolent than the pathogens responsible for typical bacterial pneumonia, the course of the illness is less acute, developing over days to weeks.

Pharmacologic Treatment

Treatment is primarily supportive, with immediate tracheal suction recommended for witnessed aspiration events along with supplemental oxygen and mechanical ventilation, if needed.

Suggested regimens for aspiration include beta-lactam derivatives combined with a beta-lactamase inhibitor, such as ampicillin-sulbactam, as these include coverage for the anaerobic bacteria that frequently cause aspiration pneumonia. Carbapenems or fluoroquinolones are reasonable alternative choices.[37] Differentiating aspiration pneumonitis from pneumonia may be difficult, and patients with more severe presentations may warrant empiric expanded coverage with broad-spectrum antibiotics.[38] Cases of aspiration pneumonia during or following hospitalization may warrant additional antibiotic coverage targeted toward methicillin-resistant *Staphylococcus aureus* (MRSA) and other more resistant pathogens.

Management of Aspiration in Pregnancy

Aspiration prophylaxis is frequently used in pregnant women who are to undergo cesarean delivery or other surgery under general anesthesia, although there are little empiric data about its effectiveness.[39] Nonparticulate antacids, H2 receptor antagonists, and proton-pump inhibitors are all viable options. An effective reduction in gastric acidity to a pH of above 2.5 has been demonstrated with the combination of antacids and H2 receptor antagonists, with more limited data available regarding the use of proton-pump inhibitors.[3] Other prophylactic measures include preoperative fasting, including 6 hours of preoperative fasting for solid food prior to the planned procedure.

Infectious Pulmonary Diseases in Pregnancy

Influenza
Epidemiology
Influenza infection is common during pregnancy and has been associated with a high risk of maternal mortality, especially late in the third trimester and with advanced maternal age. High influenza-associated mortality rates in pregnant women have occurred in historical pandemics, such as the 1918-1919 influenza pandemic, and more recent endemics, such as the H1N1 virus in 2009, where pregnant women comprised 5% of influenza-related deaths.[40]

Clinical Presentation
Influenza typically presents with systemic symptoms including fever, headache, myalgias, malaise, and upper respiratory symptoms such as rhinorrhea, sore throat, and a nonproductive cough. Severe cases may involve the lower respiratory tract infection and must be distinguished from superimposed bacterial pneumonia. In some cases, influenza can directly cause pneumonia, which can progress to ARDS and cause respiratory failure.

Influenza can also be complicated by bacterial infections, classically due to *Streptococcus pneumoniae, Staphylococcus aureus,* or *Haemophilus influenzae.*[41] MRSA is an emerging concern in post-influenza pneumonia and should be considered as a potential pathogen, especially in severe cases of pneumonia or patients with positive nares surveillance testing for MRSA.

Clinical Assessment
Physical examination findings are variable and may include postnasal discharge, cervical adenopathy, and rhonchi, wheezes, and/or rales on chest examinations. If influenza is suspected in a pregnant or recently postpartum patient, testing should be performed expeditiously to confirm the diagnosis. Polymerase chain reaction (PCR)–based tests are preferred over rapid antigen tests due to their superior sensitivity.

Pharmacologic Treatment
Suspected cases of influenza should be treated without delay while awaiting test results. The neuraminidase inhibitors, oseltamivir and zanamivir, are currently the first-line therapies for suspected or confirmed influenza infection, although there is greater clinical experience with oseltamivir. The safety of these medications during pregnancy has yet to be definitively established, although the consensus is that the potential benefits of pharmacologic intervention outweigh the risks. Antibiotics are reserved for complications such as secondary bacterial pneumonia but should not be stopped abruptly if suspicion for superimposed infection remains.[42]

Management of Influenza in Pregnancy
Current recommendations advise influenza vaccination for all persons aged 6 months or older without contraindications, which includes pregnant women or women who plan to become pregnant. Pregnant women should be given inactivated vaccines rather than live-attenuated vaccines due to concern over their safety during pregnancy. Unfortunately, rates of vaccination in pregnant women remain relatively low, with rates of 49% reported in 2017-2018.[43]

Bacterial Pneumonia
Epidemiology
Pneumonia of all types is a relatively common cause of maternal morbidity, with a reported incidence of

0.5 to 1.5 per 1000 deliveries, which is similar to the nonpregnant population.[44] Although the mortality of pneumonia during pregnancy has improved with antibiotics and modern obstetric care, pneumonia remains a significant cause of maternal death, especially among women with preexisting cardiopulmonary diseases.

Clinical Presentation

The clinical presentation of pneumonia in pregnancy does not appear to differ substantially from that in nonpregnant adults and classically begins with abrupt-onset fever, rigors, cough productive of purulent sputum, dyspnea, and pleuritic chest pain.[45] The most common reported pathogens causing antepartum pneumonia include *Streptococcus pneumoniae*, which accounts for 65% of cases of bacterial pneumonia in which a pathogen is identified, *Mycoplasma pneumoniae*, and *Haemophilus influenzae* (**Table 29.2**).[45] *Staphylococcus aureus, Legionella pneumophila, Klebsiella pneumoniae*, and *Pseudomonas* spp. are less frequently reported as causes of bacterial pneumonia in pregnancy.[44]

Clinical Assessment

Physical findings may include signs of distress, such as tachycardia or tachypnea, as well as physical examination findings of pulmonary consolidation, which may include dullness to percussion, egophony, and tactile fremitus. Often, plain film radiography of the chest will show the presence of segmental or lobar consolidation. Laboratory findings may often include leukocytosis with left shift.

Screening

Diagnostic workup typically includes chest x-ray or CT scan with appropriate shielding of the fetus and sputum Gram stain and culture from a high-quality sample, which may show gram-positive cocci in pairs and chains in the case of pneumococcal pneumonia or gram-negative coccobacilli in the case of *Haemophilus,* although the utility of routine sputum testing is somewhat controversial.[46] A PCR-based respiratory viral panel, if available, should also be performed to rule out suspected influenza or other viral causes of lower respiratory tract infection, especially during winter seasons when the prevalence of these pathogens is higher. Use of these panels may decrease the patient's exposure to unnecessary or potentially harmful antibiotics, although coinfection with both viral and bacterial pathogens is not uncommon.[42]

Blood cultures may not be required in all patients but should be obtained in all patients with chronic liver disease, active alcohol abuse, leukopenia, the presence of a pleural effusion, or who are to be admitted to an intensive care unit.[47] Urine antigen tests for pneumococcus or *Legionella* are highly specific may also be helpful for diagnosis of these specific pathogens, although tests for pneumococcus have a high false-positive rate if the patient had pneumonia in the prior few weeks.[48]

Pharmacologic Treatment

Management should include early resuscitation and antibiotic administration as well as supplemental oxygen as needed. In general, all pregnant women with a suspected bacterial pneumonia should be admitted for initiation of antibiotics, fetal monitoring, and maintenance of respiratory stability.[49] Empiric antibiotic therapy for pregnant patients should follow the same guidelines as those for nonpregnant patients, with careful attention to any potential for fetal toxicity (**Table 29.3**). Combined use of a beta-lactam agent, such as a third-generation cephalosporin, and a macrolide, such as azithromycin, remains the recommended empiric regimen for uncomplicated community-acquired pneumonia.[47] Both cephalosporins and macrolides have a favorable safety record in pregnancy. If certain risk factors are present, including chronic structural lung disease or recent broad-spectrum antibiotic use, an antipseudomonal beta-lactam such as piperacillin-tazobactam or cefepime should be considered as an empiric choice. Respiratory fluoroquinolones are an acceptable alternate empiric choice, as there are increasing data suggesting a lack of fetal harm or association with unfavorable pregnancy outcomes.[51,52] Tetracyclines should be avoided due to evidence of hepatotoxicity and adverse effects on fetal bones and teeth, although these effects are reportedly very rare with doxycycline as compared to older tetracyclines.[53] If a pathogen is isolated from sputum or blood cultures, antibiotic treatment can be tailored to the organism found, and the recommended length of antibiotic treatment is the same as in the general population.

Table 29.2 Pathogens in Community-Acquired Pneumonia

More frequently encountered	
Streptococcus pneumoniae	
Haemophilus influenzae	
Mycoplasma pneumoniae	
Viruses (rhinovirus, influenza, RSV, adenovirus, etc.)	
Less frequently encountered	**Risk factors**
Staphylococcus aureus (MSSA, MRSA)	Postinfluenza pneumonia, aspiration, structural lung disease, mechanical ventilation
Legionella pneumophila	Known outbreaks, exposure to contaminated water, immunocompromised state
Klebsiella pneumoniae	Alcoholism, diabetes mellitus, mechanical ventilation
Pseudomonas aeruginosa	Immunocompromised state, structural lung disease, recent antibiotic use, mechanical ventilation

RSV, respiratory syncytial virus; MSSA, methicillin-sensitive *Staphylococcus aureus*; MRSA, methicillin-resistant *Staphylococcus aureus*.

Management of Bacterial Pneumonia in Pregnancy

Pneumonia may cause significant hypoxemia that requires the use of supplemental oxygen. Adequate fetal oxygenation should be ensured by maintaining maternal Pao_2 of at least 65 mmHg at all times, although optimal oxygen saturation targets are not established.[44] Positive-pressure ventilation using high-flow nasal cannula or bilevel positive airway pressure (BPAP) ventilation should be considered to ensure adequate oxygenation.

As in the general population, the 23-valent pneumococcal polysaccharide vaccine should be given prior to pregnancy to adults older than 19 years with comorbidities that increase the likelihood of invasive pneumococcal disease, such as cigarette smoking, chronic heart or lung disease, diabetes mellitus, or alcohol abuse. Dual vaccination with both the 13-valent and 23-valent pneumococcal vaccines is recommended in immunocompromised patients, including those with human immunodeficiency virus (HIV) infection, solid organ transplant, hematologic malignancy, or chronic renal failure.[54] If not previously given,

administration in the second and third trimesters has not shown adverse effects, although there are no data on outcomes with PCV13 use in pregnancy.[55]

Varicella Pneumonia
Epidemiology and Risk to the Fetus

Viruses are increasingly implicated as causes of lower respiratory tract infections in both pregnant and nonpregnant adults.[56] Viral pneumonia due to varicella-zoster virus (VZV) is a rare but life-threatening illness with a mortality rate in pregnant women estimated to be 15%. With the advent of the varicella vaccine, there has been a substantial reduction in the number of varicella cases and hospitalizations in the general population.[57] Rates of varicella pneumonia among pregnant woman are not greater than the general population, but the disease appears to be more severe in pregnancy.[58-60]

Maternal varicella infection is associated with potentially lethal, although rare, congenital abnormalities, and there is a risk of fatal disseminated infection in the infant if varicella is contracted within 5 days of delivery. The risk of congenital varicella syndrome after maternal varicella infection is estimated at <1% with the syndrome associated with infection only in the first two trimesters of pregnancy.[61] Early case reports also demonstrated a higher rate of preterm labor, although this has not been substantiated in later studies.[44]

Clinical Presentation

Symptoms of pneumonia typically develop slowly within 1 to 6 days after appearance of rash. In its severe form, symptoms may resemble those of bacterial pneumonia, including high fever, dyspnea, cough, and pleuritic chest pain.

Clinical Assessment

Chest radiograph classically shows diffuse bilateral opacities that may have a nodular component. Diagnosis is largely clinical and based on the appearance of respiratory symptoms alongside typical skin lesions and known contact with varicella, but PCR testing of vesicular skin scrapings or fluid can help with confirmation of the diagnosis.[62,63]

Management of Varicella Pneumonia in Pregnancy

Prevention is of paramount importance, and all women considering pregnancy should be questioned about their varicella history with titers

Table 29.3 IDSA Community-Acquired Pneumonia Antibiotic Treatment Strategies[50]

Outpatient	Amoxicillin **or** doxycycline, **or** a macrolide (if local pneumococcal resistance is <25%) In those with chronic comorbidities, such as chronic lung, liver, or heart disease, alcoholism, or asplenia, use combination therapy with amoxicillin-clavulanate or cephalosporin **plus** a macrolide or doxycycline, **or** a respiratory fluoroquinolone alone
Inpatient, nonsevere	Respiratory fluoroquinolone **or** beta-lactam with activity against pneumococcus (ceftriaxone, ampicillin-sulbactam, cefotaxime) **plus** a macrolide
Inpatient, severe	Antipneumococcal beta-lactam **plus** azithromycin **or** a beta-lactam **plus** a respiratory fluoroquinolone If recent hospitalization with use of parenteral antibiotics and risk factors present for MRSA and/or *Pseudomonas,* add empiric coverage and de-escalate according to culture data
Special indications	For prior *Pseudomonas* isolation from the respiratory tract, use an antipneumococcal beta-lactam with antipseudomonal activity, ie, cefepime, piperacillin-tazobactam, or carbapenem, **plus** a respiratory fluoroquinolone or macrolide For prior isolation of MRSA from the respiratory tract, add coverage with vancomycin or linezolid

IDSA, Infectious Disease Society of America; MRSA, methicillin-resistant *Staphylococcus aureus.*

drawn to confirm immunity. If there is no evidence of immunity, a live attenuated varicella vaccine should be given in two doses 4 to 8 weeks apart along standard guidelines. However, the vaccine should not be administered during pregnancy because of the risk of causing congenital disease. In pregnant women shown to be nonimmune to varicella, the vaccine should be given immediately following delivery. For nonimmune pregnant women with confirmed varicella exposure, post-exposure prophylaxis with varicella-zoster immune globulin (VZIG) is recommended.[64]

Pharmacologic Treatment

It is recommended that any pregnant woman with varicella pneumonia be admitted for parenteral antiviral therapy. First-line treatment for complicated varicella infection in pregnant women, including varicella pneumonia, is intravenous acyclovir. Although there are few large studies, acyclovir use during the first trimester has not been shown to increase the risk of teratogenicity.[65]

Amniotic Fluid Embolus Syndrome

Epidemiology

Amniotic fluid embolism syndrome (AFES) is a rare but devastating complication unique to pregnancy that most often occurs within 24 hours of delivery.[76] Despite its rarity, occurring in 1.7 to 2.0 per 100,000 deliveries, AFES remains a major cause of maternal

death and morbidity, with a large proportion of survivors experiencing severe neurological deficits.[77,78] Mortality rates as high as 20% have been shown in a meta-analysis of population-based studies.[79]

Etiology

AFES was previously thought to occur due to the embolization of amniotic fluid from the fetal circulation into the pulmonary circulation, resulting in acute respiratory failure and shock. Current understanding of the pathophysiology of AFES is that the entry of amniotic fluid containing fetal cells into the maternal bloodstream evokes a systemic inflammatory response with release of endogenous mediators with vasoactive and procoagulant effects, and subsequent disseminated intravascular coagulation (DIC). The presence of amniotic fluid in the pulmonary circulation is now considered nonspecific, although mechanical obstruction of the pulmonary vasculature by fetal cells, debris, and amniotic fluid, along with elevated circulating pulmonary vasoconstrictors, may contribute to right ventricular failure, which often occurs in AFES.[80]

Clinical Presentation

Patients are at greatest risk for AFES during labor, when approximately 70% of cases occur. Most of the remaining cases occur during delivery or immediately postpartum. Clinical presentation classically includes sudden onset of severe hypoxemia and shock, evidence of DIC, and signs of neurological dysfunction including altered mental status and seizure. Acute lung injury may progress rapidly and be accompanied by acute right ventricular failure and subsequent left ventricular failure, cardiogenic pulmonary edema, and cardiogenic shock. Death may occur from multiorgan failure, hemorrhage from the placental bed, or cardiac arrest.

Clinical Assessment

The diagnosis of AFES is clinical and is a diagnosis of exclusion of other more common conditions, including pulmonary embolism, septic shock, or anaphylactic shock, and should be considered in the event of any acute cardiopulmonary collapse during labor or shortly after delivery.[80] The combination of consumptive coagulopathy, ARDS, and shock in a pregnant woman with risk factors during labor, delivery, or immediately postpartum is generally considered to be AFES until proven otherwise (**Table 29.4**). A standardized definition of AFES has been proposed, which is helpful in streamlining the clinical assessment and includes the presence of cardiorespiratory arrest or severe hypotension, overt DIC, absence of fever during labor, and timing of clinical onset during labor or within 30 minutes of placental delivery.[81] Neurological signs, although not explicitly included in the Society for Maternal-Fetal Medicine definition, are considered supportive of the diagnosis (**Table 29.5**).[82]

Management of AFES in Pregnancy

There remains no way to predict or prevent amniotic fluid embolism. A multidisciplinary team involving specialists in maternal-fetal medicine, anesthesiology, critical care, and respiratory therapy is recommended,

Table 29.4 Risk Factors for Amniotic Fluid Embolus Syndrome

Operative delivery (cesarean or vaginal)
Placenta previa or placenta accreta
Placental abruption
Amniocentesis
Trauma
Termination of pregnancy with hypertonic saline
Multiparity and/or advanced maternal age
Prolonged gestation
Male fetus
Women of ethnic minorities

Table 29.5 Research Diagnostic Criteria for Amniotic Fluid Embolus Syndrome (Society for Maternal-Fetal Medicine and Amniotic Fluid Embolism Foundation)

Proposed diagnostic criteria for amniotic fluid embolism syndrome (AFES)
All four of the following:
• Sudden onset of cardiorespiratory arrest or hypotension (SBP < 90 mm Hg) with evidence of respiratory compromise
• Documentation of overt DIC based on a score of ≥3 using International Society on Thrombosis and Haemostasis (ISTH) DIC scoring system:
• Platelet count > 100,000/mL = 0 points, <100,000 = 1 point, <50,000 = 2 points
• Prothrombin time or INR < 25% increased = 0 points, 25%-50% increase = 1 point, >50% increase = 2 points
• Fibrinogen level > 200 mg/L = 0 points, <200 mg/L = 1 point
• Clinical onset during labor or within 30 min of placental delivery
• Absence of fever (≥38.0 °C) during labor

DIC, disseminated intravascular coagulation; INR, international normalized ratio; SBP, systolic blood pressure.
Modified from Clark SL, Romero R, Dildy GA, et al. Proposed diagnostic criteria for the case definition of amniotic fluid embolism in research studies. *Am J Obstet Gynecol.* 2016;215(4):408-412.

and treatment remains supportive, including supplemental oxygen and mechanical ventilation, vasopressor and/or inotrope support to address systemic hypotension, and aggressive transfusion for blood loss that may occur as the result of systemic coagulopathy. Excess fluid administration, hyperoxia, and hyperglycemia should be avoided.[80] Continuous renal replacement therapy should also be considered in the event of acute renal failure. Immediate basic and advanced cardiovascular life support, with emphasis on high-quality chest compressions, is necessary in the event of cardiac arrest, and targeted temperature management should be considered if return of spontaneous circulation occurs after arrest. If maternal cardiac arrest occurs, the chance of survival without profound neurologic deficit is very low. Emergent fetal delivery of any fetus past the age of viability is indicated to prevent fetal death, and medical treatment of uterine atony up to uterine artery ligation or hysterectomy may be required to control hemorrhage secondary to DIC and save the life of the mother.[80]

KEY POINTS

- Overall, respiratory changes during pregnancy result in a respiratory alkalosis with slightly increased Pao_2 or arterial oxygen tension. Both are normal physiologic changes that result from the increase in ventilation that occurs primarily due to circulating progesterone.
- Asthma is the most common chronic disease occurring in pregnant women and carries potential health hazards for both mother and fetus.
- During all stages of pregnancy, it is important to maintain patients with asthma on their controller medications and to aggressively manage exacerbations.

- Pregnant women are at increased risk for aspiration of gastric contents, especially during and immediately following labor.
- Treatment for chemical pneumonitis is primarily supportive, and antibiotics are withheld unless pneumonia develops, but differentiating aspiration pneumonitis from pneumonia may be difficult.
- Influenza infection is common during pregnancy and has been associated with a high risk of maternal mortality, especially late in the third trimester.
- Pregnant women should be vaccinated with inactivated vaccines and oseltamivir and/or zanamivir should be initiated for influenza infection.

REFERENCES

(only references cited in synoptic print chapter; for a complete reference list, see ebook)

1. Garcia-Rio F, Pino JM, Gomez L, et al. Regulation of breathing and perception of dyspnea in healthy pregnant women. *Chest*. 1996;110(2):446-453.
2. Milne JA, Howie AD, Pack AI. Dyspnoea during normal pregnancy. *Br J Obstet Gynaecol*. 1978;85(4):260-263.
3. Prowse CM, Gaensler EA. Respiratory and acid-base changes during pregnancy. *Anesthesiology*. 1965;26:381-392.
4. Simon PM, Schwartzstein RM, Weiss JW, et al. Distinguishable types of dyspnea in patients with shortness of breath. *Am Rev Respir Dis*. 1990;142(5):1009-1014.
5. Gilbert R, Auchincloss JH Jr. Dyspnea of pregnancy. Clinical and physiological observations. *Am J Med Sci*. 1966;252(3):270-276.
6. LoMauro A, Aliverti A. Respiratory physiology of pregnancy: physiology masterclass. *Breathe (Sheff)*. 2015;11(4):297-301.
7. Gilroy RJ, Mangura BT, Lavietes MH. Rib cage and abdominal volume displacements during breathing in pregnancy. *Am Rev Respir Dis*. 1988;137(3):668-672.
8. Weinberger SE, Weiss ST, Cohen WR, et al. Pregnancy and the lung. *Am Rev Respir Dis*. 1980;121(3):559-581.
9. Contreras G, Gutierrez M, Beroiza T, et al. Ventilatory drive and respiratory muscle function in pregnancy. *Am Rev Respir Dis*. 1991;144(4):837-841.
10. Lee SY, Chien DK, Huang CH, et al. Dyspnea in pregnancy. *Taiwan J Obstet Gynecol*. 2017;56(4):432-436.
11. Soma-Pillay P, Nelson-Piercy C, Tolppanen H, et al. Physiological changes in pregnancy. *Cardiovasc J Afr*. 2016;27(2):89-94.
12. Bloom BM, Grundlingh J, Bestwick JP, et al. The role of venous blood gas in the emergency department: a systematic review and meta-analysis. *Eur J Emerg Med*. 2014;21(2):81-88.
13. Zeserson E, Goodgame B, Hess JD, et al. Correlation of venous blood gas and pulse oximetry with arterial blood gas in the undifferentiated critically ill patient. *J Intensive Care Med*. 2018;33(3):176-181.
14. Vogelmeier CF, Criner GJ, Martinez FJ, et al. Global Strategy for the Diagnosis, Management, and Prevention of Chronic Obstructive Lung Disease 2017 Report. GOLD Executive Summary. *Am J Respir Crit Care Med*. 2017;195(5):557-582.
15. Lutfi MF. The physiological basis and clinical significance of lung volume measurements. *Multidiscip Respir Med*. 2017;12:3.
16. American College of Obstetricians and Gynecologists' Committee on Obstetric Practice. Committee Opinion No. 656: guidelines for diagnostic imaging during pregnancy and lactation. *Obstet Gynecol*. 2016;127(2):e75-e80.

17. Tromeur C, van der Pol LM, Le Roux PY, et al. Computed tomography pulmonary angiography versus ventilation-perfusion lung scanning for diagnosing pulmonary embolism during pregnancy: a systematic review and meta-analysis. *Haematologica*. 2019;104(1):176-188.
18. Enriquez R, Griffin MR, Carroll KN, et al. Effect of maternal asthma and asthma control on pregnancy and perinatal outcomes. *J Allergy Clin Immunol*. 2007;120(3):625-630.
19. Gluck JC, Gluck PA. The effect of pregnancy on the course of asthma. *Immunol Allergy Clin North Am*. 2006;26(1):63-80.
20. Global Initative for Asthma. Global strategy for asthma management and prevention. Updated 2015. Accessed March 18, 2019. http://www.ginasthma.org/local/uploads/files/GINA_Report_2015_Aug11.pdf
21. Hamid Q. Gross pathology and histopathology of asthma. *J Allergy Clin Immunol*. 2003;111(2):431-432.
22. Tata LJ, Lewis SA, McKeever TM, et al. A comprehensive analysis of adverse obstetric and pediatric complications in women with asthma. *Am J Respir Crit Care Med*. 2007;175(10):991-997.
23. Murphy VE, Powell H, Wark PAB, et al. A prospective study of respiratory viral infection in pregnant women with and without asthma. *Chest*. 2013;144(2):420-427.
24. Murphy VE, Clifton VL, Gibson PG. Asthma exacerbations during pregnancy: incidence and association with adverse pregnancy outcomes. *Thorax*. 2006;61(2):169-176.
25. Mendola P, Laughon SK, Mannisto TI, et al. Obstetric complications among US women with asthma. *Am J Obstet Gynecol*. 2013;208(2):127.e1-127.e8.
26. Murphy VE, Wang G, Namazy JA, et al. The risk of congenital malformations, perinatal mortality and neonatal hospitalisation among pregnant women with asthma: a systematic review and meta-analysis. *Br J Obstet Gynaecol*. 2013;120(7):812-822.
27. Garne E, Hansen AV, Morris J, et al. Use of asthma medication during pregnancy and risk of specific congenital anomalies: a European case-malformed control study. *J Allergy Clin Immunol*. 2015;136(6):1496-1502.e7.
28. Kallen B, Otterblad Olausson P. Use of anti-asthmatic drugs during pregnancy. 3. Congenital malformations in the infants. *Eur J Clin Pharmacol*. 2007;63(4):383-388.
29. Lin S, Munsie JP, Herdt-Losavio ML, et al. Maternal asthma medication use and the risk of gastroschisis. *Am J Epidemiol*. 2008;168(1):73-79.
30. Cossette B, Beauchesne MF, Forget A, et al. Relative perinatal safety of salmeterol vs formoterol and fluticasone vs budesonide use during pregnancy. *Ann Allergy Asthma Immunol*. 2014;112(5):459-464.
31. Norjavaara E, de Verdier MG. Normal pregnancy outcomes in a population-based study including 2,968 pregnant women exposed to budesonide. *J Allergy Clin Immunol*. 2003;111(4):736-742.

32. Bakhireva LN, Jones KL, Schatz M, et al. Safety of leukotriene receptor antagonists in pregnancy. *J Allergy Clin Immunol.* 2007;119(3):618-625.

33. Sarkar M, Koren G, Kalra S, et al. Montelukast use during pregnancy: a multicentre, prospective, comparative study of infant outcomes. *Eur J Clin Pharmacol.* 2009;65(12):1259-1264.

34. Nelsen LM, Shields KE, Cunningham ML, et al. Congenital malformations among infants born to women receiving montelukast, inhaled corticosteroids, and other asthma medications. *J Allergy Clin Immunol.* 2012;129(1):251-254.e1-e6.

35. 35 Namazy J, Cabana MD, Scheuerle AE, et al. The Xolair Pregnancy Registry (EXPECT): the safety of omalizumab use during pregnancy. *J Allergy Clin Immunol.* 2015;135(2):407-412.

36. Madanick RD, Katz PO. *GERD and Pregnancy.* Practical Gastroenterology; 2006:30-39.

37. DiBardino DM, Wunderink RG. Aspiration pneumonia: a review of modern trends. *J Crit Care.* 2015;30(1):40-48.

38. Raghavendran K, Nemzek J, Napolitano LM, et al. Aspiration-induced lung injury. *Crit Care Med.* 2011;39(4):818-826.

39. Paranjothy S, Griffiths JD, Broughton HK, et al. Interventions at caesarean section for reducing the risk of aspiration pneumonitis. *Cochrane Database Syst Rev.* 2014;(2):CD004943.

40. Siston AM, Rasmussen SA, Honein MA, et al. Pandemic 2009 influenza A(H1N1) virus illness among pregnant women in the United States. *J Am Med Assoc.* 2010;303(15):1517-1525.

41. Morris DE, Cleary DW, Clarke SC. Secondary bacterial infections associated with influenza pandemics. *Front Microbiol.* 2017;8:1041.

42. Lee MS, Oh JY, Kang CI, et al. Guideline for antibiotic use in adults with community-acquired pneumonia. *Infect Chemother.* 2018;50(2):160-198.

43. Kahn KE, Black CL, Ding H, et al. Influenza and Tdap Vaccination Coverage Among Pregnant Women – United States, April 2018. *MMWR Morb Mortal Wkly Rep.* 2018;67(38):1055-1059.

44. Sheffield JS, Cunningham FG. Community-acquired pneumonia in pregnancy. *Obstet Gynecol.* 2009;114(4):915-922.

45. Lim WS, Macfarlane JT, Colthorpe CL. Pneumonia and pregnancy. *Thorax.* 2001;56(5):398-405.

46. Ewig S, Schlochtermeier M, Goke N, et al. Applying sputum as a diagnostic tool in pneumonia: limited yield, minimal impact on treatment decisions. *Chest.* 2002;121(5):1486-1492.

47. Mandell LA, Wunderink RG, Anzueto A, et al. Infectious Diseases Society of America/American Thoracic Society consensus guidelines on the management of community-acquired pneumonia in adults. *Clin Infect Dis.* 2007;44(suppl 2):S27-S72.

48. Athlin S, Lidman C, Lundqvist A, et al. Management of community-acquired pneumonia in immunocompetent adults: updated Swedish guidelines 2017. *Infect Dis (Lond).* 2018;50(4):247-272.

49. Goodnight WH, Soper DE. Pneumonia in pregnancy. *Crit Care Med.* 2005;33(10 suppl):S390-S397.

50. Metlay JP, Waterer GW, Long AC, et al. Diagnosis and treatment of adults with community-acquired pneumonia. An official clinical practice guideline of the American Thoracic Society and Infectious Diseases Society of America. *Am J Respir Crit Care Med.* 2019;200(7):e45-e67.

51. Yefet E, Schwartz N, Chazan B, et al. The safety of quinolones and fluoroquinolones in pregnancy: a meta-analysis. *Br J Obstet Gynaecol.* 2018;125(9):1069-1076.

52. Ziv A, Masarwa R, Perlman A, et al. Pregnancy outcomes following exposure to quinolone antibiotics – a systematic-review and meta-analysis. *Pharm Res.* 2018;35(5):109.

53. Cross R, Ling C, Day NP, et al. Revisiting doxycycline in pregnancy and early childhood – time to rebuild its reputation? *Expert Opin Drug Saf.* 2016;15(3):367-382.

54. Centers for Disease Control and Prevention. Use of 13-valent pneumococcal conjugate vaccine and 23-valent pneumococcal polysaccharide vaccine for adults with immunocompromising conditions: recommendations of the Advisory Committee on Immunization Practices (ACIP). *MMWR Morb Mortal Wkly Rep.* 2012;61(40):816-819.

55. Prevention of pneumococcal disease: recommendations of the Advisory Committee on Immunization Practices (ACIP). *MMWR Recomm Rep.* 1997;46(RR-8):1-24.

56. Burk M, El-Kersh K, Saad M, et al. Viral infection in community-acquired pneumonia: a systematic review and meta-analysis. *Eur Respir Rev.* 2016;25(140):178-188.

57. American Academy of Pediatrics Committee on Infectious Diseases. Prevention of varicella: recommendations for use of varicella vaccines in children, including a recommendation for a routine 2-dose varicella immunization schedule. *Pediatrics.* 2007;120(1):221-231.

58. Centers for Disease Control and Prevention. Varicella-related deaths among adults – United States, 1997. *MMWR Morb Mortal Wkly Rep.* 1997;46(19):409-412.

59. Esmonde TF, Herdman G, Anderson G. Chickenpox pneumonia: an association with pregnancy. *Thorax.* 1989;44(10):812-815.

60. Rogerson SJ, Nye FJ, Beeching NJ. Chickenpox pneumonia: an association with pregnancy. *Thorax.* 1990;45(3):239.

61. Smith CK, Arvin AM. Varicella in the fetus and newborn. *Semin Fetal Neonatal Med.* 2009;14(4):209-217.

62. Stranska R, Schuurman R, de Vos M, et al. Routine use of a highly automated and internally controlled real-time PCR assay for the diagnosis of herpes simplex and varicella-zoster virus infections. *J Clin Virol.* 2004;30(1):39-44.

63. Binkhamis K, Al-Siyabi T, Heinstein C, et al. Molecular detection of varicella zoster virus while keeping an eye on the budget. *J Virol Methods.* 2014;202:24-27.

64. Shrim A, Koren G, Yudin MH, et al. Management of varicella infection (chickenpox) in pregnancy. *J Obstet Gynaecol Can.* 2012;34(3):287-292.

65. Pasternak B, Hviid A. Use of acyclovir, valacyclovir, and famciclovir in the first trimester of pregnancy and the risk of birth defects. *J Am Med Assoc.* 2010;304(8):859-866.

76. Neligan PJ, Laffey JG. Clinical review: special populations – critical illness and pregnancy. *Crit Care.* 2011;15(4):227.

77. Knight M, Tuffnell D, Brocklehurst P, et al. Incidence and risk factors for amniotic-fluid embolism. *Obstet Gynecol.* 2010;115(5):910-917.

78. Fitzpatrick KE, Tuffnell D, Kurinczuk JJ, et al. Incidence, risk factors, management and outcomes of amniotic-fluid embolism: a population-based cohort and nested case-control study. *Br J Obstet Gynaecol.* 2016;123(1):100-109.

79. Benson MD. Amniotic fluid embolism mortality rate. *J Obstet Gynaecol Res.* 2017;43(11):1714-1718.

80. Society for Maternal-Fetal Medicine; Pacheco LD, Saade G, Hankins GD, Clark SL. Amniotic fluid embolism: diagnosis and management. *Am J Obstet Gynecol.* 2016;215(2):B16-B24.

81. Clark SL, Romero R, Dildy GA, et al. Proposed diagnostic criteria for the case definition of amniotic fluid embolism in research studies. *Am J Obstet Gynecol.* 2016;215(4):408-412.

82. Bonnet MP, Zlotnik D, Saucedo M, et al. Maternal death due to amniotic fluid embolism: a National study in France. *Anesth Analg.* 2018;126(1):175-182.

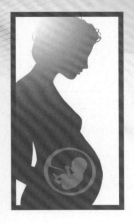

CHAPTER 30

Diabetes Mellitus in Pregnancy

Carol J. Homko, Julie A. Rosen, Perceval
Bahado-Singh, and E. Albert Reece

Diabetes mellitus is a heterogeneous disorder characterized by hyperglycemia, which is a result of relative or absolute insulin deficiency. It is estimated that diabetes mellitus affects approximately 5% of women of childbearing age in the United States and is a major cause of congenital anomalies.[1] The goal in treating patients with diabetes in pregnancy is not only a reduction in perinatal mortality but also decreases in perinatal and maternal morbidity.

CLINICAL PRESENTATION

Women with pregnancies complicated by diabetes mellitus may be separated into one of two groups **(Table 30.1)**:

1. Gestational diabetes mellitus (GDM): women diagnosed in the second or third trimester of pregnancy with diabetes that is clearly not type 1 or type 2 diabetes or other forms.
2. Preexisting diabetes: women known to have diabetes before pregnancy. For the purposes of this chapter, we will use the term "preexisting" diabetes to mean type 1 or type 2 diabetes.

In general, type 1 and type 2 can be distinguished from each other using clinical criteria, islet cell antibody studies,[10] C-peptide levels,[11] or a combination thereof.

The current, widely used definition of GDM is glucose intolerance diagnosed in the second or third trimester of pregnancy that is not clearly preexisting diabetes.[12-15]

> (e) See the eBook for expanded content, a complete reference list, and additional figures and tables.

Ninety percent of all pregnant patients with diabetes have GDM, whereas type 1 and type 2 account for the majority of the remaining 10%.[20]

Maternal Complications

Diabetic Ketoacidosis

Ketoacidosis has been reported to occur in pregnant patients with diabetes more rapidly and at lower blood glucose levels than in nonpregnant patients. It may be precipitated by stress, infection (eg, urinary tract), or omission of insulin. The use of beta-sympathomimetic agents in pregnant patients with diabetes may induce diabetic ketoacidosis (DKA) **(Figure 30.1)**.[53]

Diabetic Retinopathy

Diabetic retinopathy is classified into nonproliferative and proliferative disease stages. Within the nonproliferative stage, mild, moderate, and severe disease stages have been identified.[54] The diagnosis of severe nonproliferative retinopathy differs between the United States and other countries; however, it includes intraretinal hemorrhages, venous bleeding, and intraretinal microvascular abnormalities as findings. Proliferative disease includes neovascularization and/or vitreous or preretinal hemorrhage.

Diabetic retinopathy occurring during pregnancy should be treated in essentially the same manner as in the nonpregnant state.[55] Laser treatment can be used safely during pregnancy, when indicated. It is recommended that patients undergo careful retinal examination before conception and be treated with laser photocoagulation before pregnancy, if necessary, especially those with type 1 diabetes.

The preferred mode of delivery in patients with active proliferative retinopathy remains

Table 30.1 Classification of Diabetes in Pregnancy

Type 1 diabetes (ie, resulting from beta cell destruction, usually leading to absolute insulin deficiency)
a. Without vascular complications
b. With vascular complications (specify nephropathy, retinopathy, hypertension, arteriosclerotic heart disease, transplant, etc.)
Type 2 diabetes (ie, resulting from inadequate insulin secretion in the setting of increased insulin resistance)
a. Without vascular complications
b. With vascular complications (specify nephropathy, retinopathy, hypertension, arteriosclerotic heart disease, transplant, etc.)
Gestational diabetes (diabetes diagnosed during the second or third trimester of pregnancy and not clearly overt, eg, type 1 or type 2 diabetes)
Other diabetes (eg, genetic origin, drug or chemical induced)

Data from Ecker JL. *Pregestational Diabetes Mellitus: Obstetrical Issues and Management.* UpToDate. Topic 4806 Version 42.0. Updated January 4, 2017. Accessed May 20, 2019. https://www.uptodate.com/contents/pregestational-diabetes-mellitus-obstetrical-issues-and-management#H12665538; Cormier CM, Martinez CA, Refuerzo JS, et al. White's classification of diabetes in pregnancy in the 21st century: is it still valid? *Am J Perinatol.* 2010;27(5):349-352, and Sacks DA, Metzger BE. Classification of diabetes in pregnancy: time to reassess the alphabet. *Obstet Gynecol.* 2013;121(2 pt 1):345-348.

1. Insert two intravenous lines; obtain blood to assess levels of glucose, serum electrolytes and ketones, and arterial blood gases; and administer oxygen by face mask. Frequently assess the clinical status and follow urinary output. Repeat blood and urinary testing often.
2. Patients with DKA require simultaneous correction of fluid and electrolyte imbalance and treatment of hyperglycemia and acidosis.
   - Replacement of fluid.
     ○ Administer 1000 to 2000 mL of isotonic saline rapidly during the first hour.
     ○ If hypernatremia is present, 0.45% sodium chloride is preferred.
     ○ After the first hour, 300 to 500 mL/h is given, depending on hemodynamic status.
     ○ Normal saline is given to hypotensive patients in larger amounts. In these cases, a central line may be necessary.
   - Insulin therapy.
     ○ Administer an initial bolus of 10 to 20 U of regular insulin intravenously.
     ○ Follow this with a constant infusion of approximately 10 U/h (add 50 U of regular insulin per 500 mL of normal saline).
     ○ Larger doses of constant regular insulin infusion of 12 to 20 U/h may be required if acidosis does not begin to respond within 3 h, or if plasma glucose level does not fall by 30%.
   - Glucose administration.
     ○ Change the intravenous solution to 5% dextrose when the plasma glucose level reaches 200 to 250 mg/dL.
     ○ Simultaneously decrease the rate of the insulin infusion.
   - Potassium administration.
     ○ Hyperkalemia is usually present on administration. At this point, potassium administration is not required and, in fact, may be dangerous or even lethal because hyperkalemia may rapidly reach cardiotoxic levels.
     ○ Potassium administration is usually started after 3 to 4 h of insulin therapy, when potassium begins to fall to normal or low levels.
     ○ Add 40 mEq of potassium chloride per 1000 mL of normal saline at a rate of 10 to 20 mEq/h, as needed.
     ○ When potassium is administered, it is given with extreme caution, and that potassium and urinary output are monitored carefully.
   - Bicarbonate administration.
     ○ Add 44 mEq of sodium bicarbonate to 1L of 0.45% saline and administer intravenously only if arterial pH is less than 7.1, or serum bicarbonate is less than 5 mEq.
     ○ If the pH is less than 7, the sodium bicarbonate dose should be doubled (88 mEq).
     ○ Bicarbonate administration should be terminated if arterial pH has been corrected to 7.2.
     ○ Alkali administration in DKA is still controversial because this therapy might aggravate tissue hypoxia.

Figure 30.1 General guidelines for the treatment of diabetic ketoacidosis (DKA) in pregnant patients.

controversial. In the past, the performance of cesarean delivery was suggested to avoid the Valsalva maneuver and the risk of vitreous hemorrhage.[56] However, if well-controlled, there is no evidence to suggest that attempts at vaginal delivery should not be made.[57,58]

Diabetic Kidney Disease

A diagnosis of diabetic kidney disease (DKD) in pregnancy is made if there is persistent proteinuria of more than 300 mg/d in the first half of pregnancy.[63] Acute worsening of hypertension is very common in patients with DKD and occurs in almost 60% of cases. However, after delivery, changes in renal function, proteinuria, and hypertension return to values observed in the first trimester.

Pregnant patients with DKD require an intensive program of maternal and fetal evaluation, adequate bedrest during pregnancy, assessment of renal function and retinal status at regular intervals, blood pressure monitoring, and treatment of hypertension, when required, using methyldopa, arteriolar vasodilator, or beta-blockers. In patients taking antihypertensive medications before pregnancy, the same regimen is continued during pregnancy (with the exception of diuretics and angiotensin-converting enzyme inhibitors, which should be discontinued). A modest sodium restriction (1500 mg of Na) in all patients with significant proteinuria (>500 mg/dL) is suggested to reduce the rate of edema formation.

GESTATIONAL DIABETES MELLITUS

Screening and Clinical Assessment

Screening and diagnosis of GDM can be performed using either a one-step (2-hour, 75-g oral glucose tolerance test [OGTT]) or two-step (50 g screen followed by a 3-hour, 100-g diagnostic OGTT) approach (**Table 30.4**) (**Algorithm 30.1**).

In the United States, the GDM testing strategy uses a "two-step approach."[13,19,70] The first step is a screening test, the oral glucose challenge test, which consists of:

- A 50-g oral glucose load, followed 1 hour later by a plasma glucose determination.
- The screen is performed without regard to the time of day or interval since the last meal.

Table 30.4 Screening and Diagnostic Thresholds for the Clinical Assessment of Gestational Diabetes Mellitus

| Glucose Measure | Glucose Concentration | | | |
| | mg/dL | | mmol/L | |
	IADPSG	ACOG	IADPSG	ACOG
Oral glucose challenge test	N/A	130-140	N/A	0.55-1.5
Fasting	92	95	5.1	5.3
1 h	180	180	10.0	10.0
2 h	153	155	8.5	8.6
3 h	N/A	140	N/A	7.8

ACOG, American College of Obstetricians and Gynecologists; GDM, gestational diabetes mellitus; IADPSG, International Association of Diabetes in Pregnancy Study Groups.

- Screening is recommended at 24 to 28 weeks' gestation in average-risk women not known to have diabetes mellitus.
- Screening is recommended as soon as possible in women deemed to be a high risk for overt diabetes.

A value of plasma venous glucose between 130 and 140 mg/dL has been recommended as a threshold to indicate the need for a full diagnostic OGTT. When the plasma glucose screening test results are >185 mg/dL, patients have GDM and no further testing is required.

The diagnosis of GDM is based on an abnormal result of an OGTT during pregnancy. A minority of cases are diagnosed on the basis of high fasting glucose levels during pregnancy, in which case the OGTT does not have to be performed.

The OGTT is administered under standard conditions:

- The patient should have at least 3 days of unrestricted diet with more than 150 g of carbohydrates and should be at rest during the study.
- 100 g of glucose is given orally in at least 400 mL of water (or given as a 100-g glucose solution) after an overnight fast of 8 to 14 hours.
- Diagnosis requires that at least two of four glucose levels of the OGTT meet or exceed the upper limits of normal values (**Algorithm 30.1**)

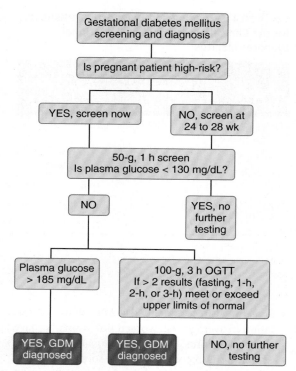

Algorithm 30.1 Decision tree: Gestational diabetes mellitus screening and diagnosis.

PREEXISTING DIABETES MELLITUS IN PREGNANCY

Preexisting diabetes is a significant health concern because uncontrolled maternal blood glucose prior to and during the first trimester of pregnancy is associated with fetal malformations, perinatal death, and maternal morbidity and mortality.[78,79]

Infant Morbidity

In the last decade the perinatal morbidity rate in pregnancies complicated by diabetes mellitus has been remarkably reduced. However, severe neonatal morbidity in infants of mothers with diabetes is still a problem that may affect even infants delivered at term,[89] including:

- Hypoglycemia
  - Plasma glucose levels <35 mg/dL in term infants and 25 mg/dL in preterm infants
  - Treatment initiated in all neonates with plasma glucose levels <40 mg/dL

- Therapy for hypoglycemia is continuous dextrose infusion at a rate of 4 to 6 mg/kg/min. The use of a bolus of a hypertonic glucose infusion should be avoided to prevent later rebound hypoglycemia[90]
  - Occasionally, hypoglycemia may persist beyond the second day of life and may require the use of glucocorticoids[91]
- Hypocalcemia[92]
  - Calcium levels ≤7 mg/dL
  - Serum calcium levels in infants are lowest on the second to third days of life
  - Hypocalcemia may be associated with "relative" neonatal hypoparathyroidism
  - Magnesium deficiency may contribute to hypoparathyroidism and hypocalcemia in infants of mothers with diabetes[93]
- Polycythemia[94]
  - Diagnosed when venous hematocrit exceeds 65%
  - Affects approximately one-third of neonates of mothers with diabetes in the first few hours of life[89]
  - Usually associated with hyperviscosity of the blood and increases the risk of microthrombus formation in multiple organs
  - Kidneys, adrenals, and lungs are the most commonly affected organs
  - Clinically, infants appear plethoric; may have convulsions, respiratory distress, tachycardia, congestive heart failure, and hyperbilirubinemia
  - Treatment consists of partial exchange transfusion with a volume expander (eg, plasma) to reduce the hematocrit to approximately 55%[89]
- Respiratory distress syndrome
- Hyperbilirubinemia
- Cardiomyopathy

MANAGEMENT OF DIABETES DURING PREGNANCY

Management of diabetes in pregnancy is directed toward reducing perinatal mortality and morbidity, a goal that may be achieved by maintaining close surveillance of the mother and fetus and stringent glucose control.

Clinical studies suggest that euglycemia can prevent congenital anomalies and maternal health complications, including diabetes-associated eye, kidney, and cardiac disease.[81,83,84,125-127] Therefore, patient management ideally begins before conception:

- At the initial visit, the patient's general medical status is assessed.
- The patient undergoes ophthalmologic evaluation, electrocardiography, and kidney function tests.
- It is generally recommended that women achieve a glycosylated hemoglobin level that is less than 1% above the upper limit of normal.
- Women should receive appropriate contraceptive therapy while preparing for pregnancy.
- For women who are not already following an intensive diabetes regimen, an extensive period of education and the institution of self-blood glucose monitoring is also necessary.

Nonpharmacologic Management

Self-Monitoring of Blood Glucose

Blood glucose measurements should be obtained at least four times a day (fasting and 1-2 hour after meals) in women with GDM, and five-to-seven times a day in women with preexisting diabetes. In addition, preprandial glucose testing is indicated in women using insulin pumps or basal-bolus insulin therapy so that premeal insulin dosages can be adjusted. In addition to this regular monitoring, patients should also test whenever they feel symptoms of either hyperglycemia or hypoglycemia. Detailed record keeping is useful to help identify glucose patterns. Ketone testing should also be performed any time the blood glucose level exceeds 200 mg/dL, during illness, or when the patient is unable to eat.

Blood glucose levels are measured in both fasted and postprandial states. The target ranges for blood glucose during pregnancy should be[129]:

- Before a meal (preprandial): 95 mg/dL or less
- 1-hour after a meal (postprandial): 140 mg/dL or less
- 2-hours after a meal (postprandial): 120 mg/dL or less

Continuous Glucose Monitoring

Continuous glucose monitoring (CGM) devices measure subcutaneous interstitial tissue glucose using an electrochemical method.

Real-time CGM systems (RT-CGM) can be extremely useful in helping women to understand how food, activity, and medications affect their blood glucose levels.

However, there remains uncertainty regarding the superiority of CGMs over traditional monitors.

Currently, there is limited evidence available to support the use of CGMs in pregnant women with type 2 diabetes, as well as women who develop GDM.

In addition, CGM systems have not been found to improve glycemic control and pregnancy outcomes when utilized before and during labor and delivery, nor do they appear to reduce the risk of severe hypoglycemia in high-risk women.[138,141]

Diet and Gestational Weight Gain

The American Pregnancy Association recommends an additional 300 to 400 kcal/d during pregnancy,[143] and a balanced diet consisting of fresh vegetables and fruits, whole grains, protein, and dairy products.

For women with GDM, it is generally accepted that carbohydrate levels should not exceed 40% to 45% of total calories. More importantly, because not all carbohydrates are similar, the healthier nutritional advice should take into consideration the type (simple versus complex carbohydrates) and quality (low versus high glycemic index) of the carbohydrates.[146-148] It is recommended that patients with GDM should consume high-quality carbohydrate foods, those that are fiber-rich complex starchy foods, which also have a low glycemic index.[146-148] This advice is supported by scientific research, particularly in obstetrics and gynecology, which has shown that foods with a low glycemic index and increased dietary fiber may have higher predictive outcomes and improved health benefits for the mother and baby.[146-148] Studies have shown that low glycemic index foods reduce insulin treatment for the mother and reduce development of macrosomia in the fetus.[146-148]

Further meal planning and nutritional advice is to limit fat intake to approximately 30% of total calories, and protein comprise the remaining 20% of total daily calories. Restricted saturated fats and cholesterol are suggested. Most patients are instructed to:

- Have three meals and one to three snacks daily.
- Last snack should be taken at bedtime.
- Bedtime snack should be composed of complex carbohydrates with proteins to maintain adequate blood glucose levels during the night, thereby avoiding nocturnal hypoglycemia.

Patient weight gains are assessed at each visit to the clinic, and caloric intake is adjusted accordingly. The aim is to prevent weight reduction and its associated ketogenic risk while ensuring optimal weight gain.

It is desirable to increase weight by 2 to 4 lb (0.9-1.7 kg) in the first trimester and 0.5-1.0 lb (200-450 g) per week thereafter until term. A total weight gain of 22 to 30 lb (10-13 kg) during normal and diabetic pregnancy is recommended.[149]

It is generally agreed that pregnancy is not the time for weight reduction; however, excessive weight gain should be firmly discouraged.

Pharmacologic Management

Insulin Administration

Insulin is the only pharmacological therapy currently recommended to treat diabetes during pregnancy. The goal of insulin therapy is to achieve blood glucose levels that are nearly identical to those observed in healthy pregnant women. Therefore, multiple injections of insulin are usually required in women with preexisting diabetes. Human insulin is the least immunogenic of all insulins and is exclusively recommended in pregnancy.

The rapid-acting insulin analogues with peak hypoglycemic action 1 to 2 hour after injection offer the potential for improved postprandial glucose control.[158-164]

Insulin requirements may change dramatically throughout the various stages of gestation:

- In the first trimester = 0.7 U/kg of body weight per day.[167]
- Third trimester = 1.0 U/kg/d.
- The three-injection scheme permits better control of the fasting blood glucose levels while minimizing the risk of middle-of-the-night hypoglycemia.[168]

Insulin Pumps

Continuous subcutaneous insulin infusion pumps have also been shown to be effective during pregnancy.[169,170] Insulin pumps deliver a continuous basal rate of insulin infusion with pulse-dose increments before meals.

Insulin Therapy in GDM

Insulin therapy should be initiated in all women with GDM who fail to maintain euglycemia with diet. We start women on a daily insulin dose of 20 U of neutral protamine Hagedorn and 10 U of regular insulin daily. Insulin doses are adjusted according to blood glucose levels, and an evening injection is added if fasting hyperglycemia persist. Some investigators have advocated the use of prophylactic insulin in GDM to reduce the risk of macrosomia. However, the advantages of this therapy must be weighed against the disadvantages of no treatment.

Oral Agents

Traditionally, insulin therapy has been considered the gold standard for management because of its efficacy in achieving tight glucose control and the fact that it does not cross the placenta. As GDM and type 2 diabetes are characterized by insulin resistance and relatively decreased insulin secretion, treatment with oral antidiabetic agents that target these defects is of potential interest.

However, outstanding questions around the long-term use of the two major oral agents prescribed, glyburide and metformin, have led several professional societies to recommend against their use as first-line therapies.[13,19,59] Glyburide and metformin also cross the placenta to the fetus and lack long-term safety data.[196-198]

ANTEPARTUM ASSESSMENT

Maternal Assessment

Ophthalmologic and renal function tests, including creatinine clearance and total urinary protein excretion, are performed in each trimester or more often, if indicated. In patients with vasculopathy, an electrocardiogram is performed at the initial visit and repeated, if clinically indicated (**Table 30.5**).

Fetal Surveillance

All pregnancies complicated by diabetes require extra assessment. The use of ultrasonography provides essential information about the fetus. A first-trimester scan is used to date the pregnancy and to establish viability and fluid volume status. A second-trimester scan is repeated at 18 to 20 weeks' gestation to rule out fetal anomalies. Subsequent ultrasound evaluations are then performed at 4- to 6-week intervals to assess fluid

Table 30.5 Overview of Antenatal Maternal Assessment in Diabetic Vasculopathy

Trimester	Cardiovascular Disease	Retinopathy	Diabetic Kidney Disease
First	• Evaluate risk factors • Control blood pressure • Consider ischemia evaluation without radiation • Perform Doppler echocardiogram	• Dilated eye exam • If severe nonproliferative or proliferative disease, evaluate monthly • Consider treatment • Control blood pressure	• Determine urine albumin excretion • Determine renal function • Control blood pressure
Second	• If positive for coronary heart disease, refer to cardiologist • If cardiomyopathy or heart failure, perform Doppler echocardiogram	• Reevaluate patients with mild disease • Control blood pressure • Consider laser treatment	• Test 24-h creatinine clearance • Evaluate for preeclampsia • Control blood pressure • 12-16 wk: AAS (100 mg/d)
Third	• If positive for coronary heart disease, refer to cardiologist • If cardiomyopathy or heart failure, perform Doppler echocardiogram	• Reevaluate patients with no or minimal disease • Reevaluate patients with mild disease • Control blood pressure • Untreated proliferative disease—consider cesarean delivery	• Test 24-h creatinine clearance • Evaluate preeclampsia • Control blood pressure • Discontinue AAS at 32-34 wk

AAS, acetylsalicylic acid.
Adapted from Leguizamón G, Trigubo D, Pereira JI, Vera MF, Fernández JA. Vascular complications in the diabetic pregnancy. *Curr Diab Rep.* 2015;15(4):22.

volume and fetal growth. Because patients with diabetes are at risk of growth aberrations (intrauterine growth restriction and macrosomia), this frequency is recommended to identify states of altered growth. Any method of fetal surveillance is ineffective unless strict control of maternal diabetes is maintained.[215]

Fetal Macrosomia

Macrosomia, arbitrarily defined as fetal weight in excess of 4000 g, or a birth weight above the 90th percentile for gestational age, occurs in approximately 10% of all pregnancies. Almost 30% of all women with diabetes deliver infants weighing more than 4000 g.[225]

Macrosomic fetuses have higher rates of perinatal morbidity and mortality, a result caused mainly by the traumatic delivery. These fetuses are at increased risk of severe fetal asphyxia due to head and neck birth trauma. Shoulder dystocia is common.

Primary cesarean delivery is performed if the estimated fetal weight is 4500 g or more. In cases of

estimated fetal weight of 4000 to 4500 g, the mode of delivery is determined individually for each patient and is based on the clinical assessment of the pelvis and the past history (eg, birth weight of previous babies). In such cases, midpelvic instrumental delivery should be avoided as much as possible.

Antepartum Fetal Testing

In pregnant patients with diabetes, stillbirth occurs with increased frequency, particularly in the third trimester.[96,227] Therefore, a program of fetal monitoring should be initiated, usually at 32 to 33 weeks. Tests include the contraction stress test (CST), nonstress test (NST), and biophysical profile.[225] The NST is most widely used for pregnancies complicated by diabetes.[228,229] However, the biophysical profile has been shown to have a lower false-abnormal test rate than either the CST or NST.[225,230] In addition, maternal assessment of fetal activity is a practical, simple, inexpensive, and valuable screening approach toward evaluation of fetal condition. Patients with diabetes are instructed to count fetal movements, beginning as early as 28 to 29 weeks of gestation, and to report any decrease in fetal movements so that further testing can be initiated if necessary.

TIMING AND MODE OF DELIVERY

It is now recognized worldwide that, if the pregnant patient with diabetes and her fetus are under stringent metabolic control and antepartum surveillance, delivery may be safely delayed in most cases until term or the onset of spontaneous labor.[225,231]

Preterm Labor

Earlier studies have found that the incidence of prematurity in diabetic pregnancies is three times higher than that in nondiabetic pregnancies.[232] Magnesium sulfate is considered the drug of choice in patients with diabetes in premature labor because it has no effect on diabetic control. In contrast, beta-sympathomimetic tocolytic agents or glucocorticosteroids have been reported to induce hyperglycemia and ketoacidosis.[233] Therefore, treatment with both medications in women with diabetes requires great caution, intensive monitoring of glucose levels, and treatment with intravenous insulin infusion as needed.

Management During Labor and Delivery

During labor and delivery, it is necessary to maintain maternal euglycemia to avoid neonatal hypoglycemia. Induced maternal hyperglycemia during labor in women with diabetes is associated with neonatal hypoglycemia.[234,235] Therefore, the goal should be to maintain glucose levels of 70 to 90 mg/dL during labor (**Algorithm 30.2**).

In patients undergoing induction of labor, the morning insulin doses should be withheld and glucose levels determined once every hour with a home glucose meter. In well-controlled patients, 1 U of insulin per hour and 3 to 6 g of glucose per hour are usually required to maintain a glucose level of 70 to 90 mg/dL. If the initial glucose level is between 80 and 120 mg/dL, 10 U of regular insulin can be added to 1000 mL of 5% dextrose in 0.5% normal saline or 5% dextrose 5% and Ringer lactate, and administered at an infusion rate of 125 mL/h.

> **During labor**
> ✓ Monitor glucose levels in 1- to 4-h intervals
>   Glycemic targets: Plasma 80 to 120 mg/dL

> **Postpartum follow-up**
> ✓ 2-h oral glucose tolerance test (75-g
>   glucose load) at 6 wk postpartum
> ✓ <140 mg/dL = normal
> ✓ 140-199 mg/dL = impaired glucose tolerance
> ✓ ≥200 mg/dL = provisionally diabetic

Algorithm 30.2 Management of patients with gestational diabetes during labor and after pregnancy.

If initial glucose levels are less than 70 mg/dL, it is recommended that, initially, 5% dextrose in water without insulin at a rate of 100 to 120 mL/h be given throughout labor.

If the patient presents in spontaneous labor and has already taken her morning intermediate-acting insulin, additional insulin may not be required throughout labor and delivery, but a continuous glucose infusion will be necessary (125 mL/h of 5% dextrose in water).

When an elective cesarean delivery is planned, the procedure should be scheduled early in the morning, when glucose levels are usually in the normal range because of the action of the intermediate-acting insulin dose given the night before. Infusion without glucose is preferred (ie, normal saline), and glucose levels are monitored frequently. If the patient is under regional anesthesia, it is easier to detect signs of hypoglycemia.

After delivery, a dramatic decrease in the insulin requirement is almost the rule because of a significant decrease in the level of placental hormones that have anti-insulin action. At this time, there is no need for stringent glucose control, and glucose levels of less than 200 mg/dL are satisfactory. In the first few days after delivery, it is preferable to give regular insulin subcutaneously before each meal on the basis of plasma glucose levels. After the patient is able to eat regular meals, she may receive one-half of the pre-pregnancy dosage of insulin, usually divided into two daily injections.

KEY POINTS

- The diagnosis of diabetes mellitus during pregnancy has certain implications for the well-being of both the mother and the fetus.
- The predominant forms of diabetes affecting pregnancy include gestational, type 1, and type 2 diabetes.
- Gestational diabetes affects up to 9% of all pregnancies and is associated with a higher incidence of cesarean delivery, preterm labor, fetal macrosomia, shoulder dystocia, preeclampsia, and admission to neonatal intensive care units.
- There remains a lack of consensus regarding timing and method of screening and diagnosis of gestational diabetes. However, in general, universal screening has yet to be recommended and, unless a patient is considered at very high risk, screening and diagnosis typically occurs between weeks 24 and 28 of pregnancy.
- Preexisting diabetes in pregnancy is primarily type 1 or type 2, although rarer forms of diabetes can affect reproductive-age women.
- Although only affecting approximately 1% to 2% of all pregnancies, preexisting diabetes in pregnancy is associated with increased risk for major birth defects, stillbirth, preterm birth, hypoglycemia, hypertensive disorders, and worsening of comorbidities (eg, DKA, retinopathy, and kidney disease).
- Advances in medical and obstetric care have dramatically improved the outlook for women with diabetes and their offspring.
- Research indicates that the majority of diabetes in pregnancy complications are associated with hyperglycemia. The achievement and maintenance of euglycemia has, therefore, become the major focus of management.
- Stringent glycemic control in pregnancy includes consistent self-monitoring of blood glucose, sometimes with the aid of continuous glucose monitors, compliance with insulin or antidiabetic medication use, and monitoring of diet and gestational weight gain.
- Antepartum assessment may include increased fetal surveillance, need to adjust timing and mode of delivery, and maintain maternal euglycemia during labor and delivery.

REFERENCES

(only references cited in synoptic print chapter; for a complete reference list, see ebook)

1. Azeez O, Kulkarni A, Kuklina EV, Kim SY, Cox S. Hypertension and diabetes in non-pregnant women of reproductive age in the United States. *Prev Chronic Dis.* 2019;16:190105.
7. Ecker JL. *Pregestational Diabetes Mellitus: Obstetrical Issues and Management.* UpToDate. Topic 4806 Version 42.0. Updated January 4, 2017. Accessed May 20, 2019. https://www.uptodate.com/contents/pregestational-diabetes-mellitus-obstetrical-issues-and-management#H12665538
8. Cormier CM, Martinez CA, Refuerzo JS, et al. White's classification of diabetes in pregnancy in the 21st century: is it still valid? *Am J Perinatol.* 2010;27(5):349-352.
9. Sacks DA, Metzger BE. Classification of diabetes in pregnancy: time to reassess the alphabet. *Obstet Gynecol.* 2013;121(2 pt 1):345-348.
10. Bonifacio E, Achenbach P. Birth and coming of age of islet autoantibodies. *Clin Exp Immunol.* 2019;198(3):294-305.
11. Leighton E, Sainsbury CA, Jones GC. A practical review of C-peptide testing in diabetes. *Diabetes Ther.* 2017;8(3):475-487.
12. *Diagnostic Criteria and Classification of Hyperglycaemia First Detected in Pregnancy.* World Health Organization; 2013:63.
13. Committee on Practice Bulletins – Obstetrics. ACOG Practice Bulletin No. 190: gestational diabetes mellitus. *Obstet Gynecol.* 2018;131(2):e49-e64.
14. International Association of Diabetes and Pregnancy Study Groups Consensus Panel; Metzger BE, Gabbe SG, Persson B, et al. International association of diabetes and pregnancy study groups recommendations on the diagnosis and classification of hyperglycemia in pregnancy. *Diabetes Care.* 2010;33(3):676-682.
15. Berger H, Gagnon R, Sermer M, et al. Diabetes in pregnancy. *J Obstet Gynaecol Can.* 2016;38(7):667-679.e1. Published correction appears in *J Obstet Gynaecol Can.* 2017;39(6):509.
19. American Diabetes Association. 2. Classification and diagnosis of diabetes: Standards of medical Care in diabetes-2020. *Diabetes Care.* 2020;43(suppl 1):S14-S31.
20. International Diabetes Federation. *IDF Diabetes Atlas.* 9th ed. International Diabetes Federation; 2019.
53. Thomas D, Gill B, Brown P, et al. Salbutamol-induced diabetic ketoacidosis. *Br Med J.* 1977;2:438.
54. Flaxel CJ, Adelman RA, Bailey ST, et al. Diabetic retinopathy preferred practice pattern°. *Ophthalmology.* 2020;127(1):P66-P145.
55. Feghali MN, Umans JG. Diabetic retinopathy. In: Reece EA, Coustan DR, eds. *Diabetes and Obesity in Women: Adolescence, Pregnancy & Menopause.* 4th ed. Lippincott Williams & Wilkins; 2018:370-380.
56. Morrison JL, Hodgson LA, Lim LL, Al-Qureshi S. Diabetic retinopathy in pregnancy: a review. *Clin Exp Ophthalmol.* 2016;44(4):321-334.
57. Mohammadi SF, Letafat-Nejad M, Ashrafi E, Delshad-Aghdam H. A survey of ophthalmologists and gynecologists regarding termination of pregnancy and choice of delivery mode in the presence of eye diseases. *J Curr Ophthalmol.* 2017;29(2):126-132.
58. Feghali M, Khoury JC, Shveiky D, Miodovnik M. Association of vaginal delivery efforts with retinal disease in women with type I diabetes. *J Matern Fetal Neonatal Med.* 2012;25(1):27-31.
59. *2018 Surveillance of Diabetes in Pregnancy: Management From Preconception to the Postnatal Period (NICE Guideline NG3).* National Institute for Health and Care Excellence (UK); 2018.
63. Bramham K, Rajasingham D. Pregnancy in diabetes and kidney disease. *J Ren Care.* 2012;38(suppl 1):78-89.

70. Blumer I, Hadar E, Hadden DR, et al. Diabetes and pregnancy: an endocrine society clinical practice guideline. *J Clin Endocrinol Metab.* 2013;98(11):4227-4249.

78. Landon MB, Mele L, Spong LY, et al. Eunice Kennedy Shriver National Institute of Child Health and Human Development (NICHD) Maternal-Fetal Medicine Units (MFMU) network. The relationship between maternal glycemia and perinatal outcomes. *Obstet Gynecol.* 2011;117:218-224.

79. Farrar D, Simmonds M, Bryant M, et al. Hyperglyemia and risk of adverse perinatal outcomes: systematic review and meta-analysis. *Br Med J.* 2016;354:14694.

81. Ornoy A, Reece EA, Pavlinkova G, Kappen C, Miller RK. Effect of maternal diabetes on the embryo, fetus and children: congenital anomalies, genetic and peifenetic changes and developmental outcomes. *Birth Defects Resc Embryo Today.* 2015;105:53-72.

83. Zhao Z, Reece EA. New concepts in diabetic embryopathy. *Clin Lab Med.* 2013;33:207-233.

84. Reece EA. Diabetes-induced birth defects: what do we know? What can we do? *Curr Diab Rep.* 2012;12(1):24-32.

89. Hay WW Jr. Care of the infant of the diabetic mother. *Curr Diab Rep.* 2012;12(1):4-15.

90. Kallem VR, Pandita A, Gupta G. Hypoglycemia: when to treat? *Clin Med Insights Pediatr.* 2017;11:1179556517748913.

91. Sweet CB, Grayson S, Polak M. Management strategies for neonatal hypoglycemia. *J Pediatr Pharmacol Ther.* 2013;18(3):199-208.

92. Hatfield L, Schwoebel A, Lynyak C. Caring for the infant of a diabetic mother. *MCN Am J Matern Child Nurs.* 2011;36(1):10-16.

93. Jain A, Agarwal R, Sankar MJ, Deorari A, Paul VK. Hypocalcemia in the newborn. *Indian J Pediatr.* 2010;77(10):1123-1128.

94. Bashir BA, Othman SA. Neonatal polycythaemia. *Sudan J Paediatr.* 2019;19(2):81-83.

96. Crimmins SD, Reddy UM. Stillbirth and diabetes. In: Reece EA, Coustan DR. *Diabetes and Obesity in Women: Adolescence, Pregnancy & Menopause.* 4th ed. Lippincott Williams & Wilkins; 2018:204-216.

125. Reece EA, Homko CJ. Why do diabetic women deliver malformed infants? *Clin Obstet Gynecol.* 2000;43(1):32-45.

126. Correa A. Pregestational diabetes mellitus and congenital heart defects. *Circulation.* 2016;133(23):2219-2221.

127. Murphy HR, Roland JM, Skinner TC, et al. Effectiveness of a regional prepregnancy care program in women with type 1 and type 2 diabetes: benefits beyond glycemic control. *Diabetes Care.* 2010;33:2514-2520.

129. American Diabetes Association. *How to Treat Gestational Diabetes: Treatment & Perspectives.* Accessed June 6, 2017. http://www.diabetes.org/diabetes-basics/gestational/how-to-treat-gestational.html#sthash.3gVZSOZQ.dpuf

138. Secher AL, Ringholm L, Andersen HU, Damm P, Mathiesen ER. The effect of real time continuous glucose monitoring in pregnant women with diabetes: a randomized controlled trial. *Diabetes Care.* 2013;36:1877-1883.

141. Cordua S, Secher AL, Ringholm L, Andersen UH, Damm P, Mathiesen ER. Real-time continuous monitoring during labor and delivery in women with type 1 diabetes-observations from a randomized severe hypoglycemia in selected pregnant women with type 1 diabetes: an observational study. *Diabet Med.* 2014;31:352-356.

143. American Pregnancy Association. *Diet During Pregnancy.* Accessed June 6, 2017. http://americanpregnancy.org/pregnancy-health/diet-during-pregnancy/

146. Zhang R, Han S, Chen GC, et al. Effects of low-glycemic-index diets in pregnancy on maternal and newborn outcomes in pregnant women: a meta-analysis of randomized controlled trials. *Eur J Nutr.* 2018;57(1):167-177.

147. Wei J, Heng W, Gao J. Effects of low glycemic index diets on gestational diabetes mellitus: a meta-analysis of randomized controlled clinical trials. *Medicine (Baltimore).* 2016;95(22):e3792.

148. Louie JC, Markovic TP, Perera N, et al. A randomized controlled trial investigating the effects of a low-glycemic index diet on pregnancy outcomes in gestational diabetes mellitus. *Diabetes Care.* 2011;34(11):2341-2346.

149. Institute of Medicine and National Research Council 2013. *Guidelines on Weight Gain and Pregnancy.* The National Academic Press; 2013. doi:10.17226/18291

158. Toledano Y, Hadar E, Hod M. Pharmacotherapy for hyperglycemia in pregnancy – the new insulins. *Diabetes Res Clin Pract.* 2018;145:59-66.

159. Doder Z, Vanechanos D, Oster M, Landgraf W, Lin S. Insulin glulisine in pregnancy – experience from clinical trials and post-marketing surveillance. *Eur Endocrinol.* 2015;11(1):17-20.

160. Lambert K, Holt RI. The use of insulin analogues in pregnancy. *Diabetes Obes Metab.* 2013;15(10):888-900.

161. Milluzzo A, Tumminia A, Scalisi NM, Frittitta L, Vigneri R, Sciacca L. Insulin degludec in the first trimester of pregnancy: report of two cases. *J Diabetes Investig.* 2017;9(3):629-631.

162. Hiranput S, Ahmed SH, Macaulay D, Azmi S. Successful outcomes with insulin degludec in pregnancy: a case series. *Diabetes Ther.* 2019;10(1):283-289.

163. Bonora BM, Avogaro A, Fadini GP. Exposure to insulin degludec during pregnancy: report of a small series and review of the literature. *J Endocrinol Invest.* 2019;42(3):345-349.

164. Keller MF, Vestgaard M, Damm P, Mathiesen ER, Ringholm L. Treatment with the long-acting insulin analog degludec during pregnancy in women with type 1 diabetes: an observational study of 22 cases. *Diabetes Res Clin Pract.* 2019;152:58-64.

167. Jovanovic L, Peterson CM. Optimal insulin delivery for the pregnant diabetic patient. *Diabetes Care.* 1982;5(suppl 2):24.

168. Homko CJ, Reece EA. Ambulatory management of the pregnant woman with diabetes. *Obstet Gynecol Clin North Am.* 1998;41:584.

169. Kallas-Koeman MM, Kong JM, Klinke JA, et al. Insulin pump use in pregnancy is associated with lower HbA1c without increasing the rate of severe hypoglycaemia or diabetic ketoacidosis in women with type 1 diabetes. *Diabetologia.* 2014;57(4):681-689.

170. Abell SK, Suen M, Pease A, et al. Pregnancy outcomes and insulin requirements in women with type 1 diabetes treated with continuous subcutaneous insulin infusion and multiple daily injections: a cohort study. *Diabetes Technol Ther.* 2017;19:280-287.

196. Silva JC, Fachin DR, Coral ML, Bertini AM. Perinatal impact of the use of metformin and glyburide for the treatment of gestational diabetes mellitus. *J Perinat Med.* 2012;40(3):225-228.

197. Camelo Castillo W, Boggess K, Stürmer T, Brookhart MA, Benjamin DK Jr, Jonsson Funk M. Association of adverse pregnancy outcomes with glyburide vs insulin in women with gestational diabetes. *JAMA Pediatr.* 2015;169(5):452-458.

198. Charles B, Norris R, Xiao X, Hague W. Population pharmacokinetics of metformin in late pregnancy. *Ther Drug Monit.* 2006;28:67-72.

215. Ahmed B, Abushama M, Khraishen M, Dudenhausen J. Role of ultrasound in the management of diabetic pregnancy. *J Matern Fetal Neonatal Med.* 2015;28:1856-1863.

225. Graves CR. Antepartum fetal surveillance and timing of delivery in the pregnancy complicated by diabetes mellitus. 2007;50:1007-1013.

227. Mathiesen ER, Ringholm L, Damn P. Still birth in diabetic pregnancy. *Best Pract Res Clin Obstet Gynaecol.* 2011;25:105-111.

228. Golde S, Plan L. Antepartum testing in diabetes. *Clin Obstet Gynecol.* 1985;28:516.

229. Phelan JP. The nonstress test: a review of 3000 tests. *Am J Obstet Gynecol.* 1981;139:7.

230. Manning FA, Morrison I, Lange IR, et al. Fetal assessment based on fetal biophysical profile scoring: experience in 12,260 referred high-risk pregnancies. *Am J Obstet Gynecol.* 1985;151:343.

231. Coustan DR. *Delivery: timing, mode and management. Diabetes and Obesity in Women: Adolescence, Pregnancy & Menopause.* 4th ed. Lippincott Williams & Wilkins; 2018:425-431.

232. Molsted-Pedersen L. Preterm labour and perinatal mortality in diabetic pregnancy: obstetric considerations. In: Sutherland HW, Stowers JM, eds. *Carbohydrate Metabolism in Pregnancy and the Newborn.* Springer-Verlag; 1979:392.

233. Diamond MP, Vaughn WK, Salyer SL, Cotton RC, Fields LM, Boehm FH. Antepartum fetal monitoring in insulin-dependent diabetic pregnancies. *Am J Obstet Gynecol.* 1985;153(5):528-533.

234. Jovanovic L, Peterson CM. Insulin and glucose requirements during the first stage of labor in insulin-dependent diabetic women. *Am J Med.* 1983;75(4):607-612.

235. Grylack LJ, Chu SS, Scanlon JW. Use of intravenous fluids before cesarean section: effects on perinatal glucose, insulin, and sodium homeostasis. *Obstet Gynecol.* 1984;63(5):654-658.

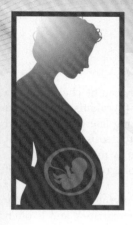

CHAPTER 31

Endocrine Disorders in Pregnancy

Rana Malek, Kashif M. Munir, and E. Albert Reece

Endocrine Changes Associated With a Normal Pregnancy

There are a number of endocrine changes that occur during normal pregnancy. Some of these changes occur through the existing maternal endocrine system, and some occur as a result of effects of placental hormones on the maternal endocrine system.

Pituitary

Lactotroph hyperplasia causes an increase in pituitary size during normal pregnancy, mainly due to estrogen stimulation of the pituitary lactotrophs. The new diagnosis of a prolactinoma in a pregnant patient is not a common problem, as substantial prolactin elevations typically result in amenorrhea and infertility. However, it is important to be aware that prolactin levels are normally elevated during pregnancy to avoid confusion in diagnosis.

Cortisol Physiology in Pregnancy

There is a two- to threefold increase in total plasma cortisol in pregnant women compared to non-pregnant women, values that match levels seen in Cushing syndrome.[3] Urinary free cortisol levels increase about 180% during pregnancy.[6]

Salt and Water Metabolism

In normal pregnancy, there is a decrease in plasma osmolality to a level of about 10 mOsmol/kg below normal.[10] This seems to result from a new steady-state setpoint caused by a decrease in the osmotic thresholds for both thirst and vasopressin suppression, similar to that seen in the syndrome of inappropriate antidiuretic hormone secretion.

See the eBook for expanded content and a complete reference list.

Calcium Metabolism

Parathyroid hormone (PTH) levels decrease to the low-normal range, sometimes even going below normal in the first trimester.[12] By the third trimester, PTH levels are in the mid-normal range with maternal calcium intake and vitamin D status influencing the levels.[13] PTH-related peptide (PTH-rp) starts to increase in the third week of gestation and is three times higher at term than at prepregnancy.[12]

In the first trimester, 1,25 (OH)2D levels start to increase and are two- to threefold higher by delivery.[16] This rise in 1,25 (OH)2D results in an increase in calcium absorption in the intestine and decrease in PTH. The rise in PTH-rp leading to a rise in 1,25(OH)2D results in increased calcium absorption from the intestine and increased renal filtered calcium load leading to hypercalciuria. The low PTH levels add to the hypercalciuria and the increased risk of kidney stones in pregnancy. Women of childbearing age are recommended to have intakes of 1000 mg calcium/day, with supplementation for women who do not meet that requirement.[25]

Thyroid

Thyroid-binding globulin (TBG) levels increase during pregnancy as a result of increased estrogen levels and lead to increases in total thyroxine (T_4) and total triiodothyroxine (T_3), peaking at approximately 16 weeks' gestation and remaining high until delivery.[26] There is often a transient rise in free T_4 (although usually within the normal range) during the first trimester of pregnancy associated with a mild decrease in thyroid-stimulating hormone (TSH). This requires different normal ranges for TSH during each trimester of pregnancy.

Human Chorionic Gonadotropin

hCG is a glycoprotein, a unique gonadotropin produced by the syncytiotrophoblast of the placenta. It is an analog of luteinizing hormone (LH). The main effect of this hormone relevant to maternal endocrine function is the thyrotropic effect, which can cause hyperthyroidism.

Human Placental Lactogen (Human Chorionic Somatomammotropin)

The major effect of human placental lactogen. on the maternal endocrine system relates to its effect on carbohydrate and fat metabolism.

Placental Growth Hormone

A placental growth hormone variant synthesized by the syncytiotrophoblast results in increased insulin-like growth factor (IGF)-1 levels during pregnancy.[30] Elevated growth hormone and IGF-1 levels may confuse the diagnostic evaluation of a patient with a possible growth hormone–secreting pituitary tumor during pregnancy.

Insulin-Like Growth Factor

Levels of IGF-1 and its binding proteins, IGFBP-1 and IGFBP-3, may be associated with fetal birthweight and predict risk of preeclampsia.[32,33]

Endocrine Disorders of Pregnancy

Thyroid Disorders

Overt hypothyroidism and hyperthyroidism have clearly been shown to have detrimental effects on the pregnancy and the fetus. It is more difficult to establish the risk to the fetus of untreated mild hypothyroidism or hyperthyroidism. Women should be screened with a TSH at the initial prenatal visit if symptoms or a history of thyroid disease, personal or family history of autoimmunity, obesity, age >30 years, or prior treatment with neck radiation are present.[26]

Goiter
Clinical Presentation

Thyroid growth is more pronounced in the presence of iodine insufficiency. It is recommended that pregnant and lactating women consume approximately 250 µg of iodine daily to avoid thyroid, cognitive, and psychomotor effects of iodine deficiency.[34]

Thyrotoxicosis
Clinical Presentation

Hyperthyroidism is the term reserved for thyrotoxicosis due to thyroid gland hyperfunction, ie, Graves disease or toxic nodular goiter.

Clinical Assessment

Thyrotoxicosis in pregnancy can be challenging to evaluate and manage. Silent thyroiditis (postpartum thyroiditis) may occur during late pregnancy and may cause transient thyrotoxicosis. Measurement of thyroid receptor antibodies may help to differentiate Graves disease from other etiologies of thyrotoxicosis.[26]

Transient gestational thyrotoxicosis is only present in the first half of pregnancy and is often associated with nausea or seen with hyperemesis gravidarum. Such patients usually do not have severe clinical features of thyrotoxicosis, and free T_4 and TSH generally return to normal by 15 to 20 weeks of gestation. Treatment with antithyroid medications is not recommended for transient gestational thyrotoxicosis. Supportive care with antiemetics, hydration, or beta-blockers may help treat symptoms.[35]

Pharmacologic Management

Radioactive iodine therapy is contraindicated in hyperthyroidism in the pregnant mother. Surgical thyroidectomy or antithyroid drug therapy are the only two therapeutic options for hyperthyroidism in pregnancy. The main indication for surgical thyroidectomy is the hyperthyroid patient who cannot tolerate thionamide therapy, or whose hyperthyroidism cannot be adequately controlled with thionamides. In the vast majority of patients, therapy with a thionamide, either PTU or MMI in the United States or carbimazole in Europe, has become the preferred therapy.

In cases of mild hyperthyroidism with symptoms of tachycardia or tremor, beta-blockers such as metoprolol or propranolol are effective in controlling symptoms in a short period of time and appear to be safe. However, long-term treatment with beta-blockers (more than 6 weeks), is not recommended, particularly during the third trimester.[37,38]

Management in Pregnancy

The mainstay of treatment for maternal hyperthyroidism is to treat the mother with a thionamide. The dose should be sufficient to keep the free T_4 level in the upper normal or mildly elevated range, which is usually accompanied by a low or suppressed TSH. PTU has traditionally been preferred over MMI. However, both PTU and MMI have potential teratogenic effects, although the birth defects with PTU appear less severe.[39] Consideration may be given to limiting the use of PTU for the first trimester of pregnancy and changing to MMI for the remainder of pregnancy. Women on preexisting thionamide therapy may consider switching to PTU once they decide on trying to conceive. If Graves hyperthyroidism is well controlled on thionamide therapy, a woman can discontinue treatment as soon as pregnancy is detected, especially if on lower doses of thionamide and treatment has persisted for >6 months, with close monitoring of thyroid function tests, at least every 4 weeks. A pregnant woman who has hyperthyroidism should be monitored at 4- to 6-week intervals during the entire pregnancy.

As the third trimester approaches, hyperthyroidism in the mother frequently improves, allowing dose reduction or discontinuation of antithyroid drug therapy. As symptomatic Graves hyperthyroidism commonly recurs in the postpartum period, careful frequent monitoring during the postpartum period with reinstitution of antithyroid therapy as soon as biochemical hyperthyroidism recurs may prevent clinically symptomatic hyperthyroidism during this time.

Measuring TSH receptor–stimulating antibodies and/or thyroid-stimulating immunoglobulins in a pregnant woman with Graves disease should be done early in pregnancy. All women with a history of Graves disease, even if not hyperthyroid during the present pregnancy, may have these circulating antibodies and should have them measured early in pregnancy and again in the third trimester.

Breastfeeding with a moderate dose of any of the thionamides appears to be safe for the infant.[42] Obtaining a radioactive iodine uptake and administering radioactive iodine therapy should be withheld until breastfeeding has been completed.

Hypothyroidism

Clinical Presentation

Iodine deficiency is a common cause of hypothyroidism. Other causes include primary thyroid gland failure resulting from radioactive iodine treatment of hyperthyroidism, surgical thyroidectomy, or Hashimoto thyroiditis. Rarely, hypothyroidism may be due to underlying pituitary disease.

Management in Pregnancy

Hypothyroidism is readily preventable by supplemental doses of dietary iodine. In addition to screening pregnant women at risk with a TSH for the presence of primary hypothyroidism, any woman on replacement L-thyroxine therapy should have their TSH and free T_4 levels monitored at least monthly during the first half of pregnancy. It has been recommended that treatment be initiated as soon as pregnancy is confirmed. Patients should be given about a 30% increase in their thyroid hormone dose and then be monitored and have their T_4 dose adjusted as necessary. TSH levels should be maintained <2.5 to 3.0 mU/L during preconception planning and during pregnancy.[26]

Women with positive TPO antibodies should be monitored by checking TSH levels every 4 weeks through mid-pregnancy, due to the increased risk of developing hypothyroidism.[26]

Postpartum Thyroid Disease

Clinical Presentation and Management in Pregnancy

In the thyrotoxic phase, disease can be confirmed by demonstrating high free T_4 and free T_3 levels with a suppressed TSH level. If the mother is not breastfeeding, a low radioactive iodine uptake may be helpful in making the diagnosis. This transient thyrotoxicosis may be followed by a transient phase of hypothyroidism. Recovery of normal thyroid function usually occurs. Beta-blocker therapy is appropriate during the hyperthyroid phase for the symptomatic patient.[48]

Thyroid Nodules

Clinical Presentation and Management in Pregnancy

A thyroid nodule discovered during pregnancy should be evaluated with an ultrasound and TSH level. If warranted, fine needle aspiration (FNA) is safe to perform during pregnancy. If FNA is performed and cytology is consistent with thyroid cancer, most women can be monitored safely with thyroid ultrasound done each trimester, without an impact on prognosis.[26] The safest time for surgery if required is the second trimester.

Pituitary Disorders

Prolactinoma

Clinical Presentation

The most common potentially serious therapeutic problem associated with pituitary gland disorders and pregnancy is the coexistence of a pituitary prolactin-producing tumor and pregnancy.

After finding an elevated serum prolactin level, a pituitary magnetic resonance image (MRI) should be done. Most commonly a microadenoma (<1 cm) but occasionally a macroadenoma (>1 cm) is demonstrated.

Management in Pregnancy

If a microprolactinoma was known to be present before the pregnancy, there is a very small risk of significant tumor growth requiring therapy during the pregnancy. Although it appears that bromocriptine is likely to be safe when taken during pregnancy, it is recommended that it be stopped as soon as the pregnancy is recognized. Monitoring prolactin levels during pregnancy is not recommended.

In a woman with a macroprolactinoma diagnosed prior to pregnancy, most endocrinologists would advise against any attempt at pregnancy until the tumor showed substantial regression following medical therapy or surgical resection. When a pregnancy occurs in a patient with a diagnosed macroprolactinoma, one must undertake frequent follow-up, including regular visual field determinations by a neuro-ophthalmologist and a follow-up MRI during the pregnancy.

Pharmacologic Treatment

The data available suggest that both bromocriptine and cabergoline are safe when given during pregnancy, although there are much less data available for use throughout pregnancy compared with use of these drugs only early in pregnancy.[2] If the tumor is less than 2 cm and not overtly impinging on the optic apparatus, it would seem reasonable to discontinue the dopamine agonist therapy and observe carefully. For a large tumor or one that is abutting the optic chiasm or invading the cavernous sinus, continue dopamine agonist therapy throughout the pregnancy and follow carefully with visual field determinations and MRI. If the tumor enlarges substantially during pregnancy or visual field abnormalities occur, one must be prepared to undertake surgical decompression of the tumor.

Other Pituitary Tumors

Clinical Presentation

Nonsecretory tumors are not commonly seen in pregnancy. Secretory pituitary tumors, such as Cushing disease and acromegaly, have been seen in pregnancy.

Management in Pregnancy

In the absence of unequivocal dramatic clinical features, the diagnosis of acromegaly or a growth hormone-secreting tumor should be delayed until the postpartum period. If a patient with known acromegaly becomes pregnant, such patients are probably best left untreated until the pregnancy is complete. The only major exception would be an increase in tumor size during pregnancy with pressure symptoms on the optic apparatus, making surgical therapy a consideration during the pregnancy.

Regarding Cushing syndrome of any type, it is best to delay biochemical evaluation until the postpartum period. The exception would be a patient with dramatic catabolic features of Cushing syndrome or a patient with ACTH-independent Cushing syndrome with a low ACTH due to an adrenal tumor. If profound pituitary Cushing disease is thought to be present, one should treat any resulting hypertension or diabetes, deferring definitive therapy until the postpartum period.

Hypopituitarism

Clinical Presentation and Management in Pregnancy

Patients with partial hypopituitarism who become pregnant should simply be monitored carefully. If they require cortisol replacement due to ACTH deficiency, slightly higher doses are often required in the third trimester and stress doses of hydrocortisone should be given during delivery.[51] Desmopressin is the preferred therapy in the rare case in which diabetes insipidus is present.

Lymphocytic Hypophysitis

Clinical Presentation

Lymphocytic hypophysitis usually presents with symptoms of a mass effect, including headaches, visual field disturbances, and a sellar/suprasellar mass visualized on MRI. Anterior pituitary hormonal deficiencies and hyperprolactinemia occur in approximately half of such patients. Diabetes insipidus is frequently present. The main differential diagnosis is an inflammatory mass and a pituitary macroadenoma.

Management in Pregnancy

Lymphocytic hypophysitis often improves spontaneously or responds to glucocorticoid therapy. Surgical therapy may sometimes be required because of the mass effect.

Sheehan Syndrome
Clinical Presentation
Sheehan syndrome is a complication of pregnancy. Sheehan syndrome is infarction of the highly vascularized pituitary gland postpartum, resulting from hypotension following massive bleeding at or around the time of delivery. Additionally, it may occur in the absence of massive bleeding, presumably secondary to vasospasm, thrombosis, or vascular compression of the anterior pituitary.[54] The key to diagnosis is the history of bleeding, the failure to lactate in the postpartum period, and failure of the resumption of menses.[55] Any patient with an obstetric hemorrhage and prolonged hypotension following delivery should have hormonal evaluation of possible hypopituitarism and be treated with stress doses of steroids until cortisol levels measured prior to treatment are available. If the diagnosis is in question, the patient can gradually be tapered off steroids after clinical improvement and undergo formal testing with a metyrapone test as well as assessment of other pituitary end-organ hormones.

Adrenal Gland Disorders

Congenital Adrenal Hyperplasia
Clinical Presentation and Management in Pregnancy
Most patients with congenital adrenal hyperplasia (CAH) have 21-hydroxylase deficiency, which may be either the salt-losing type or the simple virilizing type. Such patients are typically managed with glucocorticoids in doses adequate to clinically manage symptoms of androgen excess and reduction of 17-hydroxyprogesterone, androstenedione, and testosterone levels to levels slightly above the normal range.

Pharmacologic Treatment
Optimal management of CAH using glucocorticoid and mineralocorticoid replacement to achieve a follicular phase progesterone of <0.6 ng/mL (2 nmol/L) allows for near-normal pregnancy rates.[56] Glucocorticoid (GC) and mineralocorticoid (MC) therapy should be maintained at prepregnancy doses with monitoring of signs and symptoms of glucocorticoid deficiency and increase in dose as indicated. Similar to women with primary adrenal insufficiency (PAI), a GC dose increase of 20% to 40% may be indicated after 24 weeks and stress dosing of GC during labor is indicated.[57] Women with nonclassic CAH (NCCAH) may present later

in life with symptoms of irregular menses, infertility, or hirsutism. In those women with infertility or a history of previous miscarriage, hydrocortisone therapy is recommended.[57]

Use of dexamethasone is contraindicated in pregnancies of women with CAH.

Primary Hyperaldosteronism
Clinical Presentation
Primary hyperaldosteronism is characterized by elevated aldosterone levels in the setting of a suppressed renin. Clinical suspicion should be raised when a patient presents with hypertension and hypokalemia in the first half of pregnancy, whereas hypertension diagnosed in the second half of pregnancy is more likely to be preeclampsia.[66] The diagnosis of primary hyperaldosteronism in pregnancy is based on a suppressed renin.

Management in Pregnancy
Definitive treatment with surgery is delayed until after the pregnancy. Hypertension and hypokalemia can be managed medically with antihypertensives approved for use in pregnancy. If mineralocorticoid receptor antagonist treatment is needed, eplerenone is the preferred agent. Spironolactone is contraindicated in pregnancy.

ACTH-Independent Cushing Syndrome
Clinical Presentation
Cushing syndrome in pregnancy is rare. Clinical suspicion should be raised in the setting of hypertension, bruising, and muscle weakness[67] or pathologic fractures during pregnancy.[68] Biochemical diagnosis is best made by nighttime salivary cortisol.[69]

Management in Pregnancy
Surgery is first-line treatment for Cushing syndrome ideally done in the second trimester. Second-line treatment is medical therapy, primarily with metyrapone.

Pheochromocytoma/Paraganglioma
Clinical Presentation
Pheochromocytoma and paragangliomas are very rare.[73] Hallmark features of hypertension, headache, sweating, and palpitations are present. Diagnosis can be made by standard measurements of metanephrines in the blood or urine. Once biochemical diagnosis is confirmed, MRI is the imaging of choice in pregnant women.

Management in Pregnancy

Current treatment guidelines recommend surgical removal of the tumor laparoscopically before 24 weeks' gestation or after delivery.[74] Pregnant patients should be pretreated with alpha adrenoreceptor blockade using phenoxybenzamine or doxazosin, which can also be used to treat patients diagnosed after surgical intervention is possible.

Addison Disease

Clinical Presentation

Diagnosis is made with a 250 μg cosyntropin stimulation test. In pregnancy, higher diagnostic cutoffs for cortisol should be used: 25 μg/dL (700 nmol/L), 29 μg/dL (800 nmol/L), and 32 μg/dL (900 nmol/L) in the first, second, and third trimesters, respectively.[77]

Management and Pharmacologic Treatment in Pregnancy

Hydrocortisone is the glucocorticoid replacement of choice in pregnancy.[78] Dexamethasone is contraindicated. Women with PAI may need to have their hydrocortisone dose increased by 20% to 40% in the third trimester.[77] During labor, stress dosing of hydrocortisone should be used.[78]

Disorders of Calcium Metabolism

Vitamin D Deficiency

Clinical Presentation

Vitamin D deficiency is defined as a 25(OH)D level less than 12 ng/mL (30 nmol/L) and insufficiency as a 25(OH)D concentration of 12 to 20 ng/mL (30-50 nmol/L). Current guidelines recommend 400 to 800 IU/d for pregnant women. Some experts recommend 800 to 1000 IU 25(OH)D during preconception or pregnancy.[84]

Hyperparathyroidism

Clinical Presentation

In patients with severe hypercalcemia (calcium > 11 mg/dL or 2.75 mmol/L), or for maternal/fetal complications of hypercalcemia, surgery is the recommended treatment, ideally occurring in the second trimester.[89] Neck ultrasound is considered the imaging modality of choice.

Pharmacologic Treatment

Medical therapy for hyperparathyroidism and hypercalcemia has been described but is not the first-line therapy.[90,91]

Management in Pregnancy

PTH-rP-induced hypercalcemia or pseudohyperparathyroidism in pregnancy is caused by either placental or breast overproduction of PTH-rP in pregnancy. Treatment has included either mastectomy for mammary production[92] or delivery for placental production.[14]

Hypoparathyroidism

Clinical Presentation

Women with hypoparathyroidism must be closely monitored throughout pregnancy. Serum calcium should be maintained in the low normal range, with monitoring recommended every 3 to 4 weeks.[94] Recombinant human PTH is not recommended during pregnancy. Calcium and calcitriol are safe during pregnancy and dosing should be adjusted to reach calcium targets.

KEY POINTS

- Lactotroph hyperplasia causes pituitary size to increase during pregnancy, and prolactin levels may rise to values > 10 times the upper limit of normal for the nonpregnant state.
- Corticotropin-releasing hormone derived from the fetal-placental unit appears in the maternal circulation at very high levels, causing maternal increases in ACTH and true free cortisol levels.

- Diagnosis of Cushing syndrome during pregnancy should be made with caution.
- Plasma osmolality decreases by about 10 mOsm/kg, and renin and aldosterone levels increase three- to fourfold during normal pregnancy.
- Diagnoses of abnormalities in salt and water metabolism, ie, hyperaldosteronism, are complicated by the normal changes occurring during pregnancy.

- Maternal vitamin D requirements during pregnancy and lactation may be greater than previously thought.
- Normal pregnancy causes a mild lowering of TSH levels because of the thyrotropic effect of the high chorionic gonadotropin levels.
- Pregnancy-adjusted normal ranges for TSH should be taken into consideration when diagnosing or managing disorders of thyroid function during pregnancy.
- A placental growth hormone variant is secreted during normal pregnancy, which suppresses maternal pituitary growth hormone and increases maternal IGF-1 levels.
- Diagnosis of growth hormone deficiency or excess during pregnancy must take into consideration the effects of secretion of the placental growth hormone variant.
- As maternal hypothyroidism or hyperthyroidism may have adverse fetal effects, pregnant women should have their TSH level determined early in pregnancy.
- Thyrotoxicosis during pregnancy due to Graves hyperthyroidism may be difficult to distinguish from thyroiditis or hyperemesis gravidarum.
- Hyperthyroidism during pregnancy should be treated with antithyroid drugs in doses sufficient to achieve adequate control of maternal hyperthyroidism without causing fetal hypothyroidism.
- Pregnant women with present or past Graves disease should be screened during the early part of the third trimester for TSH receptor antibodies to determine the fetal risk for neonatal thyrotoxicosis.
- Pregnant women being treated with L-thyroxine for hypothyroidism should be monitored frequently during pregnancy as a 30% to 50% increase in L-thyroxine requirement is commonly seen.
- Women with amenorrhea and galactorrhea may have a pituitary prolactin-producing tumor, and fertility can be restored by treatment with a dopamine agonist such as bromocriptine.
- Patients with a microprolactinoma who become pregnant after taking a dopamine agonist should have the dopamine agonist stopped as soon as they learn of their pregnancy because the growth of the microprolactinoma during pregnancy is very small.
- In the unusual patient with a macroprolactinoma who becomes pregnant, the therapeutic decision must be individualized, weighing up the risks and benefits of continuing dopamine agonist therapy against follow-up therapy.
- The postpartum period, a time when the mother is dealing with the physical and emotional stresses of a new baby, is a time when thyroiditis commonly occurs, which may present as transient thyrotoxicosis or hypothyroidism.
- Presentation with headaches and amenorrhea in the postpartum period should lead one to entertain the possible diagnoses of lymphocytic hypophysitis or Sheehan syndrome.
- Pregnancy in a woman with CAH presents special ethical issues regarding possible prenatal diagnosis and/or therapeutic intervention in a potentially affected infant.

REFERENCES

(only references cited in synoptic print chapter; for a complete reference list, see ebook)

2. Cocks Eschler D, Javanmard P, Cox K, Geer EB. Prolactinoma through the female life cycle. *Endocrine*. 2018;59(1):16-29.
3. Nolten WE, Lindheimer MD, Rueckert PA, Oparil S, Ehrlich EN. Diurnal patterns and regulation of cortisol secretion in pregnancy. *J Clin Endocrinol Metab*. 1980;51(3):466-472.
6. Cousins L, Rigg L, Hollingsworth D, et al. Qualitative and quantitative assessment of the circadian rhythm of cortisol in pregnancy. *Am J Obstet Gynecol*. 1983;145(4):411-416.
10. Shakhmatova EI, Osipova NA, Natochin YV. Changes in osmolality and blood serum ion concentrations in pregnancy. *Hum Physiol*. 2000;26(1):92-95.
12. Black AJ, Topping J, Durham B, Farquharson RG, Fraser WD. A detailed assessment of alterations in bone turnover, calcium homeostasis, and bone density in normal pregnancy. *J Bone Miner Res*. 2000;15(3):557-563.
13. Kovacs CS. Maternal mineral and bone metabolism during pregnancy, lactation, and post-weaning recovery. *Physiol Rev*. 2016;96(2):449-547.
14. Eller-Vainicher C, Ossola MW, Beck-Peccoz P, Chiodini I. PTHrP-associated hypercalcemia of pregnancy resolved after delivery: a case report. *Eur J Endocrinol*. 2012;166(4):753-756.
16. Wilson SG, Retallack RW, Kent JC, Worth GK, Gutteridge DH. Serum free 1,25-dihydroxyvitamin D and the free 1,25-dihydroxyvitamin D index during a longitudinal study of human pregnancy and lactation. *Clin Endocrinol (Oxf)*. 1990;32(5):613-622.
25. Hacker AN, Fung EB, King JC. Role of calcium during pregnancy: maternal and fetal needs. *Nutr Rev*. 2012;70(7):397-409.

26. Alexander EK, Pearce EN, Brent GA, et al. 2017 Guidelines of the American Thyroid Association for the diagnosis and management of thyroid disease during pregnancy and the postpartum. *Thyroid.* 2017;27(3):315-389.

30. Perez-Ibave DC, Rodriguez-Sanchez IP, Garza-Rodriguez Mde L, Barrera-Saldaña HA. Extrapituitary growth hormone synthesis in humans. *Growth Horm IGF Res.* 2014;24(2-3):47-53.

32. Asvold BO, Eskild A, Jenum PA, Vatten LJ. Maternal concentrations of insulin-like growth factor I and insulin-like growth factor binding protein 1 during pregnancy and birth weight of offspring. *Am J Epidemiol.* 2011;174(2):129-135.

33. Liao S, Vickers MH, Taylor RS, et al. Maternal serum IGF-1, IGFBP-1 and 3, and placental growth hormone at 20weeks' gestation in pregnancies complicated by preeclampsia. *Pregnancy Hypertens.* 2017;10:149-154.

34. Pearce EN. Monitoring and effects of iodine deficiency in pregnancy: still an unsolved problem? *Eur J Clin Nutr.* 2013;67(5):481-484.

35. Pearce EN. Management of thyrotoxicosis: preconception, pregnancy, and the postpartum period. *Endocr Pract.* 2019;25(1):62-68.

37. Duan L, Ng A, Chen W, Spencer HT, Lee MS. Beta-blocker subtypes and risk of low birth weight in newborns. *J Clin Hypertens (Greenwich).* 2018;20(11):1603-1609.

38. Bateman BT, Patorno E, Desai RJ, et al. Late pregnancy beta blocker exposure and risks of neonatal hypoglycemia and bradycardia. *Pediatrics.* 2016;138(3):e20160731.

39. Andersen SL, Olsen J, Wu CS, et al. Birth defects after early pregnancy use of antithyroid drugs: a Danish nationwide study. *J Clin Endocrinol Metab.* 2013;98(11):4373-4381.

42. Garcia-Mayor RV, Larranaga A. Treatment of Graves' hyperthyroidism with thionamides-derived drugs: review. *Med Chem.* 2010;6(4):239-246.

48. Nguyen CT, Mestman JH. Postpartum thyroiditis. *Clin Obstet Gynecol.* 2019;62(2):359-364.

51. Langlois F, Lim DST, Fleseriu M. Update on adrenal insufficiency: diagnosis and management in pregnancy. *Curr Opin Endocrinol Diabetes Obes.* 2017;24(3):184-192.

54. Diri H, Karaca Z, Tanriverdi F, Unluhizarci K, Kelestimur F. Sheehan's syndrome: new insights into an old disease. *Endocrine.* 2016;51(1):22-31.

55. Kilicli F, Dokmetas HS, Acibucu F. Sheehan's syndrome. *Gynecol Endocrinol.* 2013;29(4):292-295.

56. Casteras A, De Silva P, Rumsby G, Conway GS. Reassessing fecundity in women with classical congenital adrenal hyperplasia (CAH): normal pregnancy rate but reduced fertility rate. *Clin Endocrinol (Oxf).* 2009;70(6):833-837.

57. Speiser PW, Arlt W, Auchus RJ, et al. Congenital adrenal hyperplasia due to steroid 21-hydroxylase deficiency: an endocrine society clinical practice guideline. *J Clin Endocrinol Metab.* 2018;103(11):4043-4088.

66. Riester A, Reincke M. Progress in primary aldosteronism: mineralocorticoid receptor antagonists and management of primary aldosteronism in pregnancy. *Eur J Endocrinol.* 2015;172(1):R23-R30.

67. Dong D, Li H, Xiao H. The diagnosis and management of Cushing syndrome during pregnancy. *J Obstet Gynaecol.* 2015;35(1):94-96.

68. Brue T, Amodru V, Castinetti F. Management of endocrine disease: management of Cushing's syndrome during pregnancy. Solved and unsolved questions. *Eur J Endocrinol.* 2018;178(6):R259-R266.

69. Lopes LM, Francisco RP, Galletta MA, Bronstein MD. Determination of nighttime salivary cortisol during pregnancy: comparison with values in non-pregnancy and Cushing's disease. *Pituitary.* 2016;19(1):30-38.

73. Harrington JL, Farley DR, van Heerden JA, Ramin KD. Adrenal tumors and pregnancy. *World J Surg.* 1999;23(2):182-186.

74. Lenders JW. Pheochromocytoma and pregnancy: a deceptive connection. *Eur J Endocrinol.* 2012;166(2):143-150.

77. Lebbe M, Arlt W. What is the best diagnostic and therapeutic management strategy for an Addison patient during pregnancy? *Clin Endocrinol (Oxf).* 2013;78(4):497-502.

78. Bornstein SR, Allolio B, Arlt W, et al. Diagnosis and treatment of primary adrenal insufficiency: an endocrine society clinical practice guideline. *J Clin Endocrinol Metab.* 2016;101(2):364-389.

84. Pilz S, Zittermann A, Obeid R, et al. The role of vitamin D in fertility and during pregnancy and lactation: a review of clinical data. *Int J Environ Res Public Health.* 2018;15(10):2241.

89. McCarthy A, Howarth S, Khoo S, et al. Management of primary hyperparathyroidism in pregnancy: a case series. *Endocrinol Diabetes Metab Case Rep.* 2019;2019:19-39.

90. Vera L, Oddo S, Di Iorgi N, Bentivoglio G, Giusti M. Primary hyperparathyroidism in pregnancy treated with cinacalcet: a case report and review of the literature. *J Med Case Rep.* 2016;10(1):361.

91. Ornoy A, Wajnberg R, Diav-Citrin O. The outcome of pregnancy following pre-pregnancy or early pregnancy alendronate treatment. *Reprod Toxicol.* 2006;22(4):578-579.

92. Khosla S, van Heerden JA, Gharib H, et al. Parathyroid hormone-related protein and hypercalcemia secondary to massive mammary hyperplasia. *N Engl J Med.* 1990;322(16):1157.

94. Khan AA, Clarke B, Rejnmark L, et al. Management of endocrine disease: hypoparathyroidism in pregnancy. Review and evidence-based recommendations for management. *Eur J Endocrinol.* 2019;180(2):R37-R44.

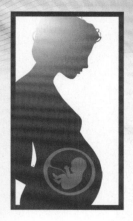

CHAPTER 32

Obesity in Pregnancy

Tania Roman and Patrick S. Ramsey

Introduction

Pregnancy is a time of significant change in a woman's life. The pregnant body undergoes a myriad of physiological changes not seen simultaneously in any other medical condition. As more women delay childbearing and new public health concerns gain strength, the care for the pregnant woman becomes more complex and challenging. One of those compelling public health issues is the rising obesity epidemic taking place around the world, specifically in developed countries. It is for this reason that physicians should be aware of the potential issues surrounding women with obesity in order to address them preconceptually and throughout the pregnancy and puerperium. This is a collaborative task requiring a multidisciplinary approach in the realm of obstetrics, public health, and general medicine.

Definition

Obesity in the United States has reached unprecedented rates affecting women of reproductive age and leading to significant maternal and perinatal complications. The Centers for Disease Control and Prevention defines adult obesity as a body mass index (BMI) ≥ 30 kg/m^2, which is calculated as weight in kilograms divided by height in meters squared. It is further stratified by class: class I (BMI 30.0-34.9 kg/m^2), class II (BMI 35.0-39.9 kg/m^2), and class III (BMI ≥ 40 kg/m^2).[1] The caveat to this standard definition is that it does not account for the physiological changes in pregnancy such as increased blood volume and fetal weight accrued over a short period of time. Thus, classification of obesity in pregnancy is based on prepregnancy BMI.

Epidemiology

Over the past 3 decades, obesity rates in the United States have increased. Based on data collected over a 1-year period, from 2015 to 2016, more than one-third of adults (39.8%) were obese, and almost one-fifth of all youths (18.5% aged 5-18 years) were obese. A breakdown by gender shows that 41.1% of women aged 20 years and older and 36.5% of women aged between 20 and 39 years were obese (**Figure 32.1**).[2] These staggering numbers do not seem to be on the decline, as these rates have been steadily increasing over the last 10 years.

The most recent data have also shown differences in obesity prevalence by race and ethnicity. Non-Hispanic black (54.8%) and Hispanic (50.6%) women have the highest rates of obesity. This was followed by non-Hispanic white (38.0%) and non-Hispanic Asian (14.8%) women. These differences reflect the disparities in maternal and neonatal health seen in the United States (**Figure 32.2**).[2]

Pathogenesis

The obesity epidemic affecting pregnant women has a vast array of clinical implications. Pregnant women with obesity have higher rates of severe maternal morbidity (SMM), defined as "unexpected outcomes of labor and delivery that result in significant short- or long-term consequences to a woman's health."[3] This includes postpartum hemorrhage requiring transfusion; thromboembolic events; and cardiovascular, respiratory, and hematological complications. The excess adipose tissue serves as an active endocrine organ that activates metabolic and inflammatory pathways leading to many pathological processes.[4,5] On a molecular level, extracellular vesicles in adipose tissue have been shown to play a role in glucose and lipid metabolism, leading to insulin resistance and metabolic syndrome.[6] Given that the amount of excess weight is linearly associated to obstetrical and fetal complications further supports the causative role of obesity in the pathogenesis of these disease processes.[7]

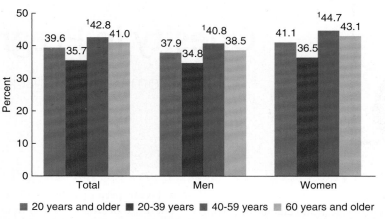

Figure 32.1 Age-adjusted prevalence of obesity among adults aged 20 years and older, by sex and race and Hispanic origin: United States, 2015-2016.[1]Significantly different from those aged 20 to 39 years.

(Reprinted from Defining Adult Overweight and Obesity. *CDC Division of Nutrition, Physical Activity, and Obesity, National Center for Chronic Disease Prevention and Health Promotion*. Page last reviewed on April 11, 2017. Accessed April 4, 2019. https://www.cdc.gov/obesity/adult/defining.html)

Clinical Presentation

Antepartum

Maternal Considerations

Recent studies have shown that prepregnancy weight (eg, maternal BMI at conception) is a stronger predictor of adverse maternal and infant outcomes than weight gain during pregnancy. A 2017 meta-analysis of 25 pooled cohort studies of 196,670 participants found that the odds ratio (OR) for any maternal or fetal adverse outcome per one standard deviation (1-SD) increase in maternal prepregnancy BMI was 1.28 (95% confidence interval [CI] 1.27-1.29) compared to 1.04 (95% CI 1.03-1.05)

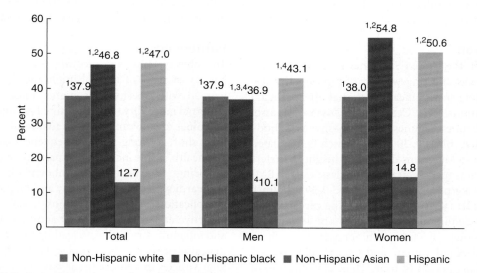

Figure 32.2 Age-adjusted prevalence of obesity among adults aged 20 years and older, by sex and race and Hispanic origin: United States, 2015 to 2016. [1]Significantly different from non-Hispanic Asian persons. [2]Significantly different from non-Hispanic white persons. [3]Significantly different from Hispanic persons. [4]Significantly different from women of same race and Hispanic origin.

(Reprinted from Defining Adult Overweight and Obesity. *CDC Division of Nutrition, Physical Activity, and Obesity, National Center for Chronic Disease Prevention and Health Promotion*. Page last reviewed on April 11, 2017. Accessed April 4, 2019. https://www.cdc.gov/obesity/adult/defining.html)

per 1-SD increase in gestational weight gain (*P* < .001 for comparison).[8] These findings emphasized the importance of preconceptual counseling to reinforce and educate women on weight loss prior to conception. However, many women may have limited access to health care or may only seek care during pregnancy or when seeking emergency services. For this reason, a majority of education and counseling regarding obesity and pregnancy will have to occur during prenatal care.

Given that earlier studies have shown an association with excess gestational weight gain and adverse maternal neonatal outcomes, the National Academy of Medicine (formerly the Institute of Medicine) provided guidelines regarding gestational weight gain (**Table 32.1**). Under these recommendations, women with obesity should gain in total 11 to 20 lbs during pregnancy. This is in sharp contrast with women in the normal range (BMI 18.5-24.9 kg/m[2]) who can gain 25 to 35 lbs during their pregnancy. Of note, the guidelines also addressed women with obesity who had multiple fetuses and recommended a weight gain of 25 to 42 lbs.[9]

Maternal Complications

Spontaneous Abortion

Obesity has been found to modestly increase the risk of early pregnancy loss. In a 2011 systematic review, including six retrospective studies and a total of 28,538 women (3800 obese [BMI ≥ 28 or 30 kg/m[2]], 3792 overweight [BMI 25-29 kg/m[2]], and 17,146 normal weight [BMI < 25 kg/m[2]]), the percentages of women with ≥1 miscarriage were 16.6% for those in the group with obesity, 11.8% for those

in the group with overweight, and 10.7% for those in the normal weight group.[10] The odds of having ≥1 miscarriage increased for women with obesity (OR 1.31, 95% CI 1.18-1.46) and women with overweight (OR 1.11, 95% CI 1.00-1.24) when compared with women with normal BMI. Furthermore, a 2018 systematic review and meta-analysis[11] of recurrent pregnancy loss (RPL), defined as three or more miscarriages, found that women with obesity had a higher risk of RPL compared to women with overweight. The meta-analysis included two prospective cohort studies of 1742 women with a history of RPL. The results showed that obesity (BMI ≥ 30 kg/m[2]) was associated with RPL (OR 1.75, 95% CI 1.24-2.47, and *P* = .001), while overweight was not associated with RPL.

Although aneuploidy is the main cause of first trimester pregnancy loss in the general population, women with obesity have been observed to have an excess loss of normal karyotype embryos.[12] One possible explanation for this is a hostile uterine environment related to the inflammatory pathways triggered by excess adipose tissue.[13] This is further supported by observations that patients with obesity who have polycystic ovary syndrome (PCOS) have a miscarriage rate of 20% to 40% higher than the baseline in the general obstetric population. Low-grade chronic inflammation commonly seen in patient with PCOS worsens during gestation and may contribute to the excess risk of miscarriage.[14]

Diabetes

Pregnancy is characterized by increased insulin resistance and decreased insulin sensitivity, both worsen with advanced gestation. These natural physiologic changes due greatly to placental

Table 32.1 National Academy of Medicine Weight Gain Recommendations for Pregnancy

Prepregnancy BMI	BMI (kg/m[2])	Total Weight Gain Range lbs (kg) Singleton Gestation	Total Weight Gain Range lbs (kg) Multiple Gestation	Rates of Weight Gain in Second and Third Trimesters Mean Range[a] lbs	kg
Normal weight	18.5-24.9	25-35 (11.5-16)	37-54 (17-25)	1 (0.8-1)	0.42 (0.35-0.50)
Overweight	25.0-29.9	15-25 (7-11.5)	31-50 (14-23)	0.6 (0.5-0.7)	0.28 (0.23-0.33)
Obese (includes all classes)	≥30.0	11-20 (5-9)	25-42 (11-19)	0.5 (0.4-0.6)	0.22 (0.17-0.27)

BMI, body mass index.
[a]Nonspecific for singleton or multiple gestation.
Modified from Institute of Medicine (US). *Weight Gain During Pregnancy: Reexamining the Guidelines*. National Academies Press; 2009.
©2009 National Academy of Science.

hormones are accentuated by obesity. Excess adipose tissue contains extracellular vesicles that have been shown to increase insulin resistance.[4,6]

The prevalence of gestational diabetes mellitus (GDM) is significantly higher in women with obesity than in the general obstetrical population, and the risk increases with increasing maternal weight and BMI. In a systematic review of studies on prepregnancy BMI and risk of GDM, the prevalence of GDM increased by 0.92% for every 1 kg/m^2 increase in BMI.[15] Pregnant women with obesity are both more likely to have diabetes at conception or develop it during pregnancy. The American College of Obstetricians and Gynecologists recommends that women with obesity who have another risk factor (ie, physical inactivity, first-degree relative with diabetes, high-risk ethnicity, history of macrosomia, previous GDM, hypertension, dyslipidemia, PCOS, hemoglobin A1C ≥5.7%, or history of cardiovascular disease) be screened when initiating prenatal care for GDM with a 1-hour glucose challenge test and screened again at 24 to 28 weeks of gestation, even if the result is normal.[16] See detailed discussion in Chapter 30.

Hypertensive Disorders

Maternal obesity has been consistently identified as an independent risk factor for gestational hypertension and preeclampsia. In a systematic review of 13 cohort studies comprising nearly 1.4 million women, the risk of preeclampsia doubled with each 5 to 7 kg/m^2 increase in prepregnancy BMI.[17] This relationship persisted in studies that excluded women with chronic hypertension, diabetes mellitus, or multiple gestations, and after adjustment for other confounders. Cohort studies of women who underwent bariatric surgery suggest that weight loss significantly reduces the occurrence of preeclampsia.[18] Given this increased risk of gestational hypertension and preeclampsia, it is important to closely monitor vital signs during every clinic visit to detect any trend in increased blood pressures from baseline. If there is a high suspicion of developing hypertensive disorder, the patient should be counseled on the symptoms of preeclampsia. A home blood pressure kit should be considered for patients to measure their blood pressure at home or work.

Hepatic Conditions

Pregnant women with obesity are more likely to be affected by nonalcoholic fatty liver disease (NAFLD) when compared to their normal weight counterparts. Up to 80% of patients with NAFLD are obese, and the severity of the disease is directly correlated with increasing BMI.[19] Most patients with NAFLD are asymptomatic and demonstrate no biochemical abnormalities. This condition is most commonly found incidentally when women have laboratory work for other causes (eg, nausea, vomiting, abdominal pain, preeclampsia panel). NAFLD is something to consider when there is an isolated mild elevation (less than two times the upper limit of normal) of liver enzymes with no other clinical symptoms or signs. Because some women may only seek routine health care during pregnancy, it is important to inform them of this finding so that they are aware of lifestyle modifications (eg, low-fat diet, exercise, weight loss) that can slow down the progression of NAFLD.

Obstructive Sleep Apnea

Obesity is a significant risk factor of obstructive sleep apnea (OSA), which, in turn, has been associated with hypertension and cardiovascular morbidity in the general population. The prevalence of OSA is increased in pregnancy and as gestation progresses. This is likely due to the elevation of the diaphragm and hormones that affect respiratory drive. Data from an inpatient sample database of 55 million women found that OSA in pregnancy increased SMM: eclampsia (OR 5.4, 95% CI 3.3-8.9), cardiomyopathy (OR 9.0, 95% CI 7.5-10.9), pulmonary embolism (OR 4.5, 95% CI 2.3-8.9), and in-hospital mortality (OR 5.3, 95% CI 2.4-11.5).[20] Pregnant women with obesity having another obesity-related comorbidity should be considered high risk for OSA. Patients should be screened for OSA and, if positive, referred for evaluation by a sleep medicine specialist.[21] Furthermore, in women with OSA consultation with anesthesiologist should be considered prior to delivery given possible difficult airway entry in case of emergency. There are several ongoing large clinical trials to assess whether management of OSA in pregnancy can reduce perinatal complications.

Fetal Assessment

Anomalies

Women with obesity are at increased risk of having offspring with congenital anomalies, including cardiac malformations, neural tube defects, orofacial defects, and limb reduction abnormalities.[22] In a

2017 population-based cohort study of 1.2 million live-born singleton infants, the risk of major congenital malformations and subgroups of specific malformations progressively increased with maternal overweight and increasing severity of obesity (**Figure 32.3**).[23] This observation is consistent with a 2009 systematic review and meta-analysis, with the addition that adjusted risk ratios were performed for maternal age, parity, early pregnancy smoking, educational level, maternal country of birth, family situation, and sex of offspring, and a sensitivity analysis was done to exclude women with preexisting diabetes and GDM. Both subanalyses showed an increased risk of anomalies with higher BMI. Compared with offspring of normal weight mothers, the adjusted risk ratios for any major congenital malformation increased with maternal BMI: 1.05 (95% CI 1.02-1.07) in mothers with overweight, 1.12 (95% CI 1.08-1.15) in mothers in obesity class I, 1.23 (95% CI 1.17-1.30) in mothers in obesity class II, and 1.37 (95% CI 1.26-1.49) in mothers in obesity class III.[24] It is possible that these data underestimate the increased risk of congenital anomalies in pregnant women with obesity because obesity presents diagnostic limitations to detect congenital anomalies using prenatal ultrasound, resulting in fewer optimal examinations and antepartum diagnoses.

Stillbirth

Pregnant women with obesity have been found to have higher rates of stillbirth. A registry-based cohort study in Sweden, which included 145, 319 women, found that the prevalence of stillbirth was 2.6/1000 in women with overweight/obesity, which is almost twice of that found in normal weight women (1.6/1000).[25] Furthermore, results from the Stillbirth Collaborative Research Network found that women with overweight (BMI 25.0-29.9 kg/m^2) and obesity (BMI $\geq$ 30 kg/m^2) were more likely to experience stillbirth than normal weight women (BMI 18-24.9 kg/m^2): OR 1.48 (95% CI 1.14-1.94) and OR 1.60 (95% CI 1.23-2.08), respectively.[26] These data are consistent with findings from a UK study,[27] where 639 stillbirths ($\geq$24 weeks) and 425 intrauterine fetal deaths (<24 weeks) were examined for associations with maternal demographic factors. A key finding was an association with increased maternal weight (BMI $\geq$ 25 kg/m^2) in the women who had a fetal loss compared to the general population. A 2014 meta-analysis of 44 publications, which included 16,274 stillbirths, found that maternal BMI was linearly correlated with fetal death, stillbirth, and perinatal death.[28] The relative risk per 5-unit increase in maternal BMI for stillbirth was 1.24 (95% CI 1.18-1.30). The absolute risk

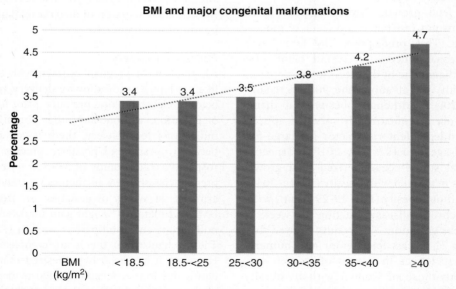

BMI and major congenital malformations

Figure 32.3 Major congenital malformations are linearly associated with increasing body mass index (BMI).

(Adapted from Persson M, Cnattingius S, Villamor E, et al. Risk of major congenital malformations in relation to maternal overweight and obesity severity: cohort study of 1.2 million singletons. *BMJ*. 2017;357:j2563.)

per 10,000 pregnancies for stillbirth was 48 (95% CI 19-23) for BMI of 25 and 48 (95% CI 46-51) for BMI of 30.[28]

Numerous hypotheses have been proposed to explain these trends. One is the increased inflammatory state that excess adipose tissue confers. However, data from the Stillbirth Collaborative Research Network looking at specific inflammatory makers (serum ferritin, C-reactive protein, white blood cell count, and histologic chorioamnionitis) and their association with stillbirth did not find an association to account for the relationship between stillbirth and obesity.[26] An alternative explanation is the potential confounders when evaluating obesity, such as concurrent diabetes and hypertensive disorders, which can, independently, lead to fetal asphyxia and death.

Perinatal death in pregnant women with obesity can be partially explained, given that high central adiposity may preclude antenatal testing and fetal monitoring and, thus, lead to a delay in the detection of fetal stress. Subsequently, this may postpone the decision to deliver or perform an emergent cesarean delivery when it is warranted. Additional discussion on fetal death in pregnancy can be found in Chapter 4.

Abnormal Fetal Growth

Maternal obesity in pregnancy is associated with abnormal fetal growth. Excess adipose tissue increases insulin resistance and leads to glucose intolerance. This predisposes the fetus, even when maternal glucose levels fall below that which are diagnostic of diabetes, to an increased risk of birth weight above the 90th percentile (**Figure 32.4**).[29] Although obesity and diabetes often occur concurrently, obesity appears to be an independent risk factor for large-for-gestational-age fetuses.[30-33] A 2018 prospective longitudinal study[34] characterized fetal growth trajectories in women with obesity (BMI > 30 kg/m²) and without obesity (BMI 19-29 kg/m²) without major chronic diseases starting at 8 weeks to 13 6/7 weeks gestation. The results showed that, as early as 21 weeks, fetal femur and humerus lengths were longer in fetuses of women with obesity than those of women without obesity. Averaged across gestation, fetal head circumference was also higher in women with obesity. Taken together, this suggests that fetal growth is

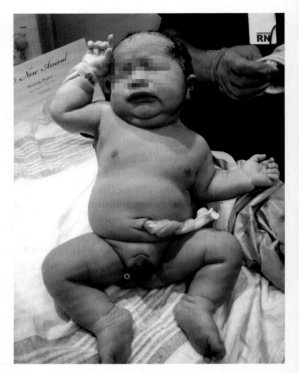

Figure 32.4 Large-for-gestational-age infant. Male infant of a mother with diabetes and obesity (body mass index of 60 kg/m²). Birth weight of 4210 g.

altered in early pregnancy in women with obesity. Additional discussion of deviant fetal growth can be found in Chapter 18.

Postterm Delivery

Although most pregnant women with obesity are likely to have an indication for delivery, such as diabetes or elevated blood pressure, prior to 41 weeks of gestation, without any other comorbidities or indications for delivery, there is an association between obesity and postterm pregnancy. A retrospective cohort study of 339,126 term singleton pregnancies showed an increasing trend in delivering at 41 weeks of gestation as prepregnancy BMI and maternal weight gain increased for both nulliparous and multiparous women ($P < .001$).[35] The mechanism for this is not completely known. However, it has been hypothesized that incorrect dating due to preconception oligo-ovulation might play a role.[36-38] Another theory is that hormonal changes associated with obesity may interfere with the onset of parturition.[39]

Management of Labor and Delivery

Timing of Delivery

Obesity by itself is not an indication for early delivery (<39 weeks of gestation), but it does play an important role when determining the gestational age for delivery. Especially in the setting of another comorbidity, such as suspected fetal macrosomia, GDM, or hypertension, it is prudent to deliver before exacerbation of any comorbidity. This decision becomes particularly important when fetal surveillance (eg, biophysical profile and nonstress test) cannot be accomplished due to maternal body habitus and central adiposity. Given that women with obesity are at a higher risk of stillbirth, if fetal surveillance is inadequate or cannot be performed, then early delivery can be considered. In women with very morbid obesity (BMI > 60 kg/m²), logistical preparations, such as ensuring proper operating room equipment and supplies, should be made. An example would be a labor and delivery bed, or surgical bed that has capacity to hold the respective maternal weight. Another important consideration is a preoperative anesthesia consult to ensure that appropriate tests or evaluation has been done prior to induction of labor or scheduled, or in the event of emergent, cesarean delivery.

Intrapartum

Maternal Considerations

A pregnant woman with obesity undergoing an induction of labor faces multiple risks compared to the general population without obesity. Risk of chorioamnionitis, arrest of dilation/descent, labor disorders, cesarean delivery, and postoperative infection are increased in the parturient with obesity. Women with obesity are less likely to undergo spontaneous labor at term and often require cervical ripening agents and intravenous oxytocin to initiate labor.[40] Induction to birth time has been noted to be longer in women with obesity, and prolongation of the latent phase is directly correlated with maternal weight such that, as BMI increases, it takes a longer time to reach active phase.[41] However, serial cervical examinations to assess labor progression and/or use of intrauterine pressure catheters predispose women to chorioamnionitis. Intrapartum infection can cause fetal heart monitoring changes indicating fetal stress, which, in turn, can lead to the decision to proceed with cesarean delivery.

Multiple studies have shown that women with obesity have higher rates of cesarean delivery.[42,43] Determining the clinical factors involved in higher cesarean rates, especially in nulliparous women with obesity, is a complex multifactorial process. Studies have evaluated the potential etiology and causes both on a pathophysiological and clinical level. One explanation for failed induction of labor is the reduced myometrial contractility in women with obesity compared with women without obesity.[44] In addition, elevated leptin and cholesterol levels have been associated with impaired contractility due to a decrease in the influx of calcium ions into the uterine smooth muscle.[45,46] There are multiple ways of performing labor induction, many different agents for cervical ripening, and numerous rates of administering oxytocin, which affect rates of cesarean delivery in pregnant women with obesity. Finally, institution-dependent decision-making and the variety of labor curves used to determine when a patient needs a cesarean delivery likely contribute to differences in cesarean rates per location.

Cesarean Delivery Technique

Obesity can present a surgical challenge during a cesarean delivery. Excess adipose tissue and a thick subcutaneous layer can make entry into the peritoneum and exposure to uterus more difficult. This, in turn, can lead to a complicated infant delivery and increased blood loss during surgery. Special attention is needed when preparing for a cesarean delivery in the pregnant patient with obesity, especially with large central obesity and increasing BMI. In addition, anesthetic considerations should be made in advance of a possible planned, or in the event of an emergent, cesarean delivery (for additional commentary see Chapter 26).

The decision whether to make a vertical versus a transverse skin incision should be individualized and based on body fat distribution and panniculus size when the patient is lying supine (**Figure 32.5**). Studies have not shown differences in wound complications based on skin incision type.[47,48] A supraumbilical incision has been described in clinical practice and in the literature.[49] This incision is usually made without moving the pannus and has been observed to facilitate exposure, visualization of lower uterine segment, and extraction of the infant. When a transverse skin incision is preferred, panniculus retractors (traditional and trademarked

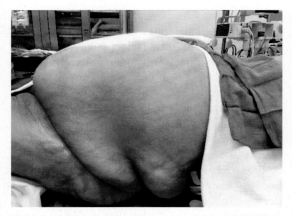

Figure 32.5 Body fat distribution in patient with obesity (body mass index of 60 kg/m²) while supine. Decision was made to proceed with supraumbilical incision.

devices) can be used to aid in lifting the pannus away from area where skin incision is planned.

Once entry of the peritoneum is made, surgical exposure can be improved with intra-abdominal O-ring retractors that can greatly enhance visualization of the uterus by moving away the bowel and omentum (**Figure 32.6**). A 2018 systematic and meta-analysis[50] of six randomized controlled trials, including 1669 women, found that the use of O-ring retractors did not reduce the risk of surgical site infections, operating time, estimated blood loss, or the need for blood transfusion. However, use of these retractors did increase the rate of adequate visualization of the operative field (relative risk 1.05 [95% CI 1.00-1.10]).

The type of uterine incision, low transverse versus vertical, should also be individually assessed and made based on visualization of the lower uterine segment and fetal gestational age and position. In the premature (especially less than 32 weeks), growth restricted, and transverse or breech fetus, a vertical uterine incision might be optimal to deliver the infant safely.

Preparation for Complications

Women with obesity who undergo long labor inductions are at increased risk of postpartum hemorrhage. If they eventually have a cesarean delivery, they are at a higher risk of uterine atony, intraoperative bleeding, and infection. It is good practice to evaluate a patient's postpartum hemorrhage risk

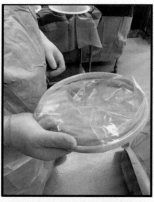

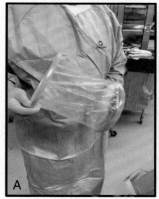

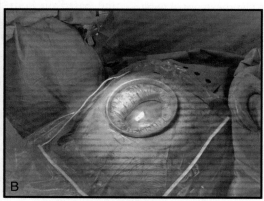

Figure 32.6 A, O-ring retractor used during cesarean delivery. Exposure to uterus is improved. **B,** O-ring retractor used in woman with obesity (body mass index of 60 kg/m²) during cesarean delivery via supraumbilical skin incision.

prior to delivery. In this manner, the care team should be aware of and prepared for a possible hemorrhage. Given the fast evolution of events, consultation with the anesthesia team prior to delivery is recommended so that they can assist in the case of an emergency.

As mentioned before, women with obesity are at higher risk of macrosomia, and shoulder dystocia should be considered if the estimated fetal weight is >90th percentile and/or protracted descent in the second stage occurs.

Postpartum

Pregnancy and the postpartum period are hypercoagulable states that place women at increased risk of venous thromboembolic events (VTE). The risk of VTE is increased fourfold to fivefold in pregnancy and the puerperium.[51] Because obesity and immobility further increase the risk of VTE, it is important to consider deep venous thrombosis prophylaxis. This can be done in several ways: (1) encouraging women to ambulate early, (2) enforcing use of sequential compression devices, (3) pharmacological management with low-molecular-weight heparin (LMWH) or unfractionated heparin. The dose for LMWH can be 40 mg daily or weight based at a dose of 0.5 mg/kg. The latter regimen is likely more effective in women with obesity.[52]

The postpartum period is also a time to reinforce continued care and follow-up. Many pregnant women with obesity experience continued glucose intolerance or hypertension. It is important to stress screening for both diabetes and hypertension at their 6-week postpartum visit. This is also an opportunity to educate patients on weight loss prior to any subsequent pregnancies. For women who had a preeclampsia, it is important to schedule a visit within a week after discharge to assess their blood pressure and to detect any lingering or new cardiovascular disease symptoms. In addition, women with obesity who had a cesarean delivery should be followed up closely, given their increased risk of seroma formation and superficial skin infections. In our institution, we follow up women with obesity 7 days after cesarean delivery for a postoperative wound assessment.

Preconception and Pregnancy Interval Counseling

Women with overweight and obesity of reproductive age should be counseled on the importance of losing weight prior to conception. In general, it is well known that obesity is associated with increased insulin resistance, diabetes, and hypertension. These conditions are exacerbated in pregnancy by presence of placental hormonal factors and the changes in maternal physiology as presented earlier. It is of paramount importance that these risks be addressed and/or discussed with women with obesity of reproductive age. This also presents opportunities in the realm of public health to increase awareness on the importance of weight control prior to conception.

For women who undergo bariatric surgery, the current recommendation is to wait at least 18 months after surgery prior to try to conceive, although recent studies have reported no differences in outcomes in women who waited 12 months after surgery compared to those who waited 18 months.[53] Women who have undergone bariatric surgery are at risk of vitamin deficiencies, in particular B_{12}, and should be supplemented accordingly during the preconception period.

KEY POINTS

- Obesity is becoming more prevalent in women of reproductive age, introducing increased morbidity in pregnancy.
- Pregnant women with obesity need to be screened early for gestational diabetes and monitored closely for the development of hypertensive disorders of pregnancy.
- Ultrasound surveillance and antenatal testing is necessary in pregnant women with obesity due to increased rate of fetal anomalies and stillbirth.
- Careful planning is needed in the peripartum period in order to decrease risk of infection, anesthesia complications, and hemorrhage in pregnant women with obesity.
- Obesity increases the risk of thromboembolic events; therefore, mechanical and/or chemical prophylaxis should be strongly considered.
- In the pregnancy interval, women with obesity should be encouraged to initiate weight loss activities and diet, and possibly consider bariatric surgery if an appropriate candidate.

REFERENCES

1. Defining Adult Overweight and Obesity. *CDC Division of Nutrition, Physical Activity, and Obesity, National Center for Chronic Disease Prevention and Health Promotion*. Page last reviewed on April 11, 2017. Accessed April 4, 2019. https://www.cdc.gov/obesity/adult/defining.html
2. Hales CM, Carroll MD, Fryar CD, et al. Prevalence of obesity among adults and youth: United States, 2015-2016. *NCHS Data Brief*. 2017;(288):1-8.
3. American College of Obstetricians and Gynecologists and the Society for Maternal – Fetal Medicine, Kilpatrick SK, Ecker JL. Severe maternal morbidity: screening and review external. *Am J Obstet Gynecol*. 2016;215(3):B17-B22.
4. Hauth JC, Clifton RG, Roberts JM, et al. Maternal insulin resistance and preeclampsia. *Am J Obstet Gynecol*. 2011;204:327.e1-327.e6.
5. Roberts JM, Bodnar LM, Patrick TE, et al. The role of obesity in preeclampsia. *Pregnancy Hypertens*. 2011;1:6-16.
6. Jayabalan N, Nair S, Nuzhat Z, et al. Cross talk between adipose tissue and placenta in obese and gestational diabetes mellitus pregnancies via exosomes. *Front Endocrinol (Lausanne)*. 2017;8:239. Published 2017 September 27.
7. Marshall NE, Guild C, Cheng YW, et al. Maternal superobesity and perinatal outcomes. *Am J Obstet Gynecol*. 2012;206:417.e1-417.e6.
8. LifeCycle Project-Maternal Obesity and Childhood Outcomes Study Group, Voerman E, Santos S, Inskip H. Association of gestational weight gain with adverse maternal and infant outcomes. *J Am Med Assoc*. 2019;321(17):1702-1715.
9. Rasmussen KM, Yaktine AL, eds. Institute of Medicine (IOM) and National Research Council Committee to reexamine IOM Pregnancy Weight Guidelines. *Weight Gain During Pregnancy: Reexamining the Guidelines National*. Academies Press; 2009.
10. Boots C, Stephenson MD. Does obesity increase the risk of miscarriage in spontaneous conception: a systematic review. *Semin Reprod Med*. 2011;29:507-513.
11. Cavalcante MB, Sarno M, Peixoto AB, et al. Obesity and recurrent miscarriage: a systematic review and meta-analysis. *J Obstet Gynaecol Res*. 2019;45:30-38.
12. Bellver J, Cruz F, Martínez MC, et al. Female overweight is not associated with a higher embryo euploidy rate in first trimester miscarriages karyotyped by hysteroembryoscopy. *Fertil Steril*. 2011;96:931-933.
13. Bellver J, Melo MA, Bosch E, et al. Obesity and poor reproductive outcome: the potential role of the endometrium. *Fertil Steril*. 2007;88:446-451.
14. Palomba S, Falbo A, Chiossi G, et al. Low-grade chronic inflammation in pregnant women with polycystic ovary syndrome: a prospective controlled clinical study. *J Clin Endocrinol Metab*. 2014;99:2942-2951.
15. Torloni MR, Betrán AP, Horta BL, et al. Prepregnancy BMI and the risk of gestational diabetes: a systematic review of the literature with meta-analysis. *Obes Rev*. 2009;10:194-203.
16. Committee on Practice Bulletins – Obstetrics. ACOG Practice Bulletin No. 190: gestational diabetes mellitus. *Obstet Gynecol*. 2018;131:e49-e64.
17. O'Brien TE, Ray JG, Chan WS. Maternal body mass index and the risk of preeclampsia: a systematic overview. *Epidemiology*. 2003;14:368-374.
18. Maggard MA, Yermilov I, Li Z, et al. Pregnancy and fertility following bariatric surgery: a systematic review. *J Am Med Assoc*. 2008;300:2286-2296.
19. Milić S, Lulić D, Štimac D. Non-alcoholic fatty liver disease and obesity: biochemical, metabolic and clinical presentations. *World J Gastroenterol*. 2014;20(28):9330-9337.
20. Louis JM, Mogos MF, Salemi JL, Redline S, Salihu HM. Obstructive sleep apnea and severe maternal-infant morbidity/mortality in the United States, 1998-2009. *Sleep*. 2014;37(5):843-849. Published 2014 May 1.
21. Louis J, Pien GW, Collop N, et al. Obstructive Sleep Apnea in Pregnancy. UpToDate. Last updated December 04, 2018. Accessed January 13, 2020. https://www.uptodate.com/contents/obstructive-sleep-apnea-in-pregnancy
22. Cai GJ, Sun XX, Zhang L, Hong Q. Association between maternal body mass index and congenital heart defects in offspring: a systematic review. *Am J Obstet Gynecol*. 2014;211:91-117.
23. Persson M, Cnattingius S, Villamor E, et al. Risk of major congenital malformations in relation to maternal overweight and obesity severity: cohort study of 1.2 million singletons. *Br Med J*. 2017;357:j2563.
24. Stothard KJ, Tennant PW, Bell R, Rankin J. Maternal overweight and obesity and the risk of congenital anomalies: a systematic review and meta-analysis. *J Am Med Assoc*. 2009;301:636-650.

25. Åmark H, Westgren M, Persson M. Prediction of stillbirth in women with overweight or obesity-A register-based cohort study. *PLoS One*. 2018;13(11):e0206940. Published 2018 Nov 19. doi:10.1371/journal.pone.0206940
26. Harrison MS, Thorsten VR, Dudley DJ, et al. Stillbirth, inflammatory markers, and obesity: results from the stillbirth collaborativer research network. *Am J Perinatol*. 2018;35(11):1071-1078.
27. Man J, Hutchinson JC, Ashworth M, et al. Stillbirth and intrauterine fetal death: contemporary demographic features of >1000 cases from an urban population. *Ultrasound Obstet Gynecol*. 2016;48:591-595.
28. Aune D, Saugstad OD, Henriksen T, Tonstad S. Maternal body mass index and the risk of fetal death, stillbirth, and infant death: a systematic review and meta-analysis. *J Am Med Assoc*. 2014;311:1536-1546.
29. ACOG Practice Bulletin No 156: obesity in pregnancy. *Obstet Gynecol*. 2015;126:e112-e126. Reaffirmed 2018.
30. The HAPO Study Cooperative Research Group. Hyperglycemia and adverse pregnancy outcomes. *N Engl J Med*. 2008;358:1991-2002.
31. HAPO Study Cooperative Research Group. Hyperglycaemia and Adverse Pregnancy Outcome (HAPO) Study: associations with maternal body mass index. *Br J Obstet Gynaecol*. 2010;117:575-584.
32. Owens LA, O'Sullivan EP, Kirwan B, et al. ATLANTIC DIP: the impact of obesity on pregnancy outcome in glucose-tolerant women. *Diabetes Care*. 2010;33:577-579.
33. Lowe WL Jr, Bain JR, Nodzenski M, et al; HAPO Study Cooperative Research Group. Maternal BMI and glycemia impact the fetal metabolome. *Diabetes Care*. 2017;40:902-910.
34. Zhang C, Hediger ML, Albert PS, et al. Association of maternal obesity with longitudinal ultrasonographic measures of fetal growth: findings from the NICHD fetal growth studies-singletons. *JAMA Pediatr*. 2018;172:24-31.
35. Halloran DR, Cheng YW, Wall TC, et al. Effect of maternal weight on postterm delivery. *J Perinatol*. 2012;32(2):85-90.
36. Bak GS, Sperling L, Källén K, et al. Prospective population-based cohort study of maternal obesity as a source of error in gestational age estimation at 11-14 weeks. *Acta Obstet Gynecol Scand*. 2016;95:1281-1287.
37. Simic M, Wåhlin IA, Marsál K, et al. Maternal obesity is a potential source of error in mid-trimester ultrasound estimation of gestational age. *Ultrasound Obstet Gynecol*. 2010;35:48-53.
38. Kullinger M, Wesström J, Kieler H, et al. Maternal and fetal characteristics affect discrepancies between pregnancy-dating methods: a population-based cross-sectional register study. *Acta Obstet Gynecol Scand*. 2017;96:86-95.
39. Frolova AI, Wang JJ, Conner SN, et al. Spontaneous labor onset and outcomes in obese women at term. *Am J Perinatol*. 2018;35(1):59-64.
40. Norman SM, Tuuli MG, Odibo AO, Caughey AB, Roehl KA, Cahill AG. The effects of obesity on the first stage of labor. *Obstet Gynecol*. 2012;120(1):130-135.
41. Wolfe KB, Rossi RA, Warshak CR. The effect of maternal obesity on the rate of failed induction of labor. *Am J Obstet Gynecol*. 2011;205:128.e1-128.e7.
42. Poobalan AS, Aucott LS, Gurung T, et al. Obesity as an independent risk factor for elective and emergency caesarean delivery in nulliparous women – systematic review and meta-analysis of cohort studies. *Obes Rev*. 2009;10:28-35.
43. Gunatilake RP, Smrtka MP, Harris B, et al. Predictors of failed trial of labor among women with an extremely obese body mass index. *Am J Obstet Gynecol*. 2013;209:562.e1-562.e5.
44. Grotegut CA, Gunatilake RP, Feng L, Heine RP, Murtha AP. The influence of maternal body mass index on myometrial oxytocin receptor expression in pregnancy. *Reprod Sci*. 2013;20(12):1471-1477.
45. Wuntakal R, Kaler M, Hollingworth T. Women with high BMI: should they be managed differently due to antagonising action of leptin in labour? *Med Hypotheses*. 2013;80(6):767-768.
46. Jie Z, Kendrick A, Quenby S, Wray S. Contractility and calcium signaling of human myometrium are profoundly affected by cholesterol manipulation: implications for labor. *Reprod Sci*. 2007;14(5):456-466.
47. Bell J, Bell S, Vahratian A, Awonuga AO. Abdominal surgical incisions and perioperative morbidity among morbidly obese women undergoing cesarean delivery. *Eur J Obstet Gynecol Reprod Biol*. 2011;154(1):16-19. Epub 2010 Sep 15.

48. McLean M, Hines R, Polinkovsky M, et al. Type of skin incision and wound complications in the obese parturient. *Am J Perinatol*. 2012;29(4):301-306. Epub 2011 Nov 21.

49. Tixier H, Thouvenot S, Coulange L, et al. Cesarean section in morbidly obese women: supra or subumbilical transverse incision? *Acta Obstet Gynecol Scand*. 2009;88:1049-1052.

50. Waring GJ, Shawer S, Hinshaw K. The use of O-ring retractors at caesarean section: a systematic review and meta analysis. *Eur J Obstet Gynecol Reprod Biol*. 2018;228:209-214.

51. Pomp ER, Lenselink AM, Rosendaal FR, Doggen CJ. Pregnancy, the postpartum period and prothrombotic defects: risk of venous thrombosis in the MEGA study. *J Thromb Haemost*. 2008;6:632-637.

52. Morgan ES, Wilson E, Watkins T, Gao F, Hunt BJ. Maternal obesity and venous thromboembolism. *Int J Obstet Anesth*. 2012;21(3):253-263.

53. Sheiner E, Edri A, Balaban E, et al. Pregnancy outcome of patients who conceive during or after the first year following bariatric surgery. *Am J Obstet Gynecol*. 2011;240:50.e1-50.e6.

CHAPTER 33

Gastrointestinal Diseases Complicating Pregnancy

Cornelia R. Graves, Washington C. Hill, Michelle Y. Owens, and Maria Jacqueline Small

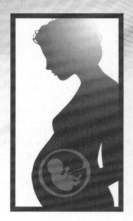

Introduction

Gastrointestinal Alterations During Normal Pregnancy

There are both mechanical and physiologic alterations in the gastrointestinal (GI) tract with the progression of pregnancy, which can pose significant challenges to the practitioner attempting a differential diagnosis of normal versus pathologic findings.[1] From a mechanical standpoint, the expanding uterus displaces the GI organs, particularly the intestines and the stomach.

These mechanical changes contribute to common aches, discomforts, and pains of pregnancy such as heartburn and gastric reflux due to displacement of the stomach and abdominal pain due to stretching of the peritoneum. However, it is vital for the practitioner to recognize that these symptoms can also indicate problems. For example, an abdominal mass can easily be missed depending on the gestational age of the fetus and the size of the uterus. In addition, the mechanical alterations of pregnancy can complicate medical interventions—ie, as the uterus expands, it causes the appendix to migrate upward, which would affect the site of a surgical incision should appendicitis be diagnosed in a pregnant patient.

From a physiologic standpoint, a major contributor to the GI changes seen in pregnancy is progesterone. An increase in progesterone levels throughout gestation leads to physiologic changes that result in a delay in gastric and gallbladder emptying; prolonged

See the eBook for expanded content, a complete reference list, and additional tables.

small bowel transit time; a decrease in gastric acid secretion; lower tone of the esophageal sphincter and in the urinary tract muscles; an increase in cholesterol synthesis and serum alkaline phosphatase concentration; changes in drug metabolism and clearance; and an increased risk for cholelithiasis, hydroureter, and hydronephrosis. All of these can result in symptoms for the pregnant woman, including reflux, dehydration, and constipation, among other sequelae.[1-3]

A newly recognized contributor to the physiologic changes of the GI system seen during pregnancy is the maternal gut microbiome.[4-6] The microbiome encompasses the microorganisms living in and on the body, which react with the host and are essential for normal immune and metabolic health. Although we are still in the early stages of discovering the importance of the maternal gut microbiome during all aspects of pregnancy and prenatal disease, several studies indicate that host-microbial interactions that impact host metabolism may be beneficial in pregnancy.

Differential Diagnosis of Abdominal Pain During Pregnancy

An understanding of the innervation of the GI tract is key to understanding the pathologies triggering pain responses[9] (**Table 33.1**). Cappell et al provide an excellent summary of the neurophysiologic pathways provoking GI pain.[10]

Nonobstetric Causes of Abdominal Pain

Clinical Presentation and Etiology

The causes of nonobstetric abdominal pain in the pregnant patient are identical to those found in the nonpregnant patient; however, clinicians must

Table 33.1 Differential Diagnosis of Nonobstetric Abdominal Pain in Pregnancy by Primary Location of Pain[9,10]

Right Upper Quadrant	Left Upper Quadrant	Epigastric	Diffuse Abdominal Pain	Lower Abdomen	Other GI Conditions	Other Conditions
Biliary colic	Splenomegaly	Pancreatitis	Bowel obstruction	Appendicitis	Porphyria	Sickle cell anemia/ vasoocclusive crises
Acute cholecystitis	Splenic infarct/rupture	Peptic ulcer disease	Perforation	Diverticulitis	Angioedema	
Acute cholangitis	Splenic abscess		Acute mesenteric ischemia	Nephrolithiasis	Celiac artery compression	Bariatric surgery
Sphincter of Oddi dysfunction	Perforated peptic ulcer	Reflux	Inflammatory bowel disease	Pyelonephritis	Chronic abdominal wall pain	
Acute hepatitis	Peptic ulcer disease	Gastritis	Viral gastroenteritis	Acute urinary retention	Abdominal migraine	
Liver abscess	Gastric volvulus	Gastroparesis	Foodborne	Ovarian cyst rupture	Aneurysm	
Budd-Chiari	Incarcerated parae- sophageal hernia		Spontaneous bacterial peritonitis	Uterine leiomyoma	Colonic pseudoobstruction/ Ogilvie syndrome	
(hepatic vein thrombosis)	Esophageal rupture		Colorectal cancer	Ovarian/adnexal mass	Eosinophilic gastroenteritis	
Portal vein throm- bosis (different from Budd-Chiari)	Esophageal stricture		Celiac disease	Endometriosis	Familial Mediterranean fever	
	Mallory-Weiss tear		Ketoacidosis		Helminthic	
	Nephrolithiasis		Adrenal insufficiency		Herpes zoster	
			Irritable bowel syndrome		Hypercalcemia	
			Constipation		Meckel diverticulum	
			Diverticulitis		Hypothyroidism	
			Lactose intolerance		Lead poisoning	
					Paroxysmal nocturnal hemoglobinuria	
					Narcotic bowel syndrome	
					Pseudoappendicitis	
					Ovarian torsion	
					Ruptured ovarian cyst	
					Endometriosis	
					Fibroid	

GI, gastrointestinal.

(Data from Kilpatrick CC, Monga M. Approach to the acute abdomen in pregnancy. *Obstet Gynecol Clin North Am.* 2007;34(3):389-402, x and Cappell MS. Gastrointestinal disorders during pregnancy. Preface. *Gastroenterol Clin North Am.* 2003;32(1):xi-xiii.)

consider physiologic changes in pregnancy that increase some pathologies during pregnancy as well as the changes in laboratory and physical exam findings.[9]

Clinical Assessment

Although diagnostic testing and management should consider the developing fetus, delay should not occur due to concerns for exposure to radiation. Most options available to the nonpregnant patient are also appropriate for the pregnant patient and delays may increase maternal morbidity and mortality. Abdominal plain films are 0.1 to 10 mGy, chest radiographs (two views) are 0.0005 to 0.01 mGy, and computed tomography (CT) scans of the abdomen are 1.3 to 35 mGy.[8] Adverse fetal outcomes have not been seen at doses below 50 mGy.[12]

One of the initial steps in the evaluation of nonobstetric abdominal pain is the distinction between the acute and chronic life-threatening conditions. In the acute setting, particularly after a trauma, point-of-care ultrasound may prove useful to facilitate evaluation for abdominal free fluid suggestive of hemoperitoneum or hematoma.

Acute, Life-Threatening Conditions

Bowel Obstruction

Bowel obstruction resulting from volvulus and adhesive disease are the most common causes of obstruction in pregnancy. Hernias and intussusception may also occur. Pregnant patients with prior history of gastric bypass surgery are particularly at risk and should be seen promptly by a surgical service when they present with abdominal pain. These patients are at high risk for hernias, volvulus, gastric rupture, and obstruction.[13] These patients may present with cramp-like pain, nausea/vomiting (N/V), and obstipation. The classic finding of peritoneal signs may be obscured due to the enlarged uterus and the relaxation of the maternal abdominal wall. Evaluation, management, and treatment are the same as in the nonpregnant state.

Perforated Peptic Ulcers

Perforated peptic ulcers are less common in pregnancy but may be found more commonly in patients following gastric surgery or those with prolonged risk factors like steroid exposure.[9,10] Clinical presentations include N/V and epigastric pain, which is often worse in the evening and postprandial. Acute, diffuse abdominal pain and associated low-grade temperature, tachycardia, and peritoneal signs should raise a high suspicion for perforated peptic ulcer. Plain upright abdominal radiograph is a fast modality for diagnosis; however, 10% to 20% of perforated duodenal ulcers will not demonstrate free air under the diaphragm.[9,10]

Ruptured Aneurysm

Visceral artery aneurysm rupture is rare in pregnancy. If they occur, the most commonly involved vessel is the splenic artery. The classic appearance presentation occurs in the setting of third trimester circulatory collapse.[14,15] Approximately 25% of patients may initially present with diffuse, abdominal pain that may radiate to the tip of the left shoulder (Kehr sign). Imaging may demonstrate the calcification in the area of aneurysmal dilation.[15]

Nausea, Vomiting, and Hyperemesis Gravidarum

Clinical Presentation

Nausea with or without vomiting is an especially common symptom during early pregnancy and the most common GI complaint, occurring in approximately 50% to 80% of pregnancies. It usually begins before 9 weeks' gestation. By mid-second trimester, most women no longer complain of these symptoms but approximately 1 to 2 per 1000 pregnant patients may experience some symptoms throughout their entire pregnancy.[16]

In its mildest form, nausea is referred to as morning sickness as most patients experience it in the morning. Symptoms are unpleasant and distressing, both physically and psychologically, but usually do not require any particular therapy. It is unknown why some patients experience no morning sickness and others are bothered by it all the time.

Clinical Assessment

The differential diagnosis of more serious nausea and vomiting of pregnancy indicative of hyperemesis gravidarum (HG) or other severe condition should include evaluations of the genitourinary and GI tracts, metabolic conditions, neurological disorders, and pregnancy-related conditions such as preeclampsia. The clinician should remember that headache, fever, abdominal pain, and tenderness are not typically seen with morning sickness.

Although most patients with serious nausea and vomiting and a few patients with HG have transient hyperthyroidism and a low thyroid-stimulating hormone or elevated free thyroxine thyroid, evaluation of thyroid function should not be part of the workup of these patients unless they have a history of thyroid disease.[26] Antithyroid medications are not necessary to treat the biochemical or transient hyperthyroidism occurring in hyperemetic pregnancies. Values return to normal when the nausea and vomiting or hyperemesis resolves or after delivery.[27]

Etiology

The exact etiology of nausea and vomiting during pregnancy and HG is unknown. The smooth muscles of the stomach relax during pregnancy due to hormonal changes, and this physiologic adaptation may play some role. Various other theories have been proposed, including a hormonal stimulus, evolutionary adaptation, and psychologic stressors and predisposition. The role of any or all of these have been studied but a clear correlation between them individually or together in the occurrence and severity of nausea and vomiting during pregnancy has not been demonstrated.[30-32]

Increased placental mass, a history of motion sickness, migraine headaches, family history, HG in a previous pregnancy, advanced molar gestation, and multifetal gestation are some of the risk factors for both nausea and vomiting during pregnancy and HG.[17,33] Another theory centers on the role of *Helicobacter pylori* in causing or predisposing a patient to the spectrum of disease from nausea and vomiting to HG; however, more research is needed to show a causal relationship between *H. pylori* and hyperemesis.[30,34]

A history of nausea or vomiting or HG in a prior pregnancy also appears to influence these conditions in subsequent pregnancies. A prospective study by Gadsby[35] found that approximately two-thirds of women who described their vomiting as severe in one pregnancy had similar symptoms in their next pregnancy, and one-half of women who described their symptoms as mild in one pregnancy found that the symptoms worsened in their next.

Management of Nausea, Vomiting, and HG in Pregnancy

The American College of Obstetricians and Gynecologists (ACOG) has recommended an evidence-based algorithm of therapeutic treatment of nausea and vomiting of pregnancy emphasizing if no improvement to move on to the next treatment option.[17]

The initial management of nausea and vomiting, whether nonpharmacologic or pharmacologic, is primarily supportive. Treatment early may prevent progression to the more serious HG, especially if the patient had it in a previous pregnancy.[39]

There are a number of accepted treatment protocols for nausea and vomiting during pregnancy and HG. The ACOG[17] in its treatment algorithm of nausea and vomiting of pregnancy also recommends thiamine, intravenously, 100 mg with the initial rehydration fluid and 100 mg daily for the next 2 to 3 days (followed by intravenous multivitamins) for women who require further intravenous hydration and have vomited for more than 3 weeks to prevent Wernicke encephalopathy.[22]

If the patient is not appropriately managed, there may be a failure of the mother and fetus to gain weight. Outpatient, hospital, or home therapy consisting of intravenous fluid hydration with 100 mL/L pyridoxine can be sufficient, along with supportive care. The management of hyperemesis in the home, although rare, can be both safe and efficacious. Furthermore, successful therapy can be achieved at a significantly reduced cost.[40]

However, when the patient's condition does not improve, hospitalization with appropriate electrolyte, caloric, and fluid management is necessary, if not mandatory. Experts emphasize nutritional support therapy is an important part of the management of nausea and vomiting.[17,41] Rehydration with intravenous fluids should be used for the patient who cannot tolerate oral fluids or when dehydration occurs. Correction of ketosis and vitamin deficiency should be strongly considered. Dextrose and vitamins should be included in the therapy when prolonged vomiting is present, and thiamine should be administered before dextrose infusion to prevent Wernicke encephalopathy.

Nasogastric or nasoduodenal enteral tube feeding should be initiated as a first-line treatment to provide nutritional support to the woman with HG who is not responsive to medical therapy and cannot maintain her weight. Total parenteral nutrition (TPN) is used when enteral tube feeding is ineffective or not tolerated. Peripherally inserted central catheters (PICCs) or lines once used frequently for TPN should not be used routinely due to the significant complications of infection and thrombosis.

PICCs should be utilized only as a last resort for nutrition because of the potential of severe maternal morbidity. Other adverse effects of persistent nausea and vomiting on pregnant women include significant psychosocial morbidity, significant financial burden, and worry about doing harm to the baby.

Nonpharmacologic Treatment

There are numerous nonpharmacologic regimens available to treat nausea and vomiting of pregnancy. These include reassurance, physical and psychological support, frequent small meals, 250 mg of ginger four times daily, kava tea, eating bland or dry foods, avoidance of foods that are unpleasant or that may trigger symptoms, adequate hydration and fluid intake, acupressure and acustimulation, and cannabis and cannabidiol use. Many of these "treatment modalities" have been studied with conflicting results and some not at all.

Pharmacologic Treatment

The standard ACOG recommendation to take prenatal vitamins containing B6 for 1 month before pregnancy, primarily in an effort to decrease neural tube defects, may also reduce the incidence and severity of nausea and vomiting of pregnancy.[17,45] When morning sickness symptoms require pharmacologic treatment, the ACOG states pyridoxine and doxylamine should be considered first-line therapy.[17]

Diclectin is a delayed-release tablet of pyridoxine and doxylamine and has been shown to be safe and effective in treating nausea and vomiting in pregnancy, although its use is associated with drowsiness, tiredness, or feeling sleepy. Other antiemetics include trimethobenzamide, metoclopramide, diphenhydramine, and the phenothiazines. However, caution should be exercised when the phenothiazines are used together with a dopamine antagonist because of an increased risk of extrapyramidal effects.

Metoclopramide, a dopamine receptor antagonist, is commonly used in the management of the spectrum of nausea and vomiting and HG during pregnancy. The use of metoclopramide during pregnancy increasing the risk of congenital malformations has been of concern. Exposure to metoclopramide in the first trimester was not associated with significantly increased risks of any of several adverse outcomes. However, metoclopramide use

is limited because of maternal side effects, including dystonia, restlessness, and somnolence, and also carries a U.S. Food and Drug Administration (FDA) black box warning due to the risks of tardive dyskinesia (repetitive and involuntary movements of the body) resulting from long-term use greater than 12 weeks.

Antihistamines have antiemetic effects through their effect on the vomiting center. Diphenhydramine, dimenhydrinate, and meclizine have been frequently used for years in the treatment of pregnant patients with nausea and vomiting.

Ondansetron is a serotonin 5-hydroxytryptamine type 3 receptor antagonist frequently used in the nonpregnant patient in the treatment of nausea and vomiting from chemotherapy and after surgery. Data on its use in pregnancy for the same indications are limited. However, a number of studies have found ondansetron when compared with metoclopramide having less side effects, and better improvement at controlling nausea and vomiting than metoclopramide or vitamin B6 combined with doxylamine.[50-52]

Adverse maternal drug-related side effects (fatigue, constipation, headache, drowsiness) are common with ondansetron, especially when used intravenously in bolus doses. There is a risk of maternal cardiac arrhythmias when this drug is used in patients who have underlying cardiac disease. The FDA recommends that ondansetron not be given intravenously in multiple doses or doses greater than 16 mg to pregnant women.

There are several conflicting studies examining the fetal safety of using ondansetron for nausea and vomiting during pregnancy. Therefore, use of ondansetron in pregnancy, especially less than 10 weeks, should be reserved for those women whose symptoms have not been adequately controlled by other methods.[55]

Droperidol (Inapsine) is a dopamine antagonist used as an antiemetic for postoperative nausea and vomiting and during chemotherapy. There is limited current information on its use during pregnancy. It can also cause QT prolongation and cardiac dysrhythmias, and use during pregnancy as an antiemetic for nausea and vomiting is not recommended. The heartburn and acid reflux experienced by patients with nausea and vomiting can be treated with acid-reducing medications and antacids containing calcium and aluminum.

Refractory HG has been successfully treated with corticosteroid therapy, but data are mixed and the exact mechanism of action remains unclear. Trials have shown statistically significant benefit,[58] no benefit,[59] and some benefit[60] of steroid use. Results are not consistent and regimens differ from study-to-study, making any meta-analysis and conclusions challenging.

Corticosteroid therapy should not be considered a first-line therapy except in cases when (1) all other causes of vomiting have been excluded; (2) vomiting has been prolonged and associated with dehydration; (3) the risks and benefits of the treatment have been clearly explained to the patient; and (4) intravenous fluid replacement and conventional antiemetics have failed. Studies have established the efficacy and safety of corticosteroid therapy for refractory hyperemesis. Methylprednisolone in tapering doses is the drug of choice.[58-60]

Although there are no established guidelines for the use of steroids, a frequently used regimen is 48 mg of methylprednisolone given orally or intravenously in three divided doses for 2 or 3 days. The ACOG and experts using this protocol recommend if there is no positive response seen within 72 hours that treatment be stopped as improvement is unlikely.[17,58,61]

Diffuse Abdominal Pain

Colonic Pseudoobstruction (Ogilvie Syndrome)

Ogilvie syndrome is a life-threatening condition that may cause colonic distention and symptoms suggestive of obstruction in the absence of an actual mechanical obstruction. The diagnosis is one of exclusion of mechanical obstruction or toxic megacolon. The severe colonic dilation can result in perforation. Treatment consists of neostigmine (contraindicated in pregnancy), colonoscopy, or surgery. Conservative measures are as effective as other treatments.[65-67]

Hemoperitoneum

Spontaneous hemoperitoneum is a rare life-threatening condition that may occur during pregnancy; the condition has been associated with endometriosis.[68]

Hereditary Angioedema

Patients with hereditary angioedema resulting from C1-inhibitor deficiency may experience severe episodes of debilitating subcutaneous and submucosal edema that may mimic an acute abdomen. Bowel wall edema may result in GI colic, NV, and diarrhea in the absence of hives. Approximately one-third of parturients will experience worsening symptom. C1-inhibitor replacement therapy is effective for acute exacerbations.[69] Androgen therapies (not recommended in pregnancy) and ultrasound may aid in the diagnosis and demonstrate bowel wall edema or ascites.[69,70]

Substance Abuse

Opioid withdrawal may result in cramp-like abdominal pain, vomiting, and diarrhea.[71]

Chronic marijuana use may result in syndrome of cannabinoid hyperemesis, characterized by cyclic vomiting and abdominal pain. Patients may report relief of symptoms with hot showers or baths.[36]

Vasoocclusive Crises

Vasoocclusive crises in sickle cell anemia may occur in response to obstruction of arterioles and splenic or mesenteric infarction. Cholelithiasis and cholecystitis are also more common in the parturient with sickle cell disease.[72]

Right Upper Quadrant Pain

Gallbladder Disease

Gallbladder disease is the second most common cause for surgery in pregnancy, following appendectomy.[8] Pregnancy increases the formation of gallstones, and pain is typically in the right upper quadrant, colicky, and associated with fat ingestion. Acute cholecystitis may result in fever, tachycardia, and leukocytosis. The presence of transaminitis and direct bilirubin suggest obstruction of the common bile duct or cholangitis. Ultrasound is the best initial diagnostic imaging tool.[12]

Hepatitis

Viral hepatitis symptoms are generally mild; however, hepatitis E may proceed to fulminant hepatic failure in pregnancy and is a global contributor to maternal mortality.[9,10,73] Other viruses such as cytomegalovirus, Epstein-Barr virus, and adenovirus may also cause maternal anorexia, nausea, jaundice, and right upper quadrant pain and should be considered in the diagnostic evaluation.

Left Upper Quadrant Pain

Spleen

Wandering spleen results from absent splenic peritoneal supports, allowing the spleen to migrate from its anatomic location. Although more common in the pediatric population, adults can be affected, and the hormonal effects of pregnancy may contribute to support ligament laxity. The syndrome classically presents with acute left upper quadrant pain and a palpable left abdominal mass. Diagnostic delay may lead to infarction, necrosis, or splenic torsion. Ultrasound may aid in the diagnosis and splenopexy is the usual treatment.[14]

Upper Abdominal Pain

Acute Pancreatitis
Pancreatitis classically manifests as upper abdominal pain that may radiate to the back in association with amylase lipase elevation. Ultrasound can aid in the diagnosis of choledocholithiasis or pseudocyst.[9,10]

Hiatal Hernias
Hiatal hernias may become clinically symptomatic during pregnancy due to the expanding uterus. Obesity may also increase the risk for a hiatal hernia. Clinical features include epigastric pain, postprandial fullness, and nausea. Symptoms of chest pain, diaphoresis, and radiation to the shoulder may appear cardiac in origin. Incarceration and ischemia may result in severe pain. Chest radiograph may demonstrate the herniation of the stomach through the hiatus of the diaphragm can establish the diagnosis. Paraesophageal hernias are at highest risk for strangulation and need repair.[9,10]

Pneumonia
Lower lobe pneumonias may cause diaphragmatic irritation and mimic conditions such as acute cholecystitis or acute abdomen. Pneumonia, however, typically presents with concomitant respiratory symptoms. A chest radiograph will appropriately aid in diagnosis.

Epigastric Pain
Peptic ulcer disease (PUD) is classically associated with epigastric pain, indigestion, and reflux. In approximately 3% of patients with type 1 diabetes, diabetic ketoacidosis may manifest as abdominal pain.[9,10]

Lower Abdominal Pain
Diverticulitis and Meckel diverticulum are rare in pregnancy as they typically affect individuals above age 45 years. Meckel diverticulum is the most common congenital malformation of the GI tract, affecting 2% of the population. Diagnostic modalities may include ultrasound, CT, or magnetic resonance imaging (MRI). Symptoms may include abdominal pain, N/V, or obstruction.[74]

Oral Cavity Complications of Pregnancy

Clinical Presentation
There are a number of normal common oral health changes and complications encountered during pregnancy. These include dental caries, pregnancy gingivitis, benign oral gingival lesions (eg, granuloma gravidarum), sialorrhea gravidarum (ptyalism), pseudosialorrhea, tooth mobility, tooth erosion, and periodontitis.[75]

Dental Caries
There is no agreement that normal pregnancy causes a decreased or increased incidence of caries. Rather, the worsening of dental caries during pregnancy is due most often to poor dental hygiene.

Pregnancy Gingivitis
Pregnancy does not cause gingivitis. The increase in gingival vascularity can result in accentuated and exaggerated gingival hyperplasia or enlargement, which is commonly referred to as pregnancy gingivitis. Once the hormonal changes of pregnancy decline, the exaggerated gingivitis due to pregnancy decreases.

Pregnancy does not increase the amount of oral calculus present on the teeth.

Granuloma Gravidarum
Pregnancy tumor, or granuloma gravidarum, forms as a result of exaggerated gingival enlargement during pregnancy.[78] They occur in approximately 1% to 5% of pregnant women. The tumors appear as localized enlargements of the hyperplastic gingiva or pedunculated growth and are typically painless, pedunculated, lobulated, red (owing to their vascularity), and soft with a smooth surface. Pregnancy tumors are pyogenic granulomas because they result from nonspecific inflammatory gingivitis secondary to poor oral hygiene, associated with deposits of plaque and calculus on the teeth. The poor teeth and gums adjacent to these lesions are responsible for the local irritation resulting in the pregnancy tumor. The preexisting inflammation, along with the hormonal effects of pregnancy on

the gingival tissues, predispose women to the development of pregnancy tumors. Consultation with a dentist is indicated.

Sialorrhea Gravidarum

Sialorrhea gravidarum, or ptyalism, is a distressful oral complication of pregnancy where the patient has excessive secretion of saliva or salivation. It can occur at any time in pregnancy but usually starts in the first trimester. Some patients unfortunately experience it their entire pregnancy. Sialorrhea is of unknown etiology but some believe it is related to the typical nausea and vomiting of pregnancy. Other causes may be smoking and other irritants, gastroesophageal reflux, cultural, psychological conditions, desire for attention, or a neurological disorder.

Pseudosialorrhea occurs when the rate of secreted saliva is normal but the patient does not swallow it due to a feeling of choking or dysphasia, customs in their culture, psychological conditions, and, rarely, neurological disease.

Patients with sialorrhea gravidarum or pseudosialorrhea complain of bad taste in their mouths and often report that swallowing the "excessive" or thickened saliva makes nausea worse, but that spitting it out is better and, therefore, may come into the office or clinic with spitting cups or jars, hand towels, and paper tissues.

Management of Oral Cavity Complications in Pregnancy

In a 2013 collaborative ACOG Committee Opinion, which was reaffirmed in 2017, maternal and child experts, dentists, and obstetrician-gynecologists emphasized the importance of oral health during pregnancy and throughout a woman's life.[82] Patients should be urged to practice good oral hygiene, and those who enter pregnancy with poor dental care should be referred and encouraged to see a dentist because prevention, diagnosis, and treatment of oral conditions are not contraindicated in pregnancy.

Prenatal care should, but frequently does not, include a good examination of the teeth by a dentist who may then consult with the obstetrician about the best treatment plan. The ACOG recommends that, at the first new obstetric visit, healthcare providers should assess a woman's oral health as part of routine counseling and should encourage all women to schedule a dental examination if it has been more than 6 months since their last examination or if they have any oral health problems. The obstetrical provider should establish a referral pattern, when needed, to a dentist knowledgeable and willing to care for pregnant patients.[84]

Nonpharmacologic Treatment

The treatment of dental problems associated with pregnancy is rarely contraindicated and, when several guidelines are used, may be performed safely.[72] If treatment is necessary but elective, it is best delayed until the second trimester, when there is the least risk of teratogenesis. Emergency treatment should be obtained whenever indicated. The supine hypotensive syndrome, which occurs most frequently during the third trimester, can be avoided by keeping the patient turned toward her side while she is in the dental chair.

Radiographs, which are often necessary to establish a proper dental diagnosis, may be taken safely during any stage of pregnancy.

There is no harm to the fetus when dental radiographs are taken with the necessary precautions, good techniques, and today's modern equipment. A local or topical anesthetic is usually recommended and is safe for both mother and fetus to help manage pain during dental procedures. Lidocaine and mepivacaine combined with epinephrine have become the local anesthetics of choice for dental work during pregnancy. Low doses of intravenous medications may be used, but should be titrated to an acceptable level before administering the local anesthesia. General anesthesia should be reserved for those patients who are hospitalized and require extensive dental surgery, and should only be administered by an anesthetist or anesthesiologist who is familiar with the risks of the procedure.[86] It is best, whenever possible, to avoid the use of an inhalation anesthetic for dental procedures during pregnancy.

Most dental procedures require no antibiotics; however, when antibiotics are necessary, tetracycline should not be given to the pregnant woman. Antibiotics frequently used by the dentist for treatment or prophylaxis therapy are penicillin, amoxicillin, cephalexin, and erythromycin.

It remains controversial whether maternal periodontal disease and progression is associated with adverse pregnancy outcomes, such as preterm birth or preeclampsia, and whether treating the disease before or during pregnancy will prevent the adverse outcome. More research and studies are needed and are ongoing.[75,89,90]

Bleeding from the gingiva, a common complaint of pregnant women, due to pregnancy gingivitis, requires no specific treatment. Gingivitis due to poor dentition and hygiene is treated by good cleaning of the teeth and by meticulous dental care.

The treatment for pregnancy tumor is complete surgical excision. The adjacent teeth should be cleaned aggressively to remove debris, plaque, and calculus. If the tumor is not completely removed, it may recur, and recurrence during a future pregnancy is not uncommon.

Gastrointestinal Reflux

Clinical Presentation

Gastroesophageal reflux occurs when contents from the stomach move into the oral pharynx. The differential diagnosis of gastroesophageal reflux disease (GERD) includes reflux, hiatal hernia, peptic ulcer disease, and myocardial infarction or other cardiac etiology.

In pregnancy, as in the nongravid state, the diagnosis of GERD can be made on symptoms alone, and further imaging or other studies are rarely indicated. The exact mechanism of reflux esophagitis in pregnancy remains unknown. However, estrogen and progesterone-mediated decreased lower esophageal sphincter tone and delayed gastric emptying, coupled with increased gastric acidity from placenta-produced gastrin, are thought to contribute to disease etiology.[91] With pregnancy progression, displacement and compression of abdominal organs potentially influence risk for reflux.

Up to 85% of pregnant women report heartburn and dyspepsia at some stage during their pregnancy, making this one of the most common symptoms in pregnancy[91,92] Fortunately, most cases are mild and self-limited, and serious complications of reflux esophagitis, such as esophageal strictures, erosion, or bleeding, are rare. Heartburn is most common in the third trimester, but may occur at any point in pregnancy.

Management of GERD in Pregnancy

Most cases of mild heartburn can be controlled with conservative measures and behavioral interventions. These include ingestion of smaller more frequent meals, limiting late night meals, elevating the head of the bed, and lying on the left side.

Furthermore, dietary restrictions (ie, reducing consumption of caffeine and spicy foods, and high-fat foods) may also minimize symptoms.

Pharmacologic and Nonpharmacologic Treatment

When medication is needed, antacids containing aluminum, magnesium, and calcium are considered first-line therapy. Care should be taken to avoid bicarbonate-containing agents, which may cause fetal and maternal metabolic acidosis and fluid overload.[92]

When symptoms are not controlled with conservative measures and antacids, histamine type 2 receptor antagonists (H2RAs) should be considered as next-line therapy. For severe symptoms refractory to other forms of therapy, proton pump inhibitors (PPIs) should be considered. Metoclopramide and sucralfate are both useful. Although H2RAs have been more widely studied in pregnancy, PPIs are also considered safe to use.

Peptic Ulcer Disease

Clinical Presentation

PUD is a disorder of the GI tract resulting from mucosal damage due to gastrin and peptic acid exposure. PUD is most commonly found in the stomach and proximal duodenum, but may also affect the lower esophagus, distal duodenum, and jejunum. This chronic disorder is characterized by exacerbations and remission. Chronic use of nonsteroidal anti-inflammatory agents (NSAIDs) and infection with *H. pylori* are among the most common etiologies of peptic ulcer disease. The symptoms of PUD are primarily dyspepsia (especially pain relieved with food), but may also include nausea and vomiting, epigastric pain, and bloating.[95]

In pregnancy, PUD is usually a benign condition, likely due to behavioral modifications that decrease symptoms (ie, reducing use of NSAIDs, reducing or eliminating smoking and alcohol consumption, and reducing use of antacids). There is no evidence of increased maternal or fetal morbidity in the presence of preexisting PUD unless it is associated with complications.

Clinical Assessment

The diagnosis of peptic ulcer disease is made by visualization of the ulcers with radiography or esophagogastroduodenoscopy (EGD). The differential diagnosis of PUD includes GERD, hiatal hernia, preeclampsia/HELLP (hemolysis, elevated liver enzymes, low platelet count) syndrome, and myocardial infarction or other cardiac condition. PUD is uncommon in pregnancy and so are its complication.[96] The exact incidence of peptic ulcer disease in pregnancy is not known, and many symptoms may be attributed to normal complaints of pregnancy. Complications of peptic ulcer disease include bleeding, perforation, penetration, and gastric outlet obstruction. Although infrequent, when these complications occur, they can be severe and require urgent intervention. Thus, a high clinical suspicion is necessary for patients with an acute abdomen and symptoms that persist or worsen despite conventional therapy.

The use of endoscopy is not contraindicated in pregnancy. In fact, EGD with sedation is safe during pregnancy and should be utilized when indicated to ensure optimal perinatal care.

Pharmacologic Treatment

Treatment includes eradication of *H. pylori* infection, when present, and secretion control with an H2RA or PPI. H2RAs, such as cimetidine, famotidine, and ranitidine, are a mainstay in the medical treatment of PUD. These agents work by decreasing the production of histamine by the parietal cells within the gastric lining. These agents cross the placenta, but no teratogenic risk has been associated with their use.[97] PPIs, such as omeprazole, lansoprazole, pantoprazole, rabeprazole, and esomeprazole, act directly on the gastric parietal cells to suppress gastric acid secretion. The use of these agents during pregnancy has not been shown to be teratogenic when used in recommended doses.[98]

Acute Appendicitis

Clinical Presentation

Acute appendicitis is the most commonly encountered general surgical problem. The classic symptoms of acute appendicitis include abdominal pain beginning in the periumbilical region and migrating to the right lower quadrant. Nausea and vomiting may be present, as well as anorexia, followed by leukocytosis and fever.

Acute appendicitis in pregnancy represents a state of increased risk for both the mother and fetus. Pregnancy complications of acute appendicitis include preterm labor and miscarriage or fetal loss. Maternal risks are largely related to complications of acute appendicitis and include peritonitis, sepsis, and death.

Clinical Assessment

Clinical diagnosis of acute appendicitis may be challenging due to the anatomic and physiologic changes of pregnancy, which may further complicate the diagnosis. Diagnosis and treatment should be rapid in order to prevent serious maternal and obstetrical complications.

The differential diagnosis for abdominal pain in pregnancy is extensive and includes both obstetrical and nonobstetrical causes. Among these are acute appendicitis, pelvic inflammatory disease, ectopic pregnancy, ovarian torsion, ovarian cyst, labor, round ligament pain, uterine leiomyoma, placental abruption, preeclampsia/HELLP syndrome, chorioamnionitis, constipation, PUD, nephrolithiasis, cholecystitis, pyelonephritis, and pancreatitis.

Imaging plays an important role in confirming the diagnosis of acute appendicitis. Graded compression ultrasonography has emerged as the initial imaging modality of choice for evaluation of abdominal pain in pregnancy. Ultrasound offers the additional benefit of providing information about other organs and structures within the abdomen and pelvis. The clinical diagnosis of suspected appendicitis is supported by identification of a noncompressible blind-ended tubular structure in the right lower quadrant with a maximal diameter greater than 6 mm.[103]

It is important to note that the inability to visualize the appendix on ultrasound does not rule out acute appendicitis. When ultrasound findings are inconclusive or unavailable, noncontrast abdominal MRI is preferred, with a reported sensitivity of 96%, specificity of 98%, and accuracy of 99% for the assessment of acute appendicitis in pregnancy.[104] The use of noncontrast CT is also considered a safe diagnostic tool in the evaluation of appendicitis.

Delays in diagnosis and treatment further exaggerate these risks. A delay of 24 hours can lead to a 66% increase of perforation.[101] Fetal loss rates and maternal morbidity and mortality are also increased in the setting of appendiceal perforation and peritonitis. Prompt diagnosis and intervention are key in the prevention of maternal and fetal morbidity and mortality.

Nonpharmacologic Treatment

The treatment of choice for acute appendicitis in pregnancy is surgical excision. Appendectomy is favored over observation due to the substantial risks of perforation, preterm labor, sepsis, septic shock, and peritonitis. Surgical removal of the appendix may be accomplished via laparotomy or laparoscopically. Considerations for the laparoscopic approach include limiting intra-abdominal pressure, trocar placement to avoid the gravid uterus, and minimizing uterine manipulation. The most important prognostic factors regarding the surgical method of appendectomy in pregnancy appear to be the skill/comfort level of the surgeon and the pregnancy health/status of the mother.[106] General considerations for surgery in pregnancy include maternal positioning to avoid hypotension by compression of the inferior vena cava by the gravid uterus and limiting anesthesia/operative time when general anesthesia is required. Antibiotics should be administered in cases complicated by perforation or extensive inflammation. Obstetric interventions such as tocolytic therapy and cesarean delivery should be reserved for their usual obstetrical indications. In the rare event of concomitant labor and acute appendicitis in an otherwise stable patient, vaginal delivery may be accomplished with surgical intervention to immediately follow.

Acute Intestinal Obstruction

Clinical Presentation

Intestinal obstruction is an infrequent but serious complication of pregnancy. The classic triad of presenting symptoms in intestinal obstruction is abdominal pain, vomiting, and constipation. Furthermore, pregnancy may dampen the peritoneal signs commonly elicited in the nonpregnant state. The most common risk factor for intestinal obstruction is history of abdominal surgery.

Clinical Assessment

The diagnosis can be elusive as the signs and symptoms of pain, nausea, vomiting, abdominal distention, and constipation overlap with normal symptoms of pregnancy. Timely diagnosis and management are of paramount importance, as acute obstruction in pregnancy is associated with significant maternal and fetal mortality rates of 6% and 26%, respectively.[108,109] Diagnostic imaging via MRI or plain abdominal radiographs (supine and upright) are considered first-line, but CT may also be useful in assessment of the bowel. Oral contrast may be considered in lieu of IV contrast to minimize fetal exposure to ionizing radiation. Radiographic or serial studies showing dilated, gas-filled loops of bowel with air-fluid levels are diagnostic.

Nonpharmacologic Treatment

Initial management during the workup of acute intestinal obstruction may be conservative with nasogastric tube placement, bowel rest, and fluid and electrolyte repletion. If conservative measures are unsuccessful, or if the patient develops fever or peritoneal signs, surgical exploration via laparotomy is warranted.[107,110] A vertical midline incision should be used to assure adequate exposure, with care taken to minimize uterine manipulation. Once the obstruction is identified and relieved, the bowel should be assessed for viability, with removal of any infarcted areas and segments that do not resume a healthy, well-perfused appearance. Acute obstruction does not require delivery at the time of intervention. Delivery is usually reserved for the usual obstetrical indications. However, each case should be assessed individually, with consideration given to the gestational age, fetal and maternal status, and other comorbidities. The need for tocolytics should be determined based on clinical symptoms.

Inflammatory Bowel Disease

Clinical Presentation

The two most common inflammatory bowel diseases (IBDs) are ulcerative colitis and Crohn disease, also called regional enteritis. Both these disorders are not uncommon in women during their reproductive years and are frequently seen either before or during pregnancy.[111-113] They can be characterized as chronic disorders that go through periods of quiescence and exacerbation, making differentiation even more difficult.[111-114] The pathologic features of these two diseases distinguish and differentiate them[111-113] (**Table 33.2**).

Ulcerative colitis is an inflammatory ulcerative pathologic process involving the mucosal lining of the colon and/or rectum. It is characteristically not transmural. A typical biopsy of ulcerative colitis lesions shows diffuse mucosal ulceration and a chronic inflammatory response consisting of polymorphonuclear cells, lymphocytes, and plasma cells. There may be abscesses of the mucosa.

Table 33.2 Pathologic Features of Common Inflammatory Bowel Diseases

Ulcerative Colitis	Crohn Disease
Mucosal layer inflammation	Transmural inflammation
Continuous	Skip areas—mouth to anus, often small bowel involvement
Rectal involvement	50% involves rectum (rectal sparing) Perianal disease

The mucosal lining is edematous and replaced by a chronic inflammatory infiltrate. As this chronic process continues over time, the bowel may become thickened. Areas of stricture, fibrosis, and stenosis develop. Intestinal obstruction and toxic dilation of the colon with resultant perforation can complicate ulcerative colitis.[111,112]

Crohn disease, on the other hand, is an inflammatory disease that may involve any area of the GI tract, but the distal small intestine, colon, and anal rectal regions are most often affected.[111,113] The pathologic process is transmural, and the granulomatous enteritis involves all layers of the bowel, mesentery, and lymph nodes. The inflammatory process consists primarily of plasma cells and lymphocytes. The bowel that is affected is edematous, thickened, hyperemic, and ulcerated. There may be adhesions of the involved portion with other loops of intestine. Intestinal obstruction, perforation, and fistula formation between loops of bowel can result. The nearby mesentery lymphadenopathy is present. The chronic inflammatory process is more granulomatous than in ulcerative colitis. Granulomas, multinucleated giant cells, and chronic ulcerations may be present. Skipped areas are common and characteristically found in removed bowel affected by regional enteritis. These are unaffected areas of the bowel located next to diseased areas.[111,113]

The clinical manifestations of IBD depend on the area of the GI tract involved. Some symptoms occur with both diseases or are more common with one or the other. Symptoms occurring with both these diseases may include soft stools, rectal bleeding, diarrhea, abdominal pain, weight loss, and urgency of defecation. Abdominal pain, diarrhea, weight loss, fever, and rectal bleeding are the most frequent symptoms occurring in ulcerative colitis. The symptoms of Crohn disease are most frequently episodic abdominal pain, fever, diarrhea, and weight loss. Perineal fistulas and scarring are more commonly present with regional enteritis and occur in one-third to one-half of the patients with this disease.[111-113]

Clinical Assessment

The clinical features and presentations of these two disorders can be quite similar, requiring sigmoidoscopy, colonoscopy, radiography, and histologic examination of a biopsy to tell the difference. The endoscopic techniques are safe during pregnancy and have replaced radiography in making a diagnosis.

Management of IBD in Pregnancy

The impact of IBDs on fertility has been studied by several authors. If the disease is in remission and a woman has never had surgery, fertility rates are equivalent to those of the general population.[115,116] Surgery, including prostatectomies and ostomies, may result in infertility secondary to inflammation of the fallopian tubes.[116]

Ulcerative colitis and regional enteritis can affect pregnancy; however, a good prognosis can be expected and IBD does not adversely affect fetal outcomes. Pregnancy, if planned, should be encouraged when the patient is in remission, although the disease or its standard treatment does not seem to dangerously affect the patient, fetus, or the newborn infant. The more inactive the disease at the time of conception, the better the prognosis for a more favorable pregnancy outcome.[111,114] The risk of exacerbation of IBD in pregnant patients is approximately 30% to 35%, not dissimilar from that in the nonpregnant patients.[116]

The worst prognosis for the pregnant woman occurs when the patient develops active disease for the first time during pregnancy. Active disease is associated with adverse pregnancy outcomes such as preterm birth and fetal growth restriction.[111,114,115] Pregnancy should, therefore, be avoided if possible while the disease is active. Active disease at the onset of pregnancy tends to remain active, and quiescent disease tends to remain quiescent. One-third of pregnant patients experience worsening of their disease, and less than a half show remission or improvement.[116]

Cesarean delivery has been recommended if severe perineal fistulas or scarring, which can occur as a complication of Crohn disease, is present.[111,114,115] Cesarean delivery is not indicated in patients simply because they have had successful restorative surgery for IBD. However, the full clinical picture, including gestational and fetal age, should be assessed.[116]

An additional consideration in the management of patients with IBD is the risk for thromboembolic events in the setting of a flare as compared to the general population. Several medical societies now include IBD in its risk factor algorithm for thromboprophylaxis in pregnancy.[117-119]

Extraintestinal manifestations of the IBDs occur in both the pregnant and the nonpregnant patient. These include nutritional and metabolic abnormalities, hematologic abnormalities, skin and mucous membrane lesions, arthritis, and eye and renal complications. Hepatic and biliary complications can also occur with the development of sclerosing cholangitis and gallstones. Systemic complications and manifestations have been reported to occur all over the body. Local complications requiring surgical and gastroenterological intervention can occur, depending on the severity of the disease. These complications include stricture, stenosis, bleeding, malignancy, abscess formation, perforation, fistulas, and perineal problems.[111-114]

Pharmacologic and Nonpharmacologic Treatment

IBD is treated by both medical and surgical measures during pregnancy. The mainstay of medical therapy for both ulcerative colitis and Crohn disease is the use of mesalamine preparations, sulfasalazine, and corticosteroids. Mesalamine is more efficacious in the treatment of ulcerative colitis than in regional enteritis. The corticosteroids most frequently used are prednisone, hydrocortisone, and prednisolone.[111,116]

Corticosteroid therapy has been used to suppress the inflammatory response present in the bowel and in treating exacerbations of Crohn disease. Doses of prednisone range from 40 to 60 mg daily for a period of several weeks to a month. The initiation or continuation of corticosteroid therapy during pregnancy is not contraindicated. Breastfeeding is likewise not contraindicated in the mother on corticosteroid therapy.

Biologics like the anti–tumor necrosis factor (TNF) agents infliximab, adalimumab, and certolizumab have been increasingly used for the management of IBD.[120] Through inhibition of TNF-α, these medications increase circulating T regulatory cells and enhance their cytokine inhibition. All except certolizumab cross the placenta. These medications have been considered safe, low risk, biologics for use during pregnancy and breastfeeding. They are not associated with an increase in birth defects, growth restriction, or preterm birth. Combination therapy with biologics and thiopurines is theoretically considered a risk for neonatal infection; however, this effect has not been consistently demonstrated. Many clinicians recommend using the lowest dosage possible near the time of delivery to avoid risks to the neonate but to optimize maternal remission.[111,116]

Medical management should include nutritional assessment and treatment. Parenteral nutrition is infrequently needed in these patients. General therapeutic measures include antidiarrheal drugs such as codeine, opium, paregoric, and diphenoxylate with atropine (Lomotil).

Surgical treatment of ulcerative colitis includes total proctocolectomy with construction of an ileostomy or ileoanal pull through.[5] Indications for surgery include perforation (with or without abscess formation), massive bleeding, and carcinoma of the colon. Patients who develop toxic megacolon and do not respond to other therapy may also be candidates for this surgical therapy. The procedure should not be done during pregnancy. Patients with ulcerative colitis who have been treated with surgery before pregnancy have no increased risk during their pregnancy. The performance of a cesarean delivery for obstetric indications only is recommended, with draping of the ileostomy out of the surgical site.[116]

Surgical therapy for Crohn disease or regional enteritis is the same as for ulcerative colitis.[116] Intractability of symptoms is the most frequent indication for surgery. Perianal complications, such as fistulas, may also lead to total proctocolectomy with ileostomy or some other variation of this surgery. There is a high recurrence rate of the disease with an internal anastomosis. Crohn disease is not cured by total proctocolectomy.

Irritable Bowel Syndrome

Irritable bowel syndrome (IBS) is a functional bowel disorder characterized by abdominal cramping and cyclic episodes of constipation, diarrhea, and flatulence in the absence of organic pathology. IBS is the most commonly diagnosed GI condition in the United States. The condition is one to two times more common in women and presents typically prior to age 50. The underlying etiology for IBS is unclear.

Clinical Presentation

Host factors associated with the condition include altered perceptions of pain, altered gut microflora, immune activation, increase in gut mucosal edema, certain food sensitivities, and neurogenic triggers resulting in hypersensitivity. IBS has also been associated with depression, anxiety, and psychosocial trauma.[121,122]

Clinical Assessment

Organic pathology should be carefully excluded prior to establishing a diagnosis of IBS. IBS typically does not begin after age 50; diarrhea does not waken patients from sleep. Hematochezia, weight loss, and anemia are not characteristic of IBS. The Rome III diagnostic criteria for IBS include recurrent abdominal pain 1 to 3 days in the previous 3 months and association with two or more symptoms: relation to stool, change in frequency, or form of stool. Rome III criteria further define subtypes of IBS related to constipation/diarrhea, mixed, and untyped IBS.

Pharmacologic and Nonpharmacologic Treatment

Treatments vary including dietary changes tailored to individual patients (eg, elimination of dairy, fatty foods, highly fermentable carbohydrates ["FODMAPS"], increase in fiber) and medications such as antispasmodics (eg, hyoscyamine), antidepressants, antidiarrheals, or laxatives.[121]

Celiac Disease

Clinical Presentation and Etiology

The disease symptoms are provoked by ingestion of gluten (storage protein for wheat, barley, and rye), and avoidance of gluten eliminates the T cell–mediated inflammatory disease activity. The most common disease symptoms are chronic diarrhea, flatulence, and weight loss. People with celiac may also demonstrate lactose intolerance, refractory anemia, and aphthous ulcers. Celiac disease (CD) is also associated with conditions such as type 1 diabetes (5%-10%), lymphocytic colitis, IBS, diarrhea, and anemia.[124] Hormonal and endocrinologic changes in pregnancy may result in the first manifestation of celiac or reactivation of the disease. Up to 20% of siblings of affected individuals may be affected and 10% in other first-degree relatives. Unexplained infertility and recurrent miscarriage are also associated with a higher risk for CD.

Clinical Assessment

Testing for CD should be prompted by the finding of iron deficiency, macrocytic anemia (from impaired absorption of potentially B12 and folic acid), and a decrease in fat soluble vitamins, such vitamin D and K deficiency.[124]

The immunoglobulin (Ig)A anti-tissue transglutimanse antibody (TTG-IgA) test is recommended to diagnose CD in individuals older than 2 years. IgA deficiency is more common in patients with CD than in nonaffected individuals and should be tested if the pretest probability of CD is high, since the TTG-IgA is more likely to be falsely negative in that setting. The diagnosis of CD is confirmed by upper endoscopy and duodenal biopsies. Even if serology is negative, biopsies should be performed if the clinical suspicion for CD is high. All testing should be performed when patients are on a gluten-containing diet.

Management of CD in Pregnancy

In pregnancy, both controlled and uncontrolled symptoms can be associated with preterm birth, intrauterine growth restriction, stillbirth, low birthweight, and small for gestational age. Elimination of gluten from the diet can decrease these risks and pregnant women with CD should be encouraged to observe a strict gluten-free diet.

Constipation

Constipation in pregnancy is only second to nausea as the most common GI complaints in pregnant women.[126]

Clinical Assessment

The ROME IV criteria constitute a useful tool to assess the presence and severity of constipation as patient perception of constipation may be different from symptoms that require medical treatment. The criteria use two or more of the following: in those having less than or equal to three stools per week, hard stools or straining, sensation of incomplete rectal evacuation, or manual maneuvers to assist in defecation or sensation of rectal blockage must occur in at least 25% of bowel movements.[127]

Nonpharmacologic Treatment

The prevention and treatment of constipation during pregnancy should consist mainly of nutrition counseling, increasing fluid intake, daily exercise, and dietary modifications to increase fiber content.[129] If these measures are unsuccessful, then osmotic laxatives, bulk-producing substances, and stool softeners may be used. Castor oil may initiate preterm uterine contractions and preterm labor and is not recommended. Laxatives most commonly recommended are the bulk-forming preparations containing fiber. The use of excess laxatives by patients to induce labor should not be condoned. The stool softener dioctyl sulfosuccinate may be used. No teratogenic effects have been reported from the use of these common laxatives, stool softeners, or bulk-forming preparations.

Diarrhea

The most common risk associated with diarrhea in pregnancy is dehydration.[130]

Clinical Presentation and Assessment

When diarrhea is persistent, profuse, bloody, or associated with other symptoms such as fever or severe abdominal pain, further investigation is warranted. If diarrhea is accompanied by nausea and vomiting of sudden onset, one should suspect viral or bacterial viral gastroenteritis. Prolonged diarrhea may be associated with chronic GI diseases such as ulcerative colitis or Crohn disease. Consultation with a gastroenterologist with diagnostic testing should be considered. Sigmoidoscopy and colonoscopy are not contraindicated in pregnancy. Most diarrhea that occurs during pregnancy is nonspecific and can be managed with a variety of nonsystemic and systemic medications. Nonsystemic medications are preferable and should be tried initially. These include kaolin with pectin (Kaopectate) and stool-bulking agents.

Systemic medications frequently prescribed include loperamide (Imodium) and diphenoxylate atropine (Lomotil). Bismuth subsalicylate (Pepto-Bismol) should be avoided in large amounts, especially during the third trimester of pregnancy due to the salicylate content, which has been associated with adverse fetal outcomes.[132]

Hemorrhoids

Clinical Presentation

Internal hemorrhoids are more likely to be associated with bleeding as they arise from the superior hemorrhoidal plexus and are often painless. External hemorrhoids, which come from the vascular complex underneath the skin of the anus, are frequently painful.

Pharmacologic and Nonpharmacologic Treatment

The goals for treatment should decrease causative factors in order to decrease symptoms. Stool softeners should be instituted to relieve constipation. Sitz baths two to three times daily can be used to treat inflamed tissue. Witch hazel pads (Tucks) and steroid creams are effective in reducing pain.

Thrombosis of external hemorrhoids causing pain requires immediate treatment. The American Gastroenterological Association recommends that surgery should be considered when less invasive procedures fail or when strangulation occurs resulting in occlusion of blood supply. Operative hemorrhoidectomy can be performed during pregnancy.

Complications After Surgery for Morbid Obesity

Clinical Presentation

Obesity, defined as a body mass index (BMI) of >30 kg/m^2, in pregnancy is associated with significant risks for both the mother and fetus. Among the maternal risks are sleep apnea, diabetes, hypertensive disorders, thromboembolic disease, miscarriage, labor dystocia, shoulder dystocia, cesarean delivery, hemorrhage, infection, and maternal mortality. Fetal risks include macrosomia, anomalies, and fetal demise. Bariatric surgery is a medically acceptable and the most effective treatment for reducing weight and improving the morbidity and mortality associated with obesity and its comorbidities, especially among morbidly obese (BMI > 40 kg/m^2) women.[135] Approximately 75% to 80% of bariatric procedures in the United States are performed on women and at least half of these women are of reproductive age.[136,137] Therefore, it is likely that more women undergoing bariatric surgery will experience postsurgical pregnancy.

Management of Complications Post–bariatric Surgery in Pregnancy

Close monitoring of nutrients is important after bariatric surgery.[138] Maintenance of adequate nutrition and micronutrients may be particularly challenging in those who have undergone malabsorptive procedures. The optimal timing of pregnancy after bariatric surgery is unknown. As weight loss is rapid and intake reduced in the first year following surgery, the ACOG recommends delaying pregnancy for a minimum of 12 to 24 months, or until weight stabilization occurs.[139] Overall, pregnancy after bariatric surgery is safe and may be associated with improved pregnancy outcomes, including decreased rates of gestational diabetes and hypertensive disorders.[136]

Total Parenteral Nutrition in Pregnancy

Pregnant patients unable to consume sufficient nutrients orally require an effective method of feeding. Alternative forms of nutrition may be particularly necessary to maintain maternal nutrition when a GI disease complicates pregnancy and can be given as enteral nutrition (tube feeding) or as TPN. TPN, parenteral nutrition, hyperalimentation, intravenous hyperalimentation, and intravenous feedings are used synonymously and interchangeably to describe the various methods of providing all required nutrients intravenously. A team of qualified, knowledgeable individuals who are familiar with the technique being used should explain it to the patient, obtain written consent, and manage the administration of the parenteral nutrition.

TPN can be complicated by death of the nonpregnant patient or by maternal and/or fetal death in the pregnant patient. An increased risk of VTE and obstetrical complications, such as preterm labor, preeclampsia, and stillbirth, have been associated with TPN. However, the disease process for which TPN is indicated may be the cause of adverse perinatal outcomes (ie, preterm labor, fetal death, small for gestation age), rather than the therapy itself. Other complications include accidental pneumothorax or hemothorax, catheter infection, various metabolic disorders, glycosuria, hypoglycemia, and, rarely, clinical sepsis. Wernicke-Korsakoff syndrome, with irreversible neurologic total abnormalities, has occurred after institution of TPN and has been reported by various authors.

It has been suggested that enteral nutrition may be preferable to parental nutrition for patients in whom gut integrity is intact due to the decreased risk for complications.

The use of TPN has mostly been limited to patients with HG.

KEY POINTS

- Nausea with or without vomiting is an especially common symptom during early pregnancy and the most common GI complaint. It usually occurs during the first trimester of pregnancy and, by mid-second trimester, most women no longer complain of these symptoms.
- HG is the abnormal condition of pregnancy associated with pernicious nausea and vomiting. Hyperemesis is both infrequent and uncommon.
- Cannabinoid hyperemesis syndrome is characterized by chronic cannabis use, cyclic episodes of nausea and vomiting, and the learned behavior of hot bathing. This complication occurs by an unknown mechanism but due to marijuana use, which should never be used in any form during pregnancy.
- A few patients with HG have transient hyperthyroidism, which in these patients is common, self-limited, and requires no therapy. Thiamine supplementation is important for patients with prolonged vomiting.
- Many pregnant women enter pregnancy with poor dental care. Their teeth are in poor condition, and numerous cavities and gingivitis are present owing to poor dental hygiene. Dental care is appropriate when necessary during pregnancy.
- Radiographs, which are often necessary to establish a proper dental diagnosis, may be safely taken during any stage of pregnancy. The maternal abdomen should be shielded with a lead apron.
- Heartburn is really a symptom of reflux esophagitis that is a common, bothersome complaint during pregnancy and occurs in as many as 70% of pregnant patients.

- Diagnostic delay should not occur during pregnancy due to concerns for exposure to radiation. This type of delay may increase maternal morbidity and mortality.
- The term inflammatory bowel disease refers to a group of idiopathic chronic inflammatory diseases of the intestinal tract. The two most commonly seen during pregnancy are ulcerative colitis and Crohn disease. There is little evidence to suggest that pregnancy has an effect on IBD and the overall maternal prognosis is good.
- IBS is a functional bowel disorder characterized by abdominal cramping and cyclic episodes of constipation, diarrhea, and flatulence in the absence of organic pathology. Treatment is tailored to the individual patient and may involve dietary restrictions, antidepressants, antidiarrheals, and laxatives.
- CD is an autoimmune disease affecting 1% of Western populations confirmed by upper endoscopy and duodenal biopsies. Symptoms are provoked by ingestion of gluten and avoidance of gluten eliminates the T cell–mediated inflammatory disease activity. The most common disease symptoms are chronic diarrhea, flatulence, and weight loss.
- Constipation is seen in over 50% of women during pregnancy with symptoms improving by the third trimester. Prolonged complaints of constipation or constipation not responsive to usual therapies requires further investigation.
- Diarrhea is not as common in pregnancy; it can be associated with maternal dehydration. Bloody diarrhea or painful diarrhea requires further investigation including consultation with a gastroenterologist.
- Hemorrhoids can be classified as internal and external. Thrombosed hemorrhoids require immediate attention. Hemorrhoidectomy is not contraindicated in pregnancy.
- TPN can be used safely in pregnancy; however, it may be associated with an increased risk of infection and venous thromboembolism.
- Enteral nutrition may decrease the risk of complications, but has not been associated with improved outcomes.

- In pregnancy, as in the nongravid state, the diagnosis of GERD can be made on symptoms alone, and further imaging or other studies are rarely indicated.
- Acute appendicitis is the most commonly encountered general surgical problem, affecting 1 in 500 to 2000 pregnancies. Imaging plays an important role in confirming the diagnosis of acute appendicitis. Graded compression ultrasonography has emerged as the initial imaging modality of choice for evaluation of abdominal pain in pregnancy.
- The treatment of choice for acute appendicitis in pregnancy is surgical excision, which may be accomplished by laparoscopy or laparotomy. Prompt diagnosis and intervention are key in the prevention of maternal and fetal morbidity and mortality.
- Intestinal obstruction is an infrequent but serious complication of pregnancy, occurring in about 1 in 2500 pregnancies. The most common risk factor for intestinal obstruction is history of abdominal surgery.
- Initial management during the workup of acute intestinal obstruction may be conservative with nasogastric tube placement, bowel rest, and fluid and electrolyte repletion. If conservative measures are unsuccessful, or if the patient develops fever or peritoneal signs, surgical exploration via laparotomy is warranted.
- Bariatric surgery is a medically acceptable treatment for obesity and its comorbidities. Approximately 75% to 80% of bariatric procedures in the United States are performed on women and at least half of these women are of reproductive age.
- The ACOG recommends delaying pregnancy for a minimum of 12 to 24 months, or until weight stabilization occurs. Nausea, vomiting, and abdominal pain in patients who have undergone bariatric surgery may be signs of serious surgical complications.
- Overall, pregnancy after bariatric surgery is safe and may be associated with improved pregnancy outcomes, including decreased rates of gestational diabetes and hypertensive disorders.

REFERENCES

(only references cited in synoptic print chapter; for a complete reference list, see ebook)

1. Tan EK, Tan EL. Alterations in physiology and anatomy during pregnancy. *Best Pract Res Clin Obstet Gynaecol.* 2013;27(6):791-802.
2. Lawson M, Kern F Jr, Everson GT. Gastrointestinal transit time in human pregnancy: prolongation in the second and third trimesters followed by postpartum normalization. *Gastroenterology.* 1985;89(5):996-999.
3. Costantine MM. Physiologic and pharmacokinetic changes in pregnancy. *Front Pharmacol.* 2014;5:65.
4. NIH HMP Working Group, Peterson J, Garges S, Giovanni M, et al. The NIH human microbiome project. *Genome Res.* 2009;19:2317-2323.
5. Baquero F, Nombela C. The microbiome as a human organ. *Clin Microbiol Infect.* 2012;18(suppl 4):2.
6. Neish AS. Microbes in gastrointestinal health and disease. *Gastroenterology.* 2009;136:65.
7. Koren O, Goodrich JK, Cullender TC, et al. Host remodeling of the gut microbiome and metabolic changes during pregnancy. *Cell.* 2012;150(3):470.
8. Kilpatrick CC, Monga M. Approach to the acute abdomen in pregnancy. *Obstet Gynecol Clin North Am.* 2007;34(3):389-402, x.
9. Cappell MS. Gastrointestinal disorders during pregnancy. *Preface Gastroenterol Clin North Am* 2003;32(1):xi-xiii.
10. Committee Opinion No. 723: guidelines for diagnostic imaging during pregnancy and lactation. *Obstet Gynecol.* 2017;130(4):e210-e216.
12. Guelinckx I, Devlieger R, Vansant G. Reproductive outcome after bariatric surgery: a critical review. *Hum Reprod Update.* 2009;15(2):189-201.
13. Sadat U, Dar O, Walsh S, Varty K. Splenic artery aneurysms in pregnancy – a systematic review. *Int J Surg.* 2008;6(3):261-265.
14. la Chapelle CF, Schutte JM, Schuitemaker NW, Steegers EA, van Roosmalen J; on behalf of the Dutch Maternal Mortality Committee. Maternal mortality attributable to vascular dissection and rupture in the Netherlands: a nationwide confidential enquiry. *Br J Obstet Gynecol.* 2012;119(1):86-93.
15. Goodwin TM. Hyperemesis gravidarum. *Obstet Gynecol Clin North Am.* 2008;35:401-417.
16. ACOG practice Bulletin No. 189: nausea and vomiting of pregnancy. *Obstet Gynecol.* 2018;131:e15-e30.
17. Oudman E, Wijnia JW, Oey M, et al. Wernicke's encephalopathy in hyperemesis gravidarum: a systematic review. *Eur J Obstet Gynecol Reprod Biol.* 2019;236:84-93.
22. Dozeman R, Kaiser FE, Cass O, Pries J. Hyperthyroidism appearing as hyperemesis gravidarum. *Arch Intern Med.* 1983;143:2202.
26. Goodwin TM, Montoro M, Mestman JH. Transient hyperthyroidism and hyperemesis gravidarum: clinical aspects. *Am J Obstet Gynecol.* 1992;167:648.
27. Lee NM, Saha S. Nausea and vomiting of pregnancy. *Gastroenterol Clin North Am.* 2011;40(2):309-334.
30. Simpson SW, Goodwin TM, Robins SB, et al. Psychological factors and hyperemesis gravidarum. *J Womens Health Gend Based Med.* 2001;10:471-477.
31. Flaxman SM, Sherman PW. Morning sickness: a mechanism for protecting mother and embryo. *Q Rev Biol.* 2000;75:113-148.
32. Whitehead SA, Andrews PL, Chamberlain GV. Characterisation of nausea and vomiting in early pregnancy: a survey of 1000 women. *J Obstet Gynaecol.* 1992;12:364-369.
33. Austin K, Wilson K, Saha S. Hyperemesis gravidarum. *Nutr Clin Pract.* 2019;34(2):226-241.
34. Gadsby R, Barnie-Adshead AM, Jagger C. A prospective study of nausea and vomiting during pregnancy. Published erratum appears in *Br J Gen Pract.* 1993;43:325. *Br J Gen Pract.* 1993;43:245-248.
35. Allen JH, de Moore GM, Heddle R, et al. Cannabinoid hyperemesis: cyclical hyperemesis in association with chronic cannabis use. *Gut.* 2004;53:1566-1570.
39. Maltepe C, Koren G. Preemptive treatment of nausea and vomiting of pregnancy: results of a randomized controlled trial. *Obstet Gynecol Int.* 2013;2013:809787.
40. Naef RW III, Chauhan SP, Roach H, et al. Treatment for hyperemesis gravidarum in the home: an alternative to hospitalization. *J Perinatol.* 1995;154:289-292.

41. Jarvis S, Nelson-Piercy C. Management of nausea and vomiting in pregnancy. *Br Med J.* 2011;342:d3606.
45. ACOG Practice Bulletin No. 187: neural tube defects. *Obstet Gynecol.* 2017;130:e279-e290.
50. Abas MN, Tan PC, Azmi N, Omar SZ. Ondansetron compared with metoclopramide for hyperemesis gravidarum: a randomized controlled trial. *Obstet Gynecol.* 2014;123:1272-1279.
51. Kashifard M, Basirat Z, Kashifard M, Golsorkhtabar-Amiri M, Moghaddamnia A. Ondansetrone or metoclopromide? Which is more effective in severe nausea and vomiting of pregnancy? A randomized trial double- blind study. *Clin Exp Obstet Gynecol.* 2013;40:127-130.
52. Oliveira LG, Capp SM, You WB, Riffenburgh RH, Carstairs SD. Ondansetron compared with doxylamine and pyridoxine for treatment of nausea in pregnancy: a randomized controlled trial. *Obstet Gynecol.* 2014;124:735-742.
55. Carstairs SD. Ondansetron use in pregnancy and birth defects: a systematic review. *Obstet Gynecol.* 2016;127(5):878-883.
58. Safari HR, Fassett MJ, Souter IC, Alsulyman OM, Goodwin TM. The efficacy of methylprednisolone in the treatment of hyperemesis gravidarum: a randomized, double-blind, controlled study. *Am J Obstet Gynecol.* 1998;179:921-924.
59. Yost NP, McIntire DD, Wians FH Jr, Ramin SM, Balko JA, Leveno KJ. A randomized, placebo-controlled trial of corticosteroids for hyperemesis due to pregnancy. *Obstet Gynecol.* 2003;102:1250-1254.
60. Boelig RC, Barton SJ, Saccone G, Kelly AJ, Edwards SJ, Berghella V. Interventions for treating hyperemesis gravidarum. *Cochrane Database Syst Rev.* 2016;(5):CD010607. doi:10.1002/14651858.CD010607.pub2
61. Badell ML, Ramin SM, Smith JA. Treatment options for nausea and vomiting during pregnancy. *Pharmacotherapy.* 2006;26(9):1273-1287.
65. Tung CS, Zighelboim I, Gardner MO. Acute colonic pseudoobstruction complicating twin pregnancy: a case report. *J Reprod Med.* 2008;53(1):52-54.
66. Chudzinski AP, Thompson EV, Ayscue JM. Acute colonic pseudoobstruction. *Clin Colon Rectal Surg.* 2015;28(2):112-117.
67. Tempfer CB, Dogan A, Hilal Z, Rezniczek GA. Acute colonic pseudoobstruction (Ogilvie's syndrome) in gynecologic and obstetric patients: case report and systematic review of the literature. *Arch Gynecol Obstet.* 2019;300(1):117-126.
68. Lier MCI, Malik RF, Ket JCF, Lambalk CB, Brosens IA, Mijatovic V. Spontaneous hemoperitoneum in pregnancy (SHiP) and endometriosis – a systematic review of the recent literature. *Eur J Obstet Gynecol Reprod Biol.* 2017;219:57-65.
69. Zuraw BL. Clinical practice. Hereditary angioedema. *N Engl J Med.* 2008;359(10):1027-1036.
70. Bowen T, Cicardi M, Bork K, et al. Hereditary angiodema: a current state-of-the-art review, VII. Canadian Hungarian 2007 International Consensus Algorithm for the Diagnosis, Therapy, and Management of Hereditary Angioedema. *Ann Allergy Asthma Immunol.* 2008;100(1 suppl 2):S30-S40.
71. Committee Opinion No. 711 summary: opioid use and opioid use disorder in pregnancy. *Obstet Gynecol.* 2017;130(2):488-489.
72. Yawn B, Buchanan G, Afenyi-Annan A, et al. Management of sickle cell disease summary of the 2014 evidence-based report by expert panel members. *J Am Med Assoc.* 2014;312(10):1033-1048.
73. Hakim M, Wang W, Bramer W, et al. The global burden of hepatitis E outbreaks: a systematic review. *Liver Int.* 2017;37:19-31.
74. Jayaram P, Mohan M, Lindow S, Konje J. Postpartum Acute Colonic Pseudo-Obstruction (Ogilvie's Syndrome): a systematic review of case reports and case series. *Eur J Obstet Gynecol Reprod Biol.* 2017;214:145-149.
75. Silk H, Douglass AB, Douglass JM, Silk L. Oral health during pregnancy. *Am Fam Physician.* 2008;77:1139-1144.
78. Regezi JA, Sciubba JJ, Jordan RCK. *Oral Pathology: Clinical Pathologic Correlations.* 7th ed. Elsevier/Saunders; 2017.
82. Committee Opinion No. 569: oral health care during pregnancy and through the lifespan. *Obstet Gynecol.* 2013;122:417-422. (Reaffirmed 2017).
84. Kurien S, Kattimani VS, Sriram R, et al. Management of pregnant patient in dentistry. *J Int Oral Health.* 2013;5(1):88-97.
86. Suresh M. *Shnider and Levinson's Anesthesia for Obstetrics.* Lippincott Williams & Wilkins; 2013.
89. Boggess KA; Society for Maternal-Fetal Medicine. Maternal oral health in pregnancy. *Obstet Gynecol.* 2008;111:976-986.

90. Macones GA, Parry S, Nelson DB, et al. Treatment of localized periodontal disease in pregnancy does not reduce the occurrence of preterm birth: results from the Periodontal Infections and Prematurity Study (PIPS). *Am J Obstet Gynecol*. 2010;202:147.e1-147.e8.

91. Ali R, Egan L. Gastroesophageal reflux disease in pregnancy. *Best Pract Res Clin Gastroenterol*. 2007;21(5):793-806.

92. Body C, Christie J. Gastrointestinal diseases in pregnancy: nausea, vomiting, hyperemesis gravidarum, gastroesophageal reflux disease, constipation, and diarrhea. *Gastroenterol Clin North Am*. 2016;45: 267-283.

95. Fashner J, Gitu A. Peptic ulcer disease. *Am Fam Physician*. 2015;91(4): 236-242.

96. Rosen C, Czuzoj-Shulman N, Mishkin DS, et al. Management and outcomes of peptic ulcer disease in pregnancy. *J Matern Fetal Neonatal Med*. 2019:1-7. doi:10.1080/14767058.2019.1637410.

97. Boregowda G, Shehata H. Gastrointestinal and liver disease in pregnancy. *Best Prac Res Clin Obstet Gynecol*. 2013;27(6):835-853.

98. Pasternak B, Hviid A. Use of proton pump inhibitors in early pregnancy and the risk of birth defects. *N Engl J Med*. 2010;363:2114-2123.

101. Walker H, Samaraee A, Mills A, et al. Laparoscopic appendectomy in pregnancy: a systematic review of the published evidence. *Int J Surg*. 2014;12:1235-1241.

103. Barloon T, Brown B, Abu-Yousef M, et al. Sonography of acute appendicitis in pregnancy. *Abdom Imaging*. 1995;20(2):149-151.

104. Burke LM, Bashir MR, Miller FH, et al. Magnetic resonance imaging of acute appendicitis in pregnancy: a 5-year multiinstitutional study. *Am J Obstet Gynecol*. 2015;213(5):693.e1-693.e6.

106. Prodromidou A, Machairas N, Kostakis I, et al. Outcomes after open and laparoscopic appendectomy during pregnancy: a meta-analysis. *Euro J Obstet Gynecol Reprod Biol*. 2018;225:40-50.

107. Ossendorp R, Silvis R, van der Bij G. Advanced colorectal cancer resulting in acute bowel obstruction during pregnancy: a case report. *Ann Med Surg*. 2016;8:18-20.

108. Perdue P, Johnson H, Stafford P. Intestinal obstruction complicating pregnancy. *Am J Surg*. 1992;164:384-388.

109. Webster P, Bailey M, Wilson J, et al. Small bowel obstruction in pregnancy is a complex surgical problem with a high risk of fetal loss. *Ann R Coll Surg Engl*. 2015;97:339-344.

110. Mukherjee R, Samanta S. Surgical emergencies in pregnancy in the era of modern diagnostics and treatment. *Taiwanese J Obstet Gynecol*. 2019;58(2):177-182.\

111. ACOG Committee Opinion No. 776: immune modulating therapies in pregnancy and lactation. *Obstet Gynecol*. 2019;133(4):e287-e295.

112. Ordas I, Eckmann L, Talamini M, Baumgart, Sandborn W. Ulcerative colitis. *Lancet*. 2012;380:1606-1619.

113. Baumgart D, Sandborn W. Crohn's disease. *Lancet*. 2012;380:1590-1605.

114. Magro F, Gionchetti P, Eliakim R, et al. Third European evidence-based consensus on diagnosis and management of ulcerative colitis. Part 1: definitions, diagnosis, extra-intestinal manifestations, pregnancy, cancer surveillance, surgery, and ileo-anal pouch disorders. *J Crohns Colitis*. 2017;11(6):649-670.

115. Beaulieu D, Kane S. Inflammatory bowel disease in pregnancy. *Gastroenterol Clin N Am*. 2011;40:399-413.

116. Mahadevan U, Robinson C, Bernasko N, et al. Inflammatory bowel disease in pregnancy clinical care pathway: a report from the American Gastroenterological Association IBD Parenthood Project Working Group. *Gastroenterology*. 2019;156:1508-1524.

117. Zitomerski N, Verhave M, Trenor C. Thrombosis and inflammatory bowel disease: a call for improved awareness and prevention. *Inflamm Bowel Dis*. 2011;17(1):458-470.

118. Nguyen G, Bernstein C, Bitton A, et al. Consensus statements on the risk, prevention and treatment of venous thromboembolism in inflammatory bowel disease: Canadian Association of Gastroenterology. *Gastroenterology*. 2014;146(3):835-848.

119. Royal College of Obstetricians and Gynecologists. *Reducing the risk of venous thromboembolism during pregnancy and the Puerperium*. Green Top Guideline No 37a. RCOG; 2015.

120. Gisbert J, Chaparro M. Safety of anti-TNF agents during pregnancy and breastfeeding in women with inflammatory bowel disease. *Am J Gastroenterol*. 2013;108:1426-1438.

121. Chey W, Kurlander J, Eswaran S. Irritable bowel syndrome A clinical review. *J Am Med Assoc*. 2015;313(9):949-958.

122. Sandler RS, Everhart JE, Donowitz M, et al. The burden of selected digestive diseases in the United States. *Gastroenterology*. 2002;122:1500.

124. Rubio-Tapia A, Hill I, Kelly C, Calderwood A, Murray J. American College of Gastroenterology clinical guideline: diagnosis and management of celiac disease. *Am J Gastroenterol*. 2013;108(5):656-677.

126. Bradley C, Kennedy CM, Turcea AM, Rao SS, Nygaard IE. Constipation in pregnancy. *Obstet Gynecol*. 2007;110:1351-1357.

127. Simren M, Palsson OS, Whitehead WE. Update on Rome IV criteria for colorectal disorders: implications for clinical practice. *Curr Gastroenterol Rep*. 2017;19(4):15.

129. Wald A. Constipation: advances in treatment and diagnosis. *J Am Med Assoc*. 2016;315(2):185-191.

130. Zielinski R, Searing K, Deibel M. Gastrointestinal distress in pregnancy. Prevalence, assessment and treatment of 5 minor discomforts. *J Perinat Neonatal Nurs*. 2015;29(1):23-31.

132. Giddings SL, Stevens AM, Leung DT. Travelers diarrhea. *Med Clin North Am*. 2016;100(2):317-330.

135. Brolin R. Update: NIH consensus conference. Gastrointestinal surgery for severe obesity. *Nutrition*. 1996;12:403-404.

136. Dolin C, Welcome A, Caughey A. Management of pregnancy in women who have undergone bariatric surgery. *Obstet Gynecol Surv*. 2016;71(12):734-740.

137. Baldreldin N, Kuller J, Rhee E, et al. Pregnancy management after bariatric surgery. *Obstet Gynecol Surv*. 2016;71(6):361-367.

138. Narayanan R, Syed A. Pregnancy following bariatric surgery – medical complications and management. *Obes Surg*. 2016;26:2523-2529.

139. American College of Obstetricians and Gynecologists. ACOG Practice Bulletin No. 105: bariatric surgery and pregnancy. *Obstet Gynecol*. 2009;113:1405-1413.

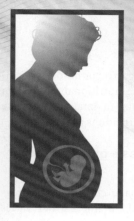

CHAPTER 34

Liver Disease in Pregnancy

Juan Ignacio Pereira and Gustavo F. Leguizamón

Introduction

Approximately 3% of all pregnancies are complicated by liver disorders.[1] These infrequent conditions pose a great diagnostic challenge for the obstetrician.

Physiological Changes in Liver in Normal Pregnancy

During normal pregnancy, many physiological and hormonal changes occur, some of which may mimic liver disease (**Table 34.1**).

Liver Diseases Unique to Pregnancy

Hyperemesis Gravidarum

Epidemiology

Although nausea and vomiting during pregnancy (NVP) affects 50% to 80% of pregnant women,[7] 90% resolve by 20 weeks of gestation. In contrast, hyperemesis gravidarum (HG) is a complication rather than a normal finding[8] and occurs in 0.3% to 3% of pregnancies.[9]

Etiology

The etiology of HG is unknown. Endocrine, infectious, psychological, and genetic factors have been proposed. History of HG in a previous pregnancy, history of motion sickness, migraine headaches, and women carrying female fetuses[8] have been identified as risk factors.

The diagnosis of HG is based on characteristic clinical findings and is achieved after the exclusion of other conditions that may also present with excessive NVP. Typical signs and symptoms include vomiting not related to other causes and an objective measure of acute starvation such as large ketonuria and weight loss.[11] Hypochloremic alkalosis, hypokalemia, hyponatremia, and mild elevation of amylase, lipase, and liver function enzymes are common laboratory abnormalities.[13] Frequently, signs of dehydration are also present, including orthostatic hypotension, tachycardia, dry skin, mood changes, and lethargy.[9] The differential diagnosis includes gastroenteritis, cholecystitis, hepatitis, biliary tract diseases, drug abuse/misuse, and migraine headaches. Infrequent causes include diabetic ketoacidosis, intracranial lesions, and intestinal obstruction.[9]

Laboratory tests commonly included in the initial assessment are complete blood count and serum metabolic panels, amylase/lipase, hCG level for evaluation of possible molar or multiple gestations, and urinalysis for ketones.[9] The 2018 ACOG guidelines recommend that serum thyroid function

Table 34.1 Physiological Changes in Maternal Circulation and Liver Function During Normal Pregnancy.

Increased	Cardiac output
	Plasma volume
	AP (due to placental/bone origin)
	Fibrinogen
	Coagulation factors I, II, V, VII, X, and XII
Decreased	Systemic vascular resistance
	Serum albumin
	Bilirubin
	GGT
Unchanged	Transaminases (AST/ALT)
	Serum bilirubin
	Direct bilirubin
	Total bile acid

ALT, alanine aminotransferase; AP, alkaline phosphatase; AST, aspartate aminotransferase; GGT, gamma-glutamyltransferase.

See the eBook for expanded content, a complete reference list, and additional tables.

studies should be obtained only in the presence of other signs of hyperthyroidism such as palpable goiter.[11] Because gastric ulcers can be a contributing factor to refractory HG, testing for *Helicobacter pylori* infection has also been recommended.[11]

Maternal-Fetal Implications

Most women with HG receiving supportive care have good outcomes. Occasionally, serious maternal complications can occur. Fetal risks include low birthweight, preterm labor, and small for gestational age infants. Recurrence risk varies from 15% to 80%.[19] Prophylactic interventions started before the onset of NVP may reduce the duration and severity of symptoms in subsequent pregnancies. Early prescription of antiemetics that proved effective in the first pregnancy is encouraged.[20]

Nonpharmacologic Treatment

Common recommendations include rest and avoidance of sensory stimuli such as odors, heat, humidity, noise, and flickering lights.[11] Taking prenatal vitamins for 1 month before pregnancy could reduce the incidence and severity of NVP.[11] Dietary modifications include avoiding spicy or fatty foods, excluding iron supplements, and eating bland or dry foods and high-protein snacks.[11]

Pharmacologic Therapies

Early treatment of NVP is recommended. Treatment of NVP with vitamin B6 (pyridoxine) alone or plus doxylamine is safe and effective and should be considered the first-line pharmacotherapy.[11] Relief of NVP with dopamine antagonists (metoclopramide, promethazine, prochlorperazine, or chlorpromazine) given orally, rectally, intramuscularly, or intravenously has been demonstrated in large groups of patients.[11] Antihistamines, such as dimenhydrinate and diphenhydramine, have been shown to be effective and are frequently used.[11] Evidence is limited on the safety and efficacy of the serotonin 5-HT3 inhibitor, ondansetron. Thus, women should be counseled weighing the risks and benefits of ondansetron use before 10 weeks.[11]

Hospitalization is recommended if oral intolerance is a concern or there is lack of response to outpatient management, a change in vital signs or in mental status, and if persistent weight loss occurs.[11] Intravenous hydration should be used. Correction of ketosis and vitamin deficiency should be considered. Dextrose and vitamins should be included.

Enteral tube feeding (nasogastric or nasoduodenal) should be used to provide nutritional support in woman with HG who cannot maintain appropriate weight, especially if malnutrition is present.[11]

Intrahepatic Cholestasis of Pregnancy

Epidemiology

The incidence of intrahepatic cholestasis of pregnancy (ICP) is between 0.2% and 2% but varies with ethnicity and geographic location. Risk factors for ICP include multiple gestations, *in vitro* fertilization, advanced maternal age, history of prior affected pregnancy, family history, and hepatitis C infection.[28,29,30] Moreover, women with ICP are more likely to develop hepatobiliary disease, including fibrosis, gallstone disease, or hepatitis.[28,29]

Etiology and Pathogenesis

The etiology of ICP appears to be related to the cholestatic effect of reproductive hormones in genetically susceptible women.[28] The transport of bile salts from the liver to the gallbladder is disrupted and there is compensatory transport from the hepatocytes into the blood.[28] Fetal complications are directly related to the toxic effect of bile acids, which accumulate in the fetal compartment.[28]

Clinical Features and Diagnosis

The classical feature of ICP is pruritus without rash or any specific dermal lesion,[29] typically occurring in the third trimester.[28] Pruritus typically affects the palms and soles but may occur anywhere, and characteristically disturbs the sleep pattern. It is often worse at night and may deteriorate as pregnancy advances.[28] Excoriation marks secondary to scratching are usually observed.[28] Systemic symptoms of cholestasis may be present, including dark urine and pale stools. Some women may also present as jaundiced but this is rarely observed.[28]

The diagnosis is confirmed after demonstration of abnormal liver function tests and especially maternal serum bile acid (SBA) levels above 10 to 14 µmol/L.[28] Liver transaminases can also be elevated.[28,29] Alkaline phosphatase is not useful in the diagnosis of ICP, because it is produced in large quantities by the placenta.[28] Bilirubin is increased in 10% of women with ICP.[28] Finally, liver ultrasound scanning is useful to rule out other causes of cholestasis, such as gallstones.[28]

Fetal Concerns

Spontaneous and iatrogenic preterm birth, meconium staining, stillbirth, and neonatal intensive care unit admission are consistently associated with this condition.[36,37] These studies reported an elevated risk of stillbirth with SBA levels greater than 40 µmol/L,[37] with the highest risk being observed when levels are greater than 100 µmol/L.[29,38,39]

Pharmacologic Treatment

ICP is commonly treated with ursodeoxycholic acid (UDCA). Randomized trials showed significant improvements in pruritus and liver function tests with UDCA therapy.[28,40,41] There is no evidence to support improved perinatal outcomes. Finally, the dose of UDCA can be titrated to symptoms and usually ranges from 500 mg to 2 g daily.[28]

Fetal Monitoring

It has been hypothesized that bile acids may cause sudden fetal death secondary to arrhythmia and vasoconstriction of placental vessels, leading to acute anoxia.[28] There is no proven effective antenatal monitoring strategy to prevent stillbirth in ICP.[28,29,43] Clinicians may find it reassuring to have regular cardiotocography, biophysical profile, and fetal growth scans.

Elective Early Delivery

To reduce the risk of stillbirth, many authors have advocated for elective early delivery.[28,30] We emphasize, however, that no randomized studies have established the optimal timing of delivery for pregnancies complicated by ICP.[28] **Algorithm 34.1** depicts a possible management approach to patients with ICP.

Postnatal Follow-Up and Preconception Counseling

The biochemical abnormalities associated with ICP typically resolve rapidly after delivery.[28] Women with ICP should have their liver function and serum bile acids checked 6 to 8 weeks postnatally.[28] Therefore, alternative methods to oral contraception should be

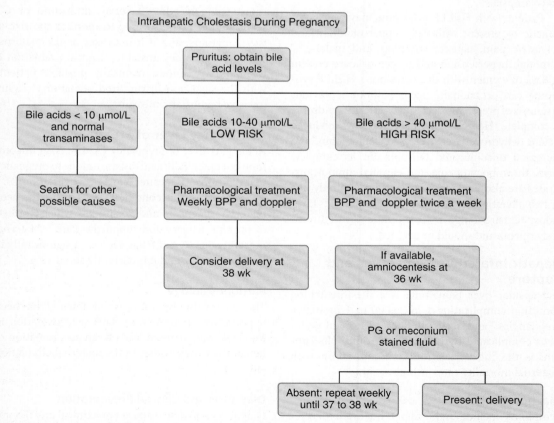

Algorithm 34.1 Management of intrahepatic cholestasis during pregnancy. BPP, biophysical profile.

advised.[45] Approximately 90% of women will have ICP recurrence in subsequent pregnancies.[28,29]

Liver Involvement in Hypertensive Disorders of Pregnancy

Preeclampsia

Hepatic involvement affects approximately 10% of women with severe preeclampsia and frequently presents with epigastric or right upper quadrant pain.[46] Transaminases are significantly increased, whereas bilirubin concentrations are rarely enhanced. Complications can include subcapsular hematoma and hepatic rupture.[30] Liver biopsy is not indicated.[1] Liver biochemical profile usually normalizes within 2 weeks of delivery.[1]

HELLP Syndrome

HELLP syndrome (hemolysis, elevated liver enzymes, and low platelet count) is characterized by hemolytic anemia, elevated liver enzymes, and low platelet count. It complicates 0.5% to 0.9% of all pregnancies,[47] and 10% of gestations with severe preeclampsia.[30]

Patients with HELLP syndrome may be asymptomatic or present with right upper quadrant and epigastric pain, nausea, vomiting, and malaise.[1,48] Although hypertension and proteinuria are present in 85% of women with this condition,[1] HELLP syndrome can occasionally occur without a previous diagnosis of preeclampsia. Usually, HELLP syndrome is complete. Hemolysis is manifested by enhanced lactate dehydrogenase, decreased haptoglobin, and increased unconjugated bilirubin. In its complete form, thrombocytopenia and elevated aminotransferases are also evident; partial forms with only one or two alterations have also been described.[1,48] Liver biopsy remains a high-risk procedure due to thrombocytopenia and should be avoided.

Hepatic Infarction, Hematoma, and Rupture

Subcapsular liver hematoma is a life-threatening condition complicating 1 in 25,000 to 1 in 40,000 pregnancies[49] and occurs in 0.9% to 1.6% of gestations complicated by HELLP syndrome.[50] Its rupture is the most catastrophic complication with maternal mortality rates as high as 50%.[51]

Diagnosis

Symptoms include right upper quadrant or epigastric pain, severe right shoulder pain, NVP, and hypotension and shock. Abdominal distention from hemoperitoneum is seen when hepatic rupture occurs.[49] Differential diagnoses are pulmonary embolism, adnexal torsion, rupture of adnexal cyst, cholelithiasis, hepatitis, pancreatitis, peptic ulcer, myocardial infarction, pyelonephritis, and nephrolithiasis.[49,52] Laboratory alterations include increased transaminases in excess of 3000 U/L, leukocytosis, pyrexia, and anemia. Clinical suspicion should prompt further evaluation. Ultrasound is a reasonable initial approach,[49] but findings need to be confirmed with either computed tomography (CT) scan or magnetic resonance imaging (MRI).[1,30,49] Complications include acute respiratory distress syndrome, acute kidney injury, and hypovolemic shock.[1]

Management of Liver Hematoma in Pregnancy

Unruptured subcapsular liver hematoma in a hemodynamically stable patient can be conservatively managed.[1,30,49] Abdominal palpation must be avoided because it can lead to the rupture and catastrophic bleeding.[49] Serial ultrasound or CT scans should be performed to monitor the size of the hematoma, and if it increases or the maternal condition becomes unstable, surgical evaluation is mandatory.[49] Hemodynamically unstable patients with the suspicion of ruptured hematoma require invasive hemostatic measures.

Acute Fatty Liver of Pregnancy

Acute fatty liver of pregnancy (AFLP) is an uncommon but potentially fatal disease unique to pregnancy that typically occurs after 30 weeks of gestation.[30,55,56] The severity of this condition underscores the need for early diagnosis and treatment, which consists of prompt delivery and supportive care.[55] Maternal mortality due to AFLP has decreased significantly in the last decades, and it is currently about 12%.[57]

Pathophysiology

The exact pathophysiology is unknown.[3] It has been hypothesized that aberrant fatty acid oxidation in the fetal compartment leads to an accumulation of hepatotoxic metabolites in the maternal circulation and liver.[3,55,58]

Diagnosis and Clinical Presentation

Diagnosis is primarily based on clinical and laboratory findings. The most common initial symptoms are nonspecific: anorexia, malaise, nausea, vomiting, and headache. Additional features may include epigastric pain, jaundice, hypertension, and disseminated intravascular coagulation (DIC).[3,30,55] AFLP and HELLP syndrome are coexistent in approximately 50% of patients.[3,30,55]

Laboratory alterations include moderate elevations in ALT and AST. Bilirubin, blood urea nitrogen, uric acid, and creatinine are also mildly elevated. Hypoglycemia is common and a valuable finding in the differential diagnosis with preeclampsia and HELLP syndrome.[3,30,55] However, the absence of hypoglycemia should not rule out AFLP.[3]

Management in Pregnancy

Delivery should not be delayed in patients whose clinical presentation and laboratory findings are consistent with AFLP. The most common life-threatening conditions include acute liver failure with encephalopathy, DIC, acute renal failure, and gastrointestinal bleeding.[55] Treatment is largely supportive.[55] Liver biopsy is rarely indicated because of the risks involved in critically ill patients.[55] Patients are expected to recover normal liver function within a week.

Offspring of women with AFLP should be monitored for manifestations of long-chain 3-hydroxyacyl coenzyme A dehydrogenase deficiency. Affected infants often show involvement of heart, liver, and skeletal muscle.[30] **Table 34.2** depicts differential features relevant to liver disorders in pregnancy.

Liver Disease Concurrent to Pregnancy

Biliary Disease

Cholelithiasis is the most common biliary condition in pregnancy. Although some pregnant patients experience uncomplicated cholelithiasis, an important proportion develops complications such as acute cholecystitis, choledocholithiasis, cholangitis, and gallstone pancreatitis.[63]

Acute cholecystitis is the second most common surgical condition in pregnancy and occurs in 1 in 6000 to 1 in 10,000 gestations.[30,64] Symptomatic gallstone disease in pregnancy is associated with increased mortality for both the mother and fetus and may result in complications such as spontaneous abortion, fetal abnormalities, preterm labor, and even death.[62,63,64]

Diagnosis

Cholelithiasis is frequently asymptomatic but may also present with right upper abdominal or epigastric pain, with colic features, that is worsened by fat-rich meals. NVP is frequently present.

Cholecystitis is a more serious condition. Although similar symptoms usually occur, fever, tachycardia, and the characteristic murphy sign (pain with abdominal palpation below the inferior costal margin at the level of the right midclavicular line, during deep inspiration) are generally present. Furthermore, increased leukocyte count and mildly elevated liver function tests could be observed. Abdominal ultrasound is a useful tool to confirm clinical suspicion of cholelithiasis. Presence of gallstones, ultrasound murphy sign, gallbladder wall thickening, and pericholecystic fluid are characteristic ultrasound finding in cholecystitis.

Management in Pregnancy

Although few patients with mild symptoms of cholelithiasis or cholecystitis can be managed conservatively, most women will benefit from surgical treatment. Medical management consists of intravenous hydration, fasting, analgesics, and antibiotics.

Most patients with established biliary disease managed conservatively will have frequent recurrences (38%-69%).[64,65]

Early cholecystectomy is the most appropriate approach in symptomatic patients with positive ultrasound findings. Both open and laparoscopic cholecystectomy are best deferred until the second trimester.[1,64]

Laparoscopic cholecystectomy in pregnant women has the advantage of reduced hospitalization, less incidence of deep vein thrombosis, decreased narcotic use, and quick return to a regular diet.[64] The following precautions should be taken during laparoscopy: (1) use an open technique for insertion of the umbilical port; (2) avoid high intraperitoneal pressures; (3) use the left lateral position to minimize aortocaval compression; (4) avoid rapid changes in patient position; and (5) use electrocautery cautiously and away from uterus.[64]

Viral Hepatitis in Pregnancy

Hepatitis A

Hepatitis A virus (HAV) is usually self-limited and does not lead to chronic infection. Fecal-oral contamination is the primary mode of infection in the United States.[68]

Table 34.2 Differential Features and Findings of Liver Disorders of Pregnancy

	AFLP	HELLP	Severe Preeclampsia
Gestational age of onset	Third trimester	Second/third trimester Postpartum	Second/third trimester Postpartum
Risk factors	Male fetus, primigravidas, multiple gestations	Previous pregnancy with HELLP Extreme ages Multiple gestations	Previous pregnancy with preeclampsia Multiple gestations Extreme ages Diabetes mellitus Autoimmune disease ART Primigravidas
Clinical features	Abdominal pain +++ Nausea/vomiting Jaundice Liver failure Hypoglycemia Coagulopathy Encephalopathy Hyperammonemia DIC	Abdominal pain ++ Vomiting Proteinuria ± Hypertension ± Headache Blurred vision Edema DIC Liver failure	Abdominal pain ++ Vomiting Proteinuria +++ Hypertension +++ Edema Renal failure Headache Blurred vision Edema Hyperreflexia
Bilirubin	5-10 mg/dL	<5 mg/dL	<5 mg/dL
AST/ALT	5-10x (300-1000 U/L)	1-100x	1-100x
Hemolysis	−	Yes	Yes
Platelet count	<100,000	<100,000	Low
Proteinuria	+	++	+++
Creatinine	Elevated	Mainly normal	Elevated
Uric acid	Elevated	Elevated	Elevated
Coagulation	Altered	Normal	Normal
Glycemia	Hypoglycemia	Normal	Normal
Imaging findings	Fatty infiltration	Mainly normal subcapsular hematomas	None
Management	Prompt delivery Supportive measures Liver transplant Monitor infant for manifestations of FAOD	Prompt delivery Platelet transfusion if platelets <50,000 and cesarean delivery is likely	Delivery if GA > 34 wk Close surveillance and steroids for lung maturation if GA < 34 wk Antihypertensive drugs Magnesium sulfate
Recurrence	+++ when LCHAD deficiency is present	Variable. Low-dose aspirin before 16th week in next pregnancy	Variable. Low-dose aspirin before 16th week in next pregnancy

AFLP, acute fatty liver of pregnancy; ART, assisted reproductive techniques; DIC, disseminated intravascular coagulation; FAOD, fatty acid oxidation deficiency; GA, gestational age; HELLP, hemolysis, elevated liver enzymes, and low platelets syndrome; LCHAD, long-chain 3-hydroxyacyl coenzyme A dehydrogenase.

HAV During Pregnancy

Maternal and fetal outcomes are excellent in developed countries.

Diagnosis requires serologic testing. The presence of HAV immunoglobulin M (IgM) is suggestive of acute infection and may persist for several months. HAV IgG predominates during convalescence and provides lifelong immunity.[68,69]

Immunization

Immunization is advised for populations presenting risk factors such as chronic liver disease, those receiving clotting factor concentrates, illegal drug users, and travelers to areas with medium to high endemicity.[68,69,71] The vaccines contain inactivated virus and are safe to use during pregnancy.[68] HAV vaccination should still be administered in addition to immunoglobulin, even in the context of postexposure prevention.

Hepatitis B

Hepatitis B virus (HBV) is a DNA virus.[68,72] It contains three antigens of clinical significance hepatitis B surface antigen (HBsAg), which circulates in the serum; hepatitis B core antigen (HBcAg), which is present only in hepatocytes; and hepatitis B e antigen (HBeAg), which indicates a high viral inoculum and active virus replication.[68] Hepatitis B is transmitted by parenteral and sexual contact.

Common risk factors include multiple sexual partners, intravenous drug use, or having sexual partners with high-risk behaviors.[68,72] Between 85% and 90% of infected adults experience complete resolution of the clinical infection and develop protective antibodies.[68] The remaining 10% to 15% becomes chronically infected, and, in a subgroup of those (15%-30%), viral replication continues and can also develop cirrhosis.[68] Vertical transmission is responsible for about half of chronic HBV infections worldwide.[74] Universal maternal screening and passive-active immunoprophylaxis of newborns have lowered transmission rates to 5% to 10%.[74]

HBV Infection in Pregnancy

When acute HBV infection occurs early in pregnancy, the rate of perinatal transmission is about 10% and increases to 60% if it occurs close to delivery.[74] Supportive care is the mainstay of therapy.[72] Maternal antiviral treatment to reduce perinatal transmission is indicated for HBsAg-positive pregnant women whose HBV DNA viral load is >200,000 IU/mL (10^6 copies/mL).[72]

Chronic HBV infection does not usually affect pregnancy outcome unless it is complicated with cirrhosis or advanced liver disease. Women with portal hypertension (PH) have increased rates of preterm labor, spontaneous abortion, and stillbirth.[74,76]

Risk of Vertical Transmission

Vertical transmission generally occurs at the time of delivery. Infants born to mothers with high viral loads are at greatest risk for infection. The risk of vertical transmission can be as high as 90%, especially if the mother was infected in the third trimester, is HbeAg positive, and has a viral load greater than 10^6 copies/mL.[72,74] Available data do not support routine cesarean delivery in women with low HBV DNA load.[72]

Screening and Diagnosis

All pregnant women should be tested for HBsAg at an early prenatal visit in each pregnancy, even if they have been previously vaccinated or screened.[72] Women not tested prenatally, those with clinical hepatitis, and those at high risk for HBV infection should be tested at the time of admission for delivery.[72] In all HBsAg-positive pregnant women, HBV DNA load should be determined to guide the use of maternal antiviral therapy during pregnancy.[72]

Prevention

HBV infection is prevented either by maternal preconception immunization or by newborn vaccination.[74] Pregnant women should be tested early in pregnancy. Unvaccinated, uninfected women at high risk of acquiring HBV infection should be vaccinated.[71,74] HBV and HBIG can be given during pregnancy and breastfeeding. All infants should be vaccinated for HBV at birth, and those born to HBsAg-positive women should receive HBV vaccine and HBIG within 12 hours of delivery.[72,74] Infants born to women whose HBsAg status is not available but there is evidence suggestive of maternal HBV infection should be managed as those born to an HBsAg-positive mother.[72]

Postvaccination serologic testing should be performed in infants born to HBsAg-positive mothers and in those infants whose mothers' HBsAg status remains unknown.[72] Anti-HBs antibody testing should not be performed before age 9 months to avoid detection of passive anti-HBs antibodies from HBIG administered at birth.[72]

Treatment of HBV Infection in Pregnancy

Antiviral therapy to reduce the risk of perinatal transmission of HBV in pregnant women with an HBV DNA load greater than 200,000 IU/mL or 10^6 copies/mL should be considered.[74,79] Tenofovir is considered the treatment of choice in pregnancy.[74,80] Patients undergoing treatment should begin at 28 to 30 weeks of gestation to allow enough time for HBV DNA levels to decline.[74] Finally, in women with cirrhosis or an advanced histologic feature, antiviral therapy should continue throughout pregnancy to prevent disease progression.[74]

Delivery and Breastfeeding

Mode of delivery does not appear to have a significant effect on HBV vertical transmission. Breastfeeding is encouraged if the infant has received appropriate immunoprophylaxis.[74]

Hepatitis C

Approximately 8% of pregnant women are infected with hepatitis C virus (HCV) worldwide.[82] The primary mode of transmission is parenteral exposure to blood during injection of illicit drugs. Other modes of transmission are vertical, occupational, and sexual intercourse.[68,82] Most pregnant women with HCV have a chronic infection.[74] Overall, vertical transmission occurs in 2% to 8% of infected mothers, but those coinfected with HIV present higher rates of perinatal infection.[68,83]

Although immunity prevails and viremia resolves in 20% to 25% of acute infections, the majority of the infected individuals develop chronic infection[84] and progressive liver damage.[82]

Vertical Transmission

Vertical transmission is the leading cause of HCV infection in children.[82] Risk factors include demonstrable viral load, exposure to maternal blood, prolonged rupture of membranes, internal fetal monitoring during labor,[84] episiotomy, and maternal coinfection with HIV.[82,84] Therefore, peripartum medical management in women with HCV should avoid when possible interventions that increase fetal exposure to maternal fluids.[82]

It is generally accepted that transmission does not occur in the setting of undetectable viral load.[84] In contrast, there is a direct relationship between increasing levels of viremia and enhanced vertical transmission.[84] Route of delivery must follow usual obstetric indications.[82,89,91] When bleeding nipple lesions are not observed, breastfeeding is not associated with increased risk of transmission.[89]

The American Academy of Pediatrics and the CDC recommend screening for anti-HCV antibodies after 18 months of age or for HCV RNA on two occasions after 1 month of the delivery.[82,93]

Screening Tests and Diagnosis

Risk-based screening for HCV in pregnancy is currently recommended[68,82] (**Table 34.4**). High-risk candidates must be tested for anti-HCV antibodies at their first prenatal visit. If negative and risk factors persist, screening should be repeated later in pregnancy.[68,82,94]

Diagnosis of HCV infection is based on detection of HCV RNA and anti-HCV antibodies.

Table 34.4 Hepatitis C in Pregnancy: Screening, Treatment, and Management

Risk Factors That May Indicate the Need for Prenatal Hepatitis C Virus Screening
• Women who ever injected illegal drugs (even once)
• Users of intranasal illicit drugs
• Women ever on long-term hemodialysis
• Women with percutaneous/parenteral exposures in unregulated setting (eg, tattoos received outside of licensed parlors or medical procedures done in settings without strict infection control policies)
• Recipients of transfusions or organ transplants before July 1992 and recipients of clotting factor concentrates produced before 1987
• Recipients of blood products from donor who later tested positive for HCV
• Women with history of incarceration
• Women seeking evaluation or care for sexually transmitted disease, including HIV
• Women with unexplained chronic liver disease (including persistently elevated ALT)

ALT, alanine aminotransferase; HCV, hepatitis C virus; HIV, human immunodeficiency virus.
Modified from Society for Maternal-Fetal Medicine (SMFM), Hughes BL, Page CM, Kuller JA. Hepatitis C in pregnancy: screening, treatment, and management. *Am J Obstet Gynecol*. 2017 Nov;217(5):B2-B12.

Treatment of HCV Infection During Pregnancy

The goal of treatment is to achieve serologic viral response, defined as undetectable HCV RNA 12 to 24 weeks after completing treatment. None of the antiviral therapies recommended for HCV infection are currently approved in pregnancy.[82] Ribavirin is teratogenic in animals.[82]

Hepatitis E

In the general population, hepatitis E virus (HEV) typically causes acute self-limited illness, with a mortality rate of about 0.2% to 1%.[101] However, during pregnancy, it can take a fulminant course, resulting in hepatic failure. In fact, HEV is the most prevalent viral cause of acute liver failure among pregnant women.[1,101] This condition can rapidly progress to acute liver failure, DIC, and encephalopathy.[101,102]

The risk of vertical transmission is 23.3% to 50%. Premature delivery, low birthweight, stillbirth, and neonatal death have been observed in 25% to 56% of infected women.[1,103,104] HEV is often self-limited in the neonate.[69,105] The risk of transmission with breastfeeding is uncertain; therefore, no sound base recommendations can be made.[69,105]

Prevention and Treatment

Pregnant women traveling to endemic areas should follow strict precautions such as washing hands frequently, avoiding nonbottled water, and ice cubes. Fruit and vegetables must be adequately washed with bottled water.[62,101] Raw or undercooked meat consumption should be avoided during pregnancy.[106]

Primary Biliary Cirrhosis and Primary Sclerosing Cholangitis

Primary biliary cirrhosis (PBC) and primary sclerosing cholangitis (PSC) are two major types of chronic cholestatic disease that lead to destruction of intrahepatic bile ducts.[1,114] Both are progressive disorders leading to end-stage liver disease over a 10- to 20-year period.[114]

Primary Biliary Cirrhosis

This condition mainly affects women (10:1)[114,115] of reproductive age.[116] The progression of the disease may ultimately lead to cirrhosis and hepatic failure.[114] Diagnosis requires two out of three of the following criteria: (1) biochemical evidence of cholestasis, (2) presence of serum AMAs (titers of 1:40), and (3) characteristic liver histology.[114] UDCA is the first-line therapy for PBC.[114,115]

Primary Sclerosing Cholangitis

PSC is an idiopathic cholestatic hepatobiliary disease characterized by chronic inflammation, progressive fibrosis, and stricturing of extrahepatic and intrahepatic bile ducts.[114,118,119] It typically progresses slowly over 10 to 15 years, leading to biliary cirrhosis and death.[114,118,120]

Pregnancy Concerns of PBC and PSC

UDCA, a pregnancy category B drug,[30] improves liver function tests and delays histological disease progression.[115] With growing evidence of UDCA safety, it appears prudent to recommend its use for PBC during pregnancy.[1,30,115,121] Cirrhosis is not a contraindication to pregnancy in compensated patients without PH.[114] It has been associated with increased rates of obstetric complications such as spontaneous abortions, premature births, and perinatal deaths.[114] Furthermore, severe maternal morbidity can occur especially among those with PH developing variceal hemorrhage, portosystemic encephalopathy, and hepatic failure.[114] Vaginal delivery with an assisted short second stage, is preferred. However, cesarean delivery is recommended in patients with large varices to avoid delivery-related increases in portal pressure and risk of variceal hemorrhage.[114] Most patients experience stable disease course during pregnancy and high risk of postpartum flares.

PSC has been associated with a 3.63-fold increase risk of preterm birth.[118] No increased risk of intrauterine growth restriction, stillbirths, congenital anomalies, or increased perinatal mortality has been reported.[118]

Budd-Chiari Syndrome

Budd-Chiari syndrome (BCS) is defined as hepatic venous outflow obstruction,[1] leading to sinusoidal congestion, liver ischemic injury, and PH.[122] The main mechanism for BCS is thrombosis. Patients with known BCS have increased risk of developing disease exacerbations during pregnancy.[1]

Clinical features of BCS include right upper quadrant pain, hepatomegaly, jaundice, and ascites. Suspicion must be followed by confirmatory Doppler ultrasound.[1,123] Treatment consists of anticoagulation, angioplasty, or stenting for hepatic vein stenosis. Maternal outcome is generally favorable in women becoming pregnant after the diagnosis and treatment of BCS,[122,124] but fetal loss of 30% before 20 weeks of gestation, as well as an increased risk for preterm birth have been reported.[124]

Cesarean delivery poses increased risk in patients with PH. Large pelvic venous collaterals and postoperative ascites are difficult to manage.[124] Therefore, in the absence of a compelling indication for cesarean delivery, vaginal delivery should be encouraged.[124]

Cirrhosis With PH

Women with cirrhosis have increased risks of spontaneous abortion, prematurity, and perinatal death.[1,125,126] PH usually worsens during pregnancy. All cirrhotic patients should undergo variceal screening[1] in the second trimester.[30] Banding before pregnancy may be appropriate for high-risk varices.[1] The greatest risk is seen in the second trimester and during delivery because of the Valsalva maneuver.[1,126] Each episode of variceal bleeding carries maternal mortality rates as high as 20% to 50%.[30]

Management of variceal bleeding focuses on endoscopic variceal ligation and supportive care for the mother and fetus.[76,128] Octreotide along with antibiotics appears to be a safe option as an adjunct treatment in acute bleeding.[30]

Patients with cirrhosis have a 10% risk of postpartum hemorrhage that may be associated to coagulopathy and thrombocytopenia due to hypersplenism.[76] Cesarean delivery carries increased risk of bleeding complications in women with PH.[30] Therefore, vaginal delivery with shortened second stage has been advocated.[30,62]

Contraception is recommended in the acute phase of disease or if liver transplant is likely to occur.[76] Pregnancy should be planned when liver disease is stable. Elective termination of pregnancy can be considered in women with severe hepatic decompensation and liver failure.[76]

Liver Transplantation

Pregnancy should be deferred for at least 1 year after liver transplantation. Although over 70% of grafted women will deliver a healthy baby,[1] pregnancy complications have been reported.

The fetal risks of exposure to cyclosporine, tacrolimus, azathioprine, sirolimus, everolimus, and corticosteroids appear to be low, and the consequences of acute cellular rejection or graft loss with their discontinuation pose a much grave prognosis.[30] Finally, mycophenalate mofetil has been associated with significant teratogenicity and should be discontinued before or during pregnancy.[1]

KEY POINTS

- Approximately 3% of all pregnancies are complicated by liver disorders.
- HG occurs in 0.3% to 3% of pregnancies and it is the most common cause of hospitalization in the first trimester. Typical signs and symptoms of HG include vomiting not related to other causes, and an objective measure of acute starvation such as large ketonuria and weight loss.
- Fetal risks of HG include low birthweight, preterm labor, and small for gestational age infants.
- Treatment of HG with vitamin B6 (pyridoxine) alone or plus doxylamine is considered the first-line pharmacotherapy. Hospitalization is recommended if oral intolerance is a concern or there is lack of response to outpatient management.

- ICP is the most common pregnancy-specific liver disease. Its classical feature is pruritus without rash or any specific dermal lesion, typically occurring in the third trimester. Pruritus typically affects the palms and soles but may occur anywhere. It is often worse at night, disturbing the sleep pattern, and may deteriorate as pregnancy advances.
- Fetal complications of ICP are directly related to the toxic effect of bile acids. An elevated risk of stillbirth was reported with SBA levels greater than 40 µmol/L, with the highest risk being observed when levels are greater than 100 µmol/L.
- ICP is commonly treated with UDCA. Randomized trials showed significant improvements in pruritus and liver function tests with UDCA.

- There is no proven effective antenatal monitoring strategy to prevent stillbirth in ICP. To reduce the risk of stillbirth, many authors have advocated for elective early delivery. However, no randomized studies have established the optimal timing of delivery for pregnancies complicated by ICP.
- Hepatic involvement affects approximately 10% of women with severe preeclampsia. Complications can include subcapsular hematoma, and hepatic rupture.
- Subcapsular liver hematoma is a life-threatening condition and occurs in 0.9% to 1.6% of gestations complicated by HELLP syndrome. Clinical suspicion should prompt further evaluation. Ultrasound is a reasonable initial approach, but findings need to be confirmed with either CT scan or MRI.
- Unruptured subcapsular liver hematoma in a hemodynamically stable patient can be conservatively managed. Even mild trauma to the liver, such as abdominal palpation, must be avoided because it can lead to the rupture and catastrophic bleeding.
- Hemodynamically unstable patients with the suspicion of ruptured hematoma require invasive hemostatic measures.
- AFLP is an uncommon but potentially fatal disease unique to pregnancy that typically occurs after 30 weeks of gestation. Maternal mortality due to AFLP is currently about 12%.
- The most common initial symptoms of AFLP are anorexia, malaise, nausea, vomiting, and headache. Additional features are epigastric pain, jaundice, hypertension, and DIC.
- AFLP and HELLP syndrome are coexistent in approximately 50% of patients. Hypoglycemia is a valuable finding in the differential diagnosis with preeclampsia and HELLP syndrome.
- Treatment is supportive. Delivery should not be delayed in patients with the suspicion of AFLP.
- Acute cholecystitis is the second most common surgical condition in pregnancy. Medical management consists of intravenous hydration, fasting, analgesics, and antibiotics. Most women will benefit from surgical treatment. Early cholecystectomy is the most appropriate approach in symptomatic patients. Both open and laparoscopic cholecystectomy are best deferred until the second trimester.

- HBV infection is caused by a DNA virus and it is transmitted by parenteral and sexual contact.
- Vertical transmission is responsible for about half of chronic HBV infections worldwide and generally occurs at the time of delivery. Infants born to mothers with high viral loads are at greatest risk for infection.
- When acute HBV infection occurs early in pregnancy, the rate of perinatal transmission is about 10% and increases to 60% if it occurs close to delivery.
- The risk of vertical transmission can be as high as 90%, especially if the mother was infected in the third trimester, is HbeAg positive, and has a viral load greater than 10^6 copies/mL.
- All pregnant women should be tested for HBsAg at an early prenatal visit in each pregnancy, even if they have been previously vaccinated or screened.
- In all HBsAg-positive pregnant women, HBV DNA load should be determined.
- HBV infection is prevented either by maternal preconception immunization or by newborn vaccination. Hepatitis B vaccine and immunoglobulin can be given during pregnancy and breastfeeding.
- All infants should be vaccinated for HBV at birth, and those born to HBsAg-positive women should receive HBV vaccine and HBIG within 12 hours of delivery. Antiviral therapy to reduce the risk of perinatal transmission of HBV in pregnant women with an HBV DNA load greater than 200,000 IU/mL or 10^6 copies/mL should be considered.
- Women with cirrhosis achieving pregnancy have increased risks of spontaneous abortion, prematurity, and perinatal death.
- All cirrhotic patients should undergo variceal screening preconception and in the second trimester. Banding before pregnancy may be appropriate for high-risk varices. The greatest risk of bleeding is seen in the second trimester and during delivery because of the Valsalva maneuver. Vaginal delivery with shortened second stage has been advocated.
- Pregnancy should be deferred for at least 1 year after liver transplantation. The fetal risks of immunosuppressants appear to be low, and the consequences of acute cellular rejection or graft loss with their discontinuation pose a much grave prognosis.

REFERENCES

(only references cited in synoptic print chapter; for a complete reference list, see ebook)

1. Joshi D, James A, Quaglia A, et al. Liver disease in pregnancy. *Lancet.* 2010;375(9714):594-605.
3. Bacak SJ, Thornburg LL. Liver failure in pregnancy. *Crit Care Clin.* 2016;32(1):61-72.
7. Niemeijer MN, Grooten IJ, Vos N, et al. Diagnostic markers for hyperemesis gravidarum: a systematic review and metaanalysis. *Am J Obstet Gynecol.* 201;211(2):150.e1-150.e15.
8. Dean CR, Shemar M, Ostrowski GAU, et al. Management of severe pregnancy sickness and hyperemesis gravidarum. *Br Med J.* 2018;363:k5000.
9. London V, Grube S, Sherer DM, et al. Hyperemesis gravidarum: a review of recent literature. *Pharmacology.* 2017;100(3-4):161-171.
11. Committee on Practice Bulletins-Obstetrics. ACOG Practice Bulletin No. 189: nausea and vomiting of pregnancy. *Obstet Gynecol.* 2018;131(1):e15-e30.
13. Lee NM, Saha S. Nausea and vomiting of pregnancy. *Gastroenterol Clin North Am.* 2011;40:309-334.
19. Dean C, Bannigan K, O'Hara M, et al. Recurrence rates of hyperemesis gravidarum in pregnancy: a systematic review protocol. *JBI Database System Rev Implement Rep.* 2017;15:2659-2665.
20. Koren G, Maltepe C. Pre-emptive therapy for severe nausea and vomiting of pregnancy and hyperemesis gravidarum. *J Obstet Gynaecol.* 2004;24:530-533.
28. Williamson C, Geenes V. Intrahepatic cholestasis of pregnancy. *Obstet Gynecol.* 2014;124(1):120-133.
29. Wood AM, Livingston EG, Hughes BL, et al. Intrahepatic cholestasis of pregnancy: a review of diagnosis and management. *Obstet Gynecol Surv.* 2018;73(2):103-109.
30. Tran TT, Ahn J, Reau NS. ACG Clinical Guideline: liver disease and pregnancy. *Am J Gastroenterol.* 2016;111(2):176-194
36. Geenes V, Chappell LC, Seed PT, et al. Association of severe intrahepatic cholestasis of pregnancy with adverse pregnancy outcomes: a prospective population-based case-control study. *Hepatology.* 2014;59:1482-1491.
37. Glantz A, Marschall HU, Mattsson LA. Intrahepatic cholestasis of pregnancy: relationships between bile acid levels and fetal complication rates. *Hepatology.* 2004;40:467-474.
38. Brouwers L, Koster MP, Page-Christiaens GC, et al. Intrahepatic cholestasis of pregnancy: maternal and fetal outcomes associ- ated with elevated bile acid levels. *Am J Obstet Gynecol.* 2015;212:100.e1-100.e7.
39. Kawakita T, Parikh LI, Ramsey PS, et al. Predictors of adverse neonatal outcomes in intrahepatic cholestasis of pregnancy. *Am J Obstet Gynecol.* 2015;213:570.e1-570.e8.
40. Chappell LC, Gurung V, Seed PT, et al. Ursodeoxycholic acid versus placebo, and early term delivery versus expectant management, in women with intrahepatic cholestasis of pregnancy: semifactorial randomised clinical trial. *Br Med J.* 2012;344:e3799.
41. Bacq Y, Sentilhes L, Reyes H, et al. Efficacy of ursodeoxycholic acid in treating intrahepatic cholestasis of pregnancy: a meta-analysis. *Gastroenterology.* 2012;143:1492-1501.
43. Puljic A, Kim E, Page J, et al. The risk of infant and fetal death by each additional week of expectant management in intrahepatic cholestasis of pregnancy by gestational age. *Am J Obstet Gynecol.* 2015;212:667.e1-667.e5.
45. Williamson C, Hems LM, Goulis DG, et al. Clinical outcome in a series of cases of obstetric cholestasis identified via a patient support group. *Br J Obstet Gynecol.* 2004;111:676-681.
46. Weinstein L. Syndrome of hemolysis, elevated liver enzymes, and low platelet count: a severe consequence of hypertension in pregnancy. *Am J Obstet Gynecol.* 1982;142(2):159-167.
47. Yoshihara M, Mayama M, Ukai M, et al. Fulminant liver failure resulting from massive hepatic infarction associated with hemolysis, elevated liver enzymes, and low platelets síndrome. *J Obstet Gynaecol Res.* 2016;42(10):1375-1378.
48. Goel A, Jamwal KD, Ramachandran A, et al. Pregnancy-related liver disorders. *J Clin Exp Hepatol.* 2014;4(2):151-162.
49. Ditisheim A, Sibai BM. Diagnosis and management of HELLP syndrome complicated by liver hematoma. *Clin Obstet Gynecol.* 2017;60(1):190-197.

50. Haddad B, Barton JR, Livingston JC, et al. Risk factors for adverse maternal outcomes among women with HELLP (hemolysis, elevated liver enzymes, and low platelet count) syndrome. *Am J Obstet Gynecol.* 2000;183:444-448.
51. Sibai BM, Ramadan MK, Usta I, et al. Maternal morbidity and mortality in 442 pregnancies with hemolysis, elevated liver enzymes, and low platelets (HELLP syndrome). *Am J Obstet Gynecol.* 1993; 169:1000-1006.
52. Chou PY, Yu CH, Chen CC, et al. Spontaneously ruptured subcapsular liver hematoma associated with hemolysis, elevated liver enzymes and low plateles (HELLP) syndrome. *Taiwan J Obstet Gynecol.* 2010;49(2):214-217.
55. Liu J, Ghaziani TT, Wolf JL. Acute fatty liver disease of pregnancy: updates in pathogenesis, diagnosis, and management. *Am J Gastroenterol.* 2017;112(6):838-846.
56. Lamprecht A, Morton A, Laurie J, et al. Acute fatty liver of pregnancy and concomitant medical conditions: a review of cases at a quaternary obstetric hospital. *Obstet Med.* 2018;11(4):178-181.
57. Xiong HF, Liu JY, Guo LM, et al. Acute fatty liver of pregnancy: over six months follow-up study of twenty-five patients. *World J Gastroenterol.* 2015;21(6):1927-1931.
58. Wajner M, Amaral AU. Mitochondrial dysfunction in fatty acid oxidation disorders: insights from human and animal studies. *Biosci Rep.* 2015;36(1):e00281.
62. Almashhrawi AA, Ahmed KT, Rahman RN, et al. Liver diseases in pregnancy: diseases not unique to pregnancy. *World J Gastroenterol.* 2013;19:7630-7638.
63. İlhan M, İlhan G, Gök AFK. The course and outcomes of complicated gallstone disease in pregnancy: experience of a tertiary center. *Turk J Obstet Gynecol.* 2016;13(4):178-182.
64. Date RS, Kaushal M, Ramesh A. A review of the management of gallstone disease and its complications in pregnancy. *Am J Surg.* 2008;196(4):599-608.
65. Hedström J, Nilsson J, Andersson R. Changing management of gallstone-related disease in pregnancy – a retrospective cohort analysis. *Scand J Gastroenterol.* 2017;52(9):1016-1021.
68. American College of Obstetricians and Gynecologists. ACOG Practice Bulletin No. 86: viral hepatitis in pregnancy. *Obstet Gynecol.* 2007;110(4):941-956.
69. Rac MW, Sheffield JS. Prevention and management of viral hepatitis in pregnancy. *Obstet Gynecol Clin North Am.* 2014;41(4):573-592.
71. ACOG Committee Opinion No. 741: maternal immunization. *Obstet Gynecol.* 2018;131(6):e214-e217.
72. Schillie S, Vellozzi C, Reingold A, et al. Prevention of hepatitis B virus infection in the United States: recommendations of the advisory committee on immunization Practices. *MMWR Recomm Rep.* 2018;67(1):1-31.
74. Shao Z, Al Tibi M, Wakim-Fleming J. Update on viral hepatitis in pregnancy. *Cleve Clin J Med.* 2017;84(3):202-206.
76. Aggarwal N, Negi N, Aggarwal A, et al. Pregnancy with portal hypertension. *J Clin Exp Hepatol.* 2014;4(2):163-171.
79. Terrault NA, Bzowej NH, Chang KM, et al; American Association for the Study of Liver Diseases. AASLD guidelines for treatment of chronic hepatitis B. *Hepatology.* 2016;63:261-283.
80. Brown RS Jr, Verna EC, Pereira MR ,et al. Hepatitis B virus and human immunodeficiency virus drugs in pregnancy: findings from the antiretroviral pregnancy registry. *J Hepatol.* 2012;57:953-959.
82. Hughes BL, Page CM, Kuller JA; Society for Maternal-Fetal Medicine (SMFM). Hepatitis C in pregnancy: screening, treatment, and management. *Am J Obstet Gynecol.* 2017;217(5):B2-B12.
83. Floreani A. Hepatitis C and pregnancy. *World J Gastroenterol.* 2013;19(40):6714-6720.
84. Prasad MR, Honegger JR. Hepatitis C virus in pregnancy. *Am J Perinatol.* 2013;30(2):149-159.
89. Dibba P, Cholankeril R, Li AA, et al. Hepatitis C in pregnancy. *Diseases.* 2018;6(2):31.
91. Connell LE, Salihu HM, Salemi JL, et al. Maternal hepatitis B and hepatitis C carrier status and perinatal outcomes. *Liver Int.* 2011;31:1163-1170.
93. Recommendations for care of children in special circumstances: hepatitis C. In: Kimberlin DW, Brady MT, Jackson MA, et al, eds. *Red Book: 2015 Report of the Committee on Infectious Diseases. American Academy of Pediatrics. Committee on Infectious Diseases; American Academy of Pediatrics.* American Academy of Pediatrics; 2015:197.

94. Joint Panel From the American Association for the Study of Liver Diseases and the Infectious Diseases Society of America. *Recommendations for Testing, Managing, and Treating Hepatitis C.* Accessed July 19, 2019. http://www.hcvguidelines.org/

101. Pérez-Gracia MT, Suay-García B, Mateos-Lindemann ML. Hepatitis E and pregnancy: current state. *Rev Med Virol.* 2017;27:e1929.

102. Kaskheli MN, Baloch S, Sheeba A, et al. Acute hepatitis E viral infection in pregnancy and maternal morbidity. *J Coll Physicians Surg Pak.* 2015;24:734-737.

103. Sayed I, Vercouter AS, Abdelwahab S, et al. Is hepatitis E virus an emerging problem in industrialized countries? *Hepatology.* 2015;62:1883-1892.

104. Chaundhry S, Verma N, Koren D. Hepatitis E infection during pregnancy. *Can Fam Physician.* 2015;61:607-608.

105. Krain LJ, Atwell JE, Nelson KE, et al. Review article: fetal and neonatal health con- sequences of vertically transmitted hepatitis E virus infection. *Am J Trop Med Hyg.* 2014;90(2):365-370.

106. Pérez-Gracia MT, García M, Suay B, et al. Current knowledge on hepatitis E. *J Clin Transl Hepatol.* 2015;3(2):117-126.

114. Marchioni Beery RM, Vaziri H, Forouhar F, et al. Primary biliary cirrhosis and primary sclerosing cholangitis: a review featuring a women's health perspective. *J Clin Transl Hepatol.* 2014;2(4):266-284.

115. Efe C, Kahramanoğlu-Aksoy E, Yilmaz B, et al. Pregnancy in women with primary biliary cirrhosis. *Autoimmun Rev.* 2014;13(9):931-935.

116. Trivedi PJ, Kumagi T, Al-Harthy N, et al. Good maternal and fetal outcomes for pregnant women' with primary biliary cirrhosis. *Clin Gastroenterol Hepatol.* 2014;12:1179-1185.e1.

118. Ludvigsson JF, Bergquist A, Ajne G, et al. A population based cohort study of pregnancy outcomes among women with primary sclerosing cholangitis. *Clin Gastroenterol Hepatol.* 2014;12(1):95-100.e1.

119. Pataia V, Dixon PH, Williamson C, et al. Pregnancy and bile acid disorders. *Am J Physiol Gastrointest Liver Physiol.* 2017;313(1):G1-G6.

120. Wellge BE, Sterneck M, Teufel A, et al. Pregnancy in primary sclerosing cholangitis. *Gut.* 2011;60(8):1117-1121.

121. Floreani A, Infantolino C, Franceschet I, et al. Pregnancy and primary biliary cirrhosis: a case-control study. *Clin Rev Allergy Immunol.* 2015;48(2-3):236-242.

122. Khan F, Rowe I, Martin B, et al. Outcomes of pregnancy in patients with known Budd-Chiari syndrome. *World J Hepatol.* 2017;9(21):945-952.

123. Merz WM, Rüland AM, Hippe V, et al. Pregnancy in Budd-Chiari syndrome: case report and proposed risk score. *Medicine (Baltimore).* 2016;95(22):e3817.

124. Rautou PE, Angermayr B, Garcia-Pagan JC, et al. Pregnancy in women with known and treated Budd-Chiari syndrome: maternal and fetal outcomes. *J Hepatol.* 2009;51(1):47-54.

125. Shaheen AA, Myers RP. The outcomes of pregnancy in patients with cirrhosis: a population-based study. *Liver Int.* 2010;30(2):275-283.

126. Rasheed SM, Abdel Monem AM, Abd Ellah AH, et al. Prognosis and determinants of pregnancy outcome among patients with post-hepatitis liver cirrhosis. *Int J Gynaecol Obstet.* 2013;121:247-251.

128. Chaudhuri K, Tan EK, Biswas A. Successful pregnancy in a woman with liver cirrhosis complicated by recurrent variceal bleeding. *J Obstet Gynaecol.* 2012;32:490-491.

CHAPTER 35

Pregnancy Complicated by Renal Disorders

Denise Trigubo, Mercedes Negri Malbrán, and
Gustavo F. Leguizamón

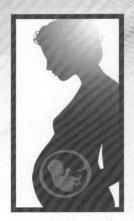

Introduction

Physiologic renal changes are cornerstone for adequate placental development, and even mildly impaired kidney function is associated with increased probability of adverse pregnancy outcomes. Furthermore, pregnancy can worsen the course of preexisting nephropathy or unmask an undiagnosed primary renal disease.

These physiological modifications must be acknowledged in order to properly diagnose and manage renal disorders during pregnancy.

Kidney growth and hydronephrosis are the most remarkable anatomical changes.

Normal pregnancy is characterized by vasodilation resulting in reduction of peripheral vascular resistance, increased cardiac output, and decreased arterial blood pressure.[8] These hemodynamic changes lead to enhancement of renal plasma flow (RPF).

The glomerular hyperfiltration and the modifications in tubular reabsorption are also responsible for changes in serum levels of analytes that may challenge the interpretation of renal and metabolic conditions (**Table 35.1**).

Clinical Assessment of Renal Function in Pregnancy

Measuring serum creatinine and 24-hour urine collection for creatinine clearance are currently the most reliable surrogates of glomerular filtration rate (GFR) and are the preferred methods to assess renal function during gestation in women with nephropathy.[9]

A serum creatinine of 1.0 mg/dL, which is considered normal in nonpregnant subjects, may reflect renal impairment during gestation.[11]

Proteinuria is usually a sign of renal injury and if persistent may represent ongoing renal damage.

Chronic Kidney Disease and Pregnancy

The prevalence of chronic kidney disease (CKD) in women of childbearing age ranges from 0.1% to 3%.[14]

Table 35.1 Normal Laboratory Values During Pregnancy

Variable	Normal Values	Average Values in pregnancy
Plasma osmolality (mOsm/kg)	275-295	275-280
Serum sodium (mEq/L)	135-145	130-148
Serum potassium (mEq/L)	3.5-5.0	3.3-5.1
Serum bicarbonate (mEq/L)	22-30	18-22
Serum creatinine (mg/dL)	1.0-1.2	0.4-0.8
Blood urea nitrogen (mg/dL)	8-10	5-8
Uric acid (mg/dL)	2.5-5.6	2-3
24-h protein excretion (mg/24 h)	<150	<300
Glomerular filtration rate (GFR)	106-132	117-182
24-h creatinine clearance (mL/min)	91-130	50-166

Values may vary throughout gestation.

e *See the eBook for expanded content, a complete reference list, and additional tables.*

Table 35.2 Chronic Kidney Disease (CKD) Stages According to Estimated Glomerular Filtration Rate (GFR)

Stage	GFR (mL/min/1.73 m²)
1	≥90 (normal or high)
2	60-89 (mildly decreased)
3a	45-59 (mildly to moderately decreased)
3b	30-44 (moderately to severely decreased)
4	15-29 (severely decreased)
5	<15 (kidney failure)

Renal disease increases the risk of adverse pregnancy outcomes, and the gestation can accelerate the progression of this condition. The degree of renal insufficiency is considered a critical prognostic factor. Two different groups of women with CKD can be identified. Early disease is defined as serum creatinine below 1.4 mg/dL, creatinine clearance greater than 70 mL/min, or stages 1 to 2 CKD.[15] On the other hand, advanced disease is characterized by serum creatinine greater than 1.4 mg/dL, creatinine clearence below 70 mL/min, and stages 3 to 5 CKD.[15]

Table 35.2 depicts CKD stages.

Impact of CKD on pregnancy outcomes

Patients with CKD have a greater risk of pregnancy complications, such as preeclampsia (PE) (odds ratio [OR] 10.3), preterm birth (OR 5.72), low birth weight (OR 4.85), cesarean delivery (OR 2.87), and perinatal death (OR 1.8).

Severe renal impairment, chronic hypertension, and proteinuria have been identified as risk factors that worsen perinatal outcomes among women with CKD.[15,16]

Furthermore, renal compromise in the context of a systemic condition, such as diabetes or systemic lupus erythematosus (SLE), presents an excess risk.

Finally, with the exception of diabetic kidney disease and autosomal dominant polycystic kidney disease, the frequency of fetal congenital malformations is not increased in pregnancies complicated with CKD.[18]

Table 35.3 depicts the outcomes in CKD.

Impact of pregnancy on CKD

Different investigators observed a strong association between advanced-stage CKD and progression of renal disease.

In fact, there is evidence to believe that GFR ≤ 40 mL/min with proteinuria ≥ 1 g/24 h are risk factors for progression of renal dysfunction during or after pregnancy.[16,19]

In conclusion, in women with early CKD and preserved renal function in early pregnancy, a significant renal deterioration is unlikely, especially if high blood pressure and proteinuria are either absent or negligible.

Pregnancy in End-Stage Renal Disease

Hemodialysis in Pregnancy

Although fertility decreases throughout the spectrum of CKD stages,[20] the incidence of pregnancy in women on dialysis has increased during the past decades.[15]

Although perinatal survival has consistently improved, maternal and fetal morbidity remains substantial. Worsening hypertension (50%-70%), polyhydramnios (40%), PE (18%-67%), intrauterine growth restriction (IUGR) (17%-77%), prematurity,

Table 35.3 Obstetrical Outcomes Across the Spectrum of Chronic Kidney Disease (CKD)

Variable		CKD Stage			
		1	**2**	**3**	**4/5**
Cesarean delivery (%)		48.4	70.1	78.4	70.0
GA at birth (weeks)		37.6 ± 2.6	35.7 ± 3.2	34.4 ± 2.4	32.6 ± 4.2
Preterm birth (%)	<37 wk	23.5	50.6	78.4	70.0
	<34 wk	7.3	20.7	37.8	44.4
Birth weight (grams)		2966.5 ± 659	2484 ± 707	2226.3 ± 582	1639 ± 870
Admission to NICU (%)		10.3	27.6	44.4	70.0
CKD upstage or need for RRT (%)		7.6	12.6	16.2	20.0

GA, gestational age; NICU, neonatal intensive care unit; RRT, renal replacement therapy.
Adapted from Piccoli GB, Cabiddu G, Attini R, et al. Risk of adverse pregnancy outcomes in women with CKD. *J Am Soc Nephrol.* 2015;26:2011-2022.

and low birth weight (50%-100%) are significantly higher than in the general population.[21]

Women who initiate dialysis during pregnancy have a higher rate of live birth (91%) than those who conceive while on hemodialysis (HD) (63%).[22]

There is a remarkable correlation between BUN levels and pregnancy-associated risks. In fact, the proportion of fetal demise, preterm delivery, and low birth weight seem to increase with BUN levels ≥50 mg/dL.[23,24]

Recent data have demonstrated that pregnancy outcomes significantly improve when the patient undergoes HD for at least 36 h/wk.[25]

Therefore, intensified HD regimes (>36 h/wk) are strongly recommended.[27]

Volume management during HD is challenging.

As a general rule, it can be considered that the normal dry weight increase during the second and third trimesters of pregnancy is 0.5 kg/wk.

Attempts should be made to minimize large fluid shifts during HD because these can be associated with hypertension as well as hypotension.

Ideally, during and after dialysis, blood pressure should not be lower than 120/70 mm Hg and should not exceed 140/90 mm Hg.[8,28]

If no other conditions, such as diabetes, are present, no dietary restrictions are made, and nutritional advice should be offered to guarantee proper protein intake (approximately 1.5-1.8 mg/kg/d). Supplements of 5 mg/d of folic acid and prenatal vitamins should be prescribed.[28,29]

Monitoring and treatment of anemia is an important consideration among pregnant women undergoing HD. To achieve a target hemoglobin level of 10 to 11 g/dL, a significant increase of the erythropoietin (EPO) dose is required. Furthermore, oral and/or intravenous iron sucrose should be supplemented as required to maintain adequate iron stores.[28]

The authors recommend renal replacement therapy (RRT) in pregnant patients with a creatinine clearance < 20 mL/min or with ongoing progressive kidney function loss, in which urea (BUN) consistently exceeds 20 mmol/L (56 mg/dL).[28]

Renal Transplantation

Following successful renal transplantation, fertility is restored and pregnancy outcomes are better than those in women with advanced stages of CKD.[20]

Although the live birth rate in pregnant women who underwent a prior renal transplant is close to 73%, maternal and fetal adverse events remain

higher than the general population.[30] In fact, the rate of PE has increased sixfold (21.5% vs 3.8%), and the risk of preterm birth is 43.1%, with a mean gestational age at delivery of 35 weeks and a mean birth weight of 2470 g.[30]

On the other hand, the overall acute rejection rate during gestation is comparable to the general population (9.4% vs 9.1%). Thus, for patients with advanced CKD and those receiving RRT who wish to conceive, it is advisable to attempt to defer pregnancy until after kidney transplantation.

The American Society of Transplantation recommends postponing pregnancy for 1 to 2 years after transplantation.[30]

Immunosuppressants commonly prescribed in patients with renal transplant are tacrolimus, cyclosporine, azathioprine, and prednisolone. These drugs are all considered to be safe during pregnancy and breastfeeding.[31]

In addition, prolonged treatment with prednisolone may be associated with maternal adrenal suppression; therefore, a stress dosage at delivery and in the first 24 to 48 hours postpartum must be administered. Azathioprine is well tolerated by both the mother and fetus at doses <2 mg/kg/d.

To achieve stable target levels of antirejection drugs in pregnancy, a 20% to 25% dose elevation may be required.[32]

Principles of Management of Pregnancy Complicated by CKD

Preconception Counseling

Preconception counseling is crucial in the setting of CKD.

Adequate metabolic control in women with diabetes, quiescent autoimmune disease for 6 months, and adequate treatment of blood pressure in women with chronic hypertension will significantly improve maternal and perinatal outcomes.

Women with CKD and preserved renal function (serum creatinine < 1.5 mg/dL, creatinine Cl > 70 mL/min, or CKD stages 1-2) are unlikely to suffer permanent deterioration. On the other hand, women with more advanced disease (serum creatinine ≥ 1.5 mg/dL, or creatinine Cl < 40 mL/min) may have a permanent loss of more than 25% of baseline renal function after pregnancy.[16,17,19,20]

Stabilization of kidney dysfunction should be accomplished before conception to increase the likelihood of success. Especially in women with advanced-stage CKD (stages 4-5), postponing conception until after renal transplantation is a reasonable option and should be discussed.

A thorough evaluation of drugs should be performed, and whenever possible, potential teratogenic agents should be withdrawn and replaced with drugs considered safe in pregnancy.[33]

Finally, and especially for women with advanced kidney disease or significant comorbidities, other alternatives for becoming a parent, such as surrogacy or adoption, should be discussed.

Antenatal Care

Medical care during the antepartum period should be delivered by a multidisciplinary team involving maternal-fetal medicine specialists, nephrologists, and neonatologists. Furthermore, it should be carried out in a tertiary care institution with neonatal intensive care and dialysis facilities.[18]

The frequency of visits should be tailored to the patient's degree of renal insufficiency and to the presence of risk factors such as proteinuria, hypertension, and a coexisting systemic disease. A reasonable approach in a stable patient would be monthly evaluation by a nephrologist and obstetrical biweekly evaluation until 32 weeks, followed by weekly visits until delivery. Because the risk of pregnancy-associated complications increases across the spectrum of kidney disease, it is recommended to intensify the frequency of medical controls in advanced stages.[18]

Intensive blood pressure control with pregnancy-safe antihypertensive drugs is essential with a blood pressure target below 140/90 mm Hg.[13,15] Abrupt changes in blood pressure and the need for a higher dose of medication should raise concern of PE.

Baseline concentrations of serum creatinine, uric acid, liver enzymes, platelet count, and urine protein excretion should be determined early in gestation for reference later on pregnancy.[13] Furthermore, evidence of hemolysis manifested by increased lactate dehydrogenase (LDH), decreased haptoglobin, or presence of schistocytes in peripheral blood smear can aid in the differential diagnosis between PE and worsening basal condition.

Although data are limited for patients with chronic renal disease, initiation of low-dose aspirin before the 16th week of gestation to prevent early-onset PE is recommended.[13,35,36]

Because patients with CKD carry a greater risk for urinary tract infections (UTIs), urine culture for asymptomatic bacteriuria (ASB) should be performed at least monthly.[20]

Considering the enhanced risk for IUGR, fetal biometry assessment should be performed every 2 to 3 weeks. If fetal growth is below the 10th percentile or the growth velocity lags behind, at least weekly Doppler evaluation should be performed to detect signs of severe placental insufficiency. We suggest complementing fetal evaluation with a non-stress test (NST) and biophysical profile (BPP) from 32 to 34 weeks onwards.

The timing of delivery should be individualized according to comorbidities.

Whenever possible, and to reduce prematurity-related complications, it is recommended to prolong pregnancy until term. The mode of delivery should be based on routine obstetric considerations.

Table 35.4 summarizes the general principles of management of pregnancy complicated by CKD.

Renal Biopsy

Kidney biopsy during pregnancy has been associated with severe bleeding complications.[18] Therefore, it should be limited to situations where proper diagnosis allows for specific treatment and safe continuation of pregnancy.[8] Because the risks will most likely outweigh the benefits, this procedure is best avoided after 30 weeks of gestation.[8,38]

Acute Kidney Injury

Acute kidney injury (AKI) in pregnancy has no uniform diagnostic criteria.[39] It is generally defined as an abrupt (within hours) decrease of renal function of varying degrees that progress from a mild increase in serum creatinine levels to overt organ failure with dialysis requirements.[38,40]

AKI is often underrecognized during pregnancy, and therefore, diagnosis is achieved only in advanced stages leading to excess maternal and perinatal morbidity and mortality.[41] Most patients fully recover renal function, but up to one-third can experience long-term renal compromise.[39]

Identifying the underlying causes of AKI is crucial to provide appropriate treatment, especially when this could mean prompt delivery of the fetus.[38]

Based on the nature of the injury and its pathophysiology, AKI is classified into three types: prerenal, intrinsic, and postrenal. Whereas the intrinsic form represents genuine renal disease, the other types are secondary to extrarenal conditions that impair GFR.[40] However, if pre- or postrenal conditions persist, they will most likely progress to intrinsic AKI.[40]

Table 35.4 Principles of Management of Pregnancy Complicated by Chronic Kidney Disease (CKD)

Preconception Counseling

- Determine renal function (SCr, CrCl, 24-h urine collection)
- Assessment of baseline disease activity (HbA1c, anti-DNA antibodies, C3, C4, etc)
- Blood pressure control
- Review medication and remove or replace teratogenic agents by drugs considered safe for pregnancy
- Assessment of pregnancy risks and consideration of other alternatives of family planning
- Initiate folic acid 4 mg daily

Antenatal Care

- Same as above in the absence of preconception counseling
- Intensify blood pressure control → target: ≤ 140/90 mm Hg
- Management of anemia → target Hb level 10-11 g/dL
- Initiate low-dose aspirin before the 16th week to prevent preeclampsia
- Monthly urine culture
- Dietary monitoring with daily protein intake of 1.5-1.8 mg/kg
- Monthly evaluation by nephrologist
- Obstetrical follow-up every 2 wk and weekly from 32 wk onwards (intensify antepartum surveillance according to CKD stage and associated comorbidities)
  - Fetal growth assessment every 2-3 wk
  - Doppler evaluation if EFW < p10
  - NST and BPP from 32-34 wk onwards

Postpartum Care

- Ensure that medication is compatible with breastfeeding

BPP, biophysical profile; CrCl, creatinine clearance; Hb, hemoglobin; NST, nonstress test; SCr, serum creatinine.

In *prerenal AKI*, the underlying cause of decreased GFR is renal hypoperfusion, without initial renal parenchyma damage.[40] In the first trimester, the most common etiologies are hyperemesis gravidarum and septic abortion. During the second half of pregnancy, obstetric emergencies, such as placental abruption or severe postpartum hemorrhage, are the most frequent causes. Although with adequate support full recovery is usually achieved, severe cases may result in irreversible acute cortical necrosis leading to permanent kidney failure.[38,42]

Furthermore, an acute obstruction of the urinary tract can cause *postrenal AKI*. During pregnancy, the most frequent etiologies are bilateral ureteral or bladder outlet obstruction secondary to a tumor or nephrolithiasis, iatrogenic injury during an emergency cesarean delivery or puerperal hysterectomy, and hydronephrosis due to uterine compression.[38]

Intrinsic renal AKI can be caused by injury to the tubules, glomeruli, interstitium, or intrarenal blood vessels. Pregnancy-related etiologies include PE, HELLP(hemolysis, elevated liver enzymes, and low platelet count) syndrome, acute fatty liver of pregnancy (AFLP), thrombotic microangiopathies like atypical hemolytic uremic syndrome (aHUS), and thrombotic thrombocytopenic purpura (TTP). **Table 35.5.**

Common Causes of AKI During Pregnancy

PE and HELLP Syndrome

The American College of Obstetricians and Gynecologists defines renal insufficiency in the context of PE as a serum creatinine level ≥ 1.1 mg/dL or as a doubling of the serum creatinine concentration in the absence of other renal disease.[13] AKI rarely complicates PE, but the frequency increases significantly if HELLP syndrome is superimposed (1% vs 15%, respectively).[43,44,45]

To prevent renal ischemia, careful empiric vascular volume resuscitation should be promptly initiated.[43] Furthermore, other comorbidities observed in PE, such as hemorrhage, coagulopathy, acute tubular necrosis (ATN), and depressed myocardial function,[43] can worsen the prognosis.

The renal and extrarenal abnormalities of PE and HELLP syndrome typically begin to resolve within 2 to 3 days postpartum, but complete recovery of GFR and heavy proteinuria can take up to 3 to 6 months.[46]

Atypical Hemolytic Uremic Syndrome

Atypical or complement-mediated HUS is defined by the presence of hemolytic anemia, thrombocytopenia, and impaired renal function, with up to a 75% risk of end-stage renal disease (ESRD).[47] It is a thrombotic microangiopathy that is caused by mutations in genes that encode for proteins in the alternative complement pathway, resulting in uncontrolled alternative complement activation.[48]

Effective treatment of aHUS with eculizumab has been reported.[47,50]

Table 35.5 Differential Diagnosis of Acute Kidney Injury Etiologies During Pregnancy

	PE/HELLP Syndrome	TTP	aHUS	AFLP	Lupus Nephritis Flare
Timing of pregnancy	>20 wk	Second/third trimester	Usually in puerperium	Third trimester	Any time
Hypertension	Almost always	Moderate likelihood	Moderate likelihood	Moderate likelihood	Almost always
Proteinuria	Almost always	Usually present with hematuria	Almost always	unusual	Almost always (active urine sediment)
Impaired renal function	50%	90%-100%	30%	60%	40%-80%
Neurologic impairment	Unusual	20%-50%	No data	30%-40%	Unusual
Fever	Absent	usual	unusual	unusual	usual
Schistocytes	50%-100%	100%	100%	15%-20%	Rare
Thrombocytopenia	Mild to severe	Moderate to severe	Moderate to severe	Mild to moderate	Mild to moderate
Elevated liver enzymes	Almost always	Rarely	Rarely	Almost always	Absent
Jaundice	Unusual	Rare	Rare	Almost always	Absent
Nausea/vomiting	Unusual	Almost always	Usual	Almost always	Absent
Abdominal pain	Usual	Usual	Usual	Usual	Absent
Treatment	Delivery of fetus	Plasma exchange	Plasmapheresis/ Eculizumab	Delivery of fetus	Immunosuppression

AFLP, acute fatty liver of pregnancy; aHUS, atypical hemolytic uremic syndrome; HELLP, hemolysis, elevated liver enzymes, and low platelet count; PE, preeclampsia; TTP, thrombotic thrombocytopenic purpura.

Thrombotic Thrombocytopenic Purpura

This is a rare hematological disorder that is usually described as a pentad consisting of microangiopathic hemolytic anemia, thrombocytopenia, fever, renal insufficiency, and mental status changes, ranging from mild confusion to a stroke-like syndrome.[51]

The etiology resides in an acquired or constitutional deficiency of a von Willebrand factor (vWF)–cleaving protease, known as ADAMTS-13. As a result, there is widespread platelet aggregation with microvascular thrombi formation leading to end-organ damage.[52]

Patients with TTP have a median platelet count between 10,000 and 30,000/mL, but severe cases present with thrombocytopenia of <1000/mL.[53]

Laboratory tests show signs of hemolysis, and the presence of schistocytes confirms the diagnosis of microangiopathic hemolytic anemia.

Furthermore, creatinine levels can be mildly to moderately increased, with mild proteinuria and hematuria.

Thrombotic thrombocytopenic purpura associated with ADAMTS-13 deficiency occurs predominantly in the second and third trimesters.[55,56] The diagnosis is based on clinical findings.

Acute Fatty Liver of Pregnancy

This infrequent entity occurs in approximately 1 out of 10,000 deliveries.[57] Women usually present in the third trimester with fatigue, vomiting, headache, and clinical signs of PE, such as hypertension and increased level of transaminases. Up to 60% of cases are associated with AKI.[57] Typical laboratory findings are abnormal hematological and liver function tests such as hyperbilirubinemia, hypoglycemia, hypocholesterolemia, prolonged partial thromboplastin time, and hypofibrinogenemia.

Therapy consists of treatment of disseminated intravascular coagulation (DIC) and immediate delivery of the fetus along with supportive care and intensive monitoring. The laboratory abnormalities frequently begin to improve within one to two days after delivery.[38]

Glomerulonephritis

Primary glomerular disease as well as secondary glomerular conditions can cause acute non–pregnancy-related AKI. Treatment and diagnosis are disease specific.[43] To minimize risks of renal flares and fetal demise, women with lupus nephritis should be on remission at least for 6 months before conception. Hydroxychloroquine should be continued throughout pregnancy to reduce the risks of flares and improve pregnancy outcomes.

The key to appropriate management in pregnancy-related AKI is supportive care (volume reposition, and correction of electrolyte abnormalities) and specific treatment of the underlying condition. Dialysis should be initiated based on the usual criteria in the nonobstetric setting. Glomerulonephritis-associated PE/HELLP and AFLP resolve only after delivery.

UTIs are the most common bacterial infections in pregnancy and may present as ASB, acute cystitis, or pyelonephritis. Bacterial colonization is promoted by urinary stasis, ureterovesical reflux, and glycosuria among other normal pregnancy-induced physiological changes.[58]

ASB occurs in up to 10% of pregnant women, and if untreated, there is a 30% risk of progression to pyelonephritis.[59] Mostly ASB and pyelonephritis have been associated with adverse maternal and neonatal outcomes such as preterm birth, low birth weight, perinatal mortality, PE, and sepsis.[60-63] Therefore, routine screening with urine culture is recommended at the first prenatal visit or in early pregnancy.[64] Patients with additional risk factors, such as history of UTI, urinary tract anomalies, CKD, and diabetes mellitus, may benefit from further screening in subsequent trimesters.

Antimicrobial treatment should be based on allergy history, prevalence of local community resistance, and community guidelines.[58] For ASB, cystitis, or pyelonephritis, a urine culture should be performed 1 to 2 weeks after completion of antibiotic treatment. Antimicrobial prophylaxis with cephalexin or low-dose nitrofurantoin is advised in patients with recurrent cystitis (≥3 episodes)[65] or after recovery from pyelonephritis.

Acute antepartum pyelonephritis complicates approximately 0.5% to 2% of all pregnancies. If untreated, this condition significantly increases the risk of several complications such as anemia (OR, 2.6), septicemia (OR, 56.5), acute pulmonary insufficiency (OR, 12.5), acute renal dysfunction (OR, 16.5), and spontaneous preterm birth (OR, 1.3).[61] Risk factors include untreated lower UTI, black or Hispanic descent, young, less educated, nulliparous, late initiation of prenatal care, and smoking during pregnancy.[61]

The typical clinical presentation consists of fever, unilateral costovertebral angle pain, and nausea/vomiting. Urinalysis shows hematuria, proteinuria, nitrites, and pyuria. Pyelonephritis treatment consists of parenteral antibiotics and intravenous fluids. Hospitalization is usually recommended because of the risk of progression to overt septicemia, preterm contractions, and, occasionally, respiratory complications.

In fact, if preterm labor occurs during treatment, caution must be exerted on the selection of the tocolytic agent.

The choice of antibiotics must be guided by the local microbiology and susceptibility data.

Parenteral treatment should be continued until the patient is afebrile for 48 hours, and oral antibiotic treatment, based the initial culture sensitivity, should follow for 14 days.

Conclusions

Although obstetric outcomes have markedly improved in last decades, pregnancy still poses considerable risk to maternal and fetal health in patients with renal disease. Given the complexity of kidney disease, maternal-fetal specialists and nephrologists should work together to optimize pregnancy control. Preconception assessment is essential to determine baseline disease and to plan the optimal timing for conception. In situations where pregnancy is contraindicated, other options, such as surrogacy or adoption, could be discussed. Follow-up should be tailored on a case-by-case basis, but in general, it is recommended to intensify medical management in women with advanced CKD and/or high-risk factors for adverse events.

KEY POINTS

- Physiological changes during pregnancy start at approximately 6 weeks of gestation and usually regress to the non-pregnant state within one to one and a half months postpartum.
- Serum creatinine and 24-hour urine collection for creatinine clearance are the preferred methods to assess renal function during gestation in women with nephropathy.
- During normal pregnancy, urinary protein excretion rises, and values greater than 300 mg/24 h are considered abnormal.
- Women with CKD can be classified into two groups: early disease (creatinine < 1.4 mg/dL, creatinine clearance > 70 mL/min and stage 1-2 CKD) and advanced disease (creatinine > 1.4 mg/dL, creatinine clearance < 70 mL/min or stage 3-5 CKD).
- Women with CKD have a significantly increased risk of PE, preterm birth, low birth weight, cesarean delivery and perinatal death.
- Severe renal impairment, chronic hypertension, and proteinuria have been identified as risk factors that worsen perinatal outcomes among women with CKD.
- There is a strong association between advanced stage CKD and progression of renal disease. Women with GFR ≤ 40 mL/min and/or proteinuria ≥ 1 g/24 h are at greater risk.
- Women undergoing HD during pregnancy have a greater risk of hypertension, polyhydramnios, PE, IUGR, prematurity, and low birth weight.
- Women who initiate dialysis during pregnancy have a higher rate of live birth than those who conceive while on HD.
- The proportion of fetal demise, preterm delivery, and low birth weight seem to increase with BUN levels ≥ 50 mg/dL.
- Pregnancy outcomes significantly improve when the patient undergoes HD for at least 36 h/wk.
- Blood pressure should be kept between 120/70 and 140/90 mm Hg during and after dialysis.
- Women who underwent renal transplantation are at increased risk of PE and preterm birth.

- Women should postpone conception for 1 to 2 years after kidney transplantation.
- Azathioprine, tacrolimus, cyclosporine and prednisolone are all considered safe during pregnancy and breastfeeding. Mycophenolate mofetil should be discontinued 6 to 12 weeks prior to conception because of its high teratogenicity.
- Adequate metabolic control in women with diabetes, quiescent autoimmune disease for 6 months, and adequate treatment of blood pressure in women with chronic hypertension will significantly improve maternal and perinatal outcomes.
- In women with advanced kidney disease or significant comorbidities, other alternatives for becoming a parent, such as surrogacy or adoption, should be addressed.
- The frequency of visits should be tailored to the patient's degree of renal insufficiency and to the presence of risk factors such as proteinuria, hypertension, and a coexisting systemic disease.
- Intensive blood pressure control with pregnancy-safe antihypertensive drugs is essential for a blood pressure target below 140/90 mm Hg.
- Evidence of hemolysis manifested by increased LDH, decreased haptoglobin, or presence of schistocytes in peripheral blood smear can aid in the differential diagnosis between PE and worsening basal renal condition.
- Initiation of low-dose aspirin before the 16th week of gestation to prevent early-onset PE is recommended.
- Urine culture for ASB should be performed at least monthly.
- Fetal biometry assessment should be performed every 2 to 3 weeks combined with weekly Doppler evaluation whenever IUGR is detected. NST and/or BPP should be performed weekly from 32 to 34 weeks onwards.
- It is recommended to prolong pregnancy until term. The mode of delivery should be based on routine obstetric considerations.
- Acute kidney injury during pregnancy is generally defined as an abrupt decrease of renal

function that progresses from a mild increase in serum creatinine levels to overt organ failure.

- According to the nature of the injury, AKI is classified into three types: prerenal (renal hypoperfusion), intrinsic (injury to the tubules, glomeruli, interstitium, or intrarenal blood vessels), and postrenal (acute obstruction of the urinary tract).

- Common causes of AKI during pregnancy are PE and HELLP syndrome, aHUS, thrombotic thrombocytopenic purpura, acute fatty liver of pregnancy, and glomerulonephritis.

- ASB occurs in up to 10% of pregnant women, and if untreated, there is a 30% risk of progression to pyelonephritis.

- Routine screening with urine culture is recommended at the first prenatal visit or in early pregnancy.

- Antimicrobial prophylaxis with cephalexin or low-dose nitrofurantoin is advised in patients with recurrent cystitis (≥ 3 episodes).

- Acute pyelonephritis complicates 0.5% to 2% of all pregnancies, and if untreated, it increases the risk of anemia, septicemia, acute pulmonary insufficiency, acute renal dysfunction and spontaneous preterm birth.

- Treatment of pyelonephritis consists of IV fluids and parenteral antibiotics until the patient is afebrile for 48 hours. Oral antibiotic treatment should follow for 14 days.

REFERENCES

(only references cited in synoptic print chapter; for a complete reference list, see ebook)

8. Hladunewich MA. Chronic kidney disease and pregnancy. *Semin Nephrol.* 2017;37(4):337-346.

9. Nguyen MT, Maynard SE, Kimmel PL. Misapplications of commonly used kidney equations: renal physiology in practice. *Clin J Am Soc Nephrol.* 2009;4(3):528-534.

11. Fischer MJ. Chronic kidney disease and pregnancy: maternal and fetal outcomes. *Adv Chronic Kidney Dis.* 2007;14:132-145.

13. American College of Obstetricians and Gynecologists; Task Force on Hypertension in Pregnancy. Hypertension in pregnancy. Report of the American College of Obstetricians and Gynecologists' Task Force on Hypertension in Pregnancy. *Obstet Gynecol.* 2013;122(5): 1122-1131.

14. Zhang JJ, Ma XX, Hao L, et al. A systematic review and meta-analysis of outcomes of pregnancy in CKD and CKD outcomes in pregnancy. *Clin J Am Soc Nephrol.* 2015;10:1964-1978.

15. Hladunewich MA, Melamad N, Bramham K. Pregnancy across the spectrum of chronic kidney disease. *Kidney Int.* 2016;89:995-1007.

16. Imbasciati E, Gregorini G, Cabiddu G, et al. Pregnancy in CKD stages 3 to 5: fetal and maternal outcomes. *Am J Kidney Dis.* 2007;49:753-762.

17. Piccoli GB, Cabiddu G, Attini R, et al. Risk of adverse pregnancy outcomes in women with CKD. *J Am Soc Nephrol.* 2015;26:2011-2022.

18. Cabiddu G, Castellino S, Gernone G, et al. A best practice position statement on pregnancy in chronic kidney disease: the Italian Study Group on Kidney and Pregnancy. *J Nephrol.* 2016;29:277-303.

19. Jones DC, Hayslett JP. Outcome of pregnancy in women with moderate or severe renal insufficiency. *N Engl J Med.* 1996;335:226-232.

20. Hall M. Chronic renal disease and antenatal care. *Best Pract Res Clin Obstet Gynaecol.* 2019;57:15-32. pii: S1521-6934(18)30203-7.

21. Fitzpatrick A, Mohammadi F, Jesudason S. Managing pregnancy in chronic kidney disease: improving outcomes for mother and baby. *Int J Womens Health.* 2016;8:273-285.

22. Jesudason S, Grace BS, McDonald SP. Pregnancy outcomes according to dialysis commencing before or after conception in women with ESRD. *Clin J Am Soc Nephrol.* 2014;9:143-149.

23. Mackay EV. Pregnancy and renal disease: a ten-year survey. *Aus N Z J Obstet Gynaecol.* 1963;3:21-34.

24. Asamiya Y, Otsubo S, Matsuda Y, et al. The importance of low blood urea nitrogen levels in pregnant patients undergoing hemodialysis to optimize birth weight and gestational age. *Kidney Int.* 2009;75:1217-1222.

25. Hladunewich MA, Hou S, Odutayo A, et al. Intensive hemodialysis associates with improved pregnancy outcomes: a Canadian and United States cohort comparison. *J Am Soc Nephrol.* 2014;25:1103-1109.

27. Cabbidu G, Castellino S, Gernone G, et al. Best practices on pregnancy on dialysis: the Italian Study Group on Kidney and Pregnancy. *J Nephrol.* 2015;28(3):279-288.

28. Hladunewich M, Schatell D. Intensive dialysis and pregnancy. *Hemodial Int.* 2016;20:339-348.

29. Wiles K, de Oliveira L. Dialysis in pregnancy. *Best Pract Res Clin Obstet Gynaecol.* 2019;57:33-46.

30. Shah S, Venkatesan RL, Gupta A, et al. Pregnancy outcome in women with kidney transplant: metaanalysis and systemic review. *BMC Nephrol.* 2019:20(1):24.

31. Bramham K. Pregnancy in renal transplant recipients and donors. *Semin Nephrol.* 2017;37(4):370-377.

32. Vijayan M, Pavlakis M. Pregnancy and the kidney transplant recipient. *Curr Opin Nephrol Hypertens.* 2017;26(6):494-500.

33. Kidney Disease: Improving Global Outcomes (KDIGO) Transplant Work Group. KDIGO clinical practice guideline for the care of kidney transplant recipients. *Am J Transplant.* 2009;9(suppl 3):S1-S155.

35. Bujold E, Roberge S, Lacasse Y, et al. Prevention of preeclampsia and intra-uterine growth restriction with aspirin started in early pregnancy: a meta-analysis. *Obstet Gynecol.* 2010;116:402-414.

36. Roberge S, Nicolaides KH, Demers S, Villa P, Bujold E. Prevention of perinatal death and adverse perinatal outcome using low-dose aspirin: a meta-analysis. *Ultrasound Obstet Gynecol.* 2013;41:491-499.

38. Jim B, Garovic VG. Acute kidney injury in pregnancy. *Semin Nephrol.* 2017;37(4):378-385.

39. Ancharya A. Management of acute kidney injury in pregnancy for the obstetrician. *Obstet Gynecol Clin North Am.* 2016;43(4):747-765.

40. Makris K, Spanou L. Acute kidney injury: definition, pathophysiology and clinical phenotypes. *Clin Biochem Rev.* 2016;37(2):85-98.

41. Liu Y, Ma X, Zheng J, Liu X, Yan T. Pregnancy outcomes in patients with acute kidney injury during pregnancy: a systemtic review and meta-analysis. *BMC Pregnancy and Childbirth.* 2017;17:235.

42. Haseler E, Melhem N, Sinha MD. Renal disease in pregnancy: fetal, neonatal and long-term outcomes. *Best Pract Res Clin Obstet Gynaecol.* 2019;57:60-76. pii: S1521-6934(18)30208-4.

43. Van Hook JW. Acute kidney injury during pregnancy. *Clin Obstet Gynecol.* 2014;57(4):851-861.

44. Kuklina EV, Ayala C, Callaghan WM. Hypertensive disorders and severe obstetric morbidity in the United States. *Obstet Gynecol.* 2009;113(6):1299-1306.

45. Sibai BM, Ramadan MK, Usta I, Salama M, Mercer BM, Friedman SA. Maternal morbidity and mortality in 442 pregnancies with hemolysis, elevated liver enzymes, and low platelets (HELLP syndrome). *Am J Obstet Gynecol.* 1993;169:1000-1006.

46. Cornelis T, Odutayo A, Keunen J, Hladunewich M. The kidney in normal pregnancy and preeclampsia. *Semin Nephrol.* 2011;31(1):4-14.

47. Mandala EM, Gkiouzepas S, Kasimatis E, et al. Pregnancy-associated atypical hemolytic uremic syndrome (aHUS), treated with eculizumab. *Blood*. 2014;124(21):5019.

48. Bresin E, Rurali E, Caprioli J, et al. Combined complement gene mutations in atypical hemolytic uremic syndrome influence clinical phenotype. *J Am Soc Nephrol*. 2013;24:475.

50. Kelly RJ, Hochsmann B, Szer J, et al. Eculizumab in pregnant patients with paroxysmal nocturnal hemoglobinuria. *N Engl J Med*. 2015;373(11):1032-1039.

51. Shatzel JJ, Taylor JA. Syndromes of thrombotic microangiopathy. *Med Clin North Am*. 2017;101(2):395-415.

52. Tsai HM, Lian EC. Antibodies to von-Willebrand factor-cleaving protease in acute thrombotic thrombocytopenic purpura. *N Engl J Med*. 1998;339:1585-1594.

53. Scully M, Hunt BJ, Benjamin S, et al. Guidelines on the diagnosis and management of thrombotic thrombocytopenic purpura and other thrombotic microangiopathies. *Br J Haematol*. 2012;158(3):323-335.

55. Vesely SK, George JN, Lämmle B, et al. ADAMTS13 activity in thrombotic thrombocytopenic purpura-hemolytic uremic syndrome: relation to presenting features and clinical outcomes in a prospective cohort of 142 patients. *Blood* 2003;102:60-68.

56. Martin JN Jr, Bailey AP, Rehberg JF, Owens MT, Keiser SD, May WL. Thrombotic thrombocytopenic purpura in 166 pregnancies: 1955-2006. *Am J Obstet Gynecol*. 2008;199:98-104.

57. Morton A. Imitators of preeclampsia: a review. *Pregnancy Hypertens*. 2016;6(1):1-9.

58. Kalinderi K, Delkos D, Kalinderis M, Athanasiadis A, Kalogiannidis I. Urinary tract infection during pregnancy: current concepts on a common multifaceted problem. *J Obstet Gynaecol*. 2018;38(4):448-453.

59. Smaill FM, Vazquez JC. Antibiotics for asymptomatic bacteriuria in pregnancy. *Cochrane Database Syst Rev*. 2015;(8):CD000490.

60. Romero R, Oyarzun E, Mazor M, Sirtori M, Hobbins JC, Bracken M. Meta-analysis of the relationship between asymptomatic bacteriuria and preterm delivery/low birth weight. *Obstet Gynecol*. 1989;73:576-582.

61. Wing DA, Fasset MJ, Getahun D. Acute pyelonephritis in pregnancy: an 18-year retrospective analysis. *Am J Obstet Gynecol*. 2014;210:219.e1-219.e6.

62. Yan L, Jin Y, Hang H, Yan B. The association between urinary tract infection during pregnancy and preeclampsia: a meta-analysis. *Medicine (Baltimore)*. 2018;97(36):e12192.

63. Hill JB, Sheffield JS, McIntire DD, Wendel GD Jr. Acute pyelonephritis in pregnancy. *Obstet Gynecol*. 2005;105:18-23.

64. Lin K. Fajardo K; U.S. Preventive Services Task Force. Screening for asymptomatic bacteriuria in adults: evidence for the U.S Preventive Services Task Force reaffirmation recommendation statement. *Ann Intern Med*. 2008;149:W20-W24.

65. Delzell JE. Urinary tract infections during pregnancy. *Am Fam Physician*. 2000;61(3):713-720.

CHAPTER 36

Neurological Disorders in Pregnancy

Tabitha Morgan Quebedeaux and Tara Dutta

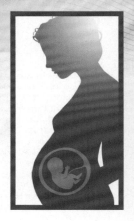

Introduction

Pregnancy predisposes women to some serious neurological problems, such as eclampsia, cerebrovascular disorders, and benign intracranial hypertension, and to a number of disorders that are relatively benign, including carpal tunnel syndrome, meralgia paresthetica, and Bell palsy. In addition, women of childbearing age with established chronic neurological problems may require special attention during pregnancy. These include epilepsy, migraine headaches, and autoimmune diseases such as multiple sclerosis (covered in Chapter 40), myasthenia gravis, and acute inflammatory demyelinating polyneuropathy (Guillain-Barré syndrome). This chapter summarizes a number of commonly encountered neurological conditions and presents current information on treatment and management in pregnancy.

Stroke

Etiology and Risk Factors for Pregnancy-Related Stroke

Pregnancy-related stroke occurs in 30/100,000 pregnancies and is increasing in frequency.[1–3] Prevalence of ischemic stroke is approximately 12/100,000 pregnancies, similar to prevalence of hemorrhagic stroke.[3] The highest risk is in the peripartum and postpartum period.[2,4] Elgendy et al queried the National Inpatient Sample in the United States and found that acute stroke (ischemic and hemorrhagic) occurred in 0.045% of pregnancy-related hospitalizations (1/2222 hospitalizations) and was associated with in-hospital mortality rate nearly 385 times higher than patients who did not experience a stroke.[5]

For ischemic stroke, hypertension, preeclampsia, diabetes, hyperlipidemia, atrial fibrillation, and obesity are among the modifiable risk factors that

are on the rise in young women of child-bearing age, while tobacco use is down trending. Migraine with aura is also associated with higher risk of stroke in women, and risk is thought to correlate with higher circulating estrogen levels.[6] Other mechanisms include arterial thrombosis secondary to hypercoagulable state, lupus, paradoxical venous thromboembolism, amniotic fluid embolism, trophoblastic embolism through a patent foramen ovale or extracardiac shunt, cervical artery dissection, vasculitis, venous infarction secondary to cerebral venous sinus thrombosis (CVT), and "reversible" cerebral vasoconstriction syndrome (RCVS). Typical presenting symptoms include aphasia, double vision, facial weakness, slurred speech, limb weakness, incoordination, sensory loss, or gait disturbance, and rarely, unexplained loss of consciousness due to basilar artery occlusion.

Management of Ischemic Stroke in Pregnancy and Postpartum

Initial management of stroke involves stabilization and consideration of acute therapies. Treating clinicians should ascertain, to the best of their ability, the time the patient was last known to be neurologically normal, pertinent medical history, and whether the patient is taking antithrombotic or anticoagulant medications. Historical or clinical features suggesting a stroke mimic (such as migraine with aura, seizure with postictal neurological deficits, or extreme hypoglycemia or hyperglycemia) should be taken into consideration. The initial decision-making should focus on stabilization and consideration of acute treatment. Hypoxia and significant glucose aberrations should be treated immediately; a rapid neurologic examination should be obtained.

A computed tomography (CT) of the head without contrast should be performed as quickly as possible to exclude the possibility of hemorrhage and evaluate for signs of established infarct or other process. If there is concern for a large vessel arterial occlusion due to symptom severity, presence of cortical signs, or sudden loss of consciousness, emergent vascular imaging should also be performed, preferably concurrently. A CT angiogram (CTA) of the head and neck will typically be the most readily available study and provide the most accurate information about the presence of a large vessel occlusion; however, if there is a significant contraindication to using iodinated contrast (eg, significant kidney disease or known contrast allergy), magnetic resonance angiogram (MRA) of the head and neck can be used as an alternative. If the head CT shows no evidence of hemorrhage or other alternative explanation for the patient's symptoms, treating physicians may consider use of alteplase for some patients (see below). Prior to alteplase administration, blood pressure must be no greater than 185/110 mm Hg and must be kept under 180/105 mm Hg in the postadministration monitoring period. IV antihypertensives, including labetalol, hydralazine, nicardipine, and clevidipine may be required to get and/or keep blood pressure within the necessary range both during and after the infusion to reduce risk of intracranial hemorrhage.

If the CTA or MRA demonstrates a large vessel arterial occlusion, the patient should be referred immediately to a stroke center with neurointerventional radiology services capable of performing mechanical thrombectomy and providing neurocritical care expertise.

With acute stroke treatment, time to treatment is critically important to reduce risk of disability from irreversible tissue death, and every effort must be made to expedite time to treatment. Once acute treatment decisions have been made, additional diagnostic workup will typically include electrocardiogram (ECG), telemetry monitoring (with particular attention to presence of atrial fibrillation, atrial cardiopathy, wall motion abnormalities, and valvular disease), and transthoracic echocardiogram. Additional studies may be indicated, particularly if the patient's medical history is not well established or if there is concern for illness such as lupus, antiphospholipid syndrome, connective tissue disease, or occult infection.

The only U.S. Food and Drug Administration (FDA)–approved medication for treatment of acute ischemic stroke in the United States as of this publication date is alteplase, a recombinant human tissue plasminogen activator (tPA), which has been shown to significantly reduce stroke-related disability. The American Heart Association (AHA) states that alteplase "may be considered in pregnancy when the anticipated benefits of treating moderate or severe stroke outweigh the anticipated increased risks of uterine bleeding" depending on the overall risk/benefit analysis as determined by the treating clinicians.[4]

For stroke occurring postpartum, risk of hemorrhagic complications with alteplase would need to be carefully considered before administration of the drug. Exclusions would include, among others, recent neuraxial anesthesia (including epidural medication delivery), cesarean delivery, or other surgery. Additionally, mechanical thrombectomy has been successfully performed in a number of obstetric patients[7,8] and should be considered for any pregnant women presenting with a disabling stroke attributable to a large vessel occlusion.

Although neither alteplase nor thrombectomy have been prospectively studied in pregnant or postpartum patients, observational and registry data suggest that these therapies are associated with similar rates of vascular reperfusion and favorable outcomes compared to women who are not pregnant or peripartum.[9,10] Leffert et al[9] created a cohort of pregnant and postpartum patients treated with reperfusion therapy (alteplase and/or mechanical thrombectomy) using the United States–based Get With The Guidelines stroke database. The 40 patients who received reperfusion therapy had similar risk-adjusted short-term outcomes (in-hospital death, independent ambulation on discharge, and discharge to home), despite a nonsignificant trend toward increased symptomatic intracranial hemorrhage and higher baseline stroke severity.

The AHA guidelines on management of acute ischemic stroke outline recommendations on this topic in more detail,[11] as well as management considerations pertinent to use of alteplase.

Prevention of Ischemic Stroke in Pregnancy

Stroke prevention in patients with prior history or deemed high risk for stroke will need close anticipatory guidance to help reduce their stroke risk factors. Counseling addressing management of hypertension, diabetes/insulin resistance, tobacco and substance use avoidance, and other modifiable risk factors is critical, preferably prior to conception when possible. Medication prophylaxis may consist of an antiplatelet agent, such as aspirin, or an anticoagulant (typically in the form of low-molecular-weight heparin), depending on the individual's underlying condition(s). Typically, individuals with prior history of stroke should be under care of a neurologist with experience in stroke management before and during pregnancy, and those with underlying hematologic or rheumatologic conditions predisposing to stroke, such as antiphospholipid syndrome or lupus, should be under care of a hematologist and/or rheumatologist as indicated. A comprehensive reference outlining management of cardiovascular disease in pregnancy, including cerebrovascular disease, was published by Mehta et al[3] and is available free to the general public online.

Cerebral Hemorrhage in Pregnancy

Etiology and Risk Factors for Intracerebral Hemorrhage in Pregnancy

Intracerebral hemorrhage (ICH) occurs in approximately 12/100,000 pregnancies[3] and carries profound morbidity and mortality. Meeks et al[12] tracked over 3 million pregnant women in three US states during pregnancy and for 24 weeks postpartum and found that risk of ICH was highest in the third trimester and remained increased during the first 12 weeks after delivery. Pregnancy-related ICH was associated with increased maternal and fetal death.[12] In a systematic review of pregnant or postpartum patients by Ascanio et al, the 43 identified patients with spontaneous ICH had a mortality rate of 48.8%, and fetal outcomes were evenly distributed between preterm or term delivery and fetal or neonatal death.[13]

Typical risk factors for ICH in pregnancy include hypertension (including gestational), preeclampsia and eclampsia, coagulopathy, age >35 years, black race, and tobacco use.[3] Presentation in pregnancy is commonly related to uncontrolled hypertension and resultant loss of integrity in the intracranial arterial wall, though vascular malformations such as arteriovenous malformations and dural arteriovenous fistulas, cerebral vein thrombosis, and metastatic lesions with propensity to hemorrhage (eg, choriocarcinoma or renal cell carcinoma) are among other possible causes.

Clinical Presentation of ICH in Pregnancy

Onset of ICH may be accompanied by a severe, abrupt-onset headache, nausea, or vomiting; profound abrupt-onset hemiparesis may occur and can progress quickly to coma.[14] Symptoms may be indistinguishable from those of ischemic stroke, though rapid progression to altered mental status and coma is more common due to rapid enlargement of hematoma, compression of brain structures, and elevation of intracranial pressure.

Clinical Assessment and Management of ICH in Pregnancy

Initial management of suspected ICH during pregnancy or the postpartum state is typically the same as that provided to a nonpregnant patient, with exception that close consultation with an obstetrics consultant is needed to help guide management and fetal monitoring. A detailed guideline recommendation on management of spontaneous ICH has been written by Hemphill et al and published by the American Heart Association[15] (**Table 36.1**).

Table 36.1 American Heart Association Blood Pressure Recommendations for Intracerebral Hemorrhage

For ICH patients presenting with SBP 150-220 mm Hg and without contraindication to acute BP treatment: • acute lowering of SBP to 140 mm Hg is safe (Class I[a]; Level of Evidence A[b])   • can be effective for improving functional outcome (Class IIa[c]; Level of Evidence B[d])   (Revised from previous guidelines)
For ICH patients presenting with SBP > 220 mm Hg: • may be reasonable to consider aggressive reduction of BP with a continuous intravenous infusion and frequent BP monitoring (Class IIb[e]; Level of Evidence C[f])   (New recommendation)

BP, blood pressure; ICH, intracerebral hemorrhage; SBP, systolic blood pressure.

[a]Conditions for which there is evidence for and/or general agreement that the procedure or treatment is useful and effective.
[b]Data derived from multiple randomized clinical trials or meta-analyses.
[c]The weight of evidence or opinion is in favor of the procedure or treatment.
[d]Data derived from a single randomized trial or nonrandomized studies.
[e]Usefulness/efficacy is less well established by evidence or opinion.
[f]Consensus opinion of experts, case studies, or standard of care.
Adapted from Hemphill JC III, Greenberg SM, Anderson CS, et al. Guidelines for the management of spontaneous intracerebral hemorrhage: a guideline for healthcare professionals from the American Heart Association/American Stroke Association. *Stroke.* 2015; 46(7):2032-2060.

Initial evaluation should include airway and hemodynamic stabilization, blood pressure measurement and initiation of rapid control, a quick neurological assessment, CT imaging to assess for hemorrhage presence, type, and size, and blood work, including a complete blood count and coagulation studies. History should be obtained about the patient's prior medical history, and with attention to hemorrhage risk factors, and current use of any antiplatelet or antithrombotic agents, as with latter, reversal therapies may be indicated.

Once blood pressure control has been initiated, typically with intravenous agent(s), additional imaging with CT angiogram may be needed to evaluate for underlying vascular malformation, aneurysm, and to assess for large vessel vasculopathy (such as might be seen in RCVS; see below). The patient should be monitored closely, preferably in a setting in which neurocritical care consultation is available. Once clinically stabilized, magnetic resonance imaging (MRI) of the brain is typically obtained to further evaluate for structural pathology, including mass lesions, ischemic stroke, and vasogenic edema (as would be seen in posterior reversible encephalopathy syndrome [PRES]; see below).

For women with a prior history of ICH, subarachnoid hemorrhage (SAH), or the other above-mentioned conditions associated with hemorrhage, anticipatory guidance before or during pregnancy may reduce risk of hemorrhagic complications. Though brain arteriovenous malformations (AVMs) were previously assumed to be associated with increased risk of hemorrhage during pregnancy, recent studies have either found no clear association or conflicting results, while others have found three times greater risk of ICH in women with AVM during pregnancy and puerperium.[16] Similarly, the frequency of aneurysm rupture is not clearly greater than that in the general population. Robba et al reviewed this topic and conducted a meta-analysis of seven retrospective studies and internal case series with 52 patients and found that the majority experienced rupture in the third trimester. Association was found with hypertension, alcohol and tobacco use, obesity, and advanced maternal age.[17] Intervention with clipping was done in all seven internal cases reviewed, all with favorable outcomes for mother and fetus.

In general, for women who have a known vascular malformation or cerebral aneurysm, consultation with a physician specializing in neurovascular

disease is suggested, as an individual patient's risk of hemorrhage may be significantly influenced by morphology of cerebrovascular lesion or other comorbid conditions.

Prevention of ICH in Pregnancy

Prevention and management of hypertension before and during pregnancy, combined with avoidance of tobacco and sympathomimetic substances, are the most critical modifiable risk factors for preventing pregnancy-related ICH. For patients with a prior history of refractory hypertension, prior ischemic or hemorrhagic stroke, underlying vasculopathy (moyamoya disease or syndrome, sickle cell disease, etc), or known vascular malformation, consultation and comanagement with a neurovascular neurologist and/or neurosurgeon is recommended.

A review of ICH management in pregnancy and postpartum period was recently published by Toossi and Moheet.[18]

Subarachnoid Hemorrhage in Pregnancy

Clinical Presentation of SAH in Pregnancy

Aneurysmal SAH is often heralded by a headache often described as "the worst headache of life" and may be accompanied by photophobia, neck stiffness, nausea, and vomiting. There is sometimes a history of less severe headache and/or syncope in the preceding days or weeks, referred to as a "sentinel bleed." Symptoms may resemble those of bacterial or viral meningitis, but the abrupt onset of headache, and (typically) absence of fever and leukocytosis should raise suspicion for the former. SAH may occur independently or in conjunction with parenchymal ICH and occurs at a similar rate in pregnant women as in the general population. Bateman and colleagues found a prevalence of 5.8/100,000 deliveries using the Nationwide Inpatient Sample of the Healthcare Cost and Utilization Project in the United States.[19]

Risk factors for intracranial aneurysm include family history, smoking, drug and alcohol use, sickle cell disease, moyamoya syndrome, sinus venous thrombosis, and connective tissue diseases such as Ehlers-Danlos or Marfan syndrome, among others. In the Bateman et al study, African Americans, Hispanics, and women of advanced maternal age were found to be at higher risk of aneurysmal SAH.[19] Pregnancy is thought to potentiate aneurysm formation, growth, and rupture, and the incidence of aneurysmal SAH is increased in pregnant patients.[20,21] The third trimester and postpartum period are thought to carry the greatest risk of rupture due to sudden and persistent elevation in intracranial pressure during parturition.[22]

Pharmacologic Management of SAH in Pregnancy

SAH increases maternal and fetal morbidity and mortality considerably, and therefore, preventative strategies through lifestyle intervention, hypertension management, and preventative aneurysm management (particularly for aneurysms >10 mm) are important. Nussbaum and colleagues recently reviewed this topic in detail and provide clinical recommendations,[23] including consideration of treatment for unruptured aneurysms that are symptomatic, enlarging, or >10 mm.

Cerebrovascular Conditions Associated With Hemorrhage in Pregnancy

Reversible Cerebral Vasoconstriction Syndrome

RCVS, sometimes referred to as "postpartum angiopathy" in the postpartum period, is a condition thought to be mediated by alteration in blood-brain barrier integrity due to endothelial dysfunction, resulting in an abrupt change in cerebrovascular arterial tone leading to vasoconstriction in one or more of the medium or large cerebral arteries, most commonly the middle cerebral arteries. Use of sympathomimetic substances, such as selective serotonin reuptake inhibitors (SSRIs), ephedrine derivatives, cannabis, and cocaine, have been associated with RCVS.

Clinical presentation of RCVS is often marked by sudden onset of thunderclap headache with or without fluctuating neurologic symptoms. Diagnosis is based on clinical suspicion and imaging of the cerebral vasculature, commonly using MRA, CTA, or conventional angiogram. Of note, the appearance of RCVS can be indistinguishable from that of vasculitis (primary angiitis of the CNS, infectious vasculitis, or systemic vasculitis affecting the CNS), so clinical presentation and absence of other typical clinical features associated with helps to distinguish RCVS.

If RCVS is suspected, based on clinical presentation and/or imaging, evaluation for underlying modifiable triggers (eg, use of SSRIs, triptan, or other sympathomimetic drug) should be undertaken, and patient may benefit from use of calcium channel blockers.

As mentioned, RCVS can be associated with SAH, ICH, ischemic stroke, and seizures and thus can have variable clinical and radiographic presentation. RCVS can occur concurrently with PRES (see below), and both can be associated with nonaneurysmal SAH, typically at the convexities. Although by definition the vasospasm associated with RCVS should resolve on imaging within several months, the term "reversible" does not always imply that it is entirely benign due to potential association with PRES and occasional complication by nonaneurysmal SAH, ICH, or ischemic stroke.

Posterior Reversible Encephalopathy Syndrome

PRES, a radiographic and clinical syndrome characterized by vasogenic edema in the white matter tracts of the brain or brainstem, is also associated with loss of autoregulatory control of the arterial cerebral vasculature. It is most commonly associated with hypertension and preeclampsia or eclampsia in the setting of pregnancy.

Typical presentation includes abrupt or gradual onset of headache, vision changes (including unilateral or bilateral cortical vision loss), other focal neurological deficits, and seizures. Blood pressure is typically, but not always, elevated, and PRES may occur in the context of preeclampsia or eclampsia. Treatment is typically targeted at lowering blood pressure and treating preeclampsia or eclampsia if concurrently present.

Cerebral Vein Thrombosis

Cerebral vein thrombosis (CVT) can occur in the setting of pregnancy or the postpartum period, with a recent meta-analysis suggesting association specifically with the puerperium.[24] Preexisting inherited thrombophilia, malignancy, smoking, dehydration, and infection are among factors that may increase risk. CVT is typically associated with a more gradual-onset headache, though presence of hemorrhage may result in sudden worsening of the pain and additional accompanying symptoms.

In cases of symptomatic CVT, management typically requires anticoagulation, regardless of presence of hemorrhage. More aggressive measures, including intracranial pressure management and, rarely, endovascular therapy, are sometimes required to reduce risk of progression to death or severe neurological disability.

Eclampsia

Etiology and Risk Factors of Eclampsia

Eclampsia is preeclampsia complicated by generalized seizures. Considered a form of hypertensive encephalopathy, it is thought to occur secondary to immune-mediated dysregulation of the vascular endothelium, resulting in loss of appropriate autoregulation in the cerebral arterioles. Identified risk factors include prior history of the condition, advanced maternal age, primiparity, hypertension, diabetes, renal disease, lupus, and other autoimmune diseases. It unfortunately remains one of the most significant causes of maternal and fetal mortality worldwide, and incidence is increasing,[25] and obesity and advanced maternal age are thought to be contributing factors.[26] Though it typically occurs after the 20th week, eclampsia can be seen up to several months postpartum.[27] One of the most feared complications of pregnancy, it can lead to both maternal and fetal death or neurologic injury rapidly.

Clinical Presentation and Diagnosis of Eclampsia in Pregnancy

Affected patients may present with generalized seizures, but before seizures develop, the condition may be heralded by symptoms including headache, nausea, vomiting, changes in mental status, visual changes, and increased deep tendon reflexes. Diagnosis is made based upon hypertension and proteinuria and/or evidence of end-organ damage (including seizures). In women affected by eclampsia, CT scan or MRI of the brain may show vasogenic edema consistent with PRES.

Pharmacologic Management and Long-Term Outcomes of Eclampsia in Pregnancy

Magnesium sulfate, the gold standard therapy, has been shown to reduce the risk of progression to eclampsia by half in women with preeclampsia, according to the Magpie trial,[28] and is superior to seizure prevention with phenytoin.[29] Fetal risks associated with preeclampsia and eclampsia include growth restriction, prematurity, and placental abruption.

Long-term outcomes following preeclampsia and eclampsia are increasingly being studied. In a systematic review and meta-analysis evaluating cardiovascular disease–related morbidity and mortality in women with a history of pregnancy complications, preeclampsia was associated with approximately 75% higher risk of cardiovascular disease–related mortality later in life.[30] Development of eclampsia during pregnancy was associated with a relative increased risk in subsequent seizure disorder in a large Canadian retrospective data linkage cohort, though the absolute risk of seizure disorder remained very low.[31] A comprehensive expert review of clinical management of eclampsia was recently published by Bartal and Sibai.[32] A detailed discussion of hypertensive disorders in pregnancy appears in Chapter 27.

Pituitary Apoplexy

Etiology, Risk Factors, and Clinical Presentation of Pituitary Apoplexy

Pituitary apoplexy is a rare but potentially life-threatening condition that is characterized by hemorrhagic infarction of the enlarging pituitary gland, probably due to increasing estrogen levels, as it outgrows its blood supply or compressed the nearby portal veins, resulting in ischemia and necrosis. Known presence of pituitary adenoma, use of anticoagulants, and trauma are risk factors. Common presenting symptoms include abrupt headache, double vision due to impairment of eye movement, bilateral vision loss, decreased level of arousal or coma, and hemodynamic instability from adrenal insufficiency.

Management of Pituitary Apoplexy in Pregnancy

Prevention in women with previously diagnosed pituitary adenoma involves consultation with specialists in endocrinology and, possibly, neurosurgery, to help determine appropriate management. Ischemic necrosis of the pituitary, referred to as Sheehan syndrome in the partum or postpartum state, may occur in the setting of a significant hemodynamic shifts, particularly hemorrhage or shock. Both conditions are considered life-threatening emergencies, as acute adrenal insufficiency and multiple hormonal deficiencies may develop paroxysmally. Emergent corticosteroid replacement with stress-dose corticosteroids, urgent endocrinologic assessment to determine pharmacologic hormonal therapy needed, and, in the case of apoplexy, sometimes neurosurgical intervention for sella decompression can be lifesaving.

A detailed review of pituitary disease in pregnancy by Petersenn and colleagues provides a more comprehensive summary, including management recommendations.[33]

Headache Syndromes in Pregnancy

Headache is a common symptom experienced by women during pregnancy and the postpartum period. While often benign, headache can occasionally signal more serious intracranial or systemic pathology, such as an enlarging meningioma or other mass, ICH, SAH, CVT, or preeclampsia as discussed previously. A review by O'Neal on this topic has been published.[34] Tension and migraine headaches are among the most common headache types seen during pregnancy.

Understanding a patient's baseline headache tendency and history is important to help gauge level of suspicion required for the latter. Additionally, preemptive counseling of women of childbearing age before pregnancy is important, as some preventative and abortive agents commonly used for conditions such as migraine can be teratogenic or carry risk for causing fetal harm. Ultimately, management of headache during pregnancy or lactation should aim to reduce risk of harm to fetus/infant while maximizing quality of life and function in mother.

Tension Headaches

Clinical Presentation of Tension Headaches

Tension headaches can be chronic or episodic with the latter occurring frequently or infrequently. Stress, cervicogenic disease, sleep deprivation, and dehydration are common triggers. Signs and symptoms of tension headaches include bilateral location, nonpulsating tightening or pressing, dull ache, pericranial tenderness, photophobia, and phonophobia.

Management of Tension Headaches

Tension headaches are typically treated conservatively during pregnancy with acetaminophen, hydration, application of gentle heat to upper back/ neck, gentle massage, and exercise. Physical therapy can be helpful, particularly in patients for whom a cervicogenic component may be responsible.

Migraine Headaches

Clinical Presentation of Migraine Headaches

Migraine headaches, which also may be chronic or episodic, tend to be more complicated and challenging to manage. Proposed pathophysiology involves activation of trigeminal nerve afferents, alteration of blood-brain barrier permeability, and aura related to cortical spreading depression. A detailed review of migraines by Ashina highlights mechanisms, definitions, symptoms, and clinical management in the general population.[35]

Family history of migraine or history of head injury are notable risk factors. Migraines are very common in women of childbearing age and may emerge for the first time during pregnancy, commonly in the first trimester. Overall, women with migraine usually experience a notable decrease in frequency during pregnancy by the second trimester, though this is more common in those with migraine without aura as compared to those with aura.[36] Frequency typically increases in the postpartum period, likely due to stress, sleep deprivation, and waning estrogen levels after parturition. The headaches may or may not be preceded by an aura of symptoms such as fatigue, poor appetite, yawning, or vision changes (e.g., scintillating scotoma or visual field deficit), are typically characterized by unilateral or bilateral pulsating or throbbing pain, and may be accompanied by multiple symptoms, including nausea or vomiting, light and noise sensitivity, motion sensitivity, and, occasionally, focal neurological symptoms such as aphasia, facial or limb weakness, numbness, or spreading paresthesias, or confusion. Symptoms may last from an hour to days or, more rarely, weeks.

Management of Migraine Headaches

Migraine management in pregnancy involves identifying underlying modifiable triggers, such as sleep deprivation, stress, dietary triggers, dehydration and using symptomatic therapy that is known to be relatively safe in pregnancy. Preventative pharmacotherapy is typically deferred if possible due to potential for adverse side effects or teratogenicity with many agents, though some women will require treatment in order to maintain quality of life. Preemptive counseling before pregnancy can be helpful for some patients, particularly with regard to lifestyle.

Acetaminophen, metoclopramide (both FDA pregnancy category B) and triptans (FDA category C) are considered reasonable symptomatic therapies for migraine headaches, with favorable safety data and supported by expert opinion.[37,38] If required for maintaining quality of life, preventative medications can be used cautiously, but experts often advise waiting until the second trimester to reduce risk of potential teratogenic effects. Propranolol; gabapentin; the tricyclic antidepressants amitriptyline, nortriptyline, and desipramine; and the serotonin-norepinephrine reuptake inhibitors duloxetine and venlafaxine are all FDA category C rated and can be considered based on discussion with patient and shared decision-making. Of note, valproic acid and topiramate should absolutely be avoided given known risk of teratogenicity. Other therapies, including occipital nerve blocks and physical therapy, can also sometimes be considered. Patients with migraine are at increased risk of miscarriage, preeclampsia, gestational hypertension, and giving birth to low-birth-weight and preterm infants[39]; thus, cardiovascular risk reduction is particularly important in this population.

Idiopathic Intracranial Hypertension

Clinical Presentation of IIH
Idiopathic intracranial hypertension (IIH) is a headache syndrome accompanied by papilledema and increased intracranial pressure in the absence of an underlying structural defect (such as CVT) or toxic cause (eg, hypervitaminosis A). The exact mechanism is unclear, although increased cerebrospinal fluid (CSF) production and impaired CSF reabsorption have both been proposed. There is an association with transverse sinus stenosis, but it is not clear whether this entity is caused by or the result of increased intracranial hypertension. Women of childbearing age, particularly those who are obese or who have experienced significant recent weight gain, are at increased risk. It may present or become exacerbated during pregnancy due to weight gain and the hemodynamic changes that occur.

The most dangerous side effect of IIH is permanent vision loss due to compression of the optic nerve sheaths. Headaches, which can be pulsating, throbbing, or aching in nature, may be focal or holocephalic, can be either intermittent or persistent, and can be accompanied by additional symptoms such as tinnitus, transient visual obscurations, and double vision (often due to unilateral or bilateral sixth cranial nerve palsy). Headache intensity may increase with cough, Valsalva, or assuming a supine position.

Diagnosis requires a careful fundoscopic examination to detect papilledema (which can be mild), and a lumbar puncture performed in the lateral recumbent position, with legs extended, demonstrating elevated opening pressure of at least 25 cm H_2O. Brain imaging, preferably with a contrast-enhanced MRI, and possibly MR venogram and angiogram, should be performed if suspected to look for supportive features (such as flattening of posterior aspects of the globes and partially empty sella syndrome) and to exclude underlying structural causes, such as hydrocephalus, mass lesion, or sinus venous thrombosis. For women who develop IIH or experience worsening during pregnancy, urgent referral to neuro-ophthalmology is essential in order to evaluate for and quantify peripheral vision loss.

Management of IIH
Treatment of IIH during pregnancy may consist of judicious, monitored weight loss and/or restricted weight gain, the carbonic anhydrase inhibitor, acetazolamide, and reducing salt intake. Although FDA category C, observational data suggest acetazolamide carries low risk of harm and is generally well tolerated. Topiramate (FDA category D) is relatively contraindicated due to potential teratogenicity. Serial lumbar punctures, optic sheath fenestration, and, more rarely, venous sinus stenting or lumbo-peritoneal or ventriculoperitoneal shunting may be done for women experiencing or at high risk for developing progressive vision loss, particularly if symptoms and intracranial hypertension have been refractory to medication and weight management strategies. Close comanagement with neurology and ophthalmology is recommended. A review of this topic in further detail has been written by Park and colleagues.[40]

Neuromuscular Disorders in Pregnancy
Women affected by chronic myopathies, such as muscular dystrophies and congenital myopathies, may experience increased difficulty with ambulation as pregnancy progresses.

Bell Palsy

Clinical Presentation of Bell Palsy

Bell (facial nerve) palsy, a condition marked by unilateral upper and lower facial weakness, occurs with increased frequency during the third trimester and postpartum period. Inflammation of the facial nerve, sometimes attributable to herpes simplex virus (HSV) or varicella-zoster virus (VZV) reactivation, is the usual culprit. Compressive vascular lesions, such as engorgement of the stylomastoid artery associated with an intracranial vascular malformation, is another rare cause. Hypertension, diabetes, and preeclampsia are known risk factors.[41]

Management of Bell Palsy

For Bell palsy, treatment with a short course of high-dose prednisone (FDA category C) may be considered if benefits are felt to outweigh risks and should be started within the first 3 to 7 days, as steroids have been shown to speed recovery.[42] Acyclovir or valacyclovir (FDA category B) should be considered if there is evidence of VZV or HSV reactivation, such as appearance of vesicles in auditory canal, but evidence does not otherwise support benefit over steroids alone. The prognosis for recovery from an incomplete Bell palsy is usually favorable; pregnancy is a negative predictor.[43,44] Ocular hydrating drops should be used frequently, and those with incomplete eye closure should use an ocular lubricant ointment and tape the eye before sleeping to reduce risk of exposure keratopathy.

Carpal Tunnel Syndrome

Clinical Presentation of CTS

Carpal tunnel syndrome (CTS, or median neuropathy at the wrist) is estimated to affect up to one half of pregnancies. It is caused by compression of the median nerve in the ventral forearm or wrist and is likely, at least in part, attributable to weight gain and edema, as well as breastfeeding postpartum. Numbness and paresthesias in the lateral palm and first three digits and weakness of grip strength are common.

Management of CTS

Conservative management of CTS is typically recommended, usually with avoidance of provocatory movements, low-salt diet, and use of wrist splints (especially at night).

Symptoms of meralgia paresthetica generally resolve within a few months after delivery.

Acute Inflammatory Demyelinating Polyneuropathy

Clinical Presentation of AIDP

Acute inflammatory demyelinating polyneuropathy (AIDP), also known as Guillain-Barré syndrome, occasionally occurs during pregnancy. The condition sometimes follows a recent infection, typically manifests with ascending weakness involving the limbs, trunk, facial, and bulbar muscles, and, when severe, may progress to neuromuscular respiratory failure due to diaphragmatic involvement. Autonomic instability, which can be severe, can occur. Deep tendon reflexes are reduced or absent. Distal paresthesias, sensory loss, and back and leg pain are common. Eye movement abnormalities and gait ataxia can also occur in the so-called Miller-Fisher variant. Other syndromes masquerading as AIDP, including botulism and tick-borne paralysis, should also be considered.

Management of AIDP

For women with AIDP, diagnostic evaluation is typically notable for CSF demonstrating a cytoalbuminologic gradient. Plasmapheresis or intravenous immunoglobulin (IVIG) can be used relatively safely during pregnancy.[45] AIDP does not seem to be associated independently with adverse maternal or neonatal risk, and in one review, almost 40% of patients were able to deliver vaginally.[45] It is recommended to avoid depolarizing neuromuscular blockade, such as succinylcholine, due to reported case of hyperkalemia and maternal death with its use.[46]

Myasthenia Gravis

Clinical Presentation of MG

Myasthenia gravis (MG) is a chronic, acquired, autoimmune disorder caused by production of antibodies against components of the neuromuscular junction. Patients may present with fatigable oculomotor and bulbar weakness, limb weakness, and, during crisis, neuromuscular respiratory failure. MG can first manifest or worsen during periods of physiologic stress, including during the pregnant or postpartum state, and can be unmasked by acute infection, certain medications, and use of anesthesia.

Clinical Assessment and Management of MG

Diagnosis of MG is typically made with serological testing demonstrating one of several antibodies to the acetylcholine receptor, though some individuals are seronegative. Preconception counseling is critical to reduce risks associated with medication-associated teratogenicity, understand risks to the infant of the disease itself, and plan for the safest birth possible. Those already on immune therapy should use two reliable forms of contraception during use and for 6 months following discontinuation of the therapy due to risks of teratogenicity associated with most of these medications. Due to the potential for exacerbation in mother and potential weakness in the neonate, women with MG are encouraged to deliver at hospitals with the ability to provide advanced maternal and neonatal care.

Pharmacologic Management of MG in Pregnancy

There are a number of medication classes that are known to adversely affect myasthenic symptoms, including magnesium products, fluoroquinolones, macrolides, aminoglycosides, and beta-blockers. Magnesium sulfate, the treatment of choice for seizure prevention in preeclampsia, inhibits acetylcholine release at the neuromuscular junction by blocking calcium entry. It should be used with significant caution when necessary. Patients in exacerbation require very close monitoring for development of bulbar weakness and neuromuscular respiratory failure and may ultimately require intubation and mechanical ventilator support. Special anesthesia considerations include avoidance of neuromuscular blocking agents whenever possible due to unpredictable effects, and, when used, steroidal agents like rocuronium and vecuronium are recommended to allow for reversal with sugammadex or neostigmine.[47]

Long-Term Outcomes of MG in Pregnancy

Transplacental passage of autoantibodies can lead to fetal skeletal muscle weakness, resulting in decreased movement, polyhydramnios, arthrogryposis multiplex congenita, or, rarely, stillbirth. Up to one-fifth of infants born to mothers with MG may demonstrate transient neonatal MG[48] and may present with hypotonia, difficulty swallowing, and respiratory weakness. Symptoms typically develop within a few hours of birth and resolve within 1 to 2 months.[49] These infants require supportive care, and most do not demonstrate any permanent sequelae.

Other Neuromuscular Disorders

Clinical Presentation of Meralgia Paresthetica, Lumbosacral Plexopathy, and Peripheral Neuropathies

Meralgia paresthetica, a neuropathy of the lateral femoral cutaneous nerve, manifests with numbness or burning pain in the lateral thigh unilaterally or bilaterally. It tends to occur with rapid weight gain or obesity, compression from tight-fitting garments or low-slung belts, and can be worsened by prolonged standing, walking, or hip flexion/extension.

Lumbosacral plexopathy and motor neuropathies of the lower extremities may occur during pregnancy or postpartum and are typically compression or stretch injuries resulting in demyelination without axonal damage. Small maternal stature, nulliparity, fetal macrosomia, prolonged second stage of labor, and fetal malpresentation are all risk factors. The pattern of weakness, which may be accompanied by sensory loss, is dependent upon the nerve or nerves involved.

Peripheral neuropathies may worsen or initially manifest during pregnancy. Diabetes is the most common cause of polyneuropathy (PN) in pregnancy, though pregnancy alone does not seem to predispose to developing polyneuropathy or precipitate worsening of preexisting PN. PN can also occur due to nutritional deficiency (see section on ataxia), particularly due to thiamine (vitamin B1) deficiency, pyridoxine (vitamin B6) deficiency, or cobalamin (vitamin B12) deficiency. These most commonly occur in the setting of hyperemesis gravidarum or other state leading to compromised nutritional intake.

Management of Other Neuromuscular Disorders

Although lumbosacral plexopathy and lower extremity motor neuropathies tend to spontaneously resolve over weeks to months, they can be extremely debilitating. It is important that caution is taken with regard to positioning and use of assistive devices during labor and/or surgery to reduce risk.

Epilepsy

Etiology and Risk Factors of Epilepsy

In 2015, approximately 3 million US adults, or about 1% of the population, had epilepsy.[50] Most women with epilepsy who do become pregnant experience an uncomplicated pregnancy and give birth to normal offspring. However, relative risks are increased for pregnancy complications and preterm delivery, and pregnant women with epilepsy have an estimated maternal death rate that is significantly higher than that of the general population.[51,52] Peripartum seizure activity also can result in maternal hypoxia, which may be harmful to the fetus.

Pregnancy may alter seizure frequency due to changes in antiepileptic drug (AED) metabolism and reduced plasma concentration, medication nonadherence, and lifestyle factors including stress and sleep deprivation.

Clinical Management of Epilepsy in Pregnancy

A woman whose seizures are chronically very well controlled on a single agent may, in conjunction with her neurologist, decide to avoid AED therapy during pregnancy. However, for those at higher risk of recurrence for whom the benefit of taking medication outweighs the risks, careful monitoring is often needed. AED levels begin to decline in the first trimester due to hormone-mediated induction of their metabolism, and both total and unbound levels may be affected.[53] More frequent monitoring and adjustment may be needed and must be individualized between the patient and her neurologist. For individuals with medically refractory epilepsy or prior history of status epilepticus, strong consideration should be made to consult with a neurologist specializing in treatment of epilepsy.

Anticonvulsant levels should be checked every 1 to 3 months, and the goal should be to maintain prepregnancy levels, with occasional exceptions. Anticonvulsant changes should be considered prior to pregnancy to optimize safety to the fetus and, in general, should not be done during pregnancy unless the overall benefit of change is felt to outweigh risks of reducing seizure control.

Long-Term Outcomes of Epilepsy in Pregnancy

Risk of major congenital malformations is significantly increased in offspring of women receiving AEDs (6.1%) as compared to women with epilepsy who do not receive AEDs (2.8%) and women without epilepsy (2.2%).[54] However, the AEDs do not all carry the same risk profile. Levetiracetam,

lamotrigine, and oxcarbazepine appear to carry the least risk, with a recent large prospective study showing no increased risk compared to offspring unexposed to AEDs.[55]

It is very clear that valproic acid use is associated with significantly increased risk of teratogenesis, including neural tube defects, reduced cognitive performance (particularly lower than expected verbal IQ),[56] autism spectrum disorders,[57,58] and hypospadias.[59] The effects are increased when used concurrently with other AEDs and are dose dependent. For this reason, valproic acid and polytherapy should be avoided in women of childbearing age at risk for pregnancy, and certainly during pregnancy, except under special circumstances.

Folic acid supplementation (0.4-4 mg daily) is recommended for all women of childbearing age due to association with significantly reduced risk of major congenital malformations and neural tube defects.[60] In women with epilepsy, its use has been associated with reduced risk of spontaneous abortion,[60] reduced risk of AED-related cognitive impairment, and higher IQ in offspring exposed to AEDs.[56]

Breastfeeding in women with epilepsy taking AEDs is encouraged with few exceptions, namely use of barbiturates and benzodiazepines, which are associated with higher risk to the infant due to sedation, lethargy, and poor feeding.

Movement Disorders in Pregnancy

Ataxia is the loss of coordinated voluntary movement and may affect the muscles controlling limb movement, eye movement, speech, and gait. It typically results from disease of the cerebellum and/or spinocerebellar tracts.

During pregnancy, the most common, preventable, and treatable cause of new-onset ataxia is thiamine (vitamin B1) deficiency. Thiamine deficiency can occur rapidly during pregnancy due to increased physiologic demand, as it is a cofactor for several enzymes critical to energy metabolism. It typically occurs in the setting of hyperemesis gravidarum and associated poor nutritional state.

Patients may also present with Wernicke encephalopathy (WE), classically described as a triad of confusion, ophthalmoplegia, and gait ataxia, though all three manifestations need not be present to make a diagnosis. In more severe cases, hypotension, hypothermia, and suppressed mental status or coma may occur.

For women with ataxia experiencing profound or persistent nausea and vomiting during pregnancy, it is important to monitor the nutritional state closely and preemptively supplement those at high risk for deficiency. Occasionally, supplementary enteral or parenteral nutrition may also be required. When ataxia is noted and WE suspected, empiric treatment should be started immediately.

Chorea Gravidarum

Clinical Presentation of CG

Chorea gravidarum (CG) is a disorder of pregnancy characterized by dance-like movements. It was originally described in association with rheumatic fever, though is now most commonly seen in association with exposure to various medications and substances, including opioids, cocaine, amphetamine, and other sympathomimetic agents, neuroleptics, and antihistamines. Lupus and other connective tissue disorders, antiphospholipid syndrome, stroke, syphilis, neuroacanthocytosis, thyrotoxicosis, Wilson disease, and encephalitis can all be associated with the disorder. When associated with history of rheumatic fever, CG often presents in the first trimester and will resolve before delivery in approximately one-third of cases. There is a 20% risk of recurrence in subsequent pregnancies.

Management of CG

Supportive management of CG helps to reduce risk of complications such as rhabdomyolysis, pain, weight loss, and hyperthermia from excess movement. Treatment with dopamine blocking and depleting agents should be deferred until at least the second trimester once organogenesis is largely complete.

Restless Leg Syndrome

Clinical Presentation of RLS

RLS is a common condition in the general population marked by an urge to move the legs, often at night. Age, obesity, smoking, multiparity, iron deficiency, and vitamin D deficiency are among risk factors that have been associated with RLS during pregnancy. Those with preexisting RLS are at higher risk of developing symptom exacerbation during pregnancy. It affects up to one-third of pregnancies, typically affecting the later stages, and often contributing to difficulty sleeping.

Management of RLS

RLS typically improves in the first month after delivery. Evaluation typically involves investigation for iron and vitamin D deficiencies and lifestyle modifications including avoidance of caffeine and alcohol. Behavioral interventions, including massage and compression stockings can be helpful. Iron supplementation may help to alleviate symptoms. Pharmacotherapy may be considered when symptoms significantly impair quality of life enough to justify potential risk of medication therapy. A collaborative guideline on treatment and was published in 2016.[61]

Parkinson Disease

Clinical Presentation of PD

Approximately half or more of pregnancies occurring in women with Parkinson disease (PD) are complicated by worsening motor symptoms, though nonmotor symptoms can also worsen. PD and pregnancy was reviewed by Seier and Hiller in 2017.[62]

Management of PD in Pregnancy

Levodopa, and nonergot dopamine agonists pramipexole, ropinirole, and rotigotine have been used successfully to treat PD during pregnancy without association with significant maternal adverse side effects or major fetal anomalies.[61] Levodopa is considered to have the most safety data available, thus currently considered the most favored treatment in pregnancy if therapy is required.

Tremor

Tremor is a common complaint in pregnancy, and normally will represent enhanced physiologic tremor, drug-induced tremor (particularly seen with SSRIs), both of which tend to be of fast frequency and low amplitude, and present particularly with sustained postures. Essential tremor, an autosomal dominant condition marked by a postural and kinetic tremor that tends to affect the upper extremities and/or head, may also emerge or worsen during pregnancy.

Neuroradiology Considerations

Elective imaging should generally be deferred until after pregnancy. For evaluation of urgent or emergent conditions, MRI is the modality of choice to provide the most accurate diagnosis for most neurological conditions and carries no known risk of fetal harm up to 3T.

Gadolinium-based contrast agents (GBCAs) cross the placenta and are considered FDA class C. Although they carry no known risk of fetal harm, they should be avoided during pregnancy, if possible, unless the clinical benefit in aiding diagnosis is felt to outweigh potential risk.

While CT does provide fetal exposure to ionizing radiation and, therefore, confers a theoretically increased—but small absolute—risk of childhood cancer, the dose exposure is felt to be low enough to confer relatively little risk. Intravenous use of iodinated contrast agents is discouraged in pregnancy unless required for evaluation of certain serious conditions. Though FDA category B, iodine has not been associated with increased risk of teratogenesis or adverse fetal outcomes. Neonatal thyroid testing is recommended for the first week after delivery due to possible risk of neonatal hypothyroidism after exposure to iodine in pregnancy. Guideline recommendations provided by the American College of Obstetricians and Gynecologists, American College of Radiology, and Society for Pediatric Radiology address this topic in further detail.[63-65] An additional discussion on radiation in pregnancy appears in Chapter 9.

KEY POINTS

- Stroke risk is increased during pregnancy. More rare etiologies, such as paradoxical venous thrombus, amniotic fluid or air embolism, trophoblastic embolism, CVT, and cervical artery dissection are seen more frequently. Emergency neurologic evaluation is essential to reduce stroke-related disability.
- Exacerbation of or reemergence of migraine after a period of quiescence is not uncommon in pregnancy and usually does not require additional investigation. Emergence of a new headache type, particularly if sudden in onset, unusually severe, poorly responsive to conservative measures, accompanied by focal neurologic deficits, papilledema, or in association with hypertension and/or proteinuria, is cause for concern and further investigation.
- Bell palsy, carpal tunnel syndrome, and meralgia paresthetica are among the most frequently seen neuromuscular disorders in pregnancy and tend to be somewhat self-limited. Lumbosacral plexopathy and lower extremity mononeuropathies can impact function and quality of life significantly. Careful positioning/padding during surgical procedures and vaginal delivery can reduce risk.
- Acute polyneuropathy in pregnancy should prompt urgent evaluation by a neurologist to assess for nutritional deficiencies, particularly thiamine deficiency. Supplementation with high-dose thiamine is recommended as soon as suspected. For patients with suspected AIDP, urgent treatment with IVIG or plasmapheresis can be used. Patients require careful monitoring for neuromuscular respiratory failure.
- MG may present for the first time during pregnancy. Crises can be managed with IVIG or plasmapheresis. While most steroid-sparing immune suppressants are relatively contraindicated in pregnancy, pyridostigmine can be continued for symptom management.
- Women with epilepsy require careful preconception counseling. AED drug levels may need to be checked much more frequently, and doses adjusted to maintain therapeutic levels. Those receiving AEDs are at increased risk for major congenital malformations compared to women not taking AEDs and women without epilepsy. Valproic acid is clearly teratogenic and should be avoided in women of childbearing potential with some occasional exceptions.
- Ataxia, chorea gravidarum, restless leg syndrome, and Parkinson disease are among the most common movement disorders affecting pregnancy. New ataxia, particularly in a woman with impaired nutrition or intractable vomiting, may be due to thiamine deficiency.

REFERENCES

1. Kuklina EV, Tong X, Bansil P, George MG, Callaghan WM. Trends in pregnancy hospitalizations that included a stroke in the United States from 1994 to 2007: reasons for concern? *Stroke.* 2011;42(9):2564-2570.
2. Swartz RH, Cayley ML, Foley N, et al. The incidence of pregnancy-related stroke: a systematic review and meta-analysis. *Int J Stroke.* 2017;12(7):687-697.
3. Mehta LS, Warnes CA, Bradley E, et al. Cardiovascular considerations in caring for pregnant patients: a scientific statement from the American Heart association. *Circulation.* 2020;141(23):e884-e903.
4. Ban L, Sprigg N, Abdul Sultan A, et al. Incidence of first stroke in pregnant and nonpregnant women of childbearing age: a population-based cohort study from england. *J Am Heart Assoc.* 2017;6(4):e004601.
5. Elgendy IY, Gad MM, Mahmoud AN, Keeley EC, Pepine CJ. Acute stroke during pregnancy and puerperium. *J Am Coll Cardiol.* 2020;75(2):180-190.
6. Rosendaal FR, Helmerhorst FM, Vandenbroucke JP. Female hormones and thrombosis. *Arterioscler Thromb Vasc Biol.* 2002;22(2):201-210.
7. Bhogal P, Aguilar M, AlMatter M, Karck U, Bäzner H, Henkes H. Mechanical thrombectomy in pregnancy: report of 2 cases and review of the literature. *Interv Neurol.* 2017;6(1-2):49-56.
8. Limaye K, Van de Walle Jones A, Shaban A, et al. Endovascular management of acute large vessel occlusion stroke in pregnancy is safe and feasible. *J Neurointerv Surg.* 2020;12(6):552-556.
9. Leffert LR, Clancy CR, Bateman BT, et al. Treatment patterns and short-term outcomes in ischemic stroke in pregnancy or postpartum period. *Am J Obstet Gynecol.* 2016;214(6):723.e1-723.e11.
10. Ladhani NNN, Swartz RH, Foley N, et al. Canadian stroke best practice consensus statement: acute stroke management during pregnancy. *Int J Stroke.* 2018;13(7):743-758.
11. Powers WJ, Rabinstein AA, Ackerson T, et al. 2018 guidelines for the early management of patients with acute ischemic stroke: a guideline for Healthcare Professionals from the American Heart association/American stroke association. *Stroke.* 2018;49(3):e46-e110.
12. Meeks JR, Bambhroliya AB, Alex KM, et al. Association of primary intracerebral hemorrhage with pregnancy and the postpartum period. *JAMA Netw Open.* 2020;3(4):e202769.
13. Ascanio LC, Maragkos GA, Young BC, Boone MD, Kasper EM. Spontaneous intracranial hemorrhage in pregnancy: a systematic review of the literature. *Neurocrit Care.* 2019;30(1):5-15.
14. Turan TN, Stern BJ. Stroke in pregnancy. *Neurol Clin.* 2004;22(4):821-840.
15. Hemphill JC III, Greenberg SM, Anderson CS, et al. Guidelines for the management of spontaneous intracerebral hemorrhage: a guideline for Healthcare Professionals from the American Heart association/American stroke association. *Stroke.* 2015;46(7):2032-2060.
16. Lee S, Kim Y, Navi BB, et al. Risk of intracranial hemorrhage associated with pregnancy in women with cerebral arteriovenous malformations. *J Neurointerv Surg.* 2020;neurintsurg-2020-016838. doi:10.1136/neurintsurg-2020-016838
17. Robba C, Bacigaluppi S, Bragazzi NL, et al. Aneurysmal subarachnoid hemorrhage in pregnancy-case series, review, and pooled data analysis. *World Neurosurg.* 2016;88:383-398.
18. Toossi S, Moheet AM. Intracerebral hemorrhage in women: a review with special attention to pregnancy and the post-partum period. *Neurocrit Care.* 2019;31(2):390-398.
19. Bateman BT, Olbrecht VA, Berman MF, Minehart RD, Schwamm LH, Leffert LR. Peripartum subarachnoid hemorrhage: nationwide data and institutional experience. *Anesthesiology.* 2012;116(2):324-333.
20. Selo-Ojeme DO, Marshman LA, Ikomi A, et al. Aneurysmal subarachnoid haemorrhage in pregnancy. *Eur J Obstet Gynecol Reprod Biol.* 2004;116(2):131-143.
21. Desai M, Wali AR, Birk HS, Santiago-Dieppa DR, Khalessi AA. Role of pregnancy and female sex steroids on aneurysm formation, growth, and rupture: a systematic review of the literature. *Neurosurg Focus.* 2019;47(1):E8.
22. Salonen Ros H, Lichtenstein P, Bellocco R, Petersson G, Cnattingius S. Increased risks of circulatory diseases in late pregnancy and puerperium. *Epidemiology.* 2001;12(4):456-460.
23. Nussbaum ES, Goddard JK, Davis AR. A systematic review of intracranial aneurysms in the pregnant patient – a clinical conundrum. *Eur J Obstet Gynecol Reprod Biol.* 2020;254:79-86.
24. Silvis SM, Lindgren E, Hiltunen S, et al. postpartum period is a risk factor for cerebral venous thrombosis. *Stroke.* 2019;50(2):501-503.
25. Khan KS, Wojdyla D, Say L, Gülmezoglu AM, Van Look PF. WHO analysis of causes of maternal death: a systematic review. *Lancet.* 2006;367(9516):1066-1074.
26. Ananth CV, Keyes KM, Wapner RJ. Pre-eclampsia rates in the United States, 1980-2010: age-period-cohort analysis. *Br Med J.* 2013;347:f6564.
27. Steegers EA, von Dadelszen P, Duvekot JJ, Pijnenborg R. Pre-eclampsia. *Lancet.* 2010;376(9741):631-644.
28. Altman D, Carroli G, Duley L, et al. Do women with pre-eclampsia, and their babies, benefit from magnesium sulphate? The Magpie Trial: a randomised placebo-controlled trial. *Lancet.* 2002;359(9321):1877-1890.
29. Lucas MJ, Leveno KJ, Cunningham FG. A comparison of magnesium sulfate with phenytoin for the prevention of eclampsia. *N Engl J Med.* 1995;333(4):201-205.
30. Grandi SM, Filion KB, Yoon S, et al. Cardiovascular disease-related morbidity and mortality in women with a history of pregnancy complications. *Circulation.* 2019;139(8):1069-1079.
31. Nerenberg KA, Park AL, Vigod SN, et al. Long-term risk of a seizure disorder after eclampsia. *Obstet Gynecol.* 2017;130(6):1327-1333.
32. Fishel Bartal M, Sibai BM. Eclampsia in the 21st century. *Am J Obstet Gynecol.* 2020;S0002-9378(20)31128-5. doi:10.1016/j.ajog.2020.09.037
33. Petersenn S, Christ-Crain M, Droste M, et al. Pituitary disease in pregnancy: special aspects of diagnosis and treatment? *Geburtshilfe Frauenheilkd.* 2019;79(4):365-374.
34. O'Neal MA. Headaches complicating pregnancy and the postpartum period. *Pract Neurol.* 2017;17(3):191-202.
35. Ashina M. Migraine. *N Engl J Med.* 2020;383(19):1866-1876.
36. Granella F, Sances G, Pucci E, Nappi RE, Ghiotto N, Napp G. Migraine with aura and reproductive life events: a case control study. *Cephalalgia.* 2000;20(8):701-707.
37. Nezvalová-Henriksen K, Spigset O, Nordeng H. Triptan exposure during pregnancy and the risk of major congenital malformations and adverse pregnancy outcomes: results from the Norwegian Mother and Child Cohort Study. *Headache.* 2010;50(4):563-575.
38. Matok I, Gorodischer R, Koren G, Sheiner E, Wiznitzer A, Levy A. The safety of metoclopramide use in the first trimester of pregnancy. *N Engl J Med.* 2009;360(24):2528-2535.
39. Skajaa N, Szépligeti SK, Xue F, et al. Pregnancy, birth, neonatal, and postnatal neurological outcomes after pregnancy with migraine. *Headache.* 2019;59(6):869-879.
40. Park DSJ, Park JSY, Sharma S, Sharma RA. Idiopathic intracranial hypertension in pregnancy. *J Obstet Gynaecol Can.* 2021;S1701-2163(20)31041-0. doi:10.1016/j.jogc.2020.12.019
41. Guidon AC, Massey EW. Neuromuscular disorders in pregnancy. *Neurol Clin.* 2012;30(3):889-911.
42. Gronseth GS, Paduga R. Evidence-based guideline update: steroids and antivirals for bell palsy. Report of the guideline development subcommittee of the American academy of neurology. *Neurology.* 2012;79(22):2209-2213.
43. Phillips KM, Heiser A, Gaudin R, Hadlock TA, Jowett N. Onset of bell's palsy in late pregnancy and early puerperium is associated with worse long-term outcomes. *Laryngoscope.* 2017;127(12):2854-2859.
44. Geddes A, Barry J, Thomas C. Increased incidence of Bell's palsy with worse outcomes in pregnancy. *Br J Oral Maxillofac Surg.* 2018;56(7):646-647.
45. Chan LY, Tsui MH, Leung TN. Guillain-Barré syndrome in pregnancy. *Acta Obstet Gynecol Scand.* 2004;83(4):319-325.
46. Feldman JM. Cardiac arrest after succinylcholine administration in a pregnant patient recovered from Guillain-Barré syndrome. *Anesthesiology.* 1990;72(5):942-944.
47. Kveraga R, Pawlowski J. *Anesthesia for the Patient With Myasthenia Gravis.* UpToDate. Accessed July 29, 2019. https://www.uptodate.com/contents/anesthesia-for-the-patient-with-myasthenia-gravis
48. Plauché WC. Myasthenia gravis in mothers and their newborns. *Clin Obstet Gynecol.* 1991;34(1):82-99.
49. Ahlsten G, Lefvert AK, Osterman PO, Stålberg E, Säfwenberg J. Follow-up study of muscle function in children of mothers with myasthenia gravis during pregnancy. *J Child Neurol.* 1992;7(3):264-269.
50. Zack MM, Kobau R. National and state estimates of the numbers of adults and children with active epilepsy – United States, 2015. *MMWR Morb Mortal Wkly Rep.* 2017;66(31):821-825.

51. Christensen J, Vestergaard M, Olsen J, Sidenius P. Validation of epilepsy diagnoses in the Danish national hospital register. *Epilepsy Res.* 2007;75(2-3):162-170.

52. MacDonald SC, Bateman BT, McElrath TF, Hernández-Díaz S. Mortality and morbidity during delivery hospitalization among pregnant women with epilepsy in the United States. *JAMA Neurol.* 2015;72(9):981-988.

53. Tomson T, Landmark CJ, Battino D. Antiepileptic drug treatment in pregnancy: changes in drug disposition and their clinical implications. *Epilepsia.* 2013;54(3):405-414.

54. Shorvon SD, Tomson T, Cock HR. The management of epilepsy during pregnancy--progress is painfully slow. *Epilepsia.* 2009;50(5):973-974.

55. Vossler DG. Comparative risk of major congenital malformations with 8 different antiepileptic drugs: a prospective cohort study of the EURAP registry. *Epilepsy Curr.* 2019;19(2):83-85.

56. Meador KJ, Baker GA, Browning N, et al. Fetal antiepileptic drug exposure and cognitive outcomes at age 6 years (NEAD study): a prospective observational study. *Lancet Neurol.* 2013;12(3):244-252.

57. Bromley RL, Mawer G, Clayton-Smith J, Baker GA. Autism spectrum disorders following in utero exposure to antiepileptic drugs. *Neurology.* 2008;71(23):1923-1924.

58. Christensen J, Grønborg TK, Sørensen MJ, et al. Prenatal valproate exposure and risk of autism spectrum disorders and childhood autism. *J Am Med Assoc.* 2013;309(16):1696-1703.

59. Jentink J, Loane MA, Dolk H, et al. Valproic acid monotherapy in pregnancy and major congenital malformations. *N Engl J Med.* 2010;362(23):2185-2193.

60. Pittschieler S, Brezinka C, Jahn B, et al. Spontaneous abortion and the prophylactic effect of folic acid supplementation in epileptic women undergoing antiepileptic therapy. *J Neurol.* 2008;255(12):1926-1931.

61. Garcia-Borreguero D, Silber MH, Winkelman JW, et al. Guidelines for the first-line treatment of restless legs syndrome/Willis-Ekbom disease, prevention and treatment of dopaminergic augmentation: a combined task force of the IRLSSG, EURLSSG, and the RLS-foundation. *Sleep Med.* 2016;21:1-11.

62. Seier M, Hiller A. Parkinson's disease and pregnancy: an updated review. *Parkinsonism Relat Disord.* 2017;40:11-17.

63. American College of Obstetricians and Gynecologists. Committee Opinion No. 723: guidelines for diagnostic imaging during pregnancy and lactation. *Obstet Gynecol.* 2017;130(4):e210-e216.

64. American College of Radiology. *ACR Practice Parameter for Performing and Interpreting Magnetic Resonance Imaging (MRI).* 2017. Accessed July 25, 2019. https://www.acr.org/-/media/ACR/Files/Practice-Parameters/MR-Perf-Interpret.pdf

65. American College of Radiology. *ACR–SPR Practice Parameter for Imaging Pregnant or Potentially Pregnant Adolescents and Women With Ionizing Radiation.* American College of Radiology; 2018. Accessed July 25, 2019. https://www.acr.org/-/media/acr/files/practice-parameters/pregnant-pts.pdf

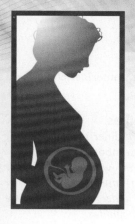

CHAPTER 37

Thromboembolic Disorders of Pregnancy

Audrey A. Merriam, Christian M. Pettker, and Michael J. Paidas

Clinical Presentation

Clinical Risk Factors for Venous Thromboembolism in Pregnancy

Vascular stasis, hypercoagulability, and vascular trauma (Virchow triad) remain the three prime antecedents to thrombosis. Clinical risk factors specific to obstetrics that increase the risk for venous thromboembolism (VTE) include pregnancy, multiple gestation, preeclampsia, cesarean delivery, operative vaginal delivery, postpartum hemorrhage requiring transfusion (**Table 37.1**).[24-26] Nonobstetric risk factors for VTE include age >35 years, infection, trauma, cancer, nephrotic syndrome, obesity, surgery, hyperviscosity syndromes, immobilization, congestive heart failure, prior VTE, and the presence of acquired and inherited thrombophilias.

Pregnant women with a history of a thrombophilia and those with a prior history of thromboembolism have the highest risks of thromboembolism (**Table 37.2**).[29]

Hemostatic Changes in Pregnancy

Substantial changes must occur in local (decidual) and systemic coagulation, anticoagulant, and fibrinolytic systems to meet the hemostatic challenges of pregnancy, including avoidance of hemorrhage at implantation, placentation, and the third stage of labor.

Table 37.3 summarizes the relevant pregnancy-associated changes in the hemostatic system.[23,35,36]

The most significant pregnancy-related prothrombotic factors are listed in **Table 37.4**.

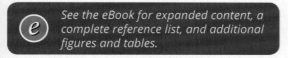

See the eBook for expanded content, a complete reference list, and additional figures and tables.

Acquired Thrombophilia

Antiphospholipid antibodies (APAs) are detected by screening for antibodies that:

- directly bind these protein epitopes (eg, *anti-β2-glycoprotein-1*, prothrombin, annexin V, activated protein C, protein S (PS), protein Z (PZ), PZ-dependent protease inhibitor, high- and low-molecular-weight kininogens, tissue-type plasminogen activator, factors Vila and XII, the complement cascade constituents, C4 and CH, and oxidized low-density lipoprotein antibodies); or
- are bound to proteins present in an anionic phospholipid matrix (eg, *anticardiolipin* and phosphatidylserine antibodies); or
- exert downstream effects on prothrombin activation in a phospholipid milieu (ie, *lupus anticoagulants*).[39]

Anti-β2-glycoprotein-1, anticardiolipin, and lupus anticoagulants are used when screening for APLS. Positive test results are as follows: anticardiolipin antibodies (IgG or IgM greater than 40 GPL [1 GPL unit is 1 µg of IgG antibody] or 40 MPL [1 MPL unit is 1 µg of IgM antibody] or greater than the 99th percentile), anti–β-2 glycoprotein-I (IgG or IgM greater than the 99th percentile), or lupus anticoagulant.[40]

Clinicians should use caution when ordering and interpreting tests in the absence of the APLS-qualifying clinical criteria listed above.

Venous thrombotic events associated with APA include deep vein thrombosis (DVT) with or without acute pulmonary embolus, whereas the most common arterial events include cerebral vascular accidents and transient ischemic attacks. At least half of patients with APA have systemic lupus erythematosus.

Table 37.1 Risk of Venous Thromboembolic Disease in Women: a Qualitative Systematic review[23]

Risk Factor	Risk per 1000 Women-Years
Pregnancy	1.23
Puerperium	3.2
Pregnancy in thrombophilic patients	40
Pregnancy and history of VTE	110

VTE, venous thromboembolism.
Data from Bremme K, Ostlund E, Almqvist I, et al. Enhanced thrombin generation and fibrinolytic activity in normal pregnancy and the puerperium. *Obstet Gynecol.* 1992;80:132-137.

A severe form of antiphospholipid antibody syndrome (APLS) is termed catastrophic APS, or CAPS, which is defined as a potentially life-threatening variant with multiple vessel thromboses leading to multiorgan failure.[44]

APAs are associated with obstetric complications in about 15% to 20% of cases including fetal loss after 9 weeks' gestation, abruptio placentae,

severe preeclampsia, and intrauterine/fetal growth restriction (FGR).

Inherited Thrombophilias
The most important risk modifier is a personal or family history of venous thrombosis.

Any woman who presents with VTE (DVT or pulmonary embolism [PE]) during pregnancy or postpartum period should undergo an appropriate workup for inherited thrombophilias.

Table 37.5 summarizes the thromboembolic risks associated with the significant known thrombophilic mutations.[61-67]

Adverse Pregnancy Outcomes and Inherited Thrombophilias
Severe Preeclampsia/Syndrome of Hemolysis, Elevated Liver Enzymes, and Low Platelets
There is no conclusive evidence of an association between inherited thrombophilias and preeclampsia.

Abruptio Placentae
At this time, there is inconclusive evidence to support an association between thrombophilias and abruptio placentae.

Table 37.2 Pregnancy-Associated Clinical Risk Factors for Venous Thromboembolism (Odds Ratios With Confidence Intervals)

	Lindqvist, 1999 (*n* = 603)	Danilenko-Dixon, 2001 (*n* = 90)	Anderson, 2003 (*n* = 1231)
Moderate-risk factors			
Age ≥35 years	1.3 (1-1.7)	–	2.0 (age >40 years)
Parity (2)	1.5 (1.1-1.9)	1.1 (0.9-1.4)	–
Parity (≥3)	2.4 (1.8-3.1)	–	–
Smoking	1.4 (1.1-1.9)	2.5 (1.3-4.7)	–
Multiple gestation	1.8 (1.1-3.0)	7 (0.4-135.5)	–
Preeclampsia	2.9 (2.1-3.9)	1 (0.14-7.1)	–
Varicose veins	–	2.4 (1.04-5.4)	4.5
Obesity	–	1.5 (0.7-3.2)	<2
Cesarean delivery	3.6 (3.0-4.3)	–	–
Obstetric hemorrhage	–	9 (1.1-71.0)	–
High-risk factors			
Spinal cord injury	–	–	>10
Major abdominal surgery ≥30 min	–	–	>10

Data from Lindqvist P, Dahlback B, Marsal K. Thrombotic risk during pregnancy: a population study. *Obstet Gynecol.* 1999;94:595-599; Danilenko-Dixon DR, Heit JA, Silverstein MD, et al. Risk factors for deep vein thrombosis and pulmonary embolism during pregnancy or postpartum: a population-based, case-control study. *Am J Obstet Gynecol.* 2001;184:104-110, and Anderson FA Jr, Spencer FA. Risk factors for venous thromboembolism. *Circulation.* 2003;107(23 suppl 1):I9-I16.

Table 37.3 Procoagulant and Anticoagulant Parameters in Pregnancy by Trimester

Variables (Mean ± SD)	Change in Pregnancy	First Trimester[a]	Second Trimester[a]	Third Trimester[a]	Normal Range
Procoagulants					
Platelet (×10⁹/L)	No change/ decrease	275 ± 64	256 ± 49	244 ± 52	150-400
Fibrinogen (g/L)	Increase	3.7 ± 0.6	4.4 ± 1.2	5.4 ± 0.8	2.1-4.2
Prothrombin complex (%)		120 ± 27	140 ± 27	130 ± 27	70-30
Soluble fibrin (nmol/L)	Increase	9.2 ± 8.6	11.8 ± 7.7	13.4 ± 5.2	<15
Thrombin-antithrombin (µg/L)	Increase	3.1 ± 1.4	5.9 ± 2.6	7.1 ± 2.4	<2.7
D-dimers (µg/L)	Increase	91 ± 24	128 ± 49	198 ± 59	<80
Plasminogen activator inhibitor-1 (AU/mL)	Increase	7.4 ± 4.9	14.9 ± 5.2	37.8 ± 19.4	<15
Plasminogen activator inhibitor-2 (µg/L)	Increase	31 ± 14	84 ± 16	160 ± 31	<5
Cardiolipin antibodies positive	Increase	2/25	2/25	3/23	0
Protein Z (µg/mL)[b]	Decrease	2.01 ± 0.76	1.47 ± 0.45	1.55 ± 0.48	–
Anticoagulants					
Antithrombin (U/mL)	No change	1.02 ± 0.10	1.07 ± 0.14	1.07 ± 0.11	0.85-1.25
Protein C (U/mL)	No change	0.92 ± 0.13	1.06 ± 0.17	0.94 ± 0.2	0.68-1.25
Protein S, total (U/mL)	Decrease	0.83 ± 0.11	0.73 ± 0.11	0.77 ± 0.10	0.70-1.70
Protein S, free (U/mL)	Decrease	0.26 ± 0.07	0.17 ± 0.04	0.14 ± 0.04	0.20-0.50
Protein S, free antigen (%)[b]	No change	–	38.9 ± 10.3	31.2 ± 7.4	–

[a]First trimester, weeks 12 to 15; second trimester, week 24; third trimester, week 35.
[b]First trimester, 0 to 14 wk; second trimester, 14 to 27 wk; third trimester, ≥27 wk.
Modified from Bremme K, Ostlund E, Almqvist I, et al. Enhanced thrombin generation and fibrinolytic activity in normal pregnancy and the puerperium. *Obstet Gynecol*. 1992;80:132-137; Paidas MJ, Ku DH, Langhoff-Roos J, Arkel YS. Inherited thrombophilias and adverse pregnancy outcome: screening and management. *Semin Perinatol*. 2005;29:150-163. ACOG Practice Bulletin No. 196: thromboembolism in pregnancy. *Obstet Gynecol*. 2018;132:e1-e17, and (b) Paidas MJ, Ku DW, Lee MJ, et al. Protein Z, protein S levels are lower in patients with thrombophilia and subsequent pregnancy complications. *J Thromb Haemost*. 2005;3:497-501.

Fetal Growth Restriction
Women with a history of FGR in a previous pregnancy do not warrant a workup for thrombophilia prior to or at the beginning of a future pregnancy.

Early and Late Fetal Loss
Women with a history of pregnancy loss or other severe pregnancy complications in a previous pregnancy do not warrant a workup for common inherited thrombophilic conditions prior to or at the beginning of a future pregnancy.

Screening
The selection of suitable patients for thrombophilia screening and the thrombophilia workup continue to evolve. At this time, suitable candidates for

Table 37.4 Most Significant Prothrombotic Changes in Pregnancy

Increased Levels of procoagulants	Diminished Fibrinolysis	Mechanical Factors
Fibrinogen	Decreased protein S	Venous distension
Factor VIII	Resistance to activated protein C	Vessel injury Compression of left iliac vein

acquired thrombophilia (ie, APS) screening include only those with a history of severe preeclampsia/HELLP (hemolysis, elevated liver enzymes, and low platelets) at <36 weeks; a history of FGR ≤5th percentile; a personal history of thrombosis; and a family history of thrombosis. Candidates for inherited thrombophilia screening include only those with a personal history of thrombosis and a family history of thrombosis. Initial thrombophilia evaluation should include protein C (functional level); PS (functional/free antigen level); antithrombin III (ATIII; functional level); factor V Leiden (by polymerase chain reaction [PCR]); prothrombin gene mutation 20210A (PCR); lupus anticoagulant; anticardiolipin antibody IgG/IgM and β2-glycoprotein-1 IgG/IgM.

Clinical Assessment

Diagnosis of Venous Thromboembolism

The diagnosis of VTE is based on history, physical examination, and diagnostic studies. The typically cited signs and symptoms of DVT include erythema, warmth, pain, edema, tenderness, and a positive Homans sign. However, among patients with these signs and symptoms, the diagnosis of DVT is confirmed in only one-third when reliable objective tests are performed.[96]

Venous ultrasound with or without color Doppler has become the primary diagnostic modality for evaluating patients at risk of DVT (**Algorithm 37.1**). The most accurate ultrasonic criterion for diagnosing venous thrombosis is noncompressibility of the venous lumen in a transverse plane under gentle probe pressure using duplex and color flow Doppler.[96]

Two other imaging modalities include magnetic resonance imaging and impedance plethysmography.

Venography remains the "gold standard" for the diagnosis of DVT; however, because it causes radiation exposure, it is not typically used in pregnancy.

Diagnosis of Acute Pulmonary Embolus

Tachypnea (>20 breaths/min) and tachycardia (>100 beats per minute) are present in 90% of

Table 37.5 Inherited Thrombophilias and Association With Venous Thromboembolism

Thrombophilia	Prevalence in European Populations (From Large Cohort Studies)	Prevalence in Patients With VTE (Range)	Relative Risk or Odds Ratio (OR) of VTE (95% CI) (Lifetime)	Reference
FVL (homozygous)	0.07%[a]	<1%[a]	80 [22-289]	47-50
FVL (heterozygous)	5.3%	6.6%-50%	2.7 [1.3-5.6]	47, 48
PGM (homozygous)	0.02%[a]	<1%	>80-fold[a]	50
PGM (heterozygous)	2.9%	7.5%	3.8 [3.0-4.9]	51
FVL/PGM (compound heterozygous)	0.17%[a]	2.0%	20.0 [11.1-36.1]	51
Antithrombin deficiency (<60% activity)	0.2%	1%-8%	17.5 [9.1-33.8]	49, 52
Protein S deficiency: <55%	0.2%	3.1%	2.4 [0.8-7.9]	53
Protein C (<60% activity)	0.2%	3%-5%	11.3 [5.7-22.3]	49, 52

CI, confidence interval; FVL, factor V Leiden; PGM, prothrombin G20201A; VTE, venous thromboembolism.
[a]Calculated based on a Hardy-Weinberg equilibrium.

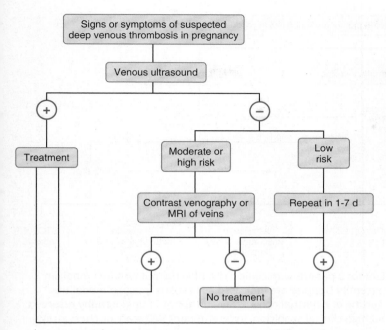

Algorithm 37.1 Management of suspected deep vein thrombosis (DVT) in pregnancy. Once a DVT is suspected, a venous ultrasound should be performed to establish the diagnosis of DVT. If positive, anticoagulation should be instituted. If negative, additional testing or repeat venous ultrasound may be indicated, depending upon the level of suspicion for the presence of DVT.

patients with PE but are nonspecific indices of risk. Symptoms such as dyspnea and pleuritic chest pain are present in up to 90% of patients with PE, whereas presyncope and syncope are rarer and indicative of massive emboli.

Electrocardiographic changes may be present in 87% of patients with proven PE who are without underlying cardiopulmonary disease; however, these findings are nonspecific. Assessment of arterial blood gases and oxygen saturation are also of limited value in PE.

More than 80% of patients with PE display sonographic imaging or Doppler abnormalities of right-ventricular size or function, including a dilated and hypokinetic right ventricle, tricuspid regurgitation, and absence of preexisting pulmonary arterial or left-heart pathology.

Laboratory assessment with D-dimer to determine a pregnant woman's risk for PE is generally not recommended as it has a lower sensitivity in pregnant patients with PE and thus it is not helpful as a test for ruling out disease. Pregnant patients with imaging confirmed PE have been found to have negative D-dimer testing (**Algorithm 37.2**).[103,106]

Chest radiography should be performed when assessment of the lower extremities for DVT is negative or when no lower extremity signs or symptoms exist. A normal chest radiograph should then prompt screening with a V/Q scan.

V/Q scanning is performed by imaging both the pulmonary vascular bed and the airspace.

A positive V/Q scan, which is considered a high or moderate probability of PE, should prompt treatment with therapeutic anticoagulation without the need for further imaging. If the V/Q scan is negative, then the diagnosis of PE is excluded. A nondiagnostic result, such as intermediate probability/equivocal test, in any patient OR a low-probability result in a patient considered to be at high risk for PE/high clinical suspicion (prior VTE, known thrombophilia, family history of thrombosis in a first-degree relative <50 years old), should trigger performance of CTPA.

For patients with an abnormal chest radiograph, or nondiagnostic V/Q imaging, CTPA is the diagnostic modality of choice. Spiral (helical) computerized tomographic angiography (spiral CT) is a technique that requires the continuous movement of a patient through a CT scanner as a contrast bolus is administered. It is of limited value with small subsegmental peripheral vessels and horizontally oriented vessels in the right middle lobe.

A positive CTPA result requires therapeutic anticoagulation. If the CTPA is nondiagnostic, further testing is required with either magnetic resonance angiography (MRA) or serial lower extremity venous ultrasound studies.

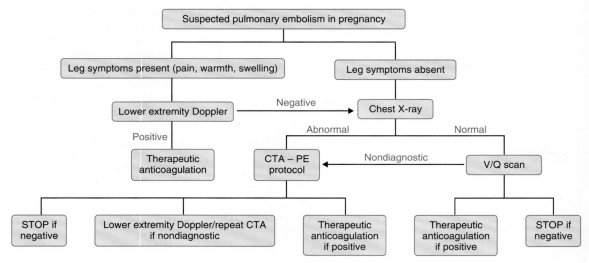

Algorithm 37.2 Management paradigm for a patient with clinical risk of acute pulmonary embolism (APE). Chest x-ray and venous lower extremity Doppler are indicated as first-line imaging modalities. V/Q scan should be performed in the setting of a normal chest x-ray and spiral CT angiography reserved for patients with negative V/Q scan and high clinical suspicion, indeterminant V/Q scan, or chest x-ray findings that would make a V/Q scan uninterpretable. Anticoagulation is indicated in the setting of: a positive spiral CT angiography; a high probability V/Q scan; a positive pulmonary angiogram; negative spiral CT and positive venous ultrasound; low or intermediate V/Q scan; and a positive venous ultrasound. CTA, computed tomography angiography; V/Q, ventilation-perfusion; PE, pulmonary embolism.

Pharmacologic Treatment

Anticoagulation Therapy

Combined heparin and aspirin administration are the best strategy for the treatment of recurrent pregnancy loss associated with APS.

Prophylaxis with heparin has been theorized to prevent recurrent pregnancy complications in the setting of inherited thrombophilias.

Management of Venous Thromboembolism in Pregnancy

While initiating anticoagulation therapy, a thrombophilia panel should be obtained. If the patient is hemodynamically stable, efforts should be made to collect the laboratory studies for a thrombophilia workup before beginning anticoagulation therapy as some of the tests become uninterpretable once treatment has begun. Women with new-onset VTE during a current pregnancy should receive therapeutic anticoagulation for the remainder of pregnancy followed by prophylactic therapy for at least 6 weeks postpartum (**Table 37.7**). Patients who have a VTE near the end of gestation should receive treatment doses for at least 20 weeks, which

may extend well into the postpartum period. During pregnancy, unfractionated heparin and low-molecular-weight heparin (LMWH) are the anticoagulants of choice. Postpartum, oral anticoagulation with warfarin may be started and is considered to be safe in breastfeeding mothers. As osteoporosis is more common with doses of heparin greater than 15,000 U/d employed for more than 6 months, all patients treated with heparin should be considered for supplementation with 1500 mg of calcium per day. Postpartum bone densitometry also may be appropriate in such patients.

The goals of therapy for an acute VTE in pregnancy are to maintain the activated partial thromboplastin time (aPTT) between 1.5- and 2.5-times control when using unfractionated heparin. The dose required may vary greatly between women secondary to interpatient differences in heparin-binding proteins during pregnancy. The aPTT should be evaluated every 4 to 6 hours during the initial phase of therapy and adjustments made in dosage as needed. Intravenous therapeutic unfractionated heparin should be continued for at least 5 to 10 days or until clinical improvement is noted.

Table 37.7 Anticoagulation in Pregnancy: Indication, Type, and Timing

Indication	Description	Antepartum	Postpartum
VTE in current pregnancy		Therapeutic LMWH/UFH from diagnosis until delivery	Therapeutic or prophylactic LMWH/UFH regimen until 6 wk postpartum depending on timing of VTE in pregnancy
High-risk thrombophilia • FVL homozygous • Prothrombin G20210A mutation homozygous • FVL/prothrombin G20210A mutation double heterozygous • Antithrombin III deficiency	History of one prior VTE	Therapeutic or prophylactic LMWH/UFH	Therapeutic or prophylactic LMWH regimen or postpartum warfarin
	No history of VTE	Prophylactic LMWH/UFH	Prophylactic LMWH or postpartum warfarin
Low-risk thrombophilia • FVL heterozygous • Prothrombin G20210A mutation heterozygous • Protein C deficiency • Protein S deficiency	History of one prior VTE	Prophylactic LMWH/UFH or surveillance without anticoagulation	Prophylactic LMWH/UFH or postpartum warfarin
	No history of VTE	Surveillance without anticoagulation or prophylactic LMWH/UFH	Surveillance without anticoagulation OR prophylactic LMWH/UFH OR postpartum warfarin if patient has *additional risk factors*
No thrombophilia	History of one prior VTE (pregnancy or estrogen related)	Prophylactic or therapeutic LMWH/UFH	Prophylactic or therapeutic LMWH/UFH for 6 wk
	History of one prior VTE (specific event, non–estrogen related)	Surveillance without anticoagulation	Surveillance without anticoagulation or prophylactic LMWH if the patient has *additional risk factors*
Two or more prior VTE episodes (thrombophilia or no thrombophilia)	On long-term anticoagulation	Therapeutic LMWH/UFH	Resumption of long-term anticoagulation therapy
	Not on long-term anticoagulation	Therapeutic or prophylactic LMWH/UFH	Therapeutic or prophylactic LMWH/UFH for 6 wk

FVL, factor V Leiden; LMWH, low-molecular-weight heparin; UFH, unfractionated heparin; VTE, venous thromboembolism.
Adapted from American College of Obstetricians and Gynecologists' Committee on Practice Bulletins—Obstetrics. ACOG Practice Bulletin No. 196: thromboembolism in pregnancy. *Obstet Gynecol.* 2018;132(1):e1-e17.

Thereafter, therapeutic doses of unfractionated heparin may be administered subcutaneously every 8 to 12 hours in order to maintain the aPTT at 1.5 to 2 times control levels 6 hours after the injection. These should be continued for the remainder of pregnancy followed by prophylactic dosages in the postpartum period, unless the event occurred near the end of gestation. Women with a VTE near the end of pregnancy should receive at least 20 weeks of therapeutic heparin.

If vaginal or cesarean delivery occurs more than 4 hours after a prophylactic dose of unfractionated heparin, the patient is not at significant risk of hemorrhagic complications. Protamine sulfate may be administered to those patients with an elevated aPTT receiving prophylactic or therapeutic unfractionated heparin who are about to deliver vaginally or by cesarean delivery (slow IV infusion of less than 20 mg/min, with no more than 50 mg given over 10 minutes). Patients can receive neuraxial anesthesia within 12 to 24 hours after their last subcutaneous dose of unfractionated heparin, depending on if they are receiving prophylactic or therapeutic dosing, respectively. Assessment of coagulation status (ie, rotational thromboelastometry) may be recommended prior to neuraxial blockade.[36]

For therapeutic dosing, the antifactor Xa level should be maintained at 0.6 to 1.0 U/mL 4 to 6 hours after injection (eg, starting with enoxaparin 1 mg/kg subcutaneously every 12 hours).

Treatment should continue for the remainder of pregnancy followed by prophylactic dosages in the postpartum period. If the event occurred near the end of gestation, therapeutic LMWH is recommended for at least 20 weeks. Patients with highly thrombogenic thrombophilias require therapeutic anticoagulation throughout pregnancy. As regional anesthesia is contraindicated within 24 hours of LMWH administration, women have the option of switching to unfractionated heparin at 36 to 37 weeks or earlier if preterm delivery is expected. For women with a planned cesarean delivery or induction date, it may be appropriate to maintain them on their therapeutic or prophylactic LMWH until 24 hours prior to admission. Patients should be counseled on both options and shared decision-making should be used to individualize treatment.

If vaginal or cesarean delivery occurs more than 12 hours from prophylactic or 24 hours from therapeutic doses of LMWH, the patient should not experience anticoagulation-related problems with delivery.

The American Society of Regional Anesthesia and Pain Medicine does not have any recommendations for neuraxial anesthesia administration in patients on the newer anticoagulants (ie, fondaparinux and rivaroxaban) in their most recent publication. If patients are on these medications, clinicians can refer to the European Society of Anesthesiology, which recommends waiting 22 to 42 hours between the last dose of these mediations and neuraxial anesthesia administration based on the half-lives of the medication.[137]

Special Considerations

Recurrent VTE
Antepartum heparin is not necessary in patients without thrombophilia and whose prior VTE is

associated with temporary risk factors. Antepartum prophylaxis is indicated in the latter group of patients. Postpartum anticoagulation is indicated in both groups.

Mechanical Heart Valves
One option is enoxaparin 1 mg/kg every 12 hours and warfarin discontinued either before or immediately after pregnancy is diagnosed. Trough levels of enoxaparin must be 0.5 IU/mL. Peak antifactor Xa levels should ideally be 0.8 to 1.0 IU/mL, but levels can safely be obtained with the upper range of the peak antifactor-Xa level being 1.5 IU/mL. Weekly peak and trough antifactor-Xa levels should be obtained.

Antithrombin Deficiency
Patients with antithrombin deficiency should receive plasma-derived or recombinant antithrombin during periods of highest thromboembolic risk, namely delivery or surgery, when anticoagulation cannot be administered due to the risk of bleeding. The baseline antithrombin level is expressed as the percentage of the normal level based on the functional ATIII assay. The goal is to increase the antithrombin levels to those found in normal human plasma (around 100%).

Postpartum Management
Prophylactic unfractionated heparin or LMWH can be restarted 4 to 6 hours after vaginal delivery or 6 to 12 hours after cesarean delivery. In patients requiring therapeutic LMWH after delivery, there should be consideration for holding their first dose until 24 hours after spinal anesthesia administration. Warfarin can be started on the first postdelivery day in combination with therapeutic doses of unfractionated heparin or LMWH for 5 days and until the international normalized ratio (INR) reaches the therapeutic range between 2.0 and 3.0 for 2 successive days. Of note, the Royal College of Obstetricians and Gynecologists recommends waiting until at least postpartum day number 5 to resume warfarin.[27] Due to the elevated risk of VTE immediately postpartum for all women, regardless of thrombophilia history, multiple professional societies recommend VTE prophylaxis for women based on clinical risk factor stratification.

KEY POINTS

- VTE is a leading cause of death in women. It is estimated that VTE complicates 1 in 1000 pregnancies, but the precise frequency of thromboembolism is probably underestimated.
- Pregnancy is associated with significant elevations in a number of clotting factors. Fibrinogen concentration is doubled, and 20% to 1000% increases in factors VII, VIII, IX, X, XII, and von Willebrand factor are observed, with maximum levels reached at term. PS decreases in pregnancy.
- The high-risk thrombophilias include ATIII deficiency, factor V Leiden homozygosity, and prothrombin gene (G20210A) mutation. Heterozygous factor V Leiden is associated with a 0.2% risk of thromboembolism associated with pregnancy, while heterozygous prothrombin gene mutation is associated with a 0.5% risk. Compound heterozygous factor V Leiden and prothrombin gene mutation is associated with a 4.6% risk of thromboembolism.
- APS is defined by the combination of VTE, obstetric complications, and APA. APAs must be present on two or more occasions at least 6 weeks apart and are immunoglobulins directed against proteins bound to negatively charged surfaces, usually anionic phospholipids.
- APAs have commonly been found in the general obstetric population, with one survey demonstrating that 2.2% of such patients have either IgM or IgG anticardiolipin antibodies, with most such women having relatively uncomplicated pregnancies.
- There is a 5% risk of VTE during pregnancy and the puerperium among patients with APA despite treatment.
- Suitable candidates for acquire thrombophilia screening include only those with a history of severe preeclampsia/HELLP at <36 weeks; a history of abruptio placentae; a history of FGR ≤5th percentile; a personal history of thrombosis; and a family history of thrombosis. Candidates for inherited thrombophilia screening include only those with a personal history of thrombosis and a family history of thrombosis.

- Initial thrombophilia evaluation should include protein C (functional level); PS (functional/free antigen level); ATIII (functional level); factor V Leiden (PCR); prothrombin gene mutation 20210A (PCR); lupus anticoagulant; anticardiolipin antibody IgG/IgM and β2-glycoprotein-I IgG/IgM.
- Heparin and aspirin administration is the best strategy for the treatment of recurrent pregnancy loss associated with APS.
- Therapeutic anticoagulation during the antepartum period should be reserved for patients with mechanical heart valves, VTE in the current pregnancy, high-risk thrombophilias (ATIII deficiency, factor V Leiden homozygosity, or prothrombin gene [G20210A] mutation) with a history of VTE or adverse pregnancy outcome.
- VTE should be treated with therapeutic anticoagulation for throughout the remainder of pregnancy, with prophylactic or therapeutic dosing extended to a minimum of 6 weeks postpartum depending on the timing of the event during gestation.
- Appropriate treatment of the APS includes prophylactic anticoagulation and aspirin in the antepartum period and prophylactic anticoagulation alone in the postpartum period.
- Dosing of therapeutic anticoagulation should be titrated to keep the PTT between 1.5 and 2.5 times control for unfractionated heparin and antifactor Xa levels between 0.6 and 1.2 U/mL for LMWH (depending on once or twice daily dosing).
- The decision to switch from LMWH to unfractionated heparin, especially for patients on therapeutic doses, should be individualized after the patients are well counseled on the risks and benefits of each option with consideration of their previous delivery history (ie preterm deliveries).
- Heparin anticoagulation may be restarted 4 to 6 hours after vaginal delivery and 6 to 12 hours after cesarean delivery. Warfarin may be started postpartum day 1.
- Therapeutic doses of LMWH or unfractionated heparin must be continued for 5 days and until

the INR reaches the therapeutic range (2.0-3.0) for 2 successive days.

- Heparin anticoagulation has been associated with thrombocytopenia (3%) and osteoporosis and, thus, patients should be managed with periodic platelet counts and calcium supplementation.
- Fetal surveillance of patients on anticoagulation during pregnancy should include fetal growth evaluation every 4 to 6 weeks beginning at 20 weeks and fetal testing

with nonstress tests and/or biophysical profiles beginning at 36 weeks, or earlier if clinically indicated.

- Antepartum heparin is not necessary in patients without thrombophilia and prior VTE associated with a temporary risk factor.
- Two useful agents in pregnancy when heparin cannot be administered are danaparoid, a low-molecular-weight heparinoid; and fondaparinux, a synthetic heparin pentasaccharide.

REFERENCES

(only references cited in synoptic print chapter; for a complete reference list, see ebook)

23. Bremme K, Ostlund E, Almqvist I, et al. Enhanced thrombin generation and fibrinolytic activity in normal pregnancy and the puerperium. *Obstet Gynecol.* 1992;80:132-137.
24. Lindqvist P, Dahlback B, Marsal K. Thrombotic risk during pregnancy: a population study. *Obstet Gynecol.* 1999;94:595-599.
25. Danilenko-Dixon DR, Heit JA, Silverstein MD, et al. Risk factors for deep vein thrombosis and pulmonary embolism during pregnancy or postpartum: a population-based, case-control study. *Am J Obstet Gynecol.* 2001;184:104-110.
26. Anderson FA Jr, Spencer FA. Risk factors for venous thromboembolism. *Circulation.* 2003;107(23 suppl 1):I9-I16.
27. Nelson-Piercy C, MacCallum P, Mackillop L. *Reducing the Risk of Thrombosis and Embolism During Pregnancy and the Puerperium (Greentop Guideline No. 37a).* Royal College of Obstetricians and Gynaecologists; 2015:1-40.
29. Romero A, Alonso C, Rincon M, et al. Risk of venous thromboembolic disease in women: a qualitative systematic review. *Eur J Obstet Gynecol Reprod Biol.* 2005;121:8-17.
33. Paidas MJ, Ku DW, Lee MJ, et al. Protein Z, protein S levels are lower in patients with thrombophilia and subsequent pregnancy complications. *J Thromb Haemost.* 2005;3:497-501.
35. Paidas MJ, Ku DH, Langhoff-Roos J, Arkel YS. Inherited thrombophilias and adverse pregnancy outcome: screening and management. *Semin Perinatol.* 2005;29:150-163.
36. ACOG Practice Bulletin No. 196: thromboembolism in pregnancy. *Obstet Gynecol.* 2018;132:e1-e17.
39. Galli M, Lucian D, Bertolini G, Barbui T. Anti-beta 2-glycoprotein I, antiprothrombin antibodies, and the risk of thrombosis in the antiphospholipid syndrome. *Blood.* 2003;102:2717-2723.
40. Miyakis S, Lockshin MD, Atsumi T, et al. International consensus statement on an update of the classification criteria for definite antiphospholipid syndrome (APS). *J Thromb Haemost.* 2006;4(2):295-306.

44. Cervera R, Piette JC, Font JK, et al; Euro-Phospholipid Project Group. Antiphospholipid syndrome: clinical and immunologic manifestations and patterns of disease expression in a cohort of 1000 patients. *Arthritis Rheum.* 2002;46:1019-1027.
61. Juul K, Tybjaerg-Hansen A, Steffensen R, et al. Factor V leiden: the Copenhagen city heart study and 2 meta-analyses. *Blood.* 2002;100:3-10.
62. Price DT, Ridker PM. Factor V Leiden mutation and the risks for thromboembolic disease: a clinical perspective. *Ann Intern Med.* 1997;127:895-903.
63. Franco RF, Reitsma PH. Genetic risk factors of venous thrombosis. *Hum Genet.* 2001;109:369-384.
64. Aznar J, Vaya A, Estelles A, et al. Risk of venous thrombosis in carriers of the prothrombin G20210A variant and factor V Leiden and their interaction with oral contraceptives. *Haematologica.* 2000;85:1271-1276.
65. Emmerich J, Rosendaal FR, Cattaneo M, et al. Combined effect of factor V Leiden and prothrombin 20210A on the risk of venous thromboembolism – pooled analysis of 8 case-control studies including 2310 cases and 3204 controls. Study Group for Pooled-Analysis in Venous Thromboembolism. *Thromb Haemost.* 2001;86:809-816.
66. Vossen CY, Conard J, Fontcuberta J, et al. Familial thrombophilia and lifetime risk of venous thrombosis. *J Thromb Haemost.* 2004;2:1526-1532.
67. Goodwin AJ, Rosendaal FR, Kottke-Marchant K, Bovill EG. A review of the technical, diagnostic, and epidemiologic considerations for protein S assays. *Arch Pathol Lab Med.* 2002;126:1349-1366.
96. Dempfle C. Minor transplacental passage of fondaparinux in vivo. *N Engl J Med.* 2004;350:1914-1915.
103. Green RM, Meyer TJ, Dunn M, Glassroth J. Pulmonary embolism in younger adults. *Chest.* 1992;01:1507-1511.
106. Leung AN, Bull TM, Jaeschke R, et al. American Thoracic Society documents: an official American Thoracic Society/Society of Thoracic Radiology clinical practice guideline – evaluation of suspected pulmonary embolism in pregnancy. *Radiology.* 2012;262(2):635-646.
137. Leffert LR, Dubois HM, Butwick AJ, et al. Neuraxial anesthesia in obstetric patients receiving thromboprophylaxis with unfractionated or low-molecular-weight heparin: a systematic review of spinal epidural hematoma. *Anesth Anal.* 2017;125:223-231.

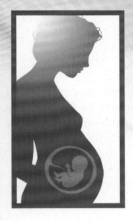

CHAPTER 38

Hematological Disorders of Pregnancy

Mae-Lan Winchester and Carl P. Weiner

Introduction

Multiple physiologic adaptations occur to help women cope with the added demands of pregnancy. Because of these rapid changes, pregnancy increases a woman's risk of developing any number of hematologic disorders.

Anemia

Etiology

The specific values of hemoglobin (Hb) and hematocrit (HCT) change during pregnancy, with cutoffs of Hb 11 g/dL and HCT 33% in the first trimester, 10.5 g/dL and 32% in the second trimester, and 11 g/dL and 33% in the third trimester considered normal. Anemia is considered moderate when the Hb is <10 g/dL and severe when it is <7 g/dL at any point during pregnancy.[3]

Risk factors for anemia in pregnancy include younger age, iron-poor diet, short-interval pregnancy, and heavy menses. Anemia due to iron deficiency in pregnancy accounts for at least 85% of all cases.[5]

The impact of anemia on the pregnancy depends upon the severity and cause of the condition.

Clinical Assessment of Anemia in Pregnancy

All pregnant women should be screened for anemia at the first prenatal visit according to CDC and American College of Obstetricians and Gynecologists (ACOG) guidelines.[12] An immediate and comprehensive laboratory investigation into

the cause of anemia is not cost-effective, given that the vast majority of pregnant women will have iron deficiency anemia.

The laboratory evaluation begins with testing for iron deficiency. Measuring serum ferritin is all that is necessary. *Importantly, iron supplementation should be withheld for 24 to 48 hours before testing.*

Further testing may be necessary based on findings in the maternal history, from laboratory tests that suggest another condition, or if testing for iron deficiency is negative.

Microcytic Anemias

Microcytosis is defined by a mean corpuscular volume (MCV) < 80 fL. Causes of microcytic anemia include iron deficiency, anemia of chronic inflammation, thalassemias, and sideroblastic anemia.

Iron Deficiency

Iron deficiency is the most common cause of anemia during pregnancy and is the diagnosis when the ferritin is low and the MCV mildly decreased. Most over-the-counter and prescription prenatal vitamins contain 27 to 29 mg elemental iron.

Intravenous (IV) iron therapy may help women who either fail to respond adequately or cannot tolerate oral therapy.

One example of an IV iron protocol (iron dextran) is listed in **Table 38.2**. A firm diagnosis of severe iron deficiency should be made before administering IV iron because of this risk.

Thalassemias

The thalassemias are a group of disorders caused by an imbalance in the ratio of α- and β-hemoglobin chains. They are classified by the abnormal chain, and the specific diagnosis is made using DNA probes.

> *e* See the eBook for expanded content, a complete reference list, and additional tables.

Table 38.2 Iron Dextran Protocol

Indications: Treatment of iron deficiency anemia in patients unable to absorb oral iron

Contraindications/precautions:

Hypersensitivity to iron dextran complex
Use caution in patients with asthma, hepatic impairment, and rheumatoid arthritis

Dosing recommendations:

Test dose:
  Administer 0.5 mL IV/IM prior to starting therapy
  For the IV dose, dilute 25 mg/0.5 mL in 50 mL of NSS and infuse over 15 min
  Have epinephrine at the bedside. Watch patient for 30 min after test dose for anaphylactic reactions

Dose (mL):

$0.0476 \times$ weight (kg) $\times$ (14.8–observed Hgb) + (1 mL/5 kg to maximum of 14 mL for iron stores)
Maximum IVIV dose = 3000 mg (60 mL)
Dilute total dose in 250-1000 mL of NSS. Usual volume 500 mL
Maximum concentration = 50 mg/mL
Infuse over 1-6 h (no faster than 50 mg/min). Common infusion time over 2-3 h. Watch patient closely during first 25 mL for allergic reactions
Do not add iron dextran to TPN

Adverse effects:

CV	flushing, hypotension, cardiovascular collapse (<1%)
CNS	dizziness, fever, headache (>10%), chills (<1%)
DERM	urticaria, phlebitis (<1%), staining of skin at IM site
GI	nausea, vomiting, metallic taste, discoloration of urine (1%-10%)
RESP	diaphoresis (>10%)

Note: Diaphoresis, urticaria, fever, chills, and dizziness may be delayed 24-48 h after IV administration and 3-4 d after IM administration. Anaphylactic reactions occur generally in the first few minutes after administration

Pregnancy category: C

Monitoring: Check blood pressure every 5 min during the test dose. Watch for allergic reactions and side effects for 3-4 d. Monitor Hgb and reticulocyte count

CNS, central nervous system; CV, cardiovascular; DERM, dermatologic; GI, gastrointestinal; Hgb, hemoglobin; IM, intramuscularly; IVIV intravenously; NSS, normal saline solution; RESP, respiratory; TPN, total parenteral nutrition.

α-Thalassemias

The α-chain is encoded by four gene copies with two copies on each chromosome 16 (αα/αα). The severity of α-thalassemia depends on the number of gene copies that are deleted or defective.

β-Thalassemias

The β-thalassemias result from an underproduction of the β-globulin chains.

The severity of the β-thalassemias is determined by the quantity of β-globulin produced. β^+ indicates that some β-chains are being produced, whereas β^0 means no chains are being produced. Homozygote patients for a defective β-thalassemia gene (thalassemia major or Cooley anemia) have markedly ineffective erythropoiesis and severe hemolysis. The disease first manifests postnatally, as the fetus produces hemoglobin F, which does not use the β-globulin chain. Postnatally, the hemoglobin type switches from hemoglobin F to adult type and β-thalassemia appears.

Sickle Cell Disease

Sickle cell disease (SCD) is caused by an abnormal β-globulin resulting from a point mutation replacement of glutamic acid with valine at the sixth position (hemoglobin S). In times of stress (eg, hypoxemia or infection), the abnormal β-globulin chain undergoes a conformational change causing sickling of the RBCs. The sickled RBCs have reduced deformability, causing microvascular occlusion, hemolysis, and increased susceptibility to infection.

A patient homozygous for hemoglobin S (hemoglobin SS) has sickle cell anemia. Heterozygous individuals (hemoglobin SA) have sickle cell trait. Other sickling hemoglobinopathies of importance during pregnancy include hemoglobin SCD and hemoglobin S/β-thalassemia.

Pregnancy in women with one of the three sickling disorders exposes the mother and fetus to increased complications due to vaso-occlusive disease, such as intrauterine growth restriction (IUGR), preterm labor, preeclampsia, and perinatal and maternal mortality.[25-28] Mortality among women with SCD is due to complications of the preexisting disease rather than obstetrical issues.[29]

The hallmark of SCD is sickle cell crisis during which the main complaint is severe pain in the back, chest, abdomen, and long bones. Pain crises are more frequent in the third trimester. The treatment of sickle cell crisis has changed very little over the past decade and consists of hydration, oxygenation, and pain relief. Pulmonary and urinary infections are common triggers and must be diagnosed and treated aggressively. Regular antepartum fetal testing for fetal well-being and growth is strongly recommended.

There are two complications of SCD that may be misdiagnosed during pregnancy. First, patients with SCD have a higher likelihood of a seizure disorder. Neurologic events secondary to SCD must be separated from pregnancy-associated events such as eclampsia. SCD associated neurologic events may be due to thrombosis, hemorrhage, hypoxia, or meperidine use. Imaging studies and other clinical findings may help to differentiate neurologic events from complications of SCD and pregnancy.

The second SCD complication commonly misdiagnosed during pregnancy is acute chest syndrome (ACS). ACS is the leading cause of death in SCD patients and the second most common cause of hospitalization.[33] Some 7% to 20% of pregnant patients with SCD develop ACS during pregnancy.[29] The presentation resembles pneumonia, consisting of fever, cough, chest pain, pulmonary infiltrates, hypoxemia, and leukocytosis. Differentiation between the two diseases may be impossible. Pneumonia is a potential cause of ACS and is diagnosed concomitantly in 20% of ACS patients. The exact role of infection, thrombosis, or embolism in the development of ACS remains unclear. Exchange transfusion and antibiotic therapy are recommended should a patient with SCD present with severe respiratory symptoms; consultation with a pulmonologist and/or a hematologist would be wise. General anesthesia increases the risk of ACS and, as such, should be avoided during delivery when possible.[34]

Normocytic Anemias

Normocytic anemia is diagnosed by an MCV between 80 and 100 fL and describes a group of structural, immunologic, and enzymopathic hemolytic anemias which can be exacerbated by pregnancy.

Macrocytic Anemias

Macrocytic anemia may be secondary to folate and/or vitamin B12 deficiency, or drugs that interfere with DNA synthesis. Blood levels of these nutrients should be obtained in cases of macrocytic anemia, as determined by MCV > 100 fL.

Coagulation Disorders in Pregnancy

Laboratory Workup of Coagulation

A coagulation panel should include a complete blood count (CBC), prothrombin time (PT), partial thromboplastin time (PTT), fibrinogen, and international normalized ratio (INR). Despite the significant changes in both thrombotic and thrombolytic factors during pregnancy, the results of these conventional coagulation tests may only minimally decrease or stay stable during pregnancy.

Thromboelastography (TEG) was developed in 1948 but has only become prevalent in rapid assessment of thrombosis and fibrosis within the past decade. This technology measures how quickly a clot forms, the strength of the clot, and the speed at which the clot is broken down. Results are available within minutes. Multiple studies have demonstrated that use of TEG reduces transfusion requirements and decreases morbidity when compared to conventional coagulation testing.[47-49] However, most of the available literature on TEG originates from the fields of trauma and general surgery; more research into its utility during pregnancy is needed.

Thrombocytopenia

Thrombocytopenia can have major clinical consequences for the management of the pregnant woman. Although the diagnosis of thrombocytopenia is usually made by a routine CBC, a platelet disorder should be suspected whenever a patient presents with spontaneous bleeding from mucous membranes, petechiae, easy bruising, and epistaxis. Concerns for maternal and fetal bleeding must be considered in determining a need for platelet transfusions, mode of delivery, and anesthesia.

The diagnosis of thrombocytopenia is made when the platelet count is below the lower laboratory reference limit. This value ranges among laboratories from 120,000 to 150,000/μL. However, management is not altered until the count drops below 100,000/μL. Most anesthesiologists use a minimum platelet of 80,000/μL to perform neuraxial anesthesia.[50] The "minimum" platelet count necessary for safely performing invasive procedures is listed in **Table 38.5**.[51] Platelet transfusions are rarely indicated during cesarean delivery when the count is above 50,000/μL and then only when there is evidence of abnormal function. Unnecessary platelet transfusion can lead to

Table 38.5 "Minimum" Amount of Platelets Necessary for Pregnancy-Related Procedures

Procedure	Platelet Count (/µL)
Minor surgery	>50,000
Major surgery	>80,000
Cesarean delivery	>80,000
Regional anesthesia	>80,000

From the Guidelines from the British Society of Haematology.[51] Note that these guidelines indicate 80,000/µL as a cutoff. Discuss the use of regional anesthesia with the anesthesiologist who may have a different level of comfort if the platelet count is < 100,000.

alloimmunization and worsen immune-mediated thrombocytopenia.

In a pregnant woman with no other medical or pregnancy problems, the most common causes of maternal thrombocytopenia are gestational thrombocytopenia (GT) and immune thrombocytopenic purpura (ITP).

Gestational Thrombocytopenia

GT affects approximately 8% of pregnancies and is the cause of approximately 75% of thrombocytopenia cases in pregnancy.[53,54] GT has no impact on pregnancy outcomes.

Immune Thrombocytopenia Purpura

ITP is the result of antibody-mediated destruction of platelets. Approximately 75% of pregnant women achieve remission after splenectomy.[55] However, splenectomy does not remove the perinatal risk during that pregnancy.

The goal of ITP management during pregnancy is a platelet count of at least 50,000/µL by delivery. A platelet count of less than 20,000/µL is associated with spontaneous bleeding, and some form of treatment is necessary. Treatment of asymptomatic women with platelet counts between 20,000 and 50,000/µL who will not deliver in the near future is unnecessary in most instances.

The first-line treatment of ITP is systemic corticosteroid administration.

If a patient is refractory or intolerant to corticosteroids, IV immunoglobulin (IVIG) may be administered and often stimulates a transient platelet increase within 24 hours. Approximately 80% of patients will respond to IVIG, and the duration of the response is 2 to 3 weeks.[61]

Pregnant women who fail corticosteroids and IVIG and need immediate treatment should be evaluated by a hematologist. Remaining therapeutic options include high-dose IV methylprednisolone or azathioprine, or splenectomy.

Unlike alloimmune thrombocytopenia, the fetus of a woman with ITP is at no or minimal risk of a hemorrhagic complication *in utero* and during delivery.[49] ITP is not an indication for either a fetal blood sample or a cesarean delivery. However, prudence dictates the avoidance of either vacuum or forceps vaginal delivery. The morbidity of ITP occurs in the newborn period as neonatal platelet counts may continue to decline during the first week of life.

No laboratory test can definitively differentiate GT from ITP. The diagnosis of GT is often made when no other maternal disease can be identified, and the platelet count is greater than 70,000/µL; the diagnosis of ITP is made when the platelet count is less than 100,000/µL. A platelet count of 70,000/µL is not associated with bleeding and requires no treatment. The patient may receive routine prenatal care with platelet counts checked every month or two. A platelet count below 50,000/µL with no other identifiable cause can be attributed to ITP. The diagnosis of ITP is strengthened when the maternal platelet count remains below 100,000/µL for 3 months after delivery, and/or the neonate has thrombocytopenia without traumatic delivery.[64,65]

Alloimmune Thrombocytopenic Purpura

Alloimmune thrombocytopenic purpura (ATP) is analogous to rhesus (Rh) disease. However, the behavior of the disease differs from RBC alloimmunization in two key ways. First, approximately half the affected fetuses occur in the first pregnancy. Second, there is no reliable screening method for ATP. The initial diagnosis is made when a thrombocytopenic neonate is born to a woman with a normal platelet count. The workup for ATP includes maternal and paternal platelet typing for human platelet antigen phenotype. At least 10 platelet antigens have been implicated in ATP, with human platelet antigen 1a accounting for most cases.

Because of the risk of intracranial hemorrhage (ICH), aggressive therapy is warranted to prevent severe fetal thrombocytopenia. Treatment options used include corticosteroids, IVIG administration to both the fetus and the mother, and fetal platelet transfusion. The optimal antenatal treatment paradigm appears to be noninvasive treatment using weekly IVIG in doses of 0.5 to 1.0 g/kg, starting in the early or late second trimester depending on risk stratification.[70] Fetuses who do not respond to IVIG alone will usually benefit from the addition of prednisone 1 mg/kg/d.[71]

Given the rarity of this disease, population-based screening is not routinely performed. Instead, patients are assigned risk stratification based on history. High-risk patients are those who have a sibling with an ICH that occurred during the peripartum period or an initial fetal platelet count of less than 20,000/mL[3]. Standard-risk patients are those who did not have a sibling with an ICH and whose initial platelet count lies between 20,000 and 100,000/mL[3]. Consideration to combination therapy (IVIG plus prednisone) should be given to high-risk patients.[65]

The optimal timing and mode of delivery remains uncertain. In general, a planned induction of labor can be considered in women with either a prior vaginal delivery and no history of a child with ICH.[66] However, a near-term cesarean delivery may lower the rate of severe complications especially when the fetal platelet count is unknown.

Other Causes of Thrombocytopenia

Preeclampsia is another common cause of thrombocytopenia during pregnancy. Thrombocytopenia due to preeclampsia is associated with hemolysis, and elevated hepatic transaminases appear to respond to corticosteroid treatment.[73] Two doses of 12 mg each of either dexamethasone or betamethasone given every 12 hours improves platelet counts.[74] Additional doses of dexamethasone (6 mg IV daily every 12 hours for a total two doses after the initial dose) have also been used. This strategy may help to increase the time available for fetal pulmonary maturity. The platelet counts rise within a week of delivery when the cause of thrombocytopenia is preeclampsia. Preeclampsia is not a cause of fetal thrombocytopenia.

Thrombotic thrombocytopenic purpura (TTP) is characterized by a fever, microangiopathic hemolytic anemia, thrombocytopenia, central nervous system (CNS) symptoms, and renal impairment. Atypical hemolytic uremic syndrome (aHUS) is clinically similar to TTP, only having a milder thrombocytopenia, no CNS changes, and worse renal dysfunction. The designation of "atypical" is used to differentiate HUS associated from diarrhea caused by Shiga toxin produced by *Escherichia coli* or *Streptococcus pneumoniae*. The principal treatment for TTP is plasmapheresis, which has increased survival by up to 90%.[75,76] Plasma exchange should be initiated without delay once the diagnosis is made, exchanging

Table 38.8 Differential Diagnosis for Thrombocytosis

Primary Causes
Myeloproliferative syndromes
Essential thrombocytosis
Polycythemia vera
Chronic myelogenous leukemia
Myelofibrosis
Secondary Causes
Infectious diseases
Inflammatory diseases
Rebound after recovery from thrombocytopenia
Asplenia
Iron deficiency
Parturition
Exercise

one plasma volume in the first 24 hours. If there is no or an inadequate response, corticosteroids (1-2 mg/kg/d of prednisone or equivalent) are added. Patients with aHUS should be promptly treated with anti-complement therapy (eculizumab).

Thrombocytosis

Thrombocytosis is defined as a platelet count greater than 450,000/µL. Most thrombocythemias are secondary to another process (**Table 38.8**). Most reports suggest the use of aspirin (81 mg) or a similar agent to improve pregnancy outcome.[77]

Platelet Qualitative Disorders

A common cause of qualitative platelet dysfunction is drug related, notably routine/daily aspirin ingestion. Other commonly used drugs in obstetrics that may affect platelet function include penicillin, cephalosporins, nitrofurantoin, nonsteroidal anti-inflammatory drugs (NSAIDs), calcium channel blockers, and ketanserin.[80]

Poor platelet function can also result from inherited disorders, such as Bernard-Soulier syndrome or Glanzmann thrombasthenia, which cause formation of an abnormal platelet surface glycoprotein that interferes with platelet adherence and/or aggregation. These rare diseases are treated by platelet transfusions in cases of hemorrhage. Both are identified prenatally by DNA studies.

Inherited Bleeding Disorders

Inherited disorders of some soluble clotting factors are rare and can be treated with their corresponding blood products if complicated by clinically significant bleeding (**Table 38.9**).

von Willebrand Disease

von Willebrand's factor (vWF) binds platelets to the damaged endothelium and is a necessary cofactor for stabilizing factor VIII.

The National Heart, Lung, and Blood Institute (NHLBI) recommends a panel of three tests (vWF antigen, vWF ristocetin cofactor activity, and factor VIII activity) to assess both the quantity and function of vWF.[83] Consultation with hematology is recommended as diagnosis of the various subtypes can be difficult. Studies should be repeated 1 to 2 months after delivery when the hemostatic changes during pregnancy should normalize.

Most experts suggest treatment for any woman for whom delivery is expected in the next several days, or when the factor VIII or vWF ristocetin cofactor activities fall below 0.5 IU/mL. Treatment includes either vasopressin or blood products (cryoprecipitate or fresh frozen plasma).

Vasopressin can be administered either parenterally (0.3 µg/kg intravenously over 30 minutes) or intranasally (150 µg; one spray in each nostril or, if the patient is <50 kg, one spray in one nostril). It is given at the onset of active labor to women with low vWF levels and repeated every 12 hours. Ninety percent of patients with type 1 vWF will respond to vasopressin.[84] Vasopressin is not as effective in patients with type 2A vWD, and it is contraindicated in patients with type 2B vWD because the administration of vasopressin to these patients can cause thrombocytopenia without improving clot function. Vasopressin has no effect on type 3 vWD.

The administration of blood products (plasma-derived vWF or factor VIII concentrate) is necessary for patients in whom vasopressin is ineffective or contraindicated. Antifibrinolytic agents, such as tranexamic or aminocaproic acid, may be useful adjuncts in the event of a postpartum hemorrhage in a patient with any type of vWD. Women with vWD are at high risk for secondary postpartum hemorrhage 48 to 96 hours later.

Hemophilia

Factor VIII deficiency (hemophilia A) and factor IX deficiency (hemophilia B) are both sex-linked recessive traits that affect the male children of female carriers.

The optimal mode of delivery for affected infants is still debated.

Carriers have variable factor levels. Those with levels greater than 50% are not expected to have a clinical disorder. Carrier mothers with factor levels < 50% require prophylaxis in labor and delivery and during the postpartum period. These patients are at risk for both primary and secondary postpartum hemorrhage. Factor levels should be checked daily and maintained above 50% with the use of

Table 38.9 Administration of Blood Products for Coagulation Deficiencies With Major Bleeding

Disorder	Therapeutic Material	Loading Dose	Maintenance Dose
Hemophilia A (factor VIII deficiency)	Cryoprecipitate	3.5 bags/10 kg	1.75/10 kg every 8 h for 1-2 d, then every 12 h
Hemophilia B (factor IX deficiency)	Purified factor IX	60-70 U/kg	20-40 U/kg every 24 h
vWD	Cryoprecipitate	Not usually required	1 bag/10 kg daily
Fibrinogen deficiency	Cryoprecipitate	1-2 bags/10 kg	1 bag/10 kg every other day
Prothrombin deficiency	FFP	15 mL/kg	5-10 mL/kg daily
Dysprothrombinemia	Purified prothrombin complex	20 U/kg	10 U/kg daily
Factor V deficiency	FFP	20 mL/kg	10 mL/kg q12-24 h
Factor VII deficiency	FFP	20 mL/kg	5 mL/kg q6-24 h
Factor X deficiency	FFP	20 mL/kg	5-10 mL/kg daily
Factor XI deficiency	FFP	20 mL/kg	5 mL/kg q6-24 h
Factor XIII deficiency	FFP	5 mL/kg q1-2 wk	Not usually required

FFP, fresh frozen plasma; vWD, von Willebrand disease.

recombinant factor VIII concentrate to decrease the postpartum hemorrhage risk.

Disseminated Intravascular Coagulation

Disseminated intravascular coagulation (DIC) can be acute or chronic and may be associated with bleeding, thrombosis, or both.

Clinical laboratory findings in acute DIC include prolongation of the PT and activated PTT, decreased fibrinogen, elevated fibrin split products, an abnormal platelet count, and schistocytosis on a peripheral blood smear. Hemorrhage can also trigger a decompensated DIC secondary to hypovolemia/hypoxemia. Management of DIC consists of two general steps: identifying and removing the underlying pathological process, and preventing hypovolemia and hypoxemia.

Chronic, compensated DIC can be caused by intrauterine fetal demise (IUFD) that, on rare occasions, becomes decompensated.

Heparin is useful for the treatment of DIC in specific scenarios. It inhibits the activation of the coagulation system and serves anti-inflammatory and immunomodulatory roles.

Heparin is not appropriate in the setting of placental abruption and/or preeclampsia. It is unknown whether the use of heparin will prevent the coagulopathy associated with amniotic fluid embolism (AFE).[87] Heparin is useful to treat DIC caused by IUFD. The dose of heparin described for the treatment of DIC with IUFD is 5000 to 10,000 U administered subcutaneously twice daily.

Overt DIC with onset during labor or within 30 minutes of placental delivery can lead to AFE, a relatively rare event (complicating approximately two to six in 100,000 pregnancies).[89] In addition to the presence of DIC, AFE is diagnosed when sudden cardiorespiratory arrest or hypotension with respiratory compromise and the absence of maternal fever during labor occur.

Treatment prioritizes maternal resuscitation and includes cardiovascular and respiratory support with inotropes and vasopressors, correction of DIC, and immediate delivery of the fetus > 23 weeks in the event of maternal arrest.[90]

Thrombophilias in Pregnancy

The most commonly encountered acquired thrombophilia in pregnancy is antiphospholipid antibody syndrome (APS). Screening should be considered when a patient meets certain clinical criteria (**Table 38.10**).

Table 38.10 Diagnostic Criteria for Antiphospholipid Syndrome (APS)

Definite APS is considered present if at least one of the clinical criteria and one of the laboratory criteria are met.

Clinical criteria:

- **Vascular thrombosis:** One or more clinical episodes of arterial, venous, or small-vessel thrombosis in any tissue or organ confirmed by imaging or Doppler studies or histopathology, with the exception of superficial venous thrombosis. For histopathologic confirmation, thrombosis should be present without inflammation in the vessel wall.
- **Pregnancy morbidity:**
  - One or more unexplained deaths of a morphologically normal fetus beyond the 10th week of gestation with normal fetal morphology documented by sonography or by direct examination, or
  - One or more premature births of a morphologically normal neonate at or before the 34th week of gestation because of severe preeclampsia or eclampsia, or severe placental insufficiency, or
  - Three or more unexplained consecutive spontaneous abortions before the 10th week of gestation with maternal anatomic or hormonal abnormalities and paternal and maternal chromosomal abnormalities excluded.

Laboratory criteria:

- Anticardiolipin antibody of IgG and/or IgM isotype in blood, present in medium or high titer, on two or more occasions, at least 6 wk apart, measured by a standardized enzyme-linked immunosorbent assay (ELISA) for β2-glycoprotein-I–dependent anticardiolipin antibodies.
- Lupus anticoagulant present in plasma on two or more occasions at least 6 wk apart, detected according to the International Society of Thrombosis and Hemostasis guideline/steps:
  - Prolonged phospholipid-dependent coagulation demonstrated on a screening test (activated PTT, kaolin clotting time, dilute Russell viper venom time, dilute PT, Textarin time),
  - Failure to correct the prolonged coagulation time on the screening test by mixing with normal platelet poor plasma,
  - Shortening or correction of the prolonged coagulation time on the screening test by addition of excess phospholipids,
  - Exclusion of other coagulopathies, eg, factor VIII inhibitor or heparin as appropriate.

IgG, immunoglobulin G; IgM, immunoglobulin M; PT, prothrombin time; PTT, partial thromboplastin time.

Table 38.11 Inherited Thrombophilias

"Greater" thrombophilias: consider therapeutic
  anticoagulation
Compound heterozygosity with factor V Leiden and
  prothrombin G20210A gene mutation
Homozygosity of factor V Leiden and prothrombin
  gene mutations
Antithrombin deficiency (activity levels < 70%)

"Lesser" thrombophilias: consider prophylactic
  anticoagulation
Protein C deficiency
Protein S deficiency
Factor V Leiden
Prothrombin G20210A gene mutation
Antiphospholipid antibodies

Other thrombophilias:
Hyperhomocysteinemia
Plasminogen activator inhibitor mutation

Most experts recommend the initiation of low-molecular-weight heparin combined with low-dose aspirin at time of conception to treat APS.

The inherited thrombophilias are listed in **Table 38.11**.

Controversy exists over which patients should receive a complete thrombophilia workup. The general consensus is that patients with previous history of VTE or a first-degree relative with a high-risk inherited thrombophilia should receive testing.[103]

There is also controversy regarding treatment during pregnancy. Inherited thrombophilias are generally divided into low and high risk. Low-risk thrombophilias include heterozygous factor V Leiden and prothrombin mutations, and protein C or protein S deficiencies. High-risk thrombophilias include homozygous factor V Leiden and prothrombin mutations, concurrent heterozygous factor V Leiden and prothrombin mutations, and antithrombin deficiency. Family or personal history of VTE will also affect management. Patients with low-risk thrombophilias without family or personal history of VTE are candidates for expectant management; however, in the presence of such a history, prophylactic anticoagulation should be considered. Those with high-risk thrombophilias should receive prophylactic anticoagulation regardless of personal or family history. Other risk factors such as cesarean delivery or preeclampsia should also be considered when considering the decision for anticoagulation therapy.

KEY POINTS

Anemia

- Pregnancy is subject to a disproportionate rise in plasma volume. The Centers for Disease Control and Prevention defines anemia as hemoglobin levels less than 11 g/dL in the first and third trimesters and less than 10.5 g/dL in the second.
- A basic workup depends on the reticulocyte count and mean corpuscular volume (MCV) of the complete blood count (CBC).
- The effect of anemia on pregnancy is dependent on the type and severity of anemia diagnosed.
- Iron supplementation should be withheld for 24 to 48 hours prior to testing for iron deficiency anemia.

- A clear diagnosis of severe iron deficiency should be made prior to administration of intravenous iron given the risk of anaphylaxis.
- Hemoglobinopathies in the mother are important to diagnose even if they have no effect on the pregnancy because of genetic implications.
- The increased maternal mortality in patients with sickle cell disease is due to complications from the disease itself, rather than obstetrical issues. Seven to twenty percent of women with sickle cell disease will develop acute chest syndrome during pregnancy, a commonly misdiagnosed complication and one that is a leading cause of death.

Coagulation Disorders

- Pregnancy causes a heightened activation of the coagulation system of both the procoagulant and the anticoagulant systems with a tendency toward thrombosis.
- A coagulation panel may include a complete blood count, PT, activated PTT, and fibrinogen. Newer technology using thromboelastography may become more useful in the obstetric population.

Thrombocytopenia/Platelet Disorders

- The most common cause of thrombocytopenia during pregnancy is gestational thrombocytopenia (GT), which rarely decreases platelet counts to less than 70,000/μL. GT has little clinical significance.
- Immune thrombocytopenic purpura (ITP) is another potential cause of thrombocytopenia and may be difficult to distinguish from GT. Treatment includes corticosteroids and IVIG. Ten to fifteen percent of fetuses born to mothers with ITP will have platelet counts under 50,000/μL. It is not an indication for fetal blood sampling or cesarean delivery, but caution with operative delivery should be used.
- Alloimmune thrombocytopenia purpura can be a devastating disease for the fetus/neonate. Management should be performed in conjunction with a fetal medicine specialist.
- Drugs, especially aspirin, can cause platelet dysfunction. Doses higher than 81 mg/d should be used with caution and discussed with an anesthesiologist before regional anesthesia is given.

Inherited Bleeding Disorders

- von Willebrand disease (vWD) is the most common inherited coagulopathy of clinical significance in the pregnant woman and has three types: type 1, type 2A and 2B, and type

3. Vasopressin should not be given in type 2B and type 3 vWD, and blood products should be given instead.
- Hemophilia is an X-linked disorder with implications for the male fetus. Genetic counseling and testing are important for proper management.

Disseminated Intravascular Coagulation

- Abruptio placentae is the most common cause of DIC, and prompt delivery, especially with laboratory abnormalities, should reverse changes. Heparin should not be given before delivery.
- Intrauterine fetal demise and septic abortion cause DIC, and delivery of the fetus or evacuation of the uterus should be prompt.
- Amniotic fluid embolus is a devastating complication that is treated with supportive measures.

Thrombophilias in Pregnancy

- There are many issues regarding thrombophilias in pregnancy that still need to be resolved, including impact, screening, and management issues.
- Thrombophilias can be divided into acquired and inherited. Acquired thrombophilias are diagnosed by laboratory and clinical criteria. Inherited thrombophilias are diagnosed by laboratory criteria.
- Management usually involves placing patients on heparin and aspirin. The amount of heparin (prophylactic versus therapeutic) depends on the thrombophilia and the past medical history.
- Methylenetetrahydrofolate reductase (MTHFR) gene testing is no longer recommended, given new data suggesting these mutations do not increase the risk of thrombotic events.

REFERENCES

(only references cited in synoptic print chapter; for a complete reference list, see ebook)

3. WHO. *Haemoglobin Concentrations for the Diagnosis of Anaemia and Assessment of Severity*. Vitamin and Mineral Nutrition Information System. World Health Organization; 2011.
5. Vinogradova MA, Fedorova TA, Strelnikova EV, Rogachevsky O, Shmakov RG, Polushkina ES. Anemia during pregnancy: the management and outcomes depending on the etiology. *Blood.* 2014; 124:4830.
25. Milner PF, Jones BR, Dobler J. Outcome of pregnancy in sickle-cell anemia and sickle cell-hemoglobin C disease. *Am J Obstet Gynecol.* 1980;138:239-245.
26. Smith JA, Espeland M, Bellevue R, et al. Pregnancy in sickle cell disease: experience of the cooperative study of sickle cell disease. *Obstet Gynecol.* 1996;87:199-204.
27. Cunningham FG, Pritchard JA, Mason R. Pregnancy and sickle cell hemoglobinopathies: results with and without prophylactic transfusions. *Obstet Gynecol.* 1983;62:419-424.
28. Tuck S. Pregnancy in sickle cell disease in the United Kingdom. *Br J Obstet Gynecol.* 1983;90:112-117.

29. Boga C, Ozdogu H. Pregnancy and sickle cell disease: a review of the current literature. *Crit Rev Oncol Hematol*. 2016;98:364-374.

33. Vichinsky EP, Neumayr LD, Earles AN, et al. Causes and outcomes of the acute chest syndrome in sickle cell disease: National Acute Chest Syndrome Study Group. *N Engl J Med*. 2000;342:1855-1865.

34. Eichhorn RF, Buurke EJ, Blok P, Berends MJ, Jansen CL. Sickle cell-like crisis and bone marrow necrosis associated with parvovirus B19 and heterozygosity for haemoglobins S and E. *J Intern Med*. 1999;245:103-106.

47. Holocomb J, Minei K, Scerbo M, et al. Admission rapid thromboelastography can replace conventional coagulation tests in the emergency department: experience with 1974 consecutive trauma patients. *Ann Surg*. 2012;256(3):476-486.

48. Bolinger D, Seeberg M, Tanaka K. Principles and practice of thromboelastography in clinical coagulation management and transfusion practice. *Transfus Med Rev*. 2012;26(1):1-13.

49. Estcourt LJ, Birchall J, Allard S, et al; British Committee for Standards in Haematology. Guidelines for the use of platelet transfusions. *Br J Haematol*. 2017;176:365-394.

51. Cines DB, Levine LD. Thrombocytopenia in pregnancy. *Blood*. 2017;130(21):2271-2277.

53. Win N, Rowley M, Pollard C, Beard J, Hambley H, Booker M. Severe gestational (incidental) thrombocytopenia: to treat or not to treat. *Hematolgoy*. 2005;10(1):69-72.

54. Freedman J, Musclow E, Garvey B, Abbott D. Unexplained per-parturient thrombocytopenia. *Am J Hematol*. 1986;21:397.

50. Rolbin SH, Abbott D, Musclow E, Papsin F, Lie LM, Freedman J. Epidural anesthesia in pregnant patients with low platelet counts. *Obstet Gynecol*. 1988;71(6 Pt 1):918-920.

55. Rezk M, Masood A, Dawood R, Emara M, El-sayed H. Improved pregnancy outcome following earlier splenectomy in women with immune thrombocytopenia: a 5-year observational study. *J Matern Fetal Neonatal Med*. 2018;31(18):2436-2440.

61. Gall B, Yee A, Berry B, et al. Rituximab for management of refractory pregnancy-associated idiopathic thrombocytopenic purpura. *J Obstet Gynaecol Can*. 2010;32(12):1167-1171.

66. Thude H, Schorner U, Helfricht C, Loth M, Maak B, Barz D. Neonatal alloimmune thrombocytopenia caused by human leucocyte antigen-B27 antibody. *Transfus Med*. 2006;16:143-149.

70. Radder CM, Brand A, Kanhai HH. Will it ever be possible to balance the risk of intracranial haemorrhage in fetal or neonatal alloimmune thrombocytopenia against the risk of treatment strategies to prevent it? *Vox Sang*. 2003;84:318-325.

73. O'Brien JM, Milligan DA, Barton JR. Impact of high-dose corticosteroid therapy for patients with HELLP (hemolysin, elevated liver enzymes, and low platelet count) syndrome. *Am J Obstet Gynecol*. 2000;183:921-924.

74. Tompkins MJ, Thiagarajah S. HELLP (hemolysis, elevated liver enzymes, and low platelet count) syndrome: the benefit of corticosteroids. *Am J Obstet Gynecol*. 1999;187:304-309.

75. Ambrose A, Welham RT, Cefalo RC. TTP in early pregnancy. *Obstet Gynecol*. 1985;66:267-272.

76. Vandeherchove F, Noens L, Colardyn F, et al. TTP mimicking toxemia. *Am J Obstet Gynecol*. 1984;150:320-322.

77. Pagliaro P, Arrigoni L, Muggiasca ML, et al. Primary thrombocythemia and pregnancy: treatment and outcome in fifteen cases. *Am J Hematol*. 1998;57:181.

80. Hoffman R, ed. *Hoffman's Hematology: Basic Principles and Practice*. 3rd ed. Churchill Livingstone; 2000.

83. Nichols WL, Hultin MB, James AH, et al. von Willebrand disease (VWD): evidence-based diagnosis and management guidelines, the National Heart, Lung, and Blood Institute Expert Panel Report (USA). *Haemophilia*. 2008;14(2):171-232.

84. Davies J, Kadir RA. Mode of delivery and cranial bleeding in newborns with haemophilia: a systematic review and meta-analysis of the literature. *Haemophilia*. 2016;22(1):32-38.

89. Knight M, Berg C, Brocklehurst P, et al. Amniotic fluid embolism incidence, risk factors, and outcomes: a review and recommendations. *BMC Pregnancy Childbirth*. 2012;12:7.

90. Pacheco LD, Saade G, Hankins GD, Clark SL; Society for Maternal-Fetal Medicine (SMFM). Amniotic fluid embolism: diagnosis and management. *Am J Obstet Gynecol*. 2016;215:B16-B24.

87. Strickland MA, Bates GW, Whitworth NS, Martin JN. Amniotic fluid embolism: prophylaxis with heparin and aspirin. *South Med J*. 1985;78:377-379.

12. American College of Obstetricians and Gynecologists. ACOG Practice Bulletin No. 95: anemia in pregnancy. *Obstet Gynecol*. 2008;112:201-207.

64. Berkowitz RL, Lesser ML, McFarland JG, et al. Antepartum treatment without early cordocentesis for standard-risk alloimmune thrombocytopenia: a randomized controlled trial. *Obstet Gynecol*. 2007;110(2 Pt 1):249-255. doi:10.1097/01.AOG.0000270302.80336.dd

65. Berkowitz RL, Kolb EA, McFarland JG, et al. Parallel randomized trials of risk-based therapy for fetal alloimmune thrombocytopenia. *Obstet Gynecol*. 2006;107:91-96. doi:10.1097/01.AOG.0000192404.25780.68

71. Bussel JB, Berkowitz RL, Lynch L, et al. Antenatal management of alloimmune thrombocytopenia: a randomized trial in fifty-five maternal-fetal pairs. *Am J Obstet Gynecol*. 1999;174:1414-1423.

103. Lockwood CJ. Inherited thrombophilias in pregnant patients: detection and treatment paradigm. *Obstet Gynecol*. 2002;99(2):333-341. doi:10.1016/s0029-7844(01)01760-4

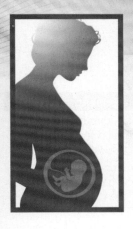

Maternal Infections, Sexually Transmitted Infections, and Human Immunodeficiency Virus Infection in Pregnancy

Meagan Elise Deming and Shyam Kottilil

The state of pregnancy is associated with increased susceptibility to and severity of several infections. First, there are physiologic changes that decrease pulmonary volumes and increase urinary stasis. Second, pregnancy is associated with significant immune modulations necessary for the allowance of fetal antigens.

Beyond the infectious complications that may increase maternal morbidity and mortality, management of infections in pregnant women are complicated by safety concerns.

Immunization should be an integral part of practice for obstetrician-gynecologists to protect adults, pregnant women, and newborns from preventable diseases. Pregnant women are a special population requiring unique recommendations for immunization, as the state of pregnancy is one of both vulnerability and opportunity for disease prevention.

Vaccine recommendations and postexposure prophylaxis options are included in **Table 39.1**.

Up-to-date recommendations for the use of vaccines in the United States are provided by the Advisory Committee on Immunization Practices (ACIP) and are available on the Centers for Disease Control and Prevention (CDC) website.[33]

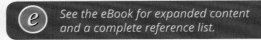

See the eBook for expanded content and a complete reference list.

Maternal Infections

Urinary Tract Infections
Urinary tract infections (UTIs) are the most common bacterial infections in pregnancy due to increased urinary stasis. Pregnancy is one of the few times asymptomatic bacteriuria should be treated due to the risk for progression to pyelonephritis and possible association with low birth weight and preterm births.[41-44]

Asymptomatic bacteriuria is defined as $\geq 10^5$ colony-forming units without dysuria, urgency, or other symptoms of a UTI.[44] If symptomatic, empiric antimicrobial therapy based on local antibiograms can begin while awaiting culture results.

Group B streptococcal (GBS) bacteriuria is associated with severe neonatal infections. Detection of GBS bacteriuria is an indication for intrapartum prophylaxis with penicillin to prevent neonatal infection. In the case of penicillin allergies, intrapartum cefazolin can be used as second-line treatment if there is a low risk for anaphylaxis, or clindamycin or vancomycin if there is a high risk for anaphylaxis.[49]

Respiratory Tract Infections
Respiratory tract infections compose nearly half of self-reported infections during pregnancy in the United States and are frequent causes of obstetric hospital admissions.[50,51] Most upper respiratory tract infections (rhinosinusitis, bronchitis) are viral.

Table 39.1 Vaccine Recommendations in Pregnancy

Vaccine	Recommendation in Pregnancy	Postexposure Management
Influenza (inactivated)	**Each pregnancy**, prior to the start of influenza season	Oseltamivir 75 mg daily through 1 wk after exposure (or vaccination and 2 wk oseltamivir if not previously vaccinated)
Tetanus-diphtheria-acellular pertussis (Tdap)	**Each pregnancy**, weeks 27-36	Pertussis: in the third trimester and within 21 d of onset of cough in index patient, azithromycin 500 mg then 250 mg days 2-5
Hepatitis A	If benefit outweighs risk (eg, travel to endemic areas, outbreak settings)	HepA vaccine (not Twinrix) up to 2 wk after exposure. IVIG may be administered in addition if high likelihood of hepatitis A virus exposure
Hepatitis B	If nonimmune and at risk for HBV infection (sexual partners with HBV, new or suspected STI, intravenous drug use, travel to endemic areas)	Antiviral therapy (eg, tenofovir) if indicated after infection
Measles/mumps/rubella (MMR)	Prior to pregnancy if nonimmune, completed at least 28 d prior to conception	Measles: IVIG if no evidence of immunity Mumps, rubella: supportive care
Meningococcal ACWY	Travel to or residence in endemic countries (sub-Saharan Africa December to June, or Mecca during the Hajj)	Vaccination and ceftriaxone 250 mg IM once
Meningococcal B	If benefit outweighs risk (eg, in outbreak settings)	
Varicella	Prior to pregnancy if nonimmune, completed at least 28 d prior to conception	VariZIG 125 IU/kg up to 10 d after exposure

HBV, hepatitis B virus; IM, intramuscular; IVIG, intravenous immunoglobulin; STI, sexually transmitted infection. Recommendations from the CDC and the ACIP.[14-18]

Influenza infections in pregnancy are associated with increased risk for hospitalization, acute respiratory distress syndrome, and death.[56-58] Preventive care for pregnant individuals (and up to 2 weeks postpartum) includes vaccination and prophylactic therapy with oseltamivir after known exposure to individuals with influenza (dosed 75 mg daily for 1 week after last known exposure).[59]

Treatment for community-acquired pneumonia is minimally changed in pregnant women compared to nonpregnant patients. For clinically stable pregnant individuals without recent hospitalization, azithromycin monotherapy (500 mg daily for 3 days) is appropriate. If hospitalized, antimicrobials should expand to include a beta-lactam antibiotic (eg, ceftriaxone or ampicillin/sulbactam) for coverage of potentially macrolide-resistant *Streptococcus pneumoniae*, and a history of recent antibiotics or hospitalization may necessitate the addition of an antipseudomonal beta-lactam (eg, piperacillin-tazobactam).[47,64]

Listeria

Listeria monocytogenes is a gram-positive rod bacterium with a predilection for causing illness in pregnancy, with estimates of a 17- to 100-fold (or higher) increased risk over the baseline adult population.[65,66]

Invasive listeriosis results in bacteremia, meningitis, and, in a survey of US cases, progression to fetal loss or neonatal death.[66,69]

Treatment includes high-dose ampicillin (minimum 2 g every 8 hours), with addition of gentamicin for synergy in severe illness (eg, meningitis). For patients with a penicillin allergy, ampicillin is substituted with trimethoprim/sulfamethoxazole (TMP/SMX) (10-20 mg/kg/d of trimethoprim component divided every 6 or every 12 hours).[72-74]

The mortality rate for HEV is 1% to 4% in nonpregnant adults and 10-fold higher in pregnancy.[78] Prevention remains in the realm of good sanitation. Pregnant travelers should be advised as to the risks of HEV and the importance of hand hygiene and clean drinking water. Management is purely supportive.

Tick-Borne Illnesses

Lyme disease, caused by the spirochete *Borrelia burgdorferi*, is a tick-borne disease usually presenting as a rash (erythema migrans) but with rare complications including Lyme carditis, neuroborreliosis, or late manifestations of arthritis.[82] No clear association exists between Lyme disease in pregnancy and adverse birth outcomes.[83]

Although rickettsial infections, such as Rocky Mountain spotted fever (RMSF), anaplasmosis, or ehrlichia, do not appear to have increased susceptibility or severity in pregnancy, these are potentially life-threatening infections.

First-line therapy is doxycycline (100 mg twice daily) and has been used successfully in a few cases of RMSF, ehrlichia, or anaplasma in pregnancy without evident sequelae in surviving cases.[84,86-88] Initiation of doxycycline should be based on clinical suspicion, as delays in diagnosis are associated with increased mortality and most confirmatory tests are not rapid. Doxycycline is the only therapy effective for *Ehrlichia chaffeensis* or Anaplasma phagocytophilum, and the alternate agent chloramphenicol, used for RMSF, is not as effective and is associated.

Sexually Transmitted Infections in Pregnancy

Syphilis

Syphilis is a chronic systemic infection caused by the spirochete *Treponema pallidum* and characterized by infrequent but severe and varied exacerbations. When left untreated, the natural history of this infection may encompass several decades. Vertical transmission of syphilis to the fetus can occur at any point in pregnancy or disease (including latent infection), with impacts ranging from significant morbidity and mortality in newborns to neonatal death.[94]

Universal screening for syphilis in pregnancy allows for treatment to protect the health of the mother and to prevent significant health problems for the infant. Women at increased risk or in high-risk areas should undergo repeat screening early in the third trimester and again at delivery.[96,97]

Although the definitive test for syphilis includes darkfield microscopy to identify *T. pallidum* spirochetes, diagnostic algorithms can use a combination of nontreponemal and treponemal tests. Nontreponemal tests are semiquantitative, nonspecific antibody-based tests, including rapid plasma regain (RPR) and venereal disease research laboratory (VDRL) titers. Treponemal tests are more specific, including enzyme immunoassays (TP-EIA) or fluorescent treponemal antibody absorption (FTA-ABS), and, with decreasing costs and ease, have become the initial rather than confirmatory tests.[98,99] Notably, treponemal tests are often positive lifelong and do not help in the diagnosis of reinfection or relapse.[100] Latent syphilis without clinical manifestations may be detected by serology.[96,101]

Penicillin G is the only recommended treatment for syphilis in pregnancy.

Chlamydia

Chlamydia trachomatis is a gram-negative, obligate intracellular bacterium whose primary site of infection in women is the cervix. The majority of women with chlamydial infections are asymptomatic. When present, symptoms may include cervicitis or dysuria due to urethritis. If progressed to involve the upper reproductive tract, chlamydia may cause pelvic inflammatory disease or additional sequelae, including ectopic pregnancy or tubal infertility.[96,102] There may further be an association with preterm labor, low birth weight, and perinatal mortality, although studies have been inconclusive.[103,104] Notably, individuals diagnosed with chlamydia before or during pregnancy (and presumably treated) had no differences in preterm births, small for gestational age fetuses, or stillbirths compared to individuals with negative chlamydia screening tests.[105]

Neonatal infection, and subsequent neonatal conjunctivitis or pneumonia, may be acquired during vaginal delivery and mandates aggressive screening for chlamydia (including retesting in the third trimester) for all pregnant individuals younger than 25 years or those who are at risk for infection.[96] Diagnosis is made using nucleic acid amplification tests (NAATs) from first-catch urine or cervical or vaginal swabs. Treatment is a single dose of azithromycin (1 g taken orally). Although doxycycline is another first-line therapy, it is contraindicated in the second and third trimesters of pregnancy. Alternate therapies in pregnancy include amoxicillin or erythromycin (**Table 39.2**). Treatment should be followed by a test of cure at 3 to 4 weeks and repeat screening after 3 months to assess for reinfection.[96]

Gonorrhea

Although initial infections are often asymptomatic, gonorrhea increases the risk of HIV acquisition and can progress to cause pelvic inflammatory disease and reproductive complications, including ectopic pregnancy and tubal infertility.[116] Disseminated, it causes fever, migratory septic arthritis, rash, tendonitis, endocarditis, or meningitis.

Pregnant individuals with gonorrhea should be treated with a single intramuscular injection of ceftriaxone (250 mg) and azithromycin (1 g) under direct observation. Sex partners should be preemptively treated, and pregnant individuals should be retested after 3 months as reinfection is common. If alternative regimens are used (eg, due to a documented beta-lactam allergy, see **Table 39.2**), a test-of-cure should be conducted 1 week later. Any case of treatment failure (detected either by test-of-cure or by persistent symptoms 3-5 days after treatment) should be referred to an infectious disease specialist.[110]

Trichomoniasis

Although not a reportable disease (and, therefore, requiring less precise incidence estimates), trichomonas is more common than chlamydia and gonorrhea combined in the United States.[117] Symptoms range from asymptomatic to severe inflammation, including purulent occasionally malodorous discharge, pruritus, dysuria, and dyspareunia. Uncommon associations may include low abdominal pain and lymphadenitis.[96]

Microscopic evaluation of vaginal discharge is a convenient evaluation that, if positive for motile trichomonads on a wet-mount slide, requires no further testing. If negative, NAATs (with the advantage of high sensitivity and specificity, as well as concurrent testing for gonorrhea or chlamydia) or rapid diagnostic kits may be used.[98]

The only effective therapy for trichomoniasis are the 5-nitroimidazole drugs, metronidazole or tinidazole, taken as a single 2-g oral dose for either drug. For those with trichomonas and HIV treatment is prolonged to 500 mg twice daily for 7 days due to reduced efficacy of the usual 2-g single dose in this population.[111]

Tinidazole has limited safety data in pregnancy and is, therefore, avoided. Metronidazole crosses the placenta, but most studies have shown no increased risk of adverse fetal events.[96,112]

Herpes Simplex Virus

Herpes simplex virus types-1 and -2 (HSV-1 and HSV-2) are alpha-herpesviruses transmitted by close contact with individuals shedding virus from mucosal surfaces, genital, or oral secretions and may infect via mucosal surfaces or skin abrasions. Able to establish a latent infection in neuronal ganglia, HSV can cause recurrent outbreaks that tend to be comparable between pregnant and non-pregnant individuals. However, primary infections in pregnant individuals, particularly in the third trimester, are associated with increased risk for disseminated disease, complications (including hepatitis), or transmission to the neonate.[113,122,123] Additionally, genital HSV is associated with increased risk for HIV acquisition and transmission.[124]

HSV-1 is responsible for either perioral lesions ("cold sores") or genital lesions, whereas HSV-2 predominantly causes genital lesions.

Primary infection with HSV during pregnancy increases the risk for disseminated disease including HSV hepatitis, an otherwise very rare cause of acute liver failure. Pregnancy is the second largest group with disseminated HSV. Neonatal herpes is predominantly acquired from contact with infected genital secretions during delivery, with high risk of transmission associated with primary or first-episode nonprimary genital infections near the time of delivery.[131,132] In rare cases, congenital infections can occur in offspring of mothers with primary HSV infection during pregnancy.[133]

Unlike more common etiologies in pregnancy (ie, hemolysis, elevated liver enzymes, low platelet count [HELLP], cholelithiasis, cholestasis, other viral hepatitides), HSV hepatitis has a safe and effective therapy in the form of intravenous acyclovir.[113,115] For pregnant individuals with painful ulceration without a history of HSV, empiric therapy with acyclovir (400 mg three times daily) or valacyclovir (1 g twice daily) can begin while awaiting laboratory results.

Treatment for disseminated HSV, encephalitis, hepatitis, or severe genital infections includes intravenous acyclovir given in doses of 5 to 10 mg/kg every 8 hours pending clinical improvement, followed by oral acyclovir to complete at least a 10-day treatment course.

Table 39.2 Sexually Transmitted Infections Treatment Regimens

Infection and References		Recommended	Alternative
Syphilis[93-100]	Primary, secondary, or early latent[a]	Penicillin G 2.4 million units IM single dose	For penicillin-allergic patients, desensitization is recommended
	Late latent or unknown duration	Penicillin G 2.4 million units IM × 3 doses at 1-wk intervals	
	Neurosyphilis	Aqueous crystalline penicillin G 18-24 million units daily (either 3-4 million units every 4 h or a continuous infusion). Duration 10-14 d	
Chlamydia[93]		Azithromycin 1 g PO single dose	• Amoxicillin 500 mg PO every 8 h for 7 d • Erythromycin base 500 mg PO four times daily for 7 d • Erythromycin base 250 mg PO four times daily for 14 d • Erythromycin ethylsuccinate 800 mg PO four times daily for 7 d • Erythromycin ethylsuccinate 400 mg PO four times daily for 14 d
Gonorrhea[93,106-110]		Ceftriaxone 250 mg IM single dose AND azithromycin 1 g PO single dose	If allergic to cephalosporins: azithromycin 2 g PO single dose AND gentamicin 240 mg IM single dose, with test of cure 1 wk later
Trichomoniasis[96,98,111,112]		Metronidazole 2 g PO single dose	With HIV: metronidazole 500 mg twice daily for 7 d
Herpes simplex virus[113-115]	Primary	Acyclovir 400 mg PO three times daily for 7-10 d	Valacyclovir 1 g PO twice daily for 7-10 d
	Suppression[b]	Acyclovir 400 mg PO three times daily until delivery	Valacyclovir 500 mg PO twice daily until delivery
	Severe or disseminated disease	Acyclovir 5-10 mg/kg IV every 8 h until clinical improvement, then PO to complete a minimum 10 d	

HIV, human immunodeficiency virus; IM, intramuscular; IV, intravenous; PO, orally; STI, sexually transmitted infection Virus.
Recommendations from the CDC STI treatment guidelines.[96]
[a]Early latent syphilis can be diagnosed if documented seroconversion within the past year, clear symptoms of primary or secondary syphilis, or only possible exposure was within the past year.
[b]For every individual with any episode of genital herpes during pregnancy, suppression should begin at 36 weeks to reduce the risk of neonatal transmission.

HIV in Pregnancy

The use of antiretroviral drugs and risk reduction in delivery and postpartum has dramatically reduced the incidence of perinatal HIV transmission in the United States and Europe.

Susceptibility to HIV infection is increased during pregnancy and in the postpartum period, and acute HIV infection in pregnancy increases the risk of transmission to the fetus.[139,143] Therefore, efforts should be made to screen for risks for HIV acquisition, reduce those risks as able, and diagnose infections early.

Current guidelines emphasize that all people living with HIV should be on ART with the goal of reducing and sustaining the plasma viral load to undetectable levels.[139,145] Suppression of HIV viral loads prevents transmission,[154] and for pregnant individuals this includes preventing MTCT.[136] Earlier viral suppression results in reduced risk of transmission, so individuals not on therapy should be started as early as possible in pregnancy, even before resistance results are available. If acute viral load is suspected during labor, zidovudine should be started with the option of ART for the infant while awaiting results.[139]

With the dramatic improvement in diversity and safety of antiretrovirals for HIV, complete ART regimens can and should be taken by all pregnant individuals with HIV. There may be a small risk of premature delivery associated with combination ART, particularly those regimens containing protease inhibitors.[155,156] However, these risks are small and confounded both by the adverse pregnancy outcomes associated with HIV itself and the diversity of combinations of antiretrovirals studied.[157,158] Risks of medical therapy for HIV do not outweigh the benefits of ART for maternal health and preventing MTCT.

Antiretroviral medications as a whole do not increase the risks of birth defects.[159,160] Studies to explore a possible causal relationship between dolutegravir and neural tube defects are ongoing. Current conservative recommendations avoid dolutegravir (within Europe) or list it as an alternative regimen (in the United States) while attempting conception, if of childbearing age and not on birth control, or within the first trimester of pregnancy (up to 14 weeks gestational age by last menstrual period dating). However, after the first trimester, dolutegravir is a preferred integrase strand inhibitor.[139,145]

A list of antiretrovirals and their safety data in pregnancy are included in **Table 39.3**.

Certain ART regimens include CYP3A4 inhibitors (eg, darunavir, ritonavir, cobicistat) that have several drug-drug interactions. Importantly, the use of methergine for uterine atony should be avoided for individuals taking CYP3A4 inhibitors as this can cause severe vasoconstriction.[166] In contrast, moderate CYP3A4 inducers, including

Table 39.3 Teratogenicity Data for Antiretrovirals in Pregnancy

Antiretroviral Class	>1.5-fold Risk Excluded	>2-fold Risk Excluded	Insufficient Data
Nucleoside reverse transcriptase inhibitors (NRTIs)	Abacavir (ABC) Emtricitabine (FTC) Lamivudine (3 TC) Tenofovir disoproxil fumarate (TDF) Zidovudine (ZDV)	Didanosine[a] (ddI) Stavudine[a] (d4T)	Tenofovir alafenamide (TAF)
Non–nucleoside reverse transcriptase inhibitors (NNRTIs)	Efavirenz (EFV) Nevirapine (NVP)	Rilpivirine (RPV)	Doravirine (DOR) Etravirine (ETV)
Protease inhibitors (PIs)	Atazanavir (ATV) Lopinavir (LPV) Nelfinavir[a] (NFV)	Darunavir (DRV) Indinavir[a] (IDV)	Fosamprenavir[a] (FPV) Saquinavir[a] (SQV) Tipranavir[a] (TPV)
Integrase strand transfer inhibitors (INSTIs)	—	Dolutegravir[c] (DTG) Elvitegravir (EVG) Raltegravir (RAL)	Bictegravir (BIC)
Pharmacoenhancers	Ritonavir (RTV or r)[b]	—	Cobicistat[d] (COBI)
Entry or attachment inhibitors	—	—	Enfuvirtide (T-20) Ibalizumab (IBA) Maraviroc (MVC)

Teratogenicity based on the Antiretroviral Pregnancy Registry, an observational, prospective registry of first trimester exposures to antiretrovirals.[159] Underlined, component of preferred regimens.[139]
[a]Not recommended in pregnancy due to better alternative regimens—consider change after discussion with an HIV treatment expert.
[b]or if given in combination/r, as when combined with lopinavir (LPV/r).
[c]Alternative regimen in the first trimester due to possible association with neural tube defects; preferred regimen after 14 weeks.
[d]Not recommended in pregnancy due to reduced drug levels and breakthrough viremia—change to alternative regimen.

efavirenz, etravirine, or nevirapine, may require dose adjustments to achieve desired treatment effect.[167] Individuals on methadone who start CYP3A4 inhibitors may have reduced serum concentrations and may require increased methadone doses.

Women who are partners of individuals with HIV, who exchange sex for money, or who use intravenous drugs should be advised about strategies to reduce HIV acquisition. For the partners with HIV in serodiscordant couples, adherence to ART with undetectable HIV plasma viral loads reduces transmission to near zero.[168-170]

Preexposure prophylaxis (PrEP) is the use of antiretrovirals (not a complete ART regimen) in an uninfected individual to achieve sufficient blood and genital drug levels to prevent HIV acquisition. Currently approved PrEP therapy includes tenofovir disoproxil fumarate (TDF) with emtricitabine.

Both TDF and emtricitabine are safe in pregnant and breastfeeding women, as supported by a long history of use as components of a complete ART regimens.[159,176] The use of TDF-emtricitabine as PrEP at conception also does not affect pregnancy outcomes.[159,176] However, studies to directly assess the efficacy of PrEP in pregnancy have not yet been conducted.

It is important to note that the increased volume of distribution in pregnancy alters the pharmacokinetics of TDF, and drug concentrations have been reported to decrease by 20% to 25%.[177]

Ideally, medical management for pregnant individuals with HIV includes viral suppression in the prenatal period, throughout pregnancy, and postpartum.[183] When a person living with HIV presents late in pregnancy (ie, after 28 weeks) or only starts ART late in pregnancy, the rapid suppression of HIV viral load is a priority to reduce risk of MTCT.

If HIV viral load remains >1000 copies/mL or is unknown as delivery approaches, cesarean delivery should be scheduled at 38 weeks.[167] There is no evidence of any additional prevention benefit from cesarean delivery in these cases with low levels of viremia in the mother at the time of delivery.[192] Continuous intravenous zidovudine infusion (1-hour loading dose at 2 mg/kg body weight, followed by 2 hours of 1 mg/kg/h) over a three-hour period prior to schedule cesarean delivery appears to provide sufficient time for zidovudine to equilibrate between cord blood and maternal concentrations and prevent MTCT.[193] Management of premature rupture of membranes when a cesarean delivery had already been planned must be individualized, as it remains unclear whether cesarean delivery reduces transmission at that point.[136,167]

KEY POINTS

- Pregnant individuals are at increased risk for infection and for complications from a myriad of infections; management of infections during pregnancy are often complicated by safety concerns for both the mother and the fetus.
- Vaccinate every pregnancy to provide an essential protection from infections with increased risk to the mother, eg, influenza, or the neonate, eg, Tdap.
- Postexposure prophylaxis may protect exposed nonimmune pregnant individuals from hepatitis B, measles, varicella (chickenpox), or HIV.
- Given the predominant role of penicillin and beta-lactam antibiotics in the treatment of group B *Streptococcus*, *Listeria*, syphilis, chorioamnionitis, and other infections of

pregnancy, prenatal visits should include an evaluation of reported penicillin allergies and referral for penicillin skin testing.
- The rickettsial infections Rocky Mountain spotted fever, anaplasmosis, and ehrlichia are treated exclusively with doxycycline, without evident sequelae to the fetus.
- Transmission of syphilis to the fetus can occur even with latent infection, requiring universal screening for (and treatment) of syphilis in all pregnancies, with repeat screening early in the third trimester and at delivery for individuals at increased risk.
- Other STIs including chlamydia, gonorrhea, trichomonas, and HSV are similarly associated with increased risk to the fetus and should be screened for and treated in every pregnancy.

- Pregnancy is associated with an increased susceptibility to HIV infection, and the high viral loads of acute HIV infection are associated with increased risk of transmission.
- Prevention counseling (including the role for preexposure prophylaxis for high-risk individuals or serodiscordant couples) is essential to reduce HIV acquisition, and early

testing allows rapid initiation of therapy to protect the health of the mother and fetus.
- All individuals living with HIV should be on antiretroviral therapy (ART). ART reduces HIV-associated morbidity and mortality for the mother, is not associated with increased risks for birth defects, and the resulting viral suppression reduces mother-to-child transmission.

REFERENCES

(only references cited in synoptic print chapter; for a complete reference list, see ebook)

14. Schillie S, Vellozzi C, Reingold A, et al. Prevention of hepatitis B virus infection in the United States: recommendations of the Advisory Committee on Immunization Practices. *MMWR Recomm Rep.* 2018; 67(1):1-31.

15. Liang JL, Tiwari T, Moro P, et al. Prevention of pertussis, tetanus, and diphtheria with vaccines in the United States: recommendations of the Advisory Committee on Immunization Practices (ACIP). *MMWR Recomm Rep.* 2018;67(2):1-44.

16. McLean HQ, Fiebelkorn AP, Temte JL, Wallace GS; Centers for Disease Control and Prevention. Prevention of measles, rubella, congenital rubella syndrome, and mumps, 2013: summary recommendations of the Advisory Committee on Immunization Practices (ACIP). *MMWR Recomm Rep.* 2013;62(4):1-34.

17. Kim DK, Riley LE, Hunter P; Advisory Committee on Immunization Practices. Recommended immunization schedule for adults aged 19 years or older, United States, 2018. *Ann Intern Med.* 2018;168(3):210-220.

18. Marin M, Güris D, Chaves SS, Schmid S, Seward JF. Prevention of varicella recommendations of the advisory committee on immunization practices (ACIP). *MMWR Morb Mortal Wkly Rep.* 2007;56(RR-4):1-40.

33. Advisory Committee on Immunization Practices. *Vaccine-Specific Recommendations* [Internet]. CDC; 2020. https://www.cdc.gov/vaccines/hcp/acip-recs/vacc-specific/

41. Schnarr J, Smaill F. Asymptomatic bacteriuria and symptomatic urinary tract infections in pregnancy. *Eur J Clin Invest.* 2008;38(suppl 2):50-57.

42. Cheung KL, Lafayette RA. Renal physiology of pregnancy. *Adv Chronic Kidney Dis.* 2013;20(3):209-214.

43. Smaill F, Vazquez J. Antibiotics for asymptomatic bacteriuria in pregnancy. *Cochrane Database Syst Rev.* 2015;(8):CD000490.

44. Nicolle LE, Gupta K, Bradley SF, et al. Clinical practice guideline for the management of asymptomatic bacteriuria: 2019 update by the Infectious Diseases Society of America. *Clin Infect Dis.* 2019;68(10):e83-e110.

47. Rac H, Gould AP, Eiland LS, et al. Common bacterial and viral infections: review of management in the pregnant patient. *Ann Pharmacother.* 2019;53(6):639-651.

49. ACOG Committee on Obstetric Practice. Prevention of group B streptococcal disease in the newborn: ACOG Committee Opinion Summary, Number 782. *Obstet Gynecol.* 2019;134(1):e19-e40.

50. Collier SA, Rasmussen SA, Feldkamp ML, Honein MA. Prevalence of self-reported infection during pregnancy among control mothers in the National Birth Defects Prevention Study. *Birth Defects Res A Clin Mol Teratol.* 2009;85(3):193-201.

51. Graves CR. Pneumonia in pregnancy. *Clin Obstet Gynecol.* 2010;53(2):329-336.

56. Siston AM, Rasmussen SA, Honein MA, et al. Pandemic 2009 influenza A(H1N1) virus illness among pregnant women in the United States. *J Am Med Assoc.* 2010;303(15):1517-1525.

57. Rasmussen SA, Kissin DM, Yeung LF, et al. Preparing for influenza after 2009 H1N1: special considerations for pregnant women and newborns. *Am J Obstet Gynecol.* 2011;204(6 suppl 1):S13-S20.

58. Rasmussen SA, Jamieson DJ, Uyeki TM. Effects of influenza on pregnant women and infants. *Am J Obstet Gynecol.* 2012;207(3 suppl):S3-S8.

59. American College of Obstetricians and Gynecologists. ACOG Committee Opinion No. 753: assessment and treatment of pregnant women with suspected or confirmed influenza. *Obstet Gynecol.* 2018;132(4): e169-e173.

64. Mandell LA, Wunderink RG, Anzueto A, et al. Infectious Diseases Society of America/American Thoracic Society consensus guidelines on the management of community-acquired pneumonia in adults. *Clin Infect Dis.* 2007;44(suppl 2):S27-S72.

65. Goulet V, Hebert M, Hedberg C, et al. Incidence of listeriosis and related mortality among groups at risk of acquiring listeriosis. *Clin Infect Dis.* 2012;54(5):652-660.

66. Southwick FS, Purich DL. Intracellular pathogenesis of listeriosis. *N Engl J Med.* 1996;334(12):770-775.

69. Silk BJ, Date KA, Jackson KA, et al. Invasive listeriosis in the Foodborne Diseases Active Surveillance Network (FoodNet), 2004-2009: further targeted prevention needed for higher-risk groups. *Clin Infect Dis.* 2012;54(suppl 5):2004-2009.

72. Janakiraman V. Listeriosis in pregnancy: diagnosis, treatment, and prevention. *Rev Obstet Gynecol.* 2008;1(4):179-185.

73. Fernández Guerrero ML, Torres R, Mancebo B, et al. Antimicrobial treatment of invasive non-perinatal human listeriosis and the impact of the underlying disease on prognosis. *Clin Microbiol Infect.* 2012;18(7):690-695.

74. Committee on Obstetric Practice, American College of Obstetricians and Gynecologists. Management of pregnant women with presumptive exposure to Listeria monocytogenes. *Obstet Gynecol.* 2014;124(6):1241-1244.

78. Purcell RH, Emerson SU. Hepatitis E: an emerging awareness of an old disease. *J Hepatol.* 2008;48(3):494-503.

82. Shapiro ED. Clinical practice. Lyme disease. *N Engl J Med.* 2014;370(18):1724-1731.

83. Waddell LA, Greig J, Lindsay LR, Hinckley AF, Ogden NH. A systematic review on the impact of gestational Lyme disease in humans on the fetus and newborn. *PLoS One.* 2018;13(11):e0207067.

84. Biggs HM, Behravesh CB, Bradley KK, et al. Diagnosis and management of tickborne rickettsial diseases: Rocky Mountain spotted fever and other spotted fever group rickettsioses, ehrlichioses, and anaplasmosis – United States. *MMWR Recomm Rep.* 2016;65(2):1-44.

86. Dhand A, Nadelman RB, Aguero-Rosenfeld M, Haddad FA, Stokes DP, Horowitz HW. Human granulocytic anaplasmosis during pregnancy: case series and literature review. *Clin Infect Dis.* 2007;45(5):589-593.

87. Muffly T, McCormick TC, Cook C, Wall J. Human granulocytic ehrlichiosis complicating early pregnancy. *Infect Dis Obstet Gynecol.* 2008;2008:359172.

88. Licona-Enriquez JD, Delgado-De La Mora J, Paddock CD, Ramirez-Rodriguez CA, Del Carmen Candia-Plata M, Hernández GÁ. Case report: Rocky mountain spotted fever and pregnancy. Four cases from Sonora, Mexico. *Am J Trop Med Hyg.* 2017;97(3):795-798.

93. Centers for Disease Control and Prevention. *Sexually Transmitted Disease Surveillance 2017.* U.S. Department of Health and Human Services; 2018.

94. Cooper JM, Sánchez PJ. Congenital syphilis. *Semin Perinatol.* 2018;42(3):176-184.

95. Patton ME, Su JR, Nelson R, Weinstock H. Primary and secondary syphilis – United States, 2005-2013. *MMWR Morb Mortal Wkly Rep.* 2014;63(18):402-406.

96. Workowski KA, Bolan GA. Sexually transmitted diseases treatment guidelines, 2015. *MMWR Recomm Rep.* 2015;64(3):140.

97. Rahman MM, Hoover A, Johnson C, Peterman TA. Preventing congenital syphilis-opportunities identified by congenital syphilis case review boards. *Sex Transm Dis.* 2019;46(2):139-142.

98. Miller JM, Binnicker MJ, Campbell S, et al. A guide to utilization of the microbiology laboratory for diagnosis of infectious diseases: 2018 update by the Infectious Diseases Society of America and the American Society for Microbiology. *Clin Infect Dis.* 2018;67(6):e1-e94.

99. Centers for Disease Control and Prevention. Syphilis testing algorithms using treponemal tests for initial screening – Four laboratories, New York city, 2005-2006. *MMWR Morb Mortal Wkly Rep.* 2008;57(32):872-875.

100. Ratnam S. The laboratory diagnosis of syphilis. *Can J Infect Dis Med Microbiol.* 2005;16(1):45-51.

101. Hook EW. Syphilis. *Lancet.* 2017;389:1550-1557.

102. Rodgers AK, Wang J, Zhang Y, et al. Association of tubal factor infertility with elevated antibodies to Chlamydia trachomatis caseinolytic protease P. *Am J Obstet Gynecol.* 2010;203(5):494.e7-494.e14.

103. Adachi K, Nielsen-Saines K, Klausner JD. Chlamydia trachomatis infection in pregnancy: the global challenge of preventing adverse pregnancy and infant outcomes in sub-Saharan Africa and Asia. *Biomed Res Int.* 2016;2016:9315757.

104. Silva MJ, Florêncio GL, Gabiatti JR, Amaral RL, Eleutério Júnior J, Gonçalves AK. Perinatal morbidity and mortality associated with chlamydial infection: a meta-analysis study. *Braz J Infect Dis.* 2011;15(6):533-539.

105. Reekie J, Roberts C, Preen D, et al. Chlamydia trachomatis and the risk of spontaneous preterm birth, babies who are born small for gestational age, and stillbirth: a population-based cohort study. *Lancet Infect Dis.* 2018;18(4):452-460.

106. Ohnishi M, Golparian D, Shimuta K, et al. Is Neisseria gonorrhoeae initiating a future era of untreatable gonorrhea?: detailed characterization of the first strain with high-level resistance to ceftriaxone. *Antimicrob Agents Chemother.* 2011;55(7):3538-3545.

107. European Centre for Disease Prevention and Control. *Extensively Drug-Resistant (XDR) Neisseria Gonorrhoeae in the United Kingdom and Australia.* EDEC; 2018.

108. Terkelsen D, Tolstrup J, Johnsen CH, et al. Multidrug-resistant *Neisseria gonorrhoeae* infection with ceftriaxone resistance and intermediate resistance to azithromycin, Denmark, 2017. *Euro Surveill.* 2017;22(42):1-4.

109. Martin I, Sawatzky P, Allen V, et al. Multidrug-resistant and extensively drug-resistant Neisseria gonorrhoeae in Canada, 2012-2016. *Can Commun Dis Rep.* 2019;45(2-3):45-53.

110. Committee on Gynecologic Practice. ACOG Committee Opinion No. 645: dual therapy for gonococcal infections. *Obstet Gynecol.* 2015;126:95-99.

111. Kissinger P, Mena L, Levison J, et al. A randomized treatment trial: single versus 7 Day dose of metronidazole for the treatment of Trichomonas vaginalis among HIV-infected women. *J Acquir Immune Defic Syndr.* 2010;55(5):565-571.

112. Stringer E, Read JS, Hoffman I, Valentine M, Aboud S, Goldenberg RL. Treatment of trichomoniasis in pregnancy in sub-Saharan Africa does not appear to be associated with low birth weight or preterm birth. *S Afr Med J.* 2010;100(1):58-64.

113. McCormack AL, Rabie N, Whittemore B, Murphy T, Sitler C, Magann E. HSV hepatitis in pregnancy: a review of the literature. *Obstet Gynecol Surv.* 2019;72(2):93-98.

114. ACOG Committee on Practice Bulletins. ACOG Practice Bulletin. Clinical management guidelines for obstetrician-gynecologists. No. 82 June 2007. Management of herpes in pregnancy. *Obstet Gynecol.* 2007;109(6):1489-1498.

115. Kang A, Graves C. Herpes simplex hepatitis in pregnancy: a case report and review of the literature. *Obstet Gynecol Surv.* 1999;57(7):463-468.

116. Reekie J, Donovan B, Guy R, et al. Risk of ectopic pregnancy and tubal infertility following gonorrhea and chlamydia infections. *Clin Infect Dis.* 2019;69(9):1621-1623.

117. Sutton M, Sternberg M, Koumans EH, McQuillan G, Berman S, Markowitz L. The prevalence of Trichomonas vaginalis infection among reproductive-age women in the United States, 2001-2004. *Clin Infect Dis.* 2007;45(10):1319-1326.

122. Chase RA, Pottage JC, Haber MH, Kistler G, Jensen D, Levin S. Herpes simplex viral hepatitis in adults: two case reports and review of the literature. *Rev Infect Dis.* 1987;9(2):329-333.

123. Cowan FM, Humphrey JH, Ntozini R, Mutasa K, Morrow R, Iliff P. Maternal Herpes simplex virus type 2 infection, syphilis and risk of intrapartum transmission of HIV-1: results of a case control study. *AIDS.* 2008;22(2):193-201.

124. Fox J, Fidler S. Sexual transmission of HIV-1. *Antiviral Res.* 2010;85(1):276-285.

131. Brown ZA, Benedetti J, Ashley R, et al. Neonatal herpes simplex virus infection in relation to asymptomatic maternal infection at the time of labor. *N Engl J Med.* 1991;324(18):1247-1252.

132. Brown ZA, Wald A, Morrow RA, Selke S, Zeh J, Corey L. Effect of serologic status and cesarean delivery on transmission rates of herpes simplex virus from mother to infant. *J Am Med Assoc.* 2003;289(2):203-209.

133. Florman AL, Gershon AA, Blackett PR, Nahmias AJ. Intrauterine infection with herpes simplex virus. *J Am Med Assoc.* 1973;225(2):129-132.

136. Townsend CL, Cortina-Borja M, Peckham CS, de Ruiter A, Lyall H, Tookey PA. Low rates of mother-to-child transmission of HIV following effective pregnancy interventions in the United Kingdom and Ireland, 2000-2006. *AIDS.* 2008;22(8):973-981.

139. HHS Panel on Treatment of Pregnant Women With HIV Infection and Prevention of Perinatal Transmission. *Recommendations for the Use of Antiretroviral Drugs in Pregnant Women With HIV Infection and Interventions to Reduce Perinatal HIV Transmission in the United States* [Internet]. National Institutes of Health; 2019. https://aidsinfo.nih.gov/guidelineshtml/3/perinatal/0

143. Thomson KA, Hughes J, Baeten JM, et al. Increased risk of HIV acquisition among women throughout pregnancy and during the postpartum period: a prospective per-coital-act analysis among women with HIV-infected partners. *J Infect Dis.* 2018;218(1):16-25.

145. European AIDS Clinical Society (EACS). *EACS Guidelines. Vol. 9.1.* Brussels, Belgium; 2018.

154. Cohen MS, Chen YQ, McCauley M, et al. Antiretroviral therapy for the prevention of HIV-1 transmission. *N Engl J Med.* 2016;375(9):830-839.

155. Chen JY, Ribaudo HJ, Souda S, et al. Highly active antiretroviral therapy and adverse birth outcomes among HIV-infected women in Botswana. *J Infect Dis.* 2012;206(11):1695-1705.

156. Powis KM, Kitch D, Ogwu A, et al. Increased risk of preterm delivery among HIV-infected women randomized to protease versus nucleoside reverse transcriptase inhibitor-based HAART during pregnancy. *J Infect Dis.* 2011;204(4):506-514.

157. Townsend CL, Schulte J, Thorne C, et al. Antiretroviral therapy and preterm delivery-a pooled analysis of data from the United States and Europe. *Br J Obstet Gynaecol.* 2010;117(11):1399-1410.

158. Chagomerana MB, Miller WC, Pence BW, et al. PMTCT option B+ does not increase preterm birth risk and may prevent extreme prematurity. *J Acquir Immune Defic Syndr.* 2017;74(4):367-374.

159. Antiretroviral Pregnancy Registry Steering Committee. *Antiretroviral Pregnancy Registry Interim Report, 1 January 1989 Through 31 July 2018* [Internet]. Registry Coordinating Center; 2018. http://www.apregistry.com/

160. Williams PL, Crain MJ, Yildirim C, et al. Congenital anomalies and in utero antiretroviral exposure in human immunodeficiency virus-exposed uninfected infants. *JAMA Pediatr.* 2015;169(1):48-55.

166. Navarro J, Curran A, Burgos J, et al. Acute leg ischaemia in an HIV-infected patient receiving antiretroviral treatment. *Antivir Ther.* 2017;22(1):89-90.

167. Committee on Obstetric Practice; HIV Expert Work Group. ACOG Committee Opinion No. 751: labor and delivery management of women with human immunodeficiency virus infection. *Obstet Gynecol.* 2018;132(3):e131-e137.

168. Del Romero J, Baza MB, Río I, et al. Natural conception in HIV-serodiscordant couples with the infected partner in suppressive antiretroviral therapy: a prospective cohort study. *Medicine (Baltimore).* 2016;95(30):e4398.

169. Eshleman SH, Hudelson SE, Redd AD, et al. Treatment as prevention: characterization of partner infections in the HIV prevention trials network 052 trial. *J Acquir Immune Defic Syndr.* 2017;74(1):112-116.

170. Rodger AJ, Cambiano V, Bruun T, et al. Sexual activity without condoms and risk of HIV transmission in serodifferent couples when the HIV-positive partner is using suppressive antiretroviral therapy. *J Am Med Assoc.* 2016;316(2):171-181.

176. Mugo NR, Hong T, Celum C, et al. Pregnancy incidence and outcomes among women receiving preexposure prophylaxis for HIV prevention: a randomized clinical trial. *J Am Med Assoc.* 2014;312(4):362-371.

177. Best B, Burchett S, Li H, et al. Pharmacokinetics of tenofovir during pregnancy and postpartum. *HIV Med.* 2016;118(24):6072-6078.

183. Mandelbrot L, Tubiana R, Le Chenadec J, et al. No perinatal HIV-1 transmission from women with effective antiretroviral therapy starting before conception. *Clin Infect Dis.* 2015;61(11):1715-1725.

192. Briand N, Jasseron C, Sibiude J, et al. Cesarean section for HIV-infected women in the combination antiretroviral therapies era, 2000-2010. *Am J Obstet Gynecol.* 2013;209(4):335.e1-335.e12.

193. Rodman JH, Flynn PM, Robbins B, et al. Systemic pharmacokinetics and cellular pharmacology of zidovudine in human immunodeficiency virus type 1–infected women and newborn infants. *J Infect Dis.* 1999;180(6):1844-1850.

CHAPTER 40

Rheumatologic and Connective Tissue Disorders in Pregnancy

Gustavo F. Leguizamón and E. Albert Reece

Systemic Lupus Erythematosus

Systemic lupus erythematosus (SLE) is a chronic autoimmune disorder of unknown etiology.

The frequency of involvement of major systems is depicted in **Table 40.1**.

In 2012, the Systemic Lupus International Collaborating Clinics Group revised and modified the classification of SLE.[3] If at least four criteria are met (either simultaneously or serially), the diagnosis of SLE is achieved (**Table 40.2**) with a sensitivity of 96.7% and a specificity of 83.7%.

Assessment of SLE in Pregnancy

Laboratory Evaluation

Antinuclear antibodies (ANA) are the most sensitive screening laboratory tool for evaluating patients with the clinical suspicion of SLE.

Antibodies directed against double-stranded DNA (dsDNA) and Smith (Sm) have better specificity; however, they are only present in a minority of the patients.

In some patients, however, decreasing plasma complement together with other laboratory abnormalities, such as microscopic hematuria, decreased leukocyte count, and increasing proteinuria, is better predictors of lupus exacerbation.[6]

Table 40.3 depicts relevant clinical information for different antibodies.

Effects of Pregnancy on SLE

The impact of pregnancy on SLE has been a matter of debate.

Physiologic changes of pregnancy, such as anemia, decreased platelet count, increased urinary protein excretion secondary to increased renal blood plasma flow, and changes in facial skin pigmentation, can often lead to over diagnoses of lupus flare in pregnancy.

Table 40.4 summarizes relevant information about pregnancy influencing the natural course of SLE.

Effects of SLE on Pregnancy

SLE can affect pregnancy in different ways. It increases the risk of early and late pregnancy losses owing to hypertension, renal dysfunction, placental insufficiency, and its association with antiphospholipid syndrome (APS). Furthermore, it is an important cause of fetal and neonatal heart block. Finally, it also increases the risk of spontaneous as well as medically indicated preterm labor.

Antiphospholipid Syndrome

APS is an autoimmune disorder frequently associated with other immunologic-related diseases with significant impact on perinatal and maternal outcomes.

An international consensus has been generated to orient research efforts and aid in clinical diagnosis of APS[33] (**Table 40.5**). At least one clinical and one laboratory criterion must be met to achieve the diagnosis of APS. Clinical criteria consist of either vascular thrombosis or pregnancy complications such as one or more unexplained deaths of a morphologically normal fetus at or beyond the 10th week of gestation; one or more premature births before 34 weeks of a morphologically normal fetus that was secondary to eclampsia, severe preeclampsia, or placental insufficiency; or three or more unexplained consecutive spontaneous abortions before 10 weeks of gestation.

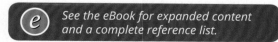

See the eBook for expanded content and a complete reference list.

Table 40.1 Frequency of Organ System Involvement in Systemic Lupus Erythematosus

System Involved	Frequency (%)
Systemic	95
Musculoskeletal	95
Cutaneous	80
Hematologic	85
Neurologic	60
Cardiopulmonary	60
Renal	50
Gastrointestinal	45
Vascular	15

Laboratory detection of lupus anticoagulant (LAC) must follow the guidelines of the International Society of Thrombosis and Haemostasis[34] including (1) prolongation of at least one phospholipid-dependent coagulation test (eg, activated partial thromboplastin time, dilute Russell viper venom time, kaolin clotting time); (2) failure to correct the initial phospholipid-dependent clotting test when mixed with normal plasma; and (3) correction of the abnormal coagulation assay when excess phospholipid is added.

Neonatal Lupus Syndrome

This rare syndrome occurs in neonates born to mothers with SLE. The occurrence of this complication is correlated with the presence of anti-SS-A/Ro and anti-SS-B/La antibodies.

One or more of the following findings are characteristic: congenital heart block (CHB), cardiomyopathy, cutaneous lesions, thrombocytopenia, and hepatobiliary disease.

Table 40.2 Classification Criteria for the Diagnosis of Systemic Lupus Erythematosus (SLE). Systemic Lupus International Collaborating Clinics Group (SLICC) Criteria. Four Criteria (At Least One Clinical and One Immunologic Item for Diagnosis)

	2012 SLICC
Cutaneous manifestations	• ACLE/SCLE • CCLE • Oral ulcers • Alopecia
Joints	Synovitis ≥2 peripheral joints (pain, tenderness, swelling, or morning stiffness ≥30 min)
Serositis	Serositis (pleuritis, typical pleurisy > 1 d, history, rub, evidence of pleural effusion, pericarditis, typical pericardial pain >1 d, ECG evidence of pericardial fusion)
Renal disorder	Renal disorder (any of the following): urine protein/creatinine ratio or urinary protein concentration of 0.5 g of protein/24 h, red blood cell casts
Hematologic disorder	• Hemolytic anemia • Leukopenia or lymphopenia (<4000/mm³, <1000/mm³ separately at least once) • Thrombocytopenia (<100,000/mm³) at least once
Immunologic abnormal	• Positive ANA • Positive anti-dsDNA (except ELISA) on ≥2 occasions • Anti-Sm • Antiphospholipid antibody (including lupus anticoagulant, false-positive RPR, anticardiolipin, anti-β2 glycoprotein-1) • Low complement (C3, C4, or CH50) • Direct Coombs test in the absence of hemolytic anemia

ACLE, acute cutaneous lupus erythematosus; ANA, antinuclear antibody; CCLE, chronic cutaneous lupus erythematosus; CH50, complement total; dsDNA, double-stranded deoxyribonucleic acid; ECG, electrocardiogram; ELISA, enzyme-linked immunosorbent assay; SCLE, subacute cutaneous lupus erythematosus; RPR, rapid plasma reagin; Sm, Smith.
Data from Hochberg MC. Updating the American College of Rheumatology revised criteria for the classification of systemic lupus erythematosus. *Arthritis Rheum*. 1997;40:1725 and Petri M, Orbai AM, Alarcon GS, et al. Derivation and validation of the systemic lupus international collaborating clinics classification criteria for systemic lupus erythematosus. *Arthritis Rheum*. 2012;64:2677e86.

Table 40.3 Antibodies of Clinical Significance in Systemic Lupus Erythematosus (SLE)

Antibody	Frequency (%)	Feature
Anti-dsDNA	60-90	Specific for SLE Associated with activity and nephritis
Anti-Sm	10-30	Specific for SLE Lupus nephritis?
Anti-La	20-40	Neonatal lupus
Anti-Ro	20-40	Neonatal lupus
Anti-RNP	10	Mixed connective tissue disorder

dsDNA, double-stranded deoxyribonucleic acid; RNP, ribonucleoprotein; Sm, Smith.

Clinical Management of SLE in Pregnancy

Preconception evaluation and counseling by a multidisciplinary team is of outmost importance to optimize maternal and perinatal outcomes in pregnant women with SLE.

A 24-hour urine collection for proteinuria and creatinine clearance should be obtained. Furthermore, blood samples for complete blood count, platelet count, serum creatinine, and liver and thyroid function tests are recommended. Disease activity should be determined on clinical grounds as well as with laboratory values such as the previously mentioned tests of renal function, ANA, C3, C4, and anti-dsDNA. A remission period of no less than 6 months is recommended prior to conception. A significant impact on pregnancy management is determined by the presence of APS; therefore, antiphospholipid antibodies and LAC need to be evaluated. Finally, anti-SS-A/SS-B antibodies need to be measured as fetal cardiac conduction anomalies will increase the risk of perinatal death, especially if they are not recognized early.

Algorithm 40.1 describes different levels of intervention in patients with SLE. Although there are no prospective randomized trials assessing the best strategy to enhance fetal and maternal well-being, some general conclusions can be made from the available information. During the first two trimesters of pregnancy, women should be evaluated every 2 weeks and then weekly during the last trimester. At each visit, a urinalysis, blood pressure measurements, maternal weight, and evaluation for signs of flare should be obtained. A 24-hour urine

Table 40.4 Effects of Pregnancy on the Natural Course of Systemic Lupus Erythematosus

- Overall, incidence of flare during pregnancy and puerperium is 26% to 34%
- Most flares (80%) are mild and controllable with medical treatment
- Women with quiescent disease at conception and 6 mo prior to becoming pregnant have better outcomes
- Patients with lupus nephritis and normal renal function usually have no long-term effects

collection for proteinuria and creatinine clearance as well as serum creatinine, urea, and uric acid should be obtained every 1 to 3 months. Serial C3 and C4 as well as anti-dsDNA should be obtained. Normally, complement levels increase during pregnancy and with preeclampsia; therefore, this measurement could help in the early diagnosis of a flare, especially when the differential diagnosis is preeclampsia.

An early ultrasound to establish heart activity and accurately date gestational age as well as an anomaly screen between 18 and 22 weeks is recommended. After 24 weeks of gestation, fetal growth should be followed with ultrasound every 4 to 6 weeks. Biophysical profile and nonstress test are advisable from 28 to 32 weeks according to individual risk factors. If fetal growth restriction is observed after 24 to 26 weeks of gestation, umbilical artery Doppler should be performed to determine fetal well-being.

Patients who are at increased risk of fetal heart block need to undergo echocardiogram in the second trimester. In general, the mode of delivery is determined by obstetric indications, and vaginal delivery should be attempted. An exception could be the delivery of the fetus with bradycardia secondary to CHB.

Pharmacologic Management

Table 40.6 depicts the maternal and fetal toxicities of frequently used drugs.

Cyclophosphamide should be avoided if an alternate drug is considered adequate treatment.

Other drugs frequently used by women with SLE that carry teratogenic potential and, therefore, should be discontinued in the preconception period include immunosuppressants (ie, mycophenolate mofetil and methotrexate), monoclonal antibodies (ie, rituximab and belimumab), antihypertensives (ie, angiotensin-converting enzyme [ACE] inhibitors

Table 40.5 International Consensus Statement on Preliminary Criteria for the Classification of the Antiphospholipid Syndrome

Clinical Criteria

Vascular thrombosis: one or more episodes of arterial, venous, or small vessel thrombosis

Complication of Pregnancy

- One or more unexplained deaths of a morphologically normal fetus at or beyond the 10th week of gestation with normal fetal morphology or
- One or more premature births of a morphologically normal neonate before 34 wk secondary to eclampsia, severe preeclampsia, or placental insufficiency or
- Three or more unexplained consecutive spontaneous abortions before 10 wk of gestation with maternal anatomic or hormonal abnormalities and paternal and maternal chromosomal causes excluded

Laboratory Criteria

- Anticardiolipin antibodies IgG or IgM present in blood at moderate or high levels (ie, >40 GPL/MPL) on two or more occasions at least 12 wk apart
- Anti-β2 glycoprotein-1 antibodies IgG or IgM present in blood on two or more occasions at least 12 wk apart
- Lupus anticoagulant antibodies detected in blood on two or more occasions at least 12 wk apart, according to the guidelines of the International Society of Thrombosis and Haemostasis

GPL, immunoglobulin G phospholipid; Ig, immunoglobulin; MPL, immunoglobulin M phospholipid.
Modified from Miyakis S, Lockshin MD, Atsumi T, et al. International consensus statement on an update of the classification criteria for definite antiphospholipid syndrome (APS). *J Thromb Haemost.* 2006;4(2):295-306.

and angiotensin II receptor blockers), antiplatelets (ie, clopidogrel and prasugrel), anticoagulants (warfarin), and the new-generation direct oral anticoagulants (ie, apixaban, dabigatran, and rivaroxaban).[57,58]

Scleroderma

Systemic sclerosis is a connective tissue disorder that affects women four times more frequently than men, with the mean age of onset in the early 1940s. This multisystem disorder is characterized by fibrosis of the skin, blood vessels, gastrointestinal tract, lungs, kidneys, and heart.

With careful planning and intensive monitoring, maternal and fetal prognoses are generally favorable.[62] Scleroderma symptoms remain unchanged or even improve during pregnancy.

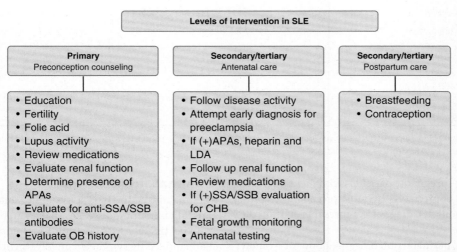

Algorithm 40.1 Levels of intervention in SLE. APAs, antiphospholipid antibodies; CHB, congenital heart block; LDA, low-dose aspirin; OB, obstetric; SLE, systemic lupus erythematosus; SSA, anti–Sjögren syndrome–related antigen A; SSB, anti–Sjögren syndrome–related antigen B.

Table 40.6 Maternal and Fetal Toxicities of Frequently Used Drugs

Drug	Major Maternal Toxicities	Fetal Toxicities	Lactation
NSAIDs	Peripartum bleeding, prolonged labor	Caution in first trimester and >32 wk. Possible association with miscarriage and malformations, premature closure of the ductus arteriosus, oligohydramnios	Compatible (nonselective COX-2 inhibitors Avoid (selective COX-2 inhibitors)
Corticosteroids Prednisone Prednisolone Prednisone	Exacerbation of diabetes and hypertension, PROM, GI discomfort, demineralization	Prematurity Avoid dexa/β-methasone for maternal indications	Compatible
Hydroxychloroquine	Well-tolerated	Well-tolerated	Compatible
Azathioprine	Well-tolerated (≤2 mg/kg/d)	Well-tolerated (≤2 mg/kg/d)	Compatible
Tacrolimus	Well-tolerated	Well-tolerated	Compatible
Anti-TNF	—	Infliximab withdrawn at 16 wk. Etanercept and adalimumab withdrawn end of the second trimester. If continued, avoid live vaccines until 7 mo of age. Certolizumab: less placental transfer, compatible throughout pregnancy	Possible (some insufficient data)
Methotrexate	Miscarriage	Avoid preconception and throughout pregnancy Fetal abnormalities (including cleft palate and hydrocephalus)	Avoid
Cyclosporine A	Well-tolerated, use lowest effective dose	Well-tolerated, use lowest effective dose	Compatible
Cyclophosphamide	Fertility	Severe fetal abnormalities	Avoid
Mycophenolate mofetil Leflunomide Biologics ACE inhibitors ARBs Antiplatelets Oral anticoagulants	—	Avoid	Avoid

ACE, angiotensin-converting enzyme; ARBs, angiotensin II receptor blockers; COX-2, cyclooxygenase-2; GI, gastrointestinal; NSAIDs, nonsteroidal anti-inflammatory drugs; PROM, prelabor rupture of membranes; TNF, tumor necrosis factor.

Among pregnant patients with scleroderma, renal crisis is probably the most problematic complication, and its diagnosis represents a difficult challenge.

Overall, perinatal outcomes are good for women who demonstrate stable disease before conception, especially for patients with localized forms.

Rheumatoid Arthritis

Rheumatoid arthritis is a systemic, autoimmune, and inflammatory disorder that primarily affects synovial tissues, with an unknown etiology. It is characterized by symmetric involvement of peripheral joints, such as metacarpophalangeal, proximal interphalangeal, wrist, and metatarsophalangeal, with characteristic cartilage destruction and eventual joint distortion.

The diagnosis is not made by a single finding, but rather by the combination of clinical and laboratory features together with the clinical course.

Pharmacologic Management of RA During Pregnancy

The goal of the treatment is to initially attain, and subsequently maintain, remission of symptoms and adequate joint function.

Methotrexate and leflunomide should be avoided during pregnancy.[60]

Ankylosing Spondylitis

Ankylosing spondylitis (AS) is an inflammatory condition with unknown etiology, strong genetic predisposition, and a remarkable association with human leukocyte antigen (HLA)-B27. It most frequently affects the axial skeleton; however, 30% of patients can develop peripheral arthritis. Its onset usually occurs during the reproductive years from adolescence to early adulthood. Characteristically, symptoms arise with insidious lumbar pain and morning stiffness. Later in the disease course, decreased spinal mobility can be observed.

Laboratory Evaluation of AS

Laboratory evaluation of AS has poor specificity and is not diagnostic. If isolated, rheumatoid factor and ANA are negative. Usually, patients are positive for HLA-B27.[73] Chest radiographs are characteristic, when the disease is well established, demonstrating evidence of symmetric erosions and sclerosis of sacroiliac joints. Furthermore, loss of the normal spine lordosis and squaring of vertebral bodies with calcification of the outer fibers of the annulus fibrosus giving the "bamboo spine" appearance can be seen.

Effect of AS on Pregnancy

Women with AS can be reassured that perinatal outcomes are not significantly affected by AS.

Management of AS During Pregnancy

Management of AS during pregnancy is oriented to maintaining functional capacity as well as to ameliorating pain. Active exercise program to preserve range of motion and nonsteroidal anti-inflammatory drugs (NSAIDs) as the first-line pharmacological intervention can be used.

Sjögren Syndrome

Sjögren syndrome (SS) is an autoimmune disease most frequently encountered in females of reproductive age and characterized by decreased lacrimal as well as salivary gland secretion leading to dry eyes and mouth. Other frequent signs and symptoms are arthralgias, myalgias, fatigue, and Raynaud phenomenon. SS can occur associated with SLE or RA or as an isolated, primary form. Upala et al[75] observed no significant associations between patients with SS and premature birth, spontaneous abortion, or stillbirth. However, they did report an increased risk of neonatal deaths. Anti-Ro/SSA antibodies are highly prevalent in women with SS, therefore, their neonates are susceptible to neonatal lupus syndrome as well as CHB. This needs to be considered during the prenatal care.

KEY POINTS

- Most patients with SLE will be positive for ANA. dsDNA and Sm antibodies are more specific but they are only present in a minority of the patients.
- Either anti-Ro (SS-A) and/or anti-La (SS-B) antibodies are present in 20% to 60% patients with the diagnosis of lupus, and they are associated with the occurrence of CHB, which most commonly presents initially between 18 and 26 weeks of gestation.
- Whether pregnancy causes exacerbation of SLE is still under debate. The incidence of flares is low among women with inactive disease at conception and higher in those with active disease.

- Moderate to severe flares during pregnancy increase maternal and perinatal morbidity and are mostly associated with lupus nephritis. Main risk factors for developing lupus flares during pregnancy or the postpartum period are active disease within 6 months of conception, active lupus nephritis at conception, and discontinuation of hydroxychloroquine.
- In women with remission of renal disease before or at early gestation, pregnancy is not associated with long-term decline in renal function.
- SLE is associated with an increased risk of poor perinatal outcome, such as early and late pregnancy loss, intrauterine growth

- restriction (IUGR), preeclampsia, preterm labor, and neonatal complications secondary to complete heart block.
- The most significant factors influencing outcome are probably activity of disease at conception, renal involvement, and the presence of APS.
- Primary APS occurs in patients without other immune disorders, and secondary APS occurs in conjunction with autoimmune disease.
- At least one clinical and one laboratory criteria must be met to achieve the diagnosis of APS.
- APS complicating SLE increases fetal risks of spontaneous abortion, stillbirth, IUGR, preeclampsia, and preterm delivery.
- Women with APS and history of stillbirth or recurrent fetal loss but no thrombotic history should receive prophylactic doses of heparin and low-dose aspirin during pregnancy and 6 weeks postpartum.
- Women with thrombotic APS should receive prophylactic anticoagulation doses of low-dose aspirin during pregnancy and continue on heparin for 6 weeks postpartum.
- During prenatal care, efforts should be directed to early detection of maternal complications, such as preeclampsia, lupus flare, renal function deterioration, and to fetal well-being including adequate growth, placental function, and normal heart rate.
- Women exposed to cyclophosphamide have a rate of permanent amenorrhea of approximately 25% and an increased incidence of infertility. Patient's age at exposure is an important risk factor. Adequate contraception is mandatory while undergoing treatment as this drug is teratogenic. Finally, cyclophosphamide should be avoided if an alternate drug is considered adequate treatment.
- Certain drugs frequently used by women with SLE that carry teratogenic potential should be discontinued in the preconception period including immunosuppressants (ie, mycophenolate mofetil and methotrexate), monoclonal antibodies (ie, rituximab and belimumab), antihypertensives (ie, ACE inhibitors and angiotensin II receptor blockers), antiplatelets (ie, clopidogrel and prasugrel), anticoagulants (warfarin), and the new-generation direct oral anticoagulants (ie, apixaban, dabigatran, and rivaroxaban).
- NSAIDs should be used with caution during the first trimester. Furthermore, these drugs should be withdrawn after 32 weeks of gestation to avoid oligohydramnios and premature closure of the ductus arteriosus.
- Corticosteroids have no teratogenic effects. When required, prednisone or prednisolone can be utilized as only 10% of these drugs cross the placenta.
- When necessary, hydroxychloroquine can be used during pregnancy. It has been shown to have no teratogenic effect or significant neonatal morbidity.
- Azathioprine can be considered in pregnancy when a cytotoxic drug is necessary. Recent studies demonstrated that it is fairly well tolerated in pregnancy.
- In general, with careful planning and intensive monitoring, maternal and fetal outcomes are good in women with scleroderma.
- Among patients with scleroderma, renal crisis is the most severe complication (acute onset of severe hypertension, rapid progression of renal impairment, daily increases in serum creatinine, and thrombocytopenia). Although ACE inhibitors have significant fetal toxicity, these drugs could be life saving and should be offered to pregnant women with scleroderma and renal crisis.
- The course of RA shows significant improvements throughout pregnancy in the majority of women. However, most relapse in the puerperium and during breastfeeding.
- The fertility rate as well as the incidence of miscarriage is not increased in women with RA. Furthermore, perinatal outcome is similar to that in the general population.
- When preconception planning is possible, either leflunomide should be stopped 2 years before conception or cholestyramine washout should be attempted in those women who desire to conceive sooner. Methotrexate should be discontinued 3 months before conception. Hydroxychloroquine and sulfasalazine can be used cautiously during pregnancy and lactation.
- AS does not generally undergo remission during pregnancy, and the few exceptions are observed in patients with involvement of the peripheral joints. Fertility and perinatal outcome are not significantly altered by the disease.

REFERENCES

(only references cited in synoptic print chapter; for a complete reference list, see ebook)

3. Petri M, Orbai AM, Alarcon GS, et al. Derivation and validation of the systemic lupus international collaborating clinics classification criteria for systemic lupus erythematosus. *Arthritis Rheum.* 2012;64:2677-2686.

6. Hahn BH. Mechanism of disease: antibodies to DNA. *N Engl J Med.* 1998;338:1359-1368.

33. Miyakis S, Lockshin MD, Atsumi T, et al. International consensus statement on an update of the classification criteria for definite antiphospholipid syndrome (APS). *J Thromb Haemost.* 2006;4:295-306.

34. Brandt JT, Triplett DA, Alving B, et al. Criteria for the diagnosis of lupus anticoagulants: an update. On behalf of the Subcommittee on Lupus Anticoagulant/Antiphospholipid Antibody of the Scientific and Standardisation Committee of the ISTH. *Thromb Haemost.* 1995;74:1185-1190.

57. Teng YKO, Bredewold EOW, Rabelink TJ, et al. An evidence-based approach to pre-pregnancy counselling for patients with systemic lupus erythematosus. *Rheumatology (Oxford).* 2018;57(10):1707-1720.

58. Andreoli L, Bertsias GK, Agmon-Levin N, et al. EULAR recommendations for women's health and the management of family planning, assisted reproduction, pregnancy and menopause in patients with systemic lupus erythematosus and/or antiphospholipid syndrome. *Ann Rheum Dis.* 2017;76(3):476-485.

60. Flint J, Panchal S, Hurrell A, et al. BSR and BHPR guideline on prescribing drugs in pregnancy and breastfeeding-Part I: standard and biologic disease modifying anti-rheumatic drugs and corticosteroids. *Rheumatology (Oxford).* 2016;55(9):1693-1697.

62. Taraborelli M, Ramoni V, Brucato A, et al. Brief report. Successful pregnancies but a higher risk of preterm births in patients with systemic sclerosis: an Italian multicenter study. *Arthritis Rheum.* 2012;64(6):1970-1977.

73. Taurog JD, Chhabra A, Colbert RA. Ankylosing spondylitis and axial spondyloarthritis. *N Engl J Med.* 2016;374(26):2563-2574.

75. Upala S, Yong WC, Sanguankeo A. Association between primary Sjögren's syndrome and pregnancy complications: a systematic review and meta-analysis. *Clin Rheumatol.* 2016;35(8):1949-1955.

CHAPTER 41

Dermatologic Disorders During Pregnancy

Marcia S. Driscoll

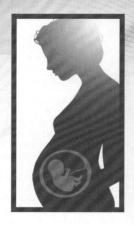

Physiologic Cutaneous Changes During Pregnancy

There are a multitude of hormonal, immunologic, and metabolic changes in the pregnant women which are manifest in the skin by pigmentary, connective tissue, adnexal, and vascular alterations. Herein, we discuss the most common physiologic cutaneous changes in pregnancy, outlined in **Table 41.1**.

Pigmentary Changes

Hyperpigmentation is the most common skin change during pregnancy.[1,2] It is believed that elevated levels of estrogen, progesterone, α- and β-melanocyte–stimulating hormone, and β-endorphins stimulate the melanocytes to produce more melanin.[3] It most often starts early in the second trimester, affects women of darker skin types more often, and occurs in anatomic areas that normally have darker pigmentation.[1,3] Anatomic areas that often darken include the areola and/or nipple and the abdominal midline, known as linea alba, which now becomes the linea nigra (**Figure 41.1**). In addition, there may be hyperpigmentation of the periumbilical area, axillae, medial thighs, and anogenital region.[3]

Facial hyperpigmentation is known as melasma, or chloasma, when occurring in the pregnant patient. This may affect as many as 26% to >50% of patients during pregnancy, occurring more often in those with dark skin type, regular sun exposure, or family history.[7,8] It typically appears as brownish or blue/gray patches that are symmetrically distributed. It can occur on the face in certain patterns: centrofacial (cheeks, forehead, upper lip, nose, and chin), malar (involving the cheeks and nose), or mandibular (affecting the ramus of the mandible).[5,8] It may persist after pregnancy. Even in women in whom chloasma fades, it may recur with hormonal stimuli, such as oral contraceptive pills, with ultraviolet light exposure, and/or with subsequent pregnancies.[2]

Early in pregnancy, initiation of broad-spectrum sunscreen with sun protection factor of 50 or more has been shown to prevent the development or worsening of melasma.[9] Drugs that inhibit tyrosinase, the key enzyme in the pathway of melanin synthesis, are important in treatment.[10] If a patient desires treatment during pregnancy or lactation, 20% azelaic acid cream twice daily to pigmented areas can be safely used due to minimal systemic absorption.[11] If a patient has persistent pigmentation in the postpartum period and is not breastfeeding, 4% hydroquinone cream alone or in combination with tretinoin and a corticosteroid cream may be more effective options.[10]

Connective Tissue Changes

The most common connective tissue alteration is striae distensae or, in pregnancy, known as striae gravidarum. Risk factors include young maternal age, personal or family history, higher maternal weight before pregnancy and before delivery, and higher birth weight.[12] Striae initially appear as pink or red/purple linear bands (striae rubra), most often on the abdomen (**Figure 41.1**), but may develop on the breasts, thighs, hips, and buttocks; onset is typically in the late second trimester and early third trimester.[1,2,3,12] Over months to years these fade to white atrophic bands (striae alba).[2,3]

ⓔ *See the eBook for expanded content and a complete reference list.*

Table 41.1 Cutaneous Physiologic Changes in Pregnancy

Pigmentary
- Melasma (chloasma)
- Linea nigra
- Hyperpigmentation of areola, nipple, periumbilical region, axillae, medial thighs, and anogenital region

Connective tissue
- Striae gravidarum
- Skin tags (acrochordons)

Adnexal (hair, eccrine and apocrine sweat glands, and sebaceous glands)
- Hirsutism
- Thickening of scalp hair during pregnancy
- Postpartum hair loss (telogen effluvium)
- Brittle nails, more rapid nail growth
- Enlargement of sebaceous glands of areola (Montgomery tubercles)
- Hyperhidrosis (increased apocrine sweat gland activity)
- Miliaria ("prickly heat")

Vascular
- Spider telangiectasias
- Palmar erythema
- Pyogenic granuloma (granuloma gravidarum, epulis gravidarum)
- Venous varicosities—legs, vulva/vagina, anus (hemorrhoids)
- Edema affecting lower extremities, sometimes face
- Gingival hyperplasia, gingivitis

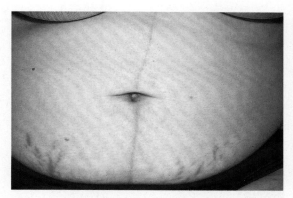

Figure 41.1 Linea nigra along with striae distensae on the abdomen.

(Reprinted from Goodheart H, Gonzalez M. Goodheart's Photoguide to Common Pediatric and Adult Skin Disorders, 4th Edition. Philadelphia: Wolters Kluwer, 2015.)

There is no optimal strategy for prevention and treatment of striae gravidarum. An additional common alteration is the development of skin tags (acrochordons). They may regress to some degree after delivery or can be treated with liquid nitrogen cryotherapy, scissor snip, or electrodesiccation.[2]

Adnexal Changes

Hirsutism may occur on the face most commonly, but also on the extremities, back, and suprapubic region due to production of placental and ovarian androgens.[17] Scalp hair may thicken due to a slowing in the progression of the hair from the growing phase (anagen) to resting phase (telogen). Within the first months postpartum, there is a prolongation of the telogen phase, and patients will note a shedding of hair (telogen effluvium). This hair loss should cease within 15 months.[17] Nails may grow more quickly and become more brittle. Sebaceous glands enlarge on the areola early in the first trimester and appear as small brownish papules (Montgomery tubercles) that regress postpartum.[2] Sebaceous gland activity on the face may be increased in the third trimester, but overall the development of acne is quite variable: it may worsen or improve.[3,17,18]

Vascular Changes

Spider telangiectasias (**Figure 41.2**) often arise between the second and fifth month of pregnancy,[17] most commonly on areas of skin drained by the superior vena cava (face, neck, arms, hands).[2,3] They present as a central area of redness (dilated afferent arteriole) with capillaries radiating outward. They typically fade after delivery. Other changes include palmar erythema, which can present as uniform mottled redness over the palms or in localized areas of the palms.[2,17] Vascular proliferation can result in gingival hyperplasia, sometimes leading to gingivitis in the presence of risk factors. Vasomotor instability may occur with episodes of facial flushing, pallor, and cutis marmorata (reticulate or lacy-appearing network of bluish erythema with intervening patches of normal skin) on exposure to cold.[2,17]

Vascular neoplasms, such as pyogenic granulomas (also known as granuloma gravidarum, epulis gravidarum), are exophytic, erythematous papules or nodules that arise in the first half of pregnancy, most commonly on the anterior mandibular or maxillary gingiva or lips (**Figure 41.3**).

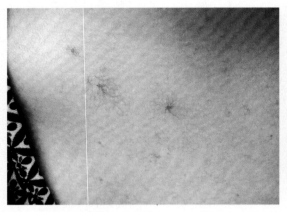

Figure 41.2 Spider telangiectasias.
(Reprinted from Goodheart H, Gonzalez M. Goodheart's Photoguide to Common Pediatric and Adult Skin Disorders, 4th Edition. Philadelphia: Wolters Kluwer, 2016.)

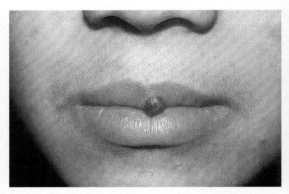

Figure 41.3 Pyogenic granuloma on the lip.
(Reprinted from Goodheart H, Gonzalez M. Goodheart's Photoguide to Common Pediatric and Adult Skin Disorders, 4th Edition. Philadelphia: Wolters Kluwer, 2017.)

Venous congestion can result in varicosities of the legs, nonpitting edema of legs, and sometimes of the face, hemorrhoids, and lower extremity purpura. Varicosities of the vestibule and vagina (Jacquemier sign) and bluish tint of the vagina (Chadwick sign) are early diagnostic signs of pregnancy.[2]

Specific Dermatoses of Pregnancy

Table 41.3 provides the current classification of the SDPs and synonyms used historically.[20] Key features of the SDPs are provided in **Table 41.4**, with a detailed description of each in the sections to follow.

Polymorphic Eruption of Pregnancy

Clinical Presentation of PEP

PEP presents in the late third trimester in primigravidae as pruritic urticarial edematous papules and plaques, typically starting within the striae distensae and/or on the lower abdomen. *Sparing of umbilical skin is a characteristic finding* (**Figure 41.4**).[2,21,22] The proximal thighs and buttocks are commonly affected.[22] It may spread to extremities and trunk (**Figure 41.5**) over days and usually spares the face, palms and soles, and mucosa.[21] The eruption last about 4 to 6 weeks and resolves spontaneously, independent of delivery.[23]

Epidemiology of PEP

PEP is the second most common of the four SDPs.[21]

Pathogenesis

The pathogenesis of PEP has not been established. It is believed to be multifactorial, with abdominal distention, hormonal milieu, and immunologic changes all playing a role.[27]

Clinical Assessment

Diagnosis of PEP is typically made based on clinical features. Laboratory testing is typically unremarkable. The most important differential diagnosis is PG, which can be distinguished by histology and direct immunofluorescence (DIF); DIF is negative in PEP. Other clinical diagnoses to consider are urticaria, AEP, contact dermatitis, drug eruption, and viral exanthem.

Table 41.3 Classification of Specific Dermatoses of Pregnancy and Historical Synonyms

Current Terminology	Historical Synonyms
Polymorphous eruption of pregnancy (PEP)	Pruritic urticarial papules and plaques of pregnancy (PUPPP)
Atopic eruption of pregnancy (AEP)	Eczema in pregnancy Papular dermatitis of Spangler Prurigo of pregnancy Pruritic folliculitis Prurigo gestationis Nurse's early prurigo
Pemphigoid gestationis (PG)	Herpes gestationis
Intrahepatic cholestasis of pregnancy (ICP)	Obstetric cholestasis Icterus gravidarum

Table 41.4 Key Features of the Specific Dermatoses of Pregnancy

	Onset	Diagnosis	Maternal Risk	Fetal Risk	Recurrence in Subsequent Pregnancies
AEP	• before third trimester	• clinical • personal or family hx of atopy	No	No	Yes
PEP	• third trimester in primigravidas • 10%-15% immediate postpartum onset	• clinical • biopsy and DIF to r/o PG	No	No	No
PG	• second and third trimester • up to 25% immediate postpartum onset • may flare postpartum especially with menses, OCPs	• biopsy and DIF	• long-term increased risk of Graves disease	• Small for gestational age • prematurity	Yes
ICP	• late second and third trimester	• Increased total serum bile acids	• early induction of labor • intrapartum hemorrhage • long-term risk for hepatobiliary disease	• prematurity • meconium staining of amniotic fluid • respiratory distress • stillbirth unusual	Yes

AEP, atopic eruption of pregnancy; DIF, direct immunofluorescence; hx, history; ICP, intrahepatic cholestasis of pregnancy; OCPs, oral contraceptive pills; PEP, polymorphic eruption of pregnancy; PG, pemphigoid gestationis; r/o, rule out.

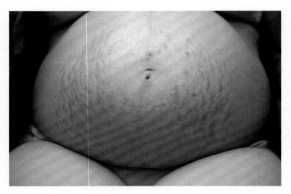

Figure 41.4 Polymorphous eruption of pregnancy showing erythematous papules within striae on abdomen and sparing of umbilical skin.

(Reprinted from Schalock PC, Hsu JT, Arndt KA. Lippincott's Primary Care Dermatology. Philadelphia: Wolters Kluwer, 2010.)

Pharmacologic and Nonpharmacologic Treatment

PEP is a self-limiting skin eruption, but symptomatic treatment is helpful. Topical corticosteroids typically of midpotency, such as 0.1% triamcinolone cream or ointment, may be used safely in pregnancy; for locations such as the face, groin, or intertriginous areas, low-potency topical steroids, such as 2.5% hydrocortisone cream or ointment, is appropriate.[22-24,29] Mild soaps, avoidance of hot showers, and use of gentle emollients with menthol may reduce pruritus.[22] Sedating oral antihistamines at bedtime may reduce pruritus; however, not all oral antihistamines are considered safe in pregnancy.[19,29] Both diphenhydramine and

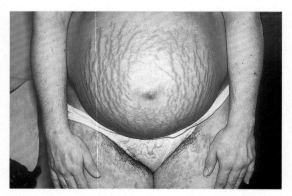

Figure 41.5 Polymorphous eruption of pregnancy showing erythematous papules and plaques of the abdominal striae, arms, and thighs.

(Reprinted from Goodheart H, Gonzalez M. Goodheart's Photoguide to Common Pediatric and Adult Skin Disorders, 4th Edition. Philadelphia: Wolters Kluwer, 2017.)

chlorpheniramine have pregnancy labeling by the US Food and Drug Administration (FDA) that states, "risk of fetal harm low based on human data" (formerly classified as Category B by the FDA).[29] In more severe cases, short courses of systemic steroids may be helpful.[22,29]

Maternal/Fetal Prognosis and Recurrence Risk

PEP will resolve over weeks without therapy, and there is no risk of harm for either the mother or fetus. Recurrence in subsequent pregnancies is unusual, except in some cases of multifetal pregnancies.[22]

Atopic Eruption of Pregnancy

Clinical Presentation

The classification of AEP comprises a group of pruritic eczematous or papular eruptions in pregnant women who have either or personal or family history of atopy, and typically presents in the first or second trimester. AEP incorporates previously-described pregnancy dermatoses (**Table 41.3**) into one group, based upon overlapping clinical and histologic features, and was the most commonly observed SDP in this study.[21] The "E-type" or eczematous presentation occurred in about two-thirds of patients with AEP. Of the 172 patients with E-type, 52 had an exacerbation of their atopic dermatitis, and 120 patients had their initial presentation (or exacerbation after a long latency period) of eczematous plaques of the face, neck, trunk, and flexural aspects of the extremities.[21] The "P-type" or papular type presented as diffuse erythematous papules, with a follicular, grouped, or exanthematous appearance on the trunk and extremities (**Figure 41.6**) or as prurigo nodules on the shins.[21]

Epidemiology

AEP is the most common of the pruritic dermatoses of pregnancy.[29]

Pathogenesis

Pregnancy-induced immunologic changes with a shift toward increased production of T-helper cell type 2 (Th2) cytokines (interleukin [IL]-4 and IL-10) may explain the development of AEP[30] because atopic dermatitis is typically initiated by increased expression of Th2 cytokines as well as Th22 and Th17 cytokines.[31]

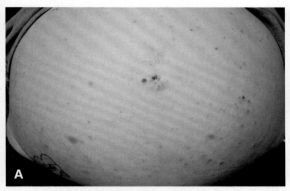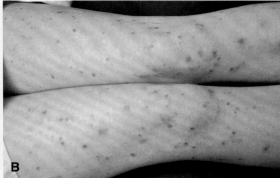

Figure 41.6 Atopic eruption of pregnancy. **A,** Excoriations on the abdomen and **(B)** excoriated papules ("P-type") on the lower extremities along with erythematous papules and small plaques ("E-type" lesions).

(Reprinted from Kroumpouzos G. Text Atlas of Obstetric Dermatology. Philadelphia: Wolters Kluwer, 2013.)

Clinical Assessment

The diagnosis is typically based on clinical findings. DIF is negative.[2,29] The differential diagnosis includes other SDPs (PEP, PG, and ICP), infectious folliculitis, drug eruption, and viral exanthem.

Pharmacologic and Nonpharmacologic Treatment

Management of AEP is similar to that of PEP: topical corticosteroids, bland emollients, gentle skin care (avoidance of hot showers and harsh soaps), and use of sedating antihistamines considered safe in pregnancy (chlorpheniramine and diphenhydramine) at bedtime as needed for itching.[22,29] More severe cases may require systemic steroids in short courses or narrow-band ultraviolet B phototherapy.[2,22,29] In the most refractory cases of AEP, cyclosporine may be considered.

Maternal/Fetal Prognosis and Recurrence Risk

There is excellent prognosis for the mother with AEP, as response to therapy is usually rapid.[2] Fetal prognosis is also excellent, except for possible subsequent development of childhood atopy.[22] There is a likely recurrence of AEP in subsequent pregnancies.[22]

Pemphigoid Gestationis

Clinical Presentation

PG is an autoimmune disorder that presents as intensely pruritic urticarial papules and plaques,

erythema multiforme–like lesions, or eczematous plaques that start on the abdomen and involve the umbilicus (**Figure 41.7**), with later progression to tense vesicles and bullae and spread to extremities and trunk (**Figure 41.8**).[25,31]

The face, palms, and soles are typically not involved. Onset is typically in the second or third trimester. The majority of patients will improve late in pregnancy, but then will flare immediately postpartum.[32] *Initial* postpartum onset occurs in about 25% of cases, usually immediately after delivery.[29] Skin lesions will clear several months postpartum,[22,33] but flares may occur with menses or oral contraceptives later in the postpartum period.[34-36] Rarely, skin lesions may persist over several years.[22]

Epidemiology

PG is a rare disorder, and the least common SDP.[37]

Pathogenesis

Although not fully elucidated, the pathogenesis of PG is considered to be similar to the autoimmune blistering disorder known as bullous pemphigoid (BP). In BP and PG, there is deposition of autoantibodies directed against two principal structural proteins found in the hemidesmosomes, which link the epidermis to the dermis. These autoantibodies subsequently cross-react to BP180 *in the skin*, which triggers complement activation, deposition of immune complexes, chemoattraction of eosinophils with subsequent degranulation, and finally skin inflammation with blistering.[24]

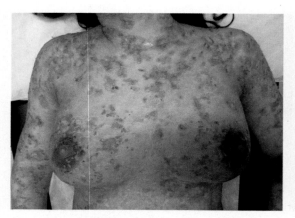

Figure 41.7 Pemphigoid gestationis with diffuse erosions on the trunk.

(Reprinted from Goodheart H, Gonzalez M. Goodheart's Photoguide to Common Pediatric and Adult Skin Disorders, 4th Edition. Philadelphia: Wolters Kluwer, 2017.)

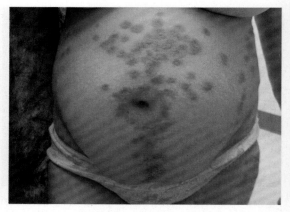

Figure 41.8 Pemphigoid gestationis with erythematous papules and plaques of the abdomen and characteristic umbilical involvement.

(Reprinted from Schalock PC, Hsu JT, Arndt KA. Lippincott's Primary Care Dermatology. Philadelphia: Wolters Kluwer, 2010.)

Clinical Assessment

Clinically, *the initial lesions of this eruption can closely resemble PEP*, as bullae may arise later in the course of PG. Therefore, lesional biopsy, perilesional DIF, and either serum enzyme-linked immunosorbent assay (ELISA) or immunoblotting directed against BP180 will establish the diagnosis.[29,33] Perilesional DIF is the gold standard as it will show linear complement component 3 (C3) deposition along the dermal-epidermal junction in 100% of patients and both C3 and IgG in 30% (**Figure 41.9**).[22] No other SDP will have a positive DIF. Histology depends on whether an early or late lesion is biopsied; early lesions may demonstrate superficial or mid-dermal edema with a perivascular mixed infiltrate of lymphocytes, histiocytes, and variable number of eosinophils.[22] Vesiculobullous lesions typically show subepidermal blister with eosinophils.[33] If there is a reason not to perform tissue biopsy for DIF, the BP180 ELISA has been found to be both highly sensitive and specific for diagnosis of PG.[33,40]

Differential diagnoses include other SDPs, urticaria, bullous lupus erythematosus, drug eruption, dermatitis herpetiformis, contact dermatitis, erythema multiforme, and viral exanthem.

Pharmacologic Treatment

In mild prebullous stages of PG, or menstrual flares occurring postpartum, mid- to high-potency topical corticosteroids may be utilized along with oral sedating antihistamines (only those considered safe in pregnancy) that are used as needed for pruritus at bedtime.[41] In the majority of cases, systemic steroids are needed to halt the formation of new blisters, and this is considered a first-line treatment.[29] Typically prednisone is initiated at a dose of 0.5 to 1.0 mg/kg/d, and the dose is titrated upwards as needed until no new blisters are noted. Prednisone is then continued at this dose for 1 to 2 weeks prior to slow tapering over weeks. As the time of delivery approaches, the dose should be increased in anticipation of flaring immediately after delivery.[22,29,39]

An additional agent utilized to treat PG which is safe for use during pregnancy, is intravenous immunoglobulin (IVIG). IVIG is used either as sole agent or in combination with systemic prednisone. Typically this has been administered at a total dose of 1 to 2 g/kg infused over 2 to 5 days and given on a monthly basis.[42-45] Other approaches include immunoapheresis (immunoadsorption)[46,47] and plasmapheresis.[48,49] Cyclosporine has also been safely utilized as a steroid-sparing agent for PG during pregnancy, but blood pressure, kidney function, and electrolytes must be closely monitored.[43,50-52] More treatment options are available in the postpartum period (after completion of breastfeeding), such

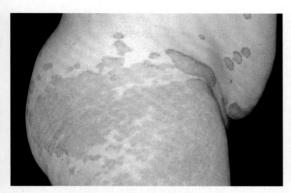

Figure 41.9 Direct immunofluorescence is positive for linear deposition of C3 ± IgG along the dermal-epidermal junction in pemphigoid gestationis. C3, component 3; IgG, immunoglobulin G.

(Reprinted from Kroumpouzos G. Text Atlas of Obstetric Dermatology. Philadelphia: Wolters Kluwer, 2013.)

as tetracycline plus nicotinamide, azathioprine, dapsone, and rituximab.[29]

Maternal/Fetal Prognosis

Women affected by PG may have an increased risk of secondary autoimmune diseases; most frequently observed is Grave disease.[53] Others include pernicious anemia and thyroiditis.

There is an enhanced risk of preterm delivery and small-for-gestational age infants, especially in women who develop PG at an earlier stage in pregnancy and with more severe skin disease.[22,54] Newborns may develop a transient vesicular or urticarial skin eruption due to passive transfer of IgG1 antibodies, which resolves over days to weeks.[24]

Recurrence Risk

PG typically recurs in subsequent pregnancies, with a mere 5% of subsequent pregnancies not affected ("skip pregnancies"). The onset of PG is usually earlier and more severe in subsequent pregnancies.[22,29]

Intrahepatic Cholestasis of Pregnancy

Clinical Presentation

ICP (obstetric cholestasis) is primarily characterized by severe pruritus during pregnancy, accompanied by the laboratory finding of elevated serum bile acids, when other causes of cholestasis have been excluded.[55] Onset is typically in the late second or third trimester with intense pruritus affecting the hands and feet, which may then become generalized; pruritus may be more severe at night.[56] Jaundice is uncommon.[57] ICP may have no accompanying skin lesions, or there may be secondary lesions associated with scratching. These may begin as minor excoriations, but, as the disorder progresses, the patient may develop prurigo nodules occurring primarily on the extremities.[29] The pruritus and any secondary skin changes typically resolve within a few days of delivery, but sometimes last 1 to 2 weeks postpartum.[24] Early induction of labor is common due to increased risk for both fetal and maternal complications.[58]

Pathogenesis

The development of ICP is likely multifactorial, with genetic, hormonal, and environmental factors playing a role.[55] Evidence for genetic predisposition stems from increased risk observed in family members, particularly first-degree relatives, and genetic defects in at least six bile canalicular transporters. The hormonal milieu of pregnancy promotes the development of ICP, with both estrogen and progesterone contributing to cholestasis. Estrogen causes cholestasis through reduction of hepatic biliary transport proteins, and estrogen reaches peak levels in the third trimester, when ICP typically has it onset. Progesterone metabolites may reach elevated levels in genetically susceptible women and serve to reduce the function of the main hepatic bile acid receptor.[57,63] Environmental factors may play a role with geographic and seasonal variation in incidence. ICP occurs more commonly in the winter months in some countries (Chile, Scandinavia), possibly related to low maternal vitamin D levels and reduced selenium intake.[64]

The cause of pruritus in ICP has not been fully explained. It has been thought that excess bile deposition in the skin was the etiology since the administration of ursodeoxycholic acid (UDCA) to lower bile acids concomitantly reduces pruritus.[65] However, the level of serum bile acids does not correlate with the severity of pruritus, and pruritus often precedes elevation in serum bile acids in ICP.[66] An elevation of sulfated progesterone metabolites is observed in patients with ICP, and one of these metabolites has been observed to correlate with itch intensity in ICP.[67] Another possible etiology is lysophosphatidic acid, a potent pruritogen, which has been shown to be elevated in the serum of women with ICP and other cholestatic liver diseases associated with pruritus and correlates with severity of itching.[68]

Clinical Assessment

Serum bile acid analysis should be performed along with other liver function tests (LFTs) in every pregnant patient with pruritus.[29] The diagnosis is made based upon the clinical presentation of pruritus along with elevation in serum bile acids and transaminases, in the absence of other disorders that can cause these abnormalities.

Severe cholestasis is generally defined as bile acids greater than 40 μmol/L.[29] If itching persists despite normal serum bile acids and LFTs, some recommend repeating these tests weekly, since as mentioned previously, pruritus may precede bile acid abnormalities in ICP. An abdominal ultrasound should be considered as well as screening for hepatitis C, as these are both risk factors for ICP.[29] Neither skin biopsy nor DIF is needed for diagnosis.

If bile acids and transaminases are repeatedly normal in the pregnant patient with severe persistent pruritus, then diagnoses other than ICP should be investigated, including systemic diseases associated with pruritus (renal, other liver disease, thyroid disease, malignancy).[56] Persistent, severe pruritus should be addressed with detailed history, review of systems, physical examination, and targeted laboratory and/or imaging studies.[56] If there is a skin eruption, then the other SDPs should be considered, although these will typically have *primary* skin lesions, not just secondary changes from scratching. If there are primary skin lesions that are not consistent with SDPs, referral to a dermatologist is appropriate for evaluation of a dermatosis unrelated to pregnancy.

Pharmacologic and Nonpharmacologic Treatment and Maternal/Fetal Risk

In ICP, both treatment and maternal/fetal risk are discussed jointly, as the primary goal of treatment is to reduce harm to the fetus and secondary goal is to reduce pruritus in the mother. The excess bile acids cross the placenta and can cause potential complications for the fetus.

Women with ICP have a significantly greater risk for spontaneous preterm birth and iatrogenic preterm birth, and babies born to women with ICP were significantly more likely to have meconium-stained amniotic fluid and respiratory distress syndrome and require admission to the neonatal intensive care unit (NICU).[72,73]

Management of pregnancy in women with ICP requires close obstetric monitoring and maternal counseling. Early induction of labor is often recommended because the risk of stillbirth seems to increase with gestational age.[58]

Recommendations vary on the timing of labor induction, as reduction of risks related to ICP need to be weighed against potential maternal/fetal consequences from early delivery (ie, low birth weight, lower Apgar scores, days in NICU, increased rate of cesarean delivery).[58] The American College of Obstetricians and Gynecologists recommends delivery at 36 0/7 to 37 0/7 weeks of gestation, or at diagnosis if diagnosed later, but earlier delivery may be appropriate depending on the clinical circumstances.[75]

Maternal prognosis is generally very good even with early induction of labor,[64] with the exception of patients with ICP having steatorrhea, who are at increased risk for intrapartum hemorrhage due to decreased absorption of vitamin K.[29] When compared to controls, later in life, patients with ICP have an increased risk for hepatobiliary disease and hepatobiliary cancer, as well as immune-mediated diseases such as diabetes mellitus, psoriasis, thyroid disease, and Crohn disease; there is an increased risk of cardiovascular disease if the patient had both a history of preeclampsia and ICP.[76,77] Maternal pruritus generally resolves after delivery.

Although emollients with menthol may mildly ease pruritus, the primary drug treatment is UDCA, also known as ursodiol. Clinical trials have thus far lacked power to demonstrate whether UDCA reduces fetal risks.[80] UDCA is typically dosed at 500 mg orally two or three times daily or 10 to 15 mg/kg/d, with reduction in pruritus occurring in 1 to 2 weeks and bile acid reduction taking several weeks.[29,80] Therapy is continued until delivery. Other medications, such as S-adenosyl-L-methionine, rifampin (added to UDCA), cholestyramine, activated charcoal, guar gum, and dexamethasone, have been used in ICP in cases refractory to UDCA, but studies of these medications included only small numbers of patients and have had mixed results.[55]

Recurrence Risk

The risk for ICP to recur in subsequent pregnancy is high, likely due to the genetic influences on its pathogenesis.[29,59]

Summary

Physiologic skin changes during pregnancy are common. Awareness of these alterations is important to appropriately counsel patients on the natural course of these alterations, and any interventions that may be appropriate for prevention or treatment.

The pregnant patient with pruritus, with or without a skin eruption, should be evaluated promptly by the obstetrician. *If a skin eruption is present*, specific dermatoses of pregnancy (SDPs) should be considered. In the case where the diagnosis is unclear, consultation with a dermatologist is appropriate to evaluate for a dermatosis that is unrelated to pregnancy. *If pruritus occurs without skin eruption or with only secondary lesions*, intrahepatic cholestasis of pregnancy (ICP) should be considered. If ICP is ruled out, then other systemic causes of pruritus should be considered (other liver disease, renal disease, thyroid disease, or malignancy).

KEY POINTS

- Hyperpigmentation is the most commonly reported skin change in pregnancy
- Melasma occurs more often in those with darker skin types, regular sun exposure, or family history
- Risk factors for striae gravidarum include young maternal age, personal or family history, elevated body mass index, and excessive weight gain during pregnancy
- No specific topical preparation is known to reliably prevent striae gravidarum
- While controversial over many years, four dermatoses are considered *specific* for pregnancy: PEP, AEP, PG, and ICP

Polymorphic Eruption of Pregnancy

- PEP typically starts on the abdomen as urticarial pruritic papules or plaques within striae, and *sparing of umbilical skin is a characteristic finding*
- PEP is common in primigravidae, with third-trimester onset, and has no fetal/maternal risk
- PEP can be treated with topical corticosteroids for milder cases; more severe cases may require systemic steroids
- PEP resolves with delivery or in 4 to 6 weeks and typically does not recur in subsequent pregnancies

Atopic Eruption of Pregnancy

- *AEP is the most common of the SDPs*
- AEP occurs prior to third trimester in patients with personal or family history of atopy
- In AEP, two-thirds of patients had eczematous lesions, one-third had papular lesions
- AEP is usually clinically diagnosed without specific laboratory or histologic findings but may have elevated serum levels of IgE
- AEP is typically treated with topical corticosteroids or systemic steroids in severe cases
- There is no maternal/fetal risk except that infant may later develop atopy
- Recurrence of AEP is likely in subsequent pregnancies

Pemphigoid Gestationis

- PG is an autoimmune blistering disorder in pregnancy, similar to BP in the nonpregnant patient, caused by autoantibodies directed against bullous pemphigoid antigen 180 (BP180) located on hemidesmosomes in the basement membrane zone of the skin
- PG starts as urticarial papules and plaques on the abdomen, *typically involving the umbilical skin*, and then progresses to tense bullae
- PG onset is typically in the second or third trimester, but initial postpartum onset occurs in about 25% of cases
- PG diagnosis is done through skin biopsy (perilesional) for DIF
- PG is treated with systemic steroids
- PG results in increased risk for preterm delivery or small-for-gestational age infants
- PG almost always recurs in subsequent pregnancy, usually earlier and more severe

Intrahepatic Cholestasis of Pregnancy

- ICP manifests as severe pruritus with elevation in serum bile acids; prompt recognition is needed due to fetal risks
- ICP onset is in late second or third trimester, with strong genetic link secondary to mutations in bile canalicular transporters in hepatocytes
- In ICP, skin lesions can be absent or secondary due to scratching

- ICP risks for the fetus include preterm delivery, meconium-stained amniotic fluid, respiratory distress and rarely stillbirth in cases where bile acid concentration is >100 µmol/L
- In ICP, early induction of labor often recommended at 36 to 37 weeks of gestation to minimize fetal risk, but varies based on specific clinical circumstances
- ICP is likely to recur in subsequent pregnancies

REFERENCES

(only references cited in synoptic print chapter; for a complete reference list, see ebook)

1. Panicker VV, Riyaz N, Balachnadran PK. A clinical study of cutaneous changes in pregnancy. *J Epidemiol Glob Health.* 2017;7:63-70.
2. Soutou B, Aractingi S. Skin disease in pregnancy. *Best Pract Res Clin Obstet Gynecol.* 2015;29:732-740.
3. Mostosko CC, Bieber AK, Pomeranz MK, et al. Physiologic changes of pregnancy: a review of the literature. *Int J Womens Dermatol.* 2017;3:219-224.
5. Bieber AK, Matires KJ, Stein JA, et al. Pigmentation and pregnancy: knowing what is normal. *Obstet Gynecol* 2017;129:168-173.
7. Ortonne JP, Arellano I, Berneburg M, et al. A global survey of the role of ultraviolet radiation and hormonal influences in the development of melasma. *J Eur Acad Dermatol Venereol.* 2009;23:1254-1262.
8. Rathore SP, Gupta S, Gupta V. Pattern and prevalence of physiological cutaneous changes in pregnancy: a study of 2000 antenatal women. *Indian J Dermatol Venereol Leprol.* 2011;77:402.
9. Lakhdar H, Zouhair K, Khadir, et al. Evaluation of the effectiveness of a broad-spectrum sunscreen in the prevention of chloasma in pregnant women. *J Eur Acad Dermatol Venereol.* 2007;21:738-742.
10. Sarkar R, Gokhale N, Godse K, et al. Medical management of melasma: a review with consensus recommendations by Indian Pigmentary Expert Group. *Indian J Dermatol.* 2017;62:558-577.
11. Graupe K, Cunliffe WJ, Gollnick HP, Zaumseil RP. Efficacy and safety of topical azelaic acid (20 percent cream): an overview of results from European clinical trials and experimental reports. *Cutis.* 1996;57:20-35.
12. Farahnik B, Park K, Kroumpouzos G, et al. Striae gravidarum: risk factors, prevention, and management. *Int J Womens Dermatol.* 2017;3:77-85.
17. Winton GB, Lewis CW. Dermatoses of pregnancy. *J Am Acad Dermatol.* 1982;6(6):977-998.
18. Elling SV, Powell FC. Physiological changes in the skin during pregnancy. *Clin Dermatol.* 1997;15:35-43.
19. Murase JE, Heller MM, Butler DC. Safety of dermatologic medications in pregnancy and lactation: Part I. Pregnancy. *J Am Acad Dermatol.* 2014;70:401.e1-401.e14.
20. Danesh M, Pomeranz MK, McMenimen E, et al. Dermatoses of pregnancy: nomenclature, misnomers, and myths. *Clin Dermatol.* 2016;34:314-319.
21. Ambros-Rudolph CN, Mullegger RR, Vaughan-Jones SA, et al. The specific dermatoses of pregnancy revisited: results of a retrospective two-center study on 505 pregnant patients. *J Am Acad Dermatol.* 2006;54:395-404.
22. Ambros-Rudolph CM. Dermatoses of pregnancy – clues to diagnosis, fetal risk, and therapy. *Ann Dermatol.* 2011;23:265-274.
23. Rudolph CM, Al-Fares S, Vaughan-Jones SA, et al. Polymorphic eruption of pregnancy: clinicopathology and potential trigger factors in 181 patients. *Br J Dermatol.* 2006;154:54-60.
24. Roth MM. Pregnancy dermatoses: diagnosis, management, and controversies. *Am J Clin Dermatol.* 2011;12:25-41.
25. Dominguez-Serrano AJ, Quiroga-Garza A, Jacobo-Baca G, et al. Polymorphic eruption of pregnancy in Mexico. *Int J Dermatol.* 2019;58:259-262.

27. Ahmadi S, Powell F. Pruritic urticarial papules and plaques of pregnancy: current status. *Austrlas J Dermatol.* 2005;46:53-58.
29. Lehrhoff S, Pomeranz MK. Specific dermatoses of pregnancy and their treatment. *Dermatol Ther.* 2013;26:274-284.
30. Garcia-Gonzalez E, Ahued-Ahued R, Arroyo E, et al. Immunology of cutaneous disorders of pregnancy. *Int J Dermatol.* 1999;38:721-729.
31. Leung DY, Guttman-Yassky E. Deciphering the complexities of atopic dermatitis: shifting paradigms in treatment approaches. *J Allergy Clin Immunol.* 2014;134:769-779.
32. Shornick JK. Dermatoses of pregnancy. *Semin Cutan Med Surg.* 1998;17:172-181.
33. Tani N, Kimura Y, Koga H, et al. Clinical and immunological profiles of 25 patients with pemphigoid gestationis. *Br J Dermatol.* 2015;172:120-129.
34. Jenkins RE, Herns S, Black MM. Clinical features and management of 87 patients with pemphigoid gestationis. *Clin Exp Dermatol.* 1999;24:255-259.
35. Lawley TJ, Stingl G, Katz SI. Fetal and maternal risk factors in herpes gestationis. *Arch Dermatol.* 1978;114:552-555.
36. Shornick JK, Bangert JL, Freeman RG, et al. Herpes gestationis: clinical and histologic features of twenty-eight cases. *J Am Acad Dermatol.* 1983;8:214-224.
37. Gan DC, Welsh B, Webster M. Successful treatment of a severe persistent case of pemphigoid gestationis with antepartum and postpartum intravenous immunoglobulin followed by azathioprine. *Australas J Dermatol.* 2012;53:66-69.
40. Al Saif F, Jouen F, Hebert V, et al. Sensitivity and specificity of BP180 NC16A enzyme-linked immunosorbent assay for the diagnosis of pemphigoid gestationis. *J Am Acad Dermatol.* 2017;76:560-562.
41. Kroumpouzos G, Cohen LM. Dermatoses of pregnancy. *J Am Acad Dermatol.* 2001;45:1-19.
42. Yang A, Uhlenhake E, Murrell DF. Pemphigoid gestationis and intravenous immunoglobulin therapy. *Int J Womens Dermatol.* 2018;4:166-169.
43. Hern S, Harman K, Bhogal BS et al. A severe persistent case of pemphigoid gestationis treated with intravenous immunoglobulins and cyclosporine. *Clin Exp Dermatol.* 1998;24:825-828.
44. Kreuter A, Harati A, Breukmann F, et al. Intravenous immunoglobulin in the treatment of persistent pemphigoid gestationis. *J Am Acad Dermatol.* 2004;51:1027-1028.
45. Rodrigues CDS, Filipe P, Solana MDM, et al. Persistent herpes gestationis treated with high dose intravenous immunoglobulin. *Acta Derm Venereol.* 2007;87:184-186.
46. Marker M, Derfler K, Monshi B, Rappersberger K. Successful immunoapheresis of bullous autoimmune diseases: pemphigus vulgaris and pemphigoid gestationis. *J Dtsch Dermatol.* 2011;9:27-31.
47. Wöhrl S, Geusau A, Karlhofer F, et al. Pemphigoid gestationis: treatment with immunoapheresis. *J Dtsch Dermatol Ges.* 2003;1:126-130.
48. Amato L, Mei S, Gallerani I, Moretti S, Fabbri P. A case of chronic herpes gestationis: persistent disease or conversion to bullous pemphigoid? *J Am Acad Dermatol.* 2003;49:302-307.
49. Van de Wiel A, Hart CH, Flinterman J, et al. Plasma exchange in the treatment of persistent pemphigoid gestationis. *Br Med J.* 1980;281:1041-1042.
50. Ozdemir O, Atalay CR, Asgarova V, et al. A resistant case of pemphigoid gestationis successfully treated with cyclosporine. *Intervent Med Appl Sci.* 2016;8:20-22.

51. Hapa A, Gurpinar A, Akan T, et al. A resistant case of pemphigus gestationis successfully treated with intravenous immunoglobulin plus cyclosporine. *Int J Dermatol.* 2014;53:e269-e271.

52. Huilaja L, Makikallio K, Hannula-Jouppi K, et al. Cyclosporine treatment in severe gestational pemphigoid. *Acta Derm Venereol.* 2015;95;593-595.

53. Shornick JK, Black MM. Secondary autoimmune disease in herpes gestationis (pemphigoid gestationis). *J Am Acad Dermatol.* 1992;26:563-566.

54. Chi CC, Wang SH, Charles-Holmes R. Pemphigoid gestationis: early onset and blister formation are associated with adverse pregnancy outcomes. *Br J Dermatol.* 2009;160:1222-1228.

55. Ovadia C, Williamson C. Intrahepatic cholestasis of pregnancy: recent advances. *Clin Dermatol.* 2016;34:327-334.

56. Mehta N, Chen KK, Kroumpouzos G. Skin disease in pregnancy: the approach of the obstetric medicine physician. *Clin Dermatol.* 2016;34:320-326.

57. Dixon PH, Williamson C. The pathophysiology of intrahepatic cholestasis of pregnancy. *Clin Res Hepatol Gastroenterol.* 2016;40:141-153.

58. Friberg AK, Zingmark V, Lyndrup J. Early induction of labor in high-risk cholestasis of pregnancy: what are the costs? *Arch Gynecol Obstet.* 2016;294:709-714.

59. Joshi D, James A, Quaglia A, et al. Liver disease in pregnancy. *Lancet.* 2010;375:594-605.

63. Menzyk T, Bator M, Derra A, et al. The role of metabolic disorders in the pathogenesis of intrahepatic cholestasis of pregnancy. *Clin Exp Hepatol.* 2018;4:217-223.

64. Reyes H, Baez ME, Gonzalez MC, et al. Selenium, zinc, and copper plasma levels in intrahepatic cholestasis of pregnancy, in normal pregnancies, and in healthy individuals, in Chile. *J Hepatol.* 2000;32:542-549.

65. Chappell LC, Gurung V, Seed PT, et al. Ursodeoxycholic acid versus placebo, and early term delivery versus expectant management in women with intrahepatic cholestasis of pregnancy: semifactorial randomised controlled trial. *Br Med J.* 2012;344:e3799.

66. Kenyon AP, Piercy CN, Girling J, et al. Pruritus may precede abnormal liver function tests in pregnant women with obstetric cholestasis: a longitudinal analysis. *Br J Obstet Gynecol.* 2001;108:1190-1192.

67. Abu-Hayyeh S, Ovadia C, Lieu T, et al. Prognostic and mechanistic potential of progesterone sulfates in intrahepatic cholestasis of pregnancy and pruritus gravidarum. *Hepatol.* 2016;63:1287-1298.

68. Kremer AE, Martens JJ, Kulik W, et al. Lysophosphatidic acid is a potential mediator of cholestatic pruritus. *Gastroenterology.* 2010;139: 1008-1018.

72. Ovadia C, Seed PT, Sklavounos A, et al. Association of adverse perinatal outcomes of intrahepatic cholestasis of pregnancy with biochemical markers: results of aggregate and individual patient data meta-analyses. *Lancet.* 2019;393:899-909.

73. Zecca E, De Luca D, Baroni S, et al. Bile acid-induced lung injury in newborn infants: a bronchoalveolar lavage fluid study. *Pediatrics.* 2008;121:e146-e149.

75. ACOG Committee Opinion No 764. Medically indicated late-preterm and early-term deliveries. *Obstet Gynecol.* 2019;133:e151-e155.

76. Marschall HU, Wikstrom SE, Ludvigssom JF, et al. Intrahepatic cholestasis of pregnancy and associated hepatobiliary disease: a population-based cohort study. *Hepatol.* 2013;58:1385-1391.

77. Wikström Shemer EA, Stephansson O, Thuresson M, et al. Intrahepatic cholestasis of pregnancy and cancer, immune-mediated and cardiovascular diseases: a population-based cohort study. *J Hepatol.* 2015;63:456-461.

80. Chappell LC, Chambers J, Dixon PH, et al. Ursodeoxycholic acid versus placebo in the treatment of women with intrahepatic cholestasis of pregnancy (ICP) to improve perinatal outcomes: protocol for a randomised controlled trial (PITCHES). *Trials.* 2018;27(19):657-667.

CHAPTER 42

Cancer and Other Neoplasms in Pregnancy

Gautam Gorantla Rao

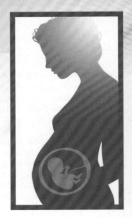

Benign Masses in Pregnancy

Uterine Myomas

Myomas are very common in the general population. They are a frequent cause of infertility and are less prevalent among pregnant women than among the same age group of nonpregnant women.

Clinical Presentation

Myomas can cause pain through degenerative changes or by direct compression of adjacent organs. Nongrowing myomas can cause symptoms during pregnancy as a result of the enlarging uterus which displaces them out of the pelvis. Symptoms may develop as asymptomatic myomas compress abdominal organs.

Uterine myomas can undergo central necrosis and degeneration, causing localized pain at the site. Degenerating myomas can provide a culture medium for pathogenic organisms with occasional leukocytosis and superimposed infection. Myomas are thought to increase the frequency of preterm labor and premature rupture of membranes. They have been implicated in first-trimester spontaneous abortions,[10,11] and large cervical and lower uterine segment myomas can cause obstructed labor and infertility.[9,12]

Placental abruption, postpartum hemorrhage, and retained placenta are thought to be complications of uterine myomas during pregnancy. However, several studies failed to show statistically different rates of these complications compared with the general population.[9,12]

See the eBook for expanded content, a complete reference list, and additional figures and tables.

Management of Myomas in Pregnancy

Preconception myomectomy may be considered based on the patient's age, reproductive history, size and location of the myomas, and symptoms. However, there is no good evidence that myomectomy will improve fertility or fecundity rates.[5] Most of the symptoms can be managed medically in pregnant women.

There are very few studies and no randomized trials available on the safety of myomectomy in pregnancy.[14-16] Myomectomy during pregnancy is best avoided in all but the most extreme circumstances, such as torsion of a pedunculated myoma or when a malignancy is suspected. The 2013 Committee Opinion by the American College of Obstetricians and Gynecologists recommends that women with previous myomectomy which caused significant compromise of the uterine integrity undergo cesarean delivery rather than a trial of labor and vaginal delivery due to small but catastrophic risk of uterine rupture.[17]

Pharmacologic Treatment

Symptomatic treatment with acetaminophen or opioid analgesics usually provides relief. Several studies have shown that nonsteroidal anti-inflammatory drugs can be used successfully in pregnancy for management of the symptoms.[2,18] However, these drugs have known fetal risks and should be used with caution during pregnancy.[19] Hydration and antibiotics can be used if infection is suspected.

Adnexal Masses in Pregnancy

Corpus Luteum Cysts

Clinical Presentation

Corpus luteum cysts can complicate pregnancy if they undergo torsion or spontaneous rupture.

Nonpharmacologic Treatment
Asymptomatic corpus luteum cysts typically regress during the second trimester and are completely absent by the third trimester. If a corpus luteum cyst is removed before 9 weeks' gestation, exogenous progesterone is administered.

Luteoma
Clinical Presentation
Luteomas of pregnancy are solid tumors that are characterized by hypertrophy of ovarian stroma. This hypertrophy may be secondary to stimulation by human chorionic gonadotropin (hCG). They are frequently bilateral and multinodular. Elevated levels of testosterone accompany luteomas in at least 25% of cases, although other hormones may be responsible for maternal virilization.[27-29] When maternal virilization is present, female fetuses are at risk of virilization. The female fetus is usually not at significant risk of labioscrotal fusion because placental aromatization of maternal androgens is not usually overwhelmed by androgen production until fusion is complete.[30,31] There does not appear to be any association between luteomas and multifetal gestation or gestational trophoblastic disease.

Nonpharmacologic Treatment
Expectant management is recommended.[32] Luteomas can occasionally recur; therefore, preconception counseling is necessary for women with a history of luteoma.[33]

Hyperreactio Luteinalis
Clinical Presentation
Hyperreactio luteinalis is a benign, nonneoplastic enlargement of theca lutein cysts, most likely due to stimulation by hCG.[34] Hyperreactio luteinalis is strongly associated with conditions that produce abnormally elevated hCG, such as multifetal gestation, gestational trophoblastic disease, and ovarian hyperstimulation syndrome.[35] Hyperreactio luteinalis is usually bilateral and multicystic with stromal edema. Ovarian enlargement can be massive. Although maternal androgen excess is occasionally present, virilization of female fetuses rarely occurs.[36,37] Life-threatening ascites, electrolyte abnormalities, thromboembolism, intravascular depletion, hemoconcentration, renal failure, and pleural effusion with respiratory difficulties may be present when hyperreactio luteinalis complicates ovarian hyperstimulation syndrome or gestational trophoblastic disease.

Nonpharmacologic Treatment
In addition to supportive measures, uterine evacuation may be necessary to reverse hCG-induced ovarian stimulation in such cases. In milder cases, expectant management is appropriate because hyperreactio luteinalis and theca lutein cysts usually resolve shortly after delivery.

Cancers in Pregnancy
The most common neoplasms in pregnancy include melanoma, breast cancer, cervical cancer, lymphomas, and leukemias.[39,40]

Screening
Serum tumor markers are an essential tool for diagnosing and monitoring patients with cancer but use of these markers should be done with caution during pregnancy. Levels of tumor markers, such as members of the cancer antigen (CA) family, may be affected by the pregnancy and may vary due to gestational age and pregnancy-related conditions.

Management of Cancer in Pregnancy
Termination of a pregnancy affected by maternal neoplasia is rarely indicated. Although a fear expressed by pregnant patients is that the cancer might spread to the placenta and fetus, information collected during the past 2 decades suggests that transplacental metastasis is extremely unusual, and metastases to the fetus are rare. The most common malignancy to be associated with fetal and placenta metastases is malignant melanoma. However, the reported number of cases in the literature of such an event is fewer than 30.[52]

Occasionally, iatrogenic preterm birth should be considered as an alternative management strategy in treating pregnant patients with cancer. This strategy requires that sophisticated newborn special care units be available for maintaining premature infants. Antenatal corticosteroid therapy has been shown to decrease complications related to organ immaturity such as respiratory distress syndrome, intraventricular hemorrhage, and necrotizing enterocolitis. Fetal interventions to promote maturation are most effective if delivery occurs from 2 to 7 days after the initiation of therapy. Tests of fetal lung maturity, such as the lecithin/sphingomyelin (L/S) ratio, could be considered in determining the timing of delivery.[53]

Nonpharmacologic Treatment

Surgery in Pregnancy

Patients may undergo successful surgical procedures when they are pregnant without jeopardizing the fetus. The timing of surgery for malignancy in pregnancy is based upon the balance of potential risks and benefits for mother and baby. In general, surgery should be delayed until the second trimester, which seems to be the safest time in terms of avoiding patients going into labor. Spontaneous abortion sometimes occurs when surgery is performed in the first trimester. After viability, fetal heart rate should be documented by Doppler or ultrasound just before and after the procedure.

Maternal surgery in the third trimester may be associated with a risk of premature labor and altered uteroplacental perfusion, putting the fetus at risk of hypoxia, brain injury, intrauterine fetal demise, and premature delivery which is, itself, associated with significant short-term and long-term risks to the neonate, including mortality.

In preparing the patient for a surgical procedure, simple technical considerations may have an important impact on the success of the operation. For example, placing the patient in a lateral position to avoid vena cava and aortic compression is an important factor in considering the anesthetic consequences of surgery.[55,56] In addition, there are many concerns about general anesthesia during pregnancy.

Laparoscopic surgery, if indicated, can be performed safely during pregnancy. General recommendations include, auscultation of fetal heart tones before and after the procedure, use of pneumatic compression devices for thromboprophylaxis, left lateral tilt of the patient to relieve pressure on the aorta and vena cava from the gravid uterus, lateral tilt of the operating table and/or use of a sponge stick in the vagina to improve visualization for pelvic procedures, careful peritoneal entry with use of Hasson technique or entry at Palmer point, lowering the insufflation pressure during surgery, avoidance of touching the uterus within the peritoneal cavity, and avoidance of routine use of tocolytics.[59]

Radiation in Pregnancy

Radiation is commonly employed in the diagnosis and management of cancers that may occur in pregnancy. Diagnostic imaging to investigate signs and symptoms of cancer malignancy should be performed during pregnancy if necessary and should not be delayed. The imaging modality should be chosen to minimize fetal radiation exposure but not at the cost of a poor study. Ultrasound is the ideal mode of imaging in pregnancy given its lack of ionizing radiation; however, ultrasound has limits as a diagnostic tool for a suspected neoplasm due to maternal body habitus and the gravid uterus. MRI with magnet strength of 3 T or less in any trimester is not associated with increased risk of harm to the fetus or in early childhood. However, maternal exposure to gadolinium, a common MRI contrast agent, should be avoided in pregnancy as it is associated with increased risk of stillbirth and neonatal death, as well as an increased risk of childhood inflammatory, rheumatologic, and infiltrative skin lesions.[60]

Deleterious effects that the fetus may experience from being exposed to radiation therapy have been recognized for many years (see Chapter 9).[61-63]

Pharmacologic Treatment

Chemotherapy and Pregnancy

Prior experience supported the concept that cytotoxic chemotherapy should not be administered to patients, especially during the first trimester of pregnancy. This was because of the high incidence of spontaneous abortion following exposure to chemotherapy and the teratogenic effects of these agents on the developing fetus.[69,70] However, as anecdotal and small series reports have accumulated, it appears that, although certain drugs must be avoided during early pregnancy, others might be life-saving and might not cause congenital anomalies in the fetus[71-74] (**Table 42.2**).

Prematurity and low birthweight are frequent complications of chemotherapy exposure in any trimester of pregnancy. However, the fear of exposure in the second and third trimesters of pregnancy resulting in congenital anomalies no longer appears to be a major concern, provided that the selection of drugs is appropriate.[69,70] The long-term neurologic consequences of intrauterine exposure to chemotherapeutic agents are yet to be established. Children who have been born after *in utero* exposure to chemotherapeutic agents during the second and third trimesters have not been noted to have significant congenital abnormalities.

Physiologic effects of pregnancy may have an impact on the efficacy and toxicity of

Table 42.2 Chemotherapeutic Agents and Reported Associated Anomalies by Trimester

Chemotherapeutic Agents	Mechanism of Action	Reported Significant Anomalies by Trimester[a]		
		First	Second	Third
Alkylating agents				
Melphalan, chlorambucil, cyclophospha-mide, triethylene thiophosphoramide, cisplatin, carboplatin, carmustine (BCNU), chloroethylcyclohexyl nitro-sourea, methyl-CCNU, busulfan	Cell cycle nonspecific; forms cross-linkages with DNA	Yes[b]	No	No
Antimetabolites				
Amethopterin (methotrexate),[c] ami-nopterin, 5-fluorouracil,[c] cytosine arab-inoside, 6-thioguanine, 5-azacytidine, hydroxyurea, hexamethylmelamine, L-asparaginase	Cell cycle specific; structural analogue of precursor purine and pyrimidine bases; lead to nonfunctional DNA and cell death	Yes[d]	No	No
Antibiotics				
Actinomycin D, doxorubicin, dauno-rubicin, bleomycin, mitomycin C, mithramycin	Cell cycle nonspecific; interferes with DNA-dependent RNA synthesis; cell death from lack of RNA and an inability to produce cell proteins	No	No	No
Vinca alkaloids				
Vincristine, vinblastine, etoposide (VP-16), teniposide (VM-26)	Cell phase specific	Yes	No	No
Glucocorticoids				
Cortisone, prednisolone, prednisone, methylprednisolone, dexamethasone	Inhibition of DNA, RNA, and protein synthesis	Yes[e]	No	No

BCNU, bis-chloroethylnitrosourea; CCNU, chloroethylnitrosourea; DNA, deoxyribonucleic acid; RNA, ribonucleic acid.
[a]Reports of anomalies are limited and should be viewed with caution.
[b]Chlorambucil syndrome: renal aplasia, cleft palate, skeletal abnormalities.
[c]Abortifacients in first trimester.
[d]Aminopterin syndrome: cranial dysostosis, hypertelorism, anomalies of the external ears, micrognathia, cleft palate.
[e]Cleft lip, cleft palate.

chemotherapeutic agents. For example, renal blood flow, glomerular filtration rate, and creatinine clearance increases may lead to increased clearance of drugs from the body.[75] It has been suggested that amniotic fluid may act as a pharmacologic third space for such drugs as methotrexate, analogous to ascites or pleural effusions, which may then increase methotrexate toxicity.[76] Gastrointestinal absorption of drugs may be decreased owing to delayed gastric motility. The distribution and kinetics of antineoplastic agents may be substantially affected by the physiologic increase in body water in a pregnant woman in association with a 15% increase in plasma volume and changes in plasma protein concentrations.[77] Drugs that cross the placenta have low molecular weight, have high lipid solubility, are nonionized, and are loosely bound to plasma proteins.[76,78,79]

Congenital anomalies have been noted in patients treated with alkylating agents in the first trimester of pregnancy but not in the second and third trimesters.[69]

Cisplatin has become the most important drug in the management of gynecologic malignancies.[80] Thus, antimetabolites other than amethopterin and aminopterin may be relatively safely used in the management of cancer during pregnancy.

Antibiotics such as actinomycin D, doxorubicin, daunorubicin, bleomycin, mitomycin C, and mithramycin have been used relatively safely in the second and third trimesters of pregnancy.

Vinca alkaloids are cell phase–specific agents that cause mitotic (cell division) arrest. These agents include vincristine, vinblastine, etoposide (VP-16), and teniposide (VM-26).

The reported rate of fetal malformations when exposed to combination chemotherapy in the first trimester (16%) is similar to that of single-agent therapy.[69,83-85] Theoretically, the incidence could be reduced to 6% by removing folate antagonists in common with radiation therapy.[71] Thus, second- and third-trimester chemotherapy appears to be safe with regards to teratogenicity in the fetus.[71] Anemia, leukopenia, and thrombocytopenia also may occur in the fetus as a result of bone marrow suppression and leukopenia, or immune suppression may lead to secondary infection.[73]

Timing of chemotherapy in relation to the anticipated delivery must be carefully assessed. Deliveries should occur when the mother is not bone marrow suppressed. Breastfeeding is discouraged in patients who are receiving cytotoxic chemotherapy, although the data supporting this are weak.[86] To date, there have been no reports of children developing leukemia after *in utero* exposure to chemotherapeutic agents.

In assessing the teratogenic effects of chemotherapeutic agents administered in pregnancy, it must be kept in mind that up to 3% of children have associated major congenital anomalies and 9% have minor anomalies in pregnancies not complicated by cancer treatments or exposure to a chemotherapeutic agent.[87]

Cervical Cancer

The cervix remains the most common site for precancerous and cancerous changes in pregnancy.

Pharmacologic and Nonpharmacologic Treatment

The identification of invasive cancer of the cervix requires prompt treatment, except for patients in the late second or third trimester, when one may briefly delay therapy until fetal viability is established.

Patients with stage IB and stage IIA cervical cancer recognized in the first trimester of pregnancy are routinely recommended to be treated with a type III radical hysterectomy and bilateral deep pelvic lymphadenectomies. This approach affords the patient the opportunity to preserve ovarian function and have a more pliable vagina compared with patients treated with radiation therapy.

Patients with more advanced cervical cancer are routinely recommended to be treated with radiation therapy concurrent with weekly cisplatin.[96-98] Intracavitary radiation follows completion of the external beam radiation regimen. At some institutions, the treatment for locally advanced cervical cancer in pregnancy is to use external beam radiation first and not to attempt to deliver the fetus prior to initiation of therapy. There are no data to suggest that delivering the fetus through an irradiated cervix affects the course of the disease.

Advanced stage cervical cancer has a particularly poor response to standard radiation therapy. A major effort in the past few years has resulted in the development of neoadjuvant chemotherapy protocols for the management of such disease.[101] It may be appropriate to consider a role for neoadjuvant chemotherapy in the management of locally advanced cervical cancer, particularly in situations where definitive treatment will be excessively delayed in order for the fetus to reach viability.

External beam radiation therapy can induce spontaneous abortion. Radiation therapy is a known abortifacient when treating pelvic malignancies. Abortion following initiation of radiation exposure occurs more rapidly in the first trimester than in the second.[103]

Human Papilloma Virus

Some forms of human papilloma virus (HPV) are associated with the development of cervical cancer. However, HPV infection itself may increase the risks of adverse pregnancy outcomes, based on limited data. Prophylactic HPV vaccination would likely reduce these risks; however, this has not yet been studied.

Cervical Intraepithelial Neoplasia
Clinical Assessment

The presence of CIN in pregnancy is usually identified by Pap smear and confirmed by colposcopically directed biopsies. It is standard practice to use colposcopy to evaluate patients with abnormal Pap smears in pregnancy and to limit the biopsy to the site that has the worst colposcopic appearance. In general, colposcopy will show the entire transformation zone, as the squamocolumnar junction tends to be present well out on the exocervix during pregnancy. Cone biopsies of the cervix are avoided, as they are associated with hemorrhage, abortion, and premature labor.[105] It is general practice to biopsy the worst colposcopically identified site and, if the cervical biopsy and Pap smear are consistent, to follow the patient throughout the pregnancy with Pap smears every 3 months.

Patients are reevaluated at approximately 36 weeks' gestation with repeat colposcopy and Pap smears to be as certain as possible that the lesion has not progressed. Cotton tip applicator sticks are used to obtain endocervical cytologic specimens in pregnancy. The preference for the cotton tip applicator stick is to avoid disrupting the fetal membranes with the wire-like tip of the cytobrush. Adenocarcinomas arising in association with carcinoma *in situ* of the exocervix are easily visualized in pregnancy and may be readily biopsied.[105] With this careful monitoring, progression of a precancerous lesion to a locally advanced cervical cancer is rare.

Management of CIN in Pregnancy

If the assessment at 36 weeks remains consistent with CIN, the patient and her physician are advised that the patient may deliver vaginally. No attempt is made routinely to perform cesarean hysterectomies in the management of CIN if further pregnancies are desired. Assessment of precancerous changes can be readily carried out at 6 weeks' postpartum.

Microinvasive Cancer of the Cervix

Clinical Presentation and Assessment

Microinvasive cancer of the cervix is defined as a lesion that has only microscopically penetrated through the basement membrane. Confirmation of the presence of stage IA1 or stage IA2 microinvasive cancer is important in distinguishing it from frankly invasive cancer. In general, patients with microinvasive cancer identified by abnormal Pap smears should undergo routine colposcopic assessment. The confirmation of the extent of disease is extremely important in pregnancy and may require a more extensive biopsy in the form of a hemicone biopsy or a cone biopsy of the cervix.

Management of Microinvasive Cervical Cancers in Pregnancy

If surgical margins are histologically free of disease on the cervical biopsy, patients may safely continue with the pregnancy as long as they are willing to be assessed with frequent Pap smears and colposcopy. Stage IA2 patients have more extensive microinvasive cancer. Once again, the issue is related to the margins of the biopsy used to establish the diagnosis and the patient's desire to preserve the pregnancy and her fertility. Those patients with stage IA1 microinvasive cancer who wish to undergo prompt therapy are usually successfully managed with a simple hysterectomy and leaving the ovaries in place. Those with stage IA2 cervical cancer are recommended to undergo a type II modified radical hysterectomy. Patients who wish to have definitive surgery performed following completion of pregnancy may be delivered vaginally with a subsequent hysterectomy (stage IA1) or may be delivered by cesarean followed by modified radical hysterectomy (stage IA2).

Breast Cancer

Incidence

Breast cancer may be difficult to diagnose during pregnancy and lactation due to the anatomic changes in the breast parenchyma associated with the preparation for lactation. Only 3% of breast cancers occur during pregnancy, but it is the second most common site for invasive cancer in a pregnant woman.[106]

Clinical Presentation

Pregnancy-associated cancers are defined as those diagnosed simultaneously or within 1 year after pregnancy. A number of studies have demonstrated that breast cancer presents at a more advanced stage because of the delay in diagnosis.[98,107-109] The median duration of symptoms before treatment is 15 months in the pregnant patient compared with 9 months in nonpregnant premenopausal women.[110]

Clinical Assessment

The breasts should be examined at the first prenatal visit and thereafter if there have been any concerns noted either by the patient or by the physician during the initial examination. With rare exceptions, any mass discovered during pregnancy should be evaluated.

An ultrasound evaluation may be helpful. If the mass is obvious, a fine needle aspiration (FNA) can be performed.[111] For most patients, an open biopsy under local anesthesia is appropriate. Sedation is not necessary and, therefore, there is no risk to the developing fetus. Because of the increased engorgement and vascularity during pregnancy, absolute hemostasis must be achieved, and a pressure dressing should be applied and left in place for 48 hours.

Open biopsy can also be performed during lactation. The breasts are emptied early in the morning of the day of surgery, and the procedure is again performed under local anesthesia. A pressure dressing is left in place for a few hours. Temporary leakage may occur during breastfeeding, but this soon disappears.

Biopsy material should be sent to the pathologist in a fresh state, and the tissue should be submitted for estrogen and progestin receptor analysis as well as DNA studies. Steroid hormone receptors may not be detected during pregnancy. Pregnancy, in fact, may depress levels of detectable estrogen and progestin receptors, resulting in a false-negative study because high circulating levels of estrogen and progesterone hormones associated with pregnancy result in many more occupied receptor sites.[112]

Management of Breast Cancer in Pregnancy

With prompt diagnosis and appropriate treatment, many patients survive the disease and desire further pregnancies. Most recurrences of breast cancer appear within the first 2 years, and pregnancy should be avoided during this period. Some studies have shown no adverse effect of a subsequent pregnancy even in patients with positive nodes or patients in whom pregnancy occurred earlier than 2 years after completion of treatment.[113-117] Abortion has not improved survival.[114]

Data now show a similar prognosis for breast cancer patients who are pregnant compared with their nonpregnant counterparts when controlled for stage.[118]

Pharmacologic and Nonpharmacologic Treatment

Once the diagnosis of carcinoma has been confirmed, prompt treatment is essential. During the first trimester, modified radical mastectomy is the treatment of choice. Breast conservation treatment poses several problems including potential fetal injury from the effects of radiation.[68] If the patient insists on breast conservation, wide local excision and axillary dissection may be performed and radiation postponed until after delivery. The alternative is termination of the pregnancy and immediate institution of radiation therapy.

During the third trimester, it may be more reasonable to complete local treatment, ie, wide local excision and axillary dissection, and to delay radiation therapy until after delivery. If the patient chooses modified radical mastectomy, this can be delayed until after delivery if the cancer was diagnosed during the third trimester. Appropriate tests should be obtained to insure maturity of the fetus before delivery. The role of sentinel node evaluation during pregnancy needs to be defined.

If axillary dissection reveals lymph node involvement, adjuvant therapy must be considered. This is standard treatment for node-positive premenopausal patients and may be considered in selected node-negative patients. Biologic response modifiers have been administered in pregnancy without adverse effects.[82,122-124]

The final decision whether to use adjuvant chemotherapy rests with the patient after she has received appropriate counseling. In cases of locally advanced cancer, the decisions are even more difficult because chemotherapy and radiotherapy may be required for palliation. In this situation, pregnancy termination would be recommended. This is a difficult decision, and there are no absolute answers. In most of these patients, life expectancy is severely limited, and a frank discussion of the issues involved is imperative.

Ovarian Cancer

Incidence

Although adnexal tumors are frequently diagnosed during pregnancy less than 5% are malignant.[125] Most ovarian cancers complicating pregnancy are either borderline malignant potential epithelial cancers or germ cell malignancies. The incidence of ovarian neoplasms recognized in pregnancy has increased with the routine use of diagnostic ultrasound in pregnancy.

Clinical Assessment

Ultrasound evaluation is a very successful way of assessing the nature of an ovarian tumor.[128] MRI is useful in further delineating the nature of the ovarian neoplasm and to aid in the differential diagnosis with other benign tumors.[127,128] **Figure 42.1** demonstrates an MRI confirming a uterine fibroid that was ultrasonographically indistinguishable from an ovarian tumor associated

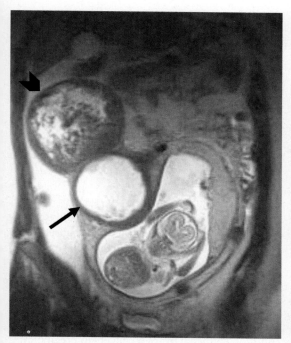

Figure 42.1 Degenerate uterine leiomyomata in pregnancy, coronal T2-weighted magnetic resonance image. There is a bilobed well-circumscribed mass arising from the right uterine wall, excluding the possibility of an adnexal mass which was originally suspected. The inferior component (arrow) is more hemorrhagic with little solid component. The superior component is less degenerate (arrowhead) with a low T2 signal wall and some internal solid component. (Courtesy of Jade Wong-You-Cheong, MD.)

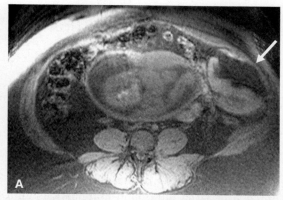

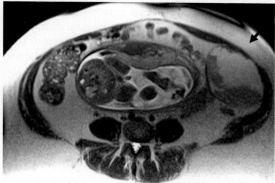

Figure 42.2 Mature cystic teratoma of left ovary in pregnancy. **A,** Axial nonfat-suppressed T2-weighted magnetic resonance image in a pregnant woman with diabetes mellitus and obesity. The left ovarian mass is heterogeneous with high signal anteriorly (arrow), similar to abdominal wall and intraabdominal fat, and low signal posteriorly and medially. **B,** Axial fat-suppressed T1-weighted magnetic resonance image shows that the anterior component (arrow) has been suppressed, similar to the abdominal wall and intraabdominal fat. This confirms the fat content and the diagnosis of mature cystic teratoma. (Courtesy of Jade Wong-You-Cheong, MD.)

with a pregnancy. **Figure 42.2** demonstrates a benign cystic teratoma diagnosed in pregnancy by MRI techniques.

Germ cell ovarian malignancies occur relatively infrequently in younger women, but must be considered in the differential diagnosis of solid or solid and cystic pelvic masses occurring in pregnancy.[129] The more rapidly growing tumors (ie, endodermal sinus tumors and embryonal carcinoma) may be associated with hemorrhage and necrosis, giving a rather inhomogeneous appearance to the mass on ultrasound or MRI scans.

Elevated levels of circulating tumor markers may help to distinguish germ cell tumors from other ovarian neoplasms. However, elevated α-fetoprotein and β-hCG titers are routine in pregnancy, and such assays may be more confusing

than informative in the preoperative evaluation of patients with pelvic masses. Similarly, serum lactic dehydrogenase (SLDH) and other liver enzyme levels may be elevated in nonpregnant women with solid adnexal tumors that prove to be dysgerminoma.[130] However, SLDH and other liver enzymes may be elevated in the pregnant state unrelated to the presence of a dysgerminoma. CA-125, an antigenic determinant made by approximately 80%

of ovarian cancers, may be elevated in early pregnancy for reasons unrelated to the presence of a malignancy.[131-133]

Nonpharmacologic Treatment

Ovarian neoplasms are usually observed in the first trimester and are operated upon in the second trimester. These lesions tend to be asymptomatic when recognized. However, torsion is a relatively frequent presentation for a germ cell malignancy of the ovary and requires prompt surgical intervention. Simple cysts of the ovary may be followed with serial ultrasound examinations until the cysts resolve. Lesions greater than 6 cm in diameter, complex cysts (ie, cysts containing both solid and cystic elements), and solid tumors are the usual indications for operative intervention in pregnancy.

In general, surgical management of ovarian neoplasms occurring in pregnancy is delayed until the second trimester, provided the patient is asymptomatic and the tumor is not suspicious for malignancy by diagnostic imaging techniques. Symptomatic patients and patients with tumors suspicious for malignancy should promptly undergo surgery to diagnose and initiate the treatment of the cancer.

Surgical Staging

Surgical staging for ovarian cancer in pregnancy should be the same as that recommended for surgical staging in the nonpregnant state. A vertical incision should be used. On entering the abdomen, any free fluid should be aspirated and sent for cytology. If no free fluid is present, washings of the paracolic spaces, the pelvis, and subdiaphragmatic spaces should be obtained. The ovarian lesion should then be removed and sent for frozen section histologic analysis. Every effort should be made to remove the tumor intact. The remaining ovary should be carefully inspected and biopsied. Any peritoneal abnormalities should be sampled. Any retroperitoneal nodularities should also be sampled. Sampling of periaortic lymph nodes should be attempted. This can be the most difficult part of the procedure in pregnancy because of the bulk of the gravid uterus.

It is inappropriate to remove both ovaries when a germ cell ovarian malignancy is diagnosed by frozen section techniques. The most common neoplasm in the contralateral ovary of a woman with a germ cell malignancy is a benign cystic teratoma. However, if both ovaries are involved with malignant growths and the patient is in the second trimester of pregnancy, each ovary should be removed, as the pregnancy will sustain itself in the second and third trimesters without ovaries being present.[105] Germ cell ovarian malignancies are almost invariably unilateral. Removing the contralateral ovary does not affect prognosis for the patient. Recent evidence suggests that occult dysgerminomas may be present in a grossly normal contralateral ovary.[134] In such a circumstance, it is not necessary to remove the entire ovary.

Pharmacologic Treatment

Nonpregnant women with microscopic dysgerminoma in the contralateral ovary have subsequently been treated with chemotherapy and have gone on to conceive normal healthy children.

Epithelial Ovarian Cancer

Clinical Presentation

Borderline malignant potential tumors are the most common epithelial ovarian cancers in pregnancy.[135]

Pharmacologic and Nonpharmacologic Treatment

Patients with stage IA and IB borderline malignant potential tumors are adequately treated with surgery alone. More advanced stage ovarian borderline malignant potential tumors are also treated surgically, with chemotherapy being reserved only for the unusual group of patients with invasive metastases in association with borderline malignant potential tumors of the ovary.[136]

Patients found to have stage I invasive cancers of the ovary are generally managed conservatively, and the pregnancy can go to term. Patients with germ cell ovarian malignancies may be given platinum-based chemotherapy in the second and third trimesters prior to the fetus reaching viability.[137] Such a strategy may be employed for common epithelial cancers as well, first recognized to be present in the second and third trimesters of pregnancy.[138]

Germ Cell Ovarian Malignancies

Clinical Presentation

Germ cell ovarian malignancies are infrequently occurring tumors that present in women in their second and third decades of life. The dysgerminoma is the most common malignancy in pregnancy.[139] Other germ cell malignancies include the embryonal carcinoma, the immature teratoma, choriocarcinoma, and mixed germ cell tumors.

Clinical Assessment

Management of dysgerminoma requires removal of the primary tumor and careful surgical staging. Dysgerminomas are the only germ cell malignancies of the ovary to frequently (5%-15%) involve both ovaries. Thus, biopsying the contralateral ovary is appropriate even if it appears to be grossly normal. Dysgerminomas also can spread to the para-aortic nodes. Every effort should be made to sample the para-aortic lymph nodes surgically at the time of the extirpation for the dysgerminoma.

Management of Germ Cell Ovarian Malignancies in Pregnancy

Pregnant women should be given the chance to maintain the pregnancy if a dysgerminoma is present. A cesarean delivery is used to deliver the fetus at the time of fetal viability.

Management of embryonal carcinoma, the immature teratoma, choriocarcinoma, and mixed germ cell tumors is based on both the stage of disease and the presence or absence of circulating oncofetal proteins that can be used as markers for response to therapy.

Pharmacologic and Nonpharmacologic Treatment

Dysgerminomas are exquisitely sensitive to radiation therapy and chemotherapy.[129] Vincristine, actinomycin D, and cyclophosphamide (VAC) and bleomycin, etoposide, and platinum (BEP) are extremely effective regimens for the management of dysgerminomas.[140] Stage IA dysgerminoma may be treated very effectively with surgery alone.[129] Advanced-stage dysgerminoma should be treated with postoperative chemotherapy.[129] Chemotherapy may be given in the second or third trimester. BEP and VAC chemotherapy regimens require only short-term administration and are given every 3 to 4 weeks. A second-look procedure may also be performed at that surgery.

The endodermal sinus tumor is the most virulent of all the germ cell ovarian malignancies and was associated with a 2-year survival of 12% to 19% in the prechemotherapy era. Our current recommendation for this disease is the BEP regimen.

Embryonal carcinoma, the immature teratoma, choriocarcinoma, and mixed germ cell tumors require aggressive therapy in the form of resection of all viable tumor followed by intense combination chemotherapy.[129] Pregnant women found to have these tumors in the second and third trimesters of pregnancy should be offered the opportunity of receiving chemotherapy during pregnancy as a way of being treated and not terminating the pregnancy.

Sex Cord-Stromal Tumors

Clinical Presentation

Sex cord-stromal tumors are rare tumors that may complicate pregnancy. The granulosa theca cell tumor is the most common member of this category and is associated with estrogen production.[141] The Sertoli-Leydig cell tumor is rare and is associated with androgen production.

Pharmacologic and Nonpharmacologic Treatment

Young and colleagues[142] reported on 36 sex cord-stromal tumors diagnosed in pregnancy. Treatment was limited to removing the tumor. Only one of these patients had subsequent recurrence.

Advanced-stage sex cord-stromal tumors require more aggressive chemotherapy. Our current recommendation in the nonpregnant state is a carboplatin and paclitaxel combination.

Hodgkin Disease

Clinical Presentation

Hodgkin disease has not been reported to be affected by the pregnancy.[146-148] Peripheral lymphadenopathy is the most common presenting symptom for patients with Hodgkin disease. Between 60% and 80% of Hodgkin disease, patients have enlarged cervical lymph nodes. In addition, patients may be asymptomatic or may have a history of fever, night sweats, weight loss, malaise, and pruritus.[149]

Clinical Assessment

Staging studies recommended for a patient with Hodgkin disease are done to identify extranodal disease. Pregnant women may undergo ultrasound or MRI studies of the liver, spleen, and retroperitoneal lymph nodes to avoid the hazard of diagnostic imaging radiation exposure to the fetus.

Pharmacologic and Nonpharmacologic Treatment

Hodgkin disease is extremely sensitive to therapy. The cure rate for localized disease treated with radiation therapy is 80%, and patients with advanced disease treated with chemotherapy can anticipate a long-term disease-free survival of 65%.[150,151] Strategies for treating patients with stage I and stage II Hodgkin disease are usually radiotherapeutic, with reported 5-year survivals of 89% and 67%, respectively.[149] Radiation is the only modality necessary for patients with stage IIIA lymphocyte-predominant or nodular sclerosing Hodgkin disease. Stage IIIA disease with other histologic types is treated with radiation and combination chemotherapy. More advanced disease is treated with combination chemotherapy.[152]

Patients with pelvic disease or disease localized to the inguinal or abdominal region should undergo therapeutic abortion prior to radiation therapy because the standard mantle field for midline mediastinal radiation to doses of 4000 rad results in fetal exposure to a degree that is greater than acceptable (no more than 10 rad).[153] Internal radiation scatter from standard mantle fields cannot be shielded and result in a greater exposure rate to the fetus than the dose recommended for continuation of the pregnancy.[152] Disease first recognized in the third trimester is treated with localized radiation therapy once fetal maturity is achieved and the infant delivered. Patients found to have rapidly progressing disease routinely receive chemotherapy, with the decision for initiating treatment based on the trimester of pregnancy and the patient's desires.

Advanced (stage III and stage IV) Hodgkin disease has been successfully treated with the MOPP regimen—Mustargen (nitrogen mustard), Oncovin (vincristine), procarbazine, and prednisone.[149] Eighty-one percent of patients in the National Cancer Institute series with previously untreated stage III and stage IV disease were successfully managed with only 6 months of treatment.[151] Therapeutic abortion should be offered to those patients in the first half of pregnancy who are unwilling to accept an increase in risk of adverse fetal outcome potentially attributable to treatment.

Non-Hodgkin Lymphoma

Incidence
Fewer than 50 cases of non-Hodgkin lymphomas during pregnancy have been published.[72,149,154]

Clinical Presentation
The most important prognostic features for non-Hodgkin lymphoma are the histologic type and the stage of disease.[152] Non-Hodgkin lymphomas tend to be widely disseminated at the time of diagnosis and therefore require less elaborate staging than Hodgkin disease. Breast and ovarian involvement are frequent, and breast metastases have a particularly bad prognosis.[155,156]

Pharmacologic and Nonpharmacologic Treatment
Because of the aggressive nature of diffuse non-Hodgkin lymphoma, aggressive therapy should not be delayed until fetal maturity. Localized non-Hodgkin lymphoma is treated with radiation and has a 50% cure rate. Chemotherapy may also be curative in this disease.[157] Disseminated nodular lymphoma and chronic lymphocytic leukemia fall into a favorable group of disseminated non-Hodgkin lymphomas. They tend to be relatively indolent.[152] Palliative treatment results in survivals of about 5 years. The unfavorable types of non-Hodgkin lymphoma have a much shorter life expectancy, although occasional complete remissions and prolonged survival with chemotherapy have been reported.[158]

Acute Leukemia

Incidence
Acute leukemia rarely complicates pregnancy, the incidence being less than one case in 75,000 pregnancies.[75,159] The disease is usually first recognized in the second or third trimester.[160]

Clinical Presentation
Presenting symptoms are becoming easily fatigued, bleeding diathesis, or recurrent infections that reflect bone marrow failure. Specific physical findings associated with acute leukemia include sternal tenderness, skin pallor, petechiae, ecchymoses, and hepatosplenomegaly. Patients with acute lymphocytic, myelocytic, or monocytic leukemia usually have normocytic anemia, normochromic anemia, mild-to-marked thrombocytopenia, and leukocytosis.[149]

Pharmacologic and Nonpharmacologic Treatment
Pregnancy does not influence the natural history of acute leukemia.[73] Prompt diagnosis and treatment within a tertiary care center with high-risk obstetrical specialists, hematologists, and neonatologists is essential. Substantial improvement in the survival of women with acute leukemia in pregnancy has occurred with the use of chemotherapy, radiation

therapy, and supportive care, including blood products, antibiotics, and autologous bone marrow transplantation.[164] Virtually all women treated with chemotherapy in pregnancy will survive to delivery, and 87% of the fetuses will also survive.[149] Intense combination chemotherapy leads to multiple complications, including severe infections secondary to bone marrow suppression and the risk of central nervous system (CNS) leukemia. The latter is treated with whole brain radiation, intrathecal methotrexate, or cytosine arabinoside. Hyperuricemia is usually treated with allopurinol.[165]

Chronic Myelocytic Leukemia

Incidence and Etiology
Chronic myelocytic leukemia makes up 90% of the chronic leukemias complicating pregnancy.[166,167] Eighty-five percent of chronic myelocytic leukemia patients have a Philadelphia chromosome, a 9:22 translocation.[149]

Management of Chronic Myelocytic Leukemia in Pregnancy
Pregnancy does not adversely affect the natural history of chronic myelocytic leukemia. Treatment is palliative. Median survival is 45 months. All patients eventually die, most from an acute blastic crisis resembling myeloblastic leukemia.[152] The median survival is less than 1 year following the development of an acute blastic crisis.[149] Approximately 96% of pregnant women with chronic myelocytic leukemia survive to delivery. Fetal survival throughout the gestation is 84%.[149]

Gastrointestinal Cancer

Colorectal Cancers
Clinical Presentation
Cancers of the gastrointestinal tract rarely complicate pregnancy.[174] There is no evidence that pregnancy changes the natural history of colorectal cancer, the most common of these neoplasms.[175-179] Most pregnant patients with gastrointestinal cancers have rectal carcinomas. Approximately 20% of patients have carcinoma presenting in the sigmoid colon.[180]

Clinical Assessment
As most diagnoses can be made by rectal examination, symptoms should be promptly evaluated. Delay in diagnosis can be associated with intussusception, obstruction, or perforation.[179]

Management of Colorectal Cancers in Pregnancy
Early-stage colorectal cancers diagnosed in the first or second trimester should be treated with prompt surgery, and the pregnancy should be allowed to go to term.[179,182] Patients with large colorectal lesions with metastases suspected or present have been allowed to carry the pregnancy until fetal maturity and then have undergone a cesarean delivery and bowel resection, provided they remained relatively asymptomatic.[180] A systematic review of 79 studies, including 119 patients, revealed that 60% of women with colorectal cancer in pregnancy underwent vaginal delivery;[183] however, cesarean delivery may be warranted as labor may result in dystocia or hemorrhage. Lesions initially identified in the third trimester are not usually treated until fetal maturity is achieved.[182]

Nonpharmacologic Treatment
Standard therapy for curable lesions is definitive surgery, including standard bowel resections, low anterior resections, or abdominal perineal resections.[184]

Pancreatic Tumors
Pancreatic carcinoma rarely complicates pregnancy and is difficult to diagnose in the presence of pancreatitis.[185,186] Three cases of pancreatic carcinoma have been diagnosed in pregnancy, with the mothers dying soon after delivery.[185,186]

Stomach Tumors
Gastric cancers rarely complicate pregnancy, and their symptoms are similar to those normally experienced in pregnancy, including gastrointestinal discomfort, nausea, and vomiting.[187-190] Diagnosis may be made by gastroscopy, which avoids diagnostic radiation exposure.

Liver Tumors
Hepatocellular carcinomas are rare in women and usually present in postmenopausal women.

Gynecologic Malignancies

Vulvar Cancer
Clinical Presentation
Forty percent of patients with vulvar carcinoma *in situ* are under age 40 years. Thus, it can be anticipated that more women will be diagnosed in

pregnancy to have vulvar carcinoma *in situ.* Vulvar carcinoma *in situ* does not progress rapidly to invasive cancer unless associated with an immune deficiency.

Management and Nonpharmacologic Treatment of Vulvar Cancer in Pregnancy

The management of a vulvar lesion in pregnancy is a wide local excision. Definitive therapy in terms of a wide local excision or vulvectomy can be delayed in most cases until after completion of the pregnancy.

Less extensive surgery has been quite effective if the tumor is only superficially invasive. Extensive vulvectomies may be performed in pregnancy, but it is recommended to manage microinvasive cancer with wide local excision in the nonpregnant state.[197,198]

Vaginal Cancer

Carcinoma of the vagina occurs infrequently and is usually a squamous carcinoma presenting in a perimenopausal or postmenopausal woman. Its management is similar to that of cervical cancer. It was noted that the pregnancy did not have an adverse effect on clear cell carcinomas of the vagina or cervix. Perhaps this is due to the fact that clear cell carcinomas do not have estrogen and progestin receptors.[199]

Endocrine Tumors

Thyroid Cancer

Incidence

Disorders of the thyroid gland are common in pregnancy, and thyroid nodules are frequently diagnosed in pregnancy.[201] However, the thyroid is an infrequent site for cancer to develop in pregnancy. As the population delays childbearing, it is possible that more papillary adenocarcinomas of the thyroid will be diagnosed in the future, as the peak distribution for papillary adenocarcinomas occurs in women aged 30 to 34 years.[202] Anaplastic carcinomas have fulminant courses and rarely complicate pregnancy, as they occur most commonly in women over 50 years of age. Medullary carcinomas can occur in association with the multiple endocrine neoplasia type II syndrome (medullary thyroid carcinoma, pheochromocytoma, and parathyroid adenoma), are bilateral, and have only once been reported in pregnancy.[203]

Clinical Presentation

Patients at high risk of thyroid cancer include women exposed to radiation therapy to the head, neck, or chest during childhood.[204,205] Most cancers of the thyroid present as solitary nodules. Most thyroid nodules appear in the first and third trimesters of pregnancy and are benign.[206]

Clinical Assessment

The most common type of thyroid cancer to be diagnosed in pregnancy is the papillary carcinoma or mixed papillary follicular carcinoma. Prognosis is not affected by subclinical metastases to regional lymph nodes, which are present in 50% to 70% of patients.

FNA biopsies are used to diagnose thyroid cancer in pregnancy.[201,207] Radionuclide scans are contraindicated in pregnancy because of the theoretical risk of destroying the fetal thyroid. FNA biopsy is associated with a false-negative rate of only 6%.[201,208]

Management of Thyroid Cancers in Pregnancy

As the overwhelming number of thyroid cancers presenting in pregnancy is histologically well differentiated, there is no reason to terminate pregnancy or avoid future pregnancies.[209,210] Pregnancy does not appear to influence the course of well-differentiated thyroid cancer.[210,211]

Pharmacologic and Nonpharmacologic Treatment

Thyroid suppression therapy may be administered until delivery, regardless of the trimester in which the cancer was diagnosed.[202] Patients should undergo prompt surgery if metastases develop in regional lymph nodes during suppression therapy or the tumor is fixed to surrounding tissue and enlarges during suppression therapy. A subtotal thyroidectomy is usually performed, and[142] iodine should be administered postpartum to avoid the surgical complication of permanent hypoparathyroidism.[212] Extensive surgery should be avoided during pregnancy, as there is a chance of miscarriage occurring as a result.[213]

Patients diagnosed in the first two trimesters of pregnancy as having a medullary carcinoma should undergo prompt total thyroidectomy and prophylactic neck dissection, whereas those diagnosed in the third trimester can await fetal maturity before definitive surgery. Patients undergoing thyroidectomy in pregnancy are recommended to receive levothyroxine postoperatively in a dose sufficient to keep serum thyroid-stimulating hormone low.[214]

Adrenal Tumors

Incidence

Pheochromocytoma is the most common tumor arising in the adrenal gland in pregnancy.

Clinical Assessment

MRI may be used to confirm the presence, laterality, and location of the pheochromocytoma.[216] Provocative tests should not be performed because these might lead to maternal fatality.[217]

Pharmacologic and Nonpharmacologic Treatment

The management of pheochromocytoma has been surgical in the first two trimesters and delivery by cesarean followed by tumor resection in the third trimester.[179] Medical management of the disease includes preoperative adrenergic blockade with oral phenoxybenzamine to lower the blood pressure and propranolol to reduce the heart rate and prevent arrhythmias through the adrenergic receptor blockade.[218,219]

Urinary Tract Malignancies

Kidney Tumors

Renal cell carcinoma is the most common malignancy arising in the urinary tract in pregnancy.

Hematuria is the most common presenting symptom. Nephrectomy with or without radiation therapy is the standard treatment.

Bladder Cancers

Bladder cancers have infrequently been reported in pregnancy.[224-225] The most common presenting symptom is hematuria. The histologic distribution is similar to that in the nonpregnant state, with an overwhelming majority being transitional cell carcinoma followed by squamous cell and adenocarcinomas. Most cases of transitional cell bladder carcinoma during pregnancy are superficial and can be treated endoscopically, and treatment can usually be deferred until after delivery.[227]

Central Nervous System Tumors

CNS tumors rarely complicate pregnancy.[228] Patients present with headaches and visual disturbances. MRI allows for rapid evaluation without radiation exposure. The overall maternal mortality for patients with CNS tumors is 60%. Therapeutic abortions have been recommended for patients diagnosed in the first trimester as having malignant brain tumors because of the rapid course of such tumors.

KEY POINTS

- Medical management is the primary means of treatment of myoma in pregnancy.
- The hormonal changes of pregnancy, particularly the production of hCG, are associated with luteomas, theca lutein cyst, hyperreactio luteinalis, and large solitary luteinized follicular cyst of pregnancy.
- Radiation and chemotherapy are commonly employed in the routine management of cancers that may occur in pregnancy, such as cervical cancer, breast cancer, ovarian cancer, uterine cancer, vaginal carcinoma, vulvar cancer, and urinary tract malignancies.

- Surgical staging for ovarian cancer in pregnancy should be the same as that recommended in the nonpregnant state.
- Dysgerminoma is a germ cell ovarian cancer and is the most common ovarian malignancy in pregnancy.
- Six sex cord-stromal tumors, such as Sertoli-Leydig cell tumors, are rare during pregnancy.
- It is estimated that one-third of women with Hodgkin disease are pregnant or have delivered within 1 year of diagnosis.
- Non-Hodgkin lymphoma, acute leukemia, gastrointestinal cancers, and thyroid cancers are rare during pregnancy.

REFERENCES

(only references cited in synoptic print chapter; for a complete reference list, see ebook)

2. Katz VL, Dotters DJ, Drogemuller W. Complication of uterine leiomyomas in pregnancy. *Obstet Gynecol.* 1989;73:593.

5. Ezzedine D, Norwitz ER. Are women with uterine fibroids at increased risk for adverse pregnancy outcome? *Clin Obstet Gynecol.* 2016;59(1):119-127.

9. Lev-Toaff AS, Coleman BG, Arger PH, et al. Leiomyomas in pregnancy: sonographic study. *Radiology.* 1987;164:375.

10. Droegmuller W, Herbest AL, Mishell DR, Stenchever MA. *Comprehensive Gynecology.* Mosby; 1987:1059.

11. Jabiry-Zieniewicz Z, Gajewska M. The pregnancy and delivery course with pregnant women with uterine myomas. Article in Polish. *Ginekol Pol.* 2002;73(4):271.

12. Vergani P, Ghidini A, Strobelt N, et al. Do uterine leiomyomas influence pregnancy outcome? *Am J Perinatol.* 1994;11:356.

14. Exacoustos C, Rosati P. Ultrasound diagnosis of uterine myomas and complications in pregnancy. *Obstet Gynecol.* 1993;82:97.

15. Lolis DE, Kalantoridou SN, Makrydimas G, et al. Successful myomectomy during pregnancy. *Hum Reprod.* 2003;18(8):1699.

16. Burton CA, Grimes DA, March CM. Surgical management of leiomyomata during pregnancy. *Obstet Gynecol.* 1989;5:707.

17. American College of Obstetricians and Gynecologists. ACOG Committee Opinion No. 560: medically indicated late-preterm and early-term deliveries. *Obstet Gynecol.* 2013;121:908.

18. Dildy GA, Moise KJ, Smith LG, et al. Indomethacin for the treatment of symptomatic uterine leiomyoma during pregnancy. *Am J Perinatol.* 1992;9:185.

19. Norton ME, Merrill J, Cooper BAB, et al. Neonatal complications after the administration of indomethacin for preterm labor. *N Engl J Med.* 1993;329:1602.

27. Kurman RJ. *Blaustein's Pathology of the Female Genital Tract.* Springer-Verlag; 1987:495.

28. Norris HJ, Taylor HB. Virilization associated with cystic granulose tumors. *Obstet Gynecol.* 1989;34:629.

29. Choi JR, Levine D, Finberg H. Luteoma of pregnancy: sonographic findings in two cases. *J Ultrasound Med.* 2000;19(12):877.

30. Van Slooten AJ, Rechner SF, Dodds WG. Recurrent maternal virilization during pregnancy caused by benign androgen-producing ovarian lesions. *Am J Obstet Gynecol.* 1992;167:1342.

31. Joshi R, Dunaif A. Ovarian disorders of pregnancy. *Endocrinol Metab Clin North Am.* 1995;24:153.

32. Baxi L, Holub D, Hembree W. Bilateral luteomas of pregnancy in a patient with diabetes. *Am J Obstet Gynecol.* 1988;159:454.

33. Shortle BE, Warren MP, Tsin D. Recurrent androgenicity in pregnancy. *Obstet Gynecol.* 1987;70:462.

34. Schnorr JA, Miller H, Davis JR, et al. Hyperreactio luteinalis associated with pregnancy: a case report and review of the literature. *Am J Perinatol.* 1996;13:95.

35. Berkowitz RS, Goldstein DP. Chorionic tumors (review). *N Engl J Med.* 1996;335:1740.

36. Suzuki S. Comparison between spontaneous ovarian hyperstimulation syndrome and hyperreactio luteinalis. *Arch Gynecol Obstet.* 2004;269(3):227.

37. Bradshaw KD, Santos-Ramos R, Rawlins SC, et al. Endocrine studies in a pregnancy complicated by ovarian theca lutein cysts and hyperreactio luteinalis. *Obstet Gynecol.* 1986;67:66S.

39. Sokal JE, Lessmann EM. Effect of cancer chemotherapeutic agents on the human fetus. *J Am Med Assoc.* 1960;172:151.

40. Benedet JL, Boyes DA, Nichols TM, et al. Colposcopic evaluation of pregnancy patients with abnormal cervical smears. *Br J Obstet Gynaecol.* 1976;84:517.

52. Potter JF, Schoeneman M. Metastasis of maternal cancer to the placenta and fetus. *Cancer,* 1970;25:380.

53. Collaborative Group of Antenatal Steroid Therapy. Effect of antenatal dexamethasone administration on prevention of respiratory distress syndrome. *Am J Obstet Gynecol.* 1981;141:276.

55. Goodlin RC. Importance of the lateral position during labor. *Obstet Gynecol.* 1971;37:698.

56. Eckstein K, Marx GF. Aortocaval compression and uterine displacement. *Anesthesiology.* 1974;40:92.

59. Stuparich MA, Nahas S, Behbehani S. Laparoscopy in pregnancy: a primer. *J Minim Invasive Gynecol.* 2020;27(7 suppl):S1-S2.

60. Ray JG, Vermeulen MJ, Bharatha A, Montanera WJ, Park AL. Association between MRI exposure during pregnancy and fetal and childhood outcomes. *J Am Med Assoc.* 2016;316(9):952-961.

61. Streffer C, Shore R, Konermann G, Meadows A, et al. Biological effects after prenatal irradiation (embryo and fetus). A report of International Commission on Radiological Protection. *Ann ICRP.* 2003;33(1-2):5.

62. Bailey H, Bragg HJ. Effects of irradiation on fetal development. *Am J Obstet Gynecol.* 1923;5:461.

63. Brill AB, Forgotson EH. Radiation and congenital malformations. *Am J Obstet Gynecol.* 1964;90:1149.

68. Stovall M, Blackwell CR, Cundiff J, et al. Fetal dose from radiotherapy with photon beams: report of AAPM radiation therapy committee task force group No. 36. *Med Phys.* 1995;22:63.

69. Nicholson HD. Cytotoxic drugs in pregnancy. *J Obstet Gynecol Br Commonw.* 1968;75:307.

70. Sweet DL, Kinzie J. Consequences of radiotherapy and antineoplastic therapy for the fetus. *J Reprod Med.* 1976;17:241.

71. Doll DC, Ringenberg S, Yarbro JW. Antineoplastic agents and cancer. *Semin Oncol.* 1989;16:337.

72. Aviles A, Diaz-Maqueo JC, Torra V, et al. Non-Hodgkin's lymphomas and pregnancy: presentation of 16 cases. *Gynecol Oncol.* 1990;37:335.

73. Reynoso EE, Shepherd FA, Messner HA, et al. Acute leukemia during pregnancy: the Toronto leukemia study group experience with long-term follow-up of children exposed in utero to chemotherapeutic agents. *J Clin Oncol.* 1987;5:1098.

74. Aviles A, Niz J. Long-term follow-up of children born to mothers with acute leukemia during pregnancy. *Med Pediatr Oncol.* 1988;16:3.

75. Redmond GP. Physiologic changes during pregnancy and their implications for pharmacologic treatment. *Clin Invest Med.* 1985;8:317.

76. Wan SH, Huffman DH, Azarnoff DL, et al. Effect of route of administration and effusions on methotrexate pharmacokinetics. *Cancer Res.* 1974;34:3487.

77. Pirani BBK, Campbell DM, MacGillivray I. Plasma volume in normal first pregnancy. *J Obstet Gynecol Br Commonw.* 1973;80:884.

78. Muckcow JC. The fate of drugs in pregnancy. *Clin Obstet Gynecol.* 1986;13:161.

79. Powis G. Anticancer drug pharmacodynamics. *Cancer Chemother Pharmacol.* 1985;14:177.

80. Zemlickis D, Klein J, Moselhy G, et al. Cisplatin protein binding in pregnancy and the neonatal period. *Med Pediatr Oncol.* 1994;23:476.

82. Garber JE. Long-term follow-up of children exposed *in utero* to antineoplastic agents. *Semin Oncol* 1989;16:437.

83. Mulvihill JJ, McKeen EA, Rosner F, et al. Pregnancy outcome in cancer patients. *Cancer.* 1987;60:1143.

84. Jones RT, Weinterman BH. MOPP (nitrogen mustard, vincristine, procarbazine and prednisone) given during pregnancy. *Obstet Gynecol.* 1979;54:477.

85. Lowenthal RM, Funnell CF, Hope DM, et al. Normal infant after combination chemotherapy including teniposide for Burkitt's lymphoma in pregnancy. *Med Pediatr Oncol.* 1982;10:165.

86. Barber HRK. Fetal and neonatal effects of cytotoxic agents. *Obstet Gynecol.* 1981;58(5 suppl):41.

87. Krepart GV, Lotocki RJ. Chemotherapy during pregnancy. In: Allen HH, Nisker JA, eds. *Cancer in Pregnancy.* Futura Publishing; 1986:69.

96. Rose PG. Combined-modality therapy of locally advanced cervical cancer. *J Clin Oncol.* 2003;21(10 suppl):211.

97. American College of Obstetricians and Gynecologists. ACOG Practice Bulletin. Diagnosis and treatment of cervical carcinoma. No. 35, May 2002. *Int J Gynecol Obstet.* 2002;78(1):79.

98. Rose PG, Lappas PT. Pharmacoeconomics of cisplatin-based chemoradiation in cervical cancer: a review. *Expert Opin Pharmacother.* 2002;3(9):1245.

101. Sardi JE, Guillermo R, DiPaola MD, et al. A possible new trend in the management of the carcinoma of the cervix uteri. *Gynecol Oncol.* 1986;25:139.

103. Prem KA, Makowski EL, McKelvey JL. Carcinoma of the cervix associated with pregnancy. *Am J Obstet Gynecol.* 1966;95:99.

105. Schwartz PE. Cancer in pregnancy. In: Gusberg SB, Shingleton HM, Deppe G, eds. *Female Genital Cancer.* Churchill Livingstone; 1988:725.

106. Wingo PA, Tong T, Bolden S. Cancer statistics, 1995. *Cancer J Clin.* 1995;45:8-30.

107. Petrek JA, Dukoff R, Rogatko A. Prognosis of pregnancy-associated breast cancer. *Cancer.* 1991;67:869.

108. Zemlickis D, Lishner M, Degendorfer P, et al. Maternal and fetal outcome after breast cancer in pregnancy. *Am J Obstet Gynecol.* 1992;166:781.

109. Jackisch C, Schwenkhagen A, Louwen F, et al. Breast cancer in pregnancy. *Proc Ann Meet Am Soc Clin Oncol.* 1995;14:228.

110. Peters MV. The effect of pregnancy in breast cancer. In: Forrest APM, Kunkler PB, eds. *Prognostic Factors in Breast Cancer.* Williams & Wilkins; 1968:65.

111. Bottles K, Taylor RN. Diagnosis of breast masses in pregnancy and lactating women by aspiration cytology. *Obstet Gynecol.* 1985;66:76S.

112. Read LD, Greene GL, Katzenellenbogen BS. Regulation of estrogen receptor messenger ribonucleic acid and protein levels in human breast cancer cell lines by sex steroid hormones, their antagonists and growth factors. *Mol Endocrinol* 1989;3:L295.

113. Clark RM, Chua AT. Breast cancer and pregnancy: the ultimate challenge. *Clin Oncol.* 1989;1:11.

114. Danforth DN. How subsequent pregnancy affects outcome in women with prior breast cancer. *Oncology.* 1991;5:2823.

115. Dow KH. Having children after breast cancer. *Cancer Pract.* 1994;2:407.

116. Sankila R, Heinaavra S, Hakulinen T. Survival of breast cancer patients after a subsequent term pregnancy: "Health mother effect". *Am J Obstet Gynecol.* 1994;170:813.

117. Antonella S, Petrek JA. Childbearing issues in breast cancer survivors. *Cancer.* 1997;79:1271.

118. Amant F, von Minckwitz G, Han SN, et al. Prognosis of women with primary breast cancer diagnosed during pregnancy: results from an international collaborative study. *J Clin Oncol.* 2013;31(20):2532-2539. doi:10.1200/JCO.2012.45.6335

119. Guinee VF, Olsson H, Moller T, et al. Effects of pregnancy on prognosis for young women with breast cancer. *Lancet.* 1984;343:157.

121. Anderson BO, Petrek JA, Byrd DR, et al. Pregnancy influences breast cancer stage at diagnosis in women 30 and younger. *Ann Surg Oncol.* 1996;3:204.

122. Doll DC, Ringenberg S, Yarbro JW. Management of cancer during pregnancy. *Arch Intern Med.* 1988;148:2058.

123. Shapiro CL, Mayer RJ. Breast cancer during pregnancy. *Adv Oncol.* 1992;8:25.

124. Arango HA, Kalter CS, DeCesare SL, et al. Management of chemotherapy in a pregnancy complicated by a large neuroblastoma. *Obstet Gynecol.* 1994;84:665.

125. Amant F, Berveiller P, Boere IA, et al. Gynecologic cancers in pregnancy: guidelines based on a third international consensus meeting. *Ann Oncol.* 2019;30(10):1601-1612. doi:10.1093/annonc/mdz228

126. Kier R, McCarthy SM, Scoutt LM, et al. Pelvic masses in pregnancy: MR imaging. *Radiology.* 1990;176:709.

128. Chang SD, Cooperberg PL, Wong AD, et al. Limited-sequence magnetic resonance imaging in the evaluation of the ultrasonographically indeterminate pelvic mass. *Can Assoc Radiol J.* 2004;55(2):87.

129. Schwartz PE. Combination chemotherapy in the management of ovarian germ cell malignancies. *Obstet Gynecol.* 1984;64:564.

130. Schwartz PE, Morris JM. Serum lactic dehydrogenase, a tumor marker for dysgerminoma. *Obstet Gynecol.* 1988;72:511.

131. Bast RC Jr, Klug TL, St John E, et al. A radioimmunoassay using a monoclonal antibody to monitor the course of epithelial ovarian cancer. *N Engl J Med.* 1983;309:883.

132. Schwartz PE, Chambers SK, Chambers JT, et al. Circulating tumor markers in the monitoring of gynecologic malignancies. *Cancer.* 1987;60:353.

133. Niloff JM, Knapp RC, Schaetzl E, et al. CA 125 antigen levels in obstetrics and gynecologic patients. *Obstet Gynecol.* 1985;64:703.

134. Bianchi UA, Sartori E, Favall G, et al. New trends in treatment of ovarian dysgerminoma. *Gynecol Oncol.* 1986;23:246.

135. Dgani R, Shoham Z, Atar E, et al. Ovarian carcinoma during pregnancy: a study of 23 cases in Israel between the years 1960 and 1984. *Gynecol Oncol.* 1989;33:326.

136. Chambers JT, Merino MJ, Kohorn EI, Schwartz PE. Borderline ovarian tumors. *Am J Obstet Gynecol.* 1988;159:1088.

137. Malone JM, Gershenson DM, Creasy RK, et al. Endodermal sinus tumor of the ovary associated with pregnancy. *Obstet Gynecol.* 1986;68(3 suppl):86.

138. Mukhopadhyay A, Shinde A, Naik R. Ovarian cysts and cancer in pregnancy. *Best Pract Res Clin Obstet Gynaecol.* 2016;33:58-72. doi:10.1016/j.bpobgyn.2015.10.015

139. Karlen JR, Akbari A, Cook WA. Dysgerminoma associated with pregnancy. *Obstet Gynecol.* 1979;53:330.

140. Gershensen DM, Morris M, Cangir A, et al. Treatment of malignant germ cell tumors of the ovary with bleomycin, etoposide, and cisplatin. *J Clin Oncol.* 1990;8:715.

141. Schwartz PE. Sex cord-stromal tumors of the ovary. In: Piver S, ed. *Ovarian Cancer.* Churchill Livingstone; 1986:251.

142. Young RH, Dudley AG, Scully RF. Granulosa cell, Sertoli-Leydig cell and unclassified sex cord-stromal tumors associated with pregnancy. A clinicopathological analysis of thirty-six cases. *Gynecol Oncol.* 1984;18:181.

146. Sweet DL Jr. Malignant lymphoma: implications during the reproductive years and pregnancy. *J Reprod Med.* 1976;17:198.

147. Tawil E, Mercier JP, Dondavino A. Hodgkin's disease complicating pregnancy. *J Can Assoc Radiol.* 1985;36:133.

148. Ward FT, Weiss RB. Lymphoma and pregnancy. *Semin Oncol.* 1989;16:397.

149. Mitchell MS, Capizzi RL. Neoplastic disease. In: Burrow GN, Ferris TF, eds. *Medical Complications During Pregnancy.* W.B. Saunders; 1982:510.

150. Sutcliffe SB, Wrigley PFM, Peto J, et al. MVPP chemotherapy regimen for advanced Hodgkin's disease. *Br Med J.* 1978;1:679.

151. Devita VT, Simon RM, Hubbard SM, et al. Curability of advanced Hodgkin disease with chemotherapy. *Ann Intern Med.* 1980;92:587.

152. Sutcliffe SB, Chapman RM. Lymphomas and leukemias. In: Allen HH, Nisker JA, eds. *Cancer in Pregnancy.* Futura Publishing; 1986:135.

153. Meruk ML, Green JP, Nussbaum H, et al. Phantom dosimetry study of shaped cobalt-60 fields in treatment of Hodgkin's disease. *Radiology.* 1968;91:554.

154. Steiner-Salz D, Yahalon J, Samuelov A, et al. Non-Hodgkin's lymphoma associated with pregnancy. A report of 6 cases with a review of the literature. *Cancer.* 1985;56:2087.

155. Armitages JD, Feagler JR, Skoog DP. Burkitt's lymphoma during pregnancy with bilateral breast involvement. *J Am Med Assoc.* 1977;237:151.

156. Armon PJ. Burkitt's lymphoma of the ovary in association with pregnancy: two case reports. *Br J Obstet Gynaecol.* 1976;83:169.

157. Miller TP, Jones SE. Chemotherapy of localized histiocytic lymphoma. *Lancet.* 1979;1:358.

158. Devita VT Jr, Chabner B, Hubbard SP, et al. Advanced diffuse histiocytic lymphoma, a potentially curable disease. *Lancet.* 1975;1:248.

159. Yahia C, Hyman GA, Phillips LL. Acute leukemia and pregnancy. *Obstet Gynecol Surv.* 1958;13:1-21.

160. Hoover BA, Schumacher HR. Acute leukemia in pregnancy. *Am J Obstet Gynecol.* 1966;96:316.

164. Roy V, Gutteridge CN, Hysenbaum A, Newliand AC. Combination chemotherapy with conservative obstetric management in the treatment of pregnant patients with acute myeloblastic leukemia. *Clin Lab Haematol.* 1989;11:171.

165. Henderson EJ. Acute leukemia: general considerations. In: Williams WJ, Beutler E, Erslev AJ, Rundles RW, eds. *Hematology.* 2nd ed. McGraw-Hill; 1977:108.

166. McLain CR Jr. Leukemia in pregnancy. *Clin Obstet Gynecol.* 1974;17:185.

167. Moloney WC. Management of leukemia in pregnancy. *Ann N Y Acad Sci.* 1964;114:857.

168. McCulloch PB, Dent PB. Melanoma. In: Allen AA, Nisker JA, eds. *Cancer in Pregnancy.* Futura Publishing; 1986:205.

170. Colbourn DS, Nathanson L, Belilos E. Pregnancy and malignant melanoma. *Semin Oncol.* 1989;16:377.

174. Byers T, Graham S, Swanson M. Parity and colorectal cancer risk in women. *J Natl Cancer Inst.* 1982;69:1059.

175. Barber HRK, Brunschwig A. Carcinoma of the bowel. *Am J Obstet Gynecol.* 1968;100:926.

176. Zaridze DG. Environmental etiology of large bowel cancer. *J Natl Cancer Inst.* 1983;70:389.

177. Girard RM, Lamarche J, Baillot R. Carcinoma of the colon associated with pregnancy. Report of a case. *Dis Colon Rectum.* 1981;24:473.

178. Bernstein MA, Madoff RD, Caushaj PF. Colon and rectal cancer in pregnancy. *Dis Colon Rectum.* 1993;36:172.

179. Cappell MS. Colon cancer during pregnancy. *Gastroenterol Clin North Am.* 2003;32(1):34.

180. Allen HH, Nisker JA. Colorectal cancer in pregnancy. In: Allen HH, Nisker JA, eds. *Cancer in Pregnancy.* Futura Publishing; 1986:281.

182. Parry BR, Tan BK, Chan WB, et al. Rectal carcinoma during pregnancy. *Aust N Z Surg.* 1994;64:618.

183. Pellino G, Simillis C, Kontovounisios C, et al. Colorectal cancer diagnosed during pregnancy: systematic review and treatment pathways. *Eur J Gastroenterol Hepatol.* 2017;29(7):743-753. doi:10.1097/MEG.0000000000000863

184. O'Leary JA, Pratt JH, Symmonds RE. Rectal carcinoma in pregnancy. A review of 17 cases. *Obstet Gynecol.* 1967;30:862.

185. Gamberdella FR. Pancreatic cancer in pregnancy. A case report. *Am J Obstet Gynecol.* 1984;149:15.

186. Boyle JM, McLeod ME. Pancreatic cancer presenting as pancreatitis in pregnancy. Case report. *Am J Gastroenterol.* 1979;70:371.

187. Skokos CK, Lipshitz J. Adenocarcinoma of the stomach associated with pregnancy. *J Tenn Med Assoc.* 1982;75:103.

188. Sims EH, Schlater TL, Sims M, et al. Obstructing gastric carcinoma complicating pregnancy. *J Natl Med Assoc.* 1980;72:21.

189. Bowers RH, Walters W. Carcinoma of the stomach complicated by pregnancy. Report of an unusual case. *Minn Med.* 1958;41:30.

190. Dai D, Chen J, Wang S. Stomach cancer in pregnancy and breast feeding: report of 17 cases. *Chin J Surg.* 1995;33:768.

195. Schwartz PE, Naftolin F. Type 2 herpes simplex virus and vulvar carcinoma in situ. *N Engl J Med*. 1981;305:517.

197. Latimer J. Gynaecological malignancies in pregnancy. *Curr Opin Obstet Gynecol*. 2007;19(2):140-144. doi:10.1097/GCO.0b013e3280464f0c

198. Bakour SH, Jaleel H, Weaver JB, Kehoe S, Radcliffe KW. Vulvar carcinoma presenting during pregnancy, associated with recurrent bone marrow hypoplasia: a case report and literature review. *Gynecol Oncol*. 2002;87(2):207-209. doi:10.1006/gyno.2002.6802

199. Senekjian EK, Hubby M, Herbst AL. Clear cell adenocarcinoma (CCA) of the cervix and vagina associated with pregnancy. *Gynecol Oncol*. 1985;20:250.

201. Tan GH, Gharib H, Gohllner JR, et al. Management of thyroid nodules in pregnancy. *Arch Intern Med*. 1996;156:2317.

202. Stuart GCE, Temple WJ. Thyroid cancer in pregnancy. In: Allen NH, Nisker JA, eds. *Cancer in Pregnancy*. Futura Publishing; 1986:191.

203. Chodander CM, Abhyankar SC, Deodhar KP. Sipple's syndrome (multiple endocrine neoplasia) in pregnancy (case report). *Aust N Z J Obstet Gynecol*. 1982;22:243.

204. Cady B, Sedwick CE, Meissner WA. Changing clinical, pathologic, therapeutic and survival patterns in differentiated thyroid carcinoma. *Ann Surg*. 1976;184:541.

205. Cady B, Sedwick CE, Meissner WA. Risk factor analysis in differentiated thyroid cancer. *Cancer*. 1979;43:810.

206. Rosen IB, Walfish PG. Pregnancy as a predisposing factor in thyroid neoplasia. *Arch Surg*. 1986;121:1287.

207. Goldman MH, Tisch B, Chattock AG. Fine needle biopsy of a solitary nodule arising during pregnancy. *J Med Soc N J*. 1983;80:525.

208. Schwartz AE, Nieburgs HE, Davis TF. The place of fine needle biopsy in the diagnosis of nodules of the thyroid. *Surg Gynecol Obstet*. 1982;155:54.

209. Rosvoll RV, Winship T. Thyroid carcinoma and pregnancy. *Surg Gynecol Obstet*. 1965;121:1039.

210. Herzon FS, Morris DM, Segal MN, et al. Coexistent thyroid cancer and pregnancy. *Arch Otolaryngol Head Neck Surg*. 1994;120:1191.

211. Hill CS, Clark RL, Wolf M. The effect of subsequent pregnancy in patients with thyroid carcinoma. *Surg Gynecol Obstet*. 1966;122:1219.

212. Farrar WB, Cooperman M, James AG. Surgical management of papillary and follicular carcinoma of the thyroid. *Am Surg*. 1980;192:701.

213. Cunningham MP, Slaughter DP. Surgical treatment of diseases of the thyroid gland in pregnancy. *Surg Gynecol Obstet*. 1970;131:486.

214. Choe W, McDougall IR. Thyroid cancer in pregnancy women: diagnostic and therapeutic management. *Thyroid*. 1994;4:433.

216. Greenberg M, Moawad AH, Wieties BM, et al. Extraadrenal pheochromocytoma: detection during pregnancy using MR imaging. *Radiology*. 1986;161:475.

217. Ellison GT, Mansberger JA, Mansberger AR Jr. Malignant recurrent pheochromocytoma during pregnancy. Case report and review of the literature. *Surgery*. 1988;103:484.

218. Fusge TL, McKinnon WMP, Geary WL. Current surgical management of pheochromocytoma during pregnancy. *Arch Surg*. 1980;115:1224.

219. Leak D, Carroll JJ, Robinson DC, et al. Management of pheochromocytoma during pregnancy. *Obstet Gynecol Surv*. 1977;32:583.

224. Stanhope CR. Management of the obstetric patient with malignancy. In: Sciarra JJ, ed. *Gynecology and Obstetrics*. Vol 2. Harper & Row; 1984:1.

225. Keegan GT, Forkowitz MJ. Transitional cell carcinoma of the bladder during pregnancy. A case report. *Tex Med*. 1982;78:44.

226. Cruikshank SH, McNellis TM. Carcinoma of the bladder in pregnancy. *Am J Obstet Gynecol*. 1983;145:768.

227. Lakmichi MA, Zehraoui R, Dahami Z, et al. Bladder cancer in the second trimester of pregnancy: tough decisions. A case report with review of the literature. *Ther Adv Urol*. 2012;4(3):139-142. doi:10.1177/1756287212441961

228. Carmel PN. Neurologic surgery in pregnancy. In: Barber HRK, ed. *Surgical Disease in Pregnancy*. W.B. Saunders; 1974:207.

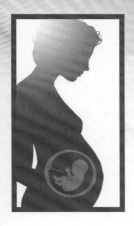

CHAPTER 43

Psychiatric Problems During and After Pregnancy

Nicole Leistikow, Patricia F. Widra, Rebecca Sokal, and Alison D. Hermann

Introduction

Perinatal depression affects nearly 20% of women throughout the peripartum,[1] making it the most common obstetric (OB) complication overall, and suicide has been identified as a leading cause of maternal mortality in industrialized nations, including the United Kingdom and the United States.[2,3] Multiple major professional organizations including the American College of Obstetricians and Gynecologists (ACOG), the American Academy of Pediatrics, and the United States Preventive Services Task Force have recommended universal depression screening procedures for pregnant and postpartum women, recognizing the essential role that obstetricians and gynecologists play as frontline clinicians in women's health care throughout the peripartum period.[4-6] ACOG has further asserted in its guidelines that OB clinicians need to be prepared to both initiate pharmacotherapy and refer patients to psychiatric treatment, if needed, as well as to put in place effective systems to prevent patients with psychiatric needs being lost to follow-up.[7] It is, therefore, essential that obstetricians and gynecologists have a basic understanding of common psychiatric illnesses and their treatments.

Changes in Approaches to Maternal Mental Illness

Replacement of the FDA Categories

The FDA drug risk categories A, B, C, D, and X were established in 1979, after an epidemic of fetal

malformations caused by thalidomide, to provide an easy-to-use standardized system that might prevent such harms in the future. Over the years, consensus developed that the categories were prone to significant misinterpretation. They were phased out by 2015 and replaced by narrative descriptions to better guide clinicians.[8] Although this change is considered a significant improvement, it nonetheless has its own limitations in that it relies on drug manufacturers to write summaries that may not be available immediately for many medications and requires greater effort by clinicians to access and weigh information about the risks of untreated illness versus the risks of medications. Despite their limitations, narrative summaries will better reflect and guide the real-life complexity of such medication decisions during pregnancy and lactation.

The Risks of Psychiatric Illness for the Mother and Fetus

Psychiatric illnesses have been linked to increased rates of congenital anomalies; OB outcomes, such as preeclampsia, preterm birth, cesarean delivery, neonatal intensive care unit (NICU) admissions, low birth weight, and small-for-gestational age fetuses; impaired mother-infant bonding; increased rates of infant neglect or abuse; and suicide and infanticide (**Table 43.1**).[11,20-26,28-31,37-40] Population groups with mental illness are less healthy than cohorts without mental illness and have increased rates of medical morbidity, including obesity, diabetes, and cardiovascular disease, which may also confer risk for some of the outcomes listed above.[41] Thus, in attempting to research the effects of medications intended to treat mental illness on fetal outcomes, the possibility of confounding by indication, or the

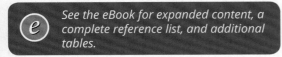

See the eBook for expanded content, a complete reference list, and additional tables.

Table 43.1 Risks of Untreated Psychiatric Illnesses in Pregnancy and Postpartum

Negative birth outcomes[20-27]	• Preeclampsia
	• Preterm labor
	• Low birth weight
	• Cesarean delivery
	• Neonatal intensive care unit admissions
Increased unhealthy maternal behaviors[24,28,29]	• Poor perinatal self-care
	• Maternal substance use (including tobacco)
	• Maternal self-harm
	• Suicide attempts
Decreased healthy maternal behaviors[11,26,28]	• Decreased adherence to safety and other recommendations (child car seats, infant safe sleep position, prenatal vitamins)
	• Impaired mother-infant bonding
	• Lower rates of pediatric preventative care
	• Lower rates of postpartum care
Increased risk in offspring for cognitive, emotional, medical, and behavioral problems[30-35]	
Increased risk of intimate partner violence[36] and decreased social support[28]	

possibility that the illness itself may be causing the outcome of interest, must be rigorously addressed.

Design Challenges in Research on Maternal Mental Illness

Due to restrictions of randomized controlled trials in pregnant women,[42] research on the effects of medications in pregnancy has relied on observational studies, which are unable to establish causation due to the limits of their design.[43,44] Additionally, publication bias has led to an underrepresentation of studies finding no association between perinatal medications and negative fetal outcomes.[45] Meta-analyses, which are higher powered to find associations by virtue of combining multiple prior studies, have no ability to change the design flaws already present in the studies they use and, therefore, may amplify confounding,[46] leading to compounded inaccuracy and false certainty.[47] Finally, the use

of pharmacy databases and filled prescriptions to denote adherence to medications is particularly problematic given high rates of women stopping psychotropic medications suddenly in pregnancy.[48] Newer statistical advances that have improved the ability to control for confounding in observational studies, such as propensity score matching, have begun to correct some of the erroneous associations found in earlier studies and should continue to advance the field.[44,47,49]

Future Challenges

The recognition of many mental illnesses as chronic relapsing-remitting illnesses associated with a wide range of potentially negative maternal and child outcomes has changed the standard of OB care to include universal screening protocols and has tipped the balance of mental illness management in favor of continuing pharmacologic treatments throughout pregnancy and postpartum for women with moderate to severe illnesses and initiating treatment in symptomatic women who are newly identified.

Despite these advances, significant challenges for OB clinicians remain. At this point, clinicians are expected not only to implement universal depression screening but also to accurately diagnose depression and initiate treatment. Meeting this new standard of care requires further clinical evaluation (discussed below), consideration of comorbid conditions, and a ruling out of important conditions based upon the differential diagnosis, such as bipolar disorders or substance use disorders, that may masquerade as depression. The clinician must additionally determine severity and consider when to initiate treatment and when to refer. While problems with access to psychiatric care necessitate that OB clinicians treat common psychiatric illnesses such as anxiety and mild to moderate unipolar depression, more severe or complicated illnesses are best managed by a psychiatrist.

Psychiatric Illness in the Perinatal Period

Mood Disorders

Depression
Epidemiology and Risk Factors
A woman's risk of depression in pregnancy is about the same as it is in the non-pregnant state, and the prevalence of depression in pregnancy is estimated

to be 6% to 17% in the United States.[50,51] Women with anxiety, stress, a prior history of depression, low social support, unintended pregnancy, lower income, a history of domestic violence, and less education are at greater risk.[52] Postpartum, the risk of depression goes up, with as many as one in five women developing depression following childbirth.[54] The primary risk factor for postpartum depression is depression during pregnancy.[53] Additional risk factors include anxiety, low social support, high stressors, and difficult infant temperament among others.[54-56]

Clinical Presentation
OB clinicians should suspect a diagnosis of depression in patients who have two or more weeks of sustained low or irritable mood and/or loss of interest in pleasurable activities (anhedonia). To meet full diagnostic criteria for depression, one or both of these cardinal symptoms must be accompanied by additional cognitive, emotional, and neurovegetative symptoms such as a change in perception of self-worth; excessive feelings of guilt; increased difficulty concentrating or making decisions; unexpected alterations in sleep, appetite, energy, or activity level; or recurrent thoughts of death, for a total of at least five symptoms overall. Anxious and/or intrusive thoughts are more common in perinatal depression than depression at other times of life and, for many women, may be the most prominent symptom of the syndrome, especially in the postpartum. Moderate to severe depression is additionally marked by significant difficulty functioning with everyday tasks, including cognitive slowing or distraction, which may interfere with work or other responsibilities, severe fatigue or other physical impairments that interfere with activities of daily living, or impaired ability to cope with problems and/or higher emotional reactivity, which causes significant conflict in important relationships. Thoughts of not wanting to live, wishing to die, or having impulses to self-injure are not normal responses to stressors and are considered markers of severe depression.

Postpartum, depression should be distinguished from "baby blues," which are experienced by up to 85% of women. If symptoms include an inability to sleep when the baby is sleeping, a desire to flee or avoid proximity to the baby, or if the emotional lability persists beyond 2 weeks postpartum, a diagnosis of depression should be considered.

If symptoms such as confusion, disorientation, changes in personality or judgment, paranoia, or other psychotic symptoms are present, other diagnoses, such as bipolar disorder or postpartum psychosis (discussed below), should be investigated.

Clinical Assessment
The most widely used screening tool for depression in adult populations is the Patient Health Questionnaire-9 (PHQ-9), although it is not as well validated in perinatal populations, particularly in the postpartum. The PHQ-9 is a nine-item scale listing depressive symptoms based on the *Diagnostic and Statistical Manual of Mental Disorders* (*DSM–5*—American Psychiatric Association) criteria, with a score of 10 or greater considered as a positive screen.[58] The Edinburgh Postnatal Depression Scale (EPDS) was developed and is the preferred screening tool for this population where feasible. It is a 10-item self-report scale that places greater emphasis on anxiety questions and less emphasis on neurovegetative symptoms. It is freely available in more than 20 languages and has been extensively validated both during pregnancy and in the postpartum; a score greater than 12 is considered a positive screen.[59]

Management of Depression in Pregnancy
For women with mild to moderate depression, first-line treatment recommendations include a trial of evidence-based psychotherapy such as cognitive behavioral therapy (CBT) or interpersonal psychotherapy (IPT). For women with moderate to severe depression or in women for whom psychotherapy is ineffective or insufficiently effective, an antidepressant is often needed to achieve symptom relief and remission.[49]

Pharmacologic Treatment
Risks of Antidepressants Selective serotonin reuptake inhibitors (SSRIs) are the most studied class of antidepressants and are considered first-line treatment for use in pregnant and lactating women (**Table 43.3**).

Studies have consistently shown antidepressants to be associated with an increased risk for poor neonatal adaptation syndrome (PNAS), which is a transient syndrome experienced by up to 30% of exposed newborns compared to 9% of newborns who are not exposed and who do not require medical interventions.[64,65] Infants with

Table 43.3 First-Line Selective Serotonin Reuptake Inhibitors (SSRIs) in Pregnancy and Breastfeeding

Summary of Risks:

- No increased risk of fetal malformations found[62,63]
- Poor neonatal adaptation syndrome: Up to 30% of newborns may experience self-limited transient symptoms lasting 2 d to 4 wk[64,65]
- Small increased risk of persistent pulmonary hypertension of the newborn, with an absolute risk increase of 0.619 per 1000 live births and a number needed to harm of 1615 in a meta-analysis[66,67]
- Low concentrations passed into breast milk, relatively safe in breastfeeding
- Can cause nausea and diarrhea, which typically fade after 2 wk, sexual side effects, weight gain, and activation or increased anxiety, which can be dose related

Agent	Starting Dose	Therapeutic Dose (Daily)	Titration Schedule (Once a therapeutic range is reached, SSRIs may require 4-8 wk to be effective)
Sertraline	25 mg	150-200 mg	Increase by 25-50 mg every 1-2 wk
Escitalopram	5-10 mg	10-20 mg	Increase by 5-10 mg every 2-4 wk
Citalopram	10-20 mg	20-40 mg	Increase by 10 mg every 2-4 wk
Fluoxetine	10 mg	20-80 mg	Increase by 10 mg every 2-4 wk

PNAS can experience increased fussiness, jitteriness, tremors, rapid breathing, increased muscle tone, and insomnia with symptoms lasting typically 2 days to 2 weeks postbirth. Although respiratory symptoms may be present in more severe cases of PNAS, this condition should not be confused with the previously discussed and much more severe condition, PPHN. Risk of PNAS increases with concomitant exposure to benzodiazepines *in utero*.[37] Breastfeeding and skin-on-skin contact are thought to reduce PNAS symptoms for infants, but importantly, tapering off antidepressants in the third trimester does not and is not recommended.[37,38]

Risks of Untreated Depression The risks of not treating depression in pregnancy are significant and include increased morbidity and mortality for both mother and infant (**Table 43.1**). Risk of suicide, though rare in pregnancy, is a leading cause of postpartum maternal mortality in industrialized nations, and the risk of postpartum depression increases with untreated depression in pregnancy. Other risks include poorer prenatal care, lower birth weight and earlier delivery, increased risk of preeclampsia and cesarean delivery, and increased NICU admission rates.[20-23,25,27] Long-term adverse child outcomes, such as attachment problems, delays in language acquisition, and behavioral problems, have also been associated with maternal depression.[30,32,33]

Initiating Antidepressants Prior to initiating antidepressants, a brief screen to rule out bipolar illness should be completed. Alternatively, a validated screening tool, such as the Mood Disorder Questionnaire can also be used to rule out bipolar disorder.[70] All patients should be warned to watch for signs of mania or hypomania induced by antidepressants and to stop taking medications if symptoms seem to be worsening.

In addition to fetal exposure concerns described above, informed consent should include a discussion of potential maternal side effects, such as nausea and diarrhea, which typically fade after 2 weeks; sexual side effects; weight gain; and increased anxiety, which can be related to higher starting doses or faster dose increases.

Once the decision has been made to treat depression in pregnancy with medication, first-line SSRI options include sertraline, escitalopram, citalopram, fluoxetine, and fluvoxamine. These agents are preferred because they are older medications about which a substantial research base has formed. Newer agents are generally avoided unless there is clinical reason to use them such as documented prior efficacy for a particular patient and/or demonstrated failure or inability to tolerate older agents. Tricyclic antidepressants are reasonable options in pregnancy, especially if a patient has prior experience of efficacy with them, but they are not typically first-line agents due to having more side effects and more narrow therapeutic windows.[71,72]

Best practice guidelines recommend limiting the number of exposures for a fetus while considering untreated mental illness as an exposure.[73] Providers should prioritize, if known, agents with demonstrated efficacy for a particular patient over untried agents with unknown efficacy for that individual. Single agents should be titrated to their maximum dose, if needed, before adding any additional medications or embarking on a new medication trial (**Table 43.3**). Additionally, the physiologic changes of pregnancy typically cause antidepressant blood levels to drop over the course of gestation, often requiring active up-titration of doses to maintain symptom control.[74] Dose titrations are typically based on clinical observation of worsening symptoms but can be anticipated and discussed ahead of time.

For women already taking antidepressants when they become pregnant, decision-making should include a discussion of the risks of remaining on the medications (with an acknowledgment that the baby has already been exposed) versus the risks of relapse of illness. If a woman and her doctor decide to stop psychiatric mediations in pregnancy, tapering slowly, over the course of at least 1 to 2 months, is recommended to reduce the risk of relapse.[75]

Postpartum, depression should be treated promptly. Antidepressants in general are expressed in low levels in breast milk and should not be considered a contraindication to breastfeeding. The same principles are followed as in pregnancy: limiting the number of exposures to the baby, including untreated maternal depression as an exposure, and using adequate doses of older agents as first-line options.

Patients with postpartum depression should be counseled to balance the value of breastfeeding through the night with the need to prioritize sleep to stabilize mood; patients should consider enlisting support persons to provide a portion of the overnight infant care, which can include bottle feeding via expressed breast milk or formula, changing, soothing the infant, and, in general, relieving a new mother of a portion of nighttime responsibilities. If sleep remains substantially disrupted, the chances of successfully treating depression are low.

Bipolar Illness

Epidemiology and risk factors

Bipolar illness is rare, with a prevalence of about 3% in the United States. It is characterized by both manic/hypomanic and depressive episodes, with the latter typically outnumbering the former and delaying accurate diagnosis, often by years.[78,79] Women whose first episode of depression occurs during their first year postpartum have an increased risk of later being diagnosed with bipolar disorder.[80] Women with a diagnosis of bipolar illness have an increased risk of attempting suicide, above that of other psychiatric illnesses. Women with bipolar illness are also at higher risk of comorbid health conditions, such as obesity, smoking, and other substance use, as well as negative obstetrical outcomes such as induction, cesarean delivery, late preterm birth, and use of instrumentation at delivery.[84]

Bipolar illness relapse during pregnancy is common, and the risk is substantially increased by discontinuing medications.[85,86] Other predictors of illness recurrence during pregnancy include a history of prior perinatal mood disturbance, a family history of perinatal mood problems, severe illness, or recent depression or hypomania.

Postpartum, women with bipolar illness remain at high risk for relapse, which can include psychotic, manic, and depressive symptoms, sometimes requiring hospitalization.[87]

Postpartum psychosis is considered a rare variant of bipolar illness with approximately 20% of cases manifesting only in the postpartum period and 80% of cases having a chronic relapsing-remitting course.[89-92]

Clinical Presentation

Hypomanic or manic episodes are characterized by a noticeable change in functioning that occurs for a period lasting longer than 2 days with decreased need for sleep, fewer hours of sleep (typically 4 hours or less), increased energy, abnormally elevated or irritable mood, increased impulsivity, and changes in hedonic behaviors such as increased spending, risk-taking, socializing, or having more sex. For an accurate diagnosis, these periods of increased energy and change in behavior should not be in the setting of drug use or other confounding factors, such as medical conditions or medications used to treat them.

Management of Bipolar Illness in Pregnancy

Given the higher health risks associated with bipolar illness and the challenges of using mood stabilizers and antipsychotics in pregnant women, patients with bipolar disorder generally should be referred to a psychiatrist and, if available, preferably a reproductive psychiatrist. In general, the standard of care is to continue an appropriate mood stabilizer in pregnancy for those women already stabilized on medications when they become pregnant and to initiate an appropriate mood stabilizer in pregnancy for those women not already on medication who are symptomatic or at high risk of relapse.

Pharmacologic Treatment

Lithium, lamotrigine, quetiapine, and olanzapine are all reasonable choices to treat bipolar illness in pregnancy, with studies generally demonstrating tolerable risk profiles (**Table 43.5**).[96,99,102,103] Higher doses of mood stabilizers or neuroleptics may be required to maintain euthymia as pregnancy progresses due to the physiologic changes of pregnancy affecting drug blood levels. For lithium (the concentration of which is reduced by increased glomerular filtration rate and greater blood volume) and lamotrigine (the concentration of which is reduced by estrogenic induction of hepatic glucuronidation), regular blood level monitoring is recommended throughout pregnancy.[103] In general, decreasing or discontinuing mood-stabilizing medications in pregnancy is not recommended as it increases the risk for symptom relapse. Once symptoms reemerge, higher doses and additional mood-stabilizing agents may be required to achieve symptom control.

The major exception to the principle of recommending mood stabilizers in pregnancy is the use of valproate, which has been banned in several countries for use in any women of childbearing age and which the American Academy of Neurology has recommended be avoided in pregnancy if possible.[104] If valproate is the only recommended option for a pregnant patient (or in women who could become pregnant), clinicians should document their discussion of risks with the patient, including increased risks of major congenital malformations, cognitive delays and deficits, and autism,[105-107] and why other agents are not an option. Prescribers should use the lowest possible dose and recommend concurrent use of 4 mg/d of folic acid supplementation.[108]

Postpartum, patients and families should be counseled to monitor for symptoms of psychosis or mania. If medications have been avoided during pregnancy, they should be restarted immediately postpartum for prevention of relapse in high-risk patients, a strategy shown to be effective most notably with lithium.[88] Sleep preservation and consolidation of sleep hours are essential and may require increased social support for nighttime feeding assistance and/or postpartum doula/nursing services if access is available. The recommendation to breastfeed on demand should be balanced with the risks associated with sleep disruption, a major risk factor for relapse in this population. Judicious use by support persons of formula supplementation or previously expressed breast milk at night can protect sleep while preserving the benefits of breastfeeding.

Fetal medication exposure *in utero* is greater than infant exposure via breast milk, so, in general, use of mood-stabilizing medication is not considered a contraindication for breastfeeding. However, lithium may be an exception as it has significant passage into the breast milk and a narrow therapeutic index; use while breastfeeding is currently controversial among experts and an evolving area of study. Lithium use while breastfeeding may be considered a reasonable choice in psychiatrically stable mothers with a full-term healthy infant working in collaboration with a pediatrician with a plan to monitor the infant's lithium level, thyroid-stimulating hormone, and creatinine and to respond quickly to dehydration or other provocations that may cause an increase in infant serum lithium level.[103,109,112] Initial research on lamotrigine in breastfeeding is reassuring; however, there are relatively high levels transmitted into breast milk.[97] The risks of untreated illness versus the risks of treatment should continue to be discussed both with patients as well as pediatricians to ensure that patients are not getting conflicting advice.

Anxiety Disorders

Generalized Anxiety Disorder

Epidemiology, Risk Factors, and Clinical Presentation

Anxiety is common in pregnancy, with prevalence estimates ranging from 4% to 39% for any anxiety disorder including phobias, with up to 10.5% of women experiencing generalized anxiety disorder.[113] Patients with a high burden of anxiety symptoms can be identified using the Generalized Anxiety Disorder 7-item scale or items 3 to 5 on the EPDS. All women, but especially those with a history of anxiety, should receive anticipatory guidance about the somatic symptoms of pregnancy, which include physical symptoms that can overlap

Table 43.5 Common Mood Stabilizers and Second-Generation Antipsychotics During Pregnancy and Breastfeeding

Agent	Starting Dose	Dosing Range (Daily)	Specific Issues
Lamotrigine[93-95]	25 mg daily (follow 6-week titration schedule)	100-300 mg Higher doses may be needed to target the individual patient's preconception level on which they were therapeutic	• Rising estrogen levels induce metabolism across pregnancy and may be expected to cause a drop in lamotrigine levels and resulting clinical symptoms • If dosage is increased during pregnancy, taper to prepregnancy dose within 3 wk after delivery to avoid toxicity in the mother and infant (if breastfeeding) • No association with major congenital malformations[96] • Variable levels found in breast milk, no known adverse effects with typical psychiatric doses, an emerging area of research[97]
Lithium[98]	300 mg daily	900-1800 mg	• Monitor/maintain therapeutic levels due to increased renal clearance during pregnancy (therapeutic level range 0.6-1.0 mEq/L for maintenance treatment) • Elevated risk of cardiac malformations (absolute risk <1/1500) • Passed into breast milk, some concern for toxicity in newborns, an emerging area of research
Valproate[98]	500 mg daily	500-1500 mg	• Avoid in women of childbearing age unless no other alternatives • Significant increase (7×) in risk for major congenital defects associated with first trimester exposure • Associated with intrauterine growth retardation infant hepatic toxicity • Associated with increased risk of autism spectrum disorder in offspring, developmental delays • Monitor/maintain therapeutic levels due to increased hepatic clearance, which may lower maternal levels (therapeutic level range 50-125 µg/mL for maintenance treatment) • Monitor maternal liver function, coagulation labs, complete blood count • Passed into breast milk in low levels, relatively safe in breastfeeding
Quetiapine[99-101]	50 mg	200-400 mg	• No significant increased risk for cardiac or other congenital malformations when potential confounding conditions are controlled for • May increase risk of gestational diabetes • Low levels found in breast milk, considered relatively safe in breastfeeding, ongoing research
Olanzapine[99-101]	5 mg	10-20 mg	• No significant increased risk for cardiac or other congenital malformations when potential confounding conditions are controlled for • May increase risk of gestational diabetes • Low levels found in breast milk, considered relatively safe in breastfeeding, ongoing research

with anxiety symptoms such as difficulty sleeping, nausea, shortness of breath, and increased heart rate. In pregnant patients with high anxiety, OB clinicians should take care not to dismiss specific worries around the health of the baby or concerning test results. However, women with frequent checking behaviors in response to anxiety, such as excessive internet searching or reassurance seeking, should be screened for obsessive-compulsive disorder (OCD) that responds poorly and may be even worsened by frequent reassurance.

Anxiety and depression are highly comorbid in pregnancy and can signify more severe illness. Delivering prematurely and having high rates of childcare stress and perceived stress increase the risk for comorbid depression with anxiety, whereas breastfeeding self-efficacy, higher maternal self-esteem, and social support decrease this risk.[114,115]

Risks of untreated anxiety during pregnancy include low birth weight and earlier delivery, hypertensive disorders of pregnancy, postpartum depression, poor mother-infant bonding, and anxiety and behavioral problems in children (**Table 43.1**).[14,23,116-119]

Management of General Anxiety Disorder in Pregnancy

In general, treatment of anxiety in pregnancy is the same as that of major depression. Mild to moderate symptoms, which are not significantly impairing, can be treated with psychotherapy as a first-line treatment, while moderate to severe symptoms often require medication in addition to psychotherapy.

Pharmacologic and Nonpharmacologic Treatments

The gold standard pharmacologic treatment for anxiety is antidepressants, frequently at higher doses than those used in depression. Benzodiazepine use, while not contraindicated in pregnancy, should be limited if possible. Medications in this class are best used short term for severe, acute symptoms unresponsive to behavioral interventions. If the benefits of benzodiazepines in pregnancy are assessed as outweighing the risks, shorter acting and less hepatotoxic agents, such as lorazepam, are preferred over long-acting agents to reduce fetal exposure and facilitate fetal clearance.

Postpartum, inability to sleep when the baby is sleeping is a concerning symptom and should be treated aggressively. CBT for insomnia, mindfulness mediation, exercise, and improved sleep hygiene are all evidence-based treatments that can improve sleep quality and duration. If adjunctive medication for insomnia is indicated after an antidepressant has already been initiated, starting with the lowest possible dose with a support person present overnight can protect sleep while also reducing concerns of maternal sedation. If using a sedating medication in the postpartum, patients should be additionally counseled about relevant behavioral safety hazards such as co-sleeping and driving. Benzodiazepines are excreted in low levels in breast milk and not typically associated with major adverse effects in infants; they should not be considered contraindicated in breastfeeding.[121]

Panic Attacks and Panic Disorder
Epidemiology, Risk Factors, and Clinical Presentation

Panic attacks are characterized as sudden-onset (often without an identifiable trigger, and sometimes during sleep) experiences of intense anxiety or a feeling of impending doom lasting 5 to 10 minutes at their peak and accompanied by symptoms of autonomic arousal including shortness of breath, nausea, sweating, racing heartbeat, dizziness, tunnel vision, numbness, chest pain, and feelings of unreality. Panic disorder is diagnosed when a patient becomes preoccupied with worry about when the next panic attack is going to occur and develops avoidance or other behavioral changes such as reducing social activities in response to these concerns.

Management of Panic Attacks and Panic Disorders in Pregnancy

First-line treatment for isolated panic attacks and panic disorder in pregnancy is CBT, which may include exposure therapy when triggers are able to be identified.[118] Exposure therapy relies on habituation effects, reinforcing for patients that they are safe in the present despite their anxieties. Despite temporarily increasing distress during exposure periods, it is considered a safe intervention to administer in pregnancy. Panic attacks and panic disorder are often comorbid with depression and anxiety disorders; when these are present, appropriate treatments for major depression or generalized anxiety should also result in improvement of panic symptoms (see above).

Obsessive-Compulsive Disorder

Epidemiology, Risk Factors, and Clinical Presentation

Although the risk of OCD is similar during pregnancy as at other times in a woman's life, postpartum poses a time of higher risk with prevalence rising from about 2% to 9%.[125] Postpartum obsessions are common outside of clinical OCD, affecting half or more of new mothers, and include unwanted intrusive thoughts typically related to harm befalling herself and/or her infant.[126] It is essential to determine whether a woman is having normal brief postpartum obsessive thoughts, versus clinical OCD, in which "egodystonic" obsessions are extremely distressing or cause functional impairments, versus psychotic or "egosyntonic" thoughts of harming herself or her infant. The latter comport with an internal and usually psychotic belief system and represent a psychiatric emergency.

When intrusive thoughts become frequent, severe, distressing, and accompanied by avoidance behaviors or ameliorative rituals that take up significant amounts of time (checking, seeking reassurance, and cleaning are common), clinical OCD is diagnosed. Risk factors are thought to include hormonal shifts, sleep deprivation, comorbid anxiety and depression, obstetrical complications, and somatic disease.[125,128]

Women with intrusive thoughts involving harm to their baby should be screened for symptoms of a psychotic disorder to assess for safety, and partners should be enlisted to provide both collateral information and support if possible. In general, women with psychosis are considered to be at increased risk of harming themselves and/or their baby; safety risk for women with OCD is closer to that of the general population, although it depends on their level of insight. Evaluating for these differences is quite nuanced and, depending on the difficulty of the case, may require input from an experienced mental health practitioner.

Management of OCD in Pregnancy

Patients with severe OCD, or those whose safety risk is unclear, should be referred to psychiatric specialists. The gold standard treatments for OCD are CBT in the form of exposure and response prevention, a form of therapy in which patients are supported to experience their fears while refraining from compensatory rituals, and high-dose SSRIs.

Women who have obsessive-compulsive symptoms that do not rise to the level of OCD should be reassured that intrusive thoughts around fear of harm to the baby are common, especially in women with postpartum depression and anxiety; that women with these thoughts are not necessarily at increased risk of acting on them; and that the treatment for these thoughts is to stop avoiding situations that might trigger them or rituals that reinforce them and to seek treatment of any concomitant mood or anxiety disorder.

Posttraumatic Stress Disorder

Epidemiology and Risk Factors

The prevalence of posttraumatic stress disorder (PTSD) in the perinatal period varies widely depending on the population being described and method of diagnosis used, with numbers being higher in certain sociodemographic groups and higher if based on self-reported symptoms rather than clinical criteria. One recent meta-analysis found a mean prevalence of 3.3% in pregnancy and 4% postpartum among general populations, but this rose to 18.9% in pregnancy and 18.5% postpartum in high-risk samples.[129,130]

PTSD in pregnancy has been associated with negative birth outcomes such as lower birth weight for babies and preterm delivery (when comorbid with major depression) as well as problems in child development such as emotional dysregulation.[131,132] Risk factors for developing PTSD include a history of trauma, having a mood or anxiety disorder, lack of social support, high subjective distress during delivery, and having an obstetrical emergency.[130,133,134]

Clinical Presentation

PTSD is defined by the DSM–5 as significantly impairing symptoms from four different clusters including reexperiencing the event (such as nightmares or flashbacks), hyperarousal (such as increased startle reflex or hypervigilance), avoidant behaviors, and negative changes in one's thinking and mood; they must last longer than 1 month and appear in response to a traumatic experience.[135]

Management of PTSD in Pregnancy

Treatment for acutely impairing symptoms should be managed by a psychiatric specialist and preferably a trauma specialist if available. For patients who are motivated, one of the most effective treatments for PTSD is individualized trauma-focused CBT with some element of exposure. Other non–exposure-based psychotherapies such as IPT are being developed but are currently not widely available. First-line pharmacologic agents for PTSD in pregnancy and breastfeeding are SSRIs. All patients should be counseled to reduce stressors, call on social support, and protect sleep. Comorbid mood, anxiety, or substance use disorders should be treated promptly and aggressively.

Chronic Psychotic Disorders

Epidemiology, Risk Factors, and Clinical Presentation

A wide range of mental illnesses can present with psychotic symptoms including schizophrenia, schizoaffective disorder, bipolar disorder, major depression, and delusional disorder. Some disorders can present with psychotic-like symptoms (eg, OCD with poor or absent insight) and require further evaluation to determine whether the symptoms represent psychotic beliefs versus intrusive thoughts.[136] In general, the prevalence of any psychotic disorder in pregnancy or postpartum is about 1%, with the postpartum period representing a time of increased risk depending on the underlying disorder as described in the illness-specific sections above.[137]

Psychosis is a broad term referring to perceptual disturbances such as hallucinations and/or delusions, which are defined as firmly held internal beliefs that are inconsistent with reality. These symptoms occur as a result of serious mental illness, although medical causes should first be ruled out (see section on Acute Psychosis under Psychiatric Emergencies). Positive symptoms of psychosis, including hallucinations and delusions as described above, but also thought disorganization, suspiciousness, feelings of persecution, or hostility, generally come to attention more readily than the negative symptoms of psychosis, which include blunted affect, impaired abstract thinking, social withdrawal, and lack of spontaneity.

Women with chronic psychotic disorders are more likely to have unplanned pregnancies and inconsistent prenatal care and require higher levels of collaboration among mental health, OB, and pediatric teams.[138,139] They also have higher rates of emergency room visits, psychiatric hospitalizations in pregnancy.[140,141]

Evaluation of new-onset psychosis requires significant medical workup to rule out underlying medical and neurologic illnesses that may present with prominent psychotic symptoms. Etiologies to consider include infection, autoimmune disease, encephalopathy, cerebral hemorrhage, brain tumors, endocrine or metabolic disorders, electrolyte disturbances, or the effects of drugs, either prescribed, over the counter, or illicit. There may be overlap of psychotic symptoms (including visual hallucinations, confusion, and agitation) with delirium as well (see **Table 43.6** and more on delirium under Psychiatric Emergencies below).

Management of Chronic Psychotic Disorders in Pregnancy

Patients with chronic psychotic disorders should be referred to a psychiatrist. For women with chronic psychotic disorders who become pregnant, it is important to anticipate problems that may arise and plan in order to maintain the safety of the patient, infant, and medical staff throughout pregnancy, labor, and delivery; such planning may include medication, as well as behavioral, surgical, social, and legal strategies.[138]

Pharmacologic and Nonpharmacologic Treatment

In general, for those women with psychotic symptoms that are result of an underlying mood disorder, treatment focuses on achieving remission of the depression or bipolar illness. For women with schizophrenia or a psychotic illness unrelated to a mood disorder, first-line treatment is a first- or second-generation antipsychotic (SGA) with preference given to that agent, if any, that has a history of previous efficacy for the individual patient. For women without prior medication trials, quetiapine or olanzapine are among the more studied SGAs in pregnancy with reassuring safety profiles.

Women whose psychotic symptoms are well managed on medications are at high risk for

Table 43.6 Differentiating Psychosis From Delirium in the Perinatal Period

Symptom	Psychotic Disorder	Postpartum Psychosis	Delirium
Unstable vital signs			+
Metabolic derangements			+
Hallucinations	+	+ (Screen for command hallucinations)	+
Paranoia	+	+	+
Waxing and waning level of consciousness		+	+
Waxing and waning psychotic symptoms		+	+
Suicidal thoughts	+	+	+
Homicidal thoughts	+	+	+
Confusion/disorientation		+	+
Agitation	+	+	+

relapse or breakthrough symptoms if medications are discontinued during pregnancy or if there is a failure to adjust dose to account for physiologic changes of pregnancy.[74,138] Therefore, medications are typically continued in pregnancy with dose increases as required based on clinical symptoms.

Eating Disorders

Epidemiology and Risk Factors

Eating disorders often come to clinical attention during pregnancy when weight and eating habits are being closely monitored. The most common eating disorders are anorexia nervosa, with a prevalence among US women of 0.9%; bulimia nervosa, with a prevalence of 1.5%; and binge eating disorder, with a prevalence of 3.5%.[146] All have been associated with adverse child outcomes, including increased risk of miscarriage, preterm delivery, lower birth weight, cesarean delivery, and hyperemesis gravidarum (**Table 43.7**).[148,150,152] After delivery, there is increased risk of slower growth rates, difficult temperament, and eating problems in the infant.[150,153,154] Additionally, eating disorders are often comorbid with other psychiatric illnesses including depression, anxiety, substance abuse, and PTSD, which have also been associated with poor pregnancy outcomes.

Clinical Presentation

Anorexia nervosa has one of the highest mortality rates of any psychiatric illness and is associated with a number of severe medical complications, including but not limited to bradycardia, hypotension, orthostasis, cardiac atrophy, electrolyte abnormalities, amenorrhea/infertility, and osteoporosis.[155-157] It is characterized by restricting food intake to achieve low body weight, intense fear of gaining weight, engaging in behaviors that interfere with weight gain despite being at a low weight, and distorted body image.[135] Anorexia nervosa can further be classified into "restricting type," in which people solely restrict caloric intake, and "binge-purge type," in which they have cycles of bingeing and purging but maintain a low body weight.[135]

Bulimia nervosa is characterized by recurrent episodes (at least one time per week for 3 months) of uncontrollable binge eating with inappropriate compensatory behavior to prevent weight gain. Women with bulimia may be of normal weight, underweight, or overweight. Compensatory behaviors can include self-induced vomiting; misuse of laxatives, diuretics, enemas, or other medications; and excessive exercise.[135] Hypokalemia, if found in an otherwise healthy young woman with normal kidney function, is highly specific for covert bulimia.[158]

Binge eating disorder is characterized by recurrent episodes of binge eating occurring at least once a week for 3 months. Binge eating is defined as eating more rapidly than normal, eating until uncomfortably full, eating large amounts of food when not physically hungry, eating alone due to embarrassment over how much one is eating, and feeling disgusted with oneself afterward.[135] Binge

Table 43.7 Risks of Specific Eating Disorders During Pregnancy

	Anorexia Nervosa	Bulimia Nervosa	Binge Eating Disorder
Hyperemesis gravidarum[147]		+	
Gestational hypertension[148]			+
Gestational diabetes[148,149]		+	+
Preeclampsia[149]			+
Premature birth[148]	+		
Small-for-gestational age[148,149]	+		
Large-for-gestational age[148-150]			+
Intrauterine growth restriction[148]	+		
Low birth weight[148,149]	+		
Higher birth weight[148-150]			+
Induced delivery[149]		+	+
Prolonged labor[148,151]			+
Cesarean delivery[149]	+		+
Resuscitation of the neonate[148]		+	
Low Apgar scores[148]		+	

eating disorder is associated with an increased risk of metabolic syndrome.[39]

Management of Eating Disorders in Pregnancy

Women who have eating disorders should be comanaged with a team of eating disorder specialists in dietetics and mental health. Psychotherapy is standard treatment of eating disorders, while medications are used to treat comorbidities, including depression and anxiety. Strong social support is also important for eating disorder recovery.

The role of the obstetrician should include routinely calculating pre-pregnancy body mass index and screening patients for a current or history of eating disorders, as well as depression and substance abuse. If a patient is identified as at risk for an active eating disorder, they should be referred for treatment. It is important to closely monitor weight and vital signs at prenatal appointments. It is helpful to query the patient about her preferences for weight measurements (eg, allowing the patient to face away from the scale or not informing her of the result unless it requires intervention). It is also important to address body image and attitudes toward weight gain during pregnancy.

Psychiatric Emergencies

Acute psychosis or mania during pregnancy, postpartum psychosis, delirium with or without agitation, acute suicidality, and homicidality in the peripartum period are considered psychiatric emergencies and can be secondary to multiple different underlying illnesses. OB clinicians must be prepared to rapidly identify and competently assess the safety risk of the patient and her child. In these cases, acute assessment primarily focuses on determining whether the perinatal psychiatric disorder is appropriate for outpatient treatment or whether the patient needs referral for emergent management.[159] Such an assessment almost always includes obtaining collateral information from family and other contacts such as other medical and mental health clinicians. As delineated in the Health Insurance Portability and Accountability Act of 1996, in order to optimally manage psychiatric emergencies, clinicians may need to disclose and share information, even without the patient's consent, to minimize risks to a patient's health or safety.[160]

Acute Psychosis and Mania during Pregnancy

Clinical Presentation of Acute Psychosis

A variety of medical or mental illnesses can present with psychotic symptoms; however, these illnesses are only considered to be psychiatric emergencies if there is an acute change from baseline symptoms and if that change confers a safety risk. Relevant factors to consider include the patient's level of insight, the nature of the specific beliefs, the degree to which they affect daily activities and functioning, and the level of concern among support persons who know the patient well.

Management of Acute Psychosis in Pregnancy

Acute psychosis, no matter what the underlying cause, can include agitation, restlessness, and threatening and dangerous behavior. Management of severe agitation in a pregnant woman must emphasize safety and may require emergency medications including neuroleptics and/or benzodiazepines.

Peripartum women with acute and impairing psychotic symptoms will require treatment on an inpatient psychiatric unit, and labor and delivery requires unique coordination among the involved services as well as transfer/admission to nonpsychiatric units.[139] Early psychiatric consultation is critical in successfully managing labor and delivery in a patient with active psychotic symptoms (**Table 43.8**).

Clinical Presentation of Mania

Breakthrough or new-onset manic symptoms with or without psychosis during pregnancy are concerning and should be evaluated further to determine whether they need to be managed on an inpatient or outpatient basis. Mania can escalate quickly, in hours to days, particularly in the peripartum, and therefore must be addressed promptly and aggressively, regardless of treatment setting. Mania consists of an abnormally irritable or elevated mood, accompanied by increased energy, decreased need for sleep (which must be distinguished from difficulty sleeping associated with pregnancy discomfort or other psychiatric illnesses such as anxiety or depression which are associated with low energy), increased goal-directed activities, rapid speech, racing thoughts, and impulsivity.

Management of Mania in Pregnancy

If left unaddressed or undermanaged, symptoms of mania can become dangerous in a variety of ways, including irritability/argumentativeness leading to violence (perpetrated by or against the patient); grandiosity or impulsivity that may contribute to dangerous behaviors, such as walking into traffic or jumping from inappropriate heights; self-neglect, including dressing inappropriately for inclement weather, ignoring food and hydration needs, and failing to attend to medical or OB symptoms or injuries; and physical exhaustion. Safety evaluations for patients with mania must consider the severity of symptoms, level of insight, judgment, level of social support, and the ability of the patient to follow a prescribed treatment plan during active symptoms. If symptoms are determined to be too severe for outpatient management, the patient should be promptly transported to the emergency department. If symptoms are mild enough to be managed on an outpatient basis, the OB clinicians should promptly contact the patient's psychiatrist and coordinate a treatment and safety plan, which must include not only the patient and her medical clinicians but also key support persons in the patient's life.

Postpartum Psychosis

Epidemiology and Risk Factors

Postpartum psychosis is a rare disorder that occurs in 1 to 2 of every 1000 deliveries. After one episode of isolated postpartum psychosis, 30% to 50% of woman will experience a recurrence after another pregnancy, although this relapse risk can be effectively mitigated with appropriate prophylactic treatment.[87] Other risk factors for postpartum psychosis include a personal or family history of bipolar disorder, primiparity, and advanced maternal age; however, most episodes of postpartum psychosis occur in women with no prior history of psychiatric symptoms.[137]

Clinical Presentation

Presentation of postpartum psychosis is distinct from other psychotic disorders that may occur in the postpartum period. Onset is usually abrupt, with marked deterioration from a woman's prior level of functioning, most often within 1 to 2 weeks of delivery. It may include mood disturbances, such as depression, mania, or irritability; anxiety symptoms including obsessive thoughts,

Table 43.8 Basic Principles of Managing Agitation and Acute Psychosis in the Peripartum[139]

- Involve the psychiatric consultation team early.
- Focus on safety (both patient and infant) and determine if inpatient hospitalization is needed.
- Use emergency or acute medications as needed for safety while reducing fetal risk as much as possible (eg, avoiding vlalproate or limiting the number of agents used). Use nonpharmacologic environmental interventions (such as a private room, a support person or sitter, soothing music) when possible.
- Monitor medication dosing across delivery and consider decreasing postpartum if appropriate, due to decreased maternal blood volumes (eg, lithium or lamotrigine, if doses were increased during pregnancy).
- Determine whether substance-induced withdrawal or intoxication is playing a role and develop a plan to manage symptoms.

From Chaudhry SK, Gordon-Elliott JS, Brody BD. The cornell peripartum psychosis management tool: a case series and template. *Psychosomatics.* 2016;57:319-324.

excessive worrying, preoccupations, and intense restlessness; and cognitive disturbances, such as confusion, disorientation, and disorganized speech and thoughts.[159] Psychotic symptoms include hallucinations (visual and auditory are most common, although olfactory, gustatory, and tactile hallucination occur as well) and delusions, the content of which can have a range of potential themes (persecutory, religious, paranoid) and often involve the newborn.[133,137] Cognitive symptoms tend to be prominent in postpartum psychosis and symptoms overall tend to wax and wane over the course of hours, with periods of clear thinking and denial of symptoms. For this reason, women being assessed for postpartum psychosis require multiple serial examinations.[135]

Although rare and often inadequately recorded, there is an increased risk of infanticide with postpartum psychosis, higher during the first 3 months after delivery.[161,162] Suicide remains a leading cause of death for postpartum women.[6,7] In women experiencing severe postpartum psychiatric disorders, the risk is significantly elevated and often involves violent methods (eg, by hanging or jumping).[163] Of note, psychotic symptoms, such as agitation and confusion with impulsivity, can be dangerous and lead to life-threatening situations even without suicidal ideation.

Management of Postpartum Psychosis

If postpartum psychosis is suspected, immediate assessment is required in the appropriate setting, most often an emergency department. Initial assessment includes differentiating postpartum psychosis from delirium and other neurological and medical disorders as well as OCD and other psychiatric disorders (**Table 43.6**). This assessment includes comprehensive laboratory investigations and a complete neurological examination in addition to a thorough psychiatric evaluation.[90] Inpatient hospitalization is usually required in order to safely manage behavior and initiate treatment.

Pharmacologic and Nonpharmacologic Treatment

Medications are usually necessary. Lithium and other mood stabilizers, SGAs, benzodiazepines, and electroconvulsive therapy are useful treatments for postpartum psychosis (**Table 43.5**), with lithium having the best evidence for long-term relapse prevention as well as immediate postpartum prophylaxis.[91] Valproate is not a preferred agent given the risk of unplanned pregnancies going forward.[108,164] Antidepressants should generally be avoided in women with postpartum psychosis.

Short-term prognosis with rapid identification and treatment is generally very good. However, there is a strong association between postpartum psychosis and bipolar disorder, a relapsing and remitting chronic illness, with approximately 80% of women with first-onset psychotic symptoms in the postpartum going on to develop bipolar disorder in the future.[1,3,5] For women who have a history of postpartum psychosis, appropriate medication prophylaxis in subsequent postpartum periods can substantially reduce the risk of relapse, with lithium having the best evidence to date.[91]

Delirium

Clinical Presentation

Delirium in the perinatal period is rare but should always be considered a medical emergency. Differentiating delirium from postpartum psychosis is challenging, but critical in order to guide treatment (**Table 43.6**). Initial presentations of delirium are very similar to postpartum psychosis, including waxing and waning symptoms, varying levels of awareness, cognitive dysfunction (eg, inattention, inability to follow simple commands, or short- or long-term memory impairment), agitation or a hypoactive state, disorientation, and hallucinations of any of the senses.

Clinical Assessment

Laboratory workup and a thorough physical and neurologic examination are required for diagnosis and management. Delirium in the perinatal period, as at any other time, can be a multifactorial condition involving metabolic, infectious, toxic, hypoxic, neurologic, or hematologic causes. Intoxication or withdrawal from substances, such as benzodiazepines and alcohol, can precipitate a life-threatening delirium and typically includes elevations in heart rate, blood pressure, temperature, and seizures.

Pharmacologic and Nonpharmacologic Treatment

Initial treatment is often supportive and requires management of agitation until further treatment can be guided by identification and remediation of the underlying medical or neurologic cause. Agitation during pregnancy and postpartum is often best managed with high-potency antipsychotics (eg, haloperidol), sometimes in combination with benzodiazepines (**Table 43.8**).[159]

Suicidality

Epidemiology and Risk Factors

Suicidality, which includes suicidal thoughts and behaviors, is less common in the perinatal population than in the general population. However, for women with severe psychiatric illness, the risk of suicide is increased 70-fold in the first postpartum year.[165,166] Some studies identify suicide as the leading cause of maternal death up to 1 year postpartum.[7,90,167,168] Although often underreported on death certificates, suicidality is elevated at both 1 month and 12 months postpartum and is a significant contributor to maternal mortality.[29,159] In order to develop a better understanding of late postpartum mortality in the future, it will be crucial to reduce underreporting by including on death certificates a decedent's pregnancy within the prior year.[169]

Other risk factors for suicidality include psychiatric symptoms during pregnancy, prior suicide attempts, a history of psychiatric illness (especially bipolar disorder), abrupt discontinuation of psychiatric medications, sleep disruption, and intimate partner violence (IPV).[159,168] In fact, IPV, a notably modifiable risk factor, is associated with over 50% of suicides around the time of pregnancy.[167,170]

Clinical Presentation and Management in Pregnancy

Thoughts of wanting to die identified in the perinatal period, whether by an answer on a screening tool, a casual comment, or direct response to questioning, warrant immediate further assessment.[29] Many women with suicidal thoughts or plans do not volunteer this information but are likely to respond honestly if asked. Screening tools that can identify suicidality include the EPDS (question 10) or the PHQ-9 (question 9).[159] Further assessment of suicidality, once it is identified, includes direct questioning about intent, plans, and access to means of self-harm. The Columbia Suicide Severity Rating Scale is an important tool that can help assess suicide risk severity and distinguish acute from chronic symptoms, facilitating further clinical decision-making and intervention.

Homicidality

Epidemiology, Risk Factors, and Clinical Presentation

Multiple specific motivators of infanticide have been identified and include altruism, which often involves suicide of the mother as well; acute psychotic beliefs occurring in the setting of severe paranoia or command hallucinations; fatal child maltreatment as a result of cumulative abuse or neglect, which may be a result of psychiatric illness; an unwanted child in which the child is considered a hindrance or burden; and rarely, spousal revenge, in which the child is killed in order to harm the other parent.[162,172]

Management of Homicidality in Pregnancy

Management consists of assessing the risk of a mother acting on homicidal ideation, treating any psychotic or other psychiatric symptoms, and maintaining the safety of the woman, infant, and any others identified as at risk. When homicidal ideation is focused on the newborn or other children in the family, legal and other social services should be engaged.

Similar to suicide, maternal and neonatal death by homicide is associated with the presence of IPV.[167,168] Perinatal homicide and suicide account for more maternal deaths than other OB complications.[168] This aspect of maternal mortality reinforces the importance of screening for IPV throughout the perinatal period and developing a better understanding of its role in pregnancy-associated deaths.

KEY POINTS

- Suicide is a leading cause of preventable maternal mortality in developed nations.
- All pregnant and postpartum women should be screened for depression as part of routine obstetrical care.
- Postpartum is a time of higher risk for new onset or relapse of maternal mental illness.
- The risks of untreated maternal mental illness are significant for both mother and baby.
- The risks of SSRIs in pregnancy are generally low, with PNAS being the most common.
- Clinicians should be prepared to discuss with women the risks of untreated illness versus the risks of medications in pregnancy and while breastfeeding.
- Women with moderate to severe depression should be offered pharmacotherapy in addition to psychotherapy in pregnancy and while breastfeeding.
- Women with more severe illness, including psychotic symptoms or bipolar illness, are at higher risk of suicide and relapse during pregnancy and are generally recommended to remain on their medications or to initiate medications in pregnancy if symptomatic.
- Valproate should not be prescribed to women of childbearing age unless there is a strong justification and no available alternatives.

- If psychiatric medications are stopped during pregnancy, the risk of illness relapse is high and may result in more medications or higher doses being required to achieve stability.
- If women are on psychiatric medications in pregnancy, they may require dosage increases as early as the first trimester to counteract the physiologic changes of pregnancy that tend to result in lower drug blood levels.
- Eating disorders in pregnancy are associated with risks for the mother and child and should be screened for with appropriate referral to specialists.
- Postpartum psychosis is a rare but life-threatening medical emergency and requires immediate evaluation, typically in an emergency room.
- Postpartum psychosis may present with features similar to delirium or other psychotic illnesses, which should be investigated and ruled out.
- Pregnant women with acute mental illness may require emergency medications to maintain their safety and that of their baby.
- Benzodiazepines and high-potency antipsychotics, either first or second generation, can be used to manage acute agitation in pregnancy and postpartum.
- Pregnant and postpartum women are at higher risk of IPV and of being the victim of homicide.

REFERENCES

(only references cited in synoptic print chapter; for a complete reference list, see ebook)

1. Viguera AC, Tondo L, Koukopoulos AE, et al. Episodes of mood disorders in 2,252 pregnancies and postpartum periods. *Am J Psychiatry.* 2011;168:1179-1185.
3. Meltzer-Brody S, Howard LM, Bergink V, et al. Postpartum psychiatric disorders. *Nat Rev Dis Prim.* 2018;4:1-18.
5. Gaynes BN, Gavin N, Meltzer-Brody S, et al. Perinatal depression: prevalence, screening accuracy, and screening outcomes. *Evid Rep Technol Assess (Summ).* 2005;119:1-8.
6. Oates M. Suicide: the leading cause of maternal death. *Br J Psychiatry.* 2003;183:279-281.
7. Building U.S. Capacity to Review and Prevent Maternal Deaths. *Report From Nine Maternal Mortality Review Committees.* 2018. Accessed November 15, 2019. http://reviewtoaction.org/Report_from_Nine_MMRCs

11. Curry SJ, Krist AH, Owens DK, et al. Interventions to prevent perinatal depression. *J Am Med Assoc.* 2019;321:580.

12. Earls MF, Yogman MW, Mattson G, et al. Incorporating recognition and management of perinatal depression into pediatric practice. *Pediatrics.* 2019;143:e20183259.

13. ACOG Committee Opinion No. 757: Screening for perinatal depression. *Obstet Gynecol.* 2018;132:e208-e212.

14. Kendig S, Keats JP, Hoffman MC, et al. Consensus bundle on maternal mental health. *Obstet Gynecol.* 2017;129:422-430.

19. Food and Drug Administration, HHS. Content and format of labeling for human prescription drug and biological products; requirements for pregnancy and lactation labeling. Final rule. *Fed Regist.* 2014;79:72063-72103.

20. Kim HG, Mandell M, Crandall C, et al. Antenatal psychiatric illness and adequacy of prenatal care in an ethnically diverse inner-city obstetric population. *Arch Womens Ment Health.* 2006;9:103-107.

21. Jarde A, Morais M, Kingston D, et al. Neonatal outcomes in women with untreated antenatal depression compared with women without depression. *JAMA Psychiatry.* 2016;73:826-837.

22. Malm H, Sourander A, Gissler M, et al. Pregnancy complications following prenatal exposure to SSRIs or maternal psychiatric disorders: results from population-based National Register Data. *Am J Psychiatry.* 2015;172:1224-1232.

23. Kurki T, Hiilesmaa V, Raitasalo R, et al. Depression and anxiety in early pregnancy and risk for preeclampsia. *Obstet Gynecol.* 2000;95:487-490.

24. Gentile S. Untreated depression during pregnancy: short- and long-term effects in offspring. A systematic review. *Neuroscience.* 2017;342:154-166.

25. Latendresse G, Wong B, Dyer J, et al. Duration of maternal stress and depression: predictors of newborn admission to neonatal intensive care unit and postpartum depression. *Nurs Res.* 2015;64:331-341.

26. Stein A, Pearson RM, Goodman SH, et al. Effects of perinatal mental disorders on the fetus and child. *Lancet.* 2014;384:1800-1819. doi:10.1016/S0140-6736(14)61277-0

27. Straub H, Adams M, Kim JJ, et al. Antenatal depressive symptoms increase the likelihood of preterm birth. *Am J Obstet Gynecol.* 2012;207:329.e1-329.e4.

28. Zuckerman B, Amaro H, Bauchner H, et al. Depressive symptoms during pregnancy: relationship to poor health behaviors. *Am J Obstet Gynecol.* 1989;160:1107-1111.

29. Wisner KL, Sit DKY, McShea MC, et al. Onset timing, thoughts of self-harm, and diagnoses in postpartum women with screen-positive depression findings. *JAMA Psychiatry.* 2013;70:490.

30. Nulman I, Koren G, Rovet J, et al. Neurodevelopment of children following prenatal exposure to venlafaxine, selective serotonin reuptake inhibitors, or untreated maternal depression. *Am J Psychiatry.* 2012;169:1165-1174.

31. Center on the Developing Child at Harvard University. *Maternal Depression Can Undermine the Development of Young Children.* Working Paper No. 8. 2009. Accessed November 15, 2019. www.developingchild.harvard.edu

32. Grace SL, Evindar A, Stewart DE. The effect of postpartum depression on child cognitive development and behavior: a review and critical analysis of the literature. *Arch Womens Ment Health.* 2003;6:263-274.

33. Badovinac S, Martin J, Guérin-Marion C, et al. Associations between mother-preschooler attachment and maternal depression symptoms: a systematic review and meta-analysis. *PLoS One.* 2018;13:e0204374.

37. Salisbury AL, O'Grady KE, Battle CL, et al. The roles of maternal depression, serotonin reuptake inhibitor treatment, and concomitant benzodiazepine use on infant neurobehavioral functioning over the first postnatal month. *Am J Psychiatry.* 2016;173:147-157.

38. Warburton W, Hertzman C, Oberlander TF. A register study of the impact of stopping third trimester selective serotonin reuptake inhibitor exposure on neonatal health. *Acta Psychiatr Scand.* 2010;121:471-479.

39. Mitchell JE. Medical comorbidity and medical complications associated with binge-eating disorder. *Int J Eat Disord.* 2016;49:319-323.

40. Boyle B, Garne E, Loane M, et al. The changing epidemiology of Ebstein's anomaly and its relationship with maternal mental health conditions: a European Registry-based study. *Cardiol Young.* 2017;27:677-685.

41. Petersen I, Evans SJ, Gilbert R, et al. Selective serotonin reuptake inhibitors and congenital heart anomalies. *J Clin Psychiatry.* 2016;77:e36-e42.

43. Messerlian C, Basso O. Cohort studies in the context of obstetric and gynecologic research: a methodologic overview. *Acta Obstet Gynecol Scand.* 2018;97:371-379.

44. Andrade C. Propensity score matching in nonrandomized studies: a concept simply explained using antidepressant treatment during pregnancy as an example. *J Clin Psychiatry.* 2017;78:e162-e165.

45. Easterbrook PJ, Berlin JA, Gopalan R, et al. Publication bias in clinical research. *Lancet.* 1991;337:867-872.

46. Liu T, Nie X, Wu Z, et al. Can statistic adjustment of OR minimize the potential confounding bias for meta-analysis of case-control study? A secondary data analysis. *BMC Med Res Methodol.* 2017;17:179.

47. Flores JM, Avila-Quintero VJ, Bloch MH. Selective serotonin reuptake inhibitor use during pregnancy – Associated with but not causative of autism in offspring. *JAMA Psychiatry.* 2019;76:1225-1227.

48. Hayes RM, Wu P, Shelton RC, et al. Maternal antidepressant use and adverse outcomes: a cohort study of 228,876 pregnancies. *Am J Obstet Gynecol.* 2012;207:49.e1-49.e9.

49. D'Agostino RB. Propensity score methods for bias reduction in the comparison of a treatment to a non-randomized control group. *Stat Med.* 1998;17:2265-2281.

50. Ashley JM, Harper BD, Arms-Chavez CJ, et al. Estimated prevalence of antenatal depression in the US population. *Arch Womens Ment Health.* 2016;19:395-400.

51. Le Strat Y, Dubertret C, Le Foll B. Prevalence and correlates of major depressive episode in pregnant and postpartum women in the United States. *J Affect Disord.* 2011;135:128-138.

52. Lancaster CA, Gold KJ, Flynn HA, et al. Risk factors for depressive symptoms during pregnancy: a systematic review. *Am J Obstet Gynecol.* 2010;202:5-14.

53. Ko JY, Rockhill KM, Tong VT, et al. Trends in postpartum depressive symptoms – 27 states, 2004, 2008, and 2012. *MMWR Morb Mortal Wkly Rep.* 2017;66:153-158.

54. Beck CT. Predictors of postpartum depression: an update. *Nurs Res.* 2001;50:275-285.

55. Rich-Edwards JW, Kleinman K, Abrams A, et al. Sociodemographic predictors of antenatal and postpartum depressive symptoms among women in a medical group practice. *J Epidemiol Community Health.* 2006;60:221-227.

56. Dennis C-L. Psychosocial and psychological interventions for prevention of postnatal depression: systematic review. *Br Med J.* 2005;331:15.

59. Gibson J, McKenzie-McHarg K, Shakespeare J, et al. A systematic review of studies validating the Edinburgh Postnatal Depression Scale in antepartum and postpartum women. *Acta Psychiatr Scand.* 2009;119:350-364.

60. Yonkers KA, Wisner KL, Stewart DE, et al. The management of depression during pregnancy: a report from the American Psychiatric Association and the American College of Obstetricians and Gynecologists. *Obstet Gynecol.* 2009;114:703-713.

64. Oberlander TF, Misri S, Fitzgerald CE, et al. Pharmacologic factors associated with transient neonatal symptoms following prenatal psychotropic medication exposure. *J Clin Psychiatry.* 2004;65:230-237.

65. Steiner M, Cheung A, Eady A, et al. The effect of prenatal antidepressant exposure on neonatal adaptation. *J Clin Psychiatry.* 2013;74:e309-e320.

70. Wang HR, Woo YS, Ahn HS, et al. The validity of the mood disorder questionnaire for screening bipolar disorder: a meta-analysis. *Depress Anxiety.* 2015;32:527-538. doi:10.1002/da.22374

71. Wisner KL, Hanusa BH, Perel JM, et al. Postpartum depression. *J Clin Psychopharmacol.* 2006;26:353-360.

72. Osborne LM, Birndorf CA, Szkodny LE, et al. Returning to tricyclic antidepressants for depression during childbearing: clinical and dosing challenges. *Arch Womens Ment Health.* 2014;17:239-246.

73. Susser LC, Sansone SA, Hermann AD. Selective serotonin reuptake inhibitors for depression in pregnancy. *Am J Obstet Gynecol.* 2016;215:722-730.

74. Sit DK, Perel JM, Helsel JC, et al. Changes in antidepressant metabolism and dosing across pregnancy and early postpartum. *J Clin Psychiatry.* 2008;69:652-658.

75. Cohen LS, Altshuler LL, Harlow BL, et al. Relapse of major depression during pregnancy in women who maintain or discontinue antidepressant treatment. *J Am Med Assoc.* 2006;295:499.

78. Rowland TA, Marwaha S. Epidemiology and risk factors for bipolar disorder. *Ther Adv Psychopharmacol.* 2018;8:251-269.

79. Merikangas KR, Akiskal HS, Angst J, et al. Lifetime and 12-month prevalence of bipolar spectrum disorder in the National Comorbidity Survey replication. *Arch Gen Psychiatry.* 2007;64:543.

80. Liu X, Agerbo E, Li J, et al. Depression and anxiety in the postpartum period and risk of bipolar disorder. *J Clin Psychiatry*. 2017;78:e469-e476.

84. Khan SJ, Fersh ME, Ernst C, et al. Bipolar disorder in pregnancy and postpartum: principles of management. *Curr Psychiatry Rep*. 2016;18:13.

85. Taylor CL, van Ravesteyn LM, van denBerg MPL, et al. The prevalence and correlates of self-harm in pregnant women with psychotic disorder and bipolar disorder. *Arch Womens Ment Health*. 2016;19:909-915.

87. Wesseloo R, Kamperman AM, Munk-Olsen T, et al. Risk of postpartum relapse in bipolar disorder and postpartum psychosis: a systematic review and meta-analysis. *Am J Psychiatry*. 2016;173:117-127.

88. Bergink V, Bouvy PF, Vervoort JSP, et al. Prevention of postpartum psychosis and mania in women at high risk. *Am J Psychiatry*. 2012;169:609-615.

89. Robling SA, Paykel ES, Dunn VJ, et al. Long-term outcome of severe puerperal psychiatric illness: a 23 year follow-up study. *Psychol Med*. 2000;30:1263-1271.

90. Sit D, Rothschild AJ, Wisner KL. A review of postpartum psychosis. *J Womens Health (Larchmt)*. 2006;15:352-368.

91. Bergink V, Rasgon N, Wisner KL. Postpartum psychosis: madness, mania, and melancholia in motherhood. *Am J Psychiatry*. 2016;173:1179-1188.

92. Schöpf J, Rust B. Follow-up and family study of postpartum psychoses. Part III: characteristics of psychoses occurring exclusively in relation to childbirth. *Eur Arch Psychiatry Clin Neurosci*. 1994;244:138-140.

96. Pariente G, Leibson T, Shulman T, et al. Pregnancy outcomes following in utero exposure to lamotrigine: a systematic review and meta-analysis. *CNS Drugs*. 2017;31:439-450.

99. Huybrechts KF, Hernández-Díaz S, Patorno E, et al. Antipsychotic use in pregnancy and the risk for congenital malformations. *JAMA Psychiatry*. 2016;73:938.

102. Munk-Olsen T, Liu X, Viktorin A, et al. Maternal and infant outcomes associated with lithium use in pregnancy: an international collaborative meta-analysis of six cohort studies. *Lancet Psychiatry*. 2018;5:644-652.

103. Hermann A, Gorun A, Benudis A. Lithium use and non-use for pregnant and postpartum women with bipolar disorder. *Curr Psychiatry Rep*. 2019;21:114.

104. Harden CL, Meador KJ, Pennell PB, et al. Practice parameter update: management issues for women with epilepsy – focus on pregnancy (an evidence-based review). Teratogenesis and perinatal outcomes. Report of the Quality Standards Subcommittee and Therapeutics and Technology Assessment Subcommittee of the American Academy of Neurology and American Epilepsy Society. *Neurology*. 2009;73:133-141.

108. Andrade C. Valproate in pregnancy: recent research and regulatory responses. *J Clin Psychiatry*. 2018;79:18f12351.

109. Viguera AC, Newport DJ, Ritchie J, et al. Lithium in breast milk and nursing infants: clinical implications. *Am J Psychiatry*. 2007;164:342-345.

112. Yonkers KA, Wisner KL, Stowe Z, et al. Management of bipolar disorder during pregnancy and the postpartum period. *Am J Psychiatry*. 2004;161:608-620.

113. Goodman JH, Chenausky KL, Freeman MP. Anxiety disorders during pregnancy. *J Clin Psychiatry*. 2014;75:e1153-e1184.

114. Falah-Hassani K, Shiri R, Dennis C-L. Prevalence and risk factors for comorbid postpartum depressive symptomatology and anxiety. *J Affect Disord*. 2016;198:142-147.

115. Farr SL, Dietz PM, O'Hara MW, et al. Postpartum anxiety and comorbid depression in a population-based sample of women. *J Women's Health*. 2014;23:120-128.

116. Glasheen C, Richardson GA, Fabio A. A systematic review of the effects of postnatal maternal anxiety on children. *Arch Womens Ment Health*. 2010;13:61-74. doi:10.1007/s00737-009-0109-y.

117. Witt WP, Litzelman K, Cheng ER, et al. Measuring stress before and during pregnancy: a review of population-based studies of obstetric outcomes. *Matern Child Health J*. 2014;18:52-63.

118. Arch JJ, Dimidjian S, Chessick C. Are exposure-based cognitive behavioral therapies safe during pregnancy? *Arch Womens Ment Health*. 2012;15:445-457.

119. Thombre MK, Talge NM, Holzman C. Association between pre-pregnancy depression/anxiety symptoms and hypertensive disorders of pregnancy. *J Women's Health*. 2015;24:228-236.

121. Kelly LE, Poon S, Madadi P, et al. Neonatal benzodiazepines exposure during breastfeeding. *J Pediatr*. 2012;161:448-451.

125. Zambaldi CF, Cantilino A, Montenegro AC, et al. Postpartum obsessive-compulsive disorder: prevalence and clinical characteristics. *Compr Psychiatry*. 2009;50:503-509.

126. Collardeau F, Corbyn B, Abramowitz J, et al. Maternal unwanted and intrusive thoughts of infant-related harm, obsessive-compulsive disorder and depression in the perinatal period: study protocol. *BMC Psychiatry*. 2019;19:94.

128. Sharma V. Role of sleep deprivation in the causation of postpar/tum obsessive-compulsive disorder. *Med Hypotheses*. 2019;122:58-61.

129. Yildiz PD, Ayers S, Phillips L. The prevalence of posttraumatic stress disorder in pregnancy and after birth: a systematic review and meta-analysis. *J Affect Disord*. 2017;208:634-645.

130. Grekin R, O'Hara MW. Prevalence and risk factors of postpartum posttraumatic stress disorder: a meta-analysis. *Clin Psychol Rev*. 2014;34:389-401.

131. Bosquet Enlow M, Kitts RL, Blood E, et al. Maternal posttraumatic stress symptoms and infant emotional reactivity and emotion regulation. *Infant Behav Dev*. 2011;34:487-503.

132. Yonkers KA, Smith MV, Forray A, et al. Pregnant women with posttraumatic stress disorder and risk of preterm birth. *JAMA Psychiatry*. 2014;71:897-904.

133. Andersen LB, Melvaer LB, Videbech P, et al. Risk factors for developing post-traumatic stress disorder following childbirth: a systematic review. *Acta Obstet Gynecol Scand*. 2012;91:1261-1272. doi:10.1111/j.1600-0412.2012.01476.x

134. Brewin CR, Andrews B, Valentine JD. Meta-analysis of risk factors for posttraumatic stress disorder in trauma-exposed adults. *J Consult Clin Psychol*. 2000;68:748-766.

135. American Psychiatric Association. *Diagnostic and Statistical Manual of Mental Disorders, 5th Edition (DSM 5)*. American Psychiatric Publishing; 2013.

137. Vesga-López O, Blanco C, Keyes K, et al. Psychiatric disorders in pregnant and postpartum women in the United States. *Arch Gen Psychiatry*. 2008;65:805-815.

138. Jones I, Chandra PS, Dazzan P, et al. Bipolar disorder, affective psychosis, and schizophrenia in pregnancy and the post-partum period. *Lancet*. 2014;384:1789-1799.

139. Chaudhry SK, Gordon-Elliott JS, Brody BD. The cornell peripartum psychosis management tool: a case series and template. *Psychosomatics*. 2016;57:319-324.

140. Rochon-Terry G, Gruneir A, Seeman MV, et al. Hospitalizations and emergency department visits for psychiatric illness during and after pregnancy among women with schizophrenia. *J Clin Psychiatry*. 2016;77:541-547.

141. Taylor CL, Broadbent M, Khondoker M, et al. Predictors of severe relapse in pregnant women with psychotic or bipolar disorders. *J Psychiatr Res*. 2018;104:100-107.

146. Hudson JI, Hiripi E, Pope HG, et al. The prevalence and correlates of eating disorders in the national comorbidity survey replication. *Biol Psychiatry*. 2007;61:348-358.

148. Linna MS, Raevuori A, Haukka J, et al. Pregnancy, obstetric, and perinatal health outcomes in eating disorders. *Am J Obstet Gynecol*. 2014;211:392. e1-392.e8.

150. Bulik CM, Von Holle A, Siega-Riz AM, et al. Birth outcomes in women with eating disorders in the Norwegian Mother and Child cohort study (MoBa). *Int J Eat Disord*. 2009;42:9-18.

152. Watson HJ, Torgersen L, Zerwas S, et al. Eating disorders, pregnancy, and the postpartum period: findings from the Norwegian Mother and Child cohort study (MoBa). *Nor Epidemiol*. 2014;24:51-62.

153. Zerwas S, Von Holle A, Torgersen L, et al. Maternal eating disorders and infant temperament: findings from the Norwegian mother and child cohort study. *Int J Eat Disord*. 2012;45:546-555.

154. Reba-Harrelson L, Von Holle A, Hamer RM, et al. Patterns of maternal feeding and child eating associated with eating disorders in the Norwegian Mother and Child cohort Study (MoBa). *Eat Behav*. 2010;11:54-61.

155. Sachs KV, Harnke B, Mehler PS, et al. Cardiovascular complications of anorexia nervosa: a systematic review. *Int J Eat Disord*. 2016;49:238-248.

156. Kimmel MC, Ferguson EH, Zerwas S, et al. Obstetric and gynecologic problems associated with eating disorders. *Int J Eat Disord*. 2016;49:260-275.

157. Misra M, Golden NH, Katzman DK. State of the art systematic review of bone disease in anorexia nervosa. *Int J Eat Disord*. 2016;49:276-292.

158. Mehler PS, Walsh K. Electrolyte and acid-base abnormalities associated with purging behaviors. *Int J Eat Disord*. 2016;49:311-318.

159. Rodriguez-Cabezas L, Clark C. Psychiatric emergencies in pregnancy and postpartum. *Clin Obstet Gynecol*. 2018;61:615-627.

160. Petrik ML, Billera M, Kaplan Y, et al. Balancing patient care and confidentiality:considerationsinobtainingcollateralinformation.*JPsychiatrPract*. 2015;21:220-224.

162. Spinelli MG. Maternal infanticide associated with mental illness: prevention and the promise of saved lives. *Am J Psychiatry*. 2004;161:1548-1557.

163. Oates M. Perinatal psychiatric disorders: a leading cause of maternal morbidity and mortality. *Br Med Bull*. 2003;67:219-229.

165. Healey C, Morriss R, Henshaw C, et al. Self-harm in postpartum depression and referrals to a perinatal mental health team: an audit study. *Arch Womens Ment Health*. 2013;16:237-245.

166. Appleby L, Mortensen PB, Faragher EB. Suicide and other causes of mortality after post-partum psychiatric admission. *Br J Psychiatry*. 1998;173:209-211.

167. Palladino CL, Singh V, Campbell J, et al. Homicide and suicide during the perinatal period: findings from the national violent death reporting system. *Obstet Gynecol*. 2011;118:1056-1063.

168. Alhusen JL, Frohman N, Purcell G. Intimate partner violence and suicidal ideation in pregnant women. *Arch Womens Ment Health*. 2015;18:573.

169. Mangla K, Hoffman MC, Trumpff C, et al. Maternal self-harm deaths: an unrecognized and preventable outcome. *Am J Obstet Gynecol*. 2019;221:295-303.

170. Kiely M, El-Mohandes AAE, El-Khorazaty MN, et al. An integrated intervention to reduce intimate partner violence in pregnancy: a randomized controlled trial. *Obstet Gynecol*. 2010;115:273-283.

172. Hatters Friedman S, Resnick PJ. Child murder by mothers: patterns and prevention. *World Psychiatry*. 2007;6:137-141.

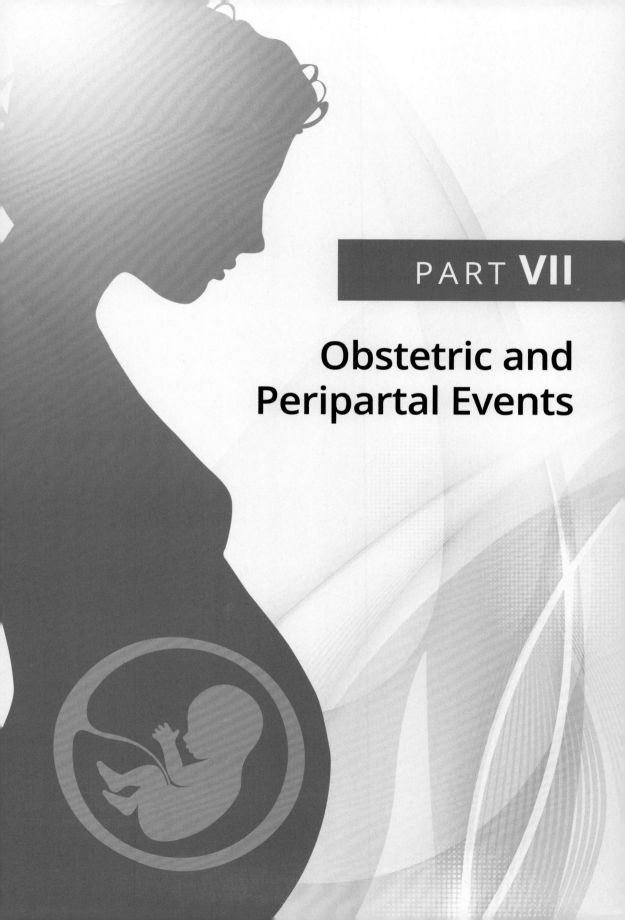

PART **VII**

Obstetric and Peripartal Events

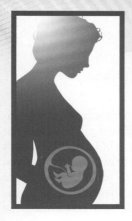

CHAPTER 44

Normal and Abnormal Labor

Anat Shmueli

Normal Cervical Dilation

By convention, full cervical dilation is considered to be 10 cm. Full dilation for most term babies is somewhat less, whereas for exceptionally large babies it may be more. This issue is of particular importance when interpreting the labor curves of very premature fetuses whose head diameter may be considerably less than 10 cm; in these cases, the curve of dilation is necessarily foreshortened.

Active Phase

These deviations in cervical dilation in the active phase can be readily identified if serial observations of cervical dilation and fetal station are plotted on square-ruled graph paper. Observation and calculation of slopes are relatively simple.[1] Paradigms exist in order to use the graphic system without the need for calculations[4-6]; some electronic medical records automate these calculations.

Usually, the cervix retracts symmetrically, but sometimes a segment lingers, particularly anteriorly, in the presence of deflexed attitudes of the head.

Normal Fetal Descent

Considerable fetal descent may sometimes occur during the latent phase. Multiparas often commence labor with the presenting part at a relatively high station, and appreciable descent takes place in the latent phase. Of utmost importance in this regard is that lack of fetal descent before active phase labor is not an evidence of a labor aberration or of fetopelvic disproportion.

Abnormal Labor

Latent Phase Dysfunction

Ignorance about the normal course of the latent phase may lead to unnecessary cesarean delivery under the erroneous assumption that continuous progress should be expected in all phases of labor or that very long labors are always abnormal.

After a dose of morphine sulfate, the patient often sleeps for several hours and awakens in active phase labor. Having had a respite from many hours of painful contractions, she may be more eager and better prepared to cope with the physical and emotional demands of the active phase.

Active Phase Dysfunction

An experienced clinician can accurately evaluate the dynamic as well as the static aspects of fetopelvic fit. In addition to determining the architectural characteristics of the pelvis, this examination should confirm the fetal position and attitude, along with the degree of cranial bone molding and caput succedaneum formation. Use of the Müller-Hillis maneuver (vaginal examination during the peak of a contraction, in advanced cervical dilation, with gentle fundal pressure applied) provides a useful assessment of the degree of descent, rotational tendencies, and attitudinal changes that are likely to occur with subsequent contractions.[23]

For example, if the protraction disorder was provoked by drugs that have the potential to inhibit contractility, oxytocin infusion may override these inhibitory influences and restore normal dilation.

Sometimes arrest disorders resolve without the need for oxytocin or operative intervention. This may occur spontaneously or as the result of an abatement of inhibitory factors. The use of maternal ambulation, warm baths, anxiolytic drugs, or psychoprophylactic techniques has advocates, but the efficacy of these techniques has not been proven.

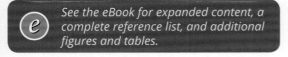

See the eBook for expanded content, a complete reference list, and additional figures and tables.

If oxytocin results in cervical dilation that is at least as rapid as before the arrest, the likelihood of eventual vaginal delivery is high. If dilation resumes at a rate slower than before the arrest, it is likely that disproportion or an insurmountable problem with uterine contractility is present.

Many clinicians believe that rupture of the membranes is effective in terminating arrest disorders, but objective data have failed to verify this.[32] It is, nevertheless, reasonable to rupture membranes when an arrest disorder has been identified. The few patients who respond do so promptly; it is therefore generally inappropriate to wait longer than approximately 60 minutes to determine whether rupture of membranes has been successful in altering the pattern of labor progress.

The Second Stage of Labor

Cephalopelvimetry

The knowledge of pelvic architecture and its relationship to labor should be used as a complementary technique to the analysis of labor curves. This approach makes it possible to explain the observed mechanism of labor and to judge the effects of labor on the fetal skull and helps to make a reasonable and informed judgment concerning the advisability of uterine stimulation or operative intervention.

If these disorders of labor occurred in the presence of a more favorable pelvic structure, spontaneous delivery would be more likely and uterine stimulation would be safer.

KEY POINTS

- A graphic analysis of dilation and descent is required to determine whether labor progress is normal.
- Intrapartum decision-making is a process of continuously reassessing the probability of safe vaginal delivery.
- Factors involved in estimating the feasibility of safe delivery include the pattern of dilation and descent; uterine contractility; fetal size, position, and attitude; and the state of fetal oxygenation.
- The first stage of labor includes the latent phase and the active phase.
- The latent phase extends from labor onset to the beginning of the active phase, which is marked by an increase in the rate of cervical dilation.
- The active phase ends with complete cervical dilation. This signals the start of the second stage of labor, which ends with delivery of the fetus.
- In a normal labor, dilation will be linear through most of the active phase.
- A prolonged latent phase is treated by stimulation with oxytocin or by maternal sedation.
- A protracted active phase is one in which dilation is progressive and linear, but at a rate below normal.

- A protracted descent is one in which active descent is progressive and linear, but at a rate below normal.
- Protraction disorders do not respond to oxytocin except when they have been caused by some inhibitory factor such as anesthesia or infection.
- Cephalopelvic disproportion, second-stage disorders, and shoulder dystocia should be considered in cases of prolonged active phase.
- A failure of descent occurs when no descent is observed from early labor to the onset of the second stage. It is the labor disorder that has the strongest association with cephalopelvic disproportion.
- The normality of dilation and descent cannot be ascertained from the pattern of uterine contractility.
- All protraction and arrest disorders may be associated with cephalopelvic disproportion, malposition, intrauterine infection, excess analgesia or anesthesia, or deficient uterine contractility.
- Most patients with arrest disorders who respond to oxytocin will do so within 3 hours of treatment.

- Artificial rupture of membranes can induce labor; however, it is not certain whether it can reliably enhance an established labor dysfunction.
- Properly administered epidural anesthesia should have little effect on the course of labor except for some lengthening of the second stage.

- It is not appropriate to terminate labor simply because an arbitrary period of time has elapsed in the second stage.
- Upright or squatting postures may enhance descent in some labors.

REFERENCES

(only references cited in synoptic print chapter; for a complete reference list, see ebook)

1. Friedman EA. Graphic analysis of labor. *Am J Obstet Gynecol.* 1954;68:1568.
4. Philpott RH, Castle WM. Cervicographs in the management of labour in primigravidae. II. The action line and treatment of abnormal labour. *J Obstet Gynaecol Br Commonw.* 1972;79:599.
5. Drouin P, Nasah BT, Nkounawa F. The value of the partogramme in the management of labor. *Obstet Gynecol.* 1979;53:741.
6. Kwast BE, Lennox CE, Farley TMM. World Health Organization partograph in management of labour. *Lancet.* 1994;343:1399.
23. Hillis DS. Diagnosis of contracted pelvis. *Ill Med J.* 1938;74:131.
32. Friedman EA, Sachtleben MR. Amniotomy and the course of labor. *Obstet Gynecol.* 1963;22:755.

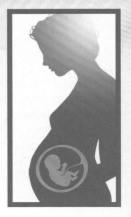

CHAPTER 45

Operative Vaginal Delivery

Eyal Krispin

Introduction

Training

The American College of Obstetricians and Gynecologists (ACOG) concludes that operative vaginal delivery (OVD) remains an important part of modern obstetric care and, under appropriate circumstances, can be used to safely avoid cesarean delivery.[13]

Case Selection and Choice of Instrument

The course of labor, maternal and fetal status, adequacy of anesthesia, exact diagnosis of the position of the fetal head (including attitude, caput, molding, asynclitism, and station of the presenting part), and, of great importance, the maternal pelvic architecture must all be assessed and integrated to arrive at a decision to attempt OVD. It is highly recommended to document this assessment, especially the clinical pelvimetry, in the maternal medical record prior to embarking on the procedure, if time permits.[16] The position of the fetal head should be ascertained at every vaginal examination during the active phase of labor, up to the time of application of an instrument, and just prior to spontaneous delivery of the head. Moreover, clinical pelvimetry should be recorded for the majority of laboring women, but especially for those diagnosed with a labor abnormality or candidates for OVD. An emerging approach includes a sonographic evaluation of the fetal head's progression during the second stage of labor aiming to predict success of vaginal delivery.[17]

(e) See the eBook for expanded content, a complete reference list, and additional tables.

Case selection can be a daunting task. There are 5 to 10 commonly used forceps from which to select (**Figure 45.1**). Vacuum proponents can select from a number of different cup designs, tailored in some cases to the position of the fetal head.

Technique

Forceps

A few points are suggested below to guide the beginner. Some of these points are not available in other sources.

The ART of forceps is an acronym that stands for application, rotation, and traction. Of these, application is the most important, as the inability to apply the forceps effectively sabotages the whole procedure. A decidedly worse circumstance is to place the forceps inaccurately and fail to recognize the error prior to either rotation or traction.

1. For a head that is at 60° left occiput anterior (**Figure 45.2**), as in the case scenario, the posterior, in this case left, blade of the forceps should be applied first. The fingers of the protecting (right) hand should extend beyond the toe of the blade and should assist in maintaining the cephalic curve of the blade in contact with the contour of the fetal skull. Once the blade has been inserted to the appropriate depth, pressure with the index and middle fingers of the right hand on top of the blade should direct it to a position slightly inferior to the posterior (left) lambdoid suture. The anterior (right) blade should be held obliquely, not vertically, with the handle in the right hand extending toward the left groin of the woman. The handle should then be lowered in contact with the woman's left thigh as the thumb of the

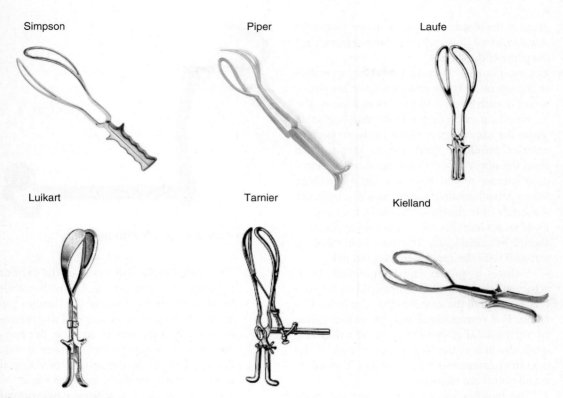

Simpson   Piper   Laufe

Luikart   Tarnier   Kielland

Figure 45.1 Forceps.

left hand advances the heel of the blade into the pelvis. Almost immediately, the right cephalic prominence of the fetal head will be encountered, and this feature of the fetal frontal bone will cause difficulty in rotating the blade into the anterior, right upper quadrant of the pelvis where it needs to be. The secret is to press

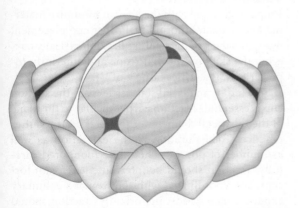

Figure 45.2 Sliding lock, a key feature of Luikart and Kielland forceps.

the handle laterally and inferiorly with the right hand, thereby bringing the blade away from the forehead of the baby. Simultaneously, the index and middle fingers of the left hand positioned under the right blade should lift it into its final position just below the anterior (right) lambdoid suture. Prior to checking the application, asynclitism (if present) should be corrected using a sliding lock, a key feature of Luikart and Kielland forceps.

2. The three standard checks proposed by Dennen presuppose the use of a fenestrated blade in order to check the depth of application.[44] No more than one fingerbreadth should be able to be inserted into the posterior aspect of the fenestra (window) of the blade. This check cannot be performed with either a solid blade or a pseudofenestrated blade. Therefore, gauging depth of insertion requires assessment of the distance between the upper border of the heel of the blade and the bony head. This distance should be <2 cm. The other two checks should be made as recommended by Dennen: the sagittal suture should bisect the

plane of the shanks, and the posterior fontanelle should be one fingerbreadth above (anterior to) the plane of the shanks.

3. Not mentioned by Dennen, but readily accessible to the operator, is the relationship of the upper aspect of each blade to the lambdoid sutures. The lambdoid suture on each side should be palpable above the upper aspect of the blade for occiput anterior positions. Furthermore, the distance from the upper aspect of the blade to the lambdoid sutures should be equal and symmetric. When either lambdoid suture cannot be palpated separately from the top of the blade, the possibility of an undesirable, brow–mastoid application should be considered. Traction should not be initiated until the application is corrected.

Once a proper application has been achieved, checked, and determined to be correct, rotation to the anterior (OA) can be undertaken. For conventional forceps with a pelvic curve, the handles should transcribe a wide arc, while the toes of the blades (out of view of the operator) transcribe a narrow arc. Two additional points are relevant:

1. The handles should not occupy the mid-sagittal plane prior to attempting rotation. Instead they should point to the maternal leg on the same side as the fetal occiput.

2. Rotation of the handles in a wide arc can be accomplished with one hand. The fingers of the other hand should be placed in the lambdoid suture adjacent to the posterior aspect of the anterior lambdoid suture to assist with and monitor the rotation.

Last but not least is traction. Modern forceps have no strain gauge attached to them, and the size and strength of modern operators vary substantially. Force can be wasted against the posterior aspect of the pubic bone, or force may be directed too far posteriorly for too long, thus putting the external anal sphincter at risk of tearing. Two very important points apply to traction on the forceps:

1. Every operator, regardless of experience, should use a Bill axis-traction handle (**Figure 45.3**) on at least a few occasions to gain an appreciation of how descent of the fetal head affects the direction of traction. This principle is illustrated diagrammatically in the 1994 ACOG Technical Bulletin.[20]

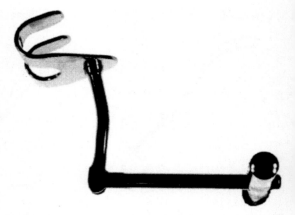

Figure 45.3 Bill axis-traction handle.

2. The control of the delivery once the occiput is under the symphysis is the responsibility of the operator. Raising the handles too high risks vaginal sulcus as well as periurethral lacerations. Failure to raise the handles enough puts the anal sphincter at risk. Forceps add 8% to the volume of the fetal head passing through the introitus. Once the fingers of the dominant hand have secured the chin of the fetus through the maternal soft tissue, the forceps should be removed, ideally in the opposite order to the way they were placed, before completing the delivery of the head. Some reports attribute morbidity to the instrument and neglect the fact that the instrument may not have been used properly to effect delivery.

Vacuum Extraction (VE)

Proper technique with the VE can minimize maternal and neonatal morbidity. Proper cup placement over the vertex of the fetal skull, symmetrically covering the skull both side-to-side and anteriorly-to-posteriorly, is a critical aspect of VE.

Excluding maternal soft tissue from the suction cup is essential. Traction perpendicular to the plane of the biparietal diameter of the fetal head requires practice. Total duration of the extraction as well as number of pop-offs should be monitored carefully. Traction should be intermittent, as with forceps, and coordinated with the woman's voluntary expulsive effort. Most importantly, traction should be associated with visible progress in descent of the fetal head.

Episiotomy

Modern obstetrics does not recommend routine episiotomy prior to OVD.

Maternal and Perinatal Outcomes After Operative Vaginal Delivery

Both forceps and vacuum extractors are acceptable and safe instruments for OVD.[13] It is important to remember that OVD is not a preference but a necessity. **Table 45.3** contains the maternal and neonatal outcomes most commonly cited as morbidity in reports on OVD.

Maternal Morbidity

VE is associated with less maternal trauma than forceps.[25] Third- and fourth-degree lacerations occurred more often with forceps than with VE.

Neonatal Morbidity

Different neonatal adverse outcomes are associated to operative vaginal deliveries. The type and frequency are related to the instrument used. During VE, traction is applied to the fetal scalp, and this may cause scalp laceration or bleeding in different potential spaces in the head (extracranial cephalohematoma and subgaleal) or intracranial hemorrhage. Other reported complications are retinal hemorrhages and brachial plexus injury.[45,47] During forceps deliveries, pressure is put on the fetal face. This may result in facial lacerations, facial nerve palsy, corneal abrasions and external ocular trauma, skull fracture, and intracranial hemorrhage. Subgaleal bleeding is a potentially life-threatening complication in the infant. Subgaleal bleeds involve the subaponeurotic layer of the scalp, can expand in all directions, and can even extend downward into the neck. Intracranial hemorrhage is significantly more prevalent in cases of VE cup pop-offs and reapplication.

A delivery complicated by a use of both instruments is at higher risk for maternal and neonatal adverse outcomes than the sum of each instrument's individual risk.[31,32] Thus, this management should be avoided and a failure of one instrument should prompt decision for cesarean delivery.

Operative Vaginal Delivery Versus Cesarean Delivery

Women who deliver by OVD have increased probability of vaginal delivery compared to those who

Table 45.3 Maternal and Neonatal Morbidity From Operative Vaginal Delivery

Maternal	Neonatal	
Short term	*Short term*	
Deep perineal lacerations (third- and fourth-degree)	Low Apgar score	Skull fracture
Vaginal lacerations	Acidosis	Ocular injury
Cervical lacerations	Facial nerve palsy	Scalp trauma
Urinary retention	Brachial plexus palsy	Jaundice
Vulvovaginal hematomas	Intracranial hemorrhage	Cephalohematoma
Symphyseal separation	Subgaleal hemorrhage	Cervical spine injury
Lumbosacral plexopathies	—	
Long term	*Long term*	
Damage to pelvic floor resulting in	Intellectual handicap	—
Urinary incontinence	Cerebral palsy	—
Fecal incontinence	Other permanent neurologic handicap	—
Pelvic prolapse	—	—
Cystocele	—	—
Rectocele	—	—
Enterocele	—	—

Cesarean delivery is also associated with significant maternal and neonatal morbidity.

undergo cesarean delivery in a prior pregnancy.[49] As the available evidence is limited, no conclusive protocol for OVD or cesarean delivery can be recommended. Training and enabling an experienced staff will allow each case to be discussed meticulously and then evaluated for the chances of OVD success against potential risks to, in real time, determine the preferred mode of delivery.

Prenatal counseling should encompass a thorough discussion regarding the probability and risks related to OVD, specifically in primigravids. An understanding of consequences may reduce anxiety and enable better communication between the patient and her care team should OVD be needed.

Summary

Preserving the performance of indicated OVD and preventing what clearly appears to be a pathway toward extinction is an important task of present and future obstetricians. The graduate obstetrician should ensure that hard-earned skills do not diminish over time; therefore, he or she should continue to perform both indicated and elective procedures and monitor the results. Only through training and practice can we confidently offer our patients an option intermittent between spontaneous vaginal delivery and cesarean delivery, thereby increasing delivery success rates while reducing complications.

KEY POINTS

- The frequency of OVD has declined steadily over the last 40 years.
- It is advisable to write a preoperative note that includes pelvic examination findings before performing operative vaginal delivery.
- One important prerequisite for OVD is an exact knowledge of the fetal position.
- The most important check to confirm proper forceps application is to ascertain that the sagittal suture bisects the plane of the shanks.
- Forceps should be removed prior to delivery of the fetal head.
- The critical principle in vacuum extraction is proper cup placement.
- Neonatal complications are distinct according to instrument used: vacuum is related to extracranial and retinal hemorrhages, and forceps are related to facial and sculp injuries.
- At 5-year follow-up, there were no significant differences in either fecal or urinary incontinence for women delivered by forceps compared with those delivered by vacuum.
- The most important variables in classifying forceps or vacuum deliveries are fetal station and rotation.
- One of the hazards of OVD is damage to the pelvic floor.
- Selective use of episiotomy rather than routine use is advocated for OVE.
- Sequential use of vacuum and forceps should be avoided.

REFERENCES

(only references cited in synoptic print chapter; for a complete reference list, see ebook)

13. ACOG Practice Bulletin No 154: operative vaginal delivery. *Obstet Gynecol.* 2015;126(5):e56-e65.
16. Leung WC, Lam HS, Lam KW, et al. Unexpected reduction in the incidence of birth trauma and birth asphyxia related to instrumental deliveries during the study period: was this the Hawthorne effect? *Br J Obstet Gynaecol.* 2003;110:319-322.
17. Ramphul M, Ooi PV, Burke G, et al. Instrumental delivery and ultrasound: a multicentre randomised controlled trial of ultrasound assessment of the fetal head position versus standard care as an approach to prevent morbidity at instrumental delivery. *Br J Obstet Gynaecol.* 2014;121(8):1029.
20. ACOG Technical Bulletin. Operative Vaginal Delivery. ACOG Technical Bulletin No. 196. *Int J Gynaecol Obstet.* 1994;47(2):179-185.
25. O'Mahony F, Hofmeyr GJ, Menon V. Choice of instruments for assisted vaginal delivery. *Cochrane Database Syst Rev.* 2010;(11):D005455.
31. Gardella G, Taylor M, Benedetti T, et al. The effect of sequential use of vacuum and forceps for assisted vaginal delivery on neonatal and maternal outcomes. *Am J Obstet Gynecol.* 2001;185:896.
32. Demissie K, Rhoads GG, Smulian JC, et al. Operative vaginal delivery and neonatal and infant adverse outcomes: population based retrospective analysis. *Br Med J.* 2004;329:24.

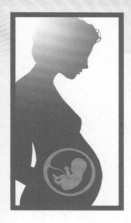

CHAPTER 46

Fetal Malpresentation

Dana R. Canfield and Robert M. Silver

Introduction

In order to discuss malpresentation, a clear understanding of the issue rests in understanding the proper terminology. *Lie* describes the orientation of the fetal spine with respect to the spine of the mother, whereas *presentation* refers to the fetal part overlying the pelvic inlet (**Figure 46.1A and B**). As a fetus grows and matures, the fetal body will generally align itself vertically so that the fetal spine runs parallel to the maternal spine, termed *longitudinal lie*. As this occurs, the fetal head will generally descend into the pelvis as the presenting part, termed *cephalic presentation*. Deviations from longitudinal lie, cephalic presentation, or both are grouped and collectively constitute *malpresentation* or breech.

There are several types of breech. Extension at the hips of one (single) or both (double) legs results in a footling breech (**Figure 46.2**). If the legs are flexed at both the hips and the knees, it is a complete breech (**Figure 46.3**). A frank breech occurs when the fetal legs are flexed at the hips and extended at the knees (**Figure 46.4**). It is important to note that for a fetus to be longitudinal and cephalic at term, several conditions must be met. First, as the delivery date approaches, the fetal head must have the space and mobility to navigate its way into the pelvis. When this has been achieved, it must engage with the pelvis as the spine remains relatively longitudinal, which involves flexion of the neck and a certain degree of immobility. Risk factors can thus be grouped by the role that they play in preventing this process.

Maternal factors that restrict the initial descent of the fetal head include abnormal placentation,

See the eBook for expanded content and a complete reference list.

myomata, Müllerian abnormalities, and syncytium. Fetal factors that inhibit flexion of the neck due to decreasing muscle tone, strength, and activity include aneuploidies, myotonic dystrophy, and skeletal abnormalities. In addition, fetal malformations, such as neck masses or hydrocephalus with macrocephaly, are associated with malpresentation. Lastly, prematurity, increasing maternal parity, and polyhydramnios increase fetal mobility by increasing the volume of amniotic fluid relative to the size of the fetus, preventing sustained engagement.

SINGLETON PREGNANCY MALPRESENTATIONS

Breech Presentation

Breech presentation is the most common type of malpresentation. The main risks of vaginal breech delivery include occlusion of the umbilical cord, delivery of the body with entrapment of the fetal head (possibly leading to brain injury or death), and trauma to fetal limbs.

A 2015 Cochrane review comparing planned cesarean with planned vaginal delivery echoed the Term Breech Trial findings by showing a reduced risk of perinatal or neonatal death (relative risk [RR] 0.29%, 95% [confidence interval] CI 0.10-0.86 for three studies including 2396 participants).[6] A meta-analysis further supported the findings, showing a twofold to fivefold higher risk of perinatal mortality and morbidity in planned vaginal delivery compared to planned cesarean delivery, with absolute risks of perinatal mortality of 0.3%, fetal neurologic morbidity of 0.7%, birth trauma of 2.4%, 5-minute Apgar scores of <7 of 2.4%, and neonatal asphyxia of 3.3 % in planned vaginal delivery groups (27 articles, 258,953 participants).[7]

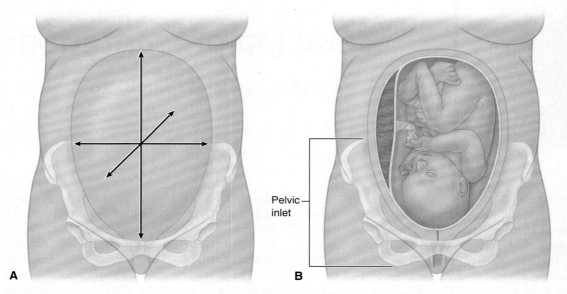

Figure 46.1 A, *Lie* refers to the orientation of the fetus with respect to the mother. **B,** *Presentation* refers to the part of the fetus coming through the pelvic inlet.

The American College of Obstetricians and Gynecologists (ACOG) released a committee opinion in 2006 recommending a case-by-case evaluation of the safety of vaginal singleton breech delivery.[8] There was an interim update to this committee opinion in 2015 which reiterated that planned vaginal delivery of a term singleton breech

Complete Breech

Figure 46.2 A fetus in footling breech presentation.

fetus may be reasonable under hospital-specific guidelines and that the decision about delivery should consider patient wishes and the experience of the healthcare clinician.

External Cephalic Version

In situations where a vaginal delivery is desired, external cephalic version (ECV) is an evidence-based, low-risk method of converting a fetus in a breech to a cephalic presentation.

Candidate Selection and Preparation for ECV

ECV does have some relative and absolute contraindications. Among the most widely cited are oligohydramnios, fetal growth restriction, abnormal fetal heart rate tracings, uterine anomaly, ruptured membranes, hypertension of pregnancy, and antepartum bleeding.

Although rare, and despite a lack of evidence, extreme caution should be used in offering ECV to women with a history of abruption and preeclampsia with severe features and should be avoided when abruption is clinically suspected. Similarly, severe fetal growth restriction or known fetal compromise should be considered absolute contraindications.[12]

In predicting the success of an ECV, there are several factors, both modifiable and nonmodifiable, that are considered favorable. Those that are

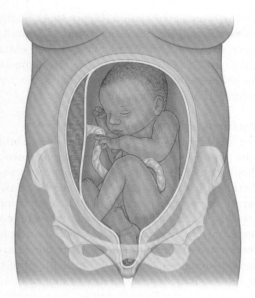

Footling Breech

Figure 46.3 A fetus in complete breech presentation.

static include multiparity, palpable fetal head, and maternal weight <65 kg,[13] as well as posterior placenta, decreased amniotic fluid volume, and a high presenting part. Neuraxial anesthesia has been proposed as a method for enhancing probability of success for ECV.

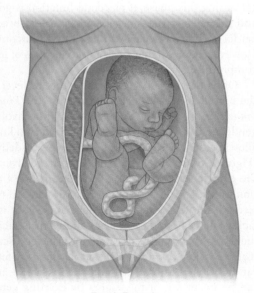

Frank Breech

Figure 46.4 A fetus in frank breech presentation.

Counseling patients about risks is critical. The most common complication is a transient abnormal fetal heart rate pattern. Rare but more serious complications include persistent pathological heart rate pattern (0.37%), placental abruption (0.12%), and vaginal bleeding (0.47%).[19]

Rate of operative delivery may be higher after ECV.[20-22] Differences in fetal heart rate patterns, lower fetoplacental ratio, and smaller head circumference may contribute to signs of "fetal distress" that prompt clinicians to intervene earlier,[20-22] while increased risk of nonengagement and asyncliticism of fetal head may also prompt operative intervention and are positive predictive factors of success in ECV.[20]

Performing ECV

Performing ECV involves exerting external pressure on the fetus through the maternal abdomen to manipulate the fetus into cephalic presentation. This generally involves applying a cephalad force to the pelvis to elevate the breeched fetus from the pelvis while the head is rotated in the direction of a forward roll (**Figure 46.5**). These forces and motions should be applied in a coordinated fashion. The procedure is typically performed by one individual, although it may be accomplished by two working together.

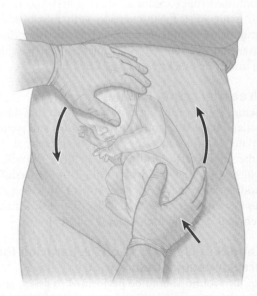

Figure 46.5 External cephalic version. As the breech is elevated from the pelvis, pressure is applied to the head in a forward roll.

Generally, three attempts at ECV are made before the venture is considered unsuccessful, although judgment is required when deciding to abandon the procedure. Between attempts, an ultrasound can be used to assess the position of the fetal head and monitor heart rate.

Following a successful procedure, induction of labor should not be initiated except in cases when delivery is indicated. This is based on a retrospective cohort study of 483 successful ECV cases demonstrating that rate of cesarean delivery is increased in both primiparous and multiparous women who deliver within 96 hours of ECV (adjusted odds ratio [OR] 2.54).[23] This may relate to a lack of engagement of the fetal head in the immediate post-ECV period.

Complementary and Alternative Methods of Cephalic Version

Moxibustion is a traditional Chinese method using heat created by burning herbal preparations containing *Artemisia vulgaris* to stimulate the acupoint Bladder 67 (located beside the outer corner of the fifth toenail).[24,25] This is thought to stimulate production of prostaglandins, which then stimulate uterine contractility and promote fetal movement. Moxibustion is often combined with postural techniques or acupuncture. Acupuncture has also been used alone but similarly lacks evidence to support its efficacy. Given available evidence, ECV should continue to be recommended as the first-line option for achieving cephalic version with moxibustion, acupuncture, and postural techniques (described elsewhere) designated as complementary therapies of uncertain efficacy.

Breech Vaginal Delivery

Before considering the candidacy of an individual patient, the setting must be deemed safe and appropriate. Two obstetricians should be present at the time of delivery. Ideally, both of these clinicians will be experienced in performing the procedure. Additionally, the ability to perform an emergent cesarean delivery and availability of anesthesia and neonatal resuscitations teams is essential.

Candidate Selection and Preparation for Breech Vaginal Delivery

An ultrasound should be performed to assess fetal growth and position. Estimated weight should be approximately between 1800 and 4000 g and fetal head should be in flexion. The fetus should be in a frank breech presentation (**Figure 46.4**). Footling or incomplete breech is a contraindication given an increased risk of cord prolapse and head entrapment. Additionally, a clinical pelvic examination should be performed to ensure that there is not a pathologic pelvic contraction.[28]

Performing Breech Vaginal Delivery

The delivery should occur in the dorsal lithotomy position with abundant room to maneuver. It should take place in an operating room with anesthesiologist present to administer uterine relaxing agents or if cesarean is required. When performing a vaginal breech delivery, early or aggressive intervention while the fetus delivers should be avoided. Uterine and maternal expulsive efforts alone should be used to deliver the baby up to the level of the umbilicus. There is a lack of data to suggest that an expedited delivery (breech delivery from umbilicus to delivery of head within one contraction) leads to improved neonatal outcomes; a Cochrane review from 2015 found only one study that examined this approach and excluded it based on methodological problems.[29] In contrast, aggressive attempts to rapidly deliver the breeched fetus can increase the risk of a nuchal arm, resulting in head entrapment or fetal trauma. It can be especially difficult to be patient during the maternal expulsive efforts because there is often cord compression and fetal bradycardia. Experience and judgment are critical during this phase; if placental function is good and the fetus is well oxygenated, transient bradycardia is not associated with adverse outcomes. However, cesarean may be required in cases of fetal compromise.

Once the breech is delivered to the level of the umbilicus, the clinician should use the *Pinard maneuver* to deliver the fetal legs. This involves gentle medial-to-lateral pressure on each fetal knee, allowing the knee to bend and the leg to deliver (**Figures 46.6-46.8**). Once the legs are delivered, the clinician can use a towel to place gentle traction on the fetal hips using a slight downward trajectory. The fetal back is maneuvered so that it is facing the ceiling and the fetal abdomen is facing the floor. This should continue until the fetal scapulae are visible (**Figure 46.9**). At that time, the fetus can be rotated to one side and the ipsilateral arm can be swept out of the vagina by exerting gentle pressure on the elbow from medial to lateral. Once the arm is delivered, the fetus is then rotated to the

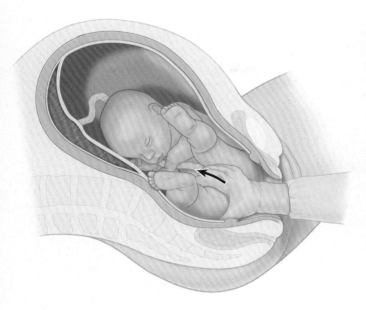

Figure 46.6 External rotation of the posterior thigh to deliver the legs via the Pinard maneuver.

opposite side and the same maneuver is performed to deliver the other arm (**Figure 46.10A**). If there is a nuchal arm, the fetus should be rotated forward (away from the arm) so that the nuchal arm can be reduced. Once both arms are delivered, the clinician should flex the fetal head from below by placing gentle pressure using fingers on the mandible and chin in the *Mauriceau-Smellie-Veit* maneuver. Simultaneously, an assistant can flex the head from

above using the *Naujok* maneuver (**Figure 46.10B**). Flexing the fetal head allows for the minimum diameter required to fit through the cervix and pelvis and facilitates delivery. Alternatively, Piper forceps can be used to deliver the head (**Figure 46.11**). Even when the delivery is uncomplicated, the infant often benefits from brief resuscitation and it is advisable to have appropriate expertise in the delivery room.

Figure 46.7 Sagittal view of external rotation of the anterior thigh, again via the Pinard maneuver.

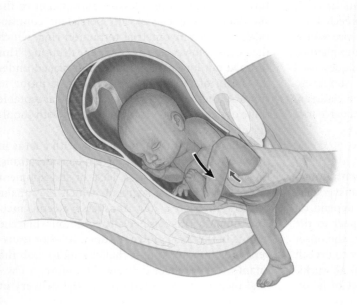

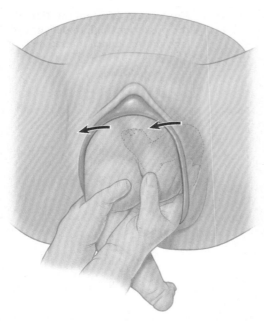

Figure 46.8 Direct view of external rotation of the anterior thigh via the Pinard maneuver.

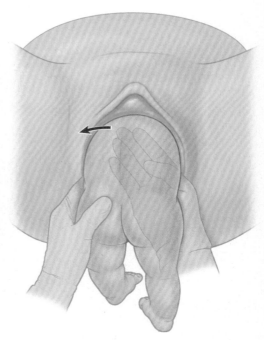

Figure 46.9 Gentle pressure is applied to the fetal sacrum when the body has been delivered to the level of the scapulae.

Clinician Training in Vaginal Breech Delivery

Clinicians have grown increasingly uncomfortable performing breech vaginal deliveries.

Simulations have been posited as a potential solution to this growing deficit of "real-world" experience by providing an opportunity for trainees to achieve a greater level of comfort with the procedure at no increased risk to patients. Clinicians may still benefit from simulated vaginal breech birth training by gaining comfort with the procedure. This may be particularly valuable in an unplanned breech delivery. In addition, the techniques used in breech vaginal delivery are quite similar to those used to deliver a breech infant via cesarean. Cesarean breech delivery is another invaluable tool for learning breech delivery.

Shoulder Presentation

Shoulder presentation is associated with transverse lie. Delivery of a term fetus in transverse lie is not possible, and management will depend on when the diagnosis is made with respect to the onset of labor. If it is discovered before the onset of labor, it can be approached similarly to breech presentation, with ECV offered at 36 to 37 weeks' gestation. When discovered after onset of labor, the patient is at risk for serious complications, including cord prolapse and uterine rupture, because the shoulder will be forced into pelvis with contractions, often forcing the arm through the cervix as the presenting part, which provides an opportunity for cord prolapse. Uterine rupture can occur, as progressive entrapment of the shoulder in the pelvis with persistent contractions creates a myometrial retraction ring, which then causes lower uterine segment thinning. This thinned out lower uterine segment, placed under the strain of repetitive contractions, is prone to rupture. Therefore, cesarean is the only acceptable route of delivery for a laboring patient with shoulder presentation.

When preparing for a cesarean with a fetus in transverse lie, there are important considerations. In some cases, there is a lack of development of the lower uterine segment, which may make delivery through a low transverse uterine incision difficult. This is especially common when the fetus is in the "back down" or dorsoinferior transverse position, making it challenging to grab the infant's feet to effect delivery. Therefore, a classical incision may be required in the delivery of

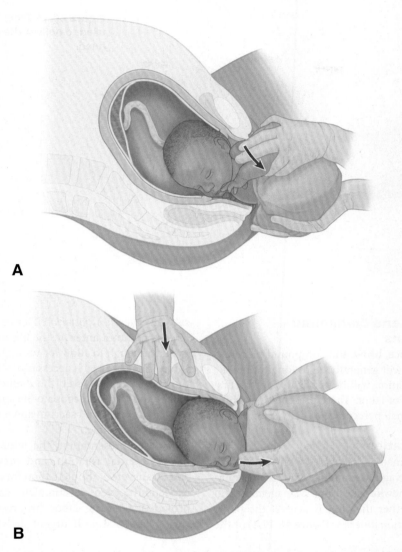

Figure 46.10 **A,** Outward rotations of the fetal arms. **B,** While the Naujok maneuver is applied from above, gentle pressure is applied to the fetal maxilla (Mauriceau-Smellie-Veit maneuver) in order to flex the fetal head.

the transverse fetus, particularly in dorsoinferior position. All patients undergoing cesarean with a transverse fetus should, therefore, be counseled about this possibility and its ramifications for future labor as part of the consent process, and the surgeon should be prepared to make a classical uterine incision.

Depending on clinician comfort, intraabdominal version techniques similar to ECV,[35,36] along with intrauterine version, may be attempted. Intrauterine version involves gently manipulating the fetus within the uterus to bring the breech to the hysterotomy and performing a breech extraction. Alternatively, if the head is more accessible, the vertex can be brought to the incision and a cephalic delivery performed. In addition, administration of an agent to relax the uterus at the time of hysterotomy may facilitate version as well as breech extraction through a low transverse incision.

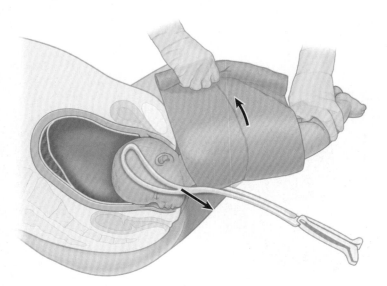

Figure 46.11 Piper forceps can be used to deliver the after-coming head.

Face, Brow, and Compound Presentations

In the case of face, brow, and compound presentations, the fetus will generally be in longitudinal lie and the presentation will be confirmed in the first or second stage of labor. These presentations complicate a very small percentage of deliveries.

Face Presentation

Typically confirmed or discovered with palpation of facial parts on a vaginal examination, face presentation can be somewhat alarming. Management will depend on whether the chin is nearest the pubic symphysis (*mentum anterior*, **Figure 46.12A**) or the sacrum (*mentum posterior*, **Figure 46.12B**). If the fetus is mentum anterior, the diameter of the head is small enough to allow for vaginal delivery. Outlet forceps may be used if necessary. In the case of mentum posterior, however, the diameter of the head will be too large to negotiate the space between the pubic symphysis and sacrum and a vaginal delivery will not be possible.

In face presentation, the fetus remains capable of internal rotation, and mentum posterior and transverse should, therefore, be managed expectantly even at complete cervical dilation provided adequate labor progression and reassuring fetal status. If urgent delivery is required

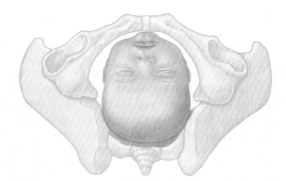

A. Mentum anterior

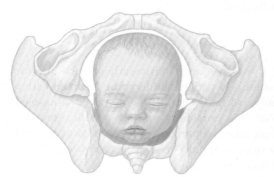

B. Mentum posterior

Figure 46.12 A, Mentum anterior. **B**, Mentum posterior.

and the fetus remains mentum posterior or transverse, a cesarean is necessary as operative vaginal delivery and vaginal manipulation are associated with high perinatal mortality rate and, thus, is contraindicated.

Brow Presentation

In brow presentation, the fetal head is partially dorsiflexed so that the anterior fontanelle is the point of reference. More than 50% of cases will convert to either a face or occiput presentation by extension or flexion of the fetal head, and, therefore, management should be expectant. However, if brow presentation persists throughout labor, vaginal delivery will occur less than one-third of the time.[1] Operative vaginal delivery and vaginal manipulation are discouraged; cesarean is recommended in the event of an arrest in the second stage of labor.

Compound Presentation

Compound presentation occurs when an extremity prolapses alongside the presenting part so that both parts present simultaneously. Complications are rare, as the presenting extremity will generally retract on its own as labor progresses, but labor dystocia and cord prolapse are both possible. In very rare cases of persistent compound presentation, blood flow to the presenting extremity can be compromised, and a case of ischemic necrosis to the presenting forearm requiring amputation has been described.[40] To prevent dystocia, cord prolapse, and limb ischemia, an attempt at reducing the extremity should be made if it prolapses below the fetal head and fails to retract. This can be done by gently pushing the extremity upward as the head is pushed down with fundal pressure.

MULTIFETAL PREGNANCIES

When considering the optimal route of delivery for multiple gestations, there are several factors to consider. These include the lie and presentation of all fetuses, especially the first or presenting fetus, the size and gestational age of the fetuses, type of multiple gestation, and placental location and function. Therefore, accurately determining placentation, fetal presentation, and fetal size by ultrasound at the onset of spontaneous labor or prior to induction is critical in planning delivery of a multiple gestation.

Cephalic/Cephalic Twins

In about 40% of twin pregnancies, both twins are in the cephalic presentation. Vaginal delivery is recommended in these cases.

Cephalic/Noncephalic Twins

In about 32% of twin pregnancies, the presenting twin (twin A) is in the cephalic presentation, while the second twin is breech, transverse, or oblique. Vaginal delivery should be offered to these patients when clinicians are experienced with breech extraction of the trailing twin. For clinicians who do not perform breech extraction, ECV can be performed after delivery of the first twin. Because rates of successful vaginal delivery are higher and complication rates are lower, breech extraction is preferred over ECV when available. If twin B is unengaged or oblique, internal podalic version may be performed on twin B by elevating the fetal vertex via external pressure on the fetal back through the maternal abdomen while internally grasping the fetal foot and rotating to a complete breech presentation.

As with singleton pregnancies, most authorities advise cesarean delivery in the case of noncephalic second twins if the fetuses are less than 2000 g or 32 weeks' gestation.

Breech/Any Position Twins

In the remaining 8% of twin pregnancies, the presenting twin (twin A) is breech. Most experts agree that due to a theoretical risk of "locked twins," cesarean delivery is preferred in cases when twin A is breech.

Triplets

Several small case series suggest that vaginal delivery is a reasonable option for carefully selected cases of triplet gestation. Considerations include cephalic presentation of twin A, >32 weeks' gestation, and estimated weights of >1800 g in all fetuses. Adequate counseling of selected patients remains essential as rare adverse events are possible. More data are needed to fully ascertain the pros, cons, and absolute risks of vaginal delivery of triplets.

KEY POINTS

- Fetal malpresentations are common and often result in cesarean delivery.
- Many cases can result in safe vaginal delivery. This is an important option for women who highly value the option of a trial of labor.
- Increased vaginal delivery of fetuses in noncephalic presentations can impact the overall rate of cesarean delivery. Most obstetric clinicians can learn to safely and effectively perform ECV of breech.
- There is little, if any, downside to trying ECV in most cases.
- Although vaginal breech delivery and breech extraction of twins have some risk, the absolute chances for serious complications are low.

- Clinician comfort with these procedures can be enhanced with simulation training, and it is important that we train subsequent generations of providers to perform these procedures.
- Given the risks associated with both malpresentation and cesarean delivery, appropriate counseling and shared decision-making remain as essential elements in any decision surrounding mode of delivery. As clinicians, it is our responsibility to facilitate these discussions with families.

REFERENCES

(only references cited in synoptic print chapter; for a complete reference list, see ebook)

1. Stitely ML, Gherman RB. Labor with abnormal presentation and position. *Obstet Gynecol Clin North Am.* 2005;32:165-179.
6. Hofmeyr GJ, Hannah M, Lawrie TA. Planned caesarean section for term breech delivery (Review). *Cochrane Database Syst Rev.* 2015;(7):CD000166.
7. Behran Y, Haileamlak A. The risks of planned vaginal breech delivery versus planned cesarean section for term breech birth: a meta-analysis including observational studies. *Br J Obstet Gynaecol.* 2016;123:49-57.
8. American College of Obstetricians and Gynecologists. ACOG Committee Opinion No. 745: mode of term singleton breech delivery. *Obstet Gynecol.* 2018;132:e60-e63.
12. Rosman AN, Guijt A, Vlemmix F, Rijnders M, Mol BW, Kok M. Contraindications for external cephalic version in breech position at term: a systematic review. *Acta Obstet Gynecol Scand.* 2013;92:137-142.
13. Kok M, Cnossen J, Gravendeel L, van der Post J, Opmeer B, Mol BW. Clinical factors to predict the outcome of external cephalic version: a metaanalysis. *Am J Obstet Gynecol.* 2008;199:630.e1-630.e7.
19. Collaris RJ, Oei SG. External cephalic version: a safe procedure? A systematic review of version-related risks. *Acta Obstet Gynecol Scand.* 2004;83:511-518.
20. de Hundt M, Velzel J, de Groot CJ, Mol BW, Kok M. Mode of delivery after successful external cephalic version: a systematic review and meta-analysis. *Obstet Gynecol.* 2004;104:155-160.
21. Kean LH, Sunwanrath C, Gargari SS, Sahota DS, James DK. A comparison of fetal behavior in breech and cephalic presentations at term. *Br J Obstet Gynaecol.* 2010;30:13-16.

22. Chan LY, Tang JL, Tsoi KF, Fok WY, Chan LW, Lau TK. Intrapartum cesarean delivery after successful external cephalic version: a meta-analysis. *Obstet Gynecol.* 2004;104:155-160.
23. Kabiri D, Elram T, Aboo-Dia M, et al. Timing of delivery after external cephalic version and the risk for cesarean delivery. *Obstet Gynecol.* 2011;118(2 pt 1):209-213.
24. Deadman P, Al-Khafaji M, Baker K. *A Manual of Acupuncture.* Journal of Chinese Medicine Publications; 1998.
25. Unschuld PU, Tessenow H, Jinsheng Z. *Huang Di Nei Jing Su Wen: An Annotated Translation of Huang Di's Inner Classic – Basic Questions.* University of California Press; 2010.
28. Kotaska A, Menticoglou S, Gagnon R, et al. SOGC clinical practice guideline. Vaginal delivery of breech presentation: no. 226, June 2009. *Int J Gynaecol Obstet.* 2009;107:169-176.
29. Hofmeyr GJ, Kulier R, West HM. Expedited versus conservative approaches for vaginal delivery in breech presentation. *Cochrane Database Systemic Rev.* 2015;(7):CD000082.
35. Shoham Z, Blickstein I, Zosmer A, Katz Z, Borenstein R. Transverse uterine incision for cesarean delivery of the transverse-lying fetus. *Eur J Obstet Gynecol Reprod Biol.* 1989;32:67-70.
36. Pelosi MA, Apuzzio J, Fricchione D, Gowda VV. The "intra-abdominal version technique" for delivery of transverse lie by low-segment cesarean section. *Am J Obstet Gynecol.* 1979;135(135):1009-1011.
40. Tebes CC, Mehta P, Calhoun DA, Richards DS. Congenital ischemic forearm necrosis associated with a compound presentation. *J Matern Fetal Med.* 1999;8:231-233.

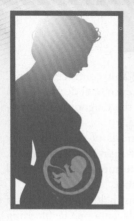

CHAPTER 47

Placental Abruption

Yinka Oyelese, Cande V. Ananth, and Anthony M. Vintzileos

Introduction

Placental abruption is an important cause of bleeding in the second half of pregnancy and is associated with greatly increased risks of stillbirth, neonatal death, preterm delivery, and long-term neurodevelopmental disability.[1-8] In addition, abruption carries increased risks for maternal hemorrhage, hypovolemia, coagulopathy, cesarean delivery, intensive care unit admissions, and even maternal death.[1-8] Emerging data suggest that women with abruption suffer from increased risk of premature death and substantial morbidity from cardiovascular and cerebrovascular complications later in life.[9,10]

Definition

It is important to distinguish abruption from the placental separation that occurs with placenta previa, as the latter condition has a different etiology and pathophysiology. Abruption may involve the entire placenta (total abruption) or just a portion of the placenta (partial abruption).[1] The term is generally used in the second half of pregnancy. If placental separation occurs in the first half of pregnancy, it is referred to as a threatened abortion.

Clinical Significance

The effects of abruption depend primarily on the extent of placental separation, the rapidity at which it separates, and the gestational age at which it occurs.[1,11,12]

Incidence

Several factors may affect the reported incidence of the condition. These include the prevalence of

different risk factors for abruption in the studied populations (see below), as well as the degree of ascertainment of the diagnosis. The observed incidence of abruption has increased for several years in the United States and Canada.[16]

A comparison of abruption rates in seven developed countries (the United States, Canada, Finland, Norway, Sweden, Denmark, and Spain) showed differing rates of abruption, ranging from 3 to 10 per 1000 births.[16] After 2000, abruption rates have declined in most of the studied Western countries, whereas rates in the United States rose until 2000 and since then have plateaued. The temporal trends in risk factors, such as the declining prevalence of smoking, may play an important role in the decreasing incidence of abruption.

Risk Factors

Risk factors for placental abruption include chronic hypertension, preeclampsia, smoking, cocaine use, abdominal trauma, polyhydramnios, oligohydramnios, extremes of maternal age, intrauterine infection, and preterm premature rupture of the membranes.[1,2,18-20]

The strongest risk factor for placental abruption is a history of abruption in a prior pregnancy.[17]

Pathophysiology

The exact etiology of placental abruption is unknown.

There is an increasing body of evidence that abruption is often the end result of long-standing defective placentation (Chapter 6), as it is associated with abnormal trophoblastic invasion and remodeling of the spiral arteries.[25,26] Rupture of maternal decidual vessels leads to dissection of the placental-decidual interface. Pathological findings consistent with abruption include indentation of the maternal surface of the placenta and a retroplacental clot.

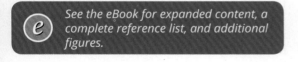

See the eBook for expanded content, a complete reference list, and additional figures.

Other findings may include intravillous or intervillous hemorrhage, hemosiderin deposition, decidual inflammation, and placental infarction.[27,28]

Importantly, whereas the diagnosis of abruption is primarily a clinical one, histopathologic findings consistent with abruption are found in a percentage of normal pregnancies. When placentas of pregnancies in preterm deliveries are examined by a pathologist, there is a higher rate of such findings than in pregnancies delivered at term.[30] These findings support the well-documented association of placental abruption with spontaneous preterm birth.[30] Abruption results in thrombin production from tissue decidual factors, provoking preterm contractions and labor. Furthermore, this may lead to degradation of metalloproteins in the membranes[30,31] and result in preterm premature rupture of the membranes.[32] In fact, at least 20% of spontaneous preterm births are the consequence of placental abruption (Chapter 49).[30]

Trauma and Abruption
Maternal trauma may lead to placental abruption. This is frequently the result of motor vehicle accidents.[34] Shearing forces as well as acceleration-deceleration forces (coup and contrecoup), which occur in a motor vehicle accident, may lead to placental abruption. In some cases, the abruption may be delayed for several hours after the accident.[1] However, trauma may also result from falls, domestic and other assault, and other accidents. Abruption may occur even in the absence of direct abdominal trauma. More rarely, abruption may follow such obstetrical interventions as external cephalic version, amnioreduction, or fetal surgery.

Clinical Presentation
Placental abruption typically presents with vaginal bleeding, abdominal pain, contractions, and fetal distress[1,3,13,35]; however, not all of these symptoms have to be present to make a diagnosis.[1] For example, abruption may present with fetal death alone. In addition, abruption may present acutely, with massive vaginal bleeding, severe abdominal pain and contractions, and fetal distress or even death, but may also present with minimal vaginal spotting, maternal abdominal discomfort, threatened preterm labor, or even backache.[1]

Clinical Assessment
The diagnosis of placental abruption is classically based on a presentation of vaginal bleeding in the second half of pregnancy, often with abdominal pain, uterine tenderness, tetanic contractions, and, frequently, fetal distress, or even fetal death.[1] When all these signs are present, the diagnosis of abruption is fairly straightforward.

Making a prompt diagnosis of abruption may lead to timely institution of appropriate treatment, prevent fetal death or severe morbidity, and avoid major morbidity to the mother.

The differential diagnosis includes other causes of bleeding in pregnancy: placenta previa; bleeding from cervical conditions, such as cervicitis, ectropion, and varices; and preterm labor. An ultrasound examination is useful in distinguishing between abruption and placenta previa.

However, a clot/hematoma arising from an abruption that overlies the internal os may be mistaken for a placenta previa.

When bleeding occurs into the myometrium, the uterus may become hard to palpation, assuming the consistency of wood. This is called a Couvelaire uterus.[1]

Fetal heart rate tracing abnormalities commonly occur in the presence of placental abruption.[1,38] Patterns that may be observed include decreased variability, late decelerations, variable decelerations, fetal tachycardia, fetal bradycardia, and a sinusoidal fetal heart rate pattern. Frequently, low-amplitude, high-frequency uterine contractions are seen on the tocograph. There is often a high basal resting uterine tone.[1]

The diagnosis of placental abruption is primarily clinical.[1]

In cases in which a sudden total abruption occurs, pathology may fail to show any significant findings.

When there is a long-standing abruption, there may be a retroplacental clot, which is useful in the differential diagnosis. In addition, the clot may lead to a depression on the maternal surface of the placenta.[27,28]

Ultrasound in the Diagnosis of Abruption
The ability of ultrasound to detect an abruption depends upon the experience and skill of the sonographer, the knowledge of the sonographer about the differing ultrasound appearances associated with abruption, whether the abruption is revealed or concealed, the amount of placental separation/bleeding, the rapidity with which the abruption occurs, and finally maternal habitus.[1,37,39]

When a sudden abruption occurs, the entire placenta separates, there may not be enough time for the placenta to develop a retroplacental clot, or other ultrasound findings. Furthermore, placental abruption may have a variety of appearances on ultrasound. These include a retroplacental clot, preplacental hematoma, subchorionic hematoma, intraplacental hematoma, and intra-amniotic hematoma.[1,39] (**Figure 47.2**) Abruption may frequently be seen as a thickened heterogeneous placenta that "jiggles" with gentle bouncing motions of the transducer on the maternal abdomen, the so-called "jello" sign.

The Kleihauer-Betke Test

The Kleihauer-Betke (K-B) test is often used to guide dosage of Rh immunoglobulin in Rh-negative women[1] and has been used to evaluate placental abruption.[1,41] This test assesses degree of fetal-maternal hemorrhage by determining the amount of fetal red blood cells transferred into the maternal circulation. However, while the K-B test is negative in the overwhelming majority of cases of placental abruption, it may also be positive in patients without abruption.

For this reason, we recommend that the K-B test not be used in the diagnosis of placental abruption.

Complications of Placental Abruption

Fetal Complications

Placental abruption is associated with increased risks for stillbirth, preterm birth, neonatal death, and both short- and long-term morbidity.[1-3,5,6,12] When greater than 50% of the placenta separates, there is a very good chance for fetal death. Higher perinatal mortality is found at earlier gestational ages. The risk of perinatal mortality across gestational ages in cases of abruption is depicted in **Figure 47.3**.[1]

Abruption is responsible for at least 20% of preterm births.[30,42]

Neonatal Complications

Pregnancies complicated by placental abruption are associated with increased perinatal mortality, morbidity, and long-term adverse outcomes for the baby.

A major contributor to the perinatal mortality associated with abruption is prematurity.[43]

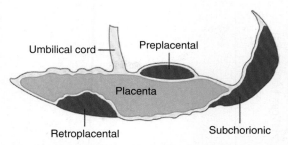

Figure 47.2 Illustration showing the different sites at which ultrasonographic evidence of abruption may be observed. Subchorionic hematomas are thought to rise from marginal abruptions. "Preplacental hemorrhage" describes both subamniotic hematoma and massive subchorial thrombosis.

(Illustration by John Yanson. Adapted from Nyberg DA, Finberg HJ. Placenta, placental membranes, and umbilical cord. In: Nyberg DA, Mahony BS, Pretorius DH, eds. *Diagnostic Ultrasound of Fetal Anomalies.* Year Book Medical Publishers; 1990. Copyright 1990, with permission from Elsevier.)

Lastly, abruption appears to be associated with increased risks of long-term neurodevelopmental deficits; however, this increased risk appears to be mediated primarily by prematurity.[4]

Maternal Complications

Abruption may lead to maternal hemorrhage, hypovolemia, increased risk for cesarean delivery, blood transfusions, hysterectomy, disseminated intravascular coagulopathy (DIC), and death.[1,2,3,5,12,13] Maternal mortality occurs in about 1% of cases of abruption. Abruption may also lead to maternal renal tubular and cortical necrosis, and thus renal failure.[1]

Management of Placental Abruption in Pregnancy

The management of abruption depends on the gestational age, the severity of the abruption, and the maternal and fetal status.[1] Importantly, perinatal death (stillbirth or neonatal death) often occurs in pregnancies in which the fetus is alive at disease presentation when there is inappropriate delay in delivery.[1,12,44] As such, extreme vigilance and prompt decision-making are crucial in cases of overt or suspected abruption. Often urgent cesarean delivery is indicated. However, in carefully selected cases, either expectant management or allowing

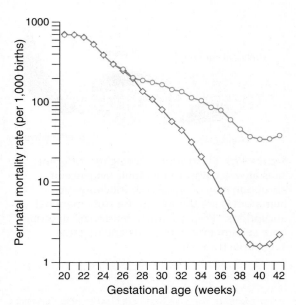

Figure 47.3 Perinatal mortality in pregnancies with and without abruption across gestation, United States, 2000 to 2002 (*N* = 11,635,328). Circles, pregnancies with abruption. Diamonds, pregnancies without abruption.

(From Oyelese Y, Ananth CV. Placental abruption. *Obstet Gynecol.* 2006;108(4):1005-1016.)

a mother to labor may be reasonable courses of action. It is also important to note that small placental abruptions with minimal symptoms, such as small amounts of vaginal bleeding/spotting, are not uncommon. When mild symptoms present at gestational ages remote from term, these pregnancies can often be managed expectantly without increased adverse outcomes (**Algorithm 47.1** and **Table 47.1**).

Abruption needs to be managed on a case-by-case basis.

However, there are some principles that may guide the management of all cases of abruption. These include prompt delivery of the baby when at term or close to term, correction of maternal hypovolemia and coagulopathy, and supportive treatment.[1]

All cases of suspected placental abruption should be admitted to labor and delivery. The anesthesia team should be informed immediately in all cases of suspected abruption, and an operating room should be available for possible urgent cesarean delivery. Intravenous access should be established immediately, preferably with two wide-bore

catheters. Intravenous crystalloid infusion should be commenced immediately in most cases. Maternal hemodynamic status should be monitored closely, with attention to the pulse and blood pressure, blood loss (preferably measured accurately), and urine output. Blood samples should be taken for complete blood count, type and screen, complete metabolic panel, and coagulation studies (fibrinogen concentration, prothrombin time and activated partial thromboplastin time). In addition, continuous fetal monitoring should be commenced. When there is evidence of coagulopathy, blood product replacement should be instituted promptly. A drug screen should be considered if use of illicit drugs such as cocaine is suspected.

In cases of term, early term, or late preterm suspected abruption, delivery is indicated.[45]

When there is any abnormal fetal heart rate tracing in a fetus at a gestational age where survival is expected, in most cases, expeditious cesarean delivery is indicated.[1,5,12,38] Often this will require a general anesthetic because a delay in delivery, such as that required to administer or top-up regional anesthesia, may result in stillbirth or delivery of a baby that is severely compromised. In selected cases in which the cervix is fully dilated, and the fetal head is sufficiently low, a forceps delivery or vacuum delivery may be performed.

In cases in which the fetal heart rate tracing is reassuring, and the patient is making quick progress in labor, without excessive bleeding and in which there is no coagulopathy, aiming at a vaginal delivery is appropriate. However, sudden complete placental separation may occur, and there must be access to immediate cesarean delivery if there is any deterioration in the fetal heart tracing or worsening of maternal condition. Regardless of a decision to allow labor to progress, there must be an extremely low threshold for resorting to cesarean delivery.[1,5,12,38]

When the fetus is dead, the goal should be a vaginal delivery if this can be safely achieved.

Even in cases with a prior cesarean, vaginal delivery is often appropriate.[46] Often, the patient is already contracting, with a tumultuous labor, which often proceeds very rapidly. However, in the face of worsening, severe hemorrhage or coagulopathy, cesarean delivery with contemporaneous replacement of blood and clotting factors is indicated.

It is important to promptly recognize and correct both hypovolemia and coagulopathy.

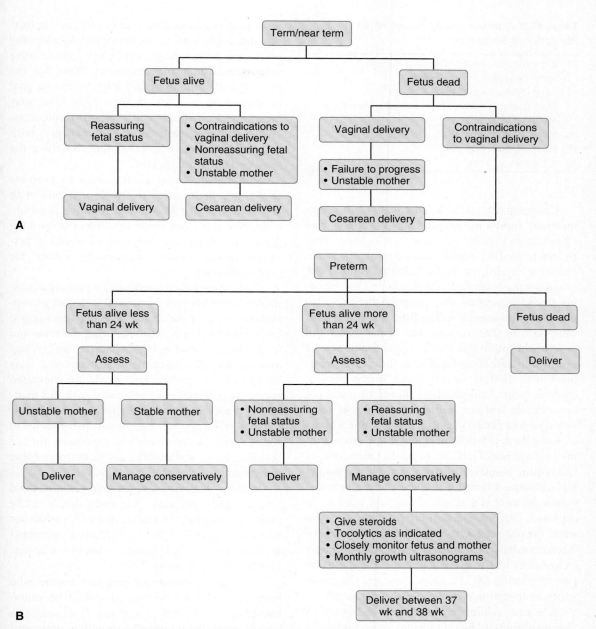

Algorithm 47.1 Algorithm for the management of placental abruption in term or near-term **(A)** and preterm births **(B)**. In all cases, complete blood count and coagulation indices should be checked; blood or blood volume should be replaced; coagulopathy should be corrected; and intake, output, and renal function should be monitored.

(From Oyelese Y, Ananth CV. Placental abruption. *Obstet Gynecol*. 2006;108(4):1005-1016.)

Importantly, abruption may often occur in the presence of preeclampsia or other hypertensive disorders of pregnancy (Chapter 27). Hypovolemia may be masked to some extent by the elevated or apparently normal blood pressure. In addition, in concealed abruption, the amount of blood loss may be significantly underestimated. Prompt replacement of volume is essential to improve tissue perfusion and prevent potentially irreversible ischemic end-organ damage.

Table 47.1 Questions to Be Asked When Abruption Is Suspected

1. Is the mother hemodynamically stable?
2. Is the fetus alive?
3. What is the gestational age?
4. Does the fetus need to be delivered immediately?
5. Are there fetal heart rate abnormalities?
6. Is the patient in labor?
7. What is the cervical status?
8. Is there coagulopathy?

Coagulopathy is a leading cause of severe maternal morbidity in placental abruption and often occurs rapidly.[47] In cases of abruption, often treatment for DIC must be started promptly. When excessive bleeding or delayed clotting is observed, coagulopathy is likely. Besides uncontrolled bleeding from the surgical site, coagulopathy may also present as abnormal bleeding from the nose, gums, venipuncture sites, rectum, and urinary tract. All cases of abruption that result in fetal death must be assumed to have coagulopathy. In these cases, treatment with clotting factors (fresh frozen plasma, cryoprecipitate, and platelets) should be instituted immediately without waiting for results of tests. Blood may be placed in a plain red-top tube with no anticoagulant. If it does not clot within 6 to 8 minutes, a diagnosis of DIC can be made. Often patients will require blood transfusions, and blood product replacement. At most US hospitals, a massive transfusion protocol is a standard and will need to be activated. Platelet transfusions may be necessary when the platelet count is less than 25,000/mm^3 or if cesarean delivery will be performed and the platelet count is less than 50,000/mm^3. An important part of treating DIC includes removing the cause, which in abruption is delivery of the placenta.[47]

Adequate volume replacement is necessary in cases of abruption. Blood pressure, pulse, and urine output should be monitored closely. A Foley catheter will be required in most cases. Urine output should be maintained at a minimum of 30 mL/hr. Cases of severe abruption with coagulopathy or severe blood loss should ideally be managed in the intensive care unit in the immediate postpartum period.

Women who are Rh negative should have a K-B test performed and should receive an appropriate dose of Rh immunoglobulin.

In carefully selected cases of abruption at preterm gestational ages (prior to 34 weeks), if both maternal and fetal conditions are reassuring and stable with no evidence of coagulopathy or severe hemorrhage, expectant conservative management may be considered.[1] This has the potential of prolonging gestation with the goal of delivering a more mature baby who may have improved short- and long-term outcomes. However, these cases must be managed with extreme vigilance, with the ability to deliver the fetus promptly if indicated.[1]

Steroids should be administered to promote fetal lung maturation in stable patients with abruption prior to 34 weeks of gestation in whom a decision has been made to attempt to prolong gestation.[1] Those cases prior to 32 weeks of gestation should receive magnesium sulfate for neuroprotection.

Often these patients will require prolonged hospitalization. However, in carefully selected asymptomatic cases in which the bleeding has stopped for at least 48 hours, with reassuring maternal and fetal status and reassuring fetal heart rate tracings and ultrasounds, outpatient management may be considered. The patient should be counseled regarding potential risks associated with this management approach, should be within a reasonable distance of the hospital, and should be counseled to return immediately should she experience further bleeding, labor, abdominal pain, or decreased fetal movements.

In cases of abruption at preterm gestations that are managed expectantly, pregnancy should not be prolonged beyond 37 weeks, due to the risks for worsening abruption and stillbirth. Amniocentesis to document fetal lung maturity should not be performed prior to delivery.[45]

It is recommended that pregnant women who have been involved in trauma should be monitored for a minimum of 4 hours. If contractions are observed, the monitoring should be prolonged to 24 hours. As such, even after prolonged monitoring, if the patient is discharged, she must be counseled to return immediately if she experiences severe abdominal pain, regular contractions, bleeding, or decreased fetal movements.

Timing of Delivery in Cases Managed Expectantly

When a partial placental abruption occurs, there is a significant risk of complete abruption, which may occur without warning and may be unpredictable.

For this reason, all cases of potential abruption must be taken seriously. When abruption is suspected after 36 weeks, because of the risk of sudden placental separation, delivery is recommended. When abruption is detected earlier, expectant management may be employed, but only if the fetal and maternal status are reassuring. In these cases, the pregnancy should not be allowed to continue beyond 37 weeks.[45]

Tocolysis in the Setting of Abruption

It has been taught in most obstetric textbooks to avoid tocolysis in cases of placental abruption. Abruption often results in painful contractions, which may then lead to further placental separation, with increased bleeding, which then provoke more contractions, a vicious cycle. Tocolysis has the potential to stop contractions, breaking the cycle. Colon and colleagues performed a randomized, double-blinded trial comparing magnesium sulfate tocolysis with intravenous normal saline for the management of non-severe preterm placental abruption.[48] They found no prolongation of pregnancy in the magnesium sulfate tocolysis group.[48] However, in cases of abruption prior to 32 weeks in which immediate delivery is not anticipated, magnesium sulfate should be administered for neuroprotection.

Abruption Found Incidentally on Ultrasound

Placental abruption may be found incidentally on ultrasound of asymptomatic women.[1]

Management should depend on gestational age, the acuteness/severity of the presentation, and fetal status. When abruption is found on ultrasound in extremely preterm gestations, expectant management is often warranted, given the significant risks for perinatal mortality and long-term morbidity in babies delivered preterm. However, these cases must be managed with extreme vigilance, with the ability to deliver the baby promptly should sudden deterioration occur.

Management of Placental Abruption in Subsequent Pregnancies

Several studies have examined the risk of recurrence of abruption in subsequent pregnancies. These studies have consistently found that women with abruptions have a many-fold increased risk for abruption in subsequent pregnancies when compared with women without abruptions.[17,49] In women with a prior abruption, rates of abruption in subsequent pregnancies is approximately 3% to 15%, compared to 0.4% to 1.3% in women without an abruption in their prior pregnancies.[17]

Women with two prior abruptions have recurrence rates of abruption in their third pregnancies as high as 30%.

Unfortunately, apart from avoiding risk factors for abruption such as smoking, cocaine use, and control of hypertension, no other interventions have proven effective in reducing the risk for abruption in subsequent pregnancies.

Because abruption carries risks for fetal and maternal morbidity and has a significant recurrence rate, pregnancies in women with prior histories of abruption should be managed as high-risk pregnancies.

There is a well-established body of evidence that the three conditions that constitute the entity known as ischemic placental disease (abruption, intrauterine growth restriction, and preeclampsia) have similar etiologies rooted in long-standing ischemic processes of the placenta, and that there is significant overlap between all three.[25] As such, women with histories of abruption may be candidates for aspirin for preeclampsia prophylaxis, and for serial growth ultrasounds in subsequent pregnancies. However, neither aspirin nor anticoagulation with heparin has been shown to decrease the risk for abruption in subsequent pregnancies in women with prior abruption.[51,52]

Summary

Placental abruption is a relatively common obstetrical complication that is associated with increased risks of death or morbidity to both the fetus and the mother. A high index of suspicion and prompt management are crucial to achieving favorable outcomes. Unfortunately, despite advances in medical technology, most cases of abruption are not predictable or preventable.

KEY POINTS

- Placental abruption is separation of a normally implanted placenta prior to delivery of the baby.
- Abruption may lead to death or serious morbidity of the fetus or mother.
- Placental abruption complicates approximately 5 to 10 in 1000 births.
- Risk factors for abruption include smoking, hypertension, previous abruption, trauma, polyhydramnios, oligohydramnios, and cocaine use.
- The strongest risk factor for abruption is an abruption in a prior pregnancy.
- Placental abruption may be revealed or concealed.
- Classical symptoms of abruption include bleeding, abdominal pain, fetal distress, and labor. Other symptoms may include backache, abdominal pain, and decreased fetal movements.
- Outcomes of abruption depend on the gestational age, the rapidity with which it occurs, and the amount of placental separation.
- Severe cases of abruption may result in coagulopathy.
- When greater than 50% of the placenta separates, the baby dies in most cases.
- At present, there are no effective methods of predicting placental abruption.

- The diagnosis of placental abruption is clinical.
- The K-B test should not be used in the diagnosis of placental abruption.
- Ultrasound is useful in the diagnosis of abruption. However, this depends on the experience, skill, and knowledge of the sonographer, and the rapidity with which the abruption occurs.
- Major goals of the management of abruption are to deliver a live baby and to correct hypovolemia and coagulopathy in the mother.
- In cases of abruption with abnormal fetal heart rate tracings, at a gestational age at which the fetus expected to survive, the baby should be delivered urgently by cesarean.
- A suspicion of abruption at term or late preterm should lead to delivery.
- When the fetus is dead and the maternal condition is stable, vaginal delivery should be the goal.
- Selected cases of abruption that occur remote from term may be managed expectantly. However, this approach should only be employed if both the maternal and fetal statuses are reassuring.
- Apart from smoking cessation, control of blood pressure, and avoiding drug use, there are no interventions to prevent abruption or its recurrence.

REFERENCES

(only references cited in synoptic print chapter; for a complete reference list, see ebook)

1. Oyelese Y, Ananth CV. Placental abruption. *Obstet Gynecol.* 2006;108:1005-1016.
2. Tikkanen M. Placental abruption: epidemiology, risk factors and consequences. *Acta Obstet Gynecol Scand.* 2011;90:140-149.
3. Downes KL, Grantz KL, Shenassa ED. Maternal, labor, delivery, and perinatal outcomes associated with placental abruption: a systematic review. *Am J Perinatol.* 2017;34:935-957.
4. Ananth CV, Friedman AM, Lavery JA, et al. Neurodevelopmental outcomes in children in relation to placental abruption. *Br J Obstet Gynaecol.* 2017;124:463-472.
5. Kayani SI, Walkinshaw SA, Preston C. Pregnancy outcome in severe placental abruption. *Br J Obstet Gynaecol.* 2003;110:679-683.
6. Downes KL, Shenassa ED, Grantz KL. Neonatal outcomes associated with placental abruption. *Am J Epidemiol.* 2017;186:1319-1328.
7. Pariente G, Wainstock T, Walfisch A, et al. Placental abruption and long-term neurological hospitalisations in the offspring. *Paediatr Perinat Epidemiol.* 2019;33:215-222.
8. Riihimäki O, Metsäranta M, Paavonen J, et al. Placental abruption and child mortality. *Pediatrics.* 2018;142(2):e20173915.

9. DeRoo L, Skjærven R, Wilcox A, et al. Placental abruption and long-term maternal cardiovascular disease mortality: a population-based registry study in Norway and Sweden. *Eur J Epidemiol.* 2016;31:501-511.
10. Ananth CV, Hansen AV, Williams MA, et al. Cardiovascular disease in relation to placental abruption: a population-based cohort study from Denmark. *Paediatr Perinat Epidemiol.* 2017;31:209-218.
11. Nkwabong E, Tiomela Goula G. Placenta abruption surface and perinatal outcome. *J Matern Fetal Neonatal Med.* 2017;30:1456-1459.
12. Onishi K. Tsuda H Fuma K, et al. The impact of the abruption severity and the onset-to-delivery time on the maternal and neonatal outcomes of placental abruption. *J Matern Fetal Neonatal Med.* 2020;33(22):3775-3783.
13. Ananth CV, Lavery JA, Vintzileos AM, et al. Severe placental abruption: clinical definition and associations with maternal complications. *Am J Obstet Gynecol.* 2016;214:272.e1-272.e9.
16. Ananth CV, Keyes KM, Hamilton A, et al. An international contrast of rates of placental abruption: an age-period-cohort analysis. *PLoS One.* 2015;10(5):e0125246.
17. Ruiter L, Ravelli ACJ, de Graaf IM, et al. Incidence and recurrence rate of placental abruption: a longitudinal linked national cohort study in the Netherlands. *Am J Obstet Gynecol.* 2015;213:573.e1-573.e8.
18. Tikkanen M, Nuutila M, Hiilesmaa V, et al. Clinical presentation and risk factors of placental abruption. *Acta Obstet Gynecol Scand.* 2006;85(6):700-705.

19. Ananth CV, Cnattingius S. Influence of maternal smoking on placental abruption in successive pregnancies: a population-based prospective cohort study in Sweden. *Am J Epidemiol.* 2007;166(3):289-295.

20. Shobeiri F, Masoumi SZ, Jenabi E. The association between maternal smoking and placenta abruption: a meta-analysis. *J Matern Fetal Neonatal Med.* 2017;30:1963-1967.

25. Ananth CV. Ischemic placental disease: a unifying concept for preeclampsia, intrauterine growth restriction, and placental abruption. *Semin Perinatol.* 2014;38:131-132.

26. Ananth CV Oyelese Y Prasad V, et al. Evidence of placental abruption as a chronic process: associations with vaginal bleeding early in pregnancy and placental lesions. *Eur J Obstet Gynecol Reprod Biol.* 2006;128:15-21.

27. Chen AL, Goldfarb IT, Scourtas AO, et al. The histologic evolution of revealed, acute abruptions. *Hum Pathol.* 2017;67:187-197.

28. Elsasser DA, Ananth CV, Prasad V, et al. New Jersey-Placental Abruption Study Investigators. Diagnosis of placental abruption: relationship between clinical and histopathological findings. *Eur J Obstet Gynecol Reprod Biol.* 2010;148(2):125-130.

30. Han CS, Schatz F, Lockwood CJ. Abruption-associated prematurity. *Clin Perinatol.* 2011;38:407-421.

31. Ananth CV, Getahun D, Peltier MR, et al. Placental abruption in term and preterm gestations: evidence for heterogeneity in clinical pathways. *Obstet Gynecol.* 2006;107:785-792.

32. Ananth CV, Oyelese Y, Srinivas N, et al. Preterm premature rupture of membranes, intrauterine infection, and oligohydramnios: risk factors for placental abruption. *Obstet Gynecol.* 2004;104:71-77.

34. Reis PM, Sander CM, Pearlman MD. Abruptio placentae after auto accidents. A case-control study. *J Reprod Med.* 2000;45(1):6-10.

35. Kasai M. Aoki S. Ogawa M, et al. Prediction of perinatal outcomes based on primary symptoms in women with placental abruption. *J Obstet Gynaecol Res.* 2015;41:850-856.

37. Shinde GR, Vaswani BP, Patange RP, et al. Diagnostic performance of ultrasonography for detection of abruption and its clinical correlation and maternal and foetal outcome. *J Clin Diagn Res.* 2016;10(8):QC04-QC07.

38. Matsuda Y, Ogawa M, Konno J, et al. Prediction of fetal acidemia in placental abruption. *BMC Pregnancy Childbirth.* 2013;13:156.

39. Fadl SA, Linnau KF, Dighe MK. Placental abruption and hemorrhage-review of imaging appearance. *Emerg Radiol.* 2019;26:87-97.

41. Atkinson AL, Santolaya-Forgas J, Matta P, et al. The sensitivity of the Kleihauer-Betke test for placental abruption. *J Obstet Gynaecol.* 2015;35:139-141.

42. Ananth CV, Vintzileos AM. Maternal-fetal conditions necessitating a medical intervention resulting in preterm birth. *Am J Obstet Gynecol.* 2006;195:1557-1563.

43. Ananth CV, VanderWeele TJ. Placental abruption and perinatal mortality with preterm delivery as a mediator: disentangling direct and indirect effects. *Am J Epidemiol.* 2011;174:99-108.

44. Atkinson AL, Santolaya-Forgas J, Blitzer DN, et al. Risk factors for perinatal mortality in patients admitted to the hospital with the diagnosis of placental abruption. *J Matern Fetal Neonatal Med.* 2015;28:594-597.

45. Gyamfi-Bannerman C; Society for Maternal-Fetal Medicine. Society for maternal-fetal medicine (SMFM) consult series #44: management of bleeding in the late preterm period. *Am J Obstet Gynecol.* 2018;218(1):B2-B8.

46. Inoue A, Kondoh E, Suginami K, et al. Vaginal delivery after placental abruption with intrauterine fetal death: a 20-year single-center experience. *J Obstet Gynaecol Res.* 2017;43(4):676-681.

47. Hall DR. Abruptio placentae and disseminated intravascular coagulopathy. *Semin Perinatol.* 2009;33(3):189-195.

48. Colón I, Berletti M, Garabedian MJ, et al. Randomized, double-blinded trial of magnesium sulfate tocolysis versus intravenous normal saline for preterm nonsevere placental abruption. *Am J Perinatol.* 2016;33(7):696-702.

49. Sakikawa M, Adachi T, Nakabayashi Y, et al. Clinical management and outcome of pregnancies complicated by previous abruption. *Hypertens Pregnancy.* 2011;30:457-464.

51. Roberge S, Bujold E, Nicolaides KH. Meta-analysis on the effect of aspirin use for prevention of preeclampsia on placental abruption and antepartum hemorrhage. *Am J Obstet Gynecol.* 2018;218(5):483-489.

52. Skeith L, Rodger M. Anticoagulants to prevent recurrent placenta-mediated pregnancy complications: is it time to put the needles away? *Thromb Res.* 2017;151(suppl 1):S38-S42.

CHAPTER 48

Cervical Insufficiency

Eran Hadar, Yinon Gilboa, and Arnon Wiznitzer

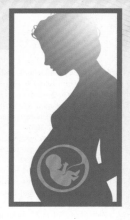

Introduction

Cervical insufficiency is commonly acknowledged as the uterine cervix's inability to retain a second-trimester gestation.[1] Medically, other than midtrimester pregnancy loss, it can also be associated with complications of habitual abortions, extreme preterm birth, chorioamnionitis, and preterm-premature ruptured membranes.

Etiology

The incidence of this phenomenon is approximately 1%.

Cervical weakness is not an all-or-none phenomenon[7,8] but rather a continuum affected by multiple structural and functional pathologies.

During a normal pregnancy, the cervical content changes, with increased water content and less collagen.[9] Equivalent, although preterm, processes occur in the pathologically weak cervix. Incompetent cervices have a higher amount of muscle tissue[10] and a smaller proportion of elastic tissue components.[11]

Congenital or acquired structural or functional abnormalities of the uterine cervix or the uterus itself can all predispose a patient to cervical insufficiency.[15-20]

Obtaining a full and detailed medical history on the presence or absence of risk factors is an important part of the evaluation in women with suspected cervical insufficiency, as it may support the diagnosis in borderline clinical scenarios and contribute to the decision on the appropriate treatment. However, if only risk factors are present and without a definitive diagnosis of cervical insufficiency, there is no indication for treatment, by either cerclage, progesterone, or any other modality.

Clinical Assessment

The diagnosis of cervical insufficiency consists of a clinical-sonographic diagnosis based on one of the following possibilities: history of second-trimester pregnancy loss in previous gestations; sonographic shortening of the cervix in the current pregnancy, with a history of a prior preterm birth; and cervical effacement and dilation detected by physical examination in the current pregnancy.

History-Defined Cervical Insufficiency

The typical presentation of cervical insufficiency will be a history of a previous single or recurrent pregnancy loss of a live fetus (although mostly nonviable at birth) occurring spontaneously during the second trimester, typically between 16 and 24 weeks' gestation.

The classic preceding description will be of an asymptomatic, or at least mildly symptomatic, advanced cervical effacement and dilatation, without additional features of labor such as contractions or bleeding.

Some instances of cervical insufficiency make the diagnosis extremely difficult and challenging.

Excluding confounders—i.e., labor, abruption, and chorioamnionitis—will be impossible.

Ultrasound-Defined Cervical Insufficiency

The diagnosis is based on a combination of obstetrical history and transvaginal ultrasound measurement of cervical length.

Sonographic surveillance of cervical length is advised every 2 to 4 weeks, up until 24 weeks to allow placement of cerclage if shortening is detected, or up until 32 to 34 weeks to administer antenatal corticosteroids, if significant shortening is detected.

e *See the eBook for expanded content, a complete reference list, and additional tables.*

Physical Examination–Defined Cervical Insufficiency

Physical examination defines this subtype alone if advanced cervical dilation and/or effacement is either viewed via speculum or palpated via vaginal examination.

Several anamnestic and contiguous features can be helpful to rule in or rule out the diagnosis of cervical insufficiency.

- Tests for cervical function—If tests for cervical function are performed they should not serve as the diagnostic basis for cervical insufficiency.
- Proactive maneuvers.
- Tocodynamometry—In order to establish the diagnosis of cervical insufficiency, tocodynamometry has to show no contractions, or at least infrequent and irregular contractions.
- Laboratory indices—Laboratory indices are essentially unchanged in cervical insufficiency and are needed to rule out other possible diagnoses.
- *In utero* "sludge"—Ultrasound examinations of cervical length during routine fetal evaluation infrequently reveal not only decreased cervical length but also demonstrate "sludge," which consists of fetal squamous cell, vernix, leukocytes, and bacteria debris.
- Innovative measures—Alternative methods to assess the cervix, such as elastography,[26] and water and collagen content,[27] are currently under investigation but are not yet in clinical use.

Treatment

Cervical insufficiency can be treated with expectant management, supplementary progesterone, and cerclage.

History-Indicated Cerclage

History-indicated or elective cerclage in women with an appropriately determined diagnosis is recommended as an elective procedure carried out in the late first trimester at 12 to 14 weeks' gestation.

Additive Supplemental Progesterone

It is debatable whether administering intramuscular 17-hydroxyprogesterone-caproate (17-OHPC) or vaginal progesterone preparations to women with a history-indicated cerclage is beneficial, as this has not been assessed by randomized clinical trials specifically designed to answer this practice question.

Ultrasound-Indicated Cerclage

Ultrasound-indicated cerclage should be performed in women with prior spontaneous preterm birth and short cervical length in the current pregnancy, measured below 25 mm, usually between 16 and 24 weeks' gestation.

Combination, Cessation, or Alternative Supplemental Progesterone

In women who are already receiving, or at least indicated to receive, supplemental progesterone, usually 17-OHPC, due to prior preterm birth, cerclage is usually added-on to progesterone once the cervix becomes short.

Progesterone Only

Another approach is to initiate vaginal progesterone as the first-line therapy or instead of 17-OHPC, if currently administered, due to a prior preterm birth, forgoing cervical suture. The evidence in favor of the progesterone-only approach is derived from an indirect meta-analysis.[37] However, this is indirect evidence, and higher-quality evidence that supports cerclage as the first-line therapy for ultrasound-defined cervical insufficiency exists.

Physical Examination–Indicated Cerclage

Physical examination–indicated cerclage, also referred to as heroic, rescue, or emergency cerclage, is considered (usually between 16 and 24 weeks' gestation), although not supported by high-quality trials.

Management

Cerclage Contraindications

If the possibility of extending pregnancy is unlikely, then cerclage is contraindicated.

The contraindications to cerclage include (1) severe and major congenital anomalies with a poor postnatal prognosis; (2) high suspicion or proven intrauterine infection; and (3) signs of labor, such as bleeding, contractions, and ruptured membranes.

When advanced dilation or extensively protruding membranes are present, the technical possibility of successfully placing cerclage is low, and the risk of infection is high.

Limits of Gestational Age for Cerclage

There is no clear upper-limit threshold for placing a cerclage in terms of the associated risks and benefits, but the ideal timeframe is often between 24 and 28 weeks' gestation. The 24-week upper limit is the common practice, and cerclage is rarely performed afterward.

Similarly, there is no clear cutoff for the lower-limit gestational age; however, it is well accepted that cerclage is not placed prior to 12 weeks' gestation due to the relatively high rate of spontaneous abortions up to this gestational age.

Pericerclage Procedures
1. Fetal evaluation
2. Amniocentesis
3. Tocolysis and antibiotics
4. Amnioreduction
5. Lifestyle adjustments

Postcerclage Follow-up
It is debatable whether to continue or not to continue cervical length follow-up after placing a cerclage.

Cerclage Complications
The procedure of cerclage is relatively safe, with severe complications being rare, as detailed in **Table 48.2**.[58]

Removal of Cerclage
Cerclage should be removed at near-term or term (ie, 36-38 weeks' gestation). Cerclage should also be removed in cases of preterm labor onset or if suspicions of infection arise.

Therefore, existing evidence suggests that cerclage should be removed following rupture of membranes, as there is no benefit in its retention, but there is the possibility of a higher rate of neonatal infections.

Cerclage Techniques
Several surgical techniques have been described for placing a cervical suture. In the McDonald suture technique, the suture is passed at the height of the cervicovaginal junction, without any tissue dissection.[63] In the Shirodkar suture, the suture is inserted

Table 48.2 Complications of Cerclage

Complication	Incidence
Cervical lacerations at delivery	1%-13%
Cesarean delivery due to labor dystocia, arrested cervical dilatation, and effacement	3%
Infectious morbidity, puerperal pyrexia, sepsis	History-indicated: rare Ultrasound-indicated: 1%-2% Physical examination–indicated: 20%-50%
Premature rupture of membranes	1/138-600

above the cervicovaginal junction by dissection of the bladder and rectum.[64] An abdominal cerclage can be placed by laparotomy, laparoscopy, or robotic assisted surgery. The suture is placed at the junction of the low uterine segment and the cervix. Abdominal cerclage is only indicated for failed prior cerclage.

Summary
The diagnosis of cervical insufficiency should be meticulously made based on anamnesis of prior pregnancy events, current cervical length shortening in women with prior spontaneous preterm birth, and unexpected early advanced cervical effacement and dilatation. The hallmark treatment for all these subtypes is cerclage, mostly by the McDonald technique, with possible combination with progesterone and other adjunctive measures.

KEY POINTS

- Cervical insufficiency is commonly acknowledged as the uterine cervix's inability to retain a second-trimester gestation; mostly a midtrimester pregnancy loss will occur, but habitual abortions, extreme preterm birth, chorioamnionitis, and preterm-premature ruptured membranes may also be the presenting scenario.
- Congenital or acquired structural or functional abnormalities of the uterine cervix or uterus can be predisposing factors. Risk factors include iatrogenic cervical damage, labor-associated cervical trauma, cervical cone procedures, collagen and elastin diseases, *in utero* diethylstilbestrol, prior early preterm birth, Mullerian anomalies, and trachelectomy.

- Cervical insufficiency is a clinical-sonographic diagnosis based on history of second-trimester pregnancy loss, prior preterm birth, and cervical effacement and dilation.
- Cervical insufficiency can be categorized into history-defined, ultrasound-defined, and physical examination–defined.
- Cervical insufficiency can be treated with expectant management, supplementary progesterone, and cerclage, which is also indicated according to history, ultrasound, and physical examination.
- Known cerclage techniques include McDonald cerclage, Shirodkar cerclage, and abdominal cerclage.

REFERENCES

(only references cited in synoptic print chapter; for a complete reference list, see ebook)

1. American College of Obstetricians and Gynecologists. ACOG Practice Bulletin No. 142: cerclage for the management of cervical insufficiency. *Obstet Gynecol.* 2014;123:372-379.

7. Iams JD, Johnson FF, Sonck J, Sachs L, Gebauer C, Samuels P. Cervical competence as a continuum: a study of ultrasonographic cervical length and obstetric performance. *Am J Obstet Gynecol.* 1995;172:1097-1103.

8. Iams JD, Goldenberg RL, Meis PJ, et al. The length of the cervix and the risk of spontaneous premature delivery. National Institute of Child Health and Human Development Maternal Fetal Medicine Unit Network. *N Engl J Med.* 1996;334:567-572.

9. Danforth DN, Veis A, Breen M, et al. The effect of pregnancy and labor on the human cervix. Changes in collagen, glycoproteins, and glycosaminoglycans. *Am J Obstet Gynecol.* 1974;120:641-651.

10. Buckingham JC, Buethe RA, Danforth DN. Collagen-muscle ratio in clinically normal and clinically incompetent cervices. *Am J Obstet Gynecol.* 1965;91:232-237.

11. Sundtoft I, Langhoff-Roos J, Sandager P, Sommer S, Uldbjerg N. Cervical collagen is reduced in non-pregnant women with a history of cervical insufficiency and a short cervix. *Acta Obstet Gynecol Scand.* 2017;96:984-990.

15. Vyas NA, Vink JS, Ghidini A, et al. Risk factors for cervical insufficiency after term delivery. *Am J Obstet Gynecol.* 2006;195:787-791.

16. Althuisius SM, Dekker GA, Hummel P, Bekedam DJ, van Geijn HP. Final results of the Cervical Incompetence Prevention Randomized Cerclage Trial (CIPRACT): therapeutic cerclage with bed rest versus bed rest alone. *Am J Obstet Gynecol.* 2001;185:1106-1112.

17. De Vos M, Nuytinck L, Verellen C, De Paepe A. Preterm premature rupture of membranes in a patient with the hypermobility type of the Ehlers-Danlos syndrome. A case report. *Fetal Diagn Ther.* 1999;14:244-247.

18. Drakeley AJ, Quenby S, Farquharson RG. Mid-trimester loss – appraisal of a screening protocol. *Hum Reprod.* 1998;13:1975-1980.

19. Fischer RL, Sveinbjornsson G, Hansen C. Cervical sonography in pregnant women with a prior cone biopsy or loop electrosurgical excision procedure. *Ultrasound Obstet Gynecol.* 2010;36:613-617.

20. Kyrgiou M, Mitra A, Arbyn M, et al. Fertility and early pregnancy outcomes after conservative treatment for cervical intraepithelial neoplasia. *Cochrane Database Syst Rev.* 2015;2015(9):CD008478.

26. Hernandez-Andrade E, Maymon E, Luewan S, et al. A soft cervix, categorized by shear-wave elastography, in women with short or with normal cervical length at 18-24 weeks is associated with a higher prevalence of spontaneous preterm delivery. *J Perinat Med.* 2018;46:489-501.

27. Feltovich H, Hall TJ, Berghella V. Beyond cervical length: emerging technologies for assessing the pregnant cervix. *Am J Obstet Gynecol.* 2012;207:345-354.

37. Conde-Agudelo A, Romero R, Da Fonseca E, et al. Vaginal progesterone is as effective as cervical cerclage to prevent preterm birth in women with a singleton gestation, previous spontaneous preterm birth, and a short cervix: updated indirect comparison meta-analysis. *Am J Obstet Gynecol.* 2018;219:10-25.

58. Melamed N, Ben-Haroush A, Chen R, Kaplan B, Yogev Y. Intrapartum cervical lacerations: characteristics, risk factors, and effects on subsequent pregnancies. *Am J Obstet Gynecol.* 2009;200:388.e1-388.e4.

63. McDonald IA. Suture of the cervix for inevitable miscarriage. *J Obstet Gynaecol Br Emp.* 1957;64:346-350.

64. O'Brien DP, Murphy JF. The shirodkar stitch. *Lancet.* 1977;310:873-874.

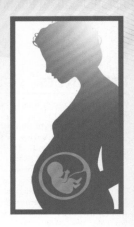

CHAPTER 49

Spontaneous Preterm Labor and Delivery

Offer Erez, Talia Lanxberg, Tal Rafaeli Yehudai, Limor Besser, Elad Laron, Nandor Gabor Than, and Arnon Wiznitzer

INTRODUCTION

Preterm birth (PTB) is a major global health problem and one of the most challenging obstetrical syndromes that affected 14.84 million (10.6%) of all live births in 2014.[1] The annual societal economic burden associated with PTB in the United States exceeded $26.2 billion in 2005,[2] and it was estimated that employer-sponsored health plans spend an extra $6 billion on preterm neonates in 2013.[3]

Preterm parturition is a syndrome resulting from multiple underlining mechanisms including intra-amniotic infection, inflammation, placental vascular disease, maternal antifetal rejection, cervical insufficiency, and progesterone deficiency,[4-6] leading to the premature activation of the common pathway of parturition, and this poses a challenge in the identification of patient at risk, as well as the development of preventive strategies and treatments.[7]

PTB is the leading cause of perinatal morbidity and mortality worldwide,[1,8] accounting for approximately 70% of neonatal and 36% of infant deaths in the United States.[9-11] Neonates born preterm are at increased risk of short-term complications, as well as long-term neonatal morbidity such as neurodevelopmental disorders and cerebral palsy.[12]

Preterm delivery can be either spontaneous or medically indicated due to maternal (ie, preeclampsia) or fetal (ie, fetal growth restriction) complications[21] regardless of the gestational age at delivery. Spontaneous PTB accounts for 75% of all preterm deliveries[24] and can be the end result of preterm labor (PTL) with intact membranes or preterm prelabor rupture of membranes (PPROM).[26] This chapter will discuss the epidemiology, underlying mechanisms of disease, clinical presentation, and management of the syndrome of spontaneous PTL with intact membranes.

Definitions

PTB is defined as a delivery occurring before 37 weeks of gestation.[27] Although the upper cutoff of 37 weeks according to menstrual age is well accepted,[27,28] there is a debate regarding the lower cutoff. The World Health Organization (WHO) includes in its definition of preterm delivery all live births before 37 weeks of gestation regardless of gestational age at delivery. Other cutoffs at 22 or 24 weeks of gestation have been proposed in which the risk for neonatal death does not exceed 50% regardless of ethnicity or race[27] (**Figure 49.2**). In the United States, the American College of Obstetricians and Gynecologists (ACOG) defines the lower cutoff for PTB at 20 0/7 weeks of gestation.[9]

Epidemiology

In 2010, approximately 15 million infants were born prematurely.[29] The overall prevalence of PTB for all live births worldwide was 11.1%, ranging from 5% to 18% depending on the geographic and demographic characteristics of the population tested.[28,31] More than 60% of preterm babies were born in South Asia, Africa, and North America.[29]

The rate of preterm deliveries in the United States increased from 11.2% in 1989 to 12.8% in 2004, then declined to 9.57% in 2014, and increased again to 10.2% in 2018.[37-39] While the rate of early (<34 weeks) PTB remained relatively constant over the past years (2.9% among singletons), the rate of late PTB (34-37 weeks) increased from 6.1% in 1990 to 7.1% in 2017.[37]

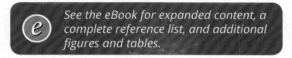

See the eBook for expanded content, a complete reference list, and additional figures and tables.

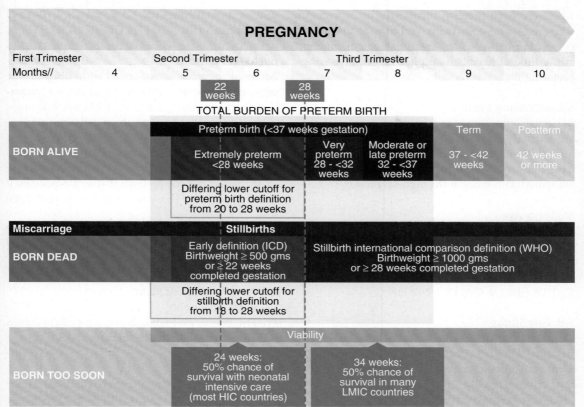

Figure 49.2 Definitions and cutoffs applied for preterm births, stillbirths, and miscarriages. HIC, high-income countries; ICD, International Classification of Diseases; LMIC, low- and middle-income countries; WHO, World Health Organization.

(Reprinted with permission from Blencowe H, Cousens S, Oestergaard MZ, et al. National, regional, and worldwide estimates of preterm birth rates in the year 2010 with time trends since 1990 for selected countries: a systematic analysis and implications. *Lancet.* 2012;379(9832):2162-2172.)

CLINICAL PRESENTATION

Risk Factors for PTB

The identification of patients at risk for preterm delivery has a significant role in its primary and secondary prevention. Because PTB is a syndrome that results from several underlying mechanisms, there is no single diagnostic test for it. Thus, the current risk assessments for spontaneous PTB include a combination of maternal factors, prior obstetrical history, and current pregnancy risks.

Maternal Risk Factors
Ethnicity
The risk for PTB is almost double among African Americans in comparison to other ethnic populations.[41] The rate of PTB among African Americans in 2016 was 13.77%, while among Pacific Islanders it was 11.5%, and among non-Hispanic whites it was 9.04%.[37] This disparity persists even after adjustment for social and medical risk factors.[42,45] Indeed, African American women living in high-income neighborhoods in Chicago still have a two-fold higher rate of PTB (at <37 weeks) than white women living in the same neighborhoods (relative risk [RR] 2.2; 95% confidence interval [CI] 1.7–2.9).[46]

African American paternal ethnicity also increases the risk for PTB (odds ratio [OR] 1.2; 95% CI 1.1–1.3), regardless of maternal race.[47]

Familial Risk
Studies suggest that there is a genetic predisposition for PTB as it is more prevalent in women

who were born preterm themselves or in women who are monozygotic twins, and there is a negative correlation between the gestational age of mother at the time of her birth and her risk of delivering preterm.[49,50]

Socioeconomic Factors

Maternal education and socioeconomic status are inversely correlated with PTB[53-56] in all ethnic groups. Women with the lowest levels of education have a nearly twofold increase in the rate of PTB compared with those at the highest levels.[58]

Maternal Age

The rate of PTB is elevated at the extremes of maternal age. Advanced maternal age (40 years and over) is independently associated with an increased risk of PTB.[59] Adolescent pregnancies have a high risk for PTB (RR 1.9; 95% CI 1.7–2.1).[59,60]

Smoking Status

Cigarette smoking is associated with increased risk for PTB. This effect persists even after adjustment for confounders, such as intrauterine growth restriction (IUGR), placental abruption, and PROM, suggesting that smoking is an independent risk factor for preterm delivery.[61]

Müllerian Anomalies

The presence of a Müllerian anomaly has been reported to be an independent risk factor for indicated preterm delivery.[24] However, the incidence of PTB is dependent on the specific type of Müllerian anomaly, with the highest rate of preterm deliveries in women with uterus didelphys, bicornis, or septated uterus.[62,66]

Cervical Surgery

Cervical procedures carry an increased risk factor for PTB that is proportional to the extent of the surgery. The frequency and severity of adverse perinatal outcomes are higher for excision than for ablation and are increased with increasing cone depth.[67-69]

Nutritional Status

Low maternal prepregnancy weight and prepregnancy overweight and obesity are associated with PTB.[88] A 2011 meta-analysis reported that underweight women have an increased overall risk of preterm delivery (RR 1.29; 95% CI 1.15–1.46) as well as spontaneous (RR 1.32; 95% CI 1.10–1.57) and indicated (RR 1.21; 95% CI 1.07–1.36) PTB.[90]

Bacterial Vaginosis

Bacterial vaginosis is associated with a higher rate of pregnancy losses in the first and second trimesters, intra-amniotic infection, PPROM, histologic chorioamnionitis, post–cesarean delivery endometritis and wound infection.[120]

The rate of bacterial vaginosis during pregnancy is 15% to 20%[98,103,104,122-128] is associated with an increased risk for preterm delivery, especially if detected prior to 16 weeks of gestation (OR 7.55; 95% CI 1.8–31.65).[129]

Professional societies do not recommend screening for the condition in women at low risk for PTB.[95,96]

Current Pregnancy Risks

Mode of Conception

Preterm delivery is higher in pregnancies conceived by assisted reproductive technology (ART).[141]

Vaginal Bleeding

Vaginal bleeding during pregnancy is a risk factor for spontaneous and indicated PTB.[104,146] Pregnancy complications, such as placenta previa and placental abruption, as well as idiopathic vaginal bleeding during the first and second trimester are associated with an increased risk for a subsequent preterm delivery.[104,146] Women who experience unexplained vaginal bleeding during the first trimester have double the risk for PTB compared with women who do not experience vaginal bleeding (OR = 2.11; 95% CI 1.43–3.10).[149]

Multifetal Gestations

In 2016, approximately 61% of multifetal gestations in the United States delivered prematurely.[40] A detailed discussion of multifetal pregnancies is the topic of Chapter 5.

Previous PTB

A previous PTB is an independent risk factor for a subsequent preterm delivery and recurrence often occurs at the same gestational age.[50,151] The frequency of recurrent spontaneous PTB is 15% to 30% after one spontaneous PTB and increases after two prior spontaneous preterm deliveries.[50] The risk for PTB in subsequent pregnancies is influenced by the number, sequence, and gestational age of prior

PTBs.[155] The risk increases as the gestational age at the time of a prior PTB declines, especially before 32 weeks of gestation.[156]

Underlying Mechanisms of Preterm Parturition Syndrome

PTL as a Syndrome

The current taxonomy of disease in obstetrics is based on the clinical presentation rather than on the underlying mechanism of disease responsible for the premature activation of the common pathway of parturition, which is defined as (1) the switch of the myometrium from the quiet phase 0 to active and contractile mode; (2) shortening and ripening of the uterine cervix; and (3) activation of the decidua and chorioamniotic membranes and their rupture. This is the consequence of anatomical, physiological, biochemical, endocrinological, immunological, and clinical events that occur in the mother and/or fetus in both term and PTL. In contrast to term labor (described in Chapter 44), in which the common pathway of parturition is physiologically activated, PTL results from a synchronous or nonsynchronous, premature pathological activation of the components of parturition. PTL is the clinical presentation of premature activation of the uterine and cervical components of the common pathway of parturition. This could be the clinical presentation of different underlying mechanisms,[5,28,158] including intrauterine infection,[159-162,167-176] uteroplacental ischemia,[177-179,182-185] uterine overdistention,[189] cervical disease,[191-193] abnormal allograft rejection,[194] allergic phenomena,[196] and endocrine disorders.[200] However, the term "preterm labor" (PTL) relates only to the clinical presentation of the disease and is not indicative to whether this condition is caused by any of the abovementioned pathological processes.

Infection and Inflammation

Infection is the only proven mechanism of disease leading to premature delivery. Microbiological and histopathological studies suggest that infection-related inflammation may account for 25% to 40% of cases of preterm deliveries.[201]

Infectious processes leading to PTB can be clinically evident (ie, pyelonephritis or chorioamnionitis); subclinical, limited to the uterus, and present as PTL or preterm PROM, resulting from bacteria that crossed through the placenta from the maternal blood and are detected in the amniotic fluid; and/or detected only after delivery in the placenta (ie, acute histologic chorioamnionitis).

Systemic Maternal Infection

Pyelonephritis, pneumonia, malaria, and other systemic maternal diseases are frequently associated with the onset of premature labor and delivery[204-207] (discussed in Chapter 39). Evidence suggests that the maternal immune response to these infectious diseases induces inflammatory processes that affect the intrauterine environment, placenta, and membranes, leading to activation of the common pathway of parturition.

Intra-amniotic Infection

The presence of bacteria or other microorganisms in the amniotic fluid, which should be sterile,[213] is associated with adverse pregnancy outcomes,[164,214-225] and identification of microorganisms during mid-trimester amniocentesis in asymptomatic patients has been associated with subsequent late miscarriage,[235] preterm delivery,[236] and even fetal demise.[159,161,203,237,246,259,171-176]

Pathogenic microorganisms can invade the amniotic fluid through several routes. The most common is ascending infection from the vagina to the cervical canal through the membranes into the amniotic cavity and subsequently infecting the membranes and the fetus.[201,238] Other routes are maternal transmission of bacteria by hematogenous[239,240] spread through the placenta or through the membranes, and finally iatrogenic introduction of bacteria into the amniotic cavity during amniocentesis of other medical intervention.[242,243]

Goncalves et al[226] reported that the overall prevalence of intra-amniotic infection in patients with PTL was 12.8% and about 50% were polymicrobial. The rate of microbial invasion of amniotic cavity (MIAC) in patients with PTL and intact membrane is gestational age dependent, ranging from as high as 45% at 23 to 26 weeks to 11.5% by 31 to 34 weeks of gestation.[244]

The most common microbial organisms isolated from the amniotic fluid of patients with PTL and intact membranes were genital mycoplasmas; followed by *Fusobacterium* species,[201] *Streptococcus agalactiae*, *Peptostreptococcus* spp., *Fusobacterium* spp., *Staphylococcus aureus*, *Gardnerella vaginalis*, *Streptococcus viridans*, and *Bacteroides* spp.[259]

Bacteria in amniotic fluid can be either planktonic (free floating) or in the form of biofilm.[260,261] Amniotic fluid sludge, which is a particulate matter identified by ultrasound near the internal os of the uterine cervix, is in fact in part of the cases a bacterial biofilm.[260,261] The identification of sludge in asymptomatic patients and in those at risk for PTB, especially when accompanied by a short sonographic cervix, is associated with an increased risk for spontaneous PTL with intact membranes, PPROM of membranes, microbial invasion of amniotic fluid, PTB, and histologic chorioamnionitis.[262,263]

The inflammatory process elicited by the presence of microbacteria in the amniotic cavity is the driving force that leads to preterm parturition in cases of MIAC.

In cases of microbial associated intra-amniotic inflammation, the inflammatory reaction in the amniotic fluid is triggered by the activation of pattern recognition receptors including toll-like receptors or RAGE in response to the presence of danger-associated molecular patterns (DAMPs) or pathogen-associated molecular patterns (ie, lipopolysaccharides).[274] The activation of pattern recognition receptors (PPRs) by microbes or their products illicits an inflammatory response, which in turn leads to the production of cytokines (IL-6 and TNFα) and matrix degrading enzymes (matrix metalloproteinase [MMP]-8) leading to the production of prostaglandins and activation of the common pathway of parturition[6] (**Figure 49.8**).

Sterile Intra-amniotic Inflammation
Inflammatory processes in the amniotic fluid in which microorganisms cannot be detected are defined as sterile intra-amniotic inflammation.

The clinical characteristics of patients with PTL who had sterile intra-amniotic inflammation are similar in terms of gestational age at delivery, amniocentesis to delivery interval, and adverse neonatal outcomes, to those reported in women with PTL and microbial associated intra-amniotic inflammation.[245,281]

Fetal Inflammatory Response Syndrome
Fetal inflammatory response syndrome (FIRS) can be considered the fetal equivalent of systemic inflammatory response syndrome, described in adults with sepsis.[287,288] FIRS is characterized by systemic activation of the fetal immune system involving all major fetal systems (ie, hematopoietic, heart, brain, lungs, kidneys, adrenals and skin).[287] Additionally, preterm neonates affected in utero by FIRS have a shorter interval from cordocentesis to delivery and a higher rate of short- and long-term complication of prematurity including respiratory distress syndrome (RDS), neonatal sepsis, pneumonia, bronchopulmonary dysplasia (BPD), intraventricular hemorrhage, periventricular leukomalacia (PVL), necrotizing enterocolitis (NEC), and cerebral palsy than those without this syndrome.[287,290-292] The rate of FIRS in pregnancies complicated by preterm parturition is about 39% and increases to 49.3% in fetuses delivered within 1 week from cordocentesis.[287,293]

Currently, there are two types of FIRS: type I and type II. Type I is considered the highest degree of intra-amniotic infection/inflammation. It describes fetuses who mounted a systemic inflammatory immune response to microorganisms, which invaded the amniotic cavity. The characteristic placental lesions of FIRS type I syndrome include histologic chorioamnionitis, evidence of umbilical cord inflammation (funisitis), and chorionic vasculitis. The presence of funisitis allows a postnatal diagnosis of neonates with FIRS type I and is associated with an increased risk for the subsequent development of cerebral palsy (OR 5.5; 95% CI, 1.2–24.5).[287,294,295]

Type II FIRS results from maternal antifetal rejection and manifests as a unique cord blood transcriptome in the affected fetuses. The clinical manifestations of FIRS type II await further research.[296]

Uteroplacental Ischemia
Placental Vascular Disease
Placental lesions consistent with maternal vascular malperfusion are present in 20% to 30% of patients who had spontaneous PTB,[177,186,302,303] and they are more prevalent after 28 weeks of gestation.[186,303] Additionally, 36% of patients with PTL and intact membranes who delivered preterm have evidence for decidual bleeding including hemosiderin depositions and retrochorionic hematoma formation.[305,306]

Role of Thrombin
The effect of decidual bleeding on the activation of premature uterine contractions and/or rupture of membranes is thought to be mediated by thrombin.[311-314,316,318,321]

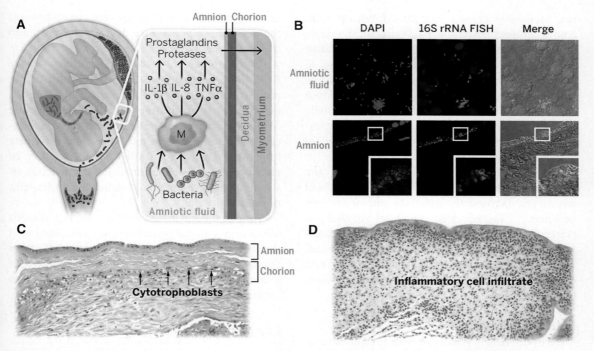

Figure 49.8 Mechanisms of microbial induced preterm labor. **A,** Bacteria from the lower genital tract gain access to the amniotic cavity and stimulate the production of chemokines and cytokines, as well as prostaglandins and reactive oxygen radicals and proteases, initiating myometrial contractility with/without membrane rupture. **B,** (Top left) Amniotic fluid containing bacteria that was retrieved by amniocentesis from a patient with preterm labor. Bacteria and nuclei stained with DAPI (4',6-diamidino-2-phenylindole) (blue). (Top middle) Bacteria identified with a probe against 16S ribosomal RNA (rRNA) using fluorescent in situ hybridization. (Bottom left and middle) Bacteria invading the amnion epithelium. Note the absence of bacteria in the subepithelial part of the amnion, suggesting that the pathway of microbial invasion is ascending into the amniotic cavity. **C,** Chorioamniotic membranes without evidence of inflammation. Amnion and chorion are identified. **D,** A similar membrane section as **(C)** from a patient with intra-amniotic infection. Inflammatory cells from the mother infiltrate the chorion and amnion. FISH, fluorescence *in situ* hybridization; rRNA, ribosomal RNA.

(Reprinted with permission from Romero R, Dey SK, Fisher SJ. Preterm labor: one syndrome, many causes. *Science.* 2014;345(6198):760-765.)

Thrombin can activate preterm parturition through several mechanisms: (1) uterotonic activities, as evidenced by experiments in which the administration of a whole blood, but not saline or heparinized blood, into a nonpregnant uterus generated uterine contractions[311,312,332]; (2) production of proinflammatory cytokines[341] associated with prostaglandins generation, premature myometrial activation, and contractions; and (3) activation of matrix degrading enzymes, such MMP-1, MMP-3, and MMP-9, which can degrade the chorioamniotic membranes leading to rupture of membranes.[342-345]

PERINATAL MORTALITY AND MORBIDITY

Perinatal Mortality

PTB is the leading cause for perinatal mortality and morbidity.

Perinatal mortality is negatively dependent on the gestational age at delivery and birthweight.[429,430] Indeed, the earlier the PTB occurs, the higher the perinatal mortality rate. This risk increases in the presence of severe SGA.[435]

Ethnic origin has its impact on the survival of preterm neonates. The overall perinatal mortality rate is double among African Americans than among whites.[437] Wallace et al[438] studied the ratio/ethnic differences in preterm perinatal mortality. Across all groups, female infants had lower risk of perinatal death compared with males, with white female infants having the lowest rates. When adjusting for infant sex, black female and male infants had 55% and 70% increased risk, respectively, for perinatal mortality compared to white female infants.

Additionally, intrauterine infection and the healthcare team's expectation that the infant will not survive increase the mortality rate of preterm neonates.[440] Factors that increase survival of preterm neonates include antenatal administration of corticosteroids and neonatal treatment with surfactant.[442-445] The preterm neonate mortality rate varies among different neonatal intensive care units (NICUs).[447]

Perinatal Morbidity

Preterm delivery is associated with specific perinatal morbidities derived from the immaturity of the neonatal organs. Neonatal morbidity is gestational age–dependent, as the earlier the delivery, the more severe the condition, especially for those born prior to 30 weeks of gestation.[448,449]

Late PTB is also associated with an increased risk for neonatal infections and respiratory morbidities.[446,450]

Prenatal administration of corticosteroids has lowered the rate of most acute neonatal morbidities. In addition, the use of recombinant surfactant has also contributed to the substantial reduction in rate of RDS. Other morbidities declined, but BPD increased between 2009 and 2012 for infants born at 26 to 27 weeks' gestation.[451]

Long-Term Consequences of Preterm Delivery

The chronic morbidity of prematurity carries a lifetime burden.

The neurological development of preterm infants is delayed; this observation is relatively common especially among extremely preterm neonates. Marlow et al reported that almost all children who were born <25 weeks of gestation had some disability at the age of 6 years: only 20% had no neurocognitive disabilities.[460] In children who were born <32 weeks of gestation, the IQ score at the age

of 7 was associated with gestational age at delivery, the presence of persistence ductus arteriosus, and the head circumference.[461]

Even among children with moderate-to-late PTB, those born at 33 to 35 weeks had a higher proportion of schooling difficulties associated with male gender and discharge from the hospital before 36 weeks' corrected age.[462] Nevertheless, adolescents who were preterm newborns with extremely low birthweight had similar self-perception of global self-worth, scholastic or job competence, or social acceptance compared with their peers with normal birthweights.[463]

Among those who did not have medical disabilities, the gestational age at birth was associated with the level of education attained, income, receipt of Social Security benefits, and the establishment of a family, but not with rates of unemployment or criminal activity.[464]

DIAGNOSIS OF PTL

An episode of premature contractions or suspected PTL is one of the leading etiologies for admission during pregnancy[466,469] ranging from 9% to 24% of all pregnant women.[466,469] However, only half of women who experience premature contractions will subsequently deliver preterm.[470]

The ACOG defines PTL based on the clinical presentation of regular uterine contractions leading to cervical changes (effacement and/or dilatation) or initial presentation with regular contractions and cervical dilatation of least 2 cm.[9] Others have proposed the definition that includes the presence of six or more uterine contractions/hour in fetal monitoring and a cervical dilatation of >3 cm with >80% effacement ascertains the diagnosis of PTL. These discrepancies reflect the elusive clinical presentation of PTL, which ranges from pelvic pressure to painful or painless uterine contractions, with or without vaginal bleeding, which may or may not lead to PTB.

Thus, today, the clinical diagnosis of PTL is based on the assessment of all the components of the common pathway of parturition, meaning signs of uterine contraction, cervical ripening and/or dilatation, as well as rupture of the chorioamniotic membranes. The initial assessment of patients with symptoms suggestive of PTL is presented in **Algorithm 49.1**. Maternal examination includes (1) fetal monitoring performed for the presence of contractions and fetal assessment; (2) speculum examination for the evidence of PROM, vaginal bleeding, or bulging membranes; (3) digital examination for cervical dilatation if rupture of the membranes or placental bleeding is excluded; and (4) abdominal ultrasound assessment for placental location, estimation of fetal weight and well-being, and amniotic fluid volume.

Sonographic Measurement of Cervical Length

Sonographic examination is needed to determine placental location, to rule out placenta previa, and to measure the cervical length as part of the assessment of the risk of impending PTB. Cervical sonography is the most objective and reliable method to assess cervical length.[442,443,500] In women presenting with an acute episode of PTL, sonographic measurement of cervical length may help to differentiate between women likely to deliver preterm. Indeed, in women with PTL, spontaneous PTB <32 weeks is unlikely if the cervical length is ≥30 mm.[494] There are several reports[494-496] suggesting that if cervical length at the time of threatened PTL is <15 mm, then the risk for impending PTB is substantially increased. A cervical length <15 mm had a 59.9%

sensitivity, 90.5% specificity, and 5.71 positive likelihood ratio for preterm delivery within 1 week from presentation; and a 46.2% sensitivity, 93.7% specificity, and 4.31 positive likelihood ratio for delivery <34 weeks.[494-496]

Fetal Fibronectin Assessment

Fetal FN (fFN), found in the basement membrane near the choriodecidual interface, is produced by fetal membranes and is likely to function as an adhesive that binds the placenta and membranes to the decidua. There is a relationship between the presence of fFN in cervicovaginal secretions and spontaneous PTB.

Clinical detection of fFN at 22 to 34 weeks at concentrations higher than 50 mg/mL is considered abnormal and indicates choriodecidual disruption. Its presence in the vagina may indicate the presence of amniotic fluid in cervicovaginal secretions.[498]

However, testing for fFN produces numerous false-positive results,[170,498] and test results were more frequently positive among multiparous than nulliparous women. To improve the accuracy of true-positive results, specimens should be obtained before any cervical manipulation and before advanced dilation or increased uterine activity has occurred.

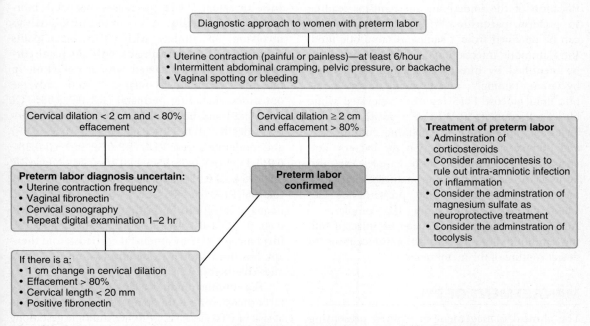

Algorithm 49.1 The initial assessment of patients with symptoms suggestive of preterm labor.

Determining the Etiology of Suspected PTL

After a diagnosis of PTL is made, assessing the underlying process(es) leading to this clinical presentation is important as it informs treatment and patient management to support best outcomes.

When vaginal bleeding is part of the presenting symptoms, clinician assessment should include the diagnosis of potential placental abruption by the presence of hypertonic uterine contractions, uterine tenderness, and, in some cases, sonographic evidence of intrauterine bleeding or blood clots, as well as the possible presence of placenta previa. In both cases, the clinician needs to estimate whether the bleeding necessitates prompt delivery and prevents the administration of tocolysis and corticosteroids.

The presence of maternal fever suggests that an infection, either systemic or intra-amniotic may underlie the PTL. The presenting clinical features of fever >37.8 °C without any other evident source, fetal tachycardia, uterine tenderness, leukocytosis, and foul-smelling amniotic fluid in case of PPROM are suggestive to chorioamnionitis. However, in most cases, intra-amniotic infection is sub-clinical, and the only clinical manifestation can be premature contractions and/or vaginal bleeding.

Amniocentesis can be a useful tool for the identification of the underlying mechanisms leading to preterm parturition.[501] Valuable information can be obtained from a sample of amniotic fluid. Intra-amniotic infection and or inflammation can be identified by direct visualization of bacteria by Gram staining[506]; measurement of low amniotic fluid glucose (<15 mg/dL)[510]; elevated white blood cell count (>50 WBCs)[270]; positive aerobic, anaerobic, and genital mycoplasma cultures[516-521]; and polymerase chain reaction for bacteria and viruses.[246,249,522] Amniotic fluid samples can also be used to test for fetal lung maturity, fetal chromosomal abnormalities, the presence of elevated thrombin-antithrombin III complexes.[313] Additionally, indigo carmine can be injected into the amniotic fluid during an amniocentesis to detect rupture of the membranes.

MANAGEMENT OF PTL

The clinical management of women presenting with PTL has the following goals: (1) prevention and reduction of complications of prematurity in the neonate by administration of corticosteroids, antibiotic treatment to prevent group B streptococcal (GBS) infections, and transfer of the patient to a hospital with adequate NICU facilities, as needed; (2) stop the process of the premature labor and, if that cannot be achieved, to prolong it enough to allow the administration of corticosteroids; (3) reduce possible neonatal neurologic sequelae; and (4) plan the mode of delivery and verify the availability of neonatal intensive care.[9]

Corticosteroid Administration

Administration of corticosteroids, primarily betamethasone or dexamethasone, is one of the most beneficial interventions in PTB because it significantly reduces neonatal morbidity and mortality[533,534] Betamethasone is given in a dose of 12 mg (6 mg betamethasone phosphate and 6 mg betamethasone) by maternal intramuscular injection with a second dose given 24 hours later. Dexamethasone is given in four 6-mg doses of dexamethasone phosphate by maternal intramuscular injection at 12-hour intervals to achieve a continuous fetal exposure for about 48 hours.[162] However, the optimal preparation and the ideal dose are still under debate.[543]

Administration of corticosteroids to women with threatened PTL decreases neonatal morbidity and mortality. A Cochrane meta-analysis involving 30 studies with 7774 participants demonstrated that treatment with antenatal corticosteroids was associated with a reduction in the most prematurity-related serious adverse outcomes, including perinatal (RR 0.72; 95% CI 0.58-0.89) and neonatal (RR 0.69; 95% CI 0.59-0.81) deaths, RDS (RR 0.66; 95% CI 0.56-0.77) and moderate/severe RDS (RR 0.59; 95% CI 0.38-0.91), IVH (RR 0.55; 95% CI 0.40-0.76), NEC (RR 0.50; 95% CI 0.32-0.78), need for mechanical ventilation (RR 0.68; 95% CI 0.56-0.84), and systemic neonatal infections in the first 48 hours of life (RR 0.60; 95% CI 0.41-0.88).[534] The reduction in the incidence of RDS by antenatal corticosteroid therapy has been shown to be effective up to 7 days after treatment.[533]

The administration of a single course of antenatal corticosteroids is the standard of care for women at risk of PTB (ie, PTL, PPROM, multiple gestation, and indicated preterm delivery due to maternal or fetal indications) within a week of presentation between 24 0/7 and 33 6/7 weeks' of gestation.[9] Moreover, the administration of corticosteroids should be considered even in women with an episode of preterm parturition at the threshold of viability between 23 0/7 and 23 6/7 who are at risk of preterm delivery within 7 days.[9] Similarly, evidence suggests that women with late PTL between 34 0/7 and 36 6/7 weeks of gestation who were not treated with corticosteroids earlier during pregnancy may benefit from a single course of betamethasone.[545] However, in the presence of clinical chorioamnionitis in the late preterm period, tocolysis and corticosteroid should not be administrated.[546]

Recommendations to use a single repeat course of antenatal corticosteroids when indicated (less than 34 0/7 weeks of gestation who are at risk of preterm delivery within 7 days, and whose prior course of antenatal corticosteroids was administered >7 days previously) are now included within the WHO recommendations on interventions to improve PTB outcomes[548] and several national clinical practice guidelines.[549,550]

Magnesium Sulfate Administration

Antenatal magnesium sulfate given to women at risk of PTB has a neuroprotective effect on the offspring.[561-563]

In October 2016, the ACOG recommended that hospitals that choose to use magnesium sulfate for fetal neuroprotection should develop specific guidelines addressing the inclusion criteria, dosage, concurrent tocolysis, and monitoring.[9]

In 2015, the WHO recommended the use of magnesium sulfate for women at risk of imminent PTB before 32 weeks of gestation for prevention of cerebral palsy.[548]

In 2019, the Society of Obstetricians and Gynaecologists of Canada published recommendations on the administration of magnesium sulfate for women with imminent PTB ≤33 6/7 weeks of gestation. For women with imminent PTB, antenatal magnesium sulfate for fetal neuroprotection should be administered as a 4-g intravenous loading dose, over 30 minutes, with or without a 1-g/hr maintenance infusion until birth and for no longer than 24 hours. For planned PTB due to fetal or maternal indications, magnesium sulfate should be started, ideally, within 4 hours before birth as a 4-g intravenous loading dose over 30 minutes.[564]

Tocolytic Therapy

The main goal of tocolytic treatment is to delay preterm delivery by 48 hours to allow the fetus/neonate to benefit from the administration of prenatal corticosteroids. Tocolytic medications carry serious maternal and fetal/neonatal side effects, which are summarized in **Table 49.5**.

Calcium Channel Blockers

Calcium channel blockers inhibit calcium flow through cell membranes and prevent the spread of intracellular calcium ions, required for the myometrium to contract in a coordinated manner.[565] The most common calcium channel blocker used for tocolysis is nifedipine.

Treatment with nifedipine was associated with an increased gestational age at birth, longer interval to delivery, and higher birthweight. There was also a reduction in perinatal morbidity such as RDS, NEC, IVH, neonatal jaundice, admission to NICU, and NICU length of stay.[567,568]

Beta-Adrenergic Receptor Agonists

Beta-adrenergic receptor agonists, or betamimetics decrease myometrial contractility.[565] Betamimetics were used to delay PTL and PTB extensively in the past, but carry significant side effects[569] (**Table 49.5**). Betamimetics should not be used for more than 48 hours due to the risk of severe maternal cardiotoxicity.

Prostaglandin Inhibitors/Cox Inhibitors

Prostaglandin inhibitors, such as nonsteroidal anti-inflammatory drugs (NSAIDs), prevent the synthesis of prostaglandins by blocking the activity of the isoenzymes cyclooxygenase 1 and 2 (COX1 and COX2). In the context of PTL, the decrease in prostaglandin production results in reduced uterine contractility.[565] Indomethacin is the most studied NSAID used for tocolysis.[572]

Indomethacin resulted in a reduction in PTB <37 weeks of gestation and an increase in gestational age at birth and birthweight.[573]

Indomethacin was associated with an increased risk of severe IVH (grade III-IV; RR 1.29; 95% CI, 1.06–1.56), NEC (RR; 1.36; 95% CI, 1.08–1.71), and PVL (RR 1.59; 95% CI 1.17–2.17).[577] Moreover, treatment with indomethacin after 32 weeks of gestation has been associated with premature closure of the ductus arteriosus and oligohydramnios.[578]

Table 49.5 Maternal and Fetal/Neonatal Side Effects and Contraindications of Tocolytic Agents

Agent or Class	Maternal Side Effects	Fetal or Newborn Adverse Effects	Contraindications
Calcium channel blockers	Dizziness, flushing, and hypotension; suppression of heart rate, contractility, and left ventricular systolic pressure when used with magnesium sulfate; and elevation of hepatic transaminases	No known adverse effects	Hypotension and preload-dependent cardiac lesions, such as aortic insufficiency
Nonsteroidal anti-inflammatory drugs	Nausea, esophageal reflux, gastritis, and emesis; platelet dysfunction is rarely of clinical significance in patients without underlying bleeding disorder	In utero constriction of ductus arteriosus[a], oligohydramnios[a], necrotizing enterocolitis in preterm newborns, and patent ductus arteriosus in newborn[b]	Platelet dysfunction or bleeding disorder, hepatic dysfunction, gastrointestinal ulcerative disease, renal dysfunction, and asthma (in women with hypersensitivity to aspirin)
Beta-adrenergic receptor agonists	Tachycardia, hypotension, tremor, palpitations, shortness of breath, chest discomfort, pulmonary edema, hypokalemia, and hyperglycemia	Fetal tachycardia	Tachycardia-sensitive maternal cardiac disease and poorly controlled diabetes mellitus
Magnesium sulfate	Causes flushing, diaphoresis, nausea, loss of deep tendon reflexes, respiratory depression, and cardiac arrest; suppresses heart rate, contractility, and left ventricular systolic pressure when used with calcium channel blockers; and produces neuromuscular blockade when used with calcium-channel blockers	Neonatal depression[c]	Myasthenia gravis

[a]Greatest risk associated with use for longer than 48 hours.
[b]Data are conflicting regarding this association.
[c]The use of magnesium sulfate in doses and duration for fetal neuroprotection alone does not appear to be associated with an increased risk of neonatal depression when correlated with cord blood magnesium levels.
Reprinted with permission from Johnson LH, Mapp DC, Rouse DJ, et al; Eunice Kennedy Shriver National Institute of Child Health and Human Development Maternal–Fetal Medicine Units Network. Association of cord blood magnesium concentration and neonatal resuscitation. *J Pediatr.* 2012;160(4):573.e1-577.e1. doi:10.1016/j.jpeds.2011.09.016 and American College of Obstetricians and Gynecologists' Committee on Practice Bulletins—Obstetrics. Practice Bulletin No. 171: management of preterm labor. *Obstet Gynecol.* 2016;128(4):e155-e164.

Oxytocin Receptor Antagonists

Oxytocin receptor antagonists inhibit the action of endogenous oxytocin on uterine tissue.[565] The most commonly used oxytocin receptor antagonist is atosiban, which is unavailable in the United States as of this writing.[569] In a Cochrane review (14 studies involving 2485 women), oxytocin receptor antagonists did not appear to have greater benefit in terms of pregnancy prolongation or neonatal outcomes than other tocolytic agents.[579]

Antibiotics

During active PTL, prophylactic antibiotic treatment against GBS infection is indicated because premature neonates are at increased risk for neonatal

GBS infection than those born at term.[9] However, antibiotics should not be routinely administered to women with PTL; it is not effective and may even be harmful to the fetus/neonate.

Treatment Following Arrest of PTL

In cases where the acute episode of PTL has been arrested, the patient management is aimed at maintaining uterine quiescence and prolonging gestation. Prolonged uterine contraction suppression does not seem to be associated with a reduction in the rate of PTB[586] here. Therefore, gestational age, cervical length, dilatation and effacement, the frequency of uterine contractions, and maternal obstetric history should be considered in the decision whether to follow up the patient in an outpatient or inpatient setting. Of note, outpatient follow-up is not associated with a better outcome in relation to the rate of PTB and birthweight.[587]

Intrapartum Management of Preterm Delivery

The management of preterm delivery is complex due to the associated maternal and fetal pathological processes present, such as intrauterine infection, hypertension, placental abruption, fetal growth restriction, and others, which require special attention and consideration.

The fetus requires continued heart trace monitoring to allow for tight control of fetal status and timely intervention in cases of compromise. Use of a fetal scalp monitor prior to 34 weeks' gestation is not recommended.

When choosing the mode of delivery, the managing physician should consider that preterm delivery can be precipitated, and the active phase of the first stage of labor and the second stage of labor can be very rapid. Currently, nonvertex preterm fetuses are delivered by cesarean due to the fear of entrapment of the head and potential difficult extraction. Small for gestational age neonates before 32 weeks are better delivered by cesarean delivery as this improves their survival. When performing the cesarean delivery, the surgeon must take into consideration the need for a nontraumatic extraction of the preterm neonate through the cesarean scar and plan accordingly. Operative vaginal delivery is contraindicated before 34 weeks of gestation and should be considered very carefully between 34 0/7 and 36 6/7 weeks.

Management Decisions at the Lower End of Viability

The improvement in neonatal care of extreme PTB infants shifted the threshold of viability toward 22 to 23 weeks of gestation. A joint workshop by the *Eunice Kennedy Shriver* National Institute of Child Health and Human Development (NICHD), Society for Maternal-Fetal Medicine (SMFM), American Academy of Pediatrics, and ACOG made several recommendations regarding management of periviable birth[588] (**Table 49.6**).

PREVENTION OF SPONTANEOUS PTB

The prevention of PTB is one of the major objectives of modern obstetrics.[593-596] However, despite all efforts, there is no specific treatment for spontaneous PTB due to the syndromic nature of preterm parturition that cannot be resolved by a single medication or intervention.

Prevention of PTB can be:

- Primary—Measures directed to all women before or during pregnancy to prevent and reduce factors associated with increased risk for preterm delivery (ie, lifestyle, environmental factors, smoking status, and periodontal disease).
- Secondary—Measures aimed at eliminating or reducing risk in women with known predisposing factors (ie, previous PTB, short cervix at the second trimester, Müllerian anomalies).
- Tertiary—Measures initiated after the parturitional process has begun with a goal of delaying or preventing preterm delivery, or improving outcomes for preterm infants (ie, administration of corticosteroids or magnesium sulfate).

In 2013 the Born Too Soon preterm prevention group and representatives of health organizations published an analysis of what would be the most effective interventions to reduce the rate of PTB in countries with very high human development index.[593] Six interventions were identified as having the greatest impact on PTB rate. The most prominent intervention was the reduction in nonmedically indicated preterm deliveries and cesarean deliveries, followed by cerclage placement, a better control of ART protocols, progesterone supplementation, and smoking cessation. In a separate study, Newnham et al[597] ranked the most effective strategies and their possible contribution to reducing

Table 49.6 General Guidance Regarding Obstetric Interventions for Threatened and Imminent Periviable Birth, According to Whether the Fetus Is Considered Potentially Viable, and the Parents' Wishes for Aggressive Intervention[a]

	Weeks of Gestation[b]		
	Less Than 22 0/7 wk	**22 0/7-22 6/7 wk**	**23 0/7 wk or More**
Antenatal corticosteroids	Not recommended	Consider if delivery at or later than 23 0/7 wk is anticipated	Recommended
Tocolytics to enhance latency for potential steroid benefit	Not recommended	Not recommended unless concurrent with antenatal steroids	Consider
Magnesium sulfate for neuroprotection	Not recommended	Not recommended	Recommended
Antibiotics for PROM to enhance latency	Consider if delivery not imminent	Consider if delivery not imminent	Recommended if delivery not imminent
Intrapartum antibiotics for GBS prophylaxis[c]	Not recommended	Not recommended	Recommended
Continuous intrapartum electronic fetal monitoring	Not recommended	Not recommended	Recommended
Cesarean delivery for fetal indication[d]	Not recommended	Not recommended	Recommended
Aggressive newborn resuscitation	Not recommended, comfort care only	Not recommended unless considered potentially viable based on individual circumstances	Recommended unless considered nonviable based on individual circumstances

GBS, group B streptococcus; PROM, prelabor rupture of membranes.

[a]Survival of infants born in the periviable period is dependent on resuscitation and support. Between 22 and 25 weeks of gestation, there may be mitigating factors (eg, intrauterine growth restriction, small fetal size, the presence of fetal malformations or aneuploidy, and pulmonary hypoplasia due to prolonged membrane rupture) that will affect the potential for survival and the determination of viability. The majority of survivors born at 25 6/7 weeks of gestation or less will incur major morbidities, regardless of gestational age at birth.

[b]Infants born before 22 0/7 weeks of gestation are generally considered nonviable. Data from recent large studies suggest survival with delivery at 22 0/7 weeks through 22 6/7 weeks to be 5% to 6%.[25,27] With survival rates of approximately 26% to 28% and higher, infants born at 23 0/7 weeks through 25 6/7 weeks of gestation are generally considered potentially viable.

[c]Group B streptococcus carrier or carrier status unknown.

[d]For example, persistently abnormal fetal heart rate patterns or biophysical testing (Category II and III).

Reprinted with permission from Raju TNK, Mercer BM, Burchfield DJ, et al. Periviable birth: executive summary of a joint workshop by the Eunice Kennedy Shriver National Institute of Child Health and Human Development, Society for Maternal-Fetal Medicine, American Academy of Pediatrics, and American College of Obstetricians and Gynecologists. *Obstet Gynecol*. 2014;123(5):1083-1096.

PTB, as summarized in **Table 49.7**, which were similar to the findings of Chang et al.[593]

Nonmedically Indicated Late-Preterm/Early-Term Birth

The restriction of nonmedically indicated late-preterm deliveries can be a major contribution for the reduction of late PTBs. Indeed, the Born Too Soon study group calculated that avoiding nonmedically indicated late PTBs can reduce the rate of PTB in 0.61% of pregnancies, which is about a 50% of the expected reduction in the rate of PTB if all the preventives measures suggested by this group were implemented.[593] The delivery of late-preterm or early-term infants is associated with increased neonatal morbidity in comparison to those delivered after 39 weeks of gestation.[598,599] Therefore, the ACOG and the SMFM published together a list for indication for late-preterm/early-term deliveries.[601]

Table 49.7 Strategies to Prevent Preterm Birth Feasible for Implementation and Likely to Be Successful in High-Resource Settings

Strategy	Possible Reduction in PTB	Level of Evidence
Judicious use of fertility treatments	63%	I
Prevention of medically indicated late-preterm/ early-term birth	55%	III-3
Progesterone supplementation	45%	I
Cervical cerclage	20%	III-1
Tobacco control— prevent smoking in pregnancy	20%	III-2
Smoke-free legislation	10%	III-3
Dedicated preterm birth prevention clinics	13%	III-2

Level I, systematic review of level II studies; level II, randomized controlled trial; level III-1, pseudo-randomized controlled trial (ie, alternate allocation or some other method); level III-2, comparative study with concurrent controls, nonrandomized experimental trial, cohort study, case-control study, interrupted time series with control group; level III-3, comparative study without concurrent controls, historical control study, two or more single-arm study, interrupted time series without a parallel control group; level IV, case series with either posttest or pretest/ posttest outcomes.
Modified from Newnham JP, Dickinson JE, Hart RJ, Pennell CE, Arrese CA, Keelan JA. Strategies to prevent preterm birth. *Front Immunol.* 2014;5:584.

Cerclage Placement

The placement of a cervical stich (cerclage) was recommended by both Chang et al and Newnham et al as one of the leading interventions in the prevention of PTB. This results from the fact that in some of the women with cervical insufficiency there is a mechanical disorder of the cervix with different degrees of severity that can be treated by cerclage placement (and see Chapter 48). Currently three types of cerclage are defined: (1) history-based/prophylactic cerclage placed in patients with a history of one or more second-trimester pregnancy losses related to painless cervical dilation and in the absence of labor or abruptio placentae, or in those with a prior cerclage due to painless cervical dilation in the second trimester; (2) physical examination–based cerclage that is targeted to patients in whom painless cervical dilation is detected during physical examination in the second trimester; and (3) sonographic short cervix (less than 25 mm) in patients with a prior PTB (<34 weeks of gestation) and a current singleton pregnancy, detected <24 weeks of gestation. Women with isolated short cervix (≤15 mm) without a prior history of PTB will not benefit from cerclage.[602] The placement of cerclage has been associated with a significant reduction in the rate of preterm delivery <37, <32, <28, and <24 weeks of gestation, as well as a reduction in the composite perinatal mortality and morbidity (RR 0.64; 95% CI 0.45–0.91).[606]

Use of Fertility Treatments

The American Society of Reproductive Medicine (ASRM) has published several guidelines of which the latest in 2017[607] focuses on the transfer of a single embryo to promote reduction of the likelihood of higher-order multiple deliveries. This trend was noted in both the percentage of ART-conceived triplets and higher-order infants (from 8.9% in 2000 to 1.4% in 2015) and twins (from 44.2% in 2000 to 33.9% in 2015).[611]

Progesterone Supplementation

Prevention of Recurrent Spontaneous PTB

Administration of progestogens to prevent recurrent pregnancy losses or PTB has been a subject of investigations and meta-analyses for several decades. Two main progestogens are currently used: synthetic 17-hydroxy progesterone caproate (17-OHPC) and natural vaginal progesterone.

The NICHD MFMU network[591] conducted a multicenter double-blind, placebo-controlled trial testing the efficacy of 17-OHPC versus placebo to reduce the rate of recurrent preterm delivery in patients with a history of spontaneous PTB. Administration of 17-OHPC reduced the rate of recurrent PTB <37 weeks (RR 0.66; 95% CI 0.54–0.81), <35 weeks (RR 0.67; 95% CI 0.48–0.93), and <32 weeks (RR 0.58; 95% CI 0.37–0.91) of gestation. Additionally, treatment with 17-OHPC improved neonatal outcomes, including lower rates of NEC, IVH, and the need for supplemental oxygen.[591]

In contrast to the results in singleton gestations, the administration of 17-OHPC for the prevention of PTB in twin[640] and triplet[642] gestations had no beneficial effects.

Effect of Progesterone in Patients With a Short Cervix

An individualized risk assessment for PTB by using sonographic cervical length and other maternal risk factors, such as age, ethnicity, body mass index, cigarette smoking, and previous cervical surgery, was developed by To et al.[656] Although only a fraction of patients who eventually delivered preterm will have a short cervix in the mid-trimester, universal cervical length screening was found to be beneficial and cost effective.[658,659] Werner et al estimate that utilization of cervical length screening in the United States would save $19 million for every 100,000 women screened.[659]

The identification of patients with a short cervix at the mid-trimester is important, as it allows the employment of preventive treatments for spontaneous PTB. Indeed, patients with a short cervix may benefit from vaginal progesterone administration to reduce the rate of spontaneous PTB,[661] while some patients with a history of previous PTB whose cervix is shortened during the index pregnancy may benefit from therapeutic cervical cerclage.[191]

Randomized clinical trials[661,664-666] and meta-analyses[667-670] have demonstrated the efficacy of vaginal progesterone supplementation in women with a short cervix at the mid-trimester to prevent spontaneous PTB.[671] Fonseca et al[661] conducted a randomized clinical trial and reported that, in women with a sonographic short cervix (≤15 mm by transvaginal ultrasound between 20 and 25 weeks of gestation), daily vaginal administration of 200 mg of micronized progesterone versus placebo (safflower oil) from 24 to 34 weeks reduced the rate of PTB <34 weeks of gestation (19.2% vs 34.4%; $P = .007$). Vaginal progesterone has also been associated with a significant reduction in the rate of RDS (RR 0.39; 95% CI 0.17–0.92; $P = .03$), any neonatal morbidity or mortality event (RR 0.57; 95% CI 0.33–0.99; $P = .04$), and birthweight <1500 g (RR 0.47; 95% CI 0.26–0.85; $P = .01$).[665]

Romero et al showed that treatment with vaginal progesterone was associated with a reduction in neonatal death (RR 0.53; 95% CI 0.35–0.81), RDS (RR 0.70; 95% CI 0.56–0.89), composite neonatal morbidity and mortality (RR 0.61; 95% CI 0.34–0.98), use of mechanical ventilation (RR 0.54; 95% CI 0.36–0.81), and birthweight <1500 g (RR 0.53; 95% CI 0.35–0.8) (all moderate-quality evidence). Nevertheless, treatment with progesterone was not associated with a significant difference in the neurodevelopmental outcomes of these children at 4 to 5 years of age.[668]

Pessary Placement

The use of the Birgit Arabin pessary for the prevention of subsequent PTB in women with a symptomatic short cervix in the second trimester with singleton or twin gestations is currently not recommended.

Clinical Care Implications

The current evidence supports the following interventions for secondary prevention of PTB[643,661,675] (**Algorithm 49.2**):

1. Administration of 17-OHPC to all women with a history of prior spontaneous PTB without a short cervix.
2. Consideration of vaginal progesterone administration to any asymptomatic woman with a short cervix (<25 mm) between 16 and 24 weeks of gestation, regardless of prior PTB, due to benefits in preventing PTB.
3. Offering of an ultrasound-indicated cerclage in women with a short cervix (<25 mm) between 16 and 24 weeks and a history of previous PTB or those with progressive shortening of the cervix during this period for the prevention of recurrent PTB.
4. Consideration of cerclage placement in women with a cervical length of <15 mm at mid-trimester and a history of PTB.

LONG-TERM MATERNAL CONSEQUENCES OF PTB

The association between PTB and subsequent maternal cardiovascular disease (CVD) is well documented,[676-682] including CVD morbidity, ischemic heart disease (IHD), CVD/IHD mortality, IHD hospitalization and mortality, and CVD/cerebrovascular disease hospitalization or death.[683]

Rich-Edwards et al[685] conducted a population-based study of Norwegian birth records and demonstrated that the hazard ratio (HR) for maternal CVD postpartum declines with advancing gestation and reaches its nadir at 39 to 41 weeks of gestation.

The comparison between the effects of a single or recurrent event of premature delivery remains under debate.[679,682,686]

Rich-Edwards et al[685] demonstrated that, in comparison to spontaneous delivery at term, indicated preterm delivery carried the highest HR for subsequent maternal cardiovascular mortality (HR of 3.7; 95% CI 2.9–4.8), followed by spontaneous PTB (HR of 1.7; 95% CI 1.5–2.0).

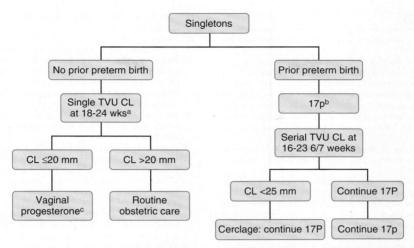

Algorithm 49.2 Algorithm of preterm birth preventive strategies. PTB, preterm birth; TVU, transvaginal ultrasound; CL, cervical length; 17P, 17 hydroxy progesterone caproid; [a]If TVU CL screening is performed. [b]17P 250 mg intramuscularly every week from 16-20 to 36 weeks. [c]eg, daily 200-mg suppository or 90-mg gel from time of diagnosis of short CL to 36 weeks.

(From Di Tommaso M, Berghella V. Cervical length for the prediction and prevention of preterm birth. *Expert Rev Obstet Gynecol.* 2013;8(4):345-355.)

KEY POINTS

- The syndrome of PTL and delivery is a leading cause for maternal and neonatal morbidity and mortality and is the result of different underlying mechanisms.
- A history of prior PTB is a leading risk factor for subsequent PTB.
- PTB is the leading cause for perinatal mortality and morbidity.
- Cervical length measurement is an effective risk assessment tool for PTB in asymptomatic women.
- The introduction of progesterone and cerclage enable secondary prevention of PTL and delivery for some patients at risk.
- Asymptomatic women with a short cervix at mid-trimester benefit from vaginal progesterone for the prevention of PTB; those with a prior PTB and a short cervix may benefit from cerclage placement.
- The use of antenatal corticosteroids, prophylactic antibiotics, and magnesium sulfate serves as tertiary preventive measures of adverse neonatal outcomes due to PTB.
- Corticosteroids are the most important intervention in women with PTL.
- Magnesium sulfate can be used for fetal neuroprotection in impending PTB prior to 34 weeks of gestation.
- Cesarean delivery can reduce neonatal morbidity and mortality in small for gestational age fetuses delivered prior to 32 weeks of gestation.
- Careful utilization of infertility treatments and the restriction of unnecessary indicated late-preterm deliveries could substantially reduce the rate of preterm deliveries.
- Meeting the universal goals of improving overall maternal and fetal health requires a joint effort of national health administrations, medical teams, and public health organizations, with management approaches tailored to the specific needs of each patient and her baby.

REFERENCES

(only references cited in synoptic print chapter; for a complete reference list, see ebook)

1. Chawanpaiboon S, Vogel JP, Moller AB, et al. Global, regional, and national estimates of levels of preterm birth in 2014: a systematic review and modelling analysis. *Lancet Glob Health.* 2019;7(1):e37-e46.
2. Institute of Medicine Committee on Understanding Premature Birth and Assuring Healthy Outcomes. The National Academies Collection: reports funded by National Institutes of Health. In: Behrman RE, Butler AS, eds. *Preterm Birth: Causes, Consequences, and Prevention.* National Academies Press (US); 2007.
3. Grosse SD, Waitzman NJ, Yang N, Abe K, Barfield WD. Employer-sponsored plan expenditures for infants born preterm. *Pediatrics.* 2017;140(4):e20171078.
4. Gotsch F, Gotsch F, Romero R, et al. The preterm parturition syndrome and its implications for understanding the biology, risk assessment, diagnosis, treatment and prevention of preterm birth. *J Matern Fetal Neonatal Med.* 2009;22(suppl 2):5-23.
5. Romero R, Espinoza J, Kusanovic JP, et al. The preterm parturition syndrome. *Br J Obstet Gynaecol.* 2006;113(suppl 3):17-42.
6. Romero R, Dey SK, Fisher SJ. Preterm labor: one syndrome, many causes. *Science.* 2014;345(6198):760-765.
7. Romero R. Prenatal medicine: the child is the father of the man. 1996. *J Matern Fetal Neonatal Med.* 2009;22(8):636-639.
8. Goldenberg RL, Culhane JF, Iams JD, Romero R. Epidemiology and causes of preterm birth. *Lancet.* 2008;371(9606):75-84.
9. American College of Obstetricians and Gynecologists' Committee on Prctice Bulletins—Obstetrics. Practice Bulletin No. 171: management of preterm labor. *Obstet Gynecol.* 2016;128(4):e155-e164.
10. Mathews TJ, MacDorman MF. Infant mortality statistics from the 2006 period linked birth/infant death data set. *Natl Vital Stat Rep.* 2010;58(17):1-31.
11. MacDorman MF, Callaghan WM, Mathews TJ, Hoyert DL, Kochanek KD. Trends in preterm-related infant mortality by race and ethnicity, United States, 1999-2004. *Int J Health Serv.* 2007;37(4):635-641.
12. Stavsky M, Mor O, Mastrolia SA, Greenbaum S, Than NG, Erez O. Cerebral palsy-trends in epidemiology and recent development in prenatal mechanisms of disease, treatment, and prevention. *Front Pediatr.* 2017;5:21.
21. Ananth CV, Getahun D, Peltier MR, Salihu HM, Vintzileos AM. Recurrence of spontaneous versus medically indicated preterm birth. *Am J Obstet Gynecol.* 2006;195(3):643-650.
24. Meis PJ, Goldenberg RL, Mercer BM, et al. The preterm prediction study: risk factors for indicated preterm births. Maternal-Fetal Medicine Units Network of the National Institute of Child Health and Human Development. *Am J Obstet Gynecol.* 1998;178(3):562-567.
26. McElrath TF, Hecht JL, Dammann O, et al. Pregnancy disorders that lead to delivery before the 28th week of gestation: an epidemiologic approach to classification. *Am J Epidemiol.* 2008;168(9):980-989.
27. World Health Organization. *Born Too Soon: The Global Action Report on Preterm Birth*; 2012.
28. Romero R, Mazor M, Munoz H, Gomez R, Galasso M, Sherer DM. The preterm labor syndrome. *Ann N Y Acad Sci.* 1994;734:414-429.
29. Blencowe H, Cousens S, Oestergaard MZ, et al. National, regional, and worldwide estimates of preterm birth rates in the year 2010 with time trends since 1990 for selected countries: a systematic analysis and implications. *Lancet.* 2012;379(9832):2162-2172.
31. Slattery MM, Morrison JJ. Preterm delivery. *Lancet.* 2002;360(9344):1489-1497.
37. Martin JA, Hamilton BE, Osterman MJK, Driscoll AK, Drake P. Births: final data for 2017. *Natl Vital Stat Rep.* 2018;67(8):1-50.
38. Martin JA, Hamilton BE, Osterman MJ, Curtin SC, Matthews TJ. Births: final data for 2013. *Natl Vital Stat Rep.* 2015;64(1):1-65.
39. Martin JA, Hamilton BE, Osterman MJK, Driscoll AK. Births: final data for 2018. *Natl Vital Stat Rep.* 2019;68(13):1-47.
40. Martin JA, Osterman MJK. Describing the increase in preterm births in the United States, 2014-2016. *NCHS Data Brief.* 2018;(312):1-8.
41. Martin JA, Hamilton BE, Osterman MJ, Driscoll AK, Mathews TJ. Births: final data for 2015. *Natl Vital Stat Rep.* 2017;66(1):1.
42. Ananth CV, Misra DP, Demissie K, Smulian JC. Rates of preterm delivery among Black women and White women in the United States

over two decades: an age-period-cohort analysis. *Am J Epidemiol.* 2001;154(7):657-665.
45. Manuck TA. Racial and ethnic differences in preterm birth: a complex, multifactorial problem. *Semin Perinatol.* 2017;41(8):511-518.
46. Collins J, David R, Simon D, Prachand N. Preterm birth among African American and white women with a lifelong residence in high-income Chicago neighborhoods: an exploratory study. *Ethn Dis.* 2007;17:113-117.
47. Simhan HN, Krohn MA. Paternal race and preterm birth. *Am J Obstet Gynecol.* 2008;198(6):644.e1-644.e6.
49. Boivin A, Luo ZC, Audibert F, et al. Risk for preterm and very preterm delivery in women who were born preterm. *Obstet Gynecol.* 2015;125(5):1177-1184.
50. Bhattacharya S, Raja EA, Mirazo ER, et al. Inherited predisposition to spontaneous preterm delivery. *Obstet Gynecol.* 2010;115(6):1125-1133.
53. Parker JD, Schoendorf KC, Kiely JL. Associations between measures of socioeconomic status and low birth weight, small for gestational age, and premature delivery in the United States. *Ann Epidemiol.* 1994;4(4):271-278.
54. Auger N, Luo ZC, Platt RW, Daniel M. Do mother's education and foreign born status interact to influence birth outcomes? Clarifying the epidemiological paradox and the healthy migrant effect. *J Epidemiol Community Health.* 2008;62(5):402-409.
55. Savitz DA, Kaufman JS, Dole N, Siega-Riz AM, Thorp JM Jr, Kaczor DT. Poverty, education, race, and pregnancy outcome. *Ethn Dis.* 2004;14(3):322-329.
56. Grjibovski A, Bygren LO, Svartbo B. Socio-demographic determinants of poor infant outcome in north-west Russia. *Paediatr Perinat Epidemiol.* 2002;16(3):255-262.
58. Donoghue D, Lincoln D, Morgan G, Beard J. Influences on the degree of preterm birth in New South Wales. *Aust N Z J Public Health.* 2013;37(6):562-567.
59. Fuchs F, Monet B, Ducruet T, Chaillet N, Audibert F. Effect of maternal age on the risk of preterm birth: a large cohort study. *PLoS One.* 2018;13(1):e0191002.
60. Fraser AM, Brockert JE, Ward RH. Association of young maternal age with adverse reproductive outcomes. *N Engl J Med.* 1995;332(17):1113-1117.
61. Kyrklund-Blomberg NB, Cnattingius S. Preterm birth and maternal smoking: risks related to gestational age and onset of delivery. *Am J Obstet Gynecol.* 1998;179(4):1051-1055.
62. Cahen-Peretz A, Sheiner E, Friger M, Walfisch A. The association between Mullerian anomalies and perinatal outcome. *J Matern Fetal Neonatal Med.* 2019;32(1):51-57.
66. Erez O, Dukler D, Novack L, et al. Trial of labor and vaginal birth after cesarean section in patients with uterine Mullerian anomalies: a population-based study. *Am J Obstet Gynecol.* 2007;196(6):537.e1-537.e11.
67. Kyrgiou M, Koliopoulos G, Martin-Hirsch P, Arbyn M, Prendiville W, Paraskevaidis E. Obstetric outcomes after conservative treatment for intraepithelial or early invasive cervical lesions: systematic review and meta-analysis. *Lancet.* 2006;367(9509):489-498.
68. Kyrgiou M, Athanasiou A, Paraskevaidi M, et al. Adverse obstetric outcomes after local treatment for cervical preinvasive and early invasive disease according to cone depth: systematic review and meta-analysis. *Br Med J.* 2016;354:i3633.
69. Kyrgiou M, Athanasiou A, Kalliala IEJ, et al. Obstetric outcomes after conservative treatment for cervical intraepithelial lesions and early invasive disease. *Cochrane Database Syst Rev.* 2017;11:CD012847.
88. Hendler I, Goldenberg RL, Mercer BM, et al. The Preterm Prediction Study: association between maternal body mass index and spontaneous and indicated preterm birth. *Am J Obstet Gynecol.* 2005;192(3):882-886.
90. Han Z, Mulla S, Beyene J, Liao G, McDonald SD. Maternal underweight and the risk of preterm birth and low birth weight: a systematic review and meta-analyses. *Int J Epidemiol.* 2011;40(1):65-101.
95. Haahr T, Ersboll AS, Karlsen MA, et al. Treatment of bacterial vaginosis in pregnancy in order to reduce the risk of spontaneous preterm delivery – a clinical recommendation. *Acta Obstet Gynecol Scand.* 2016;95(8):850-860.
96. Yudin MH, Money DM. No. 211-Screening and management of bacterial vaginosis in pregnancy. *J Obstet Gynaecol Can.* 2017;39(8):e184-e191.
98. Kurki T, Sivonen A, Renkonen OV, Savia E, Ylikorkala O. Bacterial vaginosis in early pregnancy and pregnancy outcome. *Obstet Gynecol.* 1992;80(2):173-177.

103. Hillier SL, Nugent RP, Eschenbach DA, et al. Association between bacterial vaginosis and preterm delivery of a low-birth-weight infant. The Vaginal Infections and Prematurity Study Group. *N Engl J Med.* 1995;333(26):1737-1742.

104. Meis PJ, Goldenberg RL, Mercer B, et al. The preterm prediction study: significance of vaginal infections. National Institute of Child Health and Human Development Maternal-Fetal Medicine Units Network. *Am J Obstet Gynecol.* 1995;173(4):1231-1235.

120. Vidaeff AC, Ramin SM. From concept to practice. The recent history of preterm delivery prevention. Part II: subclinical infection and hormonal effects. *Am J Perinatol.* 2006;23(2):75-84.

122. Paavonen J, Heinonen PK, Aine R, Laine S, Gronroos P. Prevalence of nonspecific vaginitis and other cervicovaginal infections during the third trimester of pregnancy. *Sex Transm Dis.* 1986;13(1):5-8.

123. Platz-Christensen JJ, Pernevi P, Hagmar B, Andersson E, Brandberg A, Wiqvist N. A longitudinal follow-up of bacterial vaginosis during pregnancy. *Acta Obstet Gynecol Scand.* 1993;72(2):99-102.

124. Sobel JD. Bacterial vaginosis. *Annu Rev Med.* 2000;51:349-356.

125. Wenman WM, Tataryn IV, Joffres MR, et al. Demographic, clinical and microbiological characteristics of maternity patients: a Canadian clinical cohort study. *Can J Infect Dis.* 2002;13(5):311-318.

126. Svare JA, Schmidt H, Hansen BB, Lose G. Bacterial vaginosis in a cohort of Danish pregnant women: prevalence and relationship with preterm delivery, low birthweight and perinatal infections. *Br J Obstet Gynaecol.* 2006;113(12):1419-1425.

127. Thorsen P, Vogel I, Molsted K, et al. Risk factors for bacterial vaginosis in pregnancy: a population-based study on Danish women. *Acta Obstet Gynecol Scand.* 2006;85(8):906-911.

128. US Preventive Services Task Force. Screening for bacterial vaginosis in pregnancy to prevent preterm delivery: US Preventive Services Task Force recommendation statement. *Ann Intern Med.* 2008;148(3):214-219.

129. Leitich H, Bodner-Adler B, Brunbauer M, Kaider A, Egarter C, Husslein P. Bacterial vaginosis as a risk factor for preterm delivery: a meta-analysis. *Am J Obstet Gynecol.* 2003;189(1):139-147.

141. American College of Obstetricians and Gynecologists' Committee on Obstetric Practice; Committee on Genetics; US Food and Drug Administration. Committee opinion No 671: perinatal risks associated with assisted reproductive technology. *Obstet Gynecol.* 2016;128(3):e61-e68.

146. Meis PJ, Michielutte R, Peters TJ, et al. Factors associated with preterm birth in Cardiff, Wales. I. Univariable and multivariable analysis. *Am J Obstet Gynecol.* 1995;173(2):590-596.

149. Szymusik I, Bartnik P, Wypych K, Kolaczkowska H, Kosinska-Kaczynska K, Wielgos M. The association of first trimester bleeding with preterm delivery. *J Perinat Med.* 2015;43(5):525-529.

151. Esplin MS, O'Brien E, Fraser A, et al. Estimating recurrence of spontaneous preterm delivery. *Obstet Gynecol.* 2008;112(3):516-523.

155. McManemy J, Cooke E, Amon E, Leet T. Recurrence risk for preterm delivery. *Am J Obstet Gynecol.* 2007;196(6):576.e1-576.e6.

156. Mercer BM, Goldenberg RL, Moawad AH, et al. The preterm prediction study: effect of gestational age and cause of preterm birth on subsequent obstetric outcome. National Institute of Child Health and Human Development Maternal-Fetal Medicine Units Network. *Am J Obstet Gynecol.* 1999;181(5 pt 1):1216-1221.

158. Romero REJ, Mazor M, Chaiworapongsa T. The preterm parturition syndrome. In: Critchley CBP, Thornton S, eds. *Preterm Birth.* RCOG Press; 2004:28-60.

159. Agrawal V, Hirsch E. Intrauterine infection and preterm labor. *Semin Fetal Neonatal Med.* 2012;17(1):12-19.

160. Burdet J, Rubio AP, Salazar AI, Ribeiro ML, Ibarra C, Franchi AM. Inflammation, infection and preterm birth. *Curr Pharm Des.* 2014;20(29):4741-4748.

161. Helmo FR, Alves EAR, Moreira RAA, et al. Intrauterine infection, immune system and premature birth. *J Matern Fetal Neonatal Med.* 2018;31(9):1227-1233.

162. Kemp MW. Preterm birth, intrauterine infection, and fetal inflammation. *Front Immunol.* 2014;5:574.

164. Park CW, Kim SM, Park JS, Jun JK, Yoon BH. Fetal, amniotic and maternal inflammatory responses in early stage of ascending intrauterine infection, inflammation restricted to chorio-decidua, in preterm gestation. *J Matern Fetal Neonatal Med.* 2014;27(1):98-105.

167. Gibbs RS, Romero R, Hillier SL, Eschenbach DA, Sweet RL. A review of premature birth and subclinical infection. *Am J Obstet Gynecol.* 1992;166(5):1515-1528.

168. Gomez R, Romero R, Galasso M, Behnke E, Insunza A, Cotton DB. The value of amniotic fluid interleukin-6, white blood cell count, and gram stain in the diagnosis of microbial invasion of the amniotic cavity in patients at term. *Am J Reprod Immunol.* 1994;32(3):200-210.

169. Oh KJ, Romero R, Park JY, Hong JS, Yoon BH. The earlier the gestational age, the greater the intensity of the intra-amniotic inflammatory response in women with preterm premature rupture of membranes and amniotic fluid infection by Ureaplasma species. *J Perinat Med.* 2019;47(5):516-527.

170. Oh KJ, Romero R, Park JY, Kang J, Hong JS, Yoon BH. A high concentration of fetal fibronectin in cervical secretions increases the risk of intra-amniotic infection and inflammation in patients with preterm labor and intact membranes. *J Perinat Med.* 2019;47(3):288-303.

171. Romero R, Avila C, Brekus CA, Morotti R. The role of systemic and intrauterine infection in preterm parturition. *Ann N Y Acad Sci.* 1991;622:355-375.

172. Romero R, Erez O, Espinoza J. Intrauterine infection, preterm labor, and cytokines. *J Soc Gynecol Investig.* 2005;12(7):463-465.

173. Romero R, Espinoza J, Gonçalves LF, Kusanovic JP, Friel L, Hassan S. The role of inflammation and infection in preterm birth. *Semin Reprod Med.* 2007;25(1):21-39.

174. Romero R, Gómez R, Chaiworapongsa T, Conoscenti G, Kim JC, Kim YM. The role of infection in preterm labour and delivery. *Paediatr Perinat Epidemiol.* 2001;15(suppl 2):41-56.

175. Romero R, Gomez-Lopez N, Winters AD, et al. Evidence that intra-amniotic infections are often the result of an ascending invasion – a molecular microbiological study. *J Perinat Med.* 2019;47(9):915-931.

176. Romero R, Shamma F, Avila C, et al. Infection and labor. VI. Prevalence, microbiology, and clinical significance of intraamniotic infection in twin gestations with preterm labor. *Am J Obstet Gynecol.* 1990;163(3):757-761.

177. Arias F, Rodriquez L, Rayne SC, Kraus FT. Maternal placental vasculopathy and infection: two distinct subgroups among patients with preterm labor and preterm ruptured membranes. *Am J Obstet Gynecol.* 1993;168(2):585-591.

178. Brosens I, Pijnenborg R, Vercruysse L, Romero R. The "Great Obstetrical Syndromes" are associated with disorders of deep placentation. *Am J Obstet Gynecol.* 2011;204(3):193-201.

179. Brosens I, Puttemans P, Benagiano G. Placental bed research. I. The placental bed: from spiral arteries remodeling to the great obstetrical syndromes. *Am J Obstet Gynecol.* 2019;221(5):437-456.

182. Kim YM, Chaemsaithong P, Romero R, et al. The frequency of acute atherosis in normal pregnancy and preterm labor, preeclampsia, small-for-gestational age, fetal death and midtrimester spontaneous abortion. *J Matern Fetal Neonatal Med.* 2015;28(17):2001-2009.

183. Kim YM, Chaemsaithong P, Romero R, et al. Placental lesions associated with acute atherosis. *J Matern Fetal Neonatal Med.* 2015;28(13):1554-1562.

184. Kovo M, Schreiber L, Bar J. Placental vascular pathology as a mechanism of disease in pregnancy complications. *Thromb Res.* 2013;131(suppl 1):S18-S21.

185. Labarrere CA, DiCarlo HL, Bammerlin E, et al. Failure of physiologic transformation of spiral arteries, endothelial and trophoblast cell activation, and acute atherosis in the basal plate of the placenta. *Am J Obstet Gynecol.* 2017;216(3):287.e1-287.e16.

186. Nijman TA, van Vliet EO, Benders MJ, et al. Placental histology in spontaneous and indicated preterm birth: a case control study. *Placenta.* 2016;48:56-62.

189. Adams Waldorf KM, Singh N, Mohan AR, et al. Uterine overdistention induces preterm labor mediated by inflammation: observations in pregnant women and nonhuman primates. *Am J Obstet Gynecol.* 2015;213(6):830.e1-830.e19.

191. Romero R, Espinoza J, Erez O, Hassan S. The role of cervical cerclage in obstetric practice: can the patient who could benefit from this procedure be identified? *Am J Obstet Gynecol.* 2006;194(1):1-9.

192. Heath VC, Southall TR, Souka AP, Elisseou A, Nicolaides KH. Cervical length at 23 weeks of gestation: prediction of spontaneous preterm delivery. *Ultrasound Obstet Gynecol.* 1998;12(5):312-317.

193. Hassan SS, Romero R, Berry SM, et al. Patients with an ultrasonographic cervical length ≤15 mm have nearly a 50% risk of early spontaneous preterm delivery. *Am J Obstet Gynecol.* 2000;182(6):1458-1467.

194. Kim CJ, Romero R, Chaemsaithong P, Kim JS. Chronic inflammation of the placenta: definition, classification, pathogenesis, and clinical significance. *Am J Obstet Gynecol.* 2015;213(4 suppl):S53-S69.

196. Holloway JA, Warner JO, Vance GH, Diaper ND, Warner JA, Jones CA. Detection of house-dust-mite allergen in amniotic fluid and umbilical-cord blood. *Lancet.* 2000;356(9245):1900-1902.

200. Allport VC, Pieber D, Slater DM, Newton R, White JO, Bennett PR. Human labour is associated with nuclear factor-kappaB activity which mediates cyclo-oxygenase-2 expression and is involved with the 'functional progesterone withdrawal'. *Mol Hum Reprod.* 2001;7(6):581-586.

201. Romero R, Mazor M, Wu YK, et al. Infection in the pathogenesis of preterm labor. *Semin Perinatol.* 1988;12(4):262-279.

203. Romero R, Sirtori M, Oyarzun E, et al. Infection and labor. V. Prevalence, microbiology, and clinical significance of intraamniotic infection in women with preterm labor and intact membranes. *Am J Obstet Gynecol.* 1989;161(3):817-824.

204. Benedetti TJ, Valle R, Ledger WJ. Antepartum pneumonia in pregnancy. *Am J Obstet Gynecol.* 1982;144(4):413-417.

205. Cunningham FG, Morris GB, Mickal A. Acute pyelonephritis of pregnancy: a clinical review. *Obstet Gynecol.* 1973;42(1):112-117.

206. Fan YD, Pastorek JG II, Miller JM Jr, Mulvey J. Acute pyelonephritis in pregnancy. *Am J Perinatol.* 1987;4(4):324-326.

207. Gilles HM, Lawson JB, Sibelas M, Voller A, Allan N. Malaria, anaemia and pregnancy. *Ann Trop Med Parasitol.* 1969;63(2):245-263.

213. Rowlands S, Danielewski JA, Tabrizi SN, Walker SP, Garland SM. Microbial invasion of the amniotic cavity in midtrimester pregnancies using molecular microbiology. *Am J Obstet Gynecol.* 2017;217(1):71.e1-71.e5.

214. Chaim W, Mazor M, Wiznitzer A. The prevalence and clinical significance of intraamniotic infection with Candida species in women with preterm labor. *Arch Gynecol Obstet.* 1992;251(1):9-15.

215. Cobo T, Palacio M, Martinez-Terron M, et al. Clinical and inflammatory markers in amniotic fluid as predictors of adverse outcomes in preterm premature rupture of membranes. *Am J Obstet Gynecol.* 2011;205(2):126.e1-126.e8.

216. Di Naro E, Cromi A, Ghezzi F, et al. Myocardial dysfunction in fetuses exposed to intraamniotic infection: new insights from tissue Doppler and strain imaging. *Am J Obstet Gynecol.* 2010;203(5):459.e1-459.e7.

217. Gomez R, Romero R, Edwin SS, David C. Pathogenesis of preterm labor and preterm premature rupture of membranes associated with intraamniotic infection. *Infect Dis Clin North Am.* 1997;11(1):135-176.

218. Horowitz S, Mazor M, Horowitz J, Porath A, Glezerman M. Antibodies to Ureaplasma urealyticum in women with intraamniotic infection and adverse pregnancy outcome. *Acta Obstet Gynecol Scand.* 1995;74(2):132-136.

219. Kacerovsky M, Musilova I, Andrys C, et al. Prelabor rupture of membranes between 34 and 37 weeks: the intraamniotic inflammatory response and neonatal outcomes. *Am J Obstet Gynecol.* 2014;210(4):325.e1-325.e10.

220. Kacerovsky M, Pliskova L, Bolehovska R, et al. The impact of the microbial load of genital mycoplasmas and gestational age on the intensity of intraamniotic inflammation. *Am J Obstet Gynecol.* 2012;206(4):342.e1-342.e8.

221. Lee SE, Romero R, Jung H, et al. The intensity of the fetal inflammatory response in intraamniotic inflammation with and without microbial invasion of the amniotic cavity. *Am J Obstet Gynecol.* 2007;197(3):294.e1-294.e6.

222. Musilova I, Andrys C, Drahosova M, et al. Intraamniotic inflammation and umbilical cord blood interleukin-6 concentrations in pregnancies complicated by preterm prelabor rupture of membranes. *J Matern Fetal Neonatal Med.* 2017;30(8):900-910.

223. Oh KJ, Lee KA, Sohn YK, et al. Intraamniotic infection with genital mycoplasmas exhibits a more intense inflammatory response than intraamniotic infection with other microorganisms in patients with preterm premature rupture of membranes. *Am J Obstet Gynecol.* 2010;203(3):211.e1-211.e8.

224. Raines DA, Wagner A, Salinas A. Intraamniotic infection and the term neonate. *Neonatal Netw.* 2017;36(6):385-387.

225. Vaisbuch E, Hassan SS, Mazaki-Tovi S, et al. Patients with an asymptomatic short cervix (≤15 mm) have a high rate of subclinical intraamniotic inflammation: implications for patient counseling. *Am J Obstet Gynecol.* 2010;202(5):433.e1-433.e8.

226. Goncalves LF, Chaiworapongsa T, Romero R. Intrauterine infection and prematurity. *Ment Retard Dev Disabil Res Rev.* 2002;8(1):3-13.

235. Giakoumelou S, Wheelhouse N, Cuschieri K, Entrican G, Howie SEM, Horne AW. The role of infection in miscarriage. *Hum Reprod Update.* 2015;22(1):116-133.

236. Gerber S, Vial Y, Hohlfeld P, Witkin SS. Detection of ureaplasma urealyticum in second-trimester amniotic fluid by polymerase chain reaction correlates with subsequent preterm labor and delivery. *J Infect Dis.* 2003;187(3):518-521.

237. Vigliani M. Chorioamnionitis and intrauterine fetal death after second-trimester amniocentesis. *Fetal Diagn Ther.* 2009;26(4):216-218.

238. Kim MJ, Romero R, Gervasi MT, et al. Widespread microbial invasion of the chorioamniotic membranes is a consequence and not a cause of intraamniotic infection. *Lab Invest.* 2009;89(8):924-936.

239. Sandu C, Folescu R, Pop E, Motoc AG. Hematogenous placental infection in acute respiratory infections. *Rom J Morphol Embryol.* 2013;54(1):157-161.

240. Payne MS, Bayatibojakhi S. Exploring preterm birth as a polymicrobial disease: an overview of the uterine microbiome. *Front Immunol.* 2014;5:595.

242. American College of Obstetricians and Gynecologists. ACOG Practice Bulletin No. 88, December 2007. Invasive prenatal testing for aneuploidy. *Obstet Gynecol.* 2007;110(6):1459.

243. Erez Y, Ben-Shushan A, Elchalal U, Ben-Meir A, Rojansky N. Maternal morbidity following routine second trimester genetic amniocentesis. *Fetal Diagn Ther.* 2007;22(3):226-228.

244. Watts DH, Krohn MA, Hillier SL, Eschenbach DA. The association of occult amniotic fluid infection with gestational age and neonatal outcome among women in preterm labor. *Obstet Gynecol.* 1992;79(3):351-357.

245. Combs CA, Gravett M, Garite TJ, et al. Amniotic fluid infection, inflammation, and colonization in preterm labor with intact membranes. *Am J Obstet Gynecol.* 2014;210(2):125.e1-125.e15.

246. DiGiulio DB, Romero R, Amogan HP, et al. Microbial prevalence, diversity and abundance in amniotic fluid during preterm labor: a molecular and culture-based investigation. *PLoS One.* 2008;3(8):e3056.

249. DiGiulio DB, Romero R, Kusanovic JP, et al. Prevalence and diversity of microbes in the amniotic fluid, the fetal inflammatory response, and pregnancy outcome in women with preterm pre-labor rupture of membranes. *Am J Reprod Immunol.* 2010;64(1):38-57.

259. Romero R, Gonzalez R, Sepulveda W, et al. Infection and labor. VIII. Microbial invasion of the amniotic cavity in patients with suspected cervical incompetence: prevalence and clinical significance. *Am J Obstet Gynecol.* 1992;167(4 pt 1):1086-1091.

260. Romero R, Kusanovic JP, Espinoza J, et al. What is amniotic fluid 'sludge'? *Ultrasound Obstet Gynecol.* 2007;30(5):793-798.

261. Romero R, Schaudinn C, Kusanovic JP, et al. Detection of a microbial biofilm in intraamniotic infection. *Am J Obstet Gynecol.* 2008;198(1):135.e1-135.e5.

262. Espinoza J, Goncalves LF, Romero R, et al. The prevalence and clinical significance of amniotic fluid 'sludge' in patients with preterm labor and intact membranes. *Ultrasound Obstet Gynecol.* 2005;25(4):346-352.

263. Kusanovic JP, Espinoza J, Romero R, et al. Clinical significance of the presence of amniotic fluid 'sludge' in asymptomatic patients at high risk for spontaneous preterm delivery. *Ultrasound Obstet Gynecol.* 2007;30(5):706-714.

270. Romero R, Quintero R, Nores J, et al. Amniotic fluid white blood cell count: a rapid and simple test to diagnose microbial invasion of the amniotic cavity and predict preterm delivery. *Am J Obstet Gynecol.* 1991;165(4 pt 1):821-830.

274. Nadeau-Vallee M, Obari D, Palacios J, et al. Sterile inflammation and pregnancy complications: a review. *Reproduction.* 2016;152(6):R277-R292.

281. Yoon BH, Romero R, Moon JB, et al. Clinical significance of intraamniotic inflammation in patients with preterm labor and intact membranes. *Am J Obstet Gynecol.* 2001;185(5):1130-1136.

287. Gomez R, Romero R, Ghezzi F, Yoon BH, Mazor M, Berry SM. The fetal inflammatory response syndrome. *Am J Obstet Gynecol.* 1998;179(1):194-202.

288. American College of Chest Physicians/Society of Critical Care Medicine Consensus Conference: definitions for sepsis and organ failure and guidelines for the use of innovative therapies in sepsis. *Crit Care Med.* 1992;20(6):864-874.

290. Sciaky-Tamir Y, Hershkovitz R, Mazor M, Shelef I, Erez O. The use of imaging technology in the assessment of the fetal inflammatory response syndrome-imaging of the fetal thymus. *Prenat Diagn.* 2015;35(5):413-419.

291. Gotsch F, Romero R, Kusanovic JP, et al. The fetal inflammatory response syndrome. *Clin Obstet Gynecol.* 2007;50(3):652-683.

292. Mastrolia SA, Erez O, Loverro G, et al. Ultrasonographic approach to diagnosis of fetal inflammatory response syndrome: a tool for at-risk fetuses? *Am J Obstet Gynecol.* 2016;215(1):9-20.

293. Romero R, Gomez R, Ghezzi F, et al. A fetal systemic inflammatory response is followed by the spontaneous onset of preterm parturition. *Am J Obstet Gynecol.* 1998;179(1):186-193.

294. Pacora P, Chaiworapongsa T, Maymon E, et al. Funisitis and chorionic vasculitis: the histological counterpart of the fetal inflammatory response syndrome. *J Matern Fetal Neonatal Med.* 2002;11(1):18-25.

295. Yoon BH, Romero R, Park JS, et al. Fetal exposure to an intra-amniotic inflammation and the development of cerebral palsy at the age of three years. *Am J Obstet Gynecol.* 2000;182(3):675-681.

296. Lee J, Romero R, Chaiworapongsa T, et al. Characterization of the fetal blood transcriptome and proteome in maternal anti-fetal rejection: evidence of a distinct and novel type of human fetal systemic inflammatory response. *Am J Reprod Immunol.* 2013;70(4):265-284.

302. Kelly R, Holzman C, Senagore P, et al. Placental vascular pathology findings and pathways to preterm delivery. *Am J Epidemiol.* 2009;170(2):148-158.

303. Lee J, Kim JS, Park J, et al. Chronic chorioamnionitis is the most common placental lesion in late preterm birth. *Placenta.* 2013;34(8):681-689.

305. Salafia CM, Lopez-Zeno JA, Sherer DM, Whittington SS, Minior VK, Vintzileos AM. Histologic evidence of old intrauterine bleeding is more frequent in prematurity. *Am J Obstet Gynecol.* 1995;173(4):1065-1070.

306. Gargano JW, Holzman CB, Senagore PK, et al. Evidence of placental haemorrhage and preterm delivery. *Br J Obstet Gynaecol.* 2010;117(4):445-455.

311. Elovitz MA, Baron J, Phillippe M. The role of thrombin in preterm parturition. *Am J Obstet Gynecol.* 2001;185(5):1059-1063.

312. Elovitz MA, Saunders T, Ascher-Landsberg J, Phillippe M. Effects of thrombin on myometrial contractions in vitro and in vivo. *Am J Obstet Gynecol.* 2000;183(4):799-804.

313. Erez O, Romer R, Vaisbuch E, et al. Changes in amniotic fluid concentration of thrombin-antithrombin III complexes in patients with preterm labor: evidence of an increased thrombin generation. *J Matern Fetal Neonatal Med.* 2009;22(11):971-982.

314. Erez O, Romero R, Vaisbuch E, et al. High tissue factor activity and low tissue factor pathway inhibitor concentrations in patients with preterm labor. *J Matern Fetal Neonatal Med.* 2010;23(1):23-33.

316. Kramer MS, Kahn SR, Rozen R, et al. Vasculopathic and thrombophilic risk factors for spontaneous preterm birth. *Int J Epidemiol.* 2009;38(3):715-723.

318. Lockwood CJ, Kayisli UA, Stocco C, et al. Abruption-induced preterm delivery is associated with thrombin-mediated functional progesterone withdrawal in decidual cells. *Am J Pathol.* 2012;181(6):2138-2148.

321. Mastrolia SA, Mazor M, Loverro G, Klaitman V, Erez O. Placental vascular pathology and increased thrombin generation as mechanisms of disease in obstetrical syndromes. *PeerJ.* 2014;2:e653.

332. Elovitz MA, Ascher-Landsberg J, Saunders T, Phillippe M. The mechanisms underlying the stimulatory effects of thrombin on myometrial smooth muscle. *Am J Obstet Gynecol.* 2000;183(3):674-681.

341. Foley JH, Conway EM. Cross talk pathways between coagulation and inflammation. *Circ Res.* 2016;118(9):1392-1408.

342. Lockwood CJ, Krikun G, Aigner S, Schatz F. Effects of thrombin on steroid-modulated cultured endometrial stromal cell fibrinolytic potential. *J Clin Endocrinol Metab.* 1996;81(1):107-112.

343. Lockwood CJ, Krikun G, Papp C, et al. The role of progestationally regulated stromal cell tissue factor and type-1 plasminogen activator inhibitor (PAI-1) in endometrial hemostasis and menstruation. *Ann N Y Acad Sci.* 1994;734:57-79.

344. Rosen T, Schatz F, Kuczynski E, Lam H, Koo AB, Lockwood CJ. Thrombin-enhanced matrix metalloproteinase-1 expression: a mechanism linking placental abruption with premature rupture of the membranes. *J Matern Fetal Neonatal Med.* 2002;11(1):11-17.

345. Han CS, Schatz F, Lockwood CJ. Abruption-associated prematurity. *Clin Perinatol.* 2011;38(3):407-421.

429. Gibson AT. Outcome following preterm birth. *Best Pract Res Clin Obstet Gynaecol.* 2007;21(5):869-882.

430. Draper ES, Manktelow B, Field DJ, James D. Prediction of survival for preterm births by weight and gestational age: retrospective population based study. *Br Med J.* 1999;319(7217):1093-1097.

435. Ray JG, Park AL, Fell DB. Mortality in infants affected by preterm birth and severe small-for-gestational age birth weight. *Pediatrics.* 2017;140(6):e20171881.

437. Gregory ECW, Drake P, Martin JA. Lack of change in perinatal mortality in the United States, 2014-2016. *NCHS Data Brief.* 2018;(316):1-8.

438. Wallace ME, Mendola P, Kim SS, et al. Racial/ethnic differences in preterm perinatal outcomes. *Am J Obstet Gynecol.* 2017;216(3):306.e1-306.e12.

440. Bottoms SF, Paul RH, Iams JD, et al. Obstetric determinants of neonatal survival: influence of willingness to perform cesarean delivery on survival of extremely low-birth-weight infants. National Institute of Child Health and Human Development Network of Maternal-Fetal Medicine Units. *Am J Obstet Gynecol.* 1997;176(5):960-966.

442. Tyson JE, Younes N, Verter J, Wright LL. Viability, morbidity, and resource use among newborns of 501- to 800-g birth weight. National Institute of child health and human development neonatal research network. *J Am Med Assoc.* 1996;276(20):1645-1651.

443. Effer SB, Moutquin JM, Farine D, et al. Neonatal survival rates in 860 singleton live births at 24 and 25 weeks gestational age. A Canadian multicentre study. *Br J Obstet Gynaecol.* 2002;109(7):740-745.

444. Ehret DEY, Edwards EM, Greenberg LT, et al. Association of antenatal steroid exposure with survival among infants receiving postnatal life support at 22 to 25 weeks' gestation. *JAMA Netw Open.* 2018;1(6):e183235.

445. Wang H, Gao X, Liu C, et al. Surfactant reduced the mortality of neonates with birth weight ⩾1500 g and hypoxemic respiratory failure: a survey from an emerging NICU network. *J Perinatol.* 2017;37(6):645-651.

446. Khashu M, Narayanan M, Bhargava S, Osiovich H. Perinatal outcomes associated with preterm birth at 33 to 36 weeks' gestation: a population-based cohort study. *Pediatrics.* 2009;123(1):109-113.

447. Vohr BR, Wright LL, Dusick AM, et al. Center differences and outcomes of extremely low birth weight infants. *Pediatrics.* 2004;113(4):781-789.

448. Manuck TA, Rice MM, Bailit JL, et al. Preterm neonatal morbidity and mortality by gestational age: a contemporary cohort. *Am J Obstet Gynecol.* 2016;215(1):103.e1-103.e14.

449. Villar J, Abalos E, Carroli G, et al. Heterogeneity of perinatal outcomes in the preterm delivery syndrome. *Obstet Gynecol.* 2004;104(1):78-87.

450. Shapiro-Mendoza CK, Tomashek KM, Kotelchuck M, et al. Effect of late-preterm birth and maternal medical conditions on newborn morbidity risk. *Pediatrics.* 2008;121(2):e223-e232.

451. Stoll BJ, Hansen NI, Bell EF, et al. Trends in care practices, morbidity, and mortality of extremely preterm neonates, 1993-2012. *J Am Med Assoc.* 2015;314(10):1039-1051.

460. Marlow N, Wolke D, Bracewell MA, Samara M. Neurologic and developmental disability at six years of age after extremely preterm birth. *N Engl J Med.* 2005;352(1):9-19.

461. Cooke RW. Perinatal and postnatal factors in very preterm infants and subsequent cognitive and motor abilities. *Arch Dis Child Fetal Neonatal Ed.* 2005;90(1):F60-F63.

462. Huddy CL, Johnson A, Hope PL. Educational and behavioural problems in babies of 32-35 weeks gestation. *Arch Dis Child Fetal Neonatal Ed.* 2001;85(1):F23-F28.

463. Saigal S, Lambert M, Russ C, Hoult L. Self-esteem of adolescents who were born prematurely. *Pediatrics.* 2002;109(3):429-433.

464. Moster D, Lie RT, Markestad T. Long-term medical and social consequences of preterm birth. *N Engl J Med.* 2008;359(3):262-273.

466. McPheeters ML, Miller WC, Hartmann KE, et al. The epidemiology of threatened preterm labor: a prospective cohort study. *Am J Obstet Gynecol.* 2005;192(4):1325-1329.

469. Gazmararian JA, Petersen R, Jamieson DJ, et al. Hospitalizations during pregnancy among managed care enrollees. *Obstet Gynecol.* 2002;100(1):94-100.

470. Vis JY, van Baaren GJ, Wilms FF, et al. Randomized comparison of nifedipine and placebo in fibronectin-negative women with symptoms of preterm labor and a short cervix (APOSTEL-I Trial). *Am J Perinatol.* 2015;32(5):451-460.

493. Westerway SC, Pedersen LH, Hyett J. Cervical length measurement: comparison of transabdominal and transvaginal approach. *Australas J Ultrasound Med.* 2015;18(1):19-26.

494. Gomez R, Romero R, Medina L, et al. Cervicovaginal fibronectin improves the prediction of preterm delivery based on sonographic cervical length in patients with preterm uterine contractions and intact membranes. *Am J Obstet Gynecol*. 2005;192(2):350-359.

495. Fuchs IB, Henrich W, Osthues K, Dudenhausen JW. Sonographic cervical length in singleton pregnancies with intact membranes presenting with threatened preterm labor. *Ultrasound Obstet Gynecol*. 2004;24(5):554-557.

496. Sotiriadis A, Papatheodorou S, Kavvadias A, Makrydimas G. Transvaginal cervical length measurement for prediction of preterm birth in women with threatened preterm labor: a meta-analysis. *Ultrasound Obstet Gynecol*. 2010;35(1):54-64.

498. Foster C, Shennan AH. Fetal fibronectin as a biomarker of preterm labor: a review of the literature and advances in its clinical use. *Biomarkers Med*. 2014;8(4):471-484.

501. Erez O, Mazor M. The role of late amniocentesis in the management of preterm parturition. *J Women's Health Care*. 2013;2:e109.

506. Romero R, Emamian M, Quintero R, et al. The value and limitations of the Gram stain examination in the diagnosis of intraamniotic infection. *Am J Obstet Gynecol*. 1988;159(1):114-119.

510. Romero R, Jimenez C, Lohda AK, et al. Amniotic fluid glucose concentration: a rapid and simple method for the detection of intraamniotic infection in preterm labor. *Am J Obstet Gynecol*. 1990;163(3):968-974.

516. Andrews WW, Hauth JC, Goldenberg RL, Gomez R, Romero R, Cassell GH. Amniotic fluid interleukin-6: correlation with upper genital tract microbial colonization and gestational age in women delivered after spontaneous labor versus indicated delivery. *Am J Obstet Gynecol*. 1995;173(2):606-612.

517. Blanchard A, Hentschel J, Duffy L, Baldus K, Cassell GH. Detection of Ureaplasma urealyticum by polymerase chain reaction in the urogenital tract of adults, in amniotic fluid, and in the respiratory tract of newborns. *Clin Infect Dis*. 1993;17(suppl 1):S148-S153.

518. Blanco JD, Gibbs RS, Malherbe H, Strickland-Cholmley M, St Clair PJ, Castaneda YS. A controlled study of genital mycoplasmas in amniotic fluid from patients with intra-amniotic infection. *J Infect Dis*. 1983;147(4):650-653.

519. Gibbs RS, Cassell GH, Davis JK, St Clair PJ. Further studies on genital mycoplasmas in intra-amniotic infection: blood cultures and serologic response. *Am J Obstet Gynecol*. 1986;154(4):717-726.

520. Gravett MG, Hummel D, Eschenbach DA, Holmes KK. Preterm labor associated with subclinical amniotic fluid infection and with bacterial vaginosis. *Obstet Gynecol*. 1986;67(2):229-237.

521. Yoneda N, Yoneda S, Niimi H, et al. Polymicrobial amniotic fluid infection with mycoplasma/ureaplasma and other bacteria induces severe intra-amniotic inflammation associated with poor perinatal Prognosis in preterm labor. *Am J Reprod Immunol*. 2016;75(2):112-125.

522. Yoon BH, Romero R, Lim JH, et al. The clinical significance of detecting Ureaplasma urealyticum by the polymerase chain reaction in the amniotic fluid of patients with preterm labor. *Am J Obstet Gynecol*. 2003;189(4):919-924.

533. Roberts D, Dalziel S. Antenatal corticosteroids for accelerating fetal lung maturation for women at risk of preterm birth. *Cochrane Database Syst Rev*. 2006;(3):CD004454.

534. Roberts D, Brown J, Medley N, Dalziel SR. Antenatal corticosteroids for accelerating fetal lung maturation for women at risk of preterm birth. *Cochrane Database Syst Rev*. 2017;3:CD004454.

543. Brownfoot FC, Gagliardi DI, Bain E, Middleton P, Crowther CA. Different corticosteroids and regimens for accelerating fetal lung maturation for women at risk of preterm birth. *Cochrane Database Syst Rev*. 2013;(8):CD006764.

545. Gyamfi-Bannerman C, Thom EA, Blackwell SC, et al. Antenatal beta-methasone for women at risk for late preterm delivery. *N Engl J Med*. 2016;374(14):1311-1320.

546. Society for Maternal-Fetal Medicine (SMFM) Publications Committee, Implementation of the use of antenatal corticosteroids in the late preterm birth period in women at risk for preterm delivery. *Am J Obstet Gynecol*. 2016;215(2):B13-B15.

548. WHO Guidelines Approved by the Guidelines Review Committee. *WHO Recommendations on Interventions to Improve Preterm Birth Outcomes*. World Health Organization; 2015.

549. National Institute for Health and Care Excellence. *Preterm Labour and Birth*. 2015. Accessed September 3, 2019. https://www.nice.org.uk/guidance/ng25

550. Committee Opinion No. 713: antenatal corticosteroid therapy for fetal maturation. *Obstet Gynecol*. 2017;130(2):e102-e109.

561. Conde-Agudelo A, Romero R. Antenatal magnesium sulfate for the prevention of cerebral palsy in preterm infants less than 34 weeks' gestation: a systematic review and metaanalysis. *Am J Obstet Gynecol*. 2009;200(6):595-609.

562. Costantine MM, Weiner SJ. Effects of antenatal exposure to magnesium sulfate on neuroprotection and mortality in preterm infants: a meta-analysis. *Obstet Gynecol*. 2009;114(2 pt 1):354-364.

563. Doyle LW, Crowther CA, Middleton P, Marret S, Rouse D. Magnesium sulphate for women at risk of preterm birth for neuroprotection of the fetus. *Cochrane Database Syst Rev*. 2009;(1):CD004661.

564. Magee LA, De Silva DA, Sawchuck D, Synnes A, von Dadelszen P. No. 376-Magnesium sulphate for fetal neuroprotection. *J Obstet Gynaecol Can*. 2019;41(4):505-522.

565. Arrowsmith S, Kendrick A, Wray S. Drugs acting on the pregnant uterus. *Obstet Gynaecol Reprod Med*. 2010;20(8):241-247.

567. Conde-Agudelo A, Romero R, Kusanovic JP. Nifedipine in the management of preterm labor: a systematic review and metaanalysis. *Am J Obstet Gynecol*. 2011;204(2):134.e1-134.e20.

568. Flenady V, Wojcieszek AM, Papatsonis DN, et al. Calcium channel blockers for inhibiting preterm labour and birth. *Cochrane Database Syst Rev*. 2014;(6):CD002255.

569. Walker KF, Thornton JG. Tocolysis and preterm labour. *Lancet*. 2016;387(10033):2068-2070.

572. Hanley M, Sayres L, Reiff ES, Wood A, Grotegut CA, Kuller JA. Tocolysis: a review of the literature. *Obstet Gynecol Surv*. 2019;74(1):50-55.

573. Reinebrant HE, Pileggi-Castro C, Romero CL, et al. Cyclo-oxygenase (COX) inhibitors for treating preterm labour. *Cochrane Database Syst Rev*. 2015;(6):CD001992.

577. Hammers AL, Sanchez-Ramos L, Kaunitz AM. Antenatal exposure to indomethacin increases the risk of severe intraventricular hemorrhage, necrotizing enterocolitis, and periventricular leukomalacia: a systematic review with metaanalysis. *Am J Obstet Gynecol*. 2015;212(4):505.e1-505. e13.

578. Vermillion ST, Scardo JA, Lashus AG, Wiles HB. The effect of indomethacin tocolysis on fetal ductus arteriosus constriction with advancing gestational age. *Am J Obstet Gynecol*. 1997;177(2):256-259.

579. Flenady V, Reinebrant HE, Liley HG, Tambimuttu EG, Papatsonis DN. Oxytocin receptor antagonists for inhibiting preterm labour. *Cochrane Database Syst Rev*. 2014;(6):CD004452.

586. Aggarwal A, Bagga R, Girish B, Kalra J, Kumar P. Effect of maintenance tocolysis with nifedipine in established preterm labour on pregnancy prolongation and neonatal outcome. *J Obstet Gynaecol*. 2018;38(2):177-184.

587. Malouf R, Redshaw M. Specialist antenatal clinics for women at high risk of preterm birth: a systematic review of qualitative and quantitative research. *BMC Pregnancy Childbirth*. 2017;17(1):51.

588. Raju TN, Mercer BM, Burchfield DJ, Joseph GF Jr. Periviable birth: executive summary of a joint workshop by the Eunice Kennedy Shriver National Institute of Child Health and Human Development, Society for Maternal-Fetal Medicine, American Academy of Pediatrics, and American College of Obstetricians and Gynecologists. *Obstet Gynecol*. 2014;123(5):1083-1096.

593. Chang HH, Larson J, Blencowe H, et al. Preventing preterm births: analysis of trends and potential reductions with interventions in 39 countries with very high human development index. *Lancet*. 2013;381(9862):223-234.

594. Howson CP, Kinney MV, McDougall L, Lawn JE. Born too soon: preterm birth matters. *Reprod Health*. 2013;10(1):S1.

595. Blencowe H, Cousens S, Chou D, et al. Born too soon: the global epidemiology of 15 million preterm births. *Reprod Health*. 2013;10(1):S2.

596. Althabe F. *Born Too Soon: The Global Action Report on Preterm Birth*. World Health Organization; 2012.

597. Newnham JP, Dickinson JE, Hart RJ, Pennell CE, Arrese CA, Keelan JA. Strategies to prevent preterm birth. *Front Immunol*. 2014;5:584.

598. Odibo IN, Bird TM, McKelvey SS, Sandlin A, Lowery C, Magann EF. Childhood respiratory morbidity after late preterm and early term delivery: a study of medicaid patients in South Carolina. *Paediatr Perinat Epidemiol*. 2016;30(1):67-75.

599. Ananth CV, Friedman AM, Gyamfi-Bannerman C. Epidemiology of moderate preterm, late preterm and early term delivery. *Clin Perinatol*. 2013;40(4):601-610.

601. ACOG Committee Opinion No. 764: medically indicated late-preterm and early-term deliveries. *Obstet Gynecol.* 2019;133(2):e151-e155.

602. To MS, Alfirevic Z, Heath VC, et al. Cervical cerclage for prevention of preterm delivery in women with short cervix: randomised controlled trial. *Lancet.* 2004;363(9424):1849-1853.

606. Berghella V, Rafael TJ, Szychowski JM, Rust OA, Owen J. Cerclage for short cervix on ultrasonography in women with singleton gestations and previous preterm birth: a meta-analysis. *Obstet Gynecol.* 2011;117(3):663-671.

607. Penzias A, Bendikson K, Butts S, et al. Guidance on the limits to the number of embryos to transfer: a committee opinion. *Fertil Steril.* 2017;107(4):901-903.

611. Sunderam S, Kissin DM, Crawford SB, et al. Assisted reproductive technology surveillance – United States, 2015. *MMWR Surveill Summ.* 2018;67(3):1-28.

629. Meis PJ, Klebanoff M, Thom E, et al. Prevention of recurrent preterm delivery by 17 alpha-hydroxyprogesterone caproate. *N Engl J Med.* 2003;348(24):2379-2385.

640. Rouse DJ, Caritis SN, Peaceman AM, et al. A trial of 17 alpha-hydroxyprogesterone caproate to prevent prematurity in twins. *N Engl J Med.* 2007;357(5):454-461.

642. Combs CA, Schuit E, Caritis SN, et al. 17-Hydroxyprogesterone caproate in triplet pregnancy: an individual patient data meta-analysis. *Br J Obstet Gynaecol.* 2016;123(5):682-690.

643. Romero R, Yeo L, Miranda J, Hassan SS, Conde-Agudelo A, Chaiworapongsa T. A blueprint for the prevention of preterm birth: vaginal progesterone in women with a short cervix. *J Perinat Med.* 2013;41(1):27-44.

656. To MS, Skentou CA, Royston P, Yu CK, Nicolaides KH. Prediction of patient-specific risk of early preterm delivery using maternal history and sonographic measurement of cervical length: a population-based prospective study. *Ultrasound Obstet Gynecol.* 2006;27(4):362-367.

658. Miller ES, Grobman WA. Cost-effectiveness of transabdominal ultrasound for cervical length screening for preterm birth prevention. *Am J Obstet Gynecol.* 2013;209(6):546.e1-546.e6.

659. Werner EF, Han CS, Pettker CM, et al. Universal cervical-length screening to prevent preterm birth: a cost-effectiveness analysis. *Ultrasound Obstet Gynecol.* 2011;38(1):32-37.

661. Fonseca EB, Celik E, Parra M, Singh M, Nicolaides KH. Progesterone and the risk of preterm birth among women with a short cervix. *N Engl J Med.* 2007;357(5):462-469.

664. Cetingoz E, Cam C, Sakallı M, Karateke A, Celik C, Sancak A. Progesterone effects on preterm birth in high-risk pregnancies: a randomized placebo-controlled trial. *Arch Gynecol Obstet.* 2011;283(3):423-429.

665. Hassan SS, Romero R, Vidyadhari D, et al. Vaginal progesterone reduces the rate of preterm birth in women with a sonographic short cervix: a multicenter, randomized, double-blind, placebo-controlled trial. *Ultrasound Obstet Gynecol.* 2011;38(1):18-31.

666. van Os MA, van der Ven AJ, Kleinrouweler CE, et al. Preventing preterm birth with progesterone in women with a short cervical length from a low-risk population: a multicenter double-blind placebo-controlled randomized trial. *Am J Perinatol.* 2015;32(10):993-1000.

667. Romero R, Nicolaides KH, Conde-Agudelo A, et al. Vaginal progesterone decreases preterm birth ≤34 weeks of gestation in women with a singleton pregnancy and a short cervix: an updated meta-analysis including data from the OPPTIMUM study. *Ultrasound Obstet Gynecol.* 2016;48(3):308-317.

668. Romero R, Conde-Agudelo A, El-Refaie W, et al. Vaginal progesterone decreases preterm birth and neonatal morbidity and mortality in women with a twin gestation and a short cervix: an updated meta-analysis of individual patient data. *Ultrasound Obstet Gynecol.* 2017;49(3):303-314.

669. Romero R, Conde-Agudelo A, Da Fonseca E, et al. Vaginal progesterone for preventing preterm birth and adverse perinatal outcomes in singleton gestations with a short cervix: a meta-analysis of individual patient data. *Am J Obstet Gynecol.* 2018;218(2):161-180.

670. Conde-Agudelo A, Romero R, Da Fonseca E, et al. Vaginal progesterone is as effective as cervical cerclage to prevent preterm birth in women with a singleton gestation, previous spontaneous preterm birth, and a short cervix: updated indirect comparison meta-analysis. *Am J Obstet Gynecol.* 2018;219(1):10-25.

671. Iams JD. Clinical practice. Prevention of preterm parturition. *N Engl J Med.* 2014;370(3):254-261.

675. Di Tommaso M, Berghella V. Cervical length for the prediction and prevention of preterm birth. *Expert Rev Obstet Gynecol.* 2013;8(4):345-355.

676. Smith GD, Whitley E, Gissler M, Hemminki E. Birth dimensions of offspring, premature birth, and the mortality of mothers. *Lancet.* 2000;356(9247):2066-2067.

677. Bonamy AK, Parikh NI, Cnattingius S, Ludvigsson JF, Ingelsson E. Birth characteristics and subsequent risks of maternal cardiovascular disease: effects of gestational age and fetal growth. *Circulation.* 2011;124(25):2839-2846.

678. Catov JM, Newman AB, Roberts JM, et al. Preterm delivery and later maternal cardiovascular disease risk. *Epidemiology.* 2007;18(6):733-739.

679. Catov JM, Wu CS, Olsen J, Sutton-Tyrrell K, Li J, Nohr EA. Early or recurrent preterm birth and maternal cardiovascular disease risk. *Ann Epidemiol.* 2010;20(8):604-609.

680. Hastie CE, Smith GC, Mackay DF, Pell JP. Maternal risk of ischaemic heart disease following elective and spontaneous pre-term delivery: retrospective cohort study of 750 350 singleton pregnancies. *Int J Epidemiol.* 2011;40(4):914-919.

681. Lykke JA, Langhoff-Roos J, Lockwood CJ, Triche EW, Paidas MJ. Mortality of mothers from cardiovascular and non-cardiovascular causes following pregnancy complications in first delivery. *Paediatr Perinat Epidemiol.* 2010;24(4):323-330.

682. Lykke JA, Paidas MJ, Damm P, Triche EW, Kuczynski E, Langhoff-Roos J. Preterm delivery and risk of subsequent cardiovascular morbidity and type-II diabetes in the mother. *Br J Obstet Gynaecol.* 2010;117(3):274-281.

683. Robbins CL, Hutchings Y, Dietz PM, Kuklina EV, Callaghan WM. History of preterm birth and subsequent cardiovascular disease: a systematic review. *Am J Obstet Gynecol.* 2014;210(4):285-297.

685. Rich-Edwards JW, Klungsoyr K, Wilcox AJ, Skjaerven R. Duration of pregnancy, even at term, predicts long-term risk of coronary heart disease and stroke mortality in women: a population-based study. *Am J Obstet Gynecol.* 2015;213(4):518.e1-518.e8.

686. Kessous R, Shoham-Vardi I, Pariente G, Holcberg G, Sheiner E. An association between preterm delivery and long-term maternal cardiovascular morbidity. *Am J Obstet Gynecol.* 2013;209(4):368.e1-368.e8.

CHAPTER 50

Prelabor Rupture of Membranes

Ali Alhousseini, Dotun Ogunyemi, Marta Szymanska, Sun Kwon Kim, and Ray Oliver Bahado-Singh

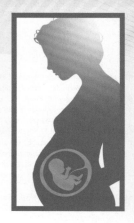

Definitions

Prelabor or premature rupture of membranes (PROM) refers to rupture of the chorioamniotic membranes before the onset of labor.[1]

Preterm PROM occurs before 37 weeks of gestation.[1] The interval between PROM and the onset of labor called the "latency period" has been proposed to last from 1 to 12 hours.[6-12] If the latency period exceeds 24 hours, it is referred to as "prolonged" PROM.[7,13,14] If PROM occurs before 23 weeks of gestation, it is referred to as "previable" PROM.[1,15] "Midtrimester" preterm PROM has been described as occurring before 28 weeks of gestation.[16] "Late preterm" PROM refers to PROM occurring after 34 and before 37 weeks of gestation.[1]

Frequency, Timing, and Site of Membrane Rupture

Site of Membrane Rupture

It is believed that spontaneous rupture of membranes (ROM) occurs at the most dependent part of the uterine cavity and in close proximity to the cervix.

Fetal Membranes and Biophysical/Biochemical Changes That Lead to PROM

The anatomic structure that includes amnion, chorion, and superficial layer of decidua represents "fetal membranes."[5,16,23]

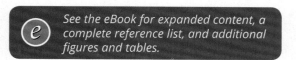

See the eBook for expanded content, a complete reference list, and additional figures and tables.

Changes in Fetal Membranes During Spontaneous Rupture

A weakening of a local area opposed to the cervix and referred to as "zone of altered morphology" (ZAM) is thought to be the site of rupture.[30-35] Causes of "altered membranes" or "changes in ZAM" are thought to include one or more biophysical or biochemical changes:

1. Increased apoptosis (programmed cell death), thinning of the trophoblast layer, and disruption of the connective tissue of the decidua[31];
2. Decrease in the density of collagen types I, III, and IV, with associated decrease in tensile strength[29];
3. Weakening of the membranes from biophysical stress related to stretch from contractions or polyhydramnios[29]; and/or
4. Biochemical changes induced by infection or bleeding (see below).

It has been proposed that two main pathophysiologic pathways lead to PROM: inflammation and oxidative stress.[36-40]

Inflammatory Pathway

Bacterial infection and sterile inflammation may lead to the production of proinflammatory cytokines, chemokines, and matrix metalloproteinases (MMPs), which damage and ultimately lead to membrane rupture.[36-38,40-43]

Oxidative Stress Pathway

A balance between antioxidants and reactive oxygen species is needed to avoid adverse outcomes such as PROM and preterm birth.[38,39]

Risk Factors for PROM

The following are risk factors linked to preterm PROM (**Algorithm 50.1**).

Previous Preterm PROM

Previous preterm PROM is a major risk factor for preterm PROM.[45-50]

Vaginal Bleeding

Vaginal bleeding is a major risk factor for preterm PROM.[44,46,47,51,52]

Possible mechanisms explaining why vaginal bleeding leads to preterm PROM are that subchorionic hematoma weakens the membrane by increasing the production of MMPs, decreasing nutrition of the amniochorion, or acting as a nidus for ascending infection.[5,53,54]

Smoking

Most studies support an association between smoking during pregnancy and preterm PROM.[5,44,46,47,50,55,56]

The risk appears to be dose dependent.[5,44,46,47,50,55,56] Women who quit smoking during pregnancy normalize their risk,[44] whereas smoking more than 10 cigarettes is a significant predictor of preterm PROM.[55,56]

Ethnicity

Women of African American origin are at increased risk for preterm PROM.[57,58]

Several studies suggested possible genetic predisposition of African American to preterm PROM.[61-64]

Sexual Intercourse

There is a controversy regarding sexual intercourse and increased risk for preterm PROM. Some studies showed increased risk if intercourse occurred within 9 days from the occurrence of preterm PROM.[49]

Other studies found no increased risk if intercourse occurred between 9 and 30 days,[66] within 1 month,[67] or at other arbitrary intervals.[44,68,69]

There is insufficient evidence to support whether sexual intercourse increases the risk of preterm PROM.

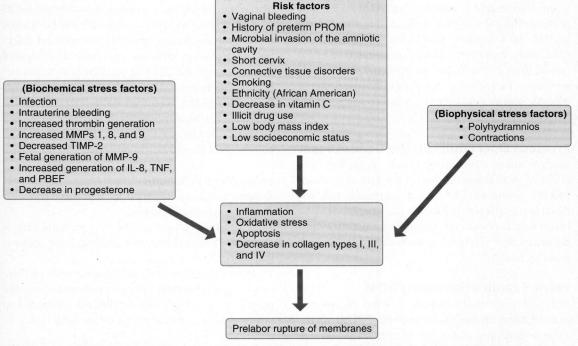

Algorithm 50.1 Risk factors for preterm PROM. IL, interleukin; MMP, matrix metalloproteinases; PBEF, pre–B-cell colony-enhancing factor; PROM, prelabor rupture of membranes; TIMP, tissue inhibitor of metalloproteinases; TNF, tumor necrosis factor.

The risk of preterm PROM may, however, be increased in women with high-risk pregnancy conditions such as cervical incompetence, preterm cervical dilation, multiple gestations, and history of preterm birth.

Vitamin C and Trace Elements

Maternal plasma concentration of less than or equal to 0.20 mg/dL was found to be associated with a higher rate of preterm PROM (14.6% [13/89]) compared to plasma concentration greater than or equal to 0.60 mg/dL (1.4% [1/69]).[74] In addition, decreased MMP activity and concentration were found in culture media in response to increased vitamin C concentrations.[75] Other studies have found decreased concentration of vitamin C in amniotic fluid of women with PROM[76] and in the fetal membranes from women with preterm PROM.[77]

Supplementation with magnesium[78] and calcium[79] was not found to be effective in preventing preterm PROM. The role of copper and zinc deficiency in PROM is not well known.[80-82]

Elevated Maternal Serum Alpha-Fetoprotein Concentration

The association of elevated maternal serum alpha-fetoprotein concentration (MSAFP) and preterm PROM has been evaluated in three studies.[83-85] Two studies found no association.[83,84] One study, however, found that elevated MSAFP (more than 2.0 multiples of median) was associated with increased risk for developing preterm PROM.[85] More evidence is needed to support this association.

Previous Operations on the Genital Tract

Studies show conflicting results regarding the effect of genital operations on the rate of preterm PROM. Some studies found increased risk for developing preterm PROM in women with a history of cervical conization and dilatation and curettage.[49,55,86] Other studies failed to show such an association.[44,86-88]

Pelvic Examinations and PROM

Although most studies report no effect of repeated examinations on the risk of preterm PROM, a reasonable position might be to minimize elective digital examinations in favor of the use of sterile speculum examination and transvaginal ultrasound as alternatives.

Colonization and Infection of the Lower Genital Tract With Selective Microorganisms

Studies support an increased risk of preterm PROM with colonization by *Chlamydia trachomatis* and *Neisseria gonorrhoeae*. There is no evidence for an increased risk for preterm PROM in colonization of the genital tract with group B streptococcus (GBS), genital mycoplasma, or the presence of bacterial vaginosis (BV) in low-risk populations.

BV and Vaginal Inflammation

Vaginal inflammation, with or without BV, appears to increase the risk of preterm PROM.[5,96,97]

The treatment of BV does not appear to be beneficial in an asymptomatic low-risk population. In high-risk populations, however, the treatment of BV may reduce the risk of preterm PROM.

Group B Streptococcus

Colonization with GBS (carrier status) is not a risk factor for spontaneous preterm delivery or preterm PROM. However, once delivery is impending, colonization is a risk factor for adverse neonatal outcomes. In patients with preterm PROM, treatment with antibiotics to prolong latency, along with GBS prophylaxis if the patient is in labor, is recommended.[100]

GBS colonization in patients with PROM is associated with increased incidence of neonatal infection, chorioamnionitis, and endometritis compared to women with PROM and negative GBS culture.[102] If a delivery is impending, treatment with antibiotics for mothers with GBS carrier status is recommended to reduce neonatal morbidity.[100] If labor arrests and delivery is no longer imminent, treatment of GBS colonization should be discontinued.[100]

Chlamydia trachomatis

Treatment is recommended for a positive endocervical *C. trachomatis* culture.

A positive culture on the first prenatal visit is associated with relative risk (RR) of 2 for preterm PROM.[104]

Positive culture of *C. trachomatis* with positive serum IgM (humoral immune response) puts the pregnancy at a high risk for PROM compared to positive culture with negative serum IgM.

Neisseria gonorrhoeae

Treatment is recommended for a positive endocervical *N. gonorrhoeae* culture. PROM is more common in women with positive culture for *N. gonorrhoeae*, than in women with negative culture. *N. gonorrhoeae* infection is associated with an increased risk of PROM[106,107] and prolonged PROM (more than 24 hours).[108]

A positive endocervical culture of *N. gonorrhoeae* is an indication for treatment even though the associated attributable risk for developing preterm PROM is unknown.

Trichomonas vaginalis

A prospective study evaluating the vaginal flora in pregnancy indicated that a positive culture of *Trichomonas vaginalis* on the first prenatal visit is associated with increased risk for developing PROM.[109]

Klebanoff et al[110] concluded that treatment of *T. vaginalis* in asymptomatic low-risk pregnant women is not recommended.

Genetic Factors

There appears to be a genetic predisposition to preterm PROM.[112-114]

Illicit Drug Use

The use of illicit drugs is a reported risk factor for preterm PROM.[116,117]

Low Body Mass Index

Low body mass index was found to be associated with preterm PROM.[44,48,117] The RR for preterm PROM in woman with low BMI (less than 19.8 kg/m^2) was 1.9 (95% confidence interval [CI] 1.3-2.8).[48]

Social Determinants of Health

Health disparities affect the risk for preterm PROM. Women who have less access to healthcare, less support for self-care, or who are under- or uninsured will have higher risk for preterm PROM.[44,116]

Biophysical and Biochemical Properties of Membranes That Rupture Prematurely

Biophysical Properties

Fetal membranes have elastic properties.[5,30,118]

Premature PROM is more likely related to acute or chronic stress factors on focal weak zones in the membrane rather than generalized weakness.[29,120-123]

Biochemical Studies

Collagen content in the fetal membranes is thought to play a major role in their tensile strength.[124,125]

Collagen breakdown is thought to play a role in the weakening and subsequent PROM.[5,124,125]

Several studies showed that PROM is associated with increased proteolytic activity.[79,124,127-145] The amniotic fluid of patients with PROM was reported to have higher proteolytic activity compared to women with intact membranes.[124] The extracellular matrix (ECM) is preserved by the maintenance of a balance between extracellular endopeptidases with MMPs and their inhibitors called tissue inhibitor of MMPs (TIMPs).[146] MMPs and TIMPs are a group of enzymes that, in concert, are responsible for the degradation of most ECM proteins during organogenesis, growth, and normal tissue turnover.[147] Increased levels of MMP-1, MMP-8,[148,149] and MMP-9[150] and decreased levels of TIMP-2[151] have been observed in the amniotic fluid of women with preterm PROM. Another protease, neutrophil elastase (NE), and its inhibitors, secretory leukocyte protease inhibitor (SLPI) and proteinase inhibitor 3, are also thought to play a role in PROM. Data indicate an increase in the concentration of NE, a decrease in the concentration of SLPI, and expression of proteinase inhibitor 3 in women with PROM[152, 153]

Romero et al[154] showed that fetuses with preterm PROM had significantly higher plasma concentration of MMP-9 compared to fetuses with preterm labor and intact membranes and proposed that the fetus may play a role in preterm PROM to speed the process of labor as a defense mechanism against insults such as infection.

Two cytokines have been evaluated in relation to PROM: pre–B-cell colony-enhancing factor (PBEF) and interleukin (IL)-8.

PBEF and IL-8 gene expression is upregulated after distension of membranes both *in vivo* and *in vitro*.[157,158] PBEF and IL-8 have been proposed to play a role against ROM, possibly through their antiapoptotic properties.[157-161]

Studies have suggested a role of increased oxidative stress and telomere reduction in PROM and preterm birth.

The specific mechanism behind a possible accelerated premature aging of fetal membranes leading to premature rupture is yet to be defined.

Compromise in the immune and mechanical properties of the fetal membranes allows for microbial invasion from the genital tract,[163] activation of the host inflammatory response leading to collagenolysis-mediated mechanical disruption,[30,164-166] and membrane weakening predisposing the membranes to preterm PROM.[23]

ROM as an Obstetrical Syndrome

Preterm PROM was classified as one of the "great obstetrical syndromes" because of the multiple pathologic processes that lead to it. Women with vaginal bleeding in the first and second trimester,[48,51,52] short cervix,[48] or positive fetal fibronectin (FFN)[48] are at increased risk for preterm PROM[82] suggesting the existence of chronic processes leading to preterm PROM.[5] The association between PROM and inflammation and infection has been well established. It has been proposed that PROM might be an adaptive response to intra-amniotic infection, as a mechanism to drain the infected amniotic cavity.[5,154] Furthermore, environmental factors, such as smoking[44] and BV,[94] have been associated with preterm PROM. These demonstrate the multiple pathologic processes and interactions that are associated with PROM justifying the categorization as an obstetrical syndrome.

Mechanisms of Disease Implicated in Preterm PROM

Intrauterine Amniotic Infection/Inflammation

Microbial invasion of the amniotic cavity (MIAC) is associated with later development of preterm PROM.[1,170] Amniotic fluid culture in the second trimester of asymptomatic pregnancies has shown that MIAC is associated with subsequent preterm PROM. The interval from time of microbial invasion to preterm PROM varied: a few hours, days or weeks.[171-173] MIAC can also occur after ROM.

Although MIAC is implicated in the development of some preterm PROM cases, not all patients demonstrate this finding.

Vascular Pathology

Bleeding in the first and second trimesters is associated with increased risk for preterm PROM.[44] Vaginal bleeding in the first and second trimester leads to separation of the chorioamnion from the decidua, thus weakening the membranes.[176] In addition, increased generation of thrombin to promote clot formation in a subchorionic bleed stimulates the release of MMPs, a further risk factor for ROM.[53,54,176-178]

Arias et al reported two common histologic lesions in the placenta of women with preterm PROM, namely vascular lesions and acute chorioamnionitis.[179] Vascular lesions reported included "failure of physiologic transformation of the spiral arteries" and atherosis.[180] These lesions are observed in other obstetrical syndromes and conditions, including preeclampsia, fetal growth restriction, abruption, and fetal death,[181] and support the inclusion of preterm PROM in this group.

Short Cervix and Uterine Cervical Pathology

Procedures affecting cervical integrity, such as conization, are associated with an elevated risk of preterm PROM.[49,55] Loss of the mucus plug may play a role in weakening the innate immune defense against ascending infection.[182-184] Cervical shortening (less than or equal to 25 mm) enhances the risk for preterm PROM (Chapter 48).[48,185,186]

Connective Tissue Disorders—Acquired or Congenital?

Acquired and genetic disorders that affect collagen synthesis and metabolism or other components of the connective tissue system may predispose women to preterm PROM. Vitamin C deficiency,[76] an affected fetus with Ehlers-Danlos syndrome,[187] and polymorphism of the MMP genes[61,63,64] are associated with increased risk for preterm PROM.

Midtrimester Fetal Heart Rate Deceleration and Subsequent Preterm PROM

Yanagihara et al[188] observed that decelerations between 24 and 27 weeks of gestation were associated with increased risk of developing preterm PROM. The subsequent occurrence of preterm PROM compared to fetuses without decelerations was 60.0% versus 37.1%, $P < .05$. The potential mechanism that would explain the association between episodic and periodic fetal heart rate deceleration in the late second and early third trimester and preterm PROM is currently unknown.

Clinical Consequences of Preterm PROM

The main consequences of preterm PROM are spontaneous preterm birth (Chapter 49), maternal and fetal infection (Chapter 39), placental abruption (Chapter 47), the oligohydramnios sequence, fetal death (Chapters 1 and 4), and maternal death.

Preterm Labor and Delivery

Preterm birth is the number one cause of neonatal morbidity and mortality,[189-192] and the most common consequence of preterm PROM is preterm delivery.[193-195]

Latency duration is inversely related to the gestational age at ROM.

Infection

Preterm PROM increases the risk of maternal, fetal, and newborn infection.[193-195] However, most women with MIAC do not have clinical evidence of infection[198] (**Table 50.1**).

What Is the Prevalence of MIAC in PROM?

Based on fluid culture, 32% (473/1462) of women with preterm PROM have MIAC,[174] whereas 34% (11/32) of women with term PROM have MIAC.[199] However, the prevalence of MIAC is likely higher than what has been reported due to two primary limitations of testing. First, use of standard bacterial culture techniques, as opposed to molecular techniques such as polymerase chain reaction (PCR), may not capture as many species and, thus, not reflect true microbial yield of fluid samples.[200,201] Second, amniocentesis is performed less frequently on women with preterm PROM in labor or in women with low amniotic fluid volume; however, these groups have a higher probability of MIAC.[202-204]

What Microorganisms Are Typically Isolated in Women With MIAC?

The most common microorganisms isolated from preterm and term PROM are genital mycoplasmas (*Ureaplasma urealyticum* and *Mycoplasma hominis*).[5,175,206-208] Other commonly isolated bacteria include GBS, *Fusobacterium* species, and *Gardnerella*

Table 50.1 Frequently Asked Questions and Answers: Infection and PPROM

Question	Answer	References
What is the prevalence of MIAC in PPROM?	34% (by culture)	174,199-201
Factors associated with increased prevalence of MIAC	Low amniotic fluid volume, earlier onset of labor (decreased latency duration)	175,202-205
What are the most common isolated microorganisms?	*Ureaplasma urealyticum, Mycoplasma hominis,* GBS, *Fusobacterium species, Gardnerella vaginalis*	5,175,206-208
Does an amniotic fluid microbiota exist in normal pregnancy?	Currently, there is no evidence	209
Consequences of MIAC	Neonatal sepsis, respiratory distress syndrome, chorioamnionitis, and endometritis	137,175,205-208, 210-213
Can intra-amniotic infection resolve without treatment?	No	175
Does antibiotic administration prevent or eradicate MIAC?	No	214,215
Can the fetus be infected *in utero*? Does this influence the latency period?	Yes. Positive fetal blood culture is associated with shorter latency period	175,216
Can the fetus mount an inflammatory response to MIAC?	Yes	37,41,154,217
Can MIAC occur before rupture of membranes?	Yes, 29%-48% of women with PPROM shortly before the onset of labor had histologic chorioamnionitis	66
Can MIAC be a consequence of PPROM?	Yes, 50% of women with PPROM and not in labor who had initial negative amniotic fluid culture had a positive culture when in labor	66,175
Is MIAC associated with histologic chorioamnionitis?	Yes	218,219

GBS, group B streptococcus; MIAC, microbial invasion of the amniotic cavity; PPROM, preterm prelabor rupture of membranes.

vaginalis in patients with preterm PROM,[5,175,206-208] and *Peptostreptococcus, Lactobacillus, Bacteroides,* and *Fusobacterium* species in patients with term PROM.[199] In addition, 26.7% (43/161) of women with preterm PROM have polymicrobial infection.[175,205-207,210-212] When quantitative microbiology has been performed, 23% (6/26) had an inoculum size greater than 10^5 colony-forming units/mL.[205]

Does an Amniotic Fluid Microbiota Exist in Normal Pregnancy?

Currently, there is no evidence for the existence of microbiota in the amniotic fluid of normal pregnancies.[209] Limitations of studies evaluating the existence of microbiota in potential low biomass locations, such as the amniotic cavity and the placenta, include the presence of bacterial DNA signal in reagents, need for appropriate technical controls, and the challenges of avoidance of contamination by the vaginal microbiota and the skin.[201,224-229] In addition, amniotic fluid has an innate immune ability against bacterial invasion and thus can suppress bacterial culture beyond measurable levels.[220-223]

What Are the Consequences of MIAC?

Infectious complications in preterm PROM include neonatal sepsis, chorioamnionitis, and endometritis. These are more common in women with MIAC compared to women without MIAC.[137,175,205-208,210-213] Neonates born to pregnancies complicated by preterm PROM with MIAC are more likely to develop respiratory distress syndrome (RDS) compared to pregnancies complicated with preterm PROM without MIAC.[212]

Is Microbial Invasion Related to the Onset of Labor in Preterm PROM?

The onset of labor in preterm PROM is associated with MIAC.

Patients with preterm PROM who showed up in labor had MIAC more frequently compared to women with preterm PROM who were not in labor.

Are There Differences in the Inoculum Size and Types of Organisms in Women in Labor Versus Those Not in Labor With Preterm PROM and MIAC?

Romero et al also showed that 55% (10/18) of women with preterm PROM who were in labor on

admission had a colony count higher than 10^5, compared to 23% (6/26) of women with preterm PROM without labor on admission ($P < .05$).[175]

The rate of polymicrobial infection was not different between the two groups.[175] Isolated *Mycoplasma* MIAC was less common in women with preterm PROM in labor (8%) compared to women not in labor (20%) on admission.[175]

Does Antibiotic Administration to Patients With Preterm PROM Prevent Subsequent Microbial Invasion or Eradicate Existing Infection at the Time of Initiation of Treatment?

The current standard of care of women with preterm PROM includes a 1-week course of antibiotics (ampicillin plus erythromycin) to prolong latency duration.[1]

However, evidence supporting the benefits of treating pregnant women complicated by MIAC with antibiotics is limited. Antibiotic treatment in women with preterm PROM with a positive amniotic fluid culture does not necessarily prevent or eradicate MIAC.

Can the Fetus Mount an Inflammatory Response to MIAC?

The fetal inflammatory response syndrome (FIRS) is characterized by elevated IL-6 levels in the fetal blood, as measured by cordocentesis, and is associated with severe neonatal morbidity[41] and shorter delivery timing.[230,231] FIRS has been observed in fetuses with preterm labor with intact membranes, preterm PROM, and fetal viral infections such as cytomegalovirus.[37] FIRS is a risk factor for short-term perinatal morbidity and mortality after adjustment for gestational age at delivery and for the development of long-term sequelae such as bronchopulmonary dysplasia (BPD) and brain injury.[37] In addition, FIRS increases fetal plasma concentrations of MMP-9,[154] which is thought to play a role in preterm PROM. Funisitis (inflammation of the umbilical cord) is a histologic manifestation of fetal inflammation[217] and is associated with increased risk for neonatal sepsis.[217]

MIAC: Cause or Consequence of PROM

MIAC can be a cause of PROM.

MIAC can also be a consequence of preterm PROM.

Correlation Between MIAC and Histologic Chorioamnionitis

Histologic chorioamnionitis is highly correlated with positive amniotic fluid culture and adverse neonatal outcomes.[218,219]

Abruptio Placentae

Abruptio placentae occurs more frequently in patients with preterm PROM compared to preterm labor with intact membranes.[233-235]

The exact mechanism of the increased occurrence of abruptio placentae in women with preterm PROM is not well defined.

Pulmonary Hypoplasia

Pulmonary hypoplasia is characterized by the poor development of fetal lung cells and airways and is associated with significant neonatal morbidity and mortality.[240] Gestational age at the time of ROM is an independent risk factor for the development of pulmonary hypoplasia.[213,240-243] The frequency of pulmonary hypoplasia with preterm PROM before 28 weeks is around 12% to 28% based on three studies.[213,240,242] The risk of pulmonary hypoplasia approaches 50% at 19 weeks and decreases to around 10% at 25 weeks.[240]

Fetal Compression Syndrome

Fetal compression is a complication of decreased amniotic fluid. It is characterized by limb and craniofacial deformities.[243,244] Two studies reported significant risk of compression deformities (12% and 46%) after 4 weeks of latency between PROM and delivery, whereas no deformities occurred if latency was less than 9 days.[245,246]

Fetal Growth Restriction

Few studies observed an association between preterm PROM and fetal growth restriction.[247-249] Additional studies would be useful for determining whether a significant relationship exists.

Fetal Death

The cause of the increased fetal death in preterm PROM may be related to cord accidents, abruption, infection, or fetal growth restriction. The rate of fetal death depends on the gestational age of occurrence of preterm PROM. The rate of fetal death is 15% when PROM occurs before 24 weeks and is 1% when PROM occurs after 24 weeks.[24]

Maternal Death

The prevalence of maternal death associated with PROM was 0.03% (1/3400) in 1982.[250] It improved from 0.2% in 1959.[251]

Diagnosis of PROM

Presenting Symptoms

The most common presentation of PROM is a leakage of fluid through the vagina or watery discharge. The timing of the initial leakage, odor, color, and consistency are useful characteristics that inform the clinician regarding latency duration, risk for infection, and other possible diagnoses such as loss of the mucus plug, cervicovaginal infection, leukorrhea, passage of meconium, intra-amniotic bleeding, and urinary incontinence.

Vaginal Examination

A sterile speculum examination allows for the visualization of a vaginal pool or obvious leakage of fluid from the cervix into the posterior fornix. Valsalva maneuver may assist in the visualization of this sign. Additionally, a speculum examination allows for collection of fluid for "nitrazine" and "ferning" tests, vaginal and cervical cultures, cervical dilation assessment, and ruling out prolapsed cord.

Arborization or ferning occurs when amniotic fluid is put on a slide and allowed to dry for at least 10 minutes (**Figure 50.2**).[252,253] The overall accuracy of this method is 95%.[254] Semen, cervical mucus, or fingerprints may lead to false-positive results.[255,256] Blood and try swabs can lead to false-negative results in 5% to 10% of cases.[253,257,258]

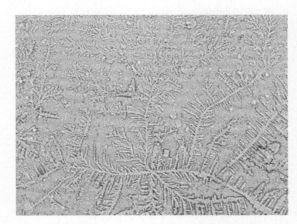

Figure 50.2 Arborization or ferning occurs when amniotic fluid is put on a slide and allowed to dry for at least 10 minutes.

Biochemical Markers Rapid Tests

Nitrazine paper changes color from yellow to blue when exposed to an alkaline pH > 7.0. The pH of amniotic fluid is around 7.0 to 7.5, whereas normal vaginal pH is 4.5 to 5.5. The accuracy of nitrazine paper in the diagnosis of PROM has been reported to be around 93.3% with up to a 10% false-negative rate.[254,259] Factors leading to false-positive nitrazine tests (range 1%-17%) include blood, semen, alkaline urine, or vaginal discharge due to BV or *Trichomonas* infection.[259]

PROM status is equivocal in 10% to 20% of women evaluated.

Noninvasive tests, using a simple dipstick, have been developed based on the detection of a specific compound found in amniotic fluid, with high sensitivity rates with low false-positive results being reported.

Insulin-like growth factor-binding protein-1 (IGFBP-1) is an excreted protein synthesized in the decidual cells and fetal liver and detected in amniotic fluid throughout pregnancy. The concentration of IGFBP-1 in amniotic fluid is 10,500 to 350,000 μg/L, whereas the concentration in maternal blood is 29 to 300 μg/L. The threshold for a positive test is >25 μg/L. Results are available in 5 minutes.[260]

The concentration of placental alpha macroglobulin-1 in amniotic fluid is 2000 to 25,000 ng/mL, whereas the concentration in maternal blood is 2.5 to 12.5 ng/mL. The threshold for a positive test is >5 ng/mL. Results are read in around 10 minutes.[260]

Other potential biochemical tests for the diagnosis of PROM include FFN, which is most commonly used for the identification of patients at risk of preterm labor and imminent delivery. The diagnostic value of FFN in PROM is less known.[261]

A false-positive FFN may be related to small amniotic fluid leakage that would be missed by traditional approach (pool, nitrazine, and ferning) or due to the release of FFN into the posterior fornix prior to the onset of labor. Positive FFN may indicate impending labor prior to ROM. Women without PROM and with positive FFN are more likely to delivery within 72 hours compared to women with negative FFN.[261,263-270] In other words, the detection of cervicovaginal FFN is not specific for PROM.

Amniotic Fluid Sampling from Vaginal Secretions

Collecting vaginal fluid facilitates the noninvasive sampling of amniotic fluid from vaginal secretions, which enables daily measurements and bedside assessment of cytokines, which is an advantage over the invasive amniocentesis.[271]

Transabdominal Dye Injection

When the diagnosis of preterm PROM is not clear, a transabdominal injection of dye (indigo carmine, Evans blue, fluorescein) into the amniotic cavity may be used for confirmation.[273-276]

Methylene blue should not be used as it may cause fetal methemoglobinemia.[277-279] A tampon in the vagina can document subsequent leakage dye in cases of PROM. The test is considered positive when the blue color can be visualized on the tampon within 30 minutes after injection.[17] Maternal urine may also turn blue and should not be confused with amniotic fluid.

Initial Assessment of Patients Presenting With Preterm PROM

INITIAL EVALUATION OF PROM

- Accurate assessment of gestational age
- Exclusion of cord prolapse
- Estimation of fetal weight and presentation
- Evaluation of the risk of infection
- Assessment of fetal well-being

Ultrasound in the Evaluation of Patients With Preterm PROM

The initial ultrasound examination aims to (1) assess fetal viability, biometry, and presentation; (2) quantify amniotic fluid volume; (3) rule out fetal anomalies if not previously performed; and (4) confirm gestational age. The reduced amniotic fluid volume and shadowing from fetal body parts limit the optimal visualization of the fetus. In women with PROM, fetal sonographic biometry underestimated true birth weight.[280-282]

Diagnosis of Intrauterine Infection in Preterm PROM

Amniocentesis

Amniocentesis is used for the evaluation of the microbiological status of the amniotic cavity and of fetal lung maturity in the patient with preterm PROM.[283] Results of amniotic fluid analysis provide a rational basis for the subsequent management of preterm PROM. Patients without evidence of infection/inflammation and lung immaturity could be managed expectantly, whereas those with evidence of infection could be managed using algorithms tailored to the gestational age (see section on Management).

The success rate of amniotic fluid retrieval by transabdominal amniocentesis varies from 49% to 96%.[170,175,210,212,284-287] The wide disparity in retrieval rates is probably attributable to differences in practice among institutions.

The traditional analyses of amniotic fluid used to detect the presence of MIAC or intra-amniotic inflammation include the following: (1) Gram stain; (2) quantitative white blood cell (WBC) count; (3) glucose concentration; and (4) microbial cultures for aerobic and anaerobic bacteria. Lower concentrations of glucose in amniotic fluid (<10 mg/dL) can serve as an additional marker for MIAC. The results of amniotic fluid culture may take days to be reported. Therefore, most centers rely on the determination of intra-amniotic inflammation because the outcome of preterm PROM in patients with intra-amniotic inflammation is similar to that in patients with MIAC proven with standard microbiological techniques.[289]

Genital mycoplasma culture and IL-6 concentration measurement improve detection of MIAC. Patients with a negative Gram stain (read by experienced personnel) and a high WBC count (more than 30 cells/μL) are at high risk of having microbial invasion with genital mycoplasmas,[290] which are not visible on Gram stain examination. Amniotic fluid IL-6 performed best in detecting MIAC, as well as in identifying patients at risk of impending preterm delivery and neonatal complications.[208] Amniotic fluid concentrations of IL-6 more than 17 ng/mL have been shown to be a sensitive test for the prospective diagnosis of acute histologic chorioamnionitis (a sensitivity of 79% [23/29] and specificity of 100% [21/21]), significant neonatal morbidity (sepsis, RDS, pneumonia, intraventricular hemorrhage, BPD, and necrotizing enterocolitis), and neonatal mortality (a sensitivity of 69% [18/26] and specificity of 79% [19/24]).[291] Other rapid tests reported for the detection of MIAC include amniotic fluid catalase,[292] alpha$_1$-antitrypsin,[137] limulus amebocyte lysate test,[293] and bacterial PCR.[294]

The risk of amniocentesis, when performed by experienced individuals, appears to be extremely low.

Ultrasound

Biophysical profile (BPP) has been used for the assessment of subclinical intra-amniotic infection. BPP test scores of 6 or less have been demonstrated to correlate with perinatal infection, with high sensitivity and specificity according to some authors.[41,297,298] However, evidence supporting the BPP as a predictor of infections is currently limited and has led to questions about its clinical use for predicting chorioamnionitis and FIRS, especially in cases of PROM.

Ultrasound findings of thymus transverse diameter measurement have recently been shown to be superior to BPP in the diagnosis of chorioamnionitis.

Advanced Sonographic Imaging

Advanced sonographic modality imaging has been described in the diagnosis of FIRS.[300]

Sonographic identification of functional and anatomical changes associated with FIRS has been reported in the heart, thymus, kidney, adrenal glands, and spleen of these fetuses.[300]

Functional echocardiographic changes associated with FIRS include a higher E/A ratio, higher velocity time integral, increased Tei index, and inverted and positive peak systolic strain and strain rate.[300] These changes are hypothesized to be due to left ventricular dysfunction. Other advanced sonographic findings associated with FIRS include decreased thymus volume, pulsatile flow in the splenic vein, and increased adrenal gland volume.[300]

Magnetic Resonance Imaging

The development of advanced magnetic resonance imaging (MRI) techniques now enables assessment of cortical folding and subtle white matter injury in the fetus. Such information about brain development may be useful with regard to the timing of delivery or therapeutic interventions such as magnesium and corticosteroid therapy. MRI may also aid in the diagnosis of pulmonary hypoplasia with PROM.

Measurements of thymic volume using MRI have also been shown to be feasible.[304]

Assessment of Fetal Well-Being

The current methods of fetal surveillance include fetal movement counts, nonstress test, and BPP or the modified BPP.

The optimal frequency or the effectiveness of different fetal assessment methods in improving neonatal and maternal outcomes is uncertain.

Management of Patients with Preterm PROM

Algorithm 50.2 provides a summary of the management strategy for patients with preterm PROM.

Does a Digital Examination Increase the Risk of Infection?

The traditional view has been that "once a cervical digital examination has been performed, the clock of infection starts to tick." The major objection to a digital examination in the setting of PROM is that it may unnecessarily increase the risk of ascending infection, and the information it provides can be obtained by sterile speculum examination.[332]

The only justification for performing a digital examination is to determine cervical status. In preterm gestation, this information rarely alters clinical management, but, in term gestation, cervical state may be a factor influencing decisions regarding induction. There is a strong relationship between the results of sterile speculum examination and digital examination of the cervix.

Preterm PROM in Maternal Genital Herpes Infection

Preterm PROM in the face of a maternal genital herpes infection represents challenging obstetric problem.

If active disease or prodromal symptoms are present at the onset of labor or when delivery is indicated, cesarean delivery is recommended.[1] Management of preterm PROM with primary HSV infection is more of a dilemma because of the increased risk of vertical transmission.

Preterm PROM in Maternal HIV Infection

Even though the duration of membrane rupture in labor correlates with risk of transmission of human immunodeficiency virus (HIV) to the newborn, there is no correlation with risk of vertical transmission in patients who receive highly active antiretroviral therapy, have a low viral load, and receive antepartum and intrapartum zidovudine. Women with HIV infection and preterm PROM should be managed in collaboration with a physician with expertise in HIV. Expectant management may be appropriate in cases with early gestational age, and low viral load on antiretroviral therapy. The American College of Obstetricians and Gynecologists (ACOG) concludes that the optimal

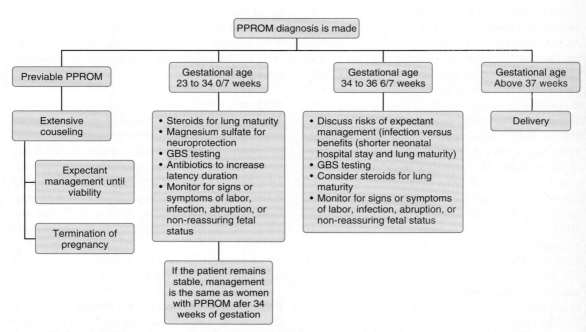

Algorithm 50.2 Management of pregnancies complicated by PPROM. GBS, group B streptococcus; PPROM, preterm prelabor rupture of membranes.

management of the patient with HIV and preterm PROM is uncertain because there are inadequate data from patients with prolonged rupture of the membranes.[1]

Previable PROM (<24 Weeks of Gestation)

The major complications of previable PROM are maternal infection, abruption, late abortion, delivery of a previable neonate, low neonatal survival rate due to sequelae of prematurity and/or pulmonary hypoplasia, deformation sequence, cord compression, neonatal sepsis, and a high risk of neurologic handicap.[341,342] Pregnancy termination is an option because of the high risk of fetal loss/severe morbidity coupled with the risk of maternal sepsis. Management of these patients requires an in-depth discussion involving the parents, neonatologists, obstetricians, and maternal-fetal medicine subspecialists with careful documentation in the medical record.

If the patient opts for expectant management, outpatient management is considered safe if the patient is stable with no evidence of infection. Outpatient monitoring is performed with the patient returning to the hospital if signs and symptoms of infection, labor, or abruption emerge. Once pregnancy reaches viability, she is admitted to hospital. Most studies of antibiotic prophylaxis with preterm PROM enrolled patients at or after 24 0/7 weeks of gestation, and there are no adequate data to assess the risks and benefits of antibiotic treatment at earlier gestational ages. ACOG practice bulletin[343] suggests that it is reasonable to offer a course of antibiotics for pregnancy prolongation to patients with previable PROM >20 weeks who choose expectant management. Antenatal corticosteroid administration, magnesium sulfate for neuroprotection, and GBS intrapartum antibiotics prophylaxis can be all be considered at 23 0/7 weeks and are recommended at 24 0/7 weeks. Tocolysis is not recommended. Cesarean delivery for fetal indication may be considered at 23 to 24 weeks, but the earliest it is recommended is at 25 0/7 weeks. None of the latter obstetrical interventions is recommended prior 23 0/7 weeks.[343]

Midtrimester ROM After Amniocentesis

Leakage of amniotic fluid after second-trimester amniocentesis should be considered as a separate entity from previable PROM. It occurs in 1.2% of patients and is usually transient in nature.[344] The risk of delayed PROM in these cases is no different from that in the general population.[345] Reaccumulation of normal amniotic fluid volume with favorable outcomes is expected.

Preterm PROM

The management goals of preterm PROM include the following: (1) excluding intra-amniotic infection/inflammation and fetal compromise and (2) instituting expectant management in patients without documented infection/inflammation or fetal compromise. Initial evaluation of the patient with preterm PROM should include an assessment of intra-amniotic infection (eg, presence of fever, uterine tenderness, purulent lochia, and maternal or fetal tachycardia), evaluation for active labor, and determination of fetal position and fetal well-being.

When Is Delivery Recommended for the Preterm Fetus in the Presence of PROM?

In a clinically stable patient with preterm PROM with reassuring maternal and fetal status, the decision regarding planned delivery versus expectant management has to be considered. The patient and family have to be counseled about the benefits and potential risks. Current consensus is that patients with PROM between 24 0/7 weeks and 34 0/7 weeks of gestation are managed expectantly if no maternal or fetal contraindications exist. The management of preterm PROM at greater than 34 0/7 weeks of gestation is more controversial. The ACOG[1] indicates that the optimal gestational age for delivery is unclear and controversial. They recommend that at 34 0/7 weeks of gestation or greater, delivery or expectant management may be considered for pregnancies complicated by preterm PROM.

If expectant management is continued beyond 34 0/7 weeks of gestation, the balance between benefits and risks should be carefully considered and discussed with the patient, and expectant management should not extend beyond 37 0/7 weeks of gestation. Likewise, the Royal College of Obstetricians and Gynecologists guidelines suggest that at 34 or 35 weeks of gestation, either planned delivery or expectant management could be considered in a shared care decision model.[347]

Intra-Amniotic Infection/Inflammation and its Management

The ACOG[356] has defined isolated maternal fever as a single oral temperature >39.0°C or two readings of an oral temperature of 38.0°C to 38.9°C that are 30 minutes apart. Suspected intra-amniotic infection is based on clinical criteria of maternal intrapartum fever and one or more of maternal leukocytosis, purulent cervical drainage, or fetal tachycardia. Confirmed intra-amniotic infection is based on a positive amniotic fluid test (Gram stain, glucose level, positive culture) or placental pathology with histologic evidence of infection or inflammation. The ACOG does contend that isolated maternal temperature >39.0°C be included in the suspected intra-amniotic infection group.

Clinical chorioamnionitis is an indication for delivery.[1] Intrapartum antibiotics also have been shown to decrease maternal febrile morbidity and length of hospital stay.[356] Induction of labor is recommended if there is no contraindication to vaginal delivery. Because of the association between dysfunctional labor and intra-amniotic infection,[356] careful labor monitoring is required.

General Management, Monitoring and Tocolysis

In all patients with preterm PROM, confirmation of dating and gestational age, ultrasound to assess estimated fetal weight and to rule out any gross fetal anomaly, and determination of fetal position and amniotic fluid volume are indicated. Initial electronic fetal heart rate and uterine activity monitoring is also indicated. The presence of regular contractions might indicate the onset of labor, which would require more intensive management and potential transfer to the labor and delivery unit. The use of tocolysis in the setting of preterm PROM is controversial.[1] Tocolysis is associated with prolongation of the latency period with an increased risk of chorioamnionitis and without significant maternal or neonatal benefits.[1]

Abruption and nonreassuring fetal status are indications for delivery.[1] GBS culture is recommended with intrapartum antibiotic prophylaxis to be initiated if the result is positive.

"Prophylactic" Antibiotic Administration

Antibiotic treatment aimed at the eradication of intra-amniotic infection should not be confused with prophylactic treatment, which is the standard of care for patients with preterm PROM, regardless of whether the inflammatory/infection state of the amniotic fluid is known. Patients between 23 and 34 weeks of gestational age without evidence of infection and inflammation are given prophylactic treatment with antibiotics. Antimicrobial therapy may prolong pregnancy by controlling microbial growth in a patient with existing MIAC and preventing secondary infection/inflammation because one-third of women with preterm PROM have a positive amniotic culture.

The ACOG suggests a 7-day course of therapy with a combination of intravenous ampicillin and erythromycin followed by oral amoxicillin and erythromycin.[1]

Should Corticosteroids Be Administered to Patients With Preterm PROM Remote From Term?

Over the decades, many studies have confirmed the benefits of antenatal corticosteroid therapy in neonates born preterm, including those with PROM.[358-360] A single course of corticosteroids is recommended for pregnant women between 24 0/7 weeks and 34 0/7 weeks of gestation and may be considered for pregnant women as early as 23 0/7 weeks of gestation who are at risk of preterm delivery within 7 days.[1,360] There is no evidence that a single course of antenatal corticosteroids is associated with increased risks of maternal or neonatal infection.[343]

However, repeat or rescue dose of corticosteroids in patients with PROM is controversial, and the ACOG states that there is insufficient evidence to recommend for or against this practice.[361]

Magnesium Sulfate for Fetal Neuroprotection in Patients With Preterm PROM

Based on a meta-analysis suggestion that prenatal administration of magnesium sulfate reduces the occurrence of cerebral palsy (RR 0.71, 95% CI 0.55-0.91).[362] to reduce the risk of cerebral palsy, the ACOG recommended the consideration of magnesium sulfate for neuroprotection before 32 weeks of gestation.[1] The recommendation for one dose for neuroprotection is as follows: 4 or 6 g as initial bolus for 20 to 30 minutes, followed by a maintenance dose of 1 to 2 g hourly for up to 24 hours.[361]

The expectant management of preterm PROM comprises (1) accelerating fetal lung maturity and improving neonatal outcomes through the administration of corticosteroids[363]; (2) therapeutic or prophylactic antibiotic administration[364,365]; (3) maternal and fetal inpatient surveillance in a tertiary medical center; and (4) magnesium sulfate for neuroprotection.

Is It Necessary to Remove a Cervical Cerclage in a Patient Who Presents With Preterm PROM?

Due to the scarcity of available studies, optimal management is controversial. Leaving the cerclage in place has been suggested to prolong pregnancy, although removing the cerclage in the presence of preterm PROM suggests a reduction in risk of infection-related complications.[366] The ACOG considers either removal or retention of cerclage as reasonable.[1]

Home Care Versus Hospital Care

The ACOG does not recommend outpatient management of preterm PROM with a viable fetus as safety has not been established through a sufficient amount of studies.[1] Home care carries the risk of delivering a preterm infant away from a tertiary center and delay in obstetric intervention if fetal distress or infection occurs. Advantages of home care include psychological benefits to the patient and decreased costs. However, the ACOG states that, because the fetus is at an increased risk of umbilical cord compression and infection may present suddenly due to frequently brief latency, hospitalization with surveillance of both the woman and her fetus is recommended once viability has been reached.[1] To date, the data collected are insufficient to recommend the outpatient management of preterm PROM with a viable fetus.[369,370]

The Role of Amnioinfusion in Preterm PROM

Amnioinfusion can potentially be of benefit by restoring the amniotic fluid volume, thereby cushioning the fetus to prevent mechanical compression of the umbilical cord and reducing fetal heart rate changes. Fetal lung hypoplasia in preterm PROM may be prevented by enabling normal amniotic fluid flow into the fetal lungs and preventing mechanical compression of the fetal thorax, which may theoretically prevent postural deformities. Furthermore, the infusion of fluid may prevent intrauterine infection, perhaps by the diluent effect on bacterial concentration, or the antibacterial effects of the infusions. Following amnioinfusion for preterm PROM, improvements in fetal ductus venosus and umbilical artery flow have been noted.[371]

During labor, use of intrapartum transcervical amnioinfusion for suspected or potential umbilical cord compression has been shown to be beneficial.

There have been recent developments that present continuous amnioinfusion therapy as a method to improve health outcomes in preterm PROM.[374]

Local anesthesia is used to prepare a subcutaneous pouch for the port capsule. Then, a needle inserts a catheter into the amniotic cavity under guided ultrasonography control. The catheter is connected to the port capsule, which is then inserted into the subcutaneous pouch. The skin is closed, and the port capsule is punctured transcutaneously by a 25-gauge needle connected to the infusion system containing the hypoosmotic saline solution like human amniotic fluid.

In conclusion, evidence in support of amnioinfusion in preterm PROM is limited, and this practice is not universally accepted in clinical practice. More research is needed regarding the potential role of amnioinfusion in reducing perinatal morbidity and mortality.

Term PROM

The management of term PROM is as follows: (1) evaluation of cord prolapse; (2) assessment for signs of infection; and (3) evaluation of fetal well-being. Induction of delivery is the management of choice if any signs of infection or fetal compromise occur. Otherwise, the primary decision is whether to induce delivery or take expectant management.[379-401]

Ninety percent of patients with term PROM will be in spontaneous labor within 24 hours.[406] Nulliparous women have a longer latency period than multiparous women.[385,391,396] There is a dilemma in managing patients with unfavorable cervix and those who do not have spontaneous labor.[400] The ACOG recommends women with PROM at 37 0/7 weeks of gestation or more to receive oxytocin infusion for induction if spontaneous labor does not present itself for those without contraindication to labor. If the patient refuses induction of labor after appropriate counseling about the risks of prolonged PROM in the presence of reassuring maternal and fetal conditions, then a course of expectant management may be acceptable.

For mechanical methods of cervical ripening, such as the Foley balloon there is a potential concern for infection, but there are insufficient data on which to base a recommendation for mechanical methods of cervical ripening in the setting of PROM.[1] The evidences for these recommendations are reviewed below.

Based on these data, we endorse a policy of immediate induction of labor in patients with term PROM. Antibiotic administration is justified before cesarean delivery for obstetric indications or for carriers of GBS.

Should There Be Routine Use of Prophylactic Antibiotics With PROM at Term in the Absence of an Indication for GBS Prophylaxis?

Whereas the current management of preterm PROM includes antibiotics prophylaxis, the current management of term PROM does not, despite known infectious risks of PROM. This is as a result of conflicting or inadequate data regarding the efficacy of antibiotics in term PROM.

The ACOG states that there is insufficient evidence to justify the routine use of prophylactic antibiotics with PROM at term in the absence of an indication for GBS prophylaxis.[1] However, the above data do suggest that prophylactic antibiotics may be beneficial in term PROM >12 hours.

Expectant Management at Home of Patients With Term PROM

The outpatient management at home of term PROM is not recommended.

The ACOG states that labor should be induced for women with PROM at 37 0/7 weeks of gestation or more if spontaneous labor does not occur near the time of presentation in those who do not have contraindication to labor. However, a course of expectant management may be acceptable for a patient who declines induction of labor as long as the clinical and fetal conditions are reassuring, and she is adequately counseled regarding the risks of prolonged PROM.[1]

Novel Treatment Techniques

Many experimental clinical studies have been conducted in order to seal the site of rupture (mostly in iatrogenic cases such as postamniocentesis). These techniques are still in the developmental stages. A recent Cochrane review Crowley et al[408] reported that there is insufficient evidence to evaluate sealing procedures in preterm PROM and recommended the conduct of well-controlled trials to assess the effect of promising interventions. A description is included because patients or their physician may inquire about these techniques.

Amniopatch

Transabdominal injection of platelets and cryoprecipitate has been evaluated to seal the membranes, similar to wound healing in vascular tissues. An ultrasound-guided amniocentesis needle is utilized to infuse platelets (0.5 units) and cryoprecipitate, which may form a plug and seal the defected site. It is thought that precise knowledge of the site of rupture is unnecessary because platelets would be activated to form a primary clot at the site of injury (rupture), followed by cryoprecipitate to stabilize the plug.[408]

Fibrin Tissue Sealant

Fibrin sealant is a mixture of fibrin, fibrinogen and thrombin. It forms a fibrin clot that may prevent the leakage of fluid at the site of rupture. Fibrin sealant is injected under ultrasound guidance at the site of rupture. Information regarding fibrin sealant success in sealing membranes is limited.

Absorbable Gelatin Sponge

Studies are conflicting regarding the use of absorbable gelatin sponge in preterm PROM.

Immunological Supplements

Limited studies suggest the use of oral immunomodulators to stimulate the healing of membranes in preterm PROM.[408,423] More studies are needed to support this approach.

Physical Barrier to Stop Leakage

A cervical cup with negative pressure was evaluated in 16 women with preterm PROM with limited favorable results.[424] More studies would be needed to explore the potential benefits of this approach.

KEY POINTS

- Preterm PROM occurs in 2% to 3.5% of pregnant women and term PROM occurs in around 10% of them.
- Biochemical and biophysical stress factors lead to focal weakness in the membranes, ultimately leading to PROM.
- The ZAM is a part of the chorioamniotic membrane located at the level of the internal cervical os. It is thought that PROM occurs due to alterations and weakness of this anatomic structure.

- MMPs were shown to degrade components of the membranes in both preterm and term PROM.
- Positive amniotic fluid cultures occur in approximately 30% of women with preterm PROM on admission and in approximately 75% of women with preterm PROM at the time of onset of labor. Positive amniotic fluid culture occurs in approximately 34% of women with term PROM on admission.
- Risk factors for preterm PROM include a history of previous spontaneous preterm delivery (with intact or ruptured membranes), vaginal bleeding in any trimester, a short cervix (≤25 mm), and smoking.
- If a pregnancy is complicated by preterm PROM and preterm delivery, the subsequent pregnancy is at a 21% risk for preterm PROM and 17% risk for term PROM.
- The main consequences of preterm PROM are: (1) preterm labor and delivery; (2) infection; (3) placental abruption; (4) fetal demise and (5) pulmonary hypoplasia.

- Fetal blood culture is positive in around 10% of mothers with preterm PROM.
- Pulmonary hypoplasia is reported to occur in around 50% of babies when PROM occurs at 19 weeks and in around 10% of newborns when PROM occurred at 25 weeks.
- Majority of women with term PROM go into spontaneous labor within 24 hours.
- Expectant management at home of patients with PROM at term is not recommended.
- In patients with preterm PROM between 23 and 34 weeks, steroids for fetal lung maturity and antibiotics for latency period prolongation are recommended. Between 23 and 32 weeks, magnesium sulfate for neuroprotection is recommended.
- In patients with late preterm PROM (between 34 and 37 weeks), expectant management to term may be considered. Late preterm steroids may also be considered if the patient is eligible.

REFERENCES

(only references cited in synoptic print chapter; for a complete reference list, see ebook)

1. American College of Obstetricians and Gynecologists' Committee on Practice Bulletins – Obstetrics. Prelabor rupture of membranes: ACOG Practice Bulletin, Number 217. *Obstet Gynecol.* 2020;135(3):e80-e97.
5. Santolaya-Forgas J, Romero R, Espinoza J, et al. Prelabor rupture of membranes. In: Hobbins JC, Reece EA, eds. *Clinical Obstetrics: The Fetus and the Mother.* Blackwell Publishing; 2007:1130-1188.
6. Hauth JC, Cunningham FG, Whalley PJ. Early labor initiation with oral PGE2 after premature rupture of the membranes at term. *Obstet Gynecol.* 1977;49(5):523-526.
7. Johnson JW, Daikoku NH, Niebyl JR, Johnson TR, Khouzami VA, Witter FR. Premature rupture of the membranes and prolonged latency. *Obstet Gynecol.* 1981;57(5):547-556.
8. Lange AP, Secher NJ, Nielsen FH, Pedersen GT. Stimulation of labor in cases of premature rupture of the membranes at or near term. A consecutive randomized study of prostaglandin E2-tablets and intravenous oxytocin. *Acta Obstet Gynecol Scand.* 1981;60(2):207-210.
9. Lebherz TB, Hellman LP, Madding R, Anctil A, Arje SL. Double-Blind study of premature rupture of the membranes. A report of 1,896 cases. *Am J Obstet Gynecol.* 1963;87:218-225.
10. Magos AL, Noble MCB, Wong Ten Yuen A, Rodeck CH. Controlled study comparing vaginal prostaglandin E2 pessaries with intravenous oxytocin for the stimulation of labour after spontaneous rupture of the membranes. *Br J Obstet Gynaecol.* 1983;90(8):726-731.
11. Tamsen L, Lyrenas S, Cnattingius S. Premature rupture of the membranes – intervention or not. *Gynecol Obstet Invest.* 1990;29(2):128-131.
12. Westergaard JG, Lange AP, Pedersen GT, Secher NJ. Use of oral oxytocics for stimulation of labor in cases of premature rupture of the membranes at term. A randomized comparative study of prostaglandin E2 tablets and demoxytocin resoriblets. *Acta Obstet Gynecol Scand.* 1983;62(2):111-116.

13. Knudsen FU, Steinrud J. Septicaemia of the newborn, associated with ruptured foetal membranes, discoloured amniotic fluid or maternal fever. *Acta Paediatr Scand.* 1976;65(6):725-731.
14. Verber IG, Pearce JM, New LC, Hamilton PA, Davies EG. Prolonged rupture of the fetal membranes and neonatal outcome. *J Perinat Med.* 1989;17(6):469-476.
15. Mercer BM. Preterm premature rupture of the membranes. *Obstet Gynecol.* 2003;101(1):178-193.
16. Tchirikov M, Schlabritz-Loutsevitch N, Maher J, et al. Mid-trimester preterm premature rupture of membranes (PPROM): etiology, diagnosis, classification, international recommendations of treatment options and outcome. *J Perinat Med.* 2018;46(5):465-488.
17. Christensen KK, Christensen P, Ingemarsson I, et al. A study of complications in preterm deliveries after prolonged premature rupture of the membranes. *Obstet Gynecol.* 1976;48(6):670-677.
23. Menon R, Richardson LS. Preterm prelabor rupture of the membranes: a disease of the fetal membranes. *Semin Perinatol.* 2017;41(7):409-419.
24. Mercer BM. Preterm premature rupture of the membranes: current approaches to evaluation and management. *Obstet Gynecol Clin North Am.* 2005;32(3):411-428.
29. Parry S, Strauss JF III. Premature rupture of the fetal membranes. *N Engl J Med.* 1998;338(10):663-670.
30. Kumar D, Moore RM, Mercer BM, Mansour JM, Redline RW, Moore JJ. The physiology of fetal membrane weakening and rupture: insights gained from the determination of physical properties revisited. *Placenta.* 2016;42:59-73.
31. Malak TM, Bell SC. Structural characteristics of term human fetal membranes: a novel zone of extreme morphological alteration within the rupture site. *Br J Obstet Gynaecol.* 1994;101(5):375-386.
32. McParland PC, Bell SC, Pringle JH, Taylor DJ. Regional and cellular localization of osteonectin/SPARC expression in connective tissue and cytotrophoblastic layers of human fetal membranes at term. *Mol Hum Reprod.* 2001;7(5):463-474.

33. McParland PC, Taylor DJ, Bell SC. Myofibroblast differentiation in the connective tissues of the amnion and chorion of term human fetal membranes-implications for fetal membrane rupture and labour. *Placenta*. 2000;21(1):44-53.

34. McParland PC, Taylor DJ, Bell SC. Mapping of zones of altered morphology and chorionic connective tissue cellular phenotype in human fetal membranes (amniochorion and decidua) overlying the lower uterine pole and cervix before labor at term. *Am J Obstet Gynecol*. 2003;189(5):1481-1488.

35. McParland P, Pringle J, Bell SC. Tenascin and the fetal membrane wound hypothesis - pro- gramming for fetal membrane rupture? *Br J Obstet Gynaecol*. 1998;105:1223-1224.

36. Goldenberg RL, Culhane JF, Iams JD, Romero R. Epidemiology and causes of preterm birth. *Lancet*. 2008;371(9606):75-84.

37. Gotsch F, Romero R, Kusanovic JP, et al. The fetal inflammatory response syndrome. *Clin Obstet Gynecol*. 2007;50(3):652-683.

38. Menon R, Papaconstantinou J. p38 Mitogen activated protein kinase (MAPK): a new therapeutic target for reducing the risk of adverse pregnancy outcomes. *Expert Opin Ther Targets*. 2016;20(12):1397-1412.

39. Myatt L, Cui X. Oxidative stress in the placenta. *Histochem Cell Biol*. 2004;122(4):369-382.

40. Romero R, Espinoza J, Gonçalves L, Kusanovic J, Friel L, Hassan S. The role of inflammation and infection in preterm birth. *Semin Reprod Med*. 2007;25(1):21-39.

41. Gomez R, Romero R, Ghezzi F, Yoon BH, Mazor M, Berry SM. The fetal inflammatory response syndrome. *Am J Obstet Gynecol*. 1998;179(1):194-202.

42. Kacerovsky M, Lenco J, Musilova I, et al. Proteomic biomarkers for spontaneous preterm birth: a systematic review of the literature. *Reprod Sci*. 2014;21(3):283-295.

43. Romero R, Miranda J, Chaiworapongsa T, et al. Prevalence and clinical significance of sterile intra-amniotic inflammation in patients with preterm labor and intact membranes. *Am J Reprod Immunol*. 2014;72(5):458-474.

44. Harger JH, Hsing AW, Tuomala RE, et al. Risk factors for preterm premature rupture of fetal membranes: a multicenter case-control study. *Am J Obstet Gynecol*. 1990;163(1 pt 1):130-137.

45. Asrat T, Lewis DF, Garite TJ, et al. Rate of recurrence of preterm premature rupture of membranes in consecutive pregnancies. *Am J Obstet Gynecol*. 1991;165(4 pt 1):1111-1115.

46. Ekwo EE, Gosselink CA, Moawad A. Unfavorable outcome in penultimate pregnancy and premature rupture of membranes in successive pregnancy. *Obstet Gynecol*. 1992;80(2):166-172.

47. Ekwo EE, Gosselink CA, Moawad A. Previous pregnancy outcomes and subsequent risk of preterm rupture of amniotic sac membranes. *Br J Obstet Gynaecol*. 1993;100(6):536-541.

48. Mercer BM, Goldenberg RL, Meis PJ, et al. The preterm prediction study: prediction of preterm premature rupture of membranes through clinical findings and ancillary testing. The National Institute of Child Health and Human Development Maternal-Fetal Medicine Units Network. *Am J Obstet Gynecol*. 2000;183(3):738-745.

49. Naeye RL. Factors that predispose to premature rupture of the fetal membranes. *Obstet Gynecol*. 1982;60(1):93-98.

50. Williams MA, Mittendorf R, Stubblefield PG, Lieberman E, Schoenbaum SC, Monson RR. Cigarettes, coffee, and preterm premature rupture of the membranes. *Am J Epidemiol*. 1992;135(8):895-903.

51. Weiss JL, Malone FD, Vidaver J, et al. Threatened abortion: a risk factor for poor pregnancy outcome, a population-based screening study. *Am J Obstet Gynecol*. 2004;190(3):745-750.

52. Yang J, Hartmann KE, Savitz DA, et al. Vaginal bleeding during pregnancy and preterm birth. *Am J Epidemiol*. 2004;160(2):118-125.

53. Mackenzie AP, Schatz F, Krikun G, Funai EF, Kadner S, Lockwood CJ. Mechanisms of abruption-induced premature rupture of the fetal membranes: thrombin enhanced decidual matrix metalloproteinase-3 (stromelysin-1) expression. *Am J Obstet Gynecol*. 2004;191(6):1996-2001.

54. Rosen T, Schatz F, Kuczynski E, Lam H, Koo AB, Lockwood CJ. Thrombin-enhanced matrix metalloproteinase-1 expression: a mechanism linking placental abruption with premature rupture of the membranes. *J Matern Fetal Neonatal Med*. 2002;11(1):11-17.

55. Evaldson G, Lagrelius A, Winiarski J. Premature rupture of the membranes. *Acta Obstet Gynecol Scand*. 1980;59(5):385-393.

56. Hadley CB, Main DM, Gabbe SG. Risk factors for preterm premature rupture of the fetal membranes. *Am J Perinatol*. 1990;7(4):374-379.

57. Meis PJ, Ernest JM, Moore ML. Causes of low birth weight births in public and private patients. *Am J Obstet Gynecol*. 1987;156(5):1165-1168.

58. Schieve LA, Handler A. Preterm delivery and perinatal death among black and white infants in a Chicago-area perinatal registry. *Obstet Gynecol*. 1996;88(3):356-363.

61. Ferrand PE, Parry S, Sammel M, et al. A polymorphism in the matrix metalloproteinase-9 promoter is associated with increased risk of preterm premature rupture of membranes in African Americans. *Mol Hum Reprod*. 2002;8(5):494-501.

62. Fortunato SJ, Lombardi SJ, Menon R. Racial disparity in membrane response to infectious stimuli: a possible explanation for observed differences in the incidence of prematurity. Community Award Paper. *Am J Obstet Gynecol*. 2004;190(6):1557-1562; discussion 1562-1563.

63. Fujimoto T, Parry S, Urbanek M, et al. A single nucleotide polymorphism in the matrix metalloproteinase-1 (MMP-1) promoter influences amnion cell MMP-1 expression and risk for preterm premature rupture of the fetal membranes. *J Biol Chem*. 2002;277(8):6296-6302.

64. Wang H, Parry S, Macones G, et al.. Functionally significant SNP MMP8 promoter haplotypes and preterm premature rupture of membranes (PPROM). *Hum Mol Genet*. 2004;13(21):2659-2669.

66. Naeye RL, Peters EC. Causes and consequences of premature rupture of fetal membranes. *Lancet*. 1980;1(8161):192-194.

67. Mills JL, Harlap S, Harley EE. Should coitus late in pregnancy be discouraged? *Lancet*. 1981;2(8238):136-138.

68. Perkins RP. Sexual behavior and response in relation to complications of pregnancy. *Am J Obstet Gynecol*. 1979;134(5):498-505.

69. Rayburn WF, Wilson EA. Coital activity and premature delivery. *Am J Obstet Gynecol*. 1980;137(8):972-974.

74. Wideman GL, Baird GH, Bolding OT. Ascorbic acid deficiency and premature rupture of fetal membranes. *Am J Obstet Gynecol*. 1964;88:592-595.

75. Vadillo Ortega F, Pfeffer Burak F, Bermejo Martínez ML, et al. Dietetic factors and premature rupture of fetal membranes. Effect of vitamin C on collagen degradation in the chorioamnion. *Ginecol Obstet Mex*. 1995;63:158-162.

76. Barrett BM, Sowell A, Gunter E, Wang M. Potential role of ascorbic acid and beta-carotene in the prevention of preterm rupture of fetal membranes. *Int J Vitam Nutr Res*. 1994;64(3):192-197.

77. Stuart EL, Evans GS, Lin YS, Powers HJ. Reduced collagen and ascorbic acid concentrations and increased proteolytic susceptibility with prelabor fetal membrane rupture in women. *Biol Reprod*. 2005;72(1):230-235.

78. Sibai BM, Villar MA, Bray E. Magnesium supplementation during pregnancy: a double-blind randomized controlled clinical trial. *Am J Obstet Gynecol*. 1989;161(1):115-119.

79. Villar J, Repke JT. Calcium supplementation during pregnancy may reduce preterm delivery in high-risk populations. *Am J Obstet Gynecol*. 1990;163(4 pt 1):1124-1131.

80. Artal R, Burgeson R, Fernandez FJ, Hobel CJ. Fetal and maternal copper levels in patients at term with and without premature rupture of membranes. *Obstet Gynecol*. 1979;53(5):608-610.

81. Kiilholma P, Grönroos M, Erkkola R, Pakarinen P, Näntö V. The role of calcium, copper, iron and zinc in preterm delivery and premature rupture of fetal membranes. *Gynecol Obstet Invest*. 1984;17(4):194-201.

82. Sikorski R, Juszkiewicz T, Paszkowski T. Zinc status in women with premature rupture of membranes at term. *Obstet Gynecol*. 1990;76(4):675-677.

83. O'Brien WF, Sternlicht D, Torres C, Knuppel RA, Montenegro R. The value of early third-trimester maternal serum alpha-fetoprotein determination. *Prenat Diagn*. 1990;10(3):183-188.

84. Waller DK, Lustig LS, Cunningham GC, Golbus MS, Hook EB. Second-trimester maternal serum alpha-fetoprotein levels and the risk of subsequent fetal death. *N Engl J Med*. 1991;325(1):6-10.

85. Simpson JL, Palomaki GE, Mercer B, et al. Associations between adverse perinatal outcome and serially obtained second- and third-trimester maternal serum alpha-fetoprotein measurements. *Am J Obstet Gynecol*. 1995;173(6):1742-1748.

86. Sagot P, Caroit Y, Winer N, Lopes P, Boog G. Obstetrical prognosis for carbon dioxide laser conisation of the uterine cervix. *Eur J Obstet Gynecol Reprod Biol*. 1995;58(1):53-58.

87. Harlap S, Davies AM. Late sequelae of induced abortion: complications and outcome of pregnancy and labor. *Am J Epidemiol*. 1975;102(3):217-224.

88. Zebitay AG, Güngör ES, Ilhan G, et al. Cervical conization and the risk of preterm birth: a population-based multicentric trial of Turkish cohort. *J Clin Diagn Res.* 2017;11(3):QC21-QC24.

95. Kurki T, Sivonen A, Renkonen OV, Savia E, Ylikorkala O. Bacterial vaginosis in early pregnancy and pregnancy outcome. *Obstet Gynecol.* 1992;80(2):173-177.

96. Romero R, Chaiworapongsa T, Kuivaniemi H, Tromp G. Bacterial vaginosis, the inflammatory response and the risk of preterm birth: a role for genetic epidemiology in the prevention of preterm birth. *Am J Obstet Gynecol.* 2004;190(6):1509-1519.

97. Simhan HN, Caritis SN, Krohn MA, Hillier SL. The vaginal inflammatory milieu and the risk of early premature preterm rupture of membranes. *Am J Obstet Gynecol.* 2005;192(1):213-218.

100. Committee Opinion No. 485: prevention of early-onset group B streptococcal disease in newborns. correction. *Obstet Gynecol.* 2018;131(2):397.

102. Newton ER, Clark M. Group B streptococcus and preterm rupture of membranes. *Obstet Gynecol.* 1988;71(2):198-202.

104. Sweet RL, Landers DV, Walker C, Schachter J. Chlamydia trachomatis infection and pregnancy outcome. *Am J Obstet Gynecol.* 1987;156(4):824-833.

106. Amstey MS, Steadman KT. Asymptomatic gonorrhea and pregnancy. *J Am Vener Dis Assoc.* 1976;3(1):14-16.

107. Edwards LE, Barrada MI, Hamann AA, Hakanson FY. Gonorrhea in pregnancy. *Am J Obstet Gynecol.* 1978;132(6):637-641.

108. Handsfield HH, Hodson WA, Holmes KK. Neonatal gonococcal infection. I. Orogastric contamination with Neisseria gonorrhoea. *J Am Med Assoc.* 1973;225(7):697-701.

109. Minkoff H, Grunebaum AN, Schwarz RH, et al. Risk factors for prematurity and premature rupture of membranes: a prospective study of the vaginal flora in pregnancy. *Am J Obstet Gynecol.* 1984;150(8):965-972.

110. Klebanoff MA, Carey JC, Hauth JC, et al. Failure of metronidazole to prevent preterm delivery among pregnant women with asymptomatic Trichomonas vaginalis infection. *N Engl J Med.* 2001;345(7):487-493.

112. Capece A, Vasieva O, Meher S, Alfirevic Z, Alfirevic A. Pathway analysis of genetic factors associated with spontaneous preterm birth and pre-labor premature rupture of membranes. *PLoS One.* 2014;9(9):e108578.

113. Manuck TA. The genomics of prematurity in an era of more precise clinical phenotyping: a review. *Semin Fetal Neonatal Med.* 2016;21(2):89-93.

114. Romero R, Friel LA, Velez Edwards DR, et al. A genetic association study of maternal and fetal candidate genes that predispose to preterm prelabor rupture of membranes (PROM). *Am J Obstet Gynecol.* 2010;203(4):361. e1-361.e30.

116. Berkowitz GS, Blackmore-Prince C, Lapinski RH, Savitz DA. Risk factors for preterm birth subtypes. *Epidemiology.* 1998;9(3):279-285.

117. Treadwell MC, Bronsteen RA, Bottoms SF. Prognostic factors and complication rates for cervical cerclage: a review of 482 cases. *Am J Obstet Gynecol.* 1991;165(3):555-558.

118. Millar LK, Stollberg J, DeBuque L, Bryant-Greenwood G. Fetal membrane distention: determination of the intrauterine surface area and distention of the fetal membranes preterm and at term. *Am J Obstet Gynecol.* 2000;182(1 pt 1):128-134.

120. Bou-Resli MN, Al-Zaid NS, Ibrahim ME. Full-term and prematurely ruptured fetal membranes. An ultrastructural study. *Cell Tissue Res.* 1981;220(2):263-278.

121. Ibrahim ME, Bou-resli MN, Al-zaid NS, Bishay LF. Intact fetal membranes. Morphological predisposal to rupture. *Acta Obstet Gynecol Scand.* 1983;62(5):481-485.

122. Lavery JP, Miller CE. The viscoelastic nature of chorioamniotic membranes. *Obstet Gynecol.* 1977;50(4):467-472.

123. Lavery JP, Miller CE. Deformation and creep in the human chorioamniotic sac. *Am J Obstet Gynecol.* 1979;134(4):366-375.

124. Kanayama N, Terao T, Kawashima Y, Horiuchi K, Fujimoto D. Collagen types in normal and prematurely ruptured amniotic membranes. *Am J Obstet Gynecol.* 1985;153(8):899-903.

125. Skinner SJ, Campos GA, Liggins GC. Collagen content of human amniotic membranes: effect of gestation length and premature rupture. *Obstet Gynecol.* 1981;57(4):487-489.

127. Bryant-Greenwood GD, Yamamoto SY. Control of peripartal collagenolysis in the human chorion-decidua. *Am J Obstet Gynecol.* 1995;172(1 pt 1):63-70.

128. Burgos H, Hsi B-L, Yeh C-JG, Faulk WP. Plasminogen binding by human amniochorion. A possible factor in premature rupture of membranes. *Am J Obstet Gynecol.* 1982;143(8):958-963.

129. Draper D, McGregor J, Hall J, et al. Elevated protease activities in human amnion and chorion correlate with preterm premature rupture of membranes. *Am J Obstet Gynecol.* 1995;173(5):1506-1512.

130. Fortunato SJ, LaFleur B, Menon R. Collagenase-3 (MMP-13) in fetal membranes and amniotic fluid during pregnancy. *Am J Reprod Immunol.* 2003;49(2):120-125.

131. Helmig R, Uldbjerg N, Ohlsson K. Secretory leukocyte protease inhibitor in the cervical mucus and in the fetal membranes. *Eur J Obstet Gynecol Reprod Biol.* 1995;59(1):95-101.

132. Jenkins DM, O'Neill M, Mattar M, France VM, Hsi B-L, Page Faulk W. Degenerative changes and detection of plasminogen in fetal membranes that rupture prematurely. *Br J Obstet Gynaecol.* 1983;90(9):841-846.

133. Lei H, Vadillo-Ortega F, Paavola LG, Strauss JF. 92-kDa gelatinase (matrix metalloproteinase-9) is induced in rat amnion immediately prior to parturition. *Biol Reprod.* 1995;53(2):339-344.

134. McGregor JA, Lawellin D, Franco-Buff A, Todd JK, Makowski EL. Protease production by microorganisms associated with reproductive tract infection. *Am J Obstet Gynecol.* 1986;154(1):109-114.

135. McGregor JA, Schoonmaker JN, Lunt BD, Lawellin DW. Antibiotic inhibition of bacterially induced fetal membrane weakening. *Obstet Gynecol.* 1990;76(1):124-128.

136. Milwidsky A, Hurwitz A, Eckstein L, Mayer M, Gutman A. Proteolytic enzymes in human fetal membranes and amniotic fluid. A comparison of normal and premature ruptured membranes. *Enzyme.* 1985;33(4):188-196.

137. O'Brien WF, Knuppel RA, Morales WJ, Angel JL, Torres CT, Amniotic fluid alpha 1-antitrypsin concentration in premature rupture of the membranes. *Am J Obstet Gynecol.* 1990;162(3):756-759.

138. Rajabi M, Dean DD, Woessner JF Jr. High levels of serum collagenase in premature labor – a potential biochemical marker. *Obstet Gynecol.* 1987;69(2):179-186.

139. Rajabi MR, Dean DD, Woessner JF Jr. Changes in active and latent collagenase in human placenta around the time of parturition. *Am J Obstet Gynecol.* 1990;163(2):499-505.

140. Sbarra AJ, Selvaraj RJ, Cetrulo CL, Feingold M, Newton E, Thomas GB. Infection and phagocytosis as possible mechanisms of rupture in premature rupture of the membranes. *Am J Obstet Gynecol.* 1985;153(1):38-43.

141. Sbarra AJ, Thomas GB, Cetrulo CL, Shakr C, Chaudhury A, Paul B. Effect of bacterial growth on the bursting pressure of fetal membranes in vitro. *Obstet Gynecol.* 1987;70(1):107-110.

142. Schoonmaker JN, Lawellin DW, Lunt B, McGregor JA. Bacteria and inflammatory cells reduce chorioamniotic membrane integrity and tensile strength. *Obstet Gynecol.* 1989;74(4):590-596.

143. Vadillo-Ortega F, González-Avila G, Furth EE, et al.. 92-kd type IV collagenase (matrix metalloproteinase-9) activity in human amniochorion increases with labor. *Am J Pathol.* 1995;146(1):148-156.

144. Vadillo-Ortega F, Hernandez A, Gonzalez-Avila G, Bermejo L, Iwata K, Strauss JF. Increased matrix metalloproteinase activity and reduced tissue inhibitor of metalloproteinases-1 levels in amniotic fluids from pregnancies complicated by premature rupture of membranes. *Am J Obstet Gynecol.* 1996;174(4):1371-1376.

145. Woessner JF Jr. Matrix metalloproteinases and their inhibitors in connective tissue remodeling. *FASEB J.* 1991;5(8):2145-2154.

146. Sabir N, Hussain T, Mangi MH, Zhao D, Zhou X. Matrix metalloproteinases: expression, regulation and role in the immunopathology of tuberculosis. *Cell Prolif.* 2019;52:e12649.

148. Maymon E, Romero R, Pacora P, et al. Evidence for the participation of interstitial collagenase (matrix metalloproteinase 1) in preterm premature rupture of membranes. *Am J Obstet Gynecol.* 2000;183(4):914-920.

149. Maymon E, Romero R, Pacora P, et al.. Human neutrophil collagenase (matrix metalloproteinase 8) in parturition, premature rupture of the membranes, and intrauterine infection. *Am J Obstet Gynecol.* 2000;183(1):94-99.

150. Maymon E, Romero R, Pacora P, et al. Evidence of in vivo differential bioavailability of the active forms of matrix metalloproteinases 9 and 2 in parturition, spontaneous rupture of membranes, and intra-amniotic infection. *Am J Obstet Gynecol.* 2000;183(4):887-894.

151. Maymon E, Romero R, Pacora P, et al. A role for the 72 kDa gelatinase (MMP-2) and its inhibitor (TIMP-2) in human parturition, premature rupture of membranes and intraamniotic infection. *J Perinat Med.* 2001;29(4):308-316.

152. Helmig BR, Romero R, Espinoza J, et al. Neutrophil elastase and secretory leukocyte protease inhibitor in prelabor rupture of membranes, parturition and intra-amniotic infection. *J Matern Fetal Neonatal Med.* 2002;12(4):237-246.

153. Tromp G, Kuivaniemi H, Romero R, et al. Genome-wide expression profiling of fetal membranes reveals a deficient expression of proteinase inhibitor 3 in premature rupture of membranes. *Am J Obstet Gynecol.* 2004;191(4):1331-1338.

154. Romero R, Chaiworapongsa T, Espinoza J, et al. Fetal plasma MMP-9 concentrations are elevated in preterm premature rupture of the membranes. *Am J Obstet Gynecol.* 2002;187(5):1125-1130.

157. Nemeth E, Millar LK, Bryant-Greenwood G. Fetal membrane distention: II. Differentially expressed genes regulated by acute distention in vitro. *Am J Obstet Gynecol.* 2000;182(1 pt 1):60-67.

158. Nemeth E, Tashima LS, Yu Z, Bryant-Greenwood GD. Fetal membrane distention: I. Differentially expressed genes regulated by acute distention in amniotic epithelial (WISH) cells. *Am J Obstet Gynecol.* 2000;182(1 pt 1):50-59.

159. Jia SH, Li Y, Parodo J, et al. Pre-B cell colony-enhancing factor inhibits neutrophil apoptosis in experimental inflammation and clinical sepsis. *J Clin Invest.* 2004;113(9):1318-1327.

160. Kettritz R, Gaido ML, Haller H, Luft FC, Jennette CJ, Falk RJ. Interleukin-8 delays spontaneous and tumor necrosis factor-alpha-mediated apoptosis of human neutrophils. *Kidney Int.* 1998;53(1):84-91.

161. Ognjanovic S, Ku TL, Bryant-Greenwood GD. Pre-B-cell colony-enhancing factor is a secreted cytokine-like protein from the human amniotic epithelium. *Am J Obstet Gynecol.* 2005;193(1):273-282.

163. DiGiulio DB, Romero R, Kusanovic JP, et al. Prevalence and diversity of microbes in the amniotic fluid, the fetal inflammatory response, and pregnancy outcome in women with preterm pre-labor rupture of membranes. *Am J Reprod Immunol.* 2010;64(1):38-57.

164. Vadillo-Ortega F, Estrada-Gutierrez G. Role of matrix metalloproteinases in preterm labour. *Br J Obstet Gynecol.* 2005;112 suppl 1:19-22.

165. Arechavaleta-Velasco F, Ogando D, Parry S, Vadillo-Ortega F. Production of matrix metalloproteinase-9 in lipopolysaccharide-stimulated human amnion occurs through an autocrine and paracrine proinflammatory cytokine-dependent system. *Biol Reprod.* 2002;67(6):1952-1958.

166. Fortunato SJ, Menon R. IL-1 beta is a better inducer of apoptosis in human fetal membranes than IL-6. *Placenta.* 2003;24(10):922-928.

170. Garite TJ, Freeman RK, Chorioamnionitis in the preterm gestation. *Obstet Gynecol.* 1982;59(5):539-545.

171. Cassell GH, Davis RO, Waites KB, et al. Isolation of mycoplasma hominis and ureaplasma urealyticum from amniotic fluid at 16-20 weeks of gestation: potential effect on outcome of pregnancy. *Sex Transm Dis.* 1983;10(4 suppl):294-302.

172. Gray DJ, Robinson HB, Malone J, Thomson RB. Adverse outcome in pregnancy following amniotic fluid isolation of ureaplasma urealyticum. *Prenat Diagn.* 1992;12(2):111-117.

173. Horowitz S, Mazor M, Romero R, Horowitz J, Glezerman M. Infection of the amniotic cavity with Ureaplasma urealyticum in the midtrimester of pregnancy. *J Reprod Med.* 1995;40(5):375-379.

174. Goncalves LF, Chaiworapongsa T, Romero R. Intrauterine infection and prematurity. *Ment Retard Dev Disabil Res Rev.* 2002;8(1):3-13.

175. Romero R, Quintero R, Oyarzun E, et al. Intraamniotic infection and the onset of labor in preterm premature rupture of the membranes. *Am J Obstet Gynecol.* 1988;159(3):661-666.

176. Gomez R, Romero R, Nien JK, et al. Idiopathic vaginal bleeding during pregnancy as the only clinical manifestation of intrauterine infection. *J Matern Fetal Neonatal Med.* 2005;18(1):31-37.

177. Curry TE Jr, Osteen KG. The matrix metalloproteinase system: changes, regulation, and impact throughout the ovarian and uterine reproductive cycle. *Endocr Rev.* 2003;24(4):428-465.

178. Stephenson CD, Lockwood CJ, Ma Y, Guller S. Thrombin-dependent regulation of matrix metalloproteinase (MMP)-9 levels in human fetal membranes. *J Matern Fetal Neonatal Med.* 2005;18(1):17-22.

179. Arias F, Rodriquez L, Rayne SC, Kraus FT. Maternal placental vasculopathy and infection: two distinct subgroups among patients with preterm labor and preterm ruptured membranes. *Am J Obstet Gynecol.* 1993;168(2):585-591.

180. Kim YM, Chaiworapongsa T, Gomez R, et al. Failure of physiologic transformation of the spiral arteries in the placental bed in preterm premature rupture of membranes. *Am J Obstet Gynecol.* 2002;187(5):1137-1142.

181. Labarrere CA, DiCarlo HL, Bammerlin E, et al. Failure of physiologic transformation of spiral arteries, endothelial and trophoblast cell activation, and acute atherosis in the basal plate of the placenta. *Am J Obstet Gynecol.* 2017;216(3):287.e1-287.e16.

182. Hein M, Helmig RB, Schønheyder HC, Ganz T, Uldbjerg N. An in vitro study of antibacterial properties of the cervical mucus plug in pregnancy. *Am J Obstet Gynecol.* 2001;185(3):586-592.

183. Hein M, Valore EV, Helmig RB, Uldbjerg N, Ganz T. Antimicrobial factors in the cervical mucus plug. *Am J Obstet Gynecol.* 2002;187(1):137-144.

184. Svinarich DM, Wolf NA, Gomez R, Gonik B, Romero R. Detection of human defensin 5 in reproductive tissues. *Am J Obstet Gynecol.* 1997;176(2):470-475.

185. Hassan S, Romero R, Hendler I, et al. A sonographic short cervix as the only clinical manifestation of intra-amniotic infection. *J Perinat Med.* 2006;34(1):13-19.

186. Rizzo G, Capponi A, Vlachopoulou A, Angelini E, Grassi C, Romanini C. Ultrasonographic assessment of the uterine cervix and interleukin-8 concentrations in cervical secretions predict intrauterine infection in patients with preterm labor and intact membranes. *Ultrasound Obstet Gynecol.* 1998;12(2):86-92.

187. Lind J, Wallenburg HC. Pregnancy and the Ehlers-Danlos syndrome: a retrospective study in a Dutch population. *Acta Obstet Gynecol Scand.* 2002;81(4):293-300.

188. Yanagihara T, Ueta M, Hanaoka U, et al. Late second-trimester nonstress test characteristics in preterm delivery before 32 weeks of gestation. *Gynecol Obstet Invest.* 2001;51(1):32-35.

189. Blencowe H, Cousens S, Oestergaard MZ, et al. National, regional, and worldwide estimates of preterm birth rates in the year 2010 with time trends since 1990 for selected countries: a systematic analysis and implications. *Lancet.* 2012;379(9832):2162-2172.

190. Liu L, Johnson HL, Cousens S, et al. Global, regional, and national causes of child mortality: an updated systematic analysis for 2010 with time trends since 2000. *Lancet.* 2012;379(9832):2151-2161.

191. Blencowe H, Cousens S, Chou D, et al. Born too soon: the global epidemiology of 15 million preterm births. *Reprod Health.* 2013;10 suppl 1:S2.

192. Shin H, Pei Z, Martinez KA, et al. The first microbial environment of infants born by C-section: the operating room microbes. *Microbiome.* 2015;3:59.

193. Cox SM, Williams ML, Leveno KJ. The natural history of preterm ruptured membranes: what to expect of expectant management. *Obstet Gynecol.* 1988;71(4):558-562.

194. Nelson LH, Anderson RL, O'Shea TM, Swain M. Expectant management of preterm premature rupture of the membranes. *Am J Obstet Gynecol.* 1994;171(2):350-356; discussion 356-358.

195. Wilson JC, Levy DL, Wilds PL. Premature rupture of membranes prior to term: consequences of nonintervention. *Obstet Gynecol.* 1982;60(5):601-606.

198. Romero R, Sirtori M, Oyarzun E, et al. Infection and labor. V. Prevalence, microbiology, and clinical significance of intraamniotic infection in women with preterm labor and intact membranes. *Am J Obstet Gynecol.* 1989;161(3):817-824.

199. Romero R, Mazor M, Morrotti R, et al. Infection and labor. VII. Microbial invasion of the amniotic cavity in spontaneous rupture of membranes at term. *Am J Obstet Gynecol.* 1992;166(1 pt 1):129-133.

200. Yoon BH, Romero R, Kim M, et al. Clinical implications of detection of Ureaplasma urealyticum in the amniotic cavity with the polymerase chain reaction. *Am J Obstet Gynecol.* 2000;183(5):1130-1137.

201. Theis KR, Romero R, Winters AD, et al. Does the human placenta delivered at term have a microbiota? Results of cultivation, quantitative real-time PCR, 16S rRNA gene sequencing, and metagenomics. *Am J Obstet Gynecol.* 2019;220(3):267.e1-267.e39.

202. Gonik B, Bottoms SF, Cotton DB. Amniotic fluid volume as a risk factor in preterm premature rupture of the membranes. *Obstet Gynecol.* 1985;65(4):456-459.

203. Park JS, Yoon BH, Romero R, et al. The relationship between oligohydramnios and the onset of preterm labor in preterm premature rupture of membranes. *Am J Obstet Gynecol.* 2001;184(3):459-462.

204. Vintzileos AM, Campbell WA, Nochimson DJ, Weinbaum PJ. Preterm premature rupture of the membranes: a risk factor for the development of abruptio placentae. *Am J Obstet Gynecol.* 1987;156(5):1235-1238.

205. Zlatnik FJ, Cruikshank DP, Petzold CR, Galask RP. Amniocentesis in the identification of inapparent infection in preterm patients with premature rupture of the membranes. *J Reprod Med.* 1984;29(9):656-660.

206. Averbuch B, Mazor M, Shoham-Vardi I, et al. Intra-uterine infection in women with preterm premature rupture of membranes: maternal and neonatal characteristics. *Eur J Obstet Gynecol Reprod Biol.* 1995;62(1):25-29.

207. Carroll SG, Papaioannou S, Ntumazah IL, Philpott-Howard J, Nicolaides KH. Lower genital tract swabs in the prediction of intrauterine infection in preterm prelabour rupture of the membranes. *Br J Obstet Gynaecol.* 1996;103(1):54-59.

208. Romero R, Yoon BH, Mazor M, et al. A comparative study of the diagnostic performance of amniotic fluid glucose, white blood cell count, interleukin-6, and gram stain in the detection of microbial invasion in patients with preterm premature rupture of membranes. *Am J Obstet Gynecol.* 1993;169(4):839-851.

209. Lim ES, Rodriguez C, Holtz LR. Amniotic fluid from healthy term pregnancies does not harbor a detectable microbial community. *Microbiome.* 2018;6(1):87.

210. Cotton DB, Hill LM, Strassner HT, Platt LD, Ledger WJ. Use of amniocentesis in preterm gestation with ruptured membranes. *Obstet Gynecol.* 1984;63(1):38-43.

212. Garite TJ, Freeman RK, Linzey EM, Braly P. The use of amniocentesis in patients with premature rupture of membranes. *Obstet Gynecol.* 1979;54(2):226-230.

213. Winn HN, Chen M, Amon E, Leet TL, Shumway JB, Mostello D. Neonatal pulmonary hypoplasia and perinatal mortality in patients with midtrimester rupture of amniotic membranes – a critical analysis. *Am J Obstet Gynecol.* 2000;182(6):1638-1644.

214. Gauthier DW, Meyer WJ, Bieniarz A. Expectant management of premature rupture of membranes with amniotic fluid cultures positive for ureaplasma urealyticum alone. *Am J Obstet Gynecol.* 1994;170(2):587-590.

215. Gomez R, Romero R, Gomez R, et al. Antibiotic administration to patients with preterm premature rupture of membranes does not eradicate intraamniotic infection. *J Matern Fetal Neonatal Med.* 2007;20(2):167-173.

216. Carroll SG, Ville Y, Greenough A, et al. Preterm prelabour amniorrhexis: intrauterine infection and interval between membrane rupture and delivery. *Arch Dis Child Fetal Neonatal Ed.* 1995;72(1):F43-F46.

217. Yoon BH, Romero R, Park JS, et al. The relationship among inflammatory lesions of the umbilical cord (funisitis), umbilical cord plasma interleukin 6 concentration, amniotic fluid infection, and neonatal sepsis. *Am J Obstet Gynecol.* 2000;183(5):1124-1129.

218. Romero R, Salafia CM, Athanassiadis AP, et al. The relationship between acute inflammatory lesions of the preterm placenta and amniotic fluid microbiology. *Am J Obstet Gynecol.* 1992;166(5):1382-1388.

219. Peng CC, Chang J-H, Lin H-Y, Cheng P-J, Su B-H. Intrauterine inflammation, infection, or both (Triple I): a new concept for chorioamnionitis. *Pediatr Neonatol.* 2018;59(3):231-237.

220. Akinbi HT, Narendran V, Pass AK, Markart P, Hoath SB. Host defense proteins in vernix caseosa and amniotic fluid. *Am J Obstet Gynecol.* 2004;191(6):2090-2096.

221. Espinoza J, Chaiworapongsa T, Romero R, et al. Antimicrobial peptides in amniotic fluid: defensins, calprotectin and bacterial/permeability-increasing protein in patients with microbial invasion of the amniotic cavity, intra-amniotic inflammation, preterm labor and premature rupture of membranes. *J Matern Fetal Neonatal Med.* 2003;13(1):2-21.

222. Otsuki K, Yoda A, Toma Y, Shimizu Y, Saito H, Yanaihara T. Lactoferrin and interleukin-6 interaction in amniotic infection. *Adv Exp Med Biol.* 1998;443:267-271.

223. Sachs BP, Stern CM. Activity and characterization of a low molecular fraction present in human amniotic fluid with broad spectrum antibacterial activity. *Br J Obstet Gynaecol.* 1979;86(2):81-86.

224. Perez-Munoz ME, Arrieta MC, Ramer-Tait AE, Walter J. A critical assessment of the "sterile womb" and "in utero colonization" hypotheses: implications for research on the pioneer infant microbiome. *Microbiome.* 2017;5:19.

225. Salter SJ, Cox MJ, Turek EM, et al. Reagent and laboratory contamination can critically impact sequence-based microbiome analyses. *BMC Biol.* 2014;12:12.

226. Weiss S, Amir A, Hyde ER, Metcalf JL, Song SJ, Knight R. Tracking down the sources of experimental contamination in microbiome studies. *Genome Biol.* 2014;15(12):564.

227. Lauder AP, Roche AM, Sherrill-Mix S, et al. Comparison of placenta samples with contamination controls does not provide evidence for a distinct placenta microbiota. *Microbiome.* 2016;4(29):1-11.

228. Kim D, Hofstaedter CE, Zhao C, et al. Optimizing methods and dodging pitfalls in microbiome research. *Microbiome.* 2017;5:14.

229. Glassing A, Dowd SE, Galandiuk S, Davis B, Chiodini RJ. Inherent bacterial DNA contamination of extraction and sequencing reagents may affect interpretation of microbiota in low bacterial biomass samples. *Gut Pathog.* 2016;8:12.

230. Berry SM, Romero R, Gomez R, et al. Premature parturition is characterized by in utero activation of the fetal immune system. *Am J Obstet Gynecol.* 1995;173(4):1315-1320.

231. Romero R, Athayde N, Gomez R, et al. The inflammatory response syndrome is characterized by the outpouring of a potent extracellular matrix degrading enzyme into the fetal circulation. *Am J Obstet Gynecol.* 1998;178:S3.

233. Ananth CV, Oyelese Y, Srinivas N, Yeo L, Vintzileos AM. Preterm premature rupture of membranes, intrauterine infection, and oligohydramnios: risk factors for placental abruption. *Obstet Gynecol.* 2004;104(1):71-77.

234. Ananth CV, Savitz DA, Williams MA. Placental abruption and its association with hypertension and prolonged rupture of membranes: a methodologic review and meta-analysis. *Obstet Gynecol.* 1996;88(2):309-318.

235. Ananth CV, Smulian JC, Demissie K, Vintzileos AM, Knuppel RA. Placental abruption among singleton and twin births in the United States: risk factor profiles. *Am J Epidemiol.* 2001;153(8):771-778.

240. Rotschild A, Ling EW, Puterman ML, Farquharson D. Neonatal outcome after prolonged preterm rupture of the membranes. *Am J Obstet Gynecol.* 1990;162(1):46-52.

241. Moessinger AC, Collins MH, Blanc WA, Rey HR, James LS. Oligohydramnios-induced lung hypoplasia: the influence of timing and duration in gestation. *Pediatr Res.* 1986;20(10):951-954.

242. Vergani P, Ghidini A, Locatelli A, et al. Risk factors for pulmonary hypoplasia in second-trimester premature rupture of membranes. *Am J Obstet Gynecol.* 1994;170(5 pt 1):1359-1364.

243. Potter EL. Bilateral renal agenesis. *J Pediatr.* 1946;29:68-76.

244. Wenstrom KD. Pulmonary hypoplasia and deformations related to premature rupture of membranes. *Obstet Gynecol Clin North Am.* 1992;19(2):397-408.

245. Blott M, Nicolaides KH, Gibb D, Greenough A, Moscoso G, Campbell S. Fetal breathing movements as predictor of favourable pregnancy outcome after oligohydramnios due to membrane rupture in second trimester. *Lancet.* 1987;2(8551):129-131.

246. Nimrod C, Varela-Gittings F, Machin G, Campbell D, Wesenberg R. The effect of very prolonged membrane rupture on fetal development. *Am J Obstet Gynecol.* 1984;148(5):540-543.

247. Bukowski R, Gahn D, Denning J, Saade G. Impairment of growth in fetuses destined to deliver preterm. *Am J Obstet Gynecol.* 2001;185(2):463-467.

248. Spinillo A, Montanari L, Sanpaolo P, Bergante C, Chiara A, Fazzi E. Fetal growth and infant neurodevelopmental outcome after preterm premature rupture of membranes. *Obstet Gynecol.* 2004;103(6):1286-1293.

249. Tamura RK, Sabbagha RE, Depp R, Vaisrub N, Dooley SL, Socol ML. Diminished growth in fetuses born preterm after spontaneous labor or rupture of membranes. *Am J Obstet Gynecol.* 1984;148(8):1105-1110.

250. Gibbs RS, Blanco JD. Premature rupture of the membranes. *Obstet Gynecol.* 1982;60(6):671-679.

251. Russell KP, Anderson GV. The aggressive management of ruptured membranes. *Am J Obstet Gynecol.* 1962;83:930-937.

252. Bennett SL, Cullen J, Sherer D, Woods J. The ferning and nitrazine tests of amniotic fluid between 12 and 41 weeks gestation. *Am J Perinatol.* 1993;10(2):101-104.

253. Reece EA, Chervenak FA, Moya FR, Hobbins JC. Amniotic fluid arborization: effect of blood, meconium, and pH alterations. *Obstet Gynecol.* 1984;64(2):248-250.

254. Friedman ML, McElin TW. Diagnosis of ruptured fetal membranes. Clinical study and review of the literature. *Am J Obstet Gynecol.* 1969;104(4):544-550.

255. Lodeiro JG, Hsieh KA, Byers JH, Feinstein S. The fingerprint, a false-positive fern test. *Obstet Gynecol.* 1989;73(5 pt 2):873-874.

256. McGregor JA, Johnson S. "Fig leaf" ferning and positive nitrazine testing: semen as a cause of misdiagnosis of premature rupture of membranes. *Am J Obstet Gynecol.* 1985;151(8):1142-1143.

257. Brookes C, Shand K, Jones WR. A reevaluation of the ferning test to detect ruptured membranes. *Aust N Z J Obstet Gynaecol.* 1986;26(4):260-264.

258. Rosemond RL, Lombardi SJ, Boehm FH. Ferning of amniotic fluid contaminated with blood. *Obstet Gynecol.* 1990;75(3 pt 1):338-340.

259. Smith RP. A technic for the detection of rupture of the membranes. A review and preliminary report. *Obstet Gynecol.* 1976;48(2):172-176.

260. Palacio M, Kühnert M, Berger R, Larios CL, Marcellin L. Meta-analysis of studies on biochemical marker tests for the diagnosis of premature rupture of membranes: comparison of performance indexes. *BMC Pregnancy Childbirth.* 2014;14(1):183.

261. Lockwood CJ, Senyei AE, Dische MR, et al. Fetal fibronectin in cervical and vaginal secretions as a predictor of preterm delivery. *N Engl J Med.* 1991;325(10):669-674.

263. Goldenberg RL, Mercer B, Meis P, Copper R, Das A, Mcnellis D. The preterm prediction study: fetal fibronectin testing and spontaneous preterm birth. NICHD Maternal Fetal Medicine Units Network. *Obstet Gynecol.* 1996;87(5 pt 1):643-648.

264. Greenhagen JB, Van Wagonera J, Dudley D, et al. Value of fetal fibronectin as a predictor of preterm delivery for a low-risk population. *Am J Obstet Gynecol.* 1996;175(4 pt 1):1054-1056.

265. Langer B, Boudier E, Schlaeder G. Cervico-vaginal fetal fibronectin: predictive value during false labor. *Acta Obstet Gynecol Scand.* 1997;76(3):218-221.

266. Leeson SC, Maresh MJA, Martindale EA. Detection of fetal fibronectin as a predictor of preterm delivery in high risk asymptomatic pregnancies. *Br J Obstet Gynaecol.* 1996;103(1):48-53.

267. Malak TM, Sizmur F, Bell SC, Taylor DJ. Fetal fibronectin in cervico-vaginal secretions as a predictor of preterm birth. *Br J Obstet Gynaecol.* 1996;103(7):648-653.

268. Morrison JC, Allbert JR, McLaughlin BN, et al. Oncofetal fibronectin in patients with false labor as a predictor of preterm delivery. *Am J Obstet Gynecol.* 1993;168(2):538-542.

269. Nageotte MP, Casal D, Senyei AE. Fetal fibronectin in patients at increased risk for premature birth. *Am J Obstet Gynecol.* 1994;170(1 pt 1):20-25.

270. Rizzo G, Capponi A, Arduini D, Lorido C, Romanini C. The value of fetal fibronectin in cervical and vaginal secretions and of ultrasonographic examination of the uterine cervix in predicting premature delivery for patients with preterm labor and intact membranes. *Am J Obstet Gynecol.* 1996;175(5):1146-1151.

271. Lee SM, Romero R, Park JS, Chaemsaithong P, Jun JK, Yoon BH. A transcervical amniotic fluid collector: a new medical device for the assessment of amniotic fluid in patients with ruptured membranes. *J Perinat Med.* 2015;43(4):381-389.

273. Atlay RD, Sutherst JR. Premature rupture of the fetal membranes confirmed by intra-amniotic injection of dye (Evans blue T-1824). *Am J Obstet Gynecol.* 1970;108(6):993-994.

274. Diaz Garzon J. Indigo carmine test of premature rupture of membranes. *Rev Colomb Obstet Ginecol.* 1969;20(5):373-376.

275. Fujimoto S, Kishida T, Sagawa T, et al. Clinical usefulness of the dye-injection method for diagnosing premature rupture of the membranes in equivocal cases. *J Obstet Gynaecol (Tokyo 1995).* 1995;21(3):215-220.

276. Meyer BA, Gonik B, Creasy RK. Evaluation of phenazopyridine hydrochloride as a tool in the diagnosis of premature rupture of the membranes. *Am J Perinatol.* 1991;8(5):297-299.

277. Cowett RM, Hakanson DO, Kocon RW, Oh W. Untoward neonatal effect of intraamniotic administration of methylene blue. *Obstet Gynecol.* 1976;48(1 suppl):74s-75s.

278. McEnerney JK, McEnerney LN. Unfavorable neonatal outcome after intraamniotic injection of methylene blue. *Obstet Gynecol.* 1983;61(3 suppl):35s-37s.

279. Troche BI. The methylene blue baby. *N Engl J Med.* 1989;320(26):1756-1757.

280. Divon MY, Chamberlain PF, Sipos L, Platt LD. Underestimation of fetal weight in premature rupture of membranes. *J Ultrasound Med.* 1984;3(12):529-531.

281. Ben-Haroush A, Yogev Y, Bar J, et al. Accuracy of sonographically estimated fetal weight in 840 women with different pregnancy complications prior to induction of labor. *Ultrasound Obstet Gynecol.* 2004;23(2):172-176.

282. Edwards A, Goff J, Baker L. Accuracy and modifying factors of the sonographic estimation of fetal weight in a high-risk population. *Aust N Z J Obstet Gynaecol.* 2001;41(2):187-190.

283. Fleischer AC, Manning FA, Jeanty P, et al. *Sonography in Obstetrics and Gynecology: Principles & Practice.* McGraw-Hill; 2001.

284. Broekhuizen FF, Gilman M, Hamilton PR. Amniocentesis for gram stain and culture in preterm premature rupture of the membranes. *Obstet Gynecol.* 1985;66(3):316-321.

285. Dudley J, Malcolm G, Ellwood D. Amniocentesis in the management of preterm premature rupture of the membranes. *Aust N Z J Obstet Gynaecol.* 1991;31(4):331-336.

286. Feinstein SJ, Vintzileos AM, Lodeiro JG, Campbell WA, Weinbaum PJ, Nochimson DJ. Amniocentesis with premature rupture of membranes. *Obstet Gynecol.* 1986;68(2):147-152.

287. Mazor M, Chen R, Ghezzi F, et al. The clinical significance of microbial invasion of the amniotic cavity with genital mycoplasmas. *Am J Obstet Gynecol.* 1997;176(1):S40.

289. Yoon BH, Romero R, Moon JB, et al. Clinical significance of intra-amniotic inflammation in patients with preterm labor and intact membranes. *Am J Obstet Gynecol.* 2001;185(5):1130-1136.

290. Yoon BH, Romero R, Park JS, et al. Microbial invasion of the amniotic cavity with Ureaplasma urealyticum is associated with a robust host response in fetal, amniotic, and maternal compartments. *Am J Obstet Gynecol.* 1998;179(5):1254-1260.

291. Yoon BH, Romero R, Kim CJ, et al. Amniotic fluid interleukin-6: a sensitive test for antenatal diagnosis of acute inflammatory lesions of preterm placenta and prediction of perinatal morbidity. *Am J Obstet Gynecol.* 1995;172(3):960-970.

292. Font GE, Gauthier DW, Meyer WJ, Myles TD, Janda W, Bieniarz A. Catalase activity as a predictor of amniotic fluid culture results in preterm labor or premature rupture of membranes. *Obstet Gynecol.* 1995;85(5):656-658.

293. Hazan Y, Mazor M, Horowitz S, Leiberman JR, Glezerman M. The diagnostic value of amniotic fluid Gram stain examination and limulus amebocyte lysate assay in patients with preterm birth. *Acta Obstet Gynecol Scand.* 1995;74(4):275-280.

294. Jalava J, Mantymaa M-L, Ekblad U, et al. Bacterial 16S rDNA polymerase chain reaction in the detection of intra-amniotic infection. *Br J Obstet Gynaecol.* 1996;103(7):664-669.

297. Vintzileos AM, Knuppel RA. Fetal biophysical assessment in premature rupture of the membranes. *Clin Obstet Gynecol.* 1995;38(1):45-58.

298. Newton ER. Preterm labor, preterm premature rupture of membranes, and chorioamnionitis. *Clin Perinatol.* 2005;32(3):571-600.

300. Mastrolia SA, Erez O, Loverro G, et al. Ultrasonographic approach to diagnosis of fetal inflammatory response syndrome: a tool for at-risk fetuses? *Am J Obstet Gynecol.* 2016;215(1):9-20.

304. Story L, Hutter J, Zhang T, et al. The use of antenatal fetal magnetic resonance imaging in the assessment of patients at high risk of preterm birth. *Eur J Obstet Gynecol Reprod Biol.* 2018;222:134-141.

332. Alexander JM, Mercer BM, Miodovnik M, et al. The impact of digital cervical examination on expectantly managed preterm rupture of membranes. *Am J Obstet Gynecol.* 2000;183(4):1003-1007.

341. Fanaroff AA, Hack M. Periventricular leukomalacia – prospects for prevention. *N Engl J Med.* 1999;341:1229-1231.

342. Hack M, Fanaroff AA. Outcomes of extremely immature infants – a perinatal dilemma. *N Engl J Med.* 1993;329:1649-1650.

343. American College of Obstetricians and Gynecologists; Society for Maternal-Fetal Medicine. Obstetric Care Consensus No. 6: periviable birth. *Obstet Gynecol.* 2017;130:e187-e199.

344. Gold RB, Goyert GL, Schwartz DB, Evans MI, Seabolt LA. Conservative management of second-trimester post-amniocentesis fluid leakage. *Obstet Gynecol.* 1989;74(5):745-747.

345. Hanson FW, Tennant FR, Zorn EM, Samuels S. Analysis of 2136 genetic amniocenteses: experience of a single physician. *Am J Obstet Gynecol.* 1985;152(4):436-443.

347. Tsakiridis I, Mamopoulos A, Chalkia-Prapa E-M, Athanasiadis A, Dagklis T. Preterm premature rupture of membranes: a review of 3 national guidelines. *Obstet Gynecol Surv.* 2018;73(6):368-375.

356. American College of Obstetricians and Gynecologists. Intrapartum management of intraamniotic infection (Committee Opinion No. 712). *Obstet Gynecol.* 2017;130(2):e95-e101.

358. Vidaeff AC, Ramin SM. Antenatal corticosteroids after preterm premature rupture of membranes. *Clin Obstet Gynecol.* 2011;54(2):337-343.

359. Harding JE, Pang J-M, Knight DB, Liggins GC. Do antenatal corticosteroids help in the setting of preterm rupture of membranes? *Am J Obstet Gynecol.* 2001;184(2):131-139.

360. Roberts D, Brown J, Medley N, Dalziel SR. Antenatal corticosteroids for accelerating fetal lung maturation for women at risk of preterm birth. *Cochrane Database Syst Rev.* 2017;3:CD004454.

361. American College of Obstetricians and Gynecologists; Committe on Practice Bulletins – Obstetrics. ACOG Practice Bulletin No. 127: management of preterm labor. *Obstet Gynecol.* 2012;119:1308-1317.

362. Doyle LW, Crowther CA, Middleton P, Marret S, Rouse D. Magnesium sulphate for women at risk of preterm birth for neuroprotection of the fetus. *Cochrane Database Syst Rev.* 2009;(1):CD004661.

363. Effect of corticosteroids for fetal maturation on perinatal outcomes: NIH consensus development panel on the effect of corticosteroids for fetal maturation on perinatal outcomes. *J Am Med Assoc.* 1995;273(5):413-418.

364. Mercer BM. Preterm premature rupture of the membranes: diagnosis and management. *Clin Perinatol.* 2004;31(4):765-782.

365. Simhan HN, Canavan TP. Preterm premature rupture of membranes: diagnosis, evaluation and management strategies. *Br J Obstet Gynaecol.* 2005;112:32-37.

366. Harger JH. Comparison of success and morbidity in cervical cerclage procedures. *Obstet Gynecol.* 1980;56(5):543-548.

369. Carlan SJ, O'Brien WF, Parsons MT, Lense JJ. Preterm premature rupture of membranes: a randomized study of home versus hospital management. *Obstet Gynecol.* 1993;81(1):61-64.

370. El Senoun GA, Dowswell T, Mousa HA. Planned home versus hospital care for preterm prelabour rupture of the membranes (PPROM) prior to 37 weeks' gestation. *Cochrane Database Syst Rev.* 2014;(4):CD008053.

371. Hofmeyr GJ, Lawrie TA. Amnioinfusion for potential or suspected umbilical cord compression in labour. *Cochrane Database Syst Rev.* 2012;(1):CD000013.

374. Göbel S, Naberezhnev Y, Seliger G, Tchirikov M. Continuous amnioinfusion via a subcutaneously implanted port system with PPROM and anhydramnios <28 +0 weeks of gestation: an international prospective randomized trial. *Ultraschall Med.* 2016;37(suppl 1):P9-P15.

379. Chua S, Arulkumaran S, Yap C, Selamat N, Ratnam SS. Premature rupture of membranes in nulliparas at term with unfavorable cervices: a double-blind randomized trial of prostaglandin and placebo. *Obstet Gynecol.* 1995;86(4):550-554.

380. Chung T, Rogers MS, Gordon H, Chang A. Prelabour rupture of the membranes at term and Unfavourable cervix; a randomized placebo-controlled trial on early intervention with intravaginal prostaglandin E2 gel. *Aust N Z J Obstet Gynaecol.* 1992;32(1):25-27.

381. Duff P, Huff RW, Gibbs RS. Management of premature rupture of membranes and unfavorable cervix in term pregnancy. *Obstet Gynecol.* 1984;63(5):697-702.

382. Ekman-Ordeberg G, Uldbjerg N, Ulmsten U. Comparison of intravenous oxytocin and vaginal prostaglandin E2 gel in women with unripe cervixes and premature rupture of the membranes. *Obstet Gynecol.* 1985;66(3):307-310.

383. Gonen R, Samberg I, Degani S. Intracervical prostaglandin E2 for induction of labor in patients with premature rupture of membranes and an unripe cervix. *Am J Perinatol.* 1994;11(06):436-438.

384. Grant JM, Serle E, Mahmood T, Sarmandal P, Conway DI. Management of prelabour rupture of the membranes in term primigravidae: report of a randomized prospective trial. *Br J Obstet Gynaecol.* 1992;99(7):557-562.

385. Hannah ME, Ohlsson A, Farine D, et al. Induction of labor compared with expectant management for prelabor rupture of the membranes at term. TERMPROM Study Group. *N Engl J Med.* 1996;334(16):1005-1010.

386. Hjertberg R, Hammarström M, Moberger B, Nordlander E, Granström L. Premature rupture of the membranes (PROM) at term in nulliparous women with a ripe cervix. *Acta Obstet Gynecol Scand.* 1996;75(1):48-53.

387. Ladfors L, Mattsson L-A, Eriksson M, Fall O. A randomised trial of two expectant managements of prelabour rupture of the membranes at 34 to 42 weeks. *Br J Obstet Gynaecol.* 1996;103(8):755-762.

388. Mahmood T, Dick MJW, Smith NC, Templeton AA. Role of prostaglandin in the management of prelabour rupture of the membranes at term. *Br J Obstet Gynaecol.* 1992;99(2):112-117.

389. Mahmood TA, Dick MJ. A randomized trial of management of pre-labor rupture of membranes at term in multiparous women using vaginal prostaglandin gel. *Obstet Gynecol.* 1995;85(1):71-74.

390. Malik N, Gittens L, Gonzalez D, Bardeguez A, Ganesh V, Apuzzio J. Clinical amnionitis and endometritis in patients with premature rupture of membranes: endocervical prostaglandin E2 gel versus oxytocin for induction of labor. *Obstet Gynecol.* 1996;88(4): 540-543.

391. Morales WJ, Lazar AJ. Expectant management of rupture of membranes at term. *South Medical Journal.* 1986;79(8):955-958.

392. Mozurkewich EL, Wolf FM. Premature rupture of membranes at term: a metaanalysis of three management schemes. *Obstet Gynecol.* 1997;89(6):1035-1043.

393. Natale R, Milne JK, Campbell MK, Potts PGG, Webster K, Halinda E. Management of premature rupture of membranes at term: randomized trial. *Am J Obstet Gynecol.* 1994;171(4):936-939.

394. Ngai SW, To WK, Lao T, Ho P. Cervical priming with oral misoprostol in pre-labor rupture of membranes at term. *Obstet Gynecol.* 1996;87(6):923-926.

395. Ray DA, Garite TJ. Prostaglandin E2 for induction of labor in patients with premature rupture of membranes at term. *Am J Obstet Gynecol.* 1992;166(3):836-843.

396. Rydhström H, Ingemarsson I. No benefit from conservative management in nulliparous women with premature rupture of the membranes (PROM) at term: a randomized study. *Acta Obstet Gynecol Scand.* 1991;70(7-8):543-547.

397. Rymer J, Parker A. A comparison of syntocinon infusion with prostaglandin vaginal pessaries when spontaneous rupture of the membranes occurs without labour after 34 weeks gestation. *Aust N Z J Obstet Gynaecol.* 1992;32(1):22-24.

398. Sperling LS, Schantz AL, Wahlin A, et al. Management of prelabor rupture of membranes at term. *Acta Obstet Gynecol Scand.* 1993;72(8): 627-632.

399. Shalev E, Peleg D, Eliyahu S, Nahum Z. Comparison of 12-and 72-hour expectant management of premature rupture of membranes in term pregnancies. *Obstet Gynecol.* 1995;85(5):766-768.

400. Wagner MV, Chin VP, Peters CJ, Drexler B, Newman LA. A comparison of early and delayed induction of labor with spontaneous rupture of membranes at term. *Obstet Gynecol.* 1989;74(1):93-97.

401. Hallak M, Bottoms SF. Induction of labor in patients with term premature rupture of membranes. *Fetal Diagn Ther.* 1999;14(3):138-142.

408. Crowley AE, Grivell RM, Dodd JM. Sealing procedures for preterm prelabour rupture of membranes. *Cochrane Database Syst Rev.* 2016;7(7):CD010218.

423. Dam P, Laha S, Bhattacharya P, Daga P. Role of amnioseal in premature rupture of membranes. *J Obstet Gynecol India.* 2011;61(3):296.

424. Vaitkiene D, Bergstrom S. Management of amniocentesis in women with oligohydramnios due to membrane rupture: evaluation of a cervical adapter. *Gynecol Obstet Invest.* 1995;40(1):28-31.

CHAPTER **51**

Prolonged Pregnancy

Eyal Krispin

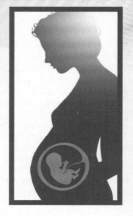

Introduction

Definitions

The American College of Obstetricians and Gynecologists (ACOG) has defined the term pregnancy as 37 0/7 to 41 6/7 weeks of gestation, and further divide term into three periods: (1) early term (37 0/7-38 6/7), (2) term (39 0/7-40 6/7), and (3) late (41 0/7-41 6/7). The ACOG classifies postterm as 42 0/7 weeks of gestation and later.

Incidence

Many factors may influence the prevalence estimates of term and postterm deliveries.

However, regardless of the variables that may influence rates of postterm pregnancy, accurate pregnancy dating remains a critical factor and perinatal mortality has been noted to increase in pregnancies with unknown dates.[14]

It is possible that some of these deaths are due to a failure to diagnose the prolonged pregnancy.

Risk Factors

The strongest risk factor for postterm pregnancy is a prior postterm pregnancy.[7]

Other noted risk factors are nulliparity, greater maternal age (35 years and older), obesity, and male fetus.[23]

Maternal Risks

Prolonged pregnancy is associated with increased maternal anxiety and morbidity. Higher rates of fetal macrosomia and uteroplacental insufficiency may result in greater need for operative vaginal delivery or cesarean delivery in both spontaneous and induced labor.[24-26]

ⓔ See the eBook for expanded content, a complete reference list, and additional tables.

Other maternal morbidities reported as associated with prolonged pregnancy include endometritis, chorioamnionitis, perineal laceration, and postpartum hemorrhage.[27]

Fetal and Neonatal Risks

Perinatal mortality reaches its nadir at 39 to 40 weeks and then increases as pregnancy exceeds 41 weeks. After 42 weeks the rate of perinatal mortality is twice the rate at term, increasing to fourfold at 43 weeks and to five- to sevenfold at 44 weeks.[28,29]

Deaths associated with postterm pregnancy occur during the antepartum, intrapartum, and neonatal period as the result of events related to uteroplacental insufficiency or to birth trauma caused by the development of fetal macrosomia. During the antepartum period, the fetus may suffer hypoxic ischemic insults resulting in stillbirth or intrauterine growth restriction and the development of the postmature syndrome.

Studies have shown that pregnancies that continue beyond 42 weeks have an increased risk of stillbirth,[30] but, when the risk of stillbirth is expressed as a function of ongoing pregnancies (stillbirth divided by total births), the mortality rate is even greater.

Most of the excessive perinatal mortality associated with a prolonged pregnancy occurs in the intrapartum and neonatal periods.[31]

Intrapartum asphyxia and meconium aspiration have been implicated in an estimated 25% of perinatal deaths.

Oligohydramnios is commonly encountered in prolonged pregnancies.

Fetal Macrosomia

The most common complication of prolonged pregnancy is fetal macrosomia, defined as newborn birth weights of 4000 to 4500 g.[35]

The clinical significance of birth weights between 4000 and 4500 g is unclear, but it has been well established that shoulder dystocia is greatest for infants weighing >4500 g.[38,39]

Macrosomia can also result in brachial plexus injuries and fractures.[35]

The diagnosis of fetal macrosomia by ultrasound is not precise, and the ACOG has concluded that ultrasound is better at ruling out macrosomia than ruling it in.[35]

Because sonographic diagnosis of fetal macrosomia has varying results based on reports in the literature, it remains unclear where the threshold for intervention should be set.

Management

The absolute goal for the management of the prolonged pregnancy is to reduce newborn morbidity and prevent stillbirth while keeping the cesarean delivery and operative vaginal delivery rates as low as possible. Although there is no clear consensus as to the most clinically correct method for the management of the prolonged pregnancy, the ACOG recommends induction of labor after 42 0/7 weeks and by 42 6/7 weeks, with earlier intervention at 41 0/7 to 42 0/7 weeks as needed.[44]

No single method of fetal assessment has proved superior in either sensitivity or specificity of fetal evaluation in the prolonged pregnancy, and as of the date of this publication, there have been no randomized controlled trials in which surveillance was compared with no surveillance.

Pregnancy Dating

The most important way to minimize the risks of postterm pregnancy is to establish accurate pregnancy dating as early as possible.

In women for whom there is uncertainty regarding their pregnancy dating, an ultrasound in the first or second trimesters should be obtained.[45-47]

The crown-rump length can determine gestational age to within 5 days.[48]

Most clinicians accept the variation in ultrasonography generally as ±7 days up to 20 weeks of gestation, ±14 days between 20 and 30 weeks of gestation, and ±21 days beyond 30 weeks of gestation. The use of ultrasound dating in these situations has significantly reduced the false diagnosis of prolonged pregnancy.[48,49]

When the ultrasound measurements differ from the last menstrual period (LMP) by more than these ranges, ultrasound estimates of estimated delivery date should be used.

Induction of Labor

Bishop scoring in prolonged pregnancy has limited applications.

A trial of labor after cesarean in prolonged pregnancies should be individually determined based on assessment of risks according to personal medical history.

Induction Protocols

Many different approaches to cervical ripening and induction of labor have been reported, and at present, there is no universally agreed upon method.[60-67]

In patients at 40 weeks or more with good pregnancy dating, consideration should be given to membrane stripping.

Both mechanical and pharmacological agents are acceptable options for labor induction in prolonged pregnancy and should be chosen according to specific patient limitations or preferences.

KEY POINTS

- Postterm pregnancy is defined as any pregnancy that continues past 42 weeks of gestation.
- Prolonged pregnancy is associated with increased maternal and fetal morbidity and mortality.
- The most common cause of the prolonged pregnancy is inaccurate dating.

- Postmaturity is a neonatal diagnosis and should be used to describe the infant with recognizable clinical features, including peeling; parchment-like skin; meconium staining of skin, membranes, and the umbilical cord; overgrown nails; well-developed creases on the palms and soles; abundance of scalp hair; little vernix or lanugo hair; scaphoid abdomen; and minimal subcutaneous fat.

- Around 20% of women cannot remember their LMP, and when there is late entry to prenatal care, there is often confusion regarding the dating of the pregnancy.
- The maternal risks from the prolonged pregnancy are associated with the increased need for operative vaginal delivery in both spontaneous and induced labor.
- Induction of labor at 41 weeks does not increase cesarean delivery rates or pregnancy cost and may reduce the incidence of stillbirth and newborn morbidity and mortality.
- Perinatal mortality reaches its nadir at 39 to 40 weeks and then increases as pregnancy exceeds 41 weeks. Multiple studies have demonstrated an increased risk of perinatal mortality after 42 weeks.
- Studies have shown that pregnancies that continue beyond 42 weeks have an increased risk of stillbirth, but when the risk of stillbirth is expressed as a function of ongoing pregnancies (stillbirth divided by total births), the mortality rate is even greater.

- Assuming that induction of labor does not carry increased perinatal risk, planned induction of labor at any gestational age should always result in fewer adverse perinatal outcomes.
- Most of the excessive perinatal mortality associated with a prolonged pregnancy occurs in the intrapartum and neonatal periods.
- Fetal conditions associated with prolonged pregnancy include intrapartum asphyxia, meconium aspiration, oligohydramnios, fetal macrosomia resulting in dystocia, and associated brachial plexus injuries and fractures.
- Given the intraobserver variability, the demonstrated poor predictive power, and the demonstrated success rates of induction protocols, Bishop scoring in the prolonged pregnancy has limited applications.
- In women for whom there is uncertainty regarding their pregnancy dating, an ultrasound in the first or second trimesters should be obtained. The crown-rump length, measured by sonography, can determine gestational age to within 5 days.

REFERENCES

(only references cited in synoptic print chapter; for a complete reference list, see ebook)

7. Oberg AS, Frisell T, Svensson AC, Iliadou AN. Maternal and fetal genetic contributions to postterm birth: familial clustering in a population-based sample of 475,429 Swedish births. *Am J Epidemiol.* 2013;177(6):531-537.

14. Ingemarsson I, Heden L. Cervical score and onset of spontaneous labor in prolonged pregnancy dated by second-trimester ultrasonic scan. *Obstet Gynecol.* 1989;74(1):102-105.

23. Morken NH, Melve KK, Skjaerven R. Recurrence of prolonged and post-term gestational age across generations: maternal and paternal contribution. *BJOG.* 2011;118(13):1630.

24. The national institute of child health and human development network of maternal-fetal medicine units. A clinical trial of induction of labor versus expectant management in postterm pregnancy. *Am J Obstet Gynecol.* 1994;170(3):716-723.

25. Hannah ME, Hannah WJ, Hellmann J, et al. Induction of labor as compared with serial antenatal monitoring in post-term pregnancy. A randomized controlled trial. The Canadian Multicenter Post-term Pregnancy Trial Group. *N Engl J Med.* 1992;326(24):1587-1592.

26. Goeree R, Hannah M, Hewson S. Cost-effectiveness of induction of labour versus serial antenatal monitoring in the Canadian Multicentre Postterm Pregnancy Trial. *Can Med Assoc J.* 1995;152(9):1445-1450.

27. Caughey AB, Stotland NE, Washington AE, Escobar GJ. Maternal and obstetric complications of pregnancy are associated with increasing gestational age at term. *Am J Obstet Gynecol.* 2007;196:155.

28. De Los Santos-Garate AM, Villa-Guillen M, Villanueva-García D, Vallejos-Ruíz ML, Murguía-Peniche MT; NEOSANO's Network. Perinatal morbidity and mortality in late-term and post-term pregnancy. NEOSANO perinatal network's experience in Mexico. *J Perinatol.* 2011;31(12):789.

29. Bruckner TA, Cheng YW, Caughey AB. Increased neonatal mortality among normal-weight births beyond 41 weeks of gestation in California. *Am J Obstet Gynecol.* 2008;199(4):421.e1.

30. Myers ER, Blumrick R, Christian AL, et al. *Management of Prolonged Pregnancy (Evidence Reports/Technology Assessments, No. 53).* Agency for Healthcare Research and Quality; 2002. Accessed July 11, 2017. https://archive.ahrq.gov/downloads/pub/evidence/pdf/prolpreg/prolpreg.pdf

31. Curtis PD, Matthews TG, Clarke TA, et al. Neonatal seizures: the Dublin Collaborative Study. *Arch Dis Child.* 1988;63(9):1065-1068.

35. American College of Obstetricians and Gynecologists' Committee on Practice Bulletins—Obstetrics. Practice Bulletin No. 173: fetal macrosomia. *Obstet Gynecol.* 2016;128(5):e195-e209.

38. Pollack RN, Hauer-Pollack G, Divon MY. Macrosomia in postdates pregnancies: the accuracy of routine ultrasonographic screening. *Am J Obstet Gynecol.* 1992;167(1):7-11.

39. Chervenak JL, Divon MY, Hirsch J, et al. Macrosomia in the postdate pregnancy: is routine ultrasonographic screening indicated? *Am J Obstet Gynecol.* 1989;161(3):753-756.

44. Middleton P, Shepherd E, Crowther CA. Induction of labour for improving birth outcomes for women at or beyond term. *Cochrane Database Syst Rev.* 2018;5(5):CD004945.

45. Bennett KA, Crane JM, O'shea P, Lacelle J, Hutchens D, Copel JA. First trimester ultrasound screening is effective in reducing postterm labor induction rates: a randomized controlled trial. *Am J Obstet Gynecol.* 2004;190:1077-1081.

46. Whitworth M, Bricker L, Neilson JP, Dowswell T. Ultrasound for fetal assessment in early pregnancy. *Cochrane Database Syst Rev.* 2010;14(4):CD007058. doi:10.1002/14651858.CD007058.pub2

47. Caughey AB, Nicholson JM, Washington AE. First-vs second-trimester ultrasound: the effect on pregnancy dating and perinatal outcomes. *Am J Obstet Gynecol.* 2008;198:703.e1-703.e5.

48. Mongelli M, Yuxin NG, Biswas A, Chew S. Accuracy of ultrasound dating formulae in the late second-trimester in pregnancies conceived with in-vitro fertilization. *Acta Radiol.* 2003;44(4):452-455.

49. Savitz DA, Terry JW Jr, Dole N, et al. Comparison of pregnancy dating by last menstrual period, ultrasound scanning, and their combination. *Am J Obstet Gynecol.* 2002;187(6):1660-1666.

60. Boulvain M, Fraser WD, Marcoux S, et al. Does sweeping of the membranes reduce the need for formal induction of labour? A randomised controlled trial. *Br J Obstet Gynaecol.* 1998;105(1):34-40.

61. Boulvain M, Irion O, Marcoux S, Fraser W. Sweeping of the membranes to prevent post-term pregnancy and to induce labour: a systematic review. *Br J Obstet Gynaecol.* 1999;106(5):481-485.

62. Cammu H, Haitsma V. Sweeping of the membranes at 39 weeks in nul-liparous women: a randomised controlled trial. *Br J Obstet Gynaecol.* 1998;105(1):41-44.

63. Crane J, Bennett K, Young D, et al. The effectiveness of sweeping membranes at term: a randomized trial. *Obstet Gynecol.* 1997;89(4):586-590.

64. el Torkey M, Grant JM. Sweeping of the membranes is an effective method of induction of labour in prolonged pregnancy: a report of a randomized trial. *Br J Obstet Gynaecol.* 1992;99(6):455-458.

65. Boulvain M, Stan CM, Irion O. Membrane sweeping for induction of labour. *Cochrane Database Syst Rev.* 2005;2005(1):CD000451. doi:10.1002/14651858.CD000451.pub2

66. de Miranda E, van der Bom JG, Bonsel GJ, Bleker OP, Rosendaal FR. Membrane sweeping and prevention of post-term pregnancy in low-risk pregnancies: a randomised controlled trial. *BJOG.* 2006;113(4):402.

67. Vaknin Z, Kurzweil Y, Sherman D. Foley catheter balloon vs locally applied prostaglandins for cervical ripening and labor induction: a systematic review and metaanalysis. *Am J Obstet Gynecol.* 2010;203(5):418.

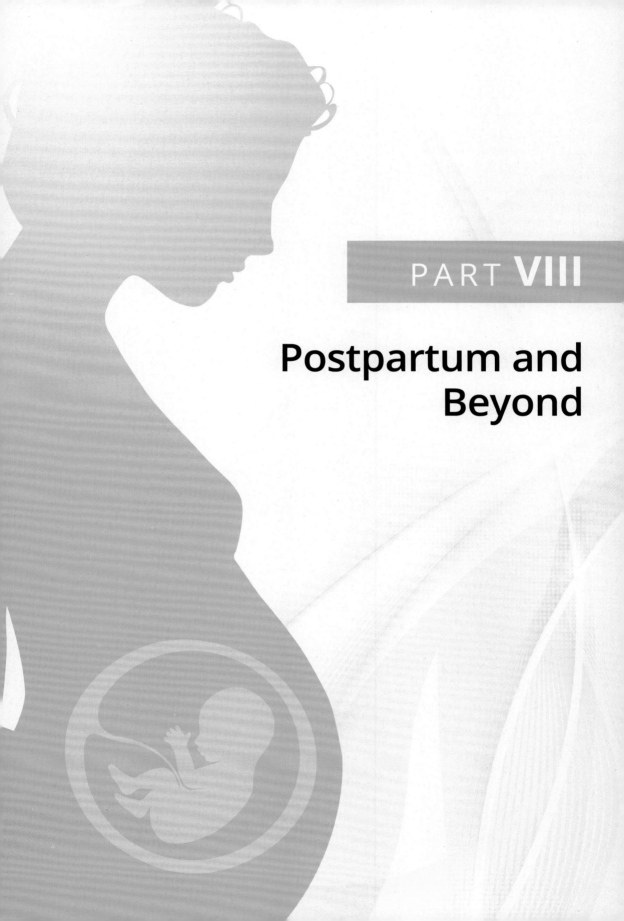

PART **VIII**

Postpartum and Beyond

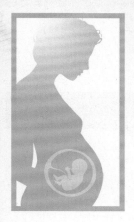

CHAPTER 52

Puerperium and Lactation: Physiology of the Reproductive System

Anat Shmueli

Reproductive System

Ultrasound evaluation of the postpartum uterus suggests a slight increase in puerperal uterine size in women who deliver via cesarean, although little difference in involution has been noted between breastfeeding and formula-feeding mothers.[1,2] Some studies suggest an increased uterine size during the puerperium in multiparous women, although others do not support this finding.[3,4] Fluid and debris may be noted in the uterine cavity of asymptomatic women in the midpuerperium.[5]

Painful postpartum uterine contractions are commonly referred to as "afterpains." This appears to be more problematic in multiparous women.[8] Breastfeeding mothers frequently note an association of afterpains with nursing episodes due to oxytocin release. Nonsteroidal anti-inflammatory agents, such as ibuprofen, may be used for analgesia.

Cervix and Vagina

Persistent heavy bleeding and a continued open cervical os should alert the physician to the possibility of retained placental fragments. Cervical dysplasia may regress in the postpartum period. Kaplan et al[10] studied 157 women with antepartum cervical squamous intraepithelial neoplasia and their subsequent postpartum course. Sixty-two percent of patients with low-grade antepartum dysplasia had regression, while only 6% experienced disease progression, although 60%

developed recurrent disease within 5 years. All 28 cases of antepartum high-grade dysplasia in this study persisted postpartum.

Hormonal Regulation

Nonlactating mothers experience ovulation on average 45 days after delivery with return of menses in many by 7 to 9 weeks postpartum. Lactating mothers experience a delayed and much more variable return to both ovulation and menstruation, which may relate to specific breastfeeding practices.[11,12] During the first 6 months after delivery, women who are amenorrheic and breastfeeding frequently ($\geq$8 times/24 hours) without giving supplements to the neonate have a less than 2% risk of pregnancy.[13-19]

Urinary System

Urinary retention with overdistention, urinary tract infection, and stress urinary incontinence are common transient problems. Dilation of the ureters may persist for 3 months or more postpartum.[23,24]

Lactation

Exclusive breastfeeding during approximately the first 6 months of life with continued breastfeeding through at least the second half of infancy is associated with reduced risk of adverse outcomes in mother and infant[25,26] (**Table 52.1**). Human milk is the recommended nutrition not only for full-term infants but also for preterm and extremely preterm infants. Environmental factors have a marked influence on breastfeeding success. Obstetric practices must be evaluated for their potential impact on lactation performance.

e   *See the eBook for expanded content and a complete reference list.*

Table 52.1 Associations Between Breastfeeding and Risk of Adverse Outcomes

| Adverse Outcome | Infant Risk | | Maternal Risk |
	During Breastfeeding	After Weaning	
Gastrointestinal and respiratory illnesses	Decreased[25]	Decreased if exclusively BF for >3 mo[25,27]	
Celiac disease	Decreased[28]	Delayed onset/possibly reduced severity[28]	
Wheezing	Decreased[29]	Decreased[29]	
Urinary infections	Decreased[25]		
Diabetes		Decreased[30,31]	Decreased[32]
Leukemia		Decreased[33,34]	
Atopic dermatitis	Decreased		
Obesity		Decreased[35,36]	
Crohn disease		Decreased[28]	
Rheumatoid arthritis		Decreased[37]	Decreased[38]
Breast cancer			Decreased[39]
Ovarian cancer			Decreased[40]
Endometrial cancer			Decreased[41]
Bone density			Temporary decrease followed by increase over baseline with resumption of menses[42,43]
Visual acuity	Increased[25]		
Cognition/psychomotor performance		Increased[44,45]	
Blood pressure and cardiovascular disease			Decreased[46]
Metabolic syndrome			Decreased[46]
Alzheimer disease			Decreased[47]

BF, breastfeeding.

Onset of Milk Production and Early Lactation Failure

Onset of copious milk production (lactogenesis stage II or LS-II) begins after delivery of the placenta and subsequent fall in progesterone.[51] The mean time for LS-II is 50 to 73 hours postpartum.[52] LS-II occurs later following stressful deliveries[53] and in primiparious,[54] obese[55-57] women with excessive gestational weight gain[58] and in women with preexisting diabetes.[52] Delayed onset of LS-II is a risk factor for premature weaning, and dyads with risk factors should be monitored closely.

Early lactation failure or partial inhibition of milk production can result from primary glandular insufficiency, retained placenta,[51] and severe postpartum hemorrhage resulting in ischemic pituitary necrosis and Sheehan syndrome.[59]

Regulation of Milk Volume

For individual women, milk volume increases or decreases in response to alterations in mammary stimulation and the degree of breast emptying.

Suckling triggers prolactin increase, which peaks at 30 minutes and returns to baseline after 2.5 to 3 hours. Relationships between milk production and prolactin levels are not straightforward. This may reflect numerical or functional differences in prolactin receptors. Milk ejection results from oxytocin-induced contraction of myoepithelial cells surrounding the alveoli. Lactiferous ducts then increase in diameter facilitating milk flow.[50,65]

Weaning and Involution of the Mammary Gland

Involution of the mammary gland is triggered by prolonged milk stasis and termination of suckling.

Composition of Human Milk

Human milk components are multifunctional, serving not only as nutrients but also in a variety of ways that promote infant health and development. Proteins, for example, are a source of peptides, amino acids, and nitrogen and are also involved in the development of the immune response (immunoglobulins), nonimmunologic defense (lactoferrin, lysozyme), growth stimulation (neural growth factor), and other functions. Carbohydrates provide nutritional support (lactose) and prevent bacterial adhesion to mucosal surfaces (oligosaccharides).[70-74] Human milk oligosaccharides (HMOs) are dietary fibers that pass through the digestive tract largely intact,[75] acting as prebiotics, and presumably promote gastric motility. Concentrations of HMOs vary over time[76-80] and this, along with variations in the type of oligosaccharides present, may be genetically determined.[72,76,77,81-83]

Human milk is commonly differentiated into colostrum, transitional, and mature milk. Colostrum, the initial milk produced in the first 3 to 7 days postpartum, is uniquely suited for the neonate. Colostrum appears to act also as an infant growth promoter.[48] Throughout lactation the specificity of secretory immunoglobulin A (sIgA), the primary antibody which defends the mucous membranes, in milk depends on the mother's antigen exposure and response. In this sense, human milk is location-specific.

Maternal Diet and Milk Composition

In general, the nutrient content of milk is more responsive to maternal diet during lactation in malnourished than in well-nourished women,[86] and current data suggest that it is not diet, but rather the maternal body composition and body mass index that may be associated with the nutritional value of human milk.[87]

Two nutrients may not be supplied in adequate amounts in milk from normal, well-nourished women: vitamin K[89] and vitamin D.[90] Routine intramuscular injection of vitamin K1 at birth provides all the vitamin K the infant needs. The American Academy of Pediatrics recommends daily supplementation with 200 IU of vitamin D to all infants unless they consume at least 500 mL/d vitamin D–fortified formula.[91]

Other nutritional deficiencies may be observed in breastfed infants of severely malnourished or diet-restricted mothers, including deficiencies in vitamin A, D, B1, B2, B3, B6, and B12, folic acid, ascorbic acid, iodine, zinc, and carnitine.[92,93] Therefore, women following a vegetarian or vegan diet should consume B12 supplements, particularly during pregnancy and lactation.

Although all human milk contains docosahexaenoic acid (DHA), 10-fold elevations can result from increased maternal dietary intake. DHA is critical for infant neurologic development.[100] Supplementation during lactation alone has not been found to improve mental functioning,[102] but may improve psychomotor functioning.[103] Conversely, milk cholesterol levels do not respond to maternal diet, and are elevated in mothers with familial hypercholesterolemia.[104]

Contaminants in Human Milk

Despite the presence of contaminants in human milk, breastfed infants are healthier than infants who are not breastfed. Much work remains to be done to identify circumstances in which the adverse effects of milk contaminants may outweigh the adverse effects of failure to provide human milk.

Exercise and Calorie Restriction Diets During Lactation

Although most women lose an average of 0.5 to 1.0 kg/mo after postpartum diuresis,[111,112] individual weight loss varies. Prenatal education regarding the realities of postpartum weight management is advisable. Failure to return to prepregnancy weight by 6 months postpartum increases the risk of obesity 1 year postpartum,[116] up to a decade later.[117] Energy required for lactation is derived from increased intake in preference to body fat mobilization.[119]

Women who desire to initiate or increase weight loss may be advised to begin moderate calorie restriction (500 kcal/d) and regular exercise after breastfeeding is well established.[123]

Exercise has no apparent impact on milk composition, excluding a temporary rise in lactate after prolonged, heavy exercise.[125] Women should be advised to consume a balanced diet during calorie restriction to protect their health.

Prenatal and Perinatal Practices and Conditions That Affect Breastfeeding

Breastfeeding should be recommended at the initial prenatal examination. Further education can be offered during prenatal care for women planning to breastfeed and those initially inclined to formula feed. Prior breast reduction or other surgery involving a periareolar incision should prompt counseling regarding the importance of communicating that information to the pediatrician and the need to monitor infant growth. Multiparous women should be questioned regarding their prior breastfeeding experiences, and any concerns should be addressed.

Cigarettes

About 50% of women resume tobacco use in the first few months after birth.[128] Infant exposure to environmental tobacco smoke is associated with increases in the incidence of respiratory allergies and in sudden infant death syndrome.[128] Nicotine and its metabolite cotinine are present in human milk. Importantly, however, neurologic deficits associated with maternal cigarette smoking in formula-fed infants were not observed in a comparison group of infants breastfed for >3 weeks.[130]

Caffeine

Rare concerns with irritability and insomnia have been reported, but are unlikely with occasional and moderate (one to two 8-ounce cups per day) consumption.

Alcohol

Contrary to previous beliefs of the beneficial effects of alcohol on breastfeeding, it has been demonstrated that alcohol to some extent inhibits lactation.[65,128] Because there is no evidence on a "safe" amount of alcohol in breast milk, alcohol exposure throughout lactation should be avoided.[133]

Substance Abuse

Substances of abuse are contraindicated during pregnancy and lactation. The exception is methadone supplied within the context of a successful maintenance program. Mothers engaging in continued substance abuse postpartum should be provided with support services for drug dependency treatment and counseled not to breastfeed.

Medication Use

Few studies examine drug use during lactation, and specialized references are required to formulate

Table 52.2 Contraindications for Breastfeeding

Condition	Contraindication
Substances of abuse (except methadone maintenance program and free of other drugs)	Absolute
Alcohol abuse	Absolute
Chemotherapeutic agents	Absolute or relative (depending on prior fetal exposure, duration of agent, and particular agent involved)
Maternal HIV	Absolute in the United States
	Relative regions with insufficient access to formula or clean water
Maternal HSV infection of nipple	Temporary cessation from involved nipple/areola until lesions resolved
Active untreated maternal tuberculosis	Temporary until after treatment established
Radioactive iodine-131 therapy	Absolute due to long half-life and potential to concentrate in thyroid and breast
Infant galactosemia	Absolute

HIV, human immunodeficiency virus; HSV, herpes simplex virus.

appropriate advice. The healthcare provider should review available information with the parents and discuss their individual situation. The age, weight, and health of the child, in addition to the amount of breast milk in the diet and any medications the child is taking, should be considered when choosing which medication is the best choice.

Maternal Health Problems

Table 52.2 lists circumstances in which breastfeeding is contraindicated. **Table 52.3** lists concerns regarding breastfeeding by women with specific diseases.

Lactation Support Strategies for Mother and Infant

Intrapartum Influences

Labor companionship and support have been associated with improved breastfeeding initiation and continuation rates.

Table 52.3 Maternal Disease and Breastfeeding Considerations

Infection	Route of Transmission	Breastfeeding Considerations
HIV	Blood and body fluids	Contraindicated in the United States and regions where safe alternatives to breast milk are available
Hepatitis A	Fecal and oral	Continued breastfeeding: encourage good hygiene
Hepatitis B	Blood and body fluids	Continued breastfeeding: infant to receive HBIG within 12 h of birth and hepatitis B vaccination
Hepatitis C	Blood and body fluids	Continued breastfeeding: no difference in transmission rate (~4%) in breastfed versus formula-fed infants. Some experts recommend temporary interruption of breastfeeding when bleeding nipples are present
Cytomegalovirus	Respiratory	Continued breastfeeding of healthy term infant
		Breastfeeding of premature infant during infection deserves individual consideration
Herpes simplex virus	Direct contact	Continued breastfeeding unless lesions on nipple/areola (see above). Cover lesions in potential contact with infant, good hygiene
Varicella virus	Respiratory, direct contact	Maternal primary infection: infant VZIG and possible vaccination depending on infant age
		Maternal shingles: continued breastfeeding, cover lesions in potential contact with infant and encourage good hygiene. Consider VZIG

HBIG, hepatitis B immunoglobulin; HIV, human immunodeficiency virus; VZIG, varicella immune globulin.

Labor Induction and Delivery Method

Studies evaluating the influence of labor induction on breastfeeding success reach varying conclusions and may be confounded by maternal confidence or intentionality. Some show lower rates of exclusive breastfeeding,[150] whereas others do not. Several studies have shown a relationship between intrapartum oxytocin administration and inhibition of breastfeeding in the immediate postpartum period. Although previously studied, the effect of epidural analgesia on breastfeeding continues to be controversial, mainly because of these studies' methodology.

Maternal-Infant Contact

Unless medically indicated, newborn interventions, such as vitamin K injection, the application of ophthalmic ointment, newborn screening, and measurements, should be delayed until after the first hour of life. In an ideal situation, these procedures can be performed in the room of the new family. The family should be encouraged to room-in with

the infant and breastfeed on demand. Rooming-in helps facilitate the acquisition of parental roles and the development of nonverbal parent-infant communication skills such as the recognition of infant hunger and satiety cues required for successful breastfeeding.

Latch and milk transfer during feeding should be assessed by trained personnel within 8 hours prior to hospital discharge (**Table 52.4**).

Common Problems in Postpartum Care

Mastitis

Mastitis occurs in approximately 10% of breastfeeding women during the first 12 weeks postpartum. *Staphylococcus aureus* is the most common organism cultured from the mastitic breast.

Signs and symptoms of mastitis include an erythematous, tender breast, fever, and flu-like symptoms such as myalgia, nausea, and headache. A localized tender knot in the breast in the absence of symptoms of infection suggests a plugged duct,

Table 52.4 Breastfeeding Information for New Parents

1. Normal milk production is quite low until after the onset of lactogenesis stage II between the first and fifth days postpartum
2. Most infants nurse 8-14 times/day in the first 1-2 wk. This decreases to 7-10 times/day by 4 wk
3. Each infant's "demand" breastfeeding frequency reflects its own developmental status and nursing skill as well as the mother's milk flow
4. After the third day of life, exclusively breastfed infants usually soak six or more diapers and have three or more stools of 1 tablespoon or greater/day
5. Infant stools normally change from dark (green or brown) to mustard yellow by the fifth day. This happens after the mother's milk "comes in and the baby begins to receive larger volumes of milk, which clears the meconium from the gastrointestinal tract"
6. Healthcare provider should be notified promptly if urine or stool patterns deviate from norms indicated in items 4 and 5 or if parents are concerned about adequacy of infant intake or maternal milk production

which can be managed with frequent nursing and warm compresses. More diffuse firmness in both breasts in the initial week postpartum is suggestive of engorgement. The presence of a fluctuant palpable and tender mass in the mastitic breast is suggestive of a breast abscess.

Mastitis is treated with a penicillinase-resistant antibiotic, such as dicloxacillin or cephalosporin, for 10 to 14 days. Breastfeeding the healthy term infant during treatment of mastitis should be continued, and drainage of the infected breast is important in recovery.

A Cochrane review published in 2015 concluded that current research is insufficient to determine whether needle aspiration is a more effective option to incision and drainage or whether an antibiotic should be routinely added to women undergoing incision and drainage for lactational breast abscesses.

KEY POINTS

- In controlled studies, lack of breastfeeding and/or earlier introduction of supplements and weaning are associated with increased risk of a variety of adverse outcomes in mothers and infants (see **Table 52.1**).
- Onset of copious milk production (stage II lactogenesis) begins after delivery of the placenta in response to the subsequent fall in circulating progesterone. Delay of lactogenesis stage II beyond 5 days postpartum should prompt evaluation.
- Failed lactogenesis can result from primary glandular insufficiency, retained placenta, or severe postpartum hemorrhage resulting in ischemic pituitary necrosis and Sheehan syndrome.
- When engorgement becomes severe, analgesics are appropriate treatment for pain, and immediate skilled assistance may be needed to achieve effective latching and efficient milk removal.
- In established lactation, milk volumes average 750 mL/d and increase or decrease in response to alterations in mammary stimulation and the degree of breast emptying.
- The nutrient content of human milk is conveyed to the infant within, and does not exist apart from, a redundant milieu of anti-infective, growth-stimulating, and anti-inflammatory agents.
- Strict vegetarians and vegans should consume vitamin B12 supplements during pregnancy and lactation for their own health and to prevent vitamin B12 deficiencies in their infants.
- In spite of the ubiquitous presence of environmental contaminants in human milk, breastfed infants are healthier than infants who are not breastfed.
- Breastfeeding women who desire to lose weight may be advised to initiate moderate caloric restriction (500 kcal/d below maintenance levels), consume a balanced diet, and undertake regular exercise after breastfeeding is well established.

- During the first 6 months postpartum, women who are amenorrheic and breastfeeding frequently (≥8 times/24 hours) have a less than 2% risk of pregnancy. Nevertheless, contraception should be offered to these women.
- Women with specific breastfeeding-related concerns, such as breast implants, prior breast surgery, inverted nipples, time constraints, or lack of confidence, should be educated regarding their particular situation.
- Advice regarding medication use during breastfeeding should be formulated only after reviewing information on that medication, exploring alternative treatments, and discussing the individual situation with the mother.
- Maternal contraindications to breastfeeding are rare and include continued use of substances of abuse, rare chemotherapeutic and other medications, and maternal HIV infection.
- Having staff trained in lactation support can help to minimize the impact of potential obstacles to breastfeeding, which may present with medically complicated pregnancies and/or medical interventions associated with delivery.
- During an uncomplicated pregnancy and delivery, the infant can be placed skin-to-skin with the mother at delivery, and breastfeeding initiation should be encouraged within the first hour after birth.
- In the initial post-cesarean period, patient-controlled analgesia with morphine or continuous extradural anesthesia is preferred over the use of meperidine because of the association of meperidine with poor infant suckling behavior in the early postpartum period.
- First-time mothers should be specifically and carefully advised of the ranges of normal for volume of colostrum, time of onset of copious milk production, frequencies of infant feeding, stooling, and urination, and the timing of meconium passage, with clear instructions to contact the care provider should the infant deviate from expected norms (**Table 52.4**).
- Breastfed infants should return to their healthcare provider in the first few days after discharge to assure that the mother's milk has come in, infant weight loss has ceased, and jaundice and dehydration are not significant.
- Evaluation of persistent breast masses should be pursued regardless of lactation status.
- Breastfeeding the healthy, term infant should be continued during treatment of mastitis with antibiotics; excellent drainage of the infected breast is important in maternal recovery.

REFERENCES

(only references cited in synoptic print chapter; for a complete reference list, see ebook)

1. Negishi H, Kishida T, Yamada H, et al. Changes in uterine size after vaginal delivery and cesarean section determined by vaginal sonography in the puerperium. *Arch Gynecol Obstet*. 1999;263(1-2):13-16.
2. Shalev J, Royburt M, Fite G, et al. Sonographic evaluation of the puerperal uterus: correlation with manual examination. *Gynecol Obstet Invest*. 2002;53(1):38-41.
3. Olayemi O, Omigbodun AA, Obajimi MO, et al. Ultrasound assessment of the effect of parity on postpartum uterine involution. *J Obstet Gynecol*. 2002;22(4):381-384.
4. Mulic-Lutvica A, Bekuretsion M, Bakos O, Axelsson O. Ultrasonic evaluation of the uterus and uterine cavity after normal, vaginal delivery. *Ultrasound Obstet Gynecol*. 2001;18(5):491-498.
5. Al-Bdour AN, Akasheh HF, Al-Husban NA. Ultrasonography of the uterus after normal vaginal delivery. *Saudi Med J*. 2004;25(1):41-44.
8. Murray A, Holdcroft A. Incidence and intensity of postpartum lower abdominal pain. *Br Med J*. 1989;298(6688):1619.
10. Kaplan KJ, Dainty LA, Dolinsky B, et al. Prognosis and recurrence risk for patients with cervical squamous intraepithelial lesions diagnosed during pregnancy. *Cancer*. 2004;102(4):228-232.
11. Howie PW, McNeilly AS. Breast-feeding and postpartum ovulation. *IPPF Med Bull*. 1982;16(2):1-3.
12. Rogers IS. Lactation and fertility. *Early Hum Dev*. 1997;49(suppl):S185-S190.
13. Lactation amenorrhea: experts recommend full breastfeeding as a child spacing method. *Network*. 1988;10(2):12.
14. Short RV, Lewis PR, Renfree MB, Shaw G. Contraceptive effects of extended lactational amenorrhoea: beyond the Bellagio Consensus. *Lancet*. 1991;337(8743):715-717.
15. Kennedy KI, Visness CM. Contraceptive efficacy of lactational amenorrhoea. *Lancet*. 1992;339(8787):227-230.
16. Perez A, Labbok MH, Queenan JT. Clinical study of the lactational amenorrhoea method for family planning. *Lancet*. 1992;339(8799):968-970.
17. Gross BA. Is the lactational amenorrhea method a part of natural family planning? Biology and policy. *Am J Obstet Gynecol*. 1991;165(6 pt 2):2014-2019.
18. World Health Organization Task Force on methods for the natural regulation of fertility. The World Health Organization Multinational Study of breast-feeding and lactational amenorrhea. III. Pregnancy during breast-feeding. *Fertil Steril*. 1999;72(3):431-440.
19. Labbok MH, Hight-Laukaran V, Peterson AE, et al. Multicenter study of the Lactational Amenorrhea Method (LAM): I. Efficacy, duration, and implications for clinical application. *Contraception*. 1997;55(6):327-336.
23. Bailey RR, Rolleston GL. Kidney length and ureteric dilatation in the puerperium. *J Obstet Gynaecol Br Commonw*. 1971;78(1):55-61.

24. Beydoun SN. Morphologic changes in the renal tract in pregnancy. *Clin Obstet Gynecol*. 1985;28(2):249-256.

25. Gartner LM, Morton J, Lawrence RA, et al. Breastfeeding and the use of human milk. *Pediatrics*. 2005;115(2):496-506.

26. Del Ciampo LA, Del Ciampo IRL. Breastfeeding and the benefits of lactation for women's health. *Rev Bras Ginecol Obstet*. 2018;40(6):354-359.

27. Wright AL, Bauer M, Naylor A, et al. Increasing breastfeeding rates to reduce infant illness at the community level. *Pediatrics*. 1998;101:837-844.

28. Akobeng AK, Ramanan AV, Buchan I, Heller RF. Effect of breastfeeding on risk of coeliac disease: a systematic review and meta-analysis of observational studies. *Arch Dis Child*. 2005;91:39-43.

29. Oddy WH, Halonen M, Martinez FD, et al. TGF-beta in human milk is associated with wheeze in infancy. *J Allergy Clin Immunol*. 2003;112:723-728.

30. Taylor JS, Kacmar JE, Nothnagle M, Lawrence RA. A systematic review of the literature associating breastfeeding with type 2 diabetes and gestational diabetes. *J Am Coll Nutr*. 2005;24:320-326.

31. Rodekamp E, Harder T, Kohlhoff R, et al. Long-term impact of breastfeeding on body weight and glucose tolerance in children of diabetic mothers: role of the late neonatal period and early infancy. *Diabetes Care*. 2005;28:1457-1462.

32. Stuebe AM, Rich-Edwards JW, Willett WC, et al. Duration of lactation and incidence of type 2 diabetes. *J Am Med Assoc*. 2005;294:2601-2610.

33. Kwan ML, Buffler PA, Abrams B, Kiley VA. Breastfeeding and the risk of childhood leukemia: a meta-analysis. *Public Health Rep*. 2004;119:521-535.

34. Martin RM, Gunnell D, Owen CG, Smith GD. Breast-feeding and childhood cancer: a systematic review with metaanalysis. *Int J Cancer*. 2005;117:1020-1031.

35. Arenz S, Ruckerl R, Koletzko B, von KR. Breast-feeding and childhood obesity – a systematic review. *Int J Obes Relat Metab Disord*. 2004;28:1247-1256.

36. Owen CG, Martin RM, Whincup PH, et al. Effect of infant feeding on the risk of obesity across the life course: a quantitative review of published evidence. *Pediatrics*. 2005;115:1367-1377.

37. Jacobsson LT, Jacobsson ME, Askling J, Knowler WC. Perinatal characteristics and risk of rheumatoid arthritis. *Br Med J*. 2003;326:1068-1069.

38. Karlson EW, Mandl LA, Hankinson SE, Grodstein F. Do breastfeeding and other reproductive factors influence future risk of rheumatoid arthritis? Results from the Nurses' Health Study. *Arthritis Rheum*. 2004;50:3458-3467.

39. Martin RM, Middleton N, Gunnell D, et al. Breast-feeding and cancer: the Boyd Orr cohort and a systematic review with meta-analysis. *J Natl Cancer Inst*. 2005;97:1446-1457.

40. Ness RB, Grisso JA, Cottreau C, et al. Factors related to inflammation of the ovarian epithelium and risk of ovarian cancer. *Epidemiology*. 2000;11:111-117.

41. Jordan SJ, Na R, Johnatty SE, et al. Breastfeeding and endometrial cancer risk: an analysis from the epidemiology of endometrial cancer consortium. *Obstet Gynecol*. 2017;129(6):1059-1067.

42. Chantry CJ, Auinger P, Byrd RS. Lactation among adolescent mothers and subsequent bone mineral density. *Arch Pediatr Adolesc Med*. 2004;158:650-656.

43. Hopkinson JM, Butte NF, Ellis K, Smith EO. Lactation delays postpartum bone mineral accretion and temporarily alters its regional distribution in women. *J Nutr*. 2000;130:777-783.

44. Drane DL, Logemann JA. A critical evaluation of the evidence on the association between type of infant feeding and cognitive development. *Paediatr Perinat Epidemiol*. 2000;14:349-356.

45. Mortensen EL, Michaelsen KF, Sanders SA, Reinsch JM. The association between duration of breastfeeding and adult intelligence. *J Am Med Assoc*. 2002;287:2365-2371.

46. Perrine CG, Nelson JM, Corbelli J, et al. Lactation and maternal cardiometabolic health. *Annu Rev Nutr*. 2016;36:627-645.

47. Fox M, Berzuini C, Knapp LA. Maternal breastfeeding history and Alzheimer's disease risk. *J Alzheimers Dis*. 2013;37(4):809-821.

48. Mosca F, Gianni ML. Human milk: composition and health benefits. *Pediatr Med Chir*. 2017;39(2):155.

50. Ramsay DT, Kent JC, Owens RA, Hartmann PE. Ultrasound imaging of milk ejection in the breast of lactating women. *Pediatrics*. 2004;113(2):361.

51. Neifert MR, McDonough SL, Neville MC. Failure of lactogenesis associated with placental retention. *Am J Obstet Gynecol*. 1981;140(4):477-478.

52. Perez-Escamilla R, Chapman DJ. Validity and public health implications of maternal perception of the onset of lactation: an international analytical overview. *J Nutr*. 2001;131(11):3021S-3024S.

53. Dewey KG. Maternal and fetal stress are associated with impaired lactogenesis in humans. *J Nutr*. 2001;131(11):3012S-3015S.

54. Hilson JA, Rasmussen KM, Kjolhede CL. High prepregnant body mass index is associated with poor lactation outcomes among white, rural women independent of psychosocial and demographic correlates. *J Hum Lact*. 2004;20(1):18.

55. Rasmussen KM, Kjolhede CL. Prepregnant overweight and obesity diminish the prolactin response to suckling in the first week postpartum. *Pediatrics*. 2004;113(5):e465-e471.

56. Donath SM, Amir LH. Does maternal obesity adversely affect breastfeeding initiation and duration? *Breastfeed Rev*. 2000;8(3):29-33.

57. Hilson JA, Rasmussen KM, Kjolhede CL. Maternal obesity and breastfeeding success in a rural population of white women. *Am J Clin Nutr*. 1997;66(6):1371-1378.

58. Preusting I, Brumley J, Odibo L, et al. Obesity as a predictor of delayed lactogenesis II. *J Hum Lact*. 2017;33(4):684-691.

59. Kelestimur F. Sheehan's syndrome. *Pituitary*. 2003;6(4):181-188.

65. Haastrup MB, Pottegård A, Damkier P. Alcohol and breastfeeding. *Basic Clin Pharmacol Toxicol*. 2014;114(2):168-173.

70. Morrow AL, Ruiz-Palacios GM, Jiang X, Newburg DS. Human-milk glycans that inhibit pathogen binding protect breast-feeding infants against infectious diarrhea. *J Nutr*. 2005;135(5):1304.

71. Morrow AL, Ruiz-Palacios GM, Altaye M, et al. Human milk oligosaccharide blood group epitopes and innate immune protection against campylobacter and calicivirus diarrhea in breast-fed infants. *Adv Exp Med Biol*. 2004;554:443.

72. Morrow AL, Ruiz-Palacios GM, Altaye M, et al. Human milk oligosaccharides are associated with protection against diarrhea in breast-fed infants. *J Pediatr*. 2004;145(3):297.

73. Clemens K, Silvia R. Physiology of oligosaccharides in lactating women and breast fed infants. *Adv Exp Med Biol*. 2000;478:241.

74. Newburg DS. Human milk glycoconjugates that inhibit pathogens. *Curr Med Chem*. 1999;6(2):117.

75. Gnoth MJ, Kunz C, Kinne-Saffran E, Rudloff S. Human milk oligosaccharides are minimally digested in vitro. *J Nutr*. 2000;130(12):3014.

76. Chaturvedi P, Warren CD, Buescher CR, et al. Survival of human milk oligosaccharides in the intestine of infants. *Adv Exp Med Biol*. 2001;501:315.

77. Erney RM, Malone WT, Skelding MB, et al. Variability of human milk neutral oligosaccharides in a diverse population. *J Pediatr Gastroenterol Nutr*. 2000;30(2):181.

78. Landberg E, Huang Y, Stromqvist M, et al. Changes in glycosylation of human bile-salt-stimulated lipase during lactation. *Arch Biochem Biophys*. 2000;377(2):246.

79. Coppa GV, Pierani P, Zampini L, et al. Oligosaccharides in human milk during different phases of lactation. *Acta Paediatr Suppl*. 1999;88(430):89.

80. Miller JB, Bull S, Miller J, McVeagh P. The oligosaccharide composition of human milk: temporal and individual variations in monosaccharide components. *J Pediatr Gastroenterol Nutr*. 1994;19(4):371.

81. Sumiyoshi W, Urashima T, Nakamura T, et al. Determination of each neutral oligosaccharide in the milk of Japanese women during the course of lactation. *Br J Nutr*. 2003;89(1):61.

82. Newburg DS, Ruiz-Palacios GM, Altaye M, et al. Innate protection conferred by fucosylated oligosaccharides of human milk against diarrhea in breastfed infants. *Glycobiology*. 2004;14(3):253.

83. Fituch CC, Palkowetz KH, Goldman AS, Schanler RJ. Concentrations of IL-10 in preterm human milk and in milk from mothers of infants with necrotizing enterocolitis. *Acta Paediatr*. 2004;93(11):1496-1500.

86. Allen LH. Multiple micronutrients in pregnancy and lactation: an overview. *Am J Clin Nutr*. 2005;81(5):1206S.

87. Bzikowska-Jura A, Czerwonogrodzka-Senczyna A, Olędzka G, et al. Maternal nutrition and body composition during breastfeeding: association with human milk composition. *Nutrients*. 2018;10(10):1379.

89. Canfield LM, Hopkinson JM, Lima AF, et al. Vitamin K in colostrum and mature human milk over the lactation period – a cross-sectional study. *Am J Clin Nutr*. 1991;53(3):730-735.

90. Lammi-Keefe CJ. Vitamins D and E in human milk. In: Jensen RG, ed. *Handbook of Milk Composition (Food Science and Technology International)*. Academic Press (Division of Harcourt Brace & Co); 1995:706-717.

91. Gartner LM, Greer FR. Prevention of rickets and vitamin D deficiency: new guidelines for vitamin D intake. *Pediatrics*. 2003;111(4 pt 1):908-910.

92. Zmora E, Gorodischer R, Bar-Ziv J. Multiple nutritional deficiencies in infants from a strict vegetarian community. *Am J Dis Child*. 1979;133(2):141-144.

93. Valentine CJ, Wagner CL. Nutritional management of the breastfeeding dyad. *Pediatr Clin North Am*. 2013;60(1):261-274.

100. Innis SM. Impact of maternal diet on human milk composition and neurological development of infants. *Am J Clin Nutr*. 2014;99(3):734S-741S.

102. Lauritzen L, Jorgensen MH, Olsen SF, et al. Maternal fish oil supplementation in lactation: effect on developmental outcome in breast-fed infants. *Reprod Nutr Dev*. 2005;45(5):535-547.

103. Jensen CL, Voigt RG, Prager TC, et al. Effects of maternal docosahexaenoic acid intake on visual function and neurodevelopment in breastfed term infants. *Am J Clin Nutr*. 2005;82(1):125-132.

104. Picciano MF. Human milk: nutritional aspects of a dynamic food. *Biol Neonate*. 1998;74(2):84-93.

111. Prentice AM, Prentice A. Energy costs of lactation. *Annu Rev Nutr*. 1988;8:63-79.

112. Butte NF, Hopkinson JM. Body composition changes during lactation are highly variable among women. *J Nutr*. 1998;128(2 suppl):381S-385S.

116. Endres LK, Straub H, McKinney C, et al. Postpartum weight retention risk factors and relationship to obesity at 1 year. *Obstet Gynecol*. 2015;125(1):144-152.

117. Rooney BL, Schauberger CW. Excess pregnancy weight gain and long-term obesity: one decade later. *Obstet Gynecol*. 2005;100(2):245-252.

119. Butte NF, Wong WW, Hopkinson JM. Energy requirements of lactating women derived from doubly labeled water and milk energy output. *J Nutr*. 2001;131(1):53-58.

123. Dalrymple KV, Flynn AC, Relph SA, et al. Lifestyle interventions in overweight and obese pregnant or postpartum women for postpartum weight management: a systematic review of the literature. *Nutrients*. 2018;10(11):1704.

125. Larson-Meyer DE. Effect of postpartum exercise on mothers and their offspring: a review of the literature. *Obes Res*. 2002;10(8):841-853.

128. Reece-Stremtan S, Marinelli KA. ABM clinical protocol #21: guidelines for breastfeeding and substance use or substance use disorder, revised 2015. *Breastfeed Med*. 2015;10(3):135-141.

130. Batstra L, Neeleman J, Hadders-Algra M. Can breast feeding modify the adverse effects of smoking during pregnancy on the child's cognitive development? *J Epidemiol Commun Health*. 2003;57(6):403-404.

133. Horst PG, Madjunkov M, Chaudry S. Alcohol: a pharmaceutical and pharmacological point of view during lactation. *J Popul Ther Clin Pharmacol*. 2016;23(2):e145-e150.

150. Zanardo V, Bertin M, Sansone L, et al. The adaptive psychological changes of elective induction of labor in breastfeeding women. *Early Hum Dev*. 2017;104:13-16.

CHAPTER 53

The Fourth Trimester

Jeannie C. Kelly and George A. Macones

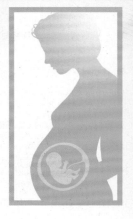

Introduction

The term, "the fourth trimester," was originally coined by pediatrician Dr Harvey Karp in his popular parenting books to describe the first 3 months of a newborn's life. This time was framed as a period of transition for the infant and focused on soothing techniques to ease and aid in adaption to an extra-uterine environment.[1] Recently, the fourth trimester has also been underscored as a critical transition for the woman as she physiologically recovers from childbirth and additionally adjusts to the physical, psychologic, emotional, and social demands of caring for a newborn.[2] During this time, she also transitions out of obstetrical care to well-woman primary care for her own medical needs, which can require challenging navigation through a complex medical system, especially if she has preexisting or newly developed health conditions. Yet, more than 40% of women have no postpartum visit with their obstetrical clinician.[2]

In the United States, birth rates have been increasing steadily for women older than 35 years, with high rates of preterm birth, cesarean delivery, and medical comorbidities compared to other developed countries. Concurrently, postpartum hospital readmission rates have risen sharply, and maternal mortality is increasing, with most cases (>40%) occurring postpartum.[2-4] Thus, the postpartum period represents a critical and medically vulnerable time, underscored by increasing obstetrical complexity and morbidity. In order to improve clinical outcomes, the postpartum period must be considered as equally crucial as prenatal care in a woman's obstetrical course with ongoing medical care.

Redefining the Fourth Trimester

In a review of cultures around the world, the postpartum period is typically defined as the time between 6 and 8 weeks after delivery, due to the resolution of postpartum lochia and other physiologic changes of pregnancy. Common postpartum rituals include organized maternal support from family members and a rest period that includes restricted activities and diets.[5] However, postpartum rituals and support groups are less defined for women in the United States outside of immigrant and ethnic/cultural group communities, leaving patients devoid of any specialized or structured care. Postpartum support thus sometimes only comprises the medical follow-up encounters between the patients and their pediatric and obstetrical clinicians.[2]

The American Academy of Pediatrics (AAP) recommends eight standard follow-up well-baby visits during the first year of an infant's life, during which screening for maternal depression is recommended at the 1-, 2-, 4-, and 6-week visits to evaluate caregiver health.[6] In contrast, traditional obstetrical medical care culminates in a single 15-minute visit at 6 weeks after delivery and must address all postpartum health concerns, including psychosocial stressors and future pregnancy planning in addition to formulating primary care and specialist follow-up plans for any medical conditions.[2] Recognizing the impractical and unfeasible challenge of this expectation, the American College of Obstetricians and Gynecologists (ACOG) and Society for Maternal-Fetal Medicine (SMFM) revised their postpartum care recommendations in 2018 to include, at minimum, an initial postpartum encounter within the first 3 weeks of delivery to address immediate delivery recovery and concerns, and a comprehensive visit no later than 12 weeks postpartum to transition out of obstetrical care (**Figure 53.1**).[2] These changes reframe the postpartum process as a sustained and active component of a woman's obstetrical care that should link seamlessly into ongoing preventative healthcare. After all, the postpartum time can also be considered the

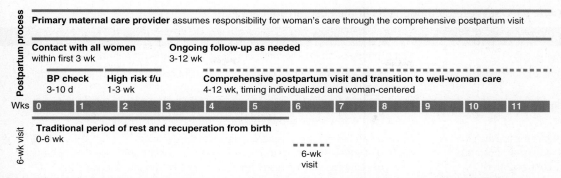

Figure 53.1 Proposed paradigm shift for postpartum visits. The American College of Obstetricians and Gynecologists' Presidential Task Force on Redefining the Postpartum Visit and the Committee on Obstetric Practice propose shifting the paradigm for postpartum care from a single 6-week visit (bottom) to a postpartum process (top). BP, blood pressure; f/u, follow-up.

interval "between pregnancies," and the ability to optimize medical comorbidities during pregnancy intervals is crucial to decrease future obstetrical disease.

Postpartum Care Planning

Formulating the birth plan, which is a document that details a woman's preferences and expectations regarding labor, delivery, and newborn care, has become a popular and routine component of prenatal counseling with maternal care clinicians.[7] This anticipatory discussion regarding the birth process is seen as an important piece of advocacy for patient autonomy in medical decision-making and presents an opportunity for the patient to openly disclose her fears and concerns. Notably, the postpartum component of most birth plans is centered around newborn care and feeding, and the plans typically conclude with discharge from the hospital. Postpartum maternal care, support, and medical follow-up visits are frequently lacking from detailed planning or discussion in current routine practices, resulting in an underutilized opportunity to maximize comprehensive maternal medical care and ensure a smooth transition to appropriate long-term care for chronic medical conditions. Increasing the proportion of women attending a postpartum visit is an objective of the Centers for Disease Control and Prevention's Healthy People 2020 initiative, and proactive postpartum guidance and planning should be started during pregnancy.[2] The positive association between preparatory counseling and maternal outcomes has been shown in randomized controlled trials to decrease rates of depression and increase rates of breastfeeding.[2]

Thus, similar to the now-ubiquitous birth plan, a Postpartum Care Plan should be discussed in detail with patients prior to delivery.

The ACOG suggests nine components to the Postpartum Care Plan and recommends reviewing each element during routine prenatal visits (**Table 53.1**).[2] Given the scope of these topics, obstetrical practices should consider utilizing routine visits with peer counselors, nurses, support staff (such as lactation consultants), and discharge planners both prior to delivery and during the delivery admission as strategies to be as comprehensive as possible. Postpartum visits should be scheduled prior to discharge from the delivery, and technology (email, text, or other apps via smart phones) should be used when possible for reminders and communication.

Common Postpartum Symptomatology

Multiple changes in maternal physiology occur after delivery, resulting in a range of symptoms that are considered normal. However, less than 50% of women reported receiving enough information regarding postpartum expectations to feel prepared.[2] These common postpartum experiences should be briefly reviewed prior to delivery with each patient so they can be anticipated, with precautions for further evaluation if they fall outside of expected parameters.

Shivering

Shivering is a common occurrence in up to 50% of women after delivery. Onset is typically within 30 minutes of delivery, lasting up to an hour in duration.[8] Many theories regarding the etiology have

Table 53.1 Suggested Components of the Postpartum Care Plan[a]

Element	Components
Care team	Name, phone number, and office or clinic address for each member of care team
Postpartum visits	Time, date, and location for postpartum visit(s); phone number to call to schedule or reschedule appointments
Infant feeding plan	Intended method of infant feeding, resources for community support (eg, WIC, Lactation Warm lines, mothers' groups), return-to-work resources
Reproductive life plan and commensurate contraception	Desired number of children and timing of next pregnancy Method of contraception, instructions for when to initiate, effectiveness, potential adverse effects, and care team member to contact with questions
Pregnancy complications	Pregnancy complications and recommended follow-up or test results (eg, glucose screening for gestational diabetes, blood pressure check for gestational hypertension), as well as risk reduction recommendations for any future pregnancies
Adverse pregnancy outcomes associated with ASCVD	Adverse pregnancy outcomes associated with ASCVD will need baseline ASCVD risk assessment, as well as discussion of need for ongoing annual assessment and need for ASCVD prevention over lifetime
Mental health	Anticipatory guidance regarding signs and symptoms of perinatal depression or anxiety; management recommendations for women with anxiety, depression, or other psychiatric issues identified during pregnancy or in the postpartum period
Postpartum problems	Recommendations for management of postpartum problems (ie, pelvic floor exercises for stress urinary incontinence, water-based lubricant for dispareunia)
Chronic health conditions	Treatment plan for ongoing physical and mental health conditions and the care team member responsible for follow-up

ASCVD, atherosclerotic cardiovascular disease; WIC, Special Supplemental Nutrition Program for Women, Infants, and Children.
[a]A Postpartum Care Plan Template is available as part of the ACOG Pregnancy Record.

been proposed, including normal physiologic consequences of childbirth and medical interventions. However, the mechanism is unclear, the process is self-limited, and no treatment is required.

Lochia

Lochia refers to the normal vaginal discharge after delivery that consists of blood, endometrial decidua, serous exudates, and physiologic cells. Lochia typically progresses through three stages[9]:

1. *Lochia rubra:* typically lasts for the first week after delivery and is red in color due to a large component of blood
2. *Lochia serosa:* typically lasts for a few weeks after lochia rubra and is thinner in consistency and lighter in color
3. *Lochia alba:* light yellow and consists of serous exudate and maternal cells

Although the total volume of lochia is about 500 mL, the normal duration is, on average, 1 month and can last up to 8 weeks postpartum in 15% of women.

Hormonal Changes

Extensive hormonal changes occur, starting with uterine separation of the placenta. Progesterone and estrogen are at their maximum levels at the end of a term pregnancy and precipitously drop with delivery, remaining low for a month afterward.[10] Some patients report hot flashes and night sweats in the first few weeks following delivery, believed to be associated with the same mechanism driven by estrogen withdrawal at the hypothalamus as in postmenopausal women.[11] Prolactin levels remain high immediately following delivery and, in the absence of progesterone, initiate milk secretion typically within 3 to 5 days. A substantial drop in human chorionic gonadotropin occurs within the first week followed by a slower rate of decline over the next month and typically disappears by 4 weeks postpartum.[10,12]

In nonlactating women, ovulation will resume, on average, within 3 months but can occur as early as 3 weeks postpartum. Most nonlactating women will resume menstruation within 12 weeks postpartum, but importantly, a large proportion (up to 71%) will ovulate prior to their first menses and thus may have a fertile period prior to onset of any symptoms indicating return of fertility. In lactating women, ovulation is delayed, with a broad variation in duration of amenorrhea that depends on maternal age, parity, duration, and frequency of breastfeeding, and is also associated with a prolonged hypoestrogenemic state.[10-12]

Hair, Skin, and Muscle Changes

Hair, skin, and muscle changes occur due to hormonal fluctuations and rapid uterine involution that occurs postpartum. Hair loss is commonly seen starting within 6 months postpartum, but this is due to the increased anagen "growing" phase present in pregnancy returning back to the normal prepregnancy telogen "resting" phase, and concludes by 1 year postpartum in the majority of patients.[13] Pregnancy striae are typically purple or red lesions that develop in up to 90% of women, commonly on the abdomen, breasts, and thighs, resulting from rapid stretching and tearing of the dermis.[14] Although the color will fade after delivery, the skin may remain lax. Additionally, the abdominal wall will improve in muscle tone but rectus diastasis can persist and may result in discomfort, postural changes, and cosmetic dissatisfaction.[15]

Pain and Discomfort

Pain and discomfort are the most common complaints postpartum, after both vaginal and cesarean deliveries.[16] Uncontrolled pain can interfere with activities of daily living, including infant care, and is associated with greater opioid use, depression, and development of chronic pain.[17] Thus, pain control with both pharmacologic and nonpharmacologic strategies in a stepwise, multimodal approach is an important consideration in the postpartum period. Uterine contractions occur with oxytocin release after delivery and in association with nursing and may be worse in multiparous women.[17] Oral nonsteroidal anti-inflammatory drugs (NSAIDs) have better evidence supporting their use for effective pain management than opioids, and the course is usually self-limited to a week.[16,17] After vaginal delivery, perineal hygiene and care, with elevation of the foot of the bed, may help with pain and discomfort. Use of perineal ice packs has been shown in meta-analysis to improve pain in the first 72 hours after delivery but does not appear to change wound inflammation/edema or healing.[17,18] Scheduled pharmacologic treatment using NSAIDs alternating with acetaminophen appear to effective in decreasing perineal pain for the majority of women but can be supplemented in a stepwise fashion with opioids if insufficient, especially for women with significant lacerations.[17] To decrease the risk of acetaminophen toxicity, opioids should be given individually and not in a combination formulation with acetaminophen. After cesarean delivery, opioids given via neuraxial regional anesthesia provide the most effective pain control but must also be augmented with other forms of analgesia as the effects wear off over time. A similar stepwise approach should be taken with scheduled alternating NSAIDs and acetaminophen, reserving opioids for breakthrough pain as needed. A local anesthetic block injected between the internal oblique and transversus muscles may also benefit postcesarean pain.[17]

There is wide variation in opioid prescribing patterns for discharge after delivery, and usually the amount does not correspond to level of pain reported or opioid requirements in the hospital.[19] The majority of women report being prescribed twice the number of opioids needed after delivery, and a minority dispose of leftover opioids appropriately.[19] Additionally, recent studies demonstrate that 1 in 300 opioid-naïve women will become persistent opioid users after postcesarean exposure (Chapter 8).[17,19] As opioid-related overdose deaths have drastically increased and the incidence of opioid use disorder continues to rise in this country, prudent prescribing of opioids is imperative to decrease rates of misuse and diversion, while at the same time appropriately treating postpartum pain.[17] Shared decision-making with the patient to determine the amount of prescribed discharge opioids, which includes discussing average pain scores and average opioid requirements after cesarean delivery, appears to improve patient satisfaction with pain control and decrease leftover opioids.[19]

Notably, about 4% to 5% of the population in the United States is "ultrafast metabolizers" of codeine and tramadol, resulting in high serum and breast milk levels of active metabolites.[17,20] Cases of breastfed infants exposed to maternal intake of codeine have been reported with oversedation, respiratory depression, and even death.[17,20] Thus, in 2017, the United States Food and Drug Administration issued a warning against codeine and tramadol in breastfeeding women.[20] However, oxycodone and hydrocodone are also metabolized by the same enzyme, and cases of infant sedation in breastfeeding mothers have also been reported.[17] Due to the wide variation in metabolism of opioids, all women prescribed opioids should have counseling regarding the risk of maternal and infant oversedation and/or toxicity, and opioids should be used for the shortest necessary time.

Breast Engorgement

Breast engorgement occurs typically within 72 hours but may occur up to 7 days after delivery. As progesterone levels fall, colostrum production of around 50 mL/d transitions to milk production of about 500 mL/d in the first 2 to 3 days after delivery.[21] During this time, the breasts becomes firm, swollen, and enlarged, with symptoms peaking at around 3 to 5 days postpartum. A self-limited fever less than 39 °C may occur and should last less than 24 hours, but any fevers should prompt evaluation for mastitis.[21,22]

In breastfeeding mothers, frequent nursing or pumping is usually sufficient for relief from breast engorgement through the peak of symptoms. Stimulation of the nipples causes a positive feedback loop to the pituitary gland, resulting in prolactin and oxytocin release. Prolactin maintains ongoing milk production, and oxytocin stimulates myoepithelial cell contraction for milk ejection from the alveoli to the areola.[21,22] However, for patients who do not elect to breastfeed due to medical contraindications or personal preference, there is no high-quality evidence to support any pharmacologic or nonpharmacologic methods that are safe and effective over expectant management for treatment of engorgement.[23] A well-fitting support garment for the breasts, ice packs, cabbage leaves, and analgesia with ibuprofen or acetaminophen appear to improve symptoms. If the nipples are not regularly stimulated and milk is not regularly removed, a negative feedback mechanism downregulates expression of prolactin receptors, diminishing milk production and suppressing lactation.[21,22]

Breastfeeding

Exclusive breastfeeding in infants is associated with lower rates of infectious morbidity, sudden infant death syndrome, childhood obesity, and diabetes. Breastfeeding mothers additionally have lower rates of breast and ovarian cancer, retained weight gain, diabetes, and cardiovascular

morbidity. Thus, the ACOG, SMFM, AAP, and the American Academy of Family Physicians all recommend exclusive breastfeeding for at least the first 6 months of life.[22,24]

Although most women will initiate breastfeeding after childbirth, more than half of women in the United States wean earlier than they desire. Additionally, breastfeeding rates are considerably affected by racial and socioeconomic disparity; low-income and African American women are significantly less likely to initiate or continue breastfeeding compared to average-income or white women.[22,24] These differences are likely due to barriers to breastfeeding grounded in structural inequity, such as lack of access to lactational support, maternity leave, and workplace support.[24,25] Disrupted lactation, where a mother is unable to meet her intended breastfeeding goals, occurs most commonly due to pain, perceived low milk supply, and problems with the newborn latch. Unplanned cessation of breastfeeding can cause substantial anxiety and stress and is associated with increased risk of postpartum depression.[22,24,25]

Breastfeeding education, promotion, and support throughout the prenatal and postnatal periods have been shown to increase initiation and duration of exclusive breastfeeding. However, knowledge among maternal healthcare clinicians varies. Implementing a comprehensive breastfeeding curriculum for clinicians has been shown to improve rates of exclusive breastfeeding to 6 months in patients. Furthermore, studies of hospitals that implement formal breastfeeding initiatives have demonstrated increased exclusive breastfeeding rates, although it remains unclear whether these interventions are applicable in the developed world and which specific elements are necessary for improved outcomes.[22,25] The ACOG has endorsed the UNICEF-World Health Organization (WHO)'s Ten Steps to Successful Breastfeeding (**Table 53.2**) as strategies that should be implemented into routine maternity care in order to improve breastfeeding rates and help mothers better meet their own breastfeeding goals.[22] In addition to these hospital guidelines, proactive face-to-face postnatal support has been shown to increase duration and exclusivity of breastfeeding over general, formal antenatal sessions after discharge from delivery admission.[24,25] Thus, ongoing, individualized lactation support after delivery should be integrated into routine postpartum care of breastfeeding women, especially

Table 53.2 Ten Hospital Practices to Encourage and Support Breastfeeding[a]

1. Have a written breastfeeding policy that is routinely communicated to all healthcare staff.

2. Train all healthcare staff in the skills necessary to implement this policy.

3. Inform all pregnant women about the benefits and management of breastfeeding.

4. Help women initiate breastfeeding within 1 h of birth.

5. Show women how to breastfeed and how to maintain lactation, even if they are separated from their newborns.

6. Give newborns no food or drink other than breast milk, unless medically indicated.

7. Practice rooming-in—allow mothers and newborns to remain together 24 h a day.

8. Encourage breastfeeding on demand.

9 Give no pacifiers or artificial nipples to breastfeeding infants.[b]

10. Foster the establishment of breastfeeding support groups and refer to them on discharge from the hospital or birth center.

[a]The 1994 report of the Healthy Mothers. Health Babies National Coalition Expert Work Group recommended that the UNICEF-WHO Baby-friendly Hospital Initiative be adapted for use in the United States as the United States Breastfeeding Health Initiative, using the adapted 10 steps above.
[b]The American Academy of Pediatrics endorsed the UNICEF-WHO Ten Steps to Successful Breastfeeding but does not support a categorical ban on pacifiers because of their role in reducing the risk of sudden infant death syndrome and their analgesic benefit during painful procedures when breastfeeding cannot provide the analgesia.
Data from Baby-Friendly USA. *Guidelines and Evaluation Criteria For Facilities Seeking Baby-Friendly Designation*. Baby Friendly USA; 2010. Retrieved October 29, 2015. https://www.babyfriendlyusa.org/get-started/the-guidelines-evaluation-criteria

as these services are covered by insurance under the Affordable Care Act. Interventions specifically aimed at decreasing the disparity in breastfeeding success among socioeconomically disadvantaged and African American women have had mixed successes and is an area that is in urgent need of further research.[24,25]

Contraindications to breastfeeding, due to infant or maternal medical conditions, and to medication exposure, are overall limited. These include infant galactosemia, maternal active illicit drug use, human immunodeficiency virus or human T-cell lymphotropic virus type I or II infections, active untreated brucellosis, varicella, or herpes simplex virus lesions on the breast(s).[22] Active, untreated tuberculosis is listed as a contraindication to breastfeeding by the AAP and ACOG due to infant and mother separation guidelines during active disease, but encouraged by the WHO.[22] Most medications are considered compatible with breastfeeding, including methadone and buprenorphine for women in recovery from opioid use disorder, and clinicians should not disrupt the breastfeeding relationship when prescribing a medication without confirming incompatibility via a lactation pharmacology resource, which is readily available from the National Institutes of Health's National Library of Medicine.[22] Often, lactating women are instructed to "pump and dump" for a set number of hours following anesthesia for surgery or undergoing radiologic studies that uses contrast, but these are common misconceptions and breastfeeding can be continued in these circumstances when the mother has recovered from her procedure enough to hold her infant.[22]

The breastfeeding relationship between a patient and her infant is vitally personal. Although the maternal and infant benefits of breastfeeding are widely known, the ability to overcome common barriers requires time, effort, and intensive social support and infrastructure. Maternal care clinicians should ensure their patients are well versed in the benefits of breastfeeding and strive to provide specialized lactation initiatives at the delivery hospital and individualized, ongoing postnatal support. Additionally, clinicians should support ongoing policy changes that support and prolong lactation in the workplace. Ultimately, the decision to initiate and continue breastfeeding is one best made by the patient for herself and her infant, after informed counseling, and should be respected.

Contraception

Discussion regarding a woman's reproductive life plans should ideally begin during the prenatal course, initially with questions regarding plans for future childbearing. This discussion can naturally progress to reviewing plans for desired family size and the evidence behind pregnancy spacing outcomes.[2] The interpregnancy interval, defined as the time between delivery and conception, is associated with increased risks for preterm birth, low birth weight, and small-for-gestational age infants when it is short (less than 18 months) or long (more than 59 months). These risks are particularly increased when the interpregnancy interval is less than 6 months, and the ACOG recommends counseling against pregnancy within this time frame.[2,26] Up to 57% of women will resume sexual activity prior to the end of the 6-week postpartum time frame, and some women will also experience return of fertility during this time. Thus, to prevent unintended short interval pregnancies, the prenatal period is an important time to formulate an anticipatory postpartum contraceptive plan.[2,26-28]

The choice of postpartum contraception may be dynamic, depending on thrombotic risk, medical comorbidities, breastfeeding status, and patient preference and previous experience.[2,26,27] However, this represents an opportune time for initiation of contraception as patients are typically highly motivated, in close contact with their maternal healthcare clinician, and have insurance coverage.[2] Although all maternal clinicians should ensure that the full range of appropriate contraception is discussed and offered to every patient, particular care should be paid to patient-centered, nonpaternalistic shared decision-making. As the United States has a history of forced sterilizations and contraception in vulnerable and marginalized populations, clinicians should take extra care that their own belief and value systems are not projected over the patient's informed decisions.

Sterilization is over 99% effective and can be performed via bilateral tubal ligation or salpingectomy, either at the time of cesarean delivery or via minilaparotomy within 48 hours after vaginal delivery.[28] As these procedures are permanent, the decision to proceed with sterilization should be made prior to delivery and has mandated waiting periods for patients with public insurance. However, up to 50% of women who desire sterilization at the time of delivery do not receive the procedure due to timing of delivery, maternal body habitus complicating surgery, and vaginal instead of cesarean delivery. These women are at high risk for unintended short interval pregnancy and, thus, should be provided other methods of highly effective contraception.[28-30]

Immediate postpartum long-acting reversible contraception (LARC) is achieved with an intrauterine device (IUD) or contraceptive implant placed in the immediate postpartum timing, either following placental delivery or prior to delivery discharge. LARC methods provide greater than 99% effectiveness with the highest continuation rates of reversible contraception, and immediate postpartum placement improves access for patients and has also been demonstrated to be cost effective.[29] However, immediate postpartum IUD placement has higher expulsion rates than placement after 6 weeks, and replacement of a failed IUD(?) may not be covered by all insurance types. Despite this, a randomized trial of immediate postpartum IUD placement demonstrated a higher rate of continuation at 6 months postpartum compared to routine 6-week postpartum placement, mostly due to lack of postpartum follow-up at 6 weeks to obtain the IUD.[31] Thus, immediate postpartum LARC should be discussed with patients as an available option prior to delivery so that appropriate plans can be made for supplies to be available.

Common Postpartum Complications

At discharge from the hospital admission for delivery, patients should be given precautions regarding common postpartum complications such as infectious and wound morbidity, abnormal bleeding patterns, mental health disorders, and urinary or bowel complications. Although a discussion of many of these complications appears in Chapter 52, a brief summary is warranted here as these conditions are pertinent to a woman's and her infant's overall health during the fourth trimester.

Mastitis

Lactational mastitis most commonly occurs within the first 3 months of delivery and is associated with reduced milk drainage, nipple trauma, milk oversupply, maternal or infant illness, and stress.[22,32,33] If untreated, a breast abscess may develop. The most common organism is *Staphylococcus aureus*, including methicillin-resistant *S. aureus* (MRSA) strains.[32] All lactating women who present with fever and flu-like symptoms should undergo breast examination for signs of mastitis, which includes a firm, warm, and erythematous area of the breast. Empiric therapy with dicloxacillin and symptomatic relief with NSAIDs is typically sufficient for treatment of most cases.[32,33] If fever persists after 48 to 72 hours, milk culture can be considered, in addition to widening antibiotic coverage to include MRSA. Frequent breastfeeding or pumping is recommended in the setting of mastitis to ensure frequent emptying of milk.[32,33]

Prolonged Bleeding/Retained Products

Vaginal bleeding past 8 weeks postpartum should prompt evaluation. Causes include return of menses, but also can be due to retained products of conception, an undiagnosed bleeding diathesis, or other rare etiologies. A careful history and physical examination, with imaging of the uterus and laboratory work if appropriate, are reasonable initial evaluations in this setting.

Wound Complications and Infections

Perineal repair breakdown is associated with operative vaginal delivery, prolonged second stage of labor, and severe perineal lacerations. Incision, drainage, and débridement are effective treatments, with resultant healing by secondary intention. Antibiotics are typically not necessary outside of cases of cellulitis, and closure of a débrided wound is typically only reserved for large defects.[34]

Cesarean wound complications of infection, hematoma, seroma, or dehiscence occurs in about 1% to 2% of deliveries and typically develops within 1 week of surgery. Obesity, uterine infection, second-stage cesarean, diabetes, and blood transfusion are associated with an increased risk of developing cesarean wound complications. Evidence-based bundles for surgical preparation and technique can decrease rates of surgical site infection.[35,36]

Postpartum endometritis is typically a polymicrobial infection that starts in the decidua and extends outward through the myometrium. Endometritis is one of the most common causes of postpartum fever, and treatment with multimicrobial coverage (typically ampicillin, gentamicin, and clindamycin) is usually sufficient for treatment and resolution of fever within 48 hours.[37,38]

Anxiety, Depression, and Mental Health Disorders

The ACOG and AAP recommend screening all women for postpartum depression, typically via the Edinburgh Postnatal Depression Scale.[2]

For maternal clinicians, anticipatory discussion regarding expected "baby blues" should take place prior to delivery, and precautions should be reviewed regarding postpartum depression and anxiety. Depression screening should take place at least at routine postpartum follow-up visits or earlier in high-risk individuals. For patients who screen positive, referral to mental health clinicians for treatment has been shown to improve symptoms and outcomes.[2] Although rare, postpartum psychosis is a serious disorder and can be life threatening for both mother and infant. Risk factors include bipolar disorder and major depression, or schizophrenia, and most commonly presents 2 weeks postpartum with the initial symptom of severe insomnia.[39] A detailed discussion of psychiatric problems after pregnancy is presented in Chapter 43.

Urinary Retention and Incontinence

Postpartum urinary retention is defined the absence of spontaneous urination 6 hours after delivery or catheter removal or with more than 150 mL of urine retained in the bladder after voiding. A prolonged second stage of labor seems to increase the risk, which appears to be due to pudendal nerve injury.[40] Most cases are self-limited and resolve within a week but in some instances can take up to 3 months. Intermittent catheterization can treat postpartum urinary retention until spontaneous resolution, and antibiotics are not routinely necessary.[40]

Postpartum incontinence of urine, flatus, or feces commonly occurs in the first year after childbirth. Almost 50% of women report urinary incontinence, and 17% report anal incontinence.[41,42] A large proportion of these women will go on to experience persistent incontinence after 1 year postpartum, thus identifying these symptoms are important for the maternal healthcare clinician in order to address them and arrange for follow-up and evaluation.

Dyspareunia/Sexual Dysfunction

Perineal trauma, emergent delivery, fatigue and sleep deprivation, and hypoestrogenemic status all contribute to a large proportion of women reporting postpartum sexual dysfunction.[43] Libido remains lower 12 months after childbirth than levels prior to pregnancy and is not usually discussed during follow-up visits with a healthcare clinician.[43] Given the common incidence in postpartum women, clinicians should offer sexual health as a topic for discussion in a safe, nonjudgmental space, as long-term symptoms can lead to psychologic difficulties. Reports of dyspareunia may need further evaluation to differentiate between abnormal scar development and a hypoestrogenemic state especially in breastfeeding mothers.[43,44] Pelvic floor therapy and increased lubrication use are helpful strategies, and vaginal estrogen is undergoing further research as treatment for lactational vaginal atrophy.[44]

Timing of Postpartum Visits

The early postpartum period is a high-risk time for women, with the majority of maternal deaths occurring during this time. Severe morbidity, such as stroke, wound infection, and exacerbation of chronic medical conditions (hypertension, epilepsy, rheumatologic and psychiatric disease), commonly occurs within the first few weeks postpartum, and obstetrical readmission rates have been rising over the last decade.[2]

The ACOG recommends contact with all patients within 3 weeks postpartum from the healthcare team. For high-risk patients, evaluation is recommended within the first 1 to 3 weeks. For patients with specific comorbidities, such as hypertensive disorders, the ACOG recommends evaluation as soon as 5 to 10 days postpartum (**Figure 53.1**).[2] Although in-person clinical visits are beneficial to evaluate for depression, wound infection, medication titration, or to provide lactation support, use of telemedicine in the form of phone calls, texts, remote monitoring devices, and smartphone applications to contact and evaluate patients has also been suggested, especially for the routine 3-week encounter, as the feasibility of attending an office visit while newly postpartum with a newborn may be logistically difficult for some patients.[2] However, depending on the patient's severity of comorbid conditions, multiple evaluations and/or office visits may be necessary throughout the postpartum period for optimization of maternal disease management and to gauge health status. During this time, the various healthcare clinicians who will continue managing ongoing conditions after discharge from maternal care should be identified, and appropriate follow-up referrals to these clinicians should also be discussed and planned with the patient and reviewed with her primary care clinician.[2]

A comprehensive postpartum visit should take place no later than 12 weeks postpartum. The ACOG recommends a full assessment of physical, social, and psychological well-being at that time and counseling regarding future pregnancy and cardiometabolic risk that may be increased due to pregnancy complications.[2] Timely follow-up with healthcare clinicians as planned for ongoing well-woman and specialist visits should be encouraged. Enabling a smooth transition out of maternal care to primary care is important to optimize maternal health and improve interpregnancy health status for any future pregnancies.

Health Disparities and Policy

Currently, postpartum care is significantly lacking more for women living in areas of high deprivation and socioeconomic need and for African American women even when controlling for socioeconomic status.[2-4] These health disparities indicate that the patients who are at highest risk for severe maternal morbidity are not receiving adequate attention or support during the most medically vulnerable time.[45] Augmenting medical care for equitable access is imperative to decreasing maternal morbidity and mortality rates, addressing disparities, and improving outcomes. The barriers to accessing postpartum care are significant, and overcoming them will require changes in healthcare policy, insurance status, and reimbursement policies.[2,45] Current global billing for obstetric, delivery, and postpartum care disincentivizes repeated visits in the postpartum period for any preexisting conditions. For example, at the time of this publication, in states without Medicaid expansion, the most vulnerable patients lose insurance status 60 days postpartum, eliminating their ability to access any medical care or transition to ongoing well-women care. This causes women with public insurance to have poorly controlled and suboptimally evaluated medical conditions that are ignored except during pregnancy, despite strong evidence to support preconception optimization of medical comorbidities as the best strategy to improve obstetrical outcomes[46]. Thus, policy changes at the level of the state government and insurance payers are necessary for optimal improvement of postpartum care.

KEY POINTS

- The fourth trimester is a critical transition for women as they physiologically recover from childbirth and adjust to the physical, psychologic, emotional, and social demands of caring for a newborn.
- Postpartum rituals and support groups are less defined for women in the United States outside of immigrant and ethnic/cultural group communities, leaving patients devoid of any specialized or structured care.
- The ACOG and SMFM recommend an initial postpartum encounter within the first 3 weeks of delivery to address immediate delivery recovery and concerns and a comprehensive visit no later than 12 weeks postpartum to transition out of obstetrical care.
- Multiple changes in maternal physiology occur after delivery, resulting in a range of symptoms that are considered normal.

- Breastfeeding education, promotion, and support throughout the prenatal and postnatal periods have been shown to increase initiation and duration of exclusive breastfeeding.
- Discussion regarding a woman's reproductive life plans should ideally begin during the prenatal course, as the interpregnancy interval—both too short (less than 6 months) or too long (more than 59 months)—can influence the success of future pregnancies.
- Patients should be given precautions regarding common postpartum complications such as infectious and wound morbidity, abnormal bleeding patterns, mental health disorders, and urinary or bowel complications.
- Augmenting medical care for equitable access is imperative to decreasing maternal morbidity and mortality rates, addressing disparities, and improving outcomes.

REFERENCES

1. Karp H. *The Happiest Baby on the Block: The New Way to Calm Crying and Help Your Baby Sleep Longer.* Bantam Books; 2002.
2. ACOG Committee Opinion No. 736: optimizing postpartum care. *Obstet Gynecol.* 2018;131:e140-e150.
3. Hamilton N, Stevens N, Lillis T, et al. The fourth trimester: toward improved postpartum health and healthcare of mothers and their families in the United States. *J Behav Med.* 2018;41:571-576.
4. Clapp A, Little SE, Zheng J, Robinson JN. A multi-state analysis of postpartum readmissions in the United States. *Am J Obstet Gynecol.* 2016;215:113. e1-113.e10.
5. Dennis C-L, Fung K, Grigoriadis S, Robinson GE, Romans S, Ross L. Traditional postpartum practices and rituals: a qualitative systematic review. *Womens Health (Lond).* 2007;3:487-502.
6. Earls MF, Yogman MW, Mattson G, et al; AAP Committee on Psychosocial Aspects of Child and Family Health. Incorporating recognition and management of perinatal depression into pediatric practice. *Pediatrics.* 2019;143(1):e20183259.
7. Lothian J. Birth plans: the good, the bad, and the future. *J Obstet Gynecol Neonatal Nurs.* 2006;35:295-303.
8. Benson MD, Haney E, Dinsmoor M, Beaumont JL. Shaking rigors in parturients. *J Reprod Med.* 2008;53:685.
9. Sherman D, Lurie S, Frenkel E, et al. Characteristics of normal lochia. *Am J Perinatol.* 1999;16:399.
10. Resnik R. The puerperium. In: Creasy RK, Resnik R, eds. *Maternal Fetal-Medicine, Principles and Practice.* W.B. Saunders; 2004:165.
11. Thurston RC, Luther JF, Wisniewski SR, et al. Prospective evaluation of nighttime hot flashes during pregnancy and postpartum. *Fertil Steril.* 2013;100:1667.
12. Jackson E, Glasier A. Return of ovulation and menses in postpartum non-lactating women: a systematic review. *Obstet Gynecol.* 2011;117:657.
13. Winton GB, Lewis CW. Dermatoses of pregnancy. *J Am Acad Dermatol.* 1982;6:977.
14. Osman H, Rubeiz N, Tamim H, Nassar AH. Risk factors for the development of striae gravidarum. *Am J Obstet Gynecol.* 2007;196:62.e1-62.e5.
15. Nahabedian MY. Management strategies for diastasis recti. *Semin Plast Surg.* 2018;32(3):147-154. doi:10.1055/s-0038-1661380

16. Declercq E, Cunningham DK, Johnson C, Sakala C. Mothers' reports of postpartum pain associated with vaginal and cesarean deliveries: results of a national survey. *Birth.* 2008;35:16-43.
17. ACOG Committee Opinion No. 742: postpartum pain management. *Obstet Gynecol.* 2018;132:e35-e43.
18. East CE, Begg L, Henshall NE, et al. Local cooling for relieving pain from perineal trauma sustained during childbirth. *Cochrane Database Syst Rev.* 2012;16:CD006304.
19. Prabhu M, McQuaid-Hanson E, Hopp S, et al. A shared decision-making intervention to guide opioid prescribing after cesarean delivery. *Obstet Gynecol.* 2017;130(1):42-46.
20. *FDA Restricts Use of Prescription Codeine Pain and Cough Medicines and Tramadol Pain Medicines in Children; Recommends Against Use in Breastfeeding Women.* Accessed on January 31, 2020. https://www.fda.gov/media/104268/download
21. Pang WW, Hartmann PE. Initiation of human lactation: secretory differentiation and secretory activation. *J Mammary Gland Biol Neoplasia.* 2007;12:211-221.
22. ACOG Committee Opinion No. 756: optimizing support for breastfeeding as part of obstetric practice. *Obstet Gynecol.* 2018;132:e187-e196.
23. Oladapo OT, Fawole B. Treatments for suppression of lactation. *Cochrane Database Syst Rev.* 2012;2012:CD005937.
24. Committee Opinion No. 570: breastfeeding in underserved women. Increasing initiation and continuation of breastfeeding. *Obstet Gynecol.* 2013;122:423-428.
25. Lewkowitz AK, López JD, Stein RI, et al. Effect of a home-based lifestyle intervention on breastfeeding initiation among socioeconomically disadvantaged African American women with overweight or obesity. *Breastfeed Med.* 2018;13(6):418-425.
26. Conde-Agudelo A, Rosas-Bermúdez A, Kafury-Goeta AC. Birth spacing and risk of adverse perinatal outcomes: a meta-analysis. *J Am Med Assoc.* 2006;295(15):1809-1823.
27. Chao S. The effect of lactation on ovulation and fertility. *Clin Perinatol.* 1987;14:39-50.
28. Committee Opinion No. 530: access to postpartum sterilization. *Obstet Gynecol.* 2012;120:212-215.
29. Committee Opinion No. 615: access to contraception. *Obstet Gynecol.* 2015;125:250-255.

30. Thurman AR, Janecek T. One-year follow-up of women with unfulfilled postpartum sterilization requests. *Obstet Gynecol.* 2010;116:1071-1077.

31. Sonalkar S, Hunter T, Gurney EP, et al. A decision analysis model of 1-year effectiveness of intended postplacental compared with intended delayed postpartum intrauterine device insertion. *Obstet Gynecol.* 2018;132:1211.

32. Stafford I, Hernandez J, Laibl V, et al. Community-acquired methicillin-resistant *Staphylococcus aureus* among patients with puerperal mastitis requiring hospitalization. *Obstet Gynecol.* 2008;112:533.

33. Foxman B, D'Arcy H, Gillespie B, et al. Lactation mastitis: occurrence and medical management among 946 breastfeeding women in the United States. *Am J Epidemiol.* 2002;155:103.

34. ACOG practice Bulletin No. 198: prevention and management of obstetric lacerations at vaginal delivery. *Obstet Gynecol Obstet Gynecol.* 2018;132:e87-e102.

35. Carter EB, Temming LA, Fowler S, et al. Evidence-based bundles and cesarean delivery surgical site infections: a systematic review and meta-analysis. *Obstet Gynecol.* 2017;130:735.

36. Temming LA, Raghuraman N, Carter EB, et al. Impact of evidence-based interventions on wound complications after cesarean delivery. *Am J Obstet Gynecol.* 2017;217:449.e1-449.e9.

37. Rosene K, Eschenbach DA, Tompkins LS, et al. Polymicrobial early postpartum endometritis with facultative and anaerobic bacteria, genital mycoplasmas, and Chlamydia trachomatis: treatment with piperacillin or cefoxitin. *J Infect Dis.* 1986;153:1028.

38. Mackeen AD, Packard RE, Ota E, Speer L. Antibiotic regimens for postpartum endometritis. *Cochrane Database Syst Rev.* 2015;2015:CD001067.

39. Wesseloo R, Kamperman AM, Munk-Olsen T, et al. Risk of postpartum relapse in bipolar disorder and postpartum psychosis: a systematic review and meta-analysis. *Am J Psychiatry.* 2016;173:117.

40. Stephansson O, Sandström A, Petersson G, et al. Prolonged second stage of labour, maternal infectious disease, urinary retention and other complications in the early postpartum period. *Br J Obstet Gynecol.* 2016;123:608.

41. MacArthur C, Wilson D, Herbison P, et al. Urinary incontinence persisting after childbirth: extent, delivery history, and effects in a 12-year longitudinal cohort study. *Br J Obstet Gynecol.* 2016;123:1022.

42. Brown S, Gartland D, Perlen S, et al. Consultation about urinary and faecal incontinence in the year after childbirth: a cohort study. *Br J Obstet Gynecol.* 2015;122:954.

43. Leeman LM, Rogers RG. Sex after childbirth: postpartum sexual function. *Obstet Gynecol.* 2012;119:647.

44. McDonald EA, Gartland D, Small R, Brown SJ. Dyspareunia and childbirth: a prospective cohort study. *Br J Obstet Gynecol.* 2015;122:672.

45. Committee Opinion No. 649: racial and ethnic disparities in obstetrics and gynecology. *Obstet Gynecol.* 2015;126:e130-e134.

46. Daw JR, Hatfield LA, Swartz K, Sommers BD. Women in the United States experience high rates of coverage 'churn' in months before and after childbirth. *Health Aff (Millwood).* 2017;36(4):598-606.

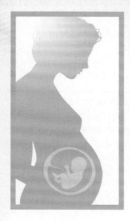

CHAPTER 54

Health Inequities in the Postpartum Period/ Pregnancy Interval Care

Ashish Premkumar, Divya Mallampati, and Melissa A. Simon

Introduction

Health disparities in the United States, both in terms of access to health care and the prevalence of adverse outcomes, continue to influence the landscape of interpregnancy and postpartum care. For the purposes of this chapter, we adhere to the definition of health disparity put forth by the National Institutes of Health, namely that certain groups face disproportionate morbidity and mortality when compared to the general population.[1]

This chapter will broadly outline key issues in the interpregnancy and postpartum periods relating to disparities in both healthcare utilization and outcomes. We limit our discussion to the United States. Our limited analytic framework is not meant to be exclusive but is meant to act as a starting point for understanding wider issues surrounding women's health after delivery, and to stimulate conversations on a global scale regarding why certain groups face adverse outcomes when compared with others.

Racism

From biases embedded into algorithms, screening tools, and predictive models utilized by clinicians to the shortage of underrepresented minorities in the clinician workforce, structural racism is embedded in every aspect of our healthcare system leading to unacceptable health outcomes.[13]

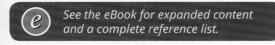 See the eBook for expanded content and a complete reference list.

Bias and systemic racism in healthcare must be addressed, given the differences in maternal mortality experienced by black women, after accounting for other sociodemographic risk factors.[16]

Common Barriers to Care

Barriers that affect minority women are grounded in social, economic, psychosocial, cultural, and historical factors (**Table 54.1**).

Healthcare Insurance Coverage

Although not a panacea to address all facets of structural racism, extending Medicaid coverage from 6 weeks to 12 months postpartum may reduce inequities in care. Medicaid expansion decreased the uninsured rate among women who gave birth in the past year, increased preconception Medicaid enrollment among low-income women, reduced racial disparities in preterm birth and low birth weight, and decreased infant mortality.[21,25,26,31]

Socioeconomic Status and Postpartum Care

Socioeconomic status (SES) is one of the key drivers affecting follow-up and retention in care in the postpartum period.[33-35] However, the effects of low SES on adverse health outcomes and retention in care in the postpartum period have yet to be fully evaluated, due, in part, to limitations in data collection as patients may switch healthcare clinicians, move out of a given medical center's catchment area, or lose health insurance altogether.

HIV Status

An important line of inquiry within disparities in postpartum follow-up has to do with women living with HIV (WLHIV).

Table 54.1 Barriers to Care

Low socioeconomic status (SES)	• Pregnancy-related Medicaid allows for coverage of all medicallynecessary and preventative services during pregnancy and up to 60 d after delivery. If an individual cannot transition to full-scope Medicaid due to income restrictions (ie, their household income exceeds the cutoff for full-scope Medicaid), then insurance coverage will not continue.[8] • Bennett and colleagues note that 51.7% of people with uncomplicated and 56.6% of people with complicated pregnancies (eg, those affected by hypertensive disorders of pregnancy) had a follow-up primary care visit within 12 mo after delivery.[9] • Clapp and colleagues note that with the passage of the Affordable Care Act (ACA), preconception Medicaid enrollment has increased in states undergoing Medicaid expansion. However, what this transition means for postpartum care is unknown.[10]
HIV status	• Siddiqui and colleagues and Mellins and colleagues note that approximately 40% of women living with HIV (WLHIV) do not engage in postpartum follow-up.[12,17] • Nonengagement with care after delivery is associated with both preconception engagement in HIV-related care and antiretroviral nonadherence.[13,18]
Immigrant status	• Proficiency in English, legal status, and ability to access health insurance may impart a lower likelihood of accessing health services and thus poorer health outcomes.[14] • Immigrant women may have better health outcomes, particularly in regard to lower incidences of preterm birth, due to immigration being undertaken by only the healthiest subpopulations from a given area (ie, "healthy immigrant" theory) or because immigrants are not exposed to the chronic racial, structural, and economic segregation that disadvantages minority women in the United States.[17,19-22] • Postpartum retention in care and exclusive breastfeeding are associated with immigration and acculturation status.[23-25]
Intimate partner violence (IPV)	• IPV is "a pattern of assaultive behavior and coercive behavior that may include physical injury, psychologic abuse, sexual assault, progressive isolation, stalking, deprivation, intimidation, and reproductive coercion."[19,26] • IPV has been associated with morbidity and mortality, particularly among racial/ethnic minorities.[27] • Postpartum depression, as well as reduced uptake of postpartum contraception, have been associated with IPV.[22,28,29]

Immigrant Status

Women who immigrate to the United States have unique health needs and considerations that may contribute to disparities in health outcomes in the postpartum and interpregnancy intervals. Important considerations, such as proficiency in English, legal status, and ability to access health insurance, may impart a lower likelihood of accessing health services, and thus poorer health outcomes.[40] Disparities in care immigrant women do experience are commonly understood through the guise of acculturation or the change in cultural norms due to a change in cultural setting.[42-47]

Data also suggest, however, that if this population is linked into care during pregnancy, they are more likely to continue in care after delivery.

It is also important to consider potential unique postpartum needs for women from different heritages.

Intimate Partner Violence

Intimate partner violence (IPV), or "a pattern of assaultive behavior and coercive behavior that may include physical injury, psychologic abuse, sexual assault, progressive isolation, stalking, deprivation, intimidation, and reproductive coercion," is a significant problem in the United States, affecting almost one out of three women during their lifetime.[18,50]

Women who experience IPV also appear to have increased morbidity and mortality, particularly in the postpartum period.

IPV has also been associated with a variety of complications in the postpartum period, including contraceptive use, that disproportionately affect certain racial/ethnic groups. Furthermore, IPV has been associated with postpartum depressive symptoms.

A related concept to IPV is reproductive and sexual coercion, or the "explicit attempts to impregnate a partner against her will, control outcomes of a pregnancy, coerce a partner to have unprotected sex, and interfere with contraceptive methods."[50] This type of abuse occurs more often in women with a prior history of IPV.

Health Behaviors

Understanding the role of health behaviors during the postpartum period in relation to adverse health outcomes is paramount (**Table 54.2**). Postpartum care has been identified as a crucial moment in which to address pregnancy complications (eg, preeclampsia, fetal anomalies, gestational diabetes mellitus), as well as chronic medical comorbidities that may impact a woman's overall health, both mentally and physically, over her life course.[5,6] Therefore, the concept of a *continuum of care*—reaching from the preconception period, through pregnancy, postpartum, and onwards—has gained traction within medical organizations dedicated to women's health such as the ACOG[6] (**Figure 54.1**). Importantly, the ACOG considers postpartum care as an "ongoing process, rather than a single encounter" that is both individualized and woman centered.

Postpartum Care

Follow-up care after delivery is highly variable, with some studies noting disparities based on maternal race/ethnicity and insurance status.

Tobacco Use

A significant proportion of women who use substances—particularly tobacco—cease use during the prenatal period (see Chapter 8); however, there are concerns regarding relapse in tobacco use after delivery.[63,65-72] SES is associated with disparity in tobacco use relapse postpartum. Importantly, craving, maternal stress, and perception of maternal agency were found to lie on the causal pathway from SES to relapse.[71]

Breastfeeding

Rates of breastfeeding in the United States have gradually increased over the last decade, with 25% of infants exclusively breastfed at 6 months of age and 57.6% fed any breastmilk at 6 months.[73,74] Despite these statistics, women face considerable challenges in initiating breastfeeding, exclusively breastfeeding, and continuing the practice. The intent and decision to breastfeed is influenced by attitude, convenience, and perceived barriers.[30] Studies have demonstrated that women who are multiparous, have a high school education or less, have smoked during pregnancy, have family or friends who have not breastfed, or have experienced problems with breastfeeding in the past are more likely not to breastfeed.[75] More importantly, racial, socioeconomic, and structural barriers have demonstrated influences on the breastfeeding practices of women and their infants.

Table 54.2 Health Behaviors

Postpartum care	• Overall engagement with postpartum care is low, with roughly half of people attending a visit.[29,42] • However, this finding may be mitigated by racial/ethnic background of the patient, location of health care services in relation to patient's residence, and household income.[35,57,58]
Tobacco use	• People who use tobacco are known to be at an elevated risk of relapse in the postpartum period. • Targeted behavioral interventions specific to pregnancy and postpartum have been shown to reduce the risk of relapse in the postpartum period, although not among people of low socioeconomic status.[46]
Breastfeeding	• While rates of breastfeeding have increased over the past decade, race/ethnicity and socioeconomic status are associated with differential initiation and continuation rates.[30,43,59] • An association between receiving governmental nutritional interventions, such as the Special Supplemental Nutrition Program for Women, Infants, and Children (WIC), and rates of breastfeeding have been mixed in the literature, suggesting the need for targeted breastfeeding interventions through the program.[47,59-61] • Employment has been demonstrated to be negatively associated with breastfeeding continuation. However, people receiving paid maternity leave have been noted to have a higher frequency of breastfeeding continuation when compared to those without paid leave.[56,62,63]

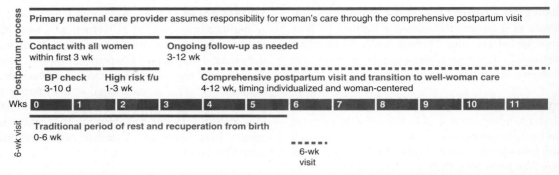

Figure 54.1 Proposed paradigm shift for postpartum visits. The American College of Obstetricians and Gynecologists' Presidential Task Force on Redefining the Postpartum Visit and the Committee on Obstetric Practice propose shifting the paradigm for postpartum care from a single 6-week visit (bottom) to a postpartum process (top). BP, blood pressure; f/u, follow-up.

There are wide variations among minority groups in terms of breastfeeding initiation and continuation rates. Asian women have the highest rates of breastfeeding among any ethnic or racial group with 86.4% ever breastfeeding and 58.6% continuing at 6 months, whereas 77.7% of non-Hispanic white women ever initiate breastfeeding and 45.1% continue at 6 months.[30] Hispanic women have high rates of breastfeeding initiation (80.6%) and continuation (46% at 6 months), yet are also more likely to supplement formula in the first 2 days of life and have lower rates of breastfeeding as compared to non-Hispanic white women.[30]

In contrast, African American and American Indian/Alaskan Native women experience lower rates of initiation, continuation, and exclusive breastfeeding.

Studies have found that mothers with higher SES have consistently higher rates of breastfeeding than mothers with a lower SES.[74] Among women who receive assistance, such as through the Special Supplemental Program for Women, Infants, and Children (WIC), the data surrounding initiation and continuation of breastfeeding are mixed. Among women whose children receive WIC benefits, rates of initiating and sustaining breastfeeding are lower than in women whose children are not receiving such benefits.[60] Women who are in WIC, however, are more likely to initiate and sustain breastfeeding if they enter the program in the prenatal period, especially if they enter in the early prenatal period.[59]

Finally, employment has been identified as a significant challenge for breastfeeding mothers. Prenatal employment has been reported as a strong predictor of a postpartum return to work, and women who are employed prior to giving birth are less likely than women who were unemployed prior to giving birth to fulfill their breastfeeding intentions.[62] Women in low-wage jobs are more likely to report a lack of support from their employers, whereas women in professional occupations are more likely to have higher rates of employer support for breastfeeding initiation and continuation.[75]

Postpartum Health Screening

Mental Health
Routine screening for postpartum depression (PPD) is essential because the mental health of mothers has an immense impact on their relationships with their children and on infant growth and physical well-being (and see Chapter 43).[81] SES has been shown to be associated with an increased risk of PPD.[82-84]

The role of race and ethnicity on the risk of PPD is not definitive. Some studies have suggested that minorities, specifically black and Hispanic women, are at a higher risk than white women,[85-87] whereas other studies note no difference in risk based on race/ethnicity alone.[82,88] However, disparities in access and receipt of mental health care among minorities are well-established.[89]

Women who experience higher psychological stressors and less control over their lives (work, family, relationships, etc) are at higher risk of having depressive symptoms in the postpartum period. Their risk of PPD also increases as the number of stressors accumulate.[91,92]

Women who experience stress due to discrimination in the healthcare system are less likely to follow treatment plans, rate care as high quality, engage in care, and have favorable mental health outcomes.[94-97]

Opportunities to Reduce Disparities

The goal of any intervention or program is to attempt to address the root cause of maternal disparities, and this includes aiming to address racism and embed racial justice into the entire perinatal care continuum. Antiracist training and curricula are essential to ensuring that all members of the healthcare team are aware of their own biases, understand historical and current racism, and are able to embed antiracist approaches into their clinical care approach and practices. In addition to training, there are several wrap-around service programs that help address social, economic, and structural factors (social determinants of health) that women face during their perinatal care trajectory.

WIC Program

The Special Supplemental Program for WIC is a national program created to ensure that women, infants, and children younger than 5 years who are from low-income backgrounds are able to access food and information on healthy eating practices.[103] This program also provides breastfeeding support and promotion, as well as healthcare referrals. Studies have linked this program to improved maternal and infant health outcomes.[104,105] As a result, WIC is an important program to assist mothers and children during a particularly vulnerable time.

While WIC services do not address the myriad of factors that can influence the lives of mothers and their children, understanding disparities that exist among participants and eligible nonparticipants is crucial. For needs that are outside of the purview of WIC services, establishing appropriate referral patterns can potentially benefit women with regard to early access to prenatal care, smoking cessation, and primary care. Providing adequate nutrition and appropriate educational tools has the potential to improve health outcomes among women and children who are part of a particularly vulnerable population.

Breastfeeding Support

In order to diminish the challenges many women face in breastfeeding, there are several programmatic, structural, and legal efforts that could help alleviate these disparities. There is a growing literature on individuals who are able to provide support to women who desire to breastfeed. Counseling therapy and interpersonal support have been demonstrated to be an important factor in enhancing both the initiation and sustainment of breastfeeding practices for women, particularly those with fewer resources.[107,108] Finally, laws and policies can enhance support for breastfeeding practices.[109]

Screening for Diabetes Postpartum

Because minority women from resource-poor backgrounds are at greatest risk of missing postpartum diabetes screening, programs have tried targeted diabetes prevention interventions, such as weight loss, exercise programs, and community outreach workers for these high-risk groups with variable results.[111]

Contraception

Unintended pregnancy is a serious problem in the United States associated with health risks to a woman, her family, and society. About one-half of all US pregnancies are unintended. A critical factor underlying this unintended pregnancy rate is a lack of access to effective family planning services.[112-114] Women with unintended pregnancies also are more likely to have poor health outcomes such as low-birth-weight infants, infant mortality, and maternal morbidity and mortality.[112,115] Empowering women to plan when they want to have children is essential, and thus, access to contraception is an important part of postpartum care.

Use of Technology in the Postpartum Period

Given its ubiquity, various forms of technology, such as mobile phones, mobile health applications, and social media, have been identified as useful tools in the postpartum period. Technology-driven interventions can enable easier communication between women and their clinicians and potentially lower the barrier of entry into postpartum care, especially for women who are socioeconomically disadvantaged or who experience disparities in information and access to care.[116,118] However, accessibility, ease-of-use, and versatility remain critical factors in patient and clinician adoption of these non-traditional methods of delivering health care and information.

Health information delivered to a mobile phone, either via text messages or mobile health applications, has been shown to influence health-related behaviors in studies involving other populations (ie, people living with HIV, adolescents).[116] While there is evidence linking birth-related events to the use of text messaging and mobile health applications, there are limited studies regarding their use in women from resource-poor settings.

The success of mobile phone–based interventions in the postpartum period, however, depends on the barriers to enrollment that women experience. Similarly, women who use mobile health applications while pregnant often note reducing use in the postpartum period, as they found the applications too expensive to continue.[118]

Another challenge to using technology-based modalities to deliver care is that there is less research on the information-seeking behavior of those who have already delivered. Even if women receive information about the postpartum period, they often express feeling confused about the care and needs of their newborn.[118] Furthermore, identifying reliable sources of information online can be difficult.

Doula, Community Health Worker, and Patient Navigator Support Programs

Doula care is increasingly recommended to support high-risk black, Indigenous, and people of color (BIPOC) women during labor to improve maternal outcomes.[121,122] A 2019 ACOG Committee Opinion endorsed by the American College of Nurse-Midwives, highlights the continuous one-to-one emotional support provided by support personnel, such as doulas, for women in labor,[124] citing evidence that the presence of these support personnel is associated with shortened labor, fewer cesarean births, and fewer reports of dissatisfaction with the labor experience.[125,126] It is posited that doulas may mitigate the effects of racism and social determinants of health in underserved populations.[127,128] However, many studies evaluating doulas have found mixed results.

Similarly, community health workers (CHWs) and patient navigators (PNs) have long been deployed to reach and navigate patients, build trust, and address health disparities in underserved areas. CHWs and PNs can connect with patients through shared culture and language, similar life experiences, and an understanding of their community members' barriers to healthcare access. They can help identify issues stemming from social determinants of health and suggest referrals to resources.

Taken together, the roles that doulas, CHWs, and PNs play in support of pregnant and postpartum women are critical to mitigation of disparities that stem from factors such as lack of support, racism, discrimination, and the social determinants of health. Thus, there is a need for more research to examinee scaling and extending the benefits that doulas, CHWs, and PNs confer to pregnant and postpartum women.

KEY POINTS

- The disparities surrounding the care and health-related outcomes of newly postpartum women extends across a variety of domains.
- Racism is a major underlying factor that drives postpartum health inequities.
- Guidelines have been published by groups like the American College of Obstetricians and Gynecologists (ACOG) and the Society for Maternal-Fetal Medicine (SMFM) that can be employed to ensure standardized enactment of care in the postpartum setting, and the most up-to-date versions of these documents should be consulted to further guide appropriate clinical screening and linkage to services.
- Healthcare clinicians within reproductive health and other allied disciplines should be familiar with the varied ways in which disparities manifest themselves and to be attentive to methods in which to reduce these disparities.
- Common barriers to care include socioeconomic, immigrant, and HIV status as well as experience of intimate partner violence and reproductive or sexual coercion.
- Women from diverse backgrounds exhibit differential health behaviors, including ability and attitudes toward breastfeeding, tobacco use, postpartum visit attendance, and screening and treatment for mental or physical health conditions.

- Programs and other innovative approaches to supporting healthy behaviors can significantly improve maternal and neonatal outcomes in the postpartum period.
- Access to contraception is an important part of postpartum care.
- Technology-based health interventions have the potential to increase women's engagement with their care after delivery, but challenges such as accessibility, ease-of-use, versatility, and discernment of reliable sources of information remain to be addressed.

- Taken together, the roles that doulas, CHWs, and PNs play in support of pregnant and postpartum women are critical to mitigation of disparities that stem from factors such as lack of support, racism, discrimination, and the social determinants of health. Thus, there is a need for more research to examinee scaling and extending the benefits that doulas, CHWs, and PNs confer to pregnant and postpartum women.

REFERENCES

(only references cited in synoptic print chapter; for a complete reference list, see ebook)

1. *NIH Health Disparities Strategic Plan and Budget Fiscal Years 2009-2013.* Accessed July 7, 2020. https://www.nimhd.nih.gov/docs/2009-2013nih_health_disparities_strategic_plan_and_budget.pdf
5. American College of Obstetricians and Gynecologists (ACOG). Committee Opinion No. 736: optimizing postpartum care. *Obstet Gynecol.* 2018;131:e140-e150.
6. American College of Obstetricians and Gynecologists (ACOG). Obstetric Care Consensus No. 8: interpregnancy care. *Obstet Gynecol.* 2019;133:e51-e72.
8. Petersen EE, Davis NL, Goodman D, et al. Racial/ethnic disparities in pregnancy-related deaths—United States, 2007-2016. *MMWR Morb Mortal Wkly Rep.* 2019;68(35):762.
9. Petersen EE, Davis NL, Goodman D, et al. Vital signs: pregnancy-related deaths, United States, 2011-2015, and strategies for prevention, 13 states, 2013-2017. *MMWR Morb Mortal Wkly Rep.* 2019;68(18):423.
10. Davis N, Smoots A, Goodman D. *Pregnancy-related Deaths: Data From 14 US Maternal Mortality Review Committees, 2008-2017.* Centers for Disease Control and Prevention; 2019.
12. Bailey ZD, Krieger N, Agénor M, Graves J, Linos N, Bassett MT. Structural racism and health inequities in the USA: evidence and interventions. *Lancet.* 2017;389(10077):1453-1463.
13. Evans MK, Rosenbaum L, Malina D, Morrissey S, Rubin EJ. Diagnosing and treating systemic racism. *N Engl J Med.* 2020;383(3):274-276.
14. Azar KM, Shen Z, Romanelli RJ, et al. Disparities in outcomes among COVID-19 patients in a large health care system in California: study examines disparities in access and outcomes for COVID-19 patients who are members of racial and ethnic minorities and socioeconomically disadvantaged groups. *Health Aff (Millwood).* 2020;38(7):1253-1262. doi:10.1377/hlthaff. 2020.00598
16. Tangel V, White RS, Nachamie AS, Pick JS. Racial and ethnic disparities in maternal outcomes and the disadvantage of peripartum black women: a multistate analysis, 2007-2014. *Am J Perinatol.* 2019;36(8):835-848.
17. Urquia ML, O'Campo PJ, Heaman MI. Revisiting the immigrant paradox in reproductive health: the roles of duration of residence and ethnicity. *Soc Sci Med.* 2012;74:1610-1621.
18. American College of Obstetricians and Gynecologists (ACOG). Committee Opinion No. 518: intimate partner violence. *Obstet Gynecol.* 2012;119:412-417.
19. Premkumar A, Debbink MP, Silver RM, et al. Association of acculturation with adverse pregnancy outcomes. *Obstet Gynecol.* 2020;135:301-309.
20. Urquia ML, Frank JW, Moineddin R, Glazier RH. Immigrants' duration of residence and adverse birth outcomes: a population-based study. *BJOG.* 2010;117:591-601.
21. Clapp MA, James KE, Kaimal AJ, Daw JR. Preconception coverage before and after the affordable care act medicaid expansions. *Obstet Gynecol.* 2018;132:1394-1400.
22. Cha S, Chapman DA, Wan W, Burton CW, Masho SW. Intimate partner violence and postpartum contraceptive use: the role of race/ethnicity and prenatal birth control counseling. *Contraception.* 2015;92:268-275.
23. Swain CA, Smith LC, Nash D, et al. Postpartum loss to HIV care and HIV viral suppression among previously diagnosed HIV-infected women with a live birth in New York state. *PLoS One.* 2016;11:e0160775.
24. Kentoffio K, Berkowitz SA, Atlas SJ, Oo SA, Percac-Lima S. Use of maternal health services: comparing refugee, immigrant and US-born populations. *Matern Child Health J.* 2016;20:2494-2501.
25. McMorrow S, Kenney G. Despite progress under the ACA, many new mothers lack insurance coverage. *Health Aff Blog.* 2018. Accessed September 13, 2020. https://www.healthaffairs.org/do/10.1377/hblog20180917.317923/abs/
26. Bhatt CB, Beck-Sagué CM. Medicaid expansion and infant mortality in the United States. *Am J Public Health.* 2018;108(4):565-567.
27. Women in the United States experience high rates of coverage 'Churn' in months before and after childbirth. *Health Aff (Millwood).* 2017;36(4):598-606.
28. Crump C, Lipsky S, Mueller BA. Adverse birth outcomes among Mexican-Americans: are US-born women at greater risk than Mexico-born women? *Ethn Health.* 1999;4:29-34.
29. Bennett WL, Chang H-Y, Levine DM, et al. Utilization of primary and obstetric care after medically complicated pregnancies: an analysis of medical claims data. *J Gen Intern Med.* 2014;29:636-645.
30. Jones KM, Power ML, Queenan JT, Schulkin J. Racial and ethnic disparities in breastfeeding. *Breastfeed Med.* 2015;10:186-196.
31. Brown CC, Moore JE, Felix HC, et al. Association of state Medicaid expansion status with low birth weight and preterm birth. *J Am Med Assoc.* 2019;321(16):1598-1609.
33. American College of Obstetricians and Gynecologists (ACOG). Importance of social determinants of health and cultural awareness in the delivery of reproductive health care. *Obstet Gynecol.* 2018;131:e43-e48.
34. Moroz L, Riley LE, D'Alton M, et al. SMFM special report: putting the "M" back in MFM. Addressing education about disparities in maternal outcomes and care. *Am J Obstet Gynecol.* 2018;218:B2-B8.
35. American College of Obstetricians and Gynecologists (ACOG). ACOG Committee Opinion No. 586: health disparities in rural women. *Obstet Gynecol.* 2014;123:384-388.
40. American College of Obstetricians and Gynecologists (ACOG). Committee Opinion No. 627: health care for unauthorized immigrants. *Obstet Gynecol.* 2015;125:755-759.
42. Abraído-Lanza AF, Echeverría SE, Flórez KR. Latino immigrants, acculturation, and health: promising new directions in research. *Ann Rev Public Health.* 2016;37:219-236.
43. Fox M, Thayer Z, Wadhwa PD. Acculturation and health: the moderating role of socio-cultural context. *Am Anthropol.* 2017;119:405-421.
44. Fox M, Thayer Z, Wadhwa PD. Assessment of acculturation in minority health research. *Soc Sci Med.* 2017;176:123-132.
45. Lopez-Class M, Castro FG, Ramirez AG. Conceptions of acculturation: a review and statement of critical issues. *Soc Sci Med.* 2011;72:1555-1562.

46. Schwartz SJ, Unger JB, Zamboanga BL, Szapocznik J. Rethinking the concept of acculturation: implications for theory and research. *Am Psychol*. 2010;65:237-251.

47. Thomson MD, Hoffman-Goetz L. Defining and measuring acculturation: a systematic review of public health studies with Hispanic populations in the United States. *Soc Sci Med*. 2009;69:983-991.

50. American College of Obstetricians and Gynecologists (ACOG). Committee Opinion No. 554: reproductive and sexual coercion. *Obstet Gynecol*. 2013;121:411-415.

56. Miller E, Decker MR, McCauley HL, et al. Pregnancy coercion, intimate partner violence and unintended pregnancy. *Contraception*. 2010;81:316-322.

57. Bromley E, Nunes A, Phipps MG. Disparities in pregnancy healthcare utilization between Hispanic and non-Hispanic white women in Rhode Island. *Matern Child Health J*. 2012;16:1576-1582.

58. Bryant A, Blake-Lamb T, Hatoum I, Kotelchuck M. Women's use of health care in the first 2 years postpartum: occurrence and correlates. *Matern Child Health J*. 2016;20:81-91.

59. Metallinos-Katsaras E, Brown L, Colchamiro R. Maternal WIC participation improves breastfeeding rates: a statewide analysis of WIC participants. *Matern Child Health J*. 2015;19:136-143.

60. Li R, Darling N, Maurice E, Barker L, Grummer-Strawn LM. Breastfeeding rates in the United States by characteristics of the child, mother, or family: the 2002 National Immunization Survey. *Pediatrics*. 2005;115:e31-e37.

61. DiBari JN, Yu SM, Chao SM, Lu MC. Use of postpartum care: predictors and barriers. *J Pregnancy*. 2014;2014:530769.

62. Attanasio L, Kozhimannil KB, McGovern P, Gjerdingen D, Johnson PJ. The impact of prenatal employment on breastfeeding intentions and breastfeeding status at 1 week postpartum. *J Hum Lact*. 2013;29:620-628.

63. Massey SH, Bublitz MH, Magee SR, et al. Maternal–fetal attachment differentiates patterns of prenatal smoking and exposure. *Addict Behav*. 2015;45:51.

65. Brandon TH, Simmons VN, Meade CD, et al. Self-help booklets for preventing postpartum smoking relapse: a randomized trial. *Am J Public Health*. 2012;102:2109-2115.

66. Massey SH, Compton MT. Psychological differences between smokers who spontaneously quit during pregnancy and those who do not: a review of observational studies and directions for future research. *Nicotine Tob Res*. 2013;15:307-319.

67. Massey SH, Neiderhiser JM, Shaw DS, Leve LD, Ganiban JM, Reiss D. Maternal self concept as a provider and cessation of substance use during pregnancy. *Addict Behav*. 2012;37:956.

68. Massey SH, Reiss D, Neiderhiser JM, Leve LD, Shaw DS, Ganiban JM. Maternal personality traits associated with patterns of prenatal smoking and exposure: implications for etiologic and prevention research. *Neurotoxicol Teratol*. 2016;53:48.

69. Massey SH, Wisner KL. Understanding pregnancy's protective effect on drug use within a developmental framework. *Am J Psychiatry*. 2018;175(3):286-287.

70. Massey SH, Decety J, Wisner KL, Wakschlag LS. Specification of change mechanisms in pregnant smokers for malleable target identification: a novel approach to a tenacious public health problem. *Front Public Health*. 2017;5:239.

71. Businelle MS, Kendzor DE, Reitzel LR, et al. Pathways linking socioeconomic status and postpartum smoking relapse. *Ann Behav Med*. 2013;45:180-191.

72. Reitzel LR, Vidrine JI, Businelle MS, et al. Preventing postpartum smoking relapse among diverse low-income women: a randomized clinical trial. *Nicotine Tob Res*. 2010;12:326-335.

73. *Breastfeeding Report Card: United States, 2018*. Centers for Disease Control and Prevention; 2018. Accessed July 7, 2020. https://www.cdc.gov/breastfeeding/pdf/2018breastfeedingreportcard.pdf

74. Darfour-Oduro SA, Kim J. WIC mothers' social environment and postpartum health on breastfeeding initiation and duration. *Breastfeed Med*. 2014;9:524-529.

75. Dagher RK, McGovern PM, Schold JD, Randall XJ. Determinants of breastfeeding initiation and cessation among employed mothers: a prospective cohort study. *BMC Pregnancy Childbirth*. 2016;16:194.

81. Doe S, LoBue S, Hamaoui A, Rezai S, Henderson CE, Mercado R. Prevalence and predictors of positive screening for postpartum depression in minority parturients in the South Bronx. *Arch Womens Ment Health*. 2017;20:291-295.

82. Dolbier CL, Rush TE, Sahadeo LS, Shaffer ML, Thorp J; Community Child Health Network Investigators. Relationships of race and socioeconomic status to postpartum depressive symptoms in rural African American and non-Hispanic white women. *Matern Child Health J*. 2013;17:1277-1287.

83. Goyal D, Gay C, Lee KA. How much does low socioeconomic status increase the risk of prenatal and postpartum depressive symptoms in first-time mothers? *Womens Health Issues*. 2010;20:96-104.

84. Pooler J, Perry DF, Ghandour RM. Prevalence and risk factors for postpartum depressive symptoms among women enrolled in WIC. *Matern Child Health J*. 2013;17:1969-1980.

85. Yonkers KA, Ramin SM, Rush AJ, et al. Onset and persistence of postpartum depression in an inner-city maternal health clinic system. *Am J Psychiatry*. 2001;158:1856-1863.

86. Abrams LS, Dornig K, Curran L. Barriers to service use for postpartum depression symptoms among low-income ethnic minority mothers in the United States. *Qual Health Res*. 2009;19:535-551.

87. Hayes DK, Ta VM, Hurwitz EL, Mitchell-Box KM, Fuddy LJ. Disparities in self-reported postpartum depression among Asian, Hawaiian, and Pacific Islander women in Hawaii: pregnancy risk Assessment Monitoring system (PRAMS), 2004-2007. *Matern Child Health J*. 2010;14:765-773.

88. Hutto HF, Kim-Godwin Y, Pollard D, Kemppainen J. Postpartum depression among White, African American, and Hispanic low-income mothers in rural southeastern North Carolina. *J Community Health Nurs*. 2011;28:41-53.

89. Glasheen C, Colpe L, Hoffman V, Warren LK. Prevalence of serious psychological distress and mental health treatment in a national sample of pregnant and postpartum women. *Matern Child Health J*. 2015;19:204-216.

91. Dagher RK, McGovern PM, Alexander BH, Dowd BE, Ukestad LK, McCaffrey DJ. The psychosocial work environment and maternal postpartum depression. *Int J Behav Med*. 2009;16:339-346.

92. Salm Ward T, Kanu FA, Robb SW. Prevalence of stressful life events during pregnancy and its association with postpartum depressive symptoms. *Arch Womens Ment Health*. 2017;20:161-171.

94. Trivedi AN, Ayanian JZ. Perceived discrimination and use of preventive health services. *J Gen Intern Med*. 2006;21:553-558.

97. Stepanikova I, Kukla L. Is perceived discrimination in pregnancy prospectively linked to postpartum depression? Exploring the role of education. *Matern Child Health J*. 2017;21:1669-1677.

103. Centers for Disease Control and Prevention. Eligibility and enrollment in the special supplemental nutrition program for women, infants, and children (WIC) – 27 states and New York city, 2007-2008. *MMWR Morb Mortal Wkly Rep*. 2013;62:189-193.

104. Sonchak L. The impact of WIC on birth outcomes: new evidence from South Carolina. *Matern Child Health J*. 2016;20:1518-1525.

105. Bitler MP, Currie J. Does WIC work? The effects of WIC on pregnancy and birth outcomes. *J Policy Anal Manage*. 2005;24:73-91.

107. Wouk K, Chetwynd E, Vitaglione T, Sullivan C. Improving access to medical lactation support and counseling: building the case for Medicaid reimbursement. *Matern Child Health J*. 2017;21:836-844.

108. Kao JC, Johnson JE, Todorova R, Zlotnick C. The positive effect of a group intervention to reduce postpartum depression on breastfeeding outcomes in low-income women. *Int J Group Psychother*. 2015;65:445-458.

109. Smith-Gagen J, Hollen R, Walker M, Cook DM, Yang W. Breastfeeding laws and breastfeeding practices by race and ethnicity. *Womens Health Issues*. 2014;24:e11-e19.

111. Mendez-Figueroa H, Daley J, Breault P, et al. Impact of an intensive follow-up program on the postpartum glucose tolerance testing rate. *Arch Gynecol Obstet*. 2014;289:1177-1183.

112. Dehlendorf C, Rodriguez MI, Levy K, Borrero S, Steinauer J. Disparities in family planning. *Am J Obstet Gynecol* 2010; 202:214-220.

113. Finer LB, Henshaw SK. Disparities in rates of unintended pregnancy in the United States, 1994 and 2001. *Perspect Sex Reprod Health*. 2006;38:90-96.

114. Frost JJ, Finer LB, Tapales A. The impact of publicly funded family planning clinic services on unintended pregnancies and government cost savings. *J Healht Care Poor Underserved*. 2008;19:778-796.

115. Rodriguez MI, Caughey AB, Edelman A, Darney PD, Foster DG. Cost-benefit analysis of state and hospital funded postpartum intrauterine contraception at a university hospital for recent immigrants to the United States. *Contraception*. 2010;82:304-308.

116. Gazmararian JA, Elon L, Yang B, Graham M, Parker R. Text4baby program: an opportunity to reach underserved pregnant and postpartum women? *Matern Child Health J.* 2014;18:223-232.

118. Guerra-Reyes L, Christie VM, Prabhakar A, Harris AL, Siek KA. Postpartum health information seeking using mobile phones: experiences of low-income mothers. *Matern Child Health J.* 2016;20:13-21.

124. Committee on Obstetric Practice. *Committee Opinion No. 687: Approaches to Limit Intervention During Labor and Birth.* 2019. Accessed August 4, 2020. https://www.acog.org/clinical-guidance/committee-opinion/articles/2019/02/approaches-to-limit-intervention-during-labor-and-birth

125. Hodnett ED, Gates S, Hofmeyr GJ, Sakala C. Continuous support for women during childbirth. *Cochrane Database Syst Rev.* 2013;7(7):CD003766.

126. Kennell J, Klaus M, McGrath S, Robertson S, Hinkley C. Continuous emotional support during labor in a US hospital: a randomized controlled trial. *J Am Med Assoc.* 1991;265(17):2197-2201.

127. Wint K, Elias TI, Mendez G, Mendez DD, Gary-Webb TL. Experiences of community doulas working with low-income, African American mothers. *Health Equity.* 2019;3(1):109-116.

128. Hardeman RR, Kozhimannil KB. Motivations for entering the doula profession: perspectives from women of color. *J Midwifery Women's Health.* 2016;61(6):773-780.

Index

Note: Page numbers followed by "f" indicate figures, "t" indicate tables, and "b" indicate boxes.